AF656610

Volume 2

Textbook of Medicinal Chemistry

As per the Latest Syllabus prescribed by Pharmacy Council of India

Fourth Edition

Volume 2

Textbook of Medicinal Chemistry

As per the Latest Syllabus prescribed by Pharmacy Council of India

Fourth Edition

V Alagarsamy MPharm PhD FIC DOMH
Professor and Principal
MNR College of Pharmacy, Sangareddy
Greater Hyderabad, Telangana

Director
MNR Foundation for Research and Innovation
Sangareddy, Greater Hyderabad, Telangana

CBSPD

CBS Publishers & Distributors Pvt Ltd

New Delhi • Bengaluru • Chennai • Kochi • Kolkata • Lucknow • Mumbai
Gujarat • Hyderabad • Jharkhand • Nagpur • Patna • Pune • Uttarakhand

Disclaimer

Science and technology are constantly changing fields. New research and experience broaden the scope of information and knowledge. The author has tried his best in giving information available to him while preparing the material for this book. Although all efforts have been made to ensure optimum accuracy of the material, yet it is quite possible some errors might have been left uncorrected. The publisher, the printer and the author will not be held responsible for any inadvertent errors or inaccuracies.

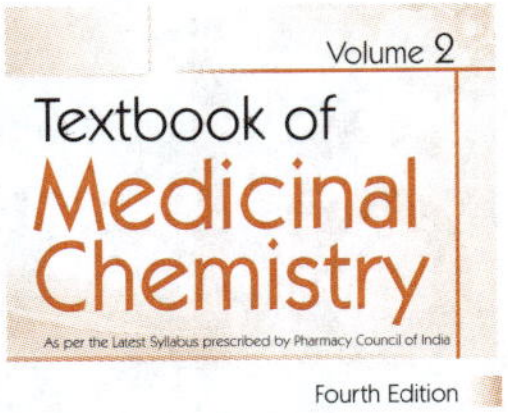

ISBN: 978-93-90709-73-1

Copyright © Author and Publisher

Fourth Edition: 2022
Reprint: 2023, 2024, 2025
Third Edition: 2016
Reprint: 2017, 2019, 2020, 2021
Second Edition: 2014
First Edition: 2009

All rights reserved. No part of this book may be reproduced or transmitted in any form or by any means, electronic or mechanical, including photocopying, recording, or any information storage and retrieval system without permission, in written from the author and the publisher.

Published by Satish Kumar Jain and produced by Varun Jain for

CBS Publishers & Distributors Pvt Ltd

4819/XI Prahlad Street, 24 Ansari Road, Daryaganj, New Delhi 110 002, India
Ph: 011-23266838, 23289259 Website: www.cbspd.com
e-mail: delhi@cbspd.com

Corporate Office: 204 FIE, Industrial Area, Patparganj, Delhi 110 092, India
Ph: 011-49344934 Fax: 011-49344935 e-mail: publishing@cbspd.com; publicity@cbspd.com

Branches

- **Bengaluru:** Seema House 2975, 17th Cross, K.R. Road, Banasankari 2nd Stage, Bengaluru 560 070, Karnataka, India
  Ph: +91-80-26771678/79 Fax: +91-80-26771680 e-mail: bangalore@cbspd.com
- **Chennai:** 18/8B, Subbarayan Street, Shenoy Nagar, Chennai 600 030, Tamil Nadu, India
  Ph: +91-44-42032115, 26681266 e-mail: chennai@cbspd.com
- **Kochi:** 42/1325, 1326, Power House Road, Opposite KSEB, Power House, Ernakulum 682018, Kochi, Kerala, India
  Ph: +91-484-4059061-65 Fax: +91-484-4059065 e-mail: kochi@cbspd.com
- **Kolkata:** 147, Hind Ceramics Compound, 1st Floor, Nilgunj Road, Belghoria, Kolkata 700056, West Bengal, India
  Ph: +91-33-25330055/56 e-mail: kolkata@cbspd.com
- **Lucknow:** Basement, Khushuma Complex, 7 Meerabai Marg (behind Jawahar Bhawan), Lucknow 226001, UP, India
  Ph: +91-522-4000032 e-mail: tiwari.lucknow@cbspd.com
- **Mumbai:** PWD Shed, Gala No. 25/26, Ramchandra Bhatt Marg, Next JJ Hospital, Gate No. 2, Opp. Union Bank of India, Noorbaug Mumbai 400009, Maharashtra, India
  Ph: +91-22-66661880/89 e-mail: mumbai@cbspd.com

Representatives

- **Gujarat** 0-9879558667
- **Hyderabad** 0-9885175004
- **Jharkhand** 0-9811541605
- **Nagpur** 0-8692091830
- **Patna** 0-9334159340
- **Pune** 0-9664372571
- **Uttarakhand** 0-9716462459

Printed at: India Binding House, Noida, UP, India

Preface to the Fourth Edition

The subject of medicinal chemistry has grown so fast and we find developments in many areas of this subject. Even though, it is a difficult task for the author to match the pace of developments of the subject, it is a great pleasure for the author and the publisher to present this revised and updated fourth edition of the *Textbook of Medicinal Chemistry*.

The enthusiastic comments received from faculty members and student community across India, as mentioned below, have inspired me to present this fourth and updated edition of the *Textbook of Medicinal Chemistry*.

- A unique book containing updated information about medicinal chemistry by complying the revised syllabus of Pharmacy Council of India (PCI).
- This book is comprehensive with all the aspects of medicinal chemistry discussed at one place.
- It is a good companion for GPAT aspirants.
- It is a favourite book for students willing to learn medicinal chemistry.
- It is presented in an attractive and easy-to-read manner.
- It is presented in student-friendly style and approach.
- It is presented in a down-to-earth fashion avoiding unnecessary complicated details.
- This is a perfect textbook.
- It helps faculty members a lot while teaching students.
- Elegant presentation of chemical structures helping students to remember and reproduce well in examinations.

Since its first edition, in 2009, *Textbook of Medicinal Chemistry*, serves as an authentic and reliable source for the medicinal chemistry aspects of the drugs. The overwhelming response to the first edition was immediate throughout the country due to its comprehensive content (especially, the classification, synthesis and drug profile and SAR). As the number of drugs available for therapeutic use is increasing day-by-day, all the chapters have been updated with newer drugs.

New to this Edition

The major goal of the author is to provide the students of pharmacy and allied health professions with a book that not only describes the chemical aspects of drugs but also reflects pharmacological aspects that are important in the field of medicine. Following are some features of the fourth edition:

- **Updated information provided** and complied with the revised PCI syllabus.
- **Attractive layout and design.**
- **Physicochemical parameters** have been explained with further information and two new chapters—Protein Binding of Drugs and Biotransformation or Metabolism of Drugs—are added under the section Physicochemical Factors in Relation to Biological Activity of Drugs.

- **New topics** like Pharmacophore Modelling, Docking and Antisense Technology are added under the section Drug Design.
- **Based on PCI syllabus, new topics** like Drugs Used in Congestive Cardiac Failure, Thyroid and Antithyroid Drugs, Antiscabies and Antipedicular Agents, Preservatives and Diagnostic Agents are introduced.
- **Several newer drugs** are incorporated in different chapters.
- **PCI syllabus-based classification of drugs** is provided for easy to study and write in examination.

I hope this new edition of the *Textbook of Medicinal Chemistry* will be welcomed by the teachers and students of pharmacy, pharmaceutical chemistry, chemistry and the related fields. You are most welcome with your valuable feedback to *authoralagarsamy@gmail.com*.

V Alagarsamy

Preface to the First Edition

Medicinal chemistry emerged as a specialized area due to the development in chemistry and biology, hence it is considered as a highly interdisciplinary science combining a wide variety of subjects such as organic chemistry, pharmacology, biochemistry, toxicology, pharmacognosy, molecular biology, genomics, proteomics, computational chemistry, physical chemistry and statistics. Now, the growth of medicinal chemistry has reached a stage where the activity-guided synthesis of compounds is possible rather than screening of synthesized compounds for different biological activities. This field also penetrates into the areas of gene therapy and biochemistry-based virtual drug receptors with the help of computer-aided molecular modelling techniques.

This book is an upshot of my vision to discover the best book on medicinal chemistry, which deals about the concise description of diseases, clear classification of drugs with their chemical structures, synthesis of each drug with different routes, mode of action, metabolism, physical and pharmacological properties along with their therapeutic uses, assay technique, dose, official dosage forms and summary of structure–activity relationship (SAR) studies. Swathing the entire features of medicinal chemistry, first of its kind, is the unique feature of this book. It facilitates the students to understand the subject more easily and interestingly.

While writing this book, I felt that the book will bring about a re-orientation in the teaching and learning process of medicinal chemistry. Academic community in India is faced with scarcity of books to cater to their needs. Numerous foreign writers' books deal well about basics and pharmacological aspects related to medicinal chemistry, but lack two major requirements, i.e. synthesis and clear classification of drugs used. Some Indian authors filled this lacuna to a certain extent by including the synthesis, but failed to give a clear classification of drugs with their chemical structure. For this, the content of this book has been carefully tailored to cater to the needs of the academicians belonging to all Indian universities, pharmacologists, clinical and industrial pharmacists by incorporating the missing links between general synthetic organic chemistry and medicinal chemistry.

This *Textbook of Medicinal Chemistry* is presented in two volumes. Volume I consists of six sections. The first section is devoted to the physicochemical properties and their relation to biological activities and the second section provides the framework of drug design, which together form the basic aspects of medicinal chemistry. The remaining sections, III to VI, deal with chemical, pharmacological, biochemical and toxicological aspects of organic medicinal compounds used in various diseases associated with different systems of the human body such as CNS, ANS, CVS and urinary system.

We hope that this special volume will be a good source of information and reference for not only graduate and postgraduate students but also basic and applied researchers in this field. Moreover, it will also be of interest to a wide range of scientists, including organic chemists, biochemists, pharmacologists and clinicians, who are interested in drug research. I welcome suggestions and constructive criticism from all corners of scientific community.

V Alagarsamy

Acknowledgements

I wish to place on record my heartfelt thanks to everyone who have made this book possible, especially my beloved teachers from first standard to doctoral programme, guides, Dr Rajani Giridhar and Dr MR Yadav.

I am immensely grateful to Dr B Suresh and Dr RK Goyal for inspiring and initiating me to write the book. I am grateful to Shri MN Raju, Chairman, and Mr Ravi Varma, Vice-chairman, MNR Educational Trust, Hyderabad, for providing constant encouragement and moral support to achieve this goal.

I express my sincere appreciation to my students, Dr V Raja Solomon (postdoctoral researcher, Canada), Dr JC Hanish Singh, Dr P Parthiban, Mr S Thiru Senthil Murugan and Ms J Rajeshwari, for helping me author this book. I also thank my colleagues, especially, Dr S Satheesh Kumar, Dr B Subba Rao, Dr K Dhanabal, Mr M Murugan, Dr MT Sulthana, Dr B Narendhar and Dr K Lahari, for their untiring support in making this book.

The friendly interaction I had experienced with the Elsevier team—Mr Subodh K Chauhan, Mr Nitin Valecha and Mr Ankush—and Televijay Technologies, Project Manager Ms Usha K Nair, offered a plenty of energy to eliminate the fatigue during the preparation of this book. If the author gets such a cooperative and energetic publication team, publishing any number of books will not be a difficult task. I thank them wholeheartedly for helping me reach this target and am requesting them to continue their service to the author community in the same intensity.

I also acknowledge the support extended by the CBS Publishing team Mr YN Arjuna (Senior Vice-President, Publishing, Editorial and Publicity) and his entire team comprising Ms Ritu Chawla (AGM Production), Ms Baljeet (graphic artist), Ms Hemlata (DTP operator), and Mr Neeraj Kumar Sharma (editor) in this revised edition.

I am also grateful to the faculty members of Faculty of Technology, Osmania University, Hyderabad, for their academic support and encouragement.

The stimulation I got from my father, mother, sister, brothers and wife to reach this target is more than analeptics, and the patience and cooperation extended by my children, Aishwarya (B Pharm) and Abhinaya, made me think of the goal without any diversion. To express my thankfulness, I pray The Almighty to bless my children with teachers like those I got in my life so that they too are inspired by their teachers and dedicate to the field of medicinal chemistry and, in turn, serve for the suffering humanity.

V Alagarsamy

Contents

SECTION V
Drugs Acting on Endocrine System

SECTION VI
Chemotherapy

SECTION VII
Miscellaneous

SECTION I

Drugs Acting on Inflammation/Allergy

CHAPTER 1

Antihistamines

INTRODUCTION

Histamine [2-(imidazol-4-yl) ethylamine], which is biosynthesized by decarboxylation of the basic amino acid histidine, is found in all organs and tissues of the human body (Table 1.1).

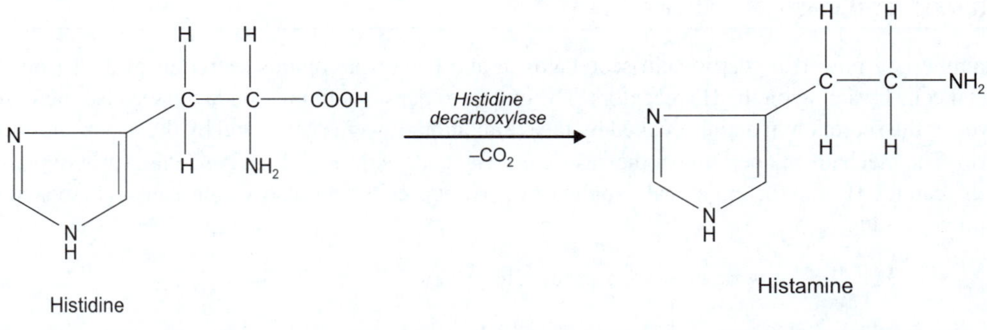

Histamine is stored in the secretory granules of mast cells (pH 5.5) as positively charged and ionically complexed with negatively charged acidic group on other secretory granules, which constitutes heparin. The principal target cells of immediate hypersensitivity reactions are mast cells and basophils to generate IgE antibodies that binds to FC receptor on the granule surface. This leads to transmembrane activation of tyrosine protein kinase, which phosphorylates and activates the phospholipase. The phosphatidyl inositol biphosphate is converted into inositol triphosphate, which triggers the intracellular release of calcium ion. The calcium ion causes exocytic release of histamine with the transfer of Na^+ ion from extracellular space. The released histamine targets the histaminergic receptors (H_1, H_2, and H_3) to elicit the actions.

Histamine is an important chemical messenger, communicating information from one cell to another, and is involved in a variety of complex biological actions. It is mainly stored in an inactive bound form, from which it is released as a result of an antigen–antibody reaction, initiated by different stimuli, such as venoms, toxins, proteolytic enzyme, detergents, food materials, and numerous chemicals. Systemically, histamine contracts smooth muscles of the lungs and the gastrointestinal system and causes vasodilation, low blood pressure, and increases the heart rate. It also causes symptoms such as itching, sneezing, watery eye, and running nose.

Histamine exerts its biological function by interacting with at least three distinctly specific receptors— H_1, H_2, and H_3. Historically, the term antihistamine has been used to describe a drug that acts on H_1- and H_2-receptors. An antihistaminic agent should ideally prevent the production or release of these autacoids by inhibiting the response of sensitized mast cells and basophils to specific antigens.

1. Antihistamines are drugs that competitively block the H_1-receptors.
2. Antihistamines antagonize the stimulant action of histamine on the smooth muscles of gastro-intestinal tract (GIT), uterus, and blood vessels, and inhibit histamine-augmented salivary secretion.
3. H_1-receptor antagonists have been used clinically to treat various allergic disorders, such as seasonal or perennial allergic rhinitis and chronic urticaria.

Release and Function of Endogenous Histamine

Histamine is released because of the interaction of an antigen with IgE antibodies on the mast cell surface and plays a central role in immediate hypersensitive reactions (Figure 1.1).

The release of histamine, in addition to the stimulation of IgE receptors, also activates the phospholipase A_2, leading to the production of host mediators, including platelet activating factors and metabolites of arachidonic acid. Leukotriene D_4 is also generated, which is a potent constrictor of smooth muscles. This mediates the constriction of bronchi.

Histamine and Gastric Acid Secretion

Histamine is a powerful gastric acid secretagogue and evokes a copious secretion of acid from the parietal cells by acting on the H_2-receptors. The output of pepsin and intrinsic factors is also increased. However, the secretion of acid is evoked by the stimulation of vagus nerve and by the enteric hormone gastrin. The mechanism operating at the gastric parietal cells is through H^+-K^+-ATPase (proton pump), which secretes H^+ ions in the apical canaliculi of parietal cells and also which can be activated by histamine (Figure 1.2).

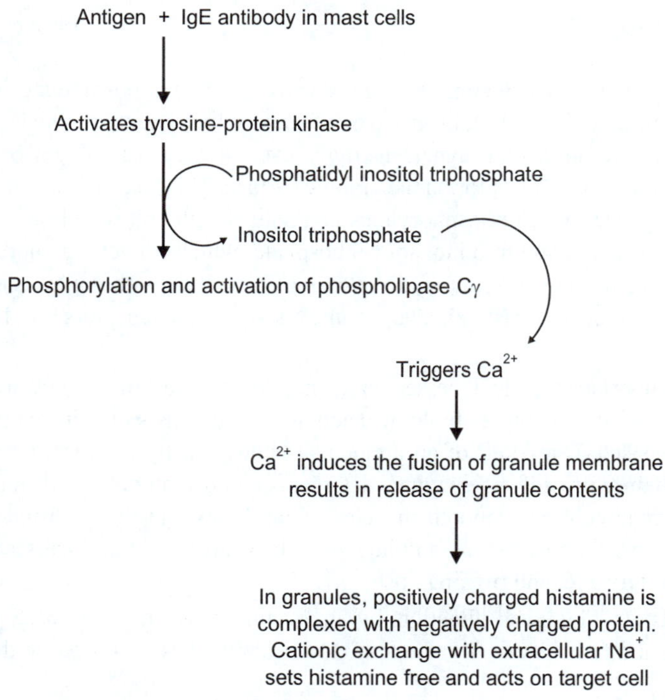

Figure 1.1: Steps involved in the release of histamine.

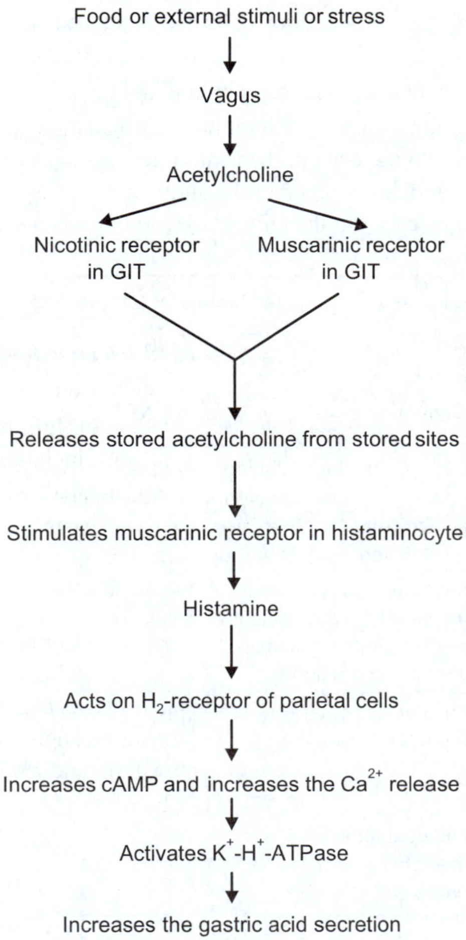

Figure 1.2: Histamine-induced gastric acid secretion.

The therapeutically available antagonists of histamine receptors are used as antiallergic drugs by targeting H_1-receptors and as antiulcers by targeting H_2-receptors.

Mode of Action of Antihistamines

After the release of histamine by the mast cells, it binds with histaminergic receptors (H_1, H_2, and H_3) to elicit a series of events that mediates the characteristic responses through second messenger systems. The histaminergic receptors are G-protein coupled type. H_1-receptors are coupled to phospholipase-C and their activation leads to the formation of inositol phosphate (IP_3) and diacylglycerol (DAG), respectively, from phospholipids in cell membrane. IP_3 causes rapid release of Ca^{2+} from endoplasmic reticulum. DAG activates the protein kinase C. Altogether, the turnover of Ca^{2+} and protein kinase-C activates Ca^{2+}/calmodulin dependent protein kinase and phospholipase A_2. The antihistaminergic drugs (H_1-antagonist) binds to the H_1-receptors and decreases the production of phospholipase-C and their activation to form IP_3 and DAG, thereby blocks the characteristic response of histamine.

Histamine on H_2-receptors produces cAMP-dependent protein kinase (cyclic adenosine monophosphate (cAMP), also known as cyclic AMP or 3′-5′-cyclic adenosine monophosphate) to elicit a response in the GIT. The H_2-antagonist reversibly binds the H_2-receptors and reduces the cAMP formation, which is responsible for the activation of proton pump and, subsequently, reduces the gastric acid formation in the GIT.

H_3-receptors are also G-protein coupled receptors, unlike H_1 and H_2, and they produce a decreased Ca^{2+} influx. H_3-receptors function as feedback inhibitors for histamine and other neurotransmitters by decreasing the calcium influx into the cells in the central nervous system (CNS), and in the GIT, they reduce the secretion of gastrin and down-regulates histamine through auto-regulatory effects. Blocking H_3-receptors antagonize these effects, but the clinical extendibility is narrow for H_3.

Table 1.1: Distribution of histamine receptors and the biological actions of histamine

Receptor	***Location***	***Biological actions of histamine***		
		General	***In CNS***	***In allergy and immune modulation***
H_1	Widespread in the neuronal system, smooth muscles, endothelium	On stimulation: Itching, pain, vasodilation, tachycardia, broncho-constriction	Controls sleep–wake cycle, temperature regulation memory	Increases release of histamine, IgE production
H_2	Gastric mucosa, smooth muscle, heart, brain	Increased gastric acidity, increased airway mucous production, increased vascular permeability	Neuroendocrine regulation	Decreases neutrophil and eosinophil chemotaxis, suppresses cellular immunity
H_3	Histaminergic neurons and mysentric plexus	Prevent excessive broncho-constriction	Presynaptic hetero-receptor decreases histamine, NA, DA, 5-H, ACh release	–
H_4	Bone marrow and eosinophils, neutrophils	Differentiation of myeloblasts and promyelocytes	–	Increases eosinophills, chemotaxis and IL-16 production

STRUCTURE–ACTIVITY RELATIONSHIP—H_1-RECEPTOR ANTAGONISTS

Based on the pharmacological profile, the H_1-antihistamines are divided into two major groups:

1. First-generation or classical antihistamines
2. Second-generation or non-sedative antihistamines

The SAR of antihistamines is discussed with reference to the first-generation antihistamines. The structural requirements (pharmacophore) for H_1-antihistamines are shown below.

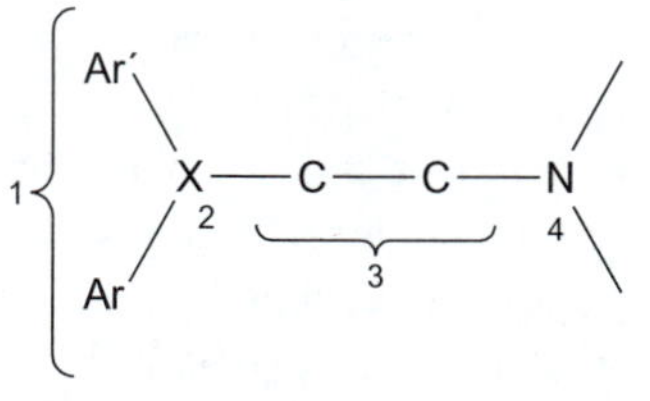

1. Aryl groups

- The diaryl substitution is essential for significant H_1-receptor affinity. It is present both in first-generation and second-generation antihistamines. The optimal antihistaminic activity depends on the co-planarity of two aryl substitutions. The active aryl substitutions are as follows:

  Ar: Phenyl, substituted phenyl and heteroaryl group like 2-pyridyl

  Ar′: Aryl or aryl methyl group
- The majority of H_1-antihistamines possess substituents in one of the aryl rings (generally in phenyl ring), and this influences the potency of the compound. The two aryl rings may be linked, e.g. promethazine, cyproheptadine, and azatidine.

2. Nature of 'X'

- The X-connecting moiety of H_1-antihistamines may be simple carbon chain or saturated carbon–oxygen moiety, which serves as a spacer group for required pharmacophore.
- Antihistamines containing a carbon atom in the connecting moiety (example pheniramine series and carbinoxamine) exhibit chirality, which leads to stereoselective binding at the receptor. Among the enantiomers, the *S* isomer shows higher H_1-receptor-binding affinity.
- The active substitutions of X are as follows: X = oxygen (amino alkyl ether analogue), X = nitrogen (ethylene diamine derivative), X = carbon (mono amino propyl analogue).
- Based on the nature of this connecting moiety and the aryl moieties, H_1-antihistamines are further divided as ethylene diamines, amino alkyl ethers, mono amino propyl analogues, etc.

3. Alkyl chain $(CH_2)_n$

- The carbon chain consists of two or three atoms in H_1-antihistamines, which leads to the distance between the central point of the diaryl ring system and the terminal nitrogen atom in the extended conformation of these compounds in the range of 5–6 Å.

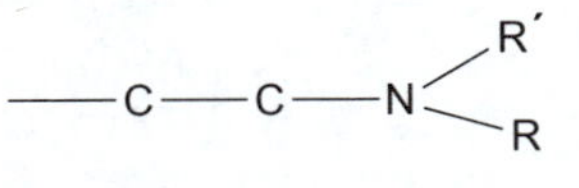

- Branching of this carbon chain leads to decrease in antihistaminic activity. (Exception is promethazine which is more potent than its non-branched counterpart.)
- If the carbon atom adjacent to the terminal nitrogen atom is branched, the possibility of asymmetry exists. However, it will not affect the binding affinity with the receptor.

4. Terminal nitrogen atom (NRR′): The terminal N-atom should be a 3° amine for maximum activity. The terminal nitrogen may be a part of heterocyclic ring, e.g. antazoline and chlorcyclizine which also retains high antihistaminic activity. The amino moiety deserves the protonation on interaction with H_1-receptor due to the basicity with pK_a 8.5–10. For preparing stable solid dosage forms through salt formation the amino moiety is important.

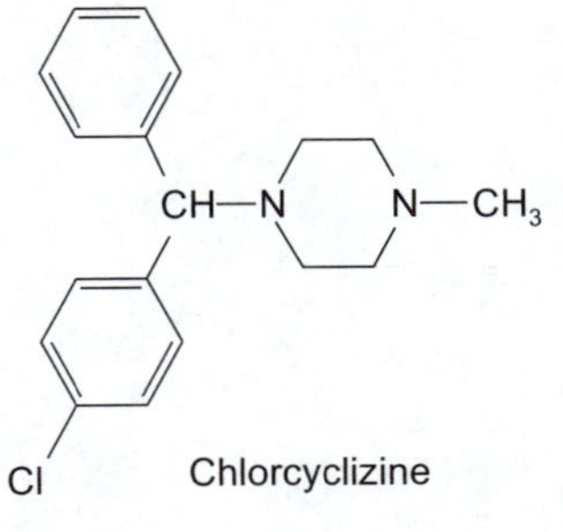

Chlorcyclizine

Note: The antihistamines exhibit a range of pharmacological activities because of their interaction with H_1-receptors distributed throughout the body, and its pharmacophore is similar to that of pharmacophore required for binding to muscarinic as well as adrenergic and serotonergic receptors, which leads to the side effects like cardiac arrhythmia, dry mouth, etc., apart from sedation.

CLASSIFICATION

I. H_1-Antagonists with Classical Structures

According to the chemical features, they are further classified as follows:

a. Ethylene diamine derivatives
b. Amino alkyl ether analogues
c. Cyclic basic chain analogues or piperazine derivatives
d. Mono amino propyl analogues
e. Tricyclic ring system or phenothiazine derivatives
f. Dibenzocycloheptenes
g. Miscellaneous agents
h. Newer agents

a. Ethylene diamine derivatives

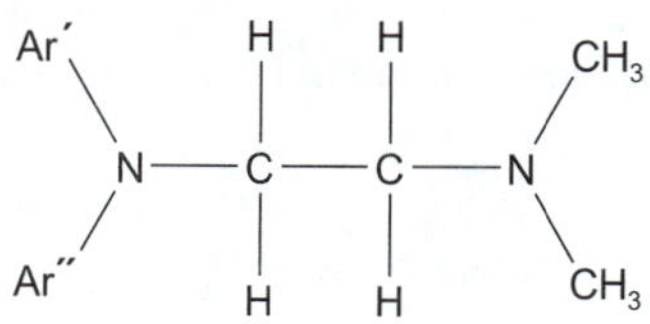

Name	Ar′	Ar″
Tripelennamine	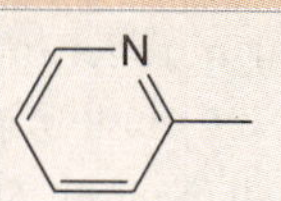	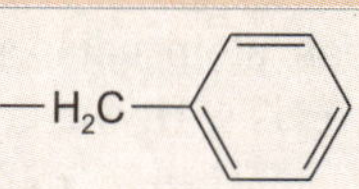
Pyrilamine	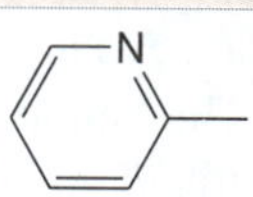	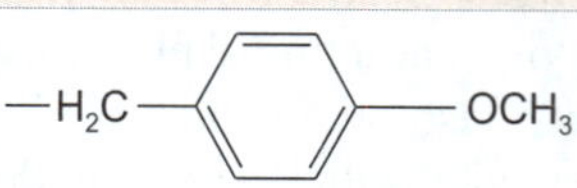
Methapyrilene	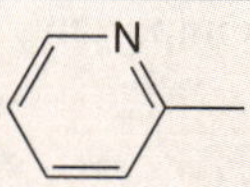	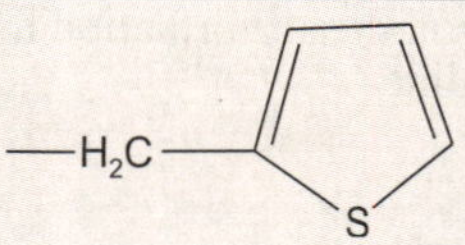
Thonzylamine	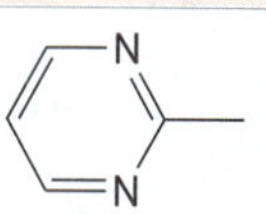	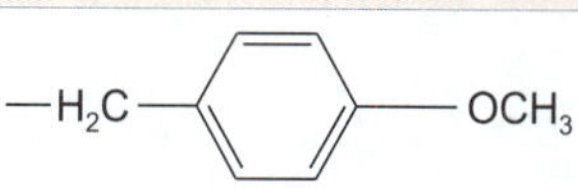
Zolamine	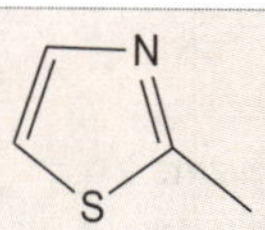	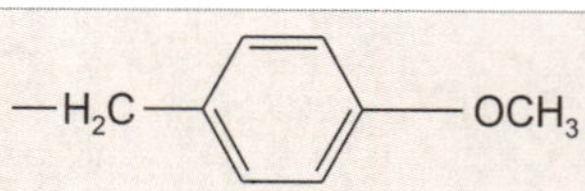

b. Amino alkyl ether analogues

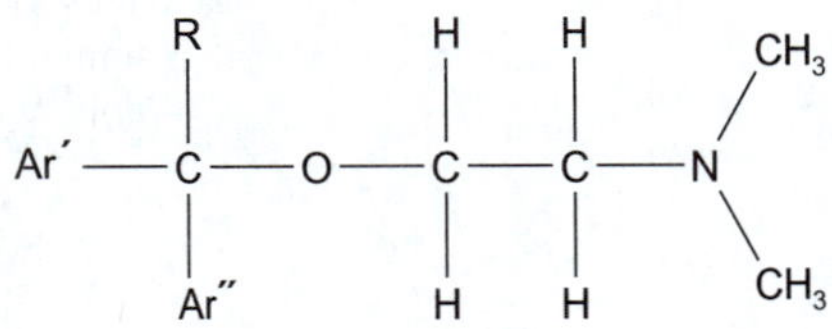

Name	Ar'	Ar''	R
Diphenhydramine	$-C_6H_5$	$-C_6H_5$	–H
Bromodiphenhydramine	$-C_6H_5$	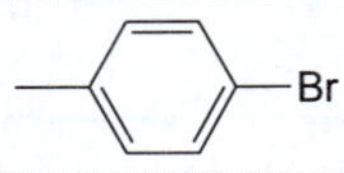	–H
Doxylamine	$-C_6H_5$	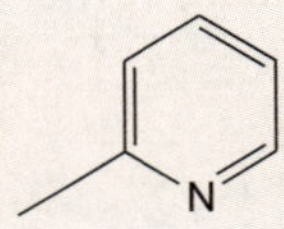	$-CH_3$
Carbinoxamine	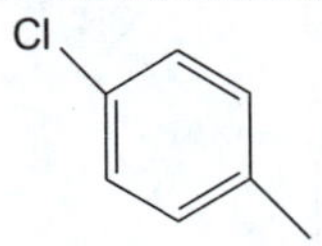	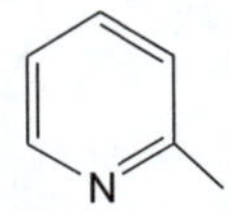	–H
Medrylamine	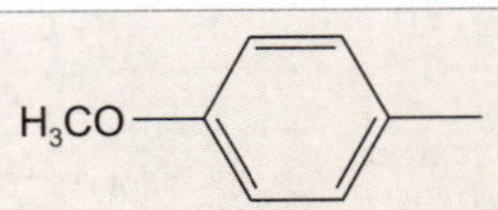	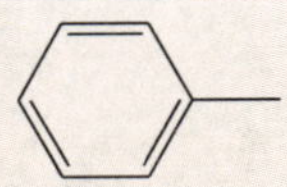	–H

Clemastine

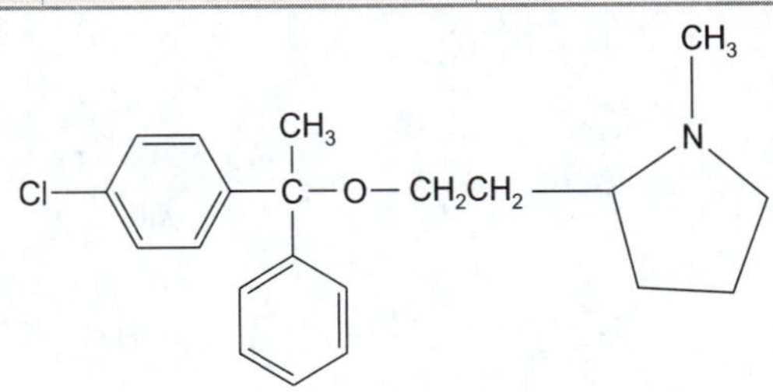

Diphenylpyraline

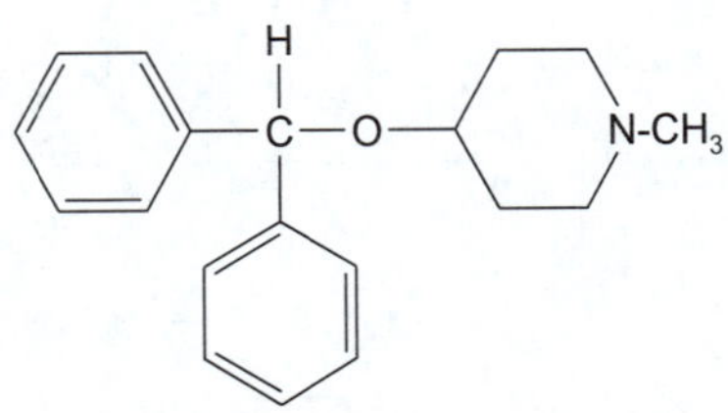

c. Cyclic basic chain analogues or piperazine derivatives

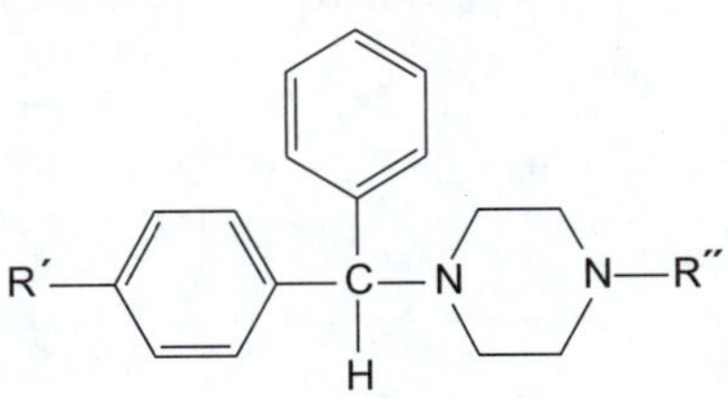

Name	***R'***	***R''***
Cyclizine	–H	$-CH_3$
Chlorcyclizine	–Cl	$-CH_3$
Meclizine	–Cl	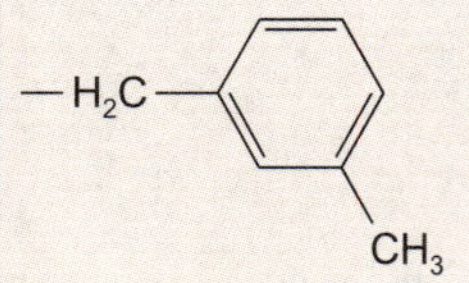
Buclizine	–Cl	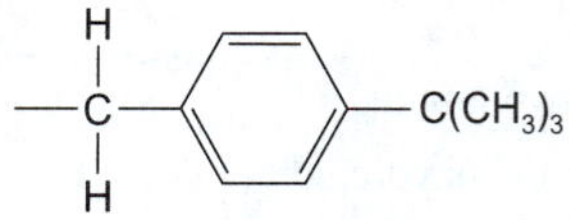

d. Mono amino propyl analogues

i. Saturated analogues

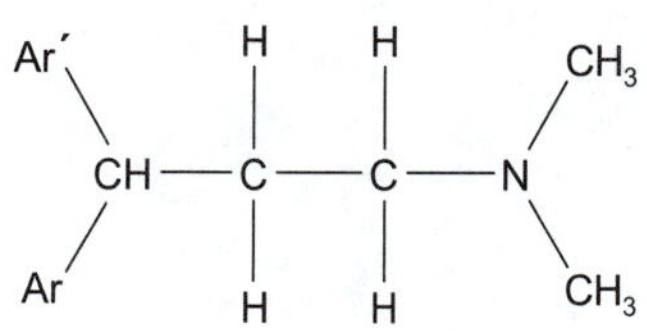

Name	***Ar***	***Ar'***
Pheniramine	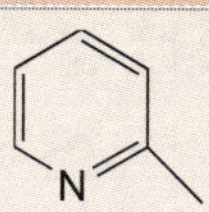	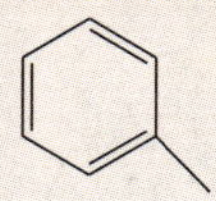
Chlorpheniramine	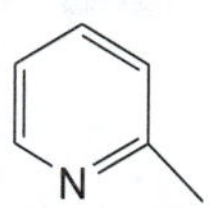	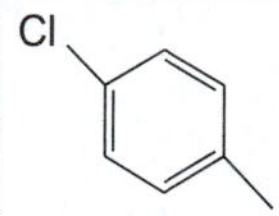
Bromopheniramine	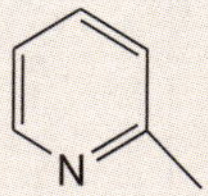	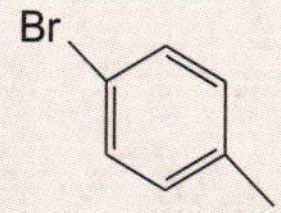

ii. Unsaturated analogues

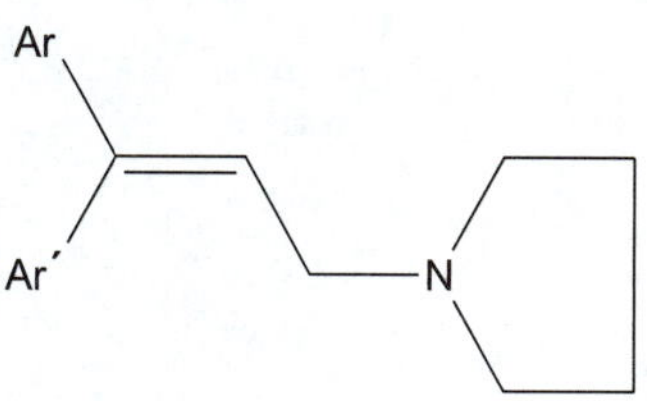

Name	***Ar***	***Ar'***
Pyrrobutamine	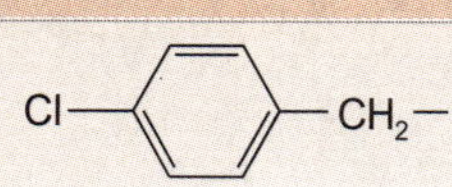	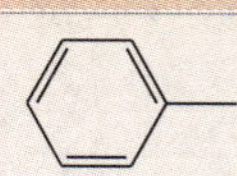
Triprolidine	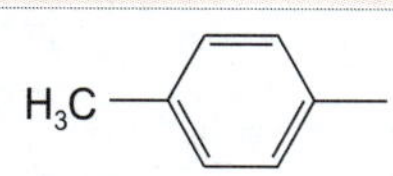	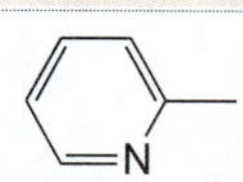

e. Tricyclic ring system or phenothiazine derivatives

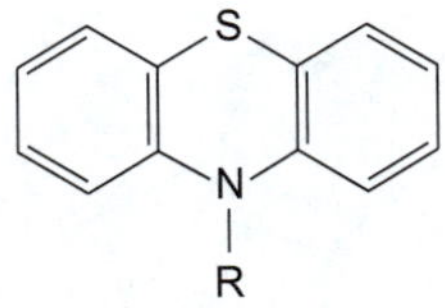

Name	*R*
Promethazine hydrochloride	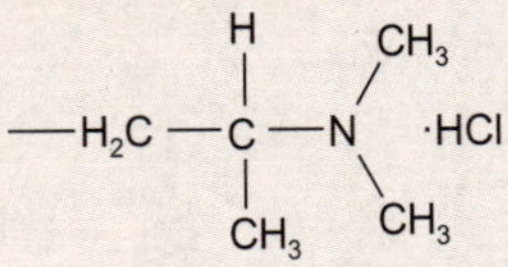
Trimeprazine	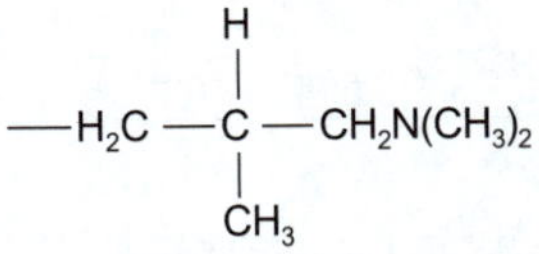
Methdilazine	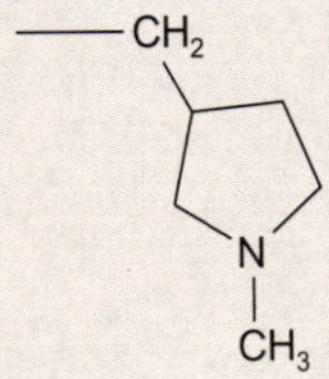

f. Dibenzocycloheptenes

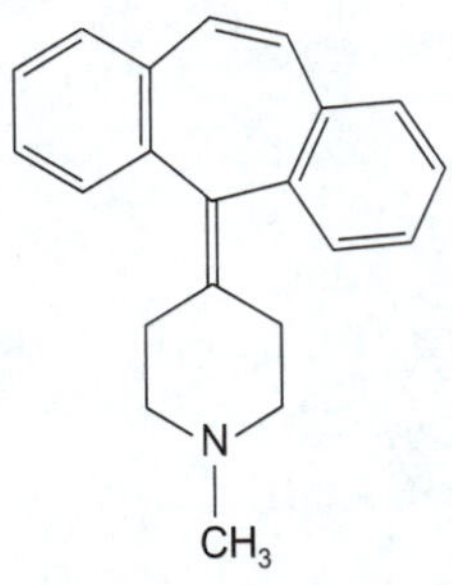

Cyproheptadine

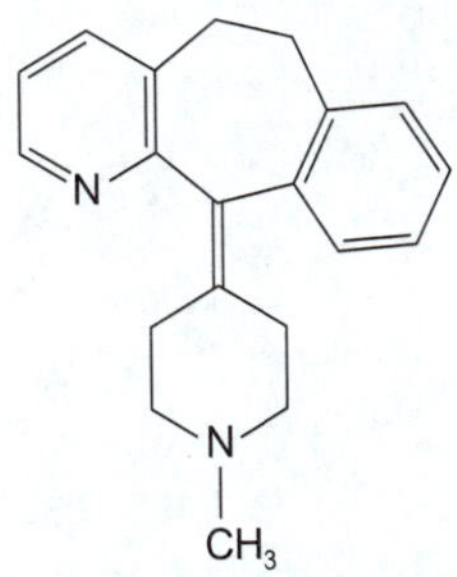

Azatadine

g. Miscellaneous agents

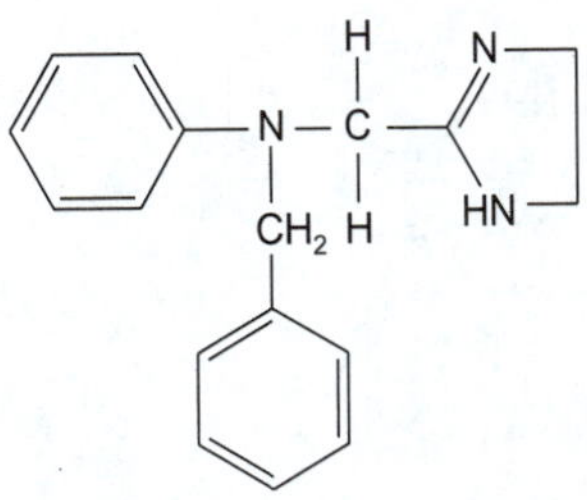

Antazoline

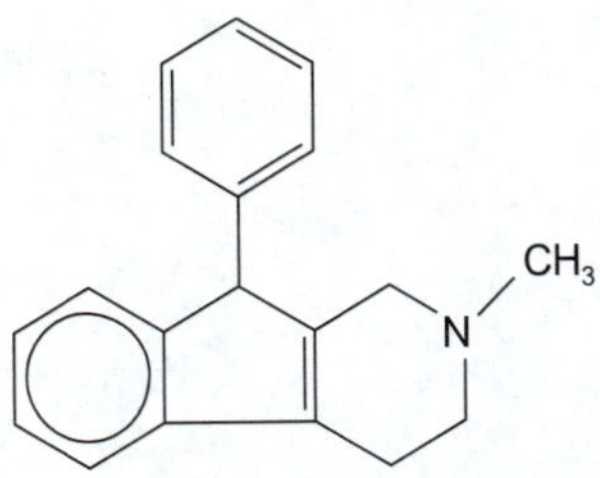

Phenindamine

h. Newer agents

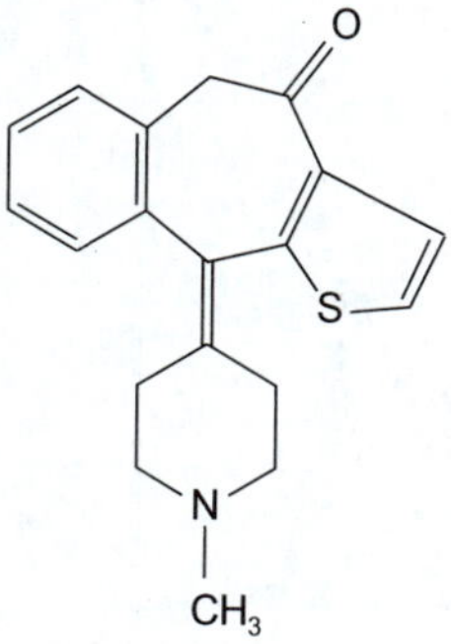

Ketotifene

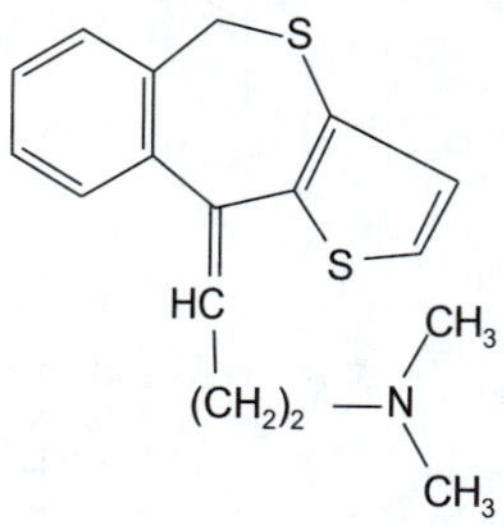

Dithiadene

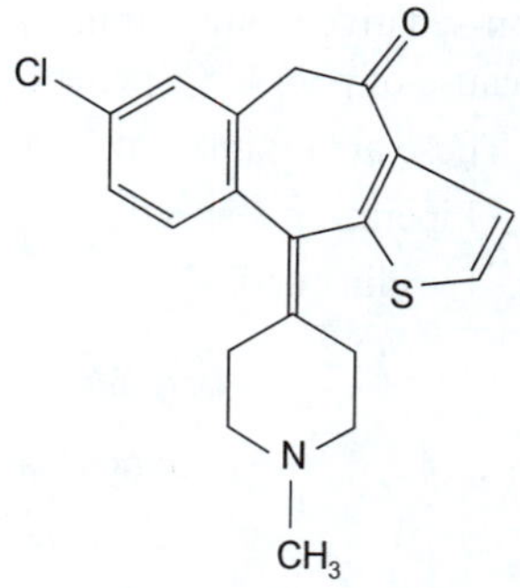

7-Chloroketotifene

II. H_1-Antagonists with Non-classical Structures

i. Azelastine

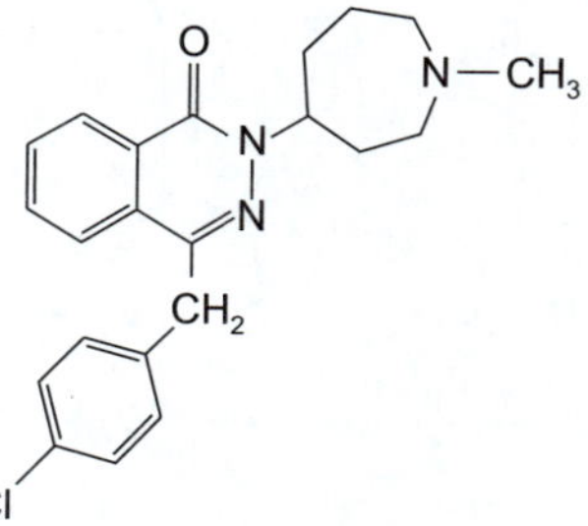

ii. Tazifylline

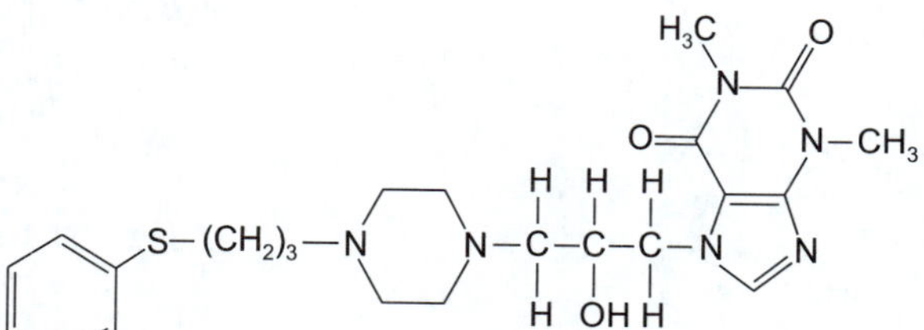

iii. Astemizole

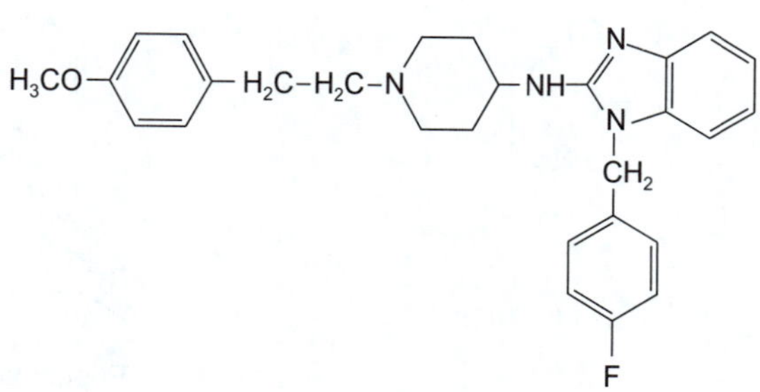

III. Non-sedative H_1-antihistamines

Non-sedative antihistamines bind only to peripheral H_1-receptors and produce with little or no sedation because of poor CNS penetration and lower affinity for central histaminic activity.

These are divided into two main classes:

1. Piperazine derivatives—cetirizine
2. Pyridine and piperidine derivatives—loratadine, fexofenadine, terfenadine, astemizole, acrivastine

i. Loratadine

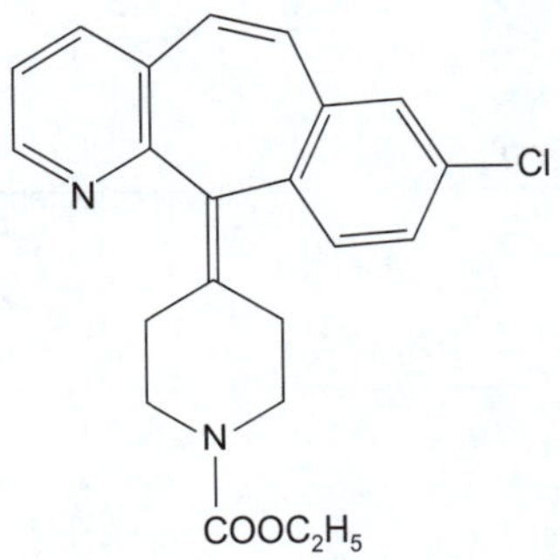

ii. Epinastine

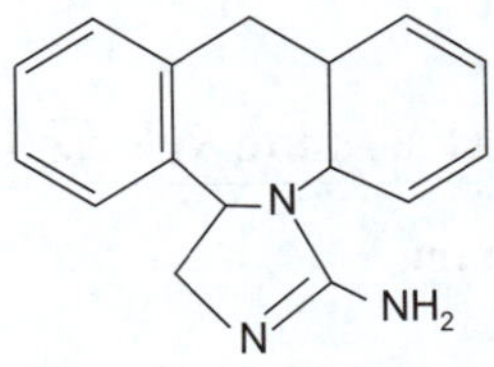

iii. Rocastine

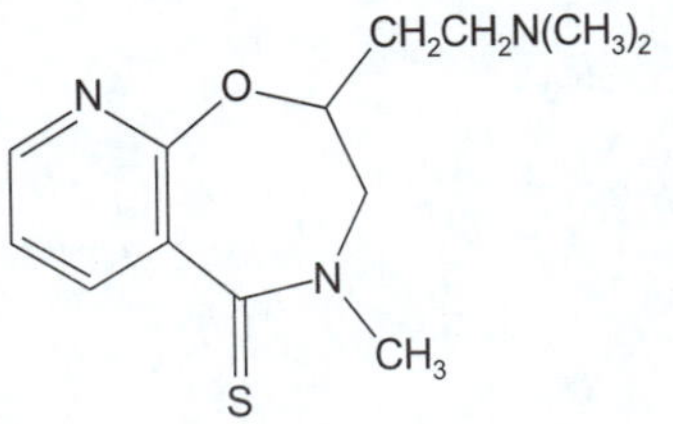

iv. Cetirizine

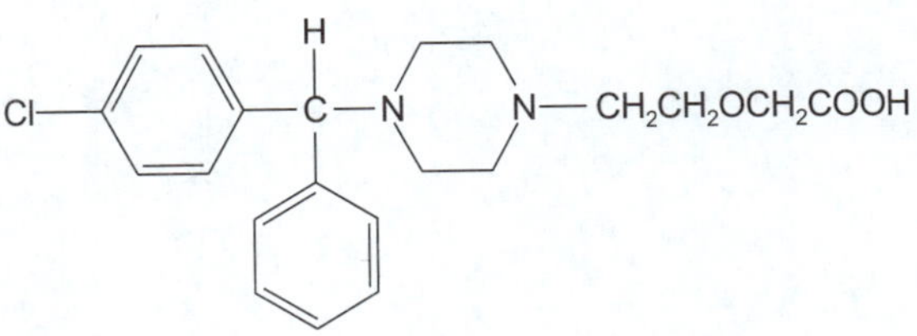

v. Fexofenadine

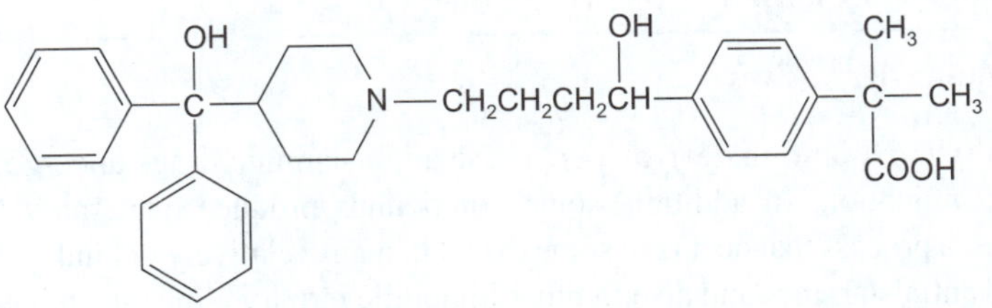

vi. Acrivastine

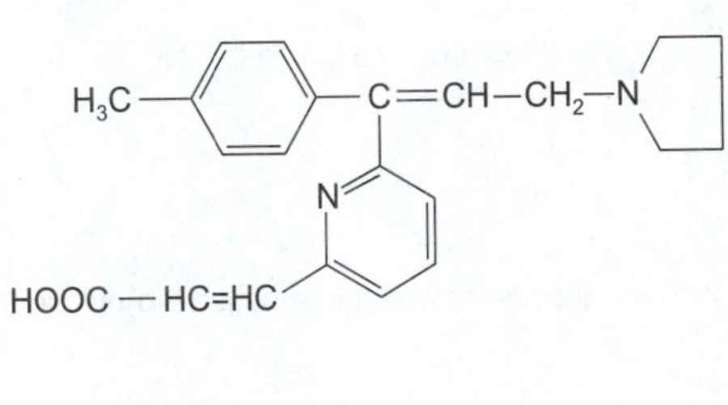

vii. Olopatadine hydrochloride

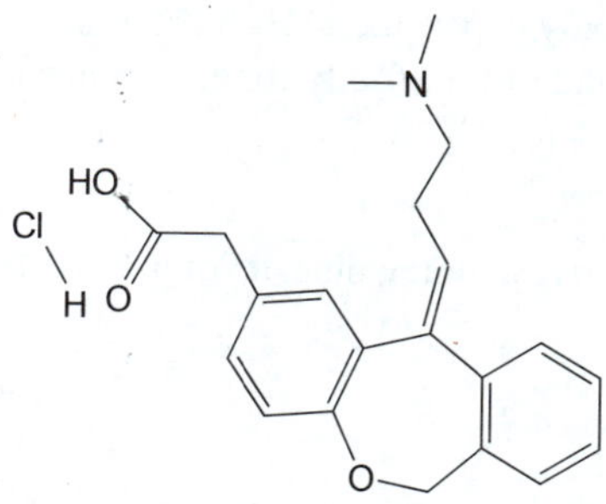

IV. Inhibition of Histamine Release (Mast Cell Stabilizers)

i. Cromolyn sodium

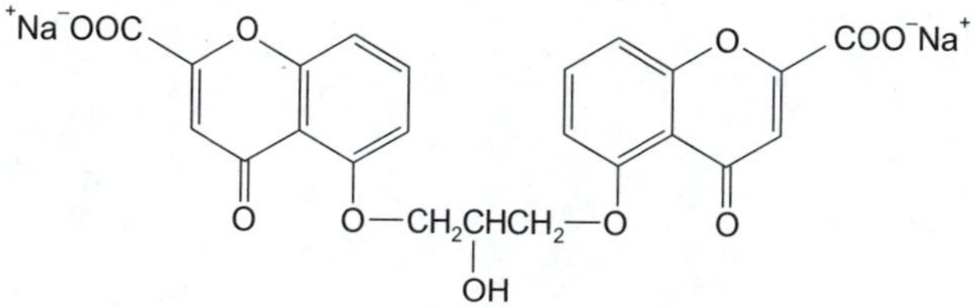

ii. Nedocromil sodium

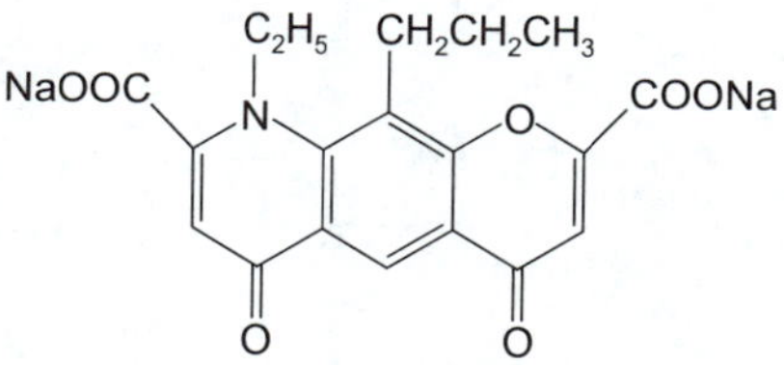

SYNTHESIS AND DRUG PROFILE

I. H_1-Antagonists with Classical Structure

a. Ethylene diamine derivatives

Metabolism of ethylene diamine derivatives: These antihistaminic drugs undergo N-demethylation and subsequent deamination. In addition, some compounds produce quaternary N-glucuronide as urinary metabolites, a process that occurs to some extent in many relatively unhindered tertiary aliphatic amines among the antihistamines and also in other lipophilic tertiary aliphatic amine drugs.

i. Tripelennamine (Pyribenzamine HCl)

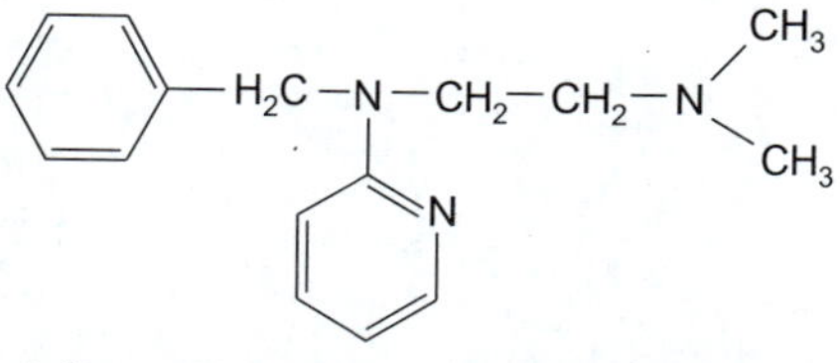

2-(Benzyl[2-(dimethylamino)ethyl]amino)pyridine

Synthesis

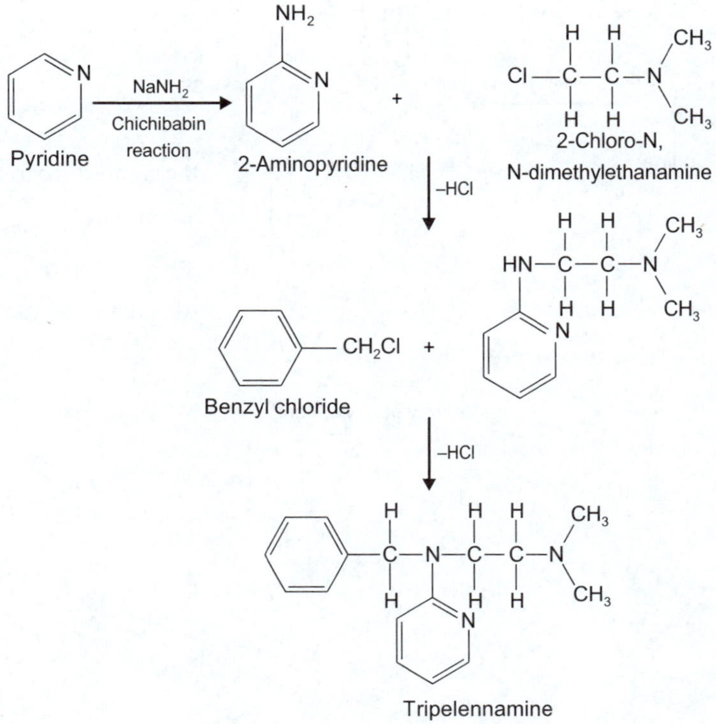

Properties and uses: It is a white, crystalline powder, soluble in water, freely soluble in alcohol and ether, but insoluble in chloroform or benzene. Tripelennamine is the first ethylenediamine developed in the American laboratories; it appears to be effective as diphenhydramine and may have the advantage of fewer and less severe side reactions. Drowsiness may occur and may impair the ability to perform tasks requiring alertness. The concurrent use of alcoholic beverage should be avoided. It is used in the treatment of allergic rhinitis, allergic conjunctivitis, angioedema, dermagraphism, and anaphylactic reactions.

Dose: Usual dose is 25–50 mg for adults consumed orally four to six times a day.

ii. Pyrilamine (Mepyramine, Anthisan)

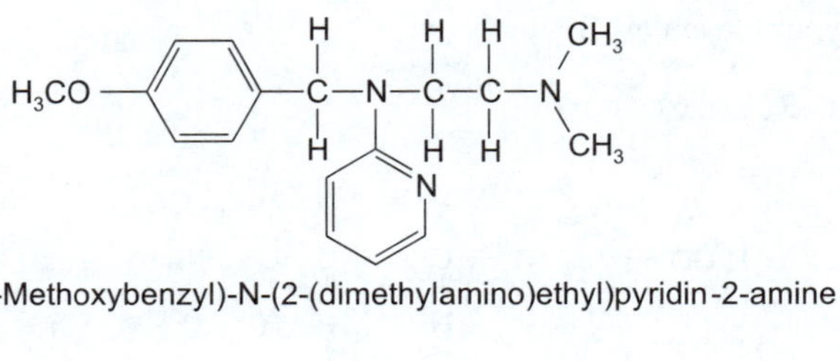

N-(4-Methoxybenzyl)-N-(2-(dimethylamino)ethyl)pyridin-2-amine

Synthesis

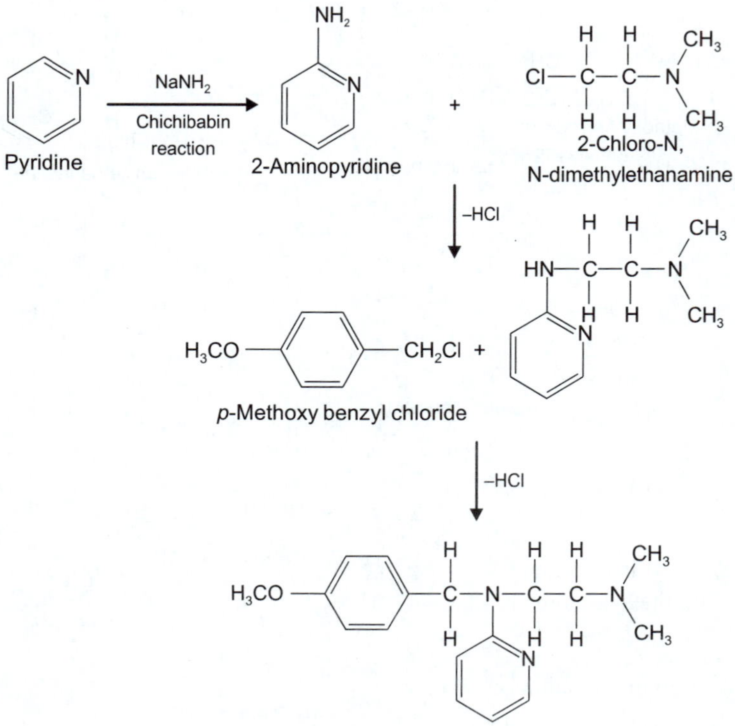

Mepyramine

Properties and uses: Mepyramine maleate is a white or slightly yellowish crystalline powder, soluble in water and in ethanol. Pyrilamine differs structurally from tripelennamine having a methoxy group in the *para* position of the benzyl radical. It differs from its more toxic and less potent precursor phenbenzamine (antergan) having a 2-pyridyl group on the nitrogen atom in the place of a phenyl group. Clinically, pyrilamine and tripelennamine are considered to be among the less potent antihistamines. It is used as an antihistaminic agent with a low incidence of sedative effects; it is also used as an antiemetic.

Assay: Dissolve the sample in anhydrous acetic acid and titrate against 0.1 M perchloric acid. Determine the end point potentiometrically.

Dose: Usual dose is 25–50 mg for adults taken orally three to four times per day.

Dosage forms: Mepyramine tablets BP.

iii. **Thonzylamine** (Resistab)

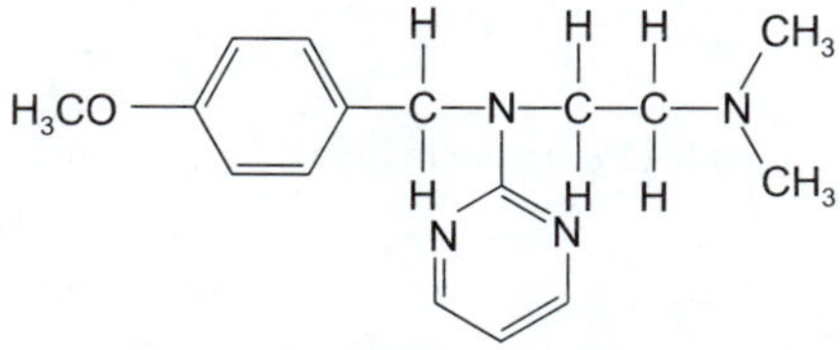

N-(4-Methoxybenzyl)-N-(2-(dimethylamino)ethyl)pyrimidin-2-amine

Synthesis

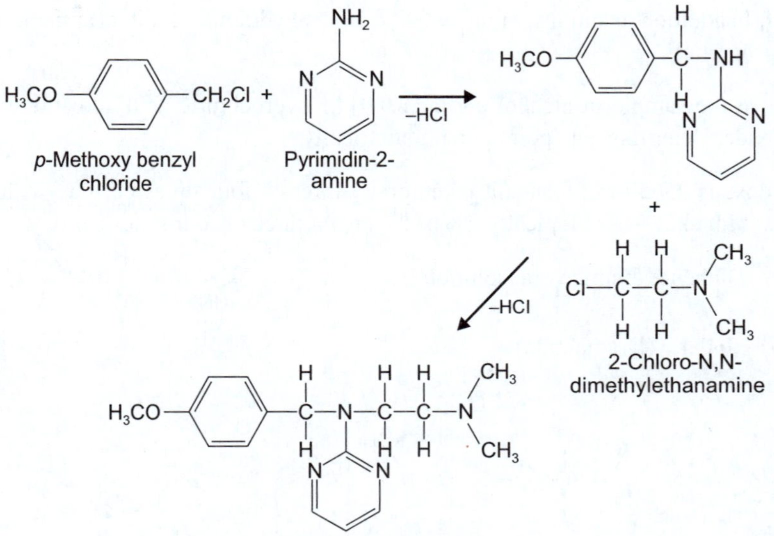

Thonzylamine

Properties and uses: It is recommended for use with streptomycin in exudative human tuberculosis. It is used in treating the symptoms of diseases, such as hay fever, urtricaria, and other mild allergic conditions.

Dose: Usual dose is 50 mg for adults consumed orally up to four times a day.

b. Amino alkyl ether analogues

i. Diphenhydramine (Benadryl, Bendylate)

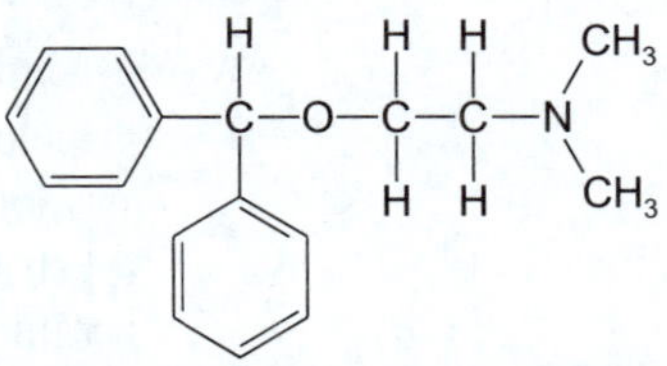

2-(Benzhydryloxy)-N,N-dimethylethanamine

Synthesis

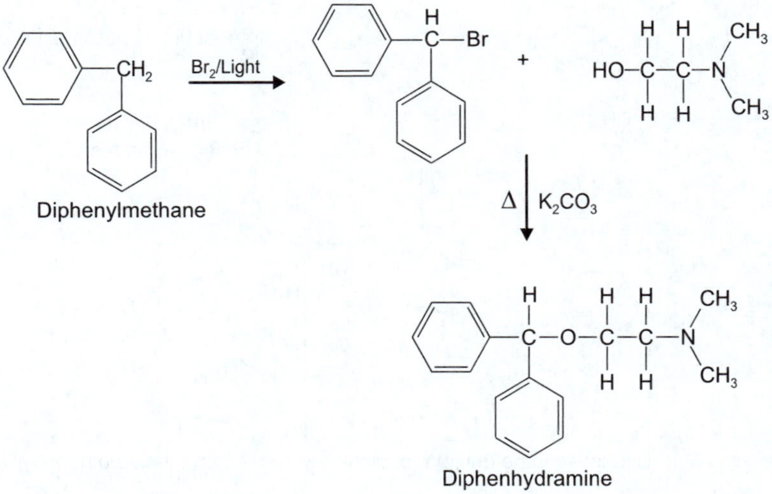

Diphenhydramine

Properties and uses: Diphenhydramine hydrochloride is a white crystalline powder, soluble in water and in alcohol. In addition to antihistaminic activity, diphenhydramine exhibits antiemetic, antitussive, and sedative properties.

Assay: Dissolve the sample in alcohol and add 0.01 M hydrochloric acid and titrate against 0.1 M sodium hydroxide. Determine end point potentiometrically.

Dose: Usual dose is 25–50 mg for adult taken orally three to four times per day with maximum of 400 mg per day; for skin—used topically 2% of the cream three or four times per day.

Dosage forms: Diphenhydramine oral solution BP.

ii. Dimenhydrinate (Dramamine)

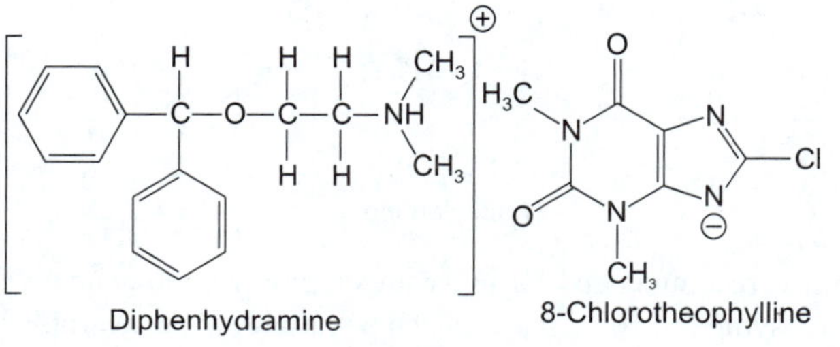

Synthesis

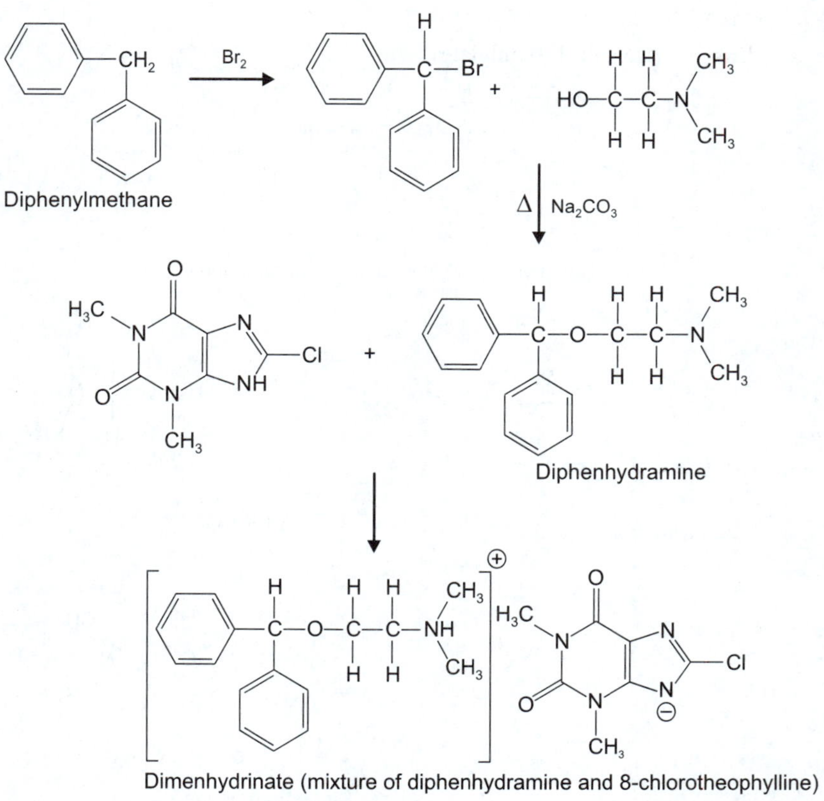

Dimenhydrinate (mixture of diphenhydramine and 8-chlorotheophylline)

Properties and uses: Dimenhydrinate is a white crystalline powder or colourless crystals, slightly soluble in water and in alcohol. Used as histamine H_1-receptor antagonist, antinauseant, in motion sickness, radiation sickness, and also in the case of nausea during pregnancy.

Assay: Dissolve the sample in anhydrous acetic acid and titrate against 0.1 M perchloric acid. Determine the end point potentiometrically.

Dose: Usual dose is taken orally as 50 mg thrice/day.

Dosage forms: Dimenhydrinate tablets BP.

iii. Bromodiphenhydramine (Ambodryl hydrochloride)

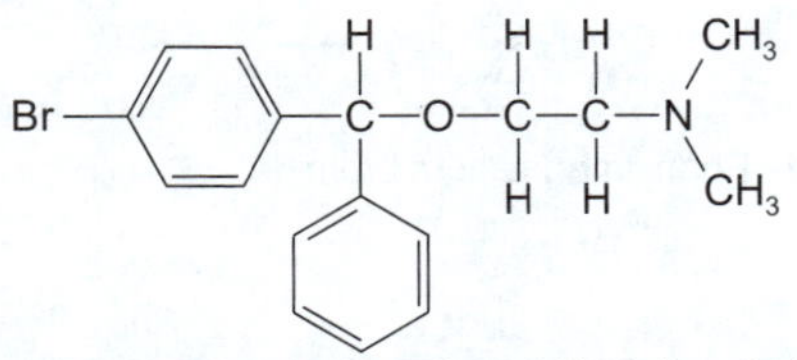

2-[(4-Bromophenyl)(phenyl)methoxy]-N,N-dimethylethanamine

Synthesis

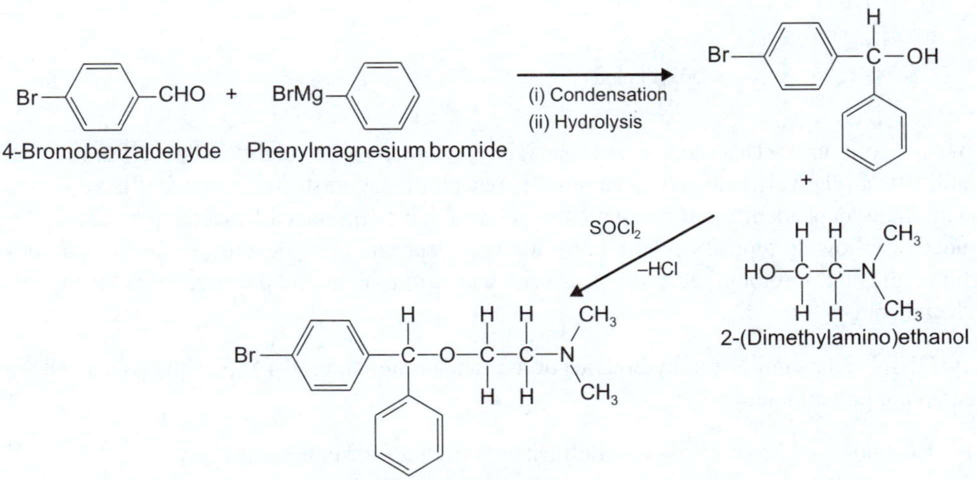

Bromodiphenhydramine

Properties and uses: It is effective for mild, local allergic reactions, physical allergy, and for minor drug reactions, characterized by pruritus.

Dose: Usual dose is 25 mg three or four times per day.

iv. Doxylamine (Decapryn succinate)

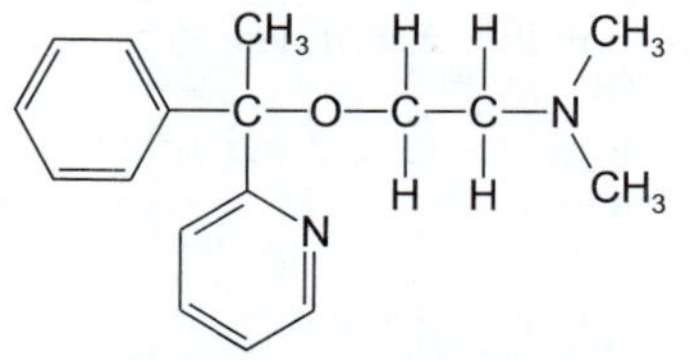

N,N-Dimethyl-2-(1-phenyl-1-(pyridin-2-yl)ethoxy)ethanamine

Synthesis

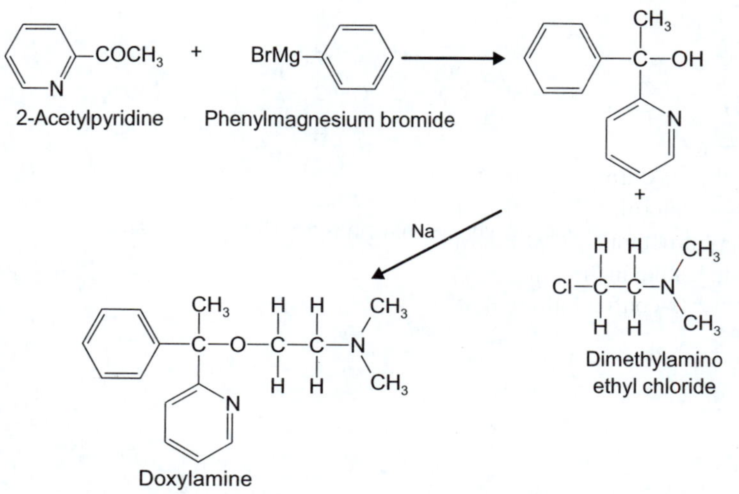

Properties and uses: Doxylamine succinate is a white powder, highly soluble in water and in alcohol. It is a relatively selective histamine H_1-receptor antagonist. *In vivo* studies have shown that concentrations dependent upon the inhibition of histamine-stimulated vascular permeability in the conjunctiva following topical ocular administration. It appears to be devoid of effects on adrenergic, dopaminergic, and serotonin receptors. It is used with antitussives and decongestants for the relief of cough and cold.

Assay: Dissolve the sample in anhydrous acetic acid and titrate against 0.1 M per chloric acid. Determine the end point potentiometrically.

Dose: Usual dose is 12.5 to 25 mg for adult taken orally four to six times per day.

v. Carbinoxamine

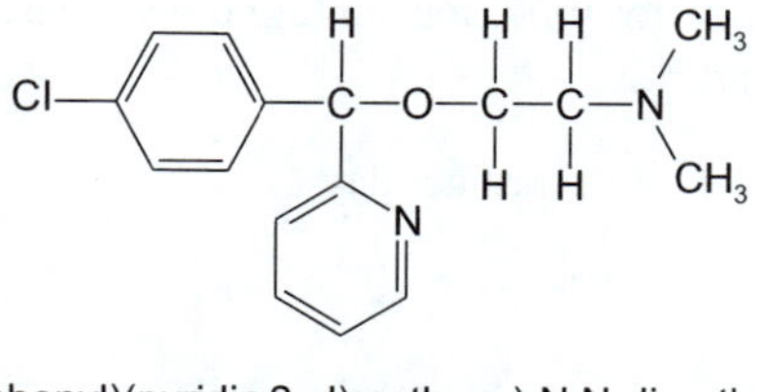

2-((4-Chlorophenyl)(pyridin-2-yl)methoxy)-N,N-dimethylethanamine

Synthesis

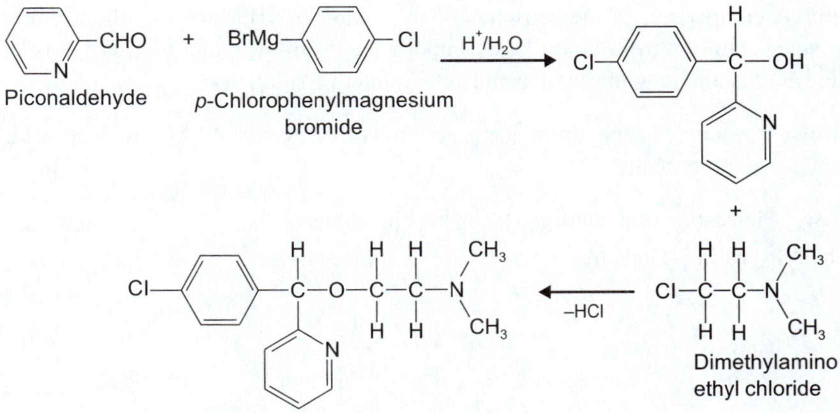

Carbinoxamine

Properties and uses: Carbinoxamine is available as white, crystalline powder with no odour, soluble in water, alcohol, chloroform, or ether. It is a potent antihistaminic and is available as the racemic mixture. It differs structurally from chlorpheniramine only in having an oxygen atom separate from the asymmetric carbon atom in the aminoethyl side chain. The levo isomer of carbinoxamine is more active than dextro isomer (*s*-configuration) of chlorpheniramine.

vi. Clemastine

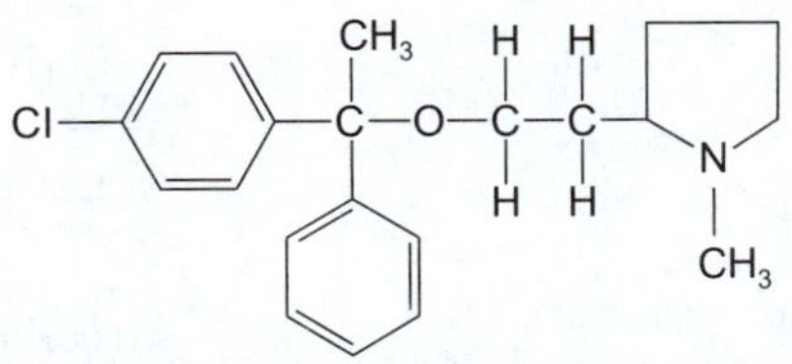

2-(2-1-(4-Chlorophenyl)-1-(phenylethoxy)ethyl)-1-methylpyrrolidine

Synthesis

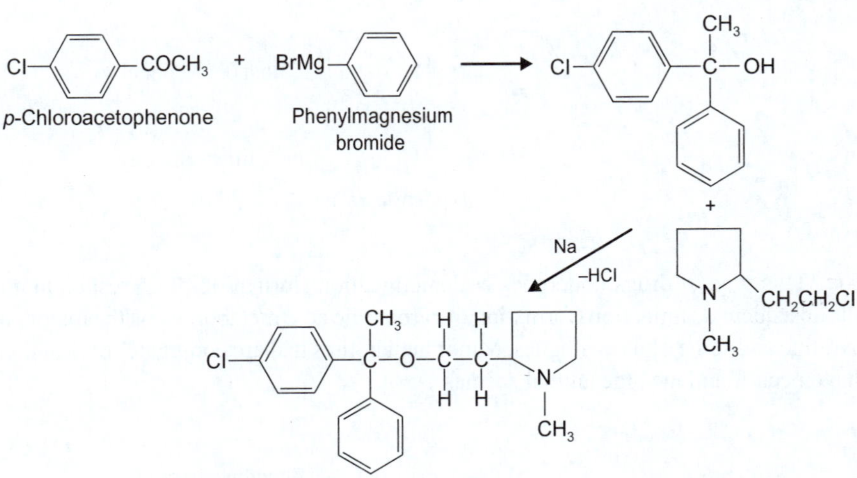

Clemastine

Properties and uses: Clemastine fumarate is a white crystalline powder, very slightly soluble in water, slightly soluble in alcohol and methanol. It has two chiral centres, each of which is (R) absolute configuration. A comparison of the activities of the antipodes indicates that the asymmetric centre close to the side chain of nitrogen is of lesser importance to antihistaminic activity. It is a long-acting ethanolamine antihistamine with sedative and anticholinergic side effects.

Assay: Dissolve the sample in anhydrous acetic acid and titrate against 0.1 M perchloric acid. Determine the end point potentiometrically.

Dosage forms: Clemastine oral solution BP, clemastine tablets BP.

vii. Diphenylpyraline (Diaben)

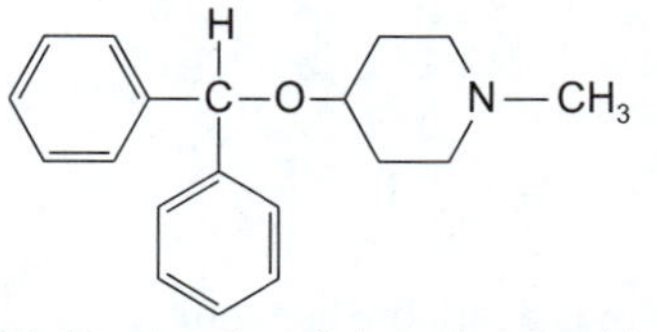

4-(Diphenylmethoxy)-1-methylpiperidine

Synthesis

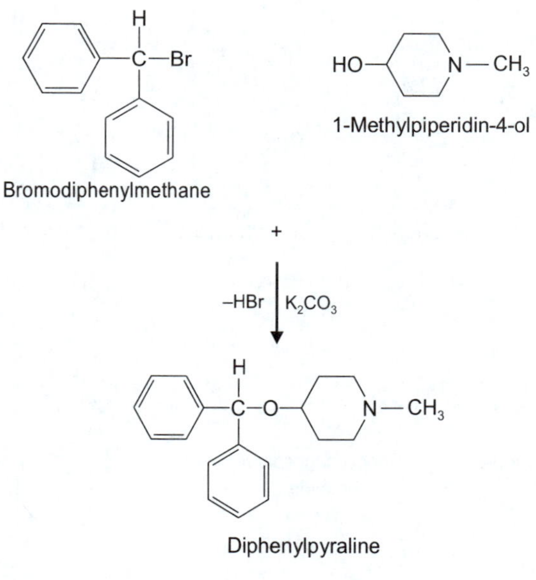

Metabolism: This type of drugs undergoes N-demethylation (formation of corresponding secondary amine) and subsequent deamination (formation of carboxylic acid metabolites) is the major pathway for diphenylpyraline and some of its analogues. Minor metabolites that are conjugates of the ether cleavage products have been found in some animal species.

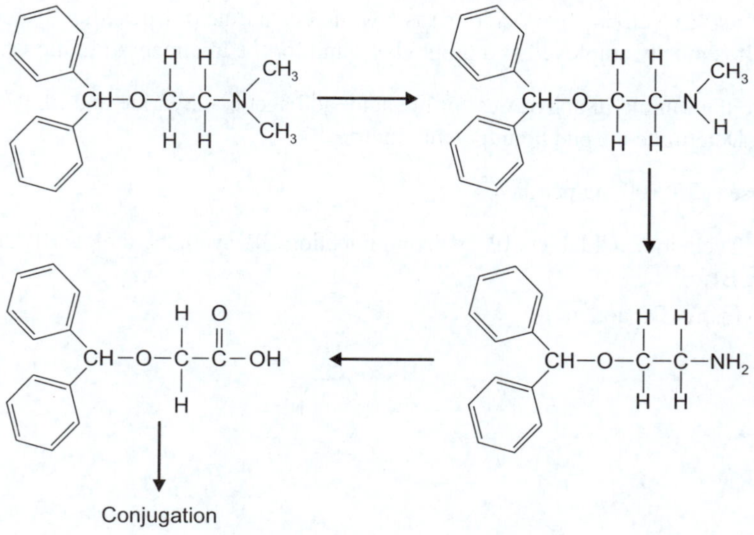

Properties and uses: Diphenylpyraline hydrochloride is a white powder, soluble in water and ethanol, practically insoluble in ether. It is structurally related to diphenhydramine with the aminoalkyl side chain incorporated in a piperidine ring. It is a potent antihistaminic agent.

Assay: Dissolve the sample in anhydrous acetic acid and add mercury(II) acetate solution and titrate against 0.1 M perchloric acid using oracet blue B solution as indicator.

Dose: Usual dose for adults taken orally is 5 mg two times per day.

c. Piperazine derivatives

i. Cyclizine (Marezine)

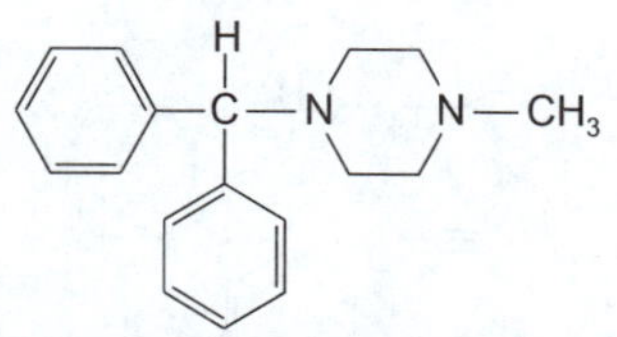

1-Benzhydryl-4-methylpiperazine

Synthesis

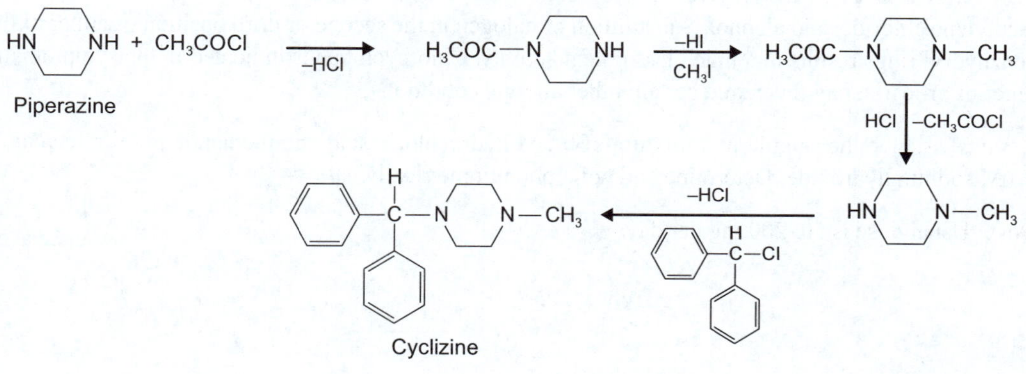

Properties and uses: Cyclizine hydrochloride is a white crystalline powder, slightly soluble in water and in alcohol. It is mostly employed as a prophylaxis and for the treatment of motion sickness.

Assay: Dissolve the sample in anhydrous formic acid, add acetic anhydride and titrate against 0.1 M perchloric acid. Determine the end point potentiometrically.

Dose: Usual dose is 25–100 mg per day.

Dosage forms: Cyclizine HCl tablets IP, cyclizine injection BP, cyclizine tablets BP, dipipanone and cyclizine tablets BP.

ii. Chlorcyclizine (Diparalene)

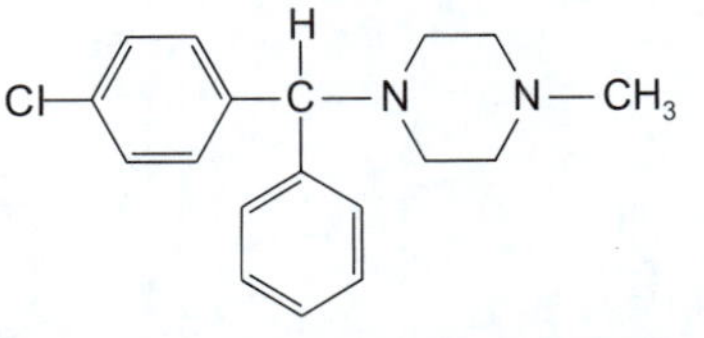

1-((4-Chlorophenyl)(phenyl)methyl)-4-methylpiperazine

Synthesis

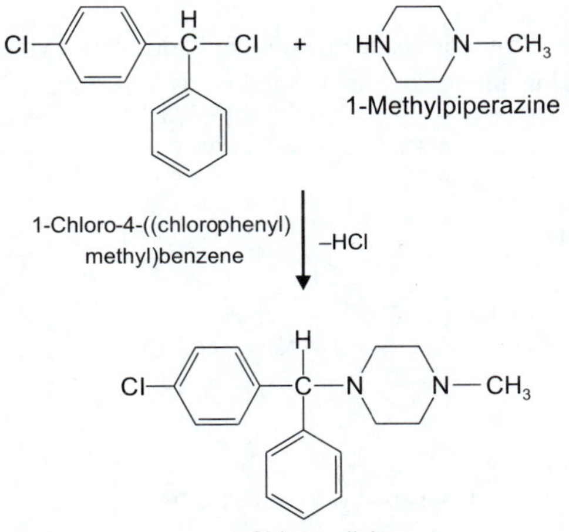

Chlorcyclizine

Properties and uses: Chlorcyclizine hydrochloride is a white crystalline powder, soluble in water, methylene chloride, and alcohol. Substitution of halogen in the second or third position of either of the benzhydryl rings results in a much less potent activity. Chlorcyclizine is indicated in the symptomatic relief of urticaria, hay fever, and certain other allergic conditions.

Assay: Dissolve the sample in a mixture of 0.1 M hydrochloric acid and methanol and titrate against 0.1 M sodium hydroxide. Determine end point potentiometrically.

Dose: Usual dose is 50–200 mg per day.

iii. Meclizine (Antivert, Bonine)

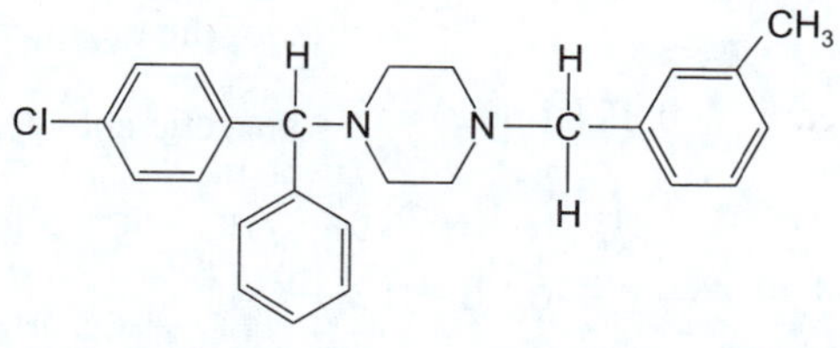

1-(*p*-Chlorophenylbenzyl)-4-(3-methylbenzyl) piperazine

Synthesis

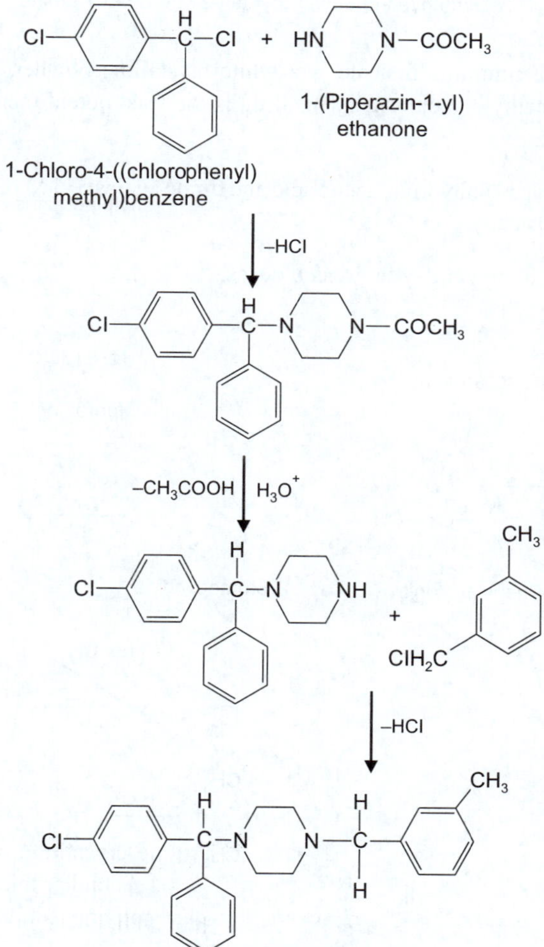

Meclizine

Properties and uses: It is a white or slightly yellowish, crystalline powder with no characteristic odour and taste. It is insoluble in water and in ether, but soluble in chloroform and alcohol. It is a moderately potent antihistaminic agent. It is used primarily as an antinauseant in the prevention and treatment of motion sickness; in the treatment of nausea and vomiting associated with vertigo and radiation sickness.

Assay: Dissolve the sample in alcohol and titrate against 0.1 M sodium hydroxide. Determine the end point potentiometrically.

Dose: Usual dose is 25–50 mg per day.

d. Monoamino propylamine derivatives

i. Saturated analogues

1. Pheniramine maleate (Avil, Polarmine)

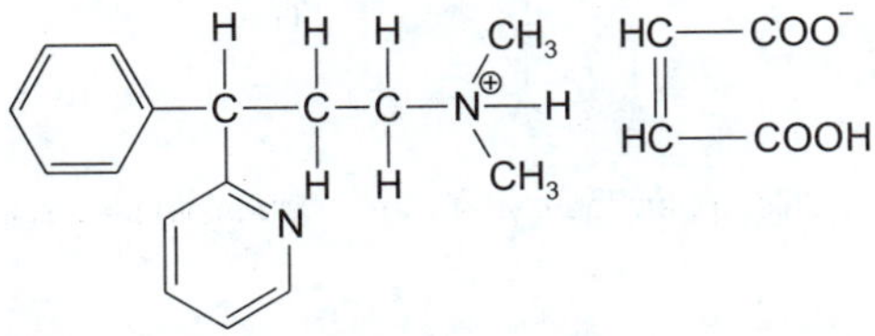

N,N-Dimethyl-3-phenyl-3-(pyridin-2-yl)propan-1-amine

Properties and uses: Pheniramine maleate is a white crystalline powder, freely soluble in water, alcohol, methanol, and methylene chloride. This drug is the least potent member of the series and is marketed as the racemate.

Assay: Dissolve the sample in anhydrous acetic acid and titrate against 0.1 M perchloric acid. Determine the end point potentiometrically.

Dose: Usual dose is 25–30 mg per day in divided doses.

Synthesis

Route I. From: 2-Phenylacetonitrile

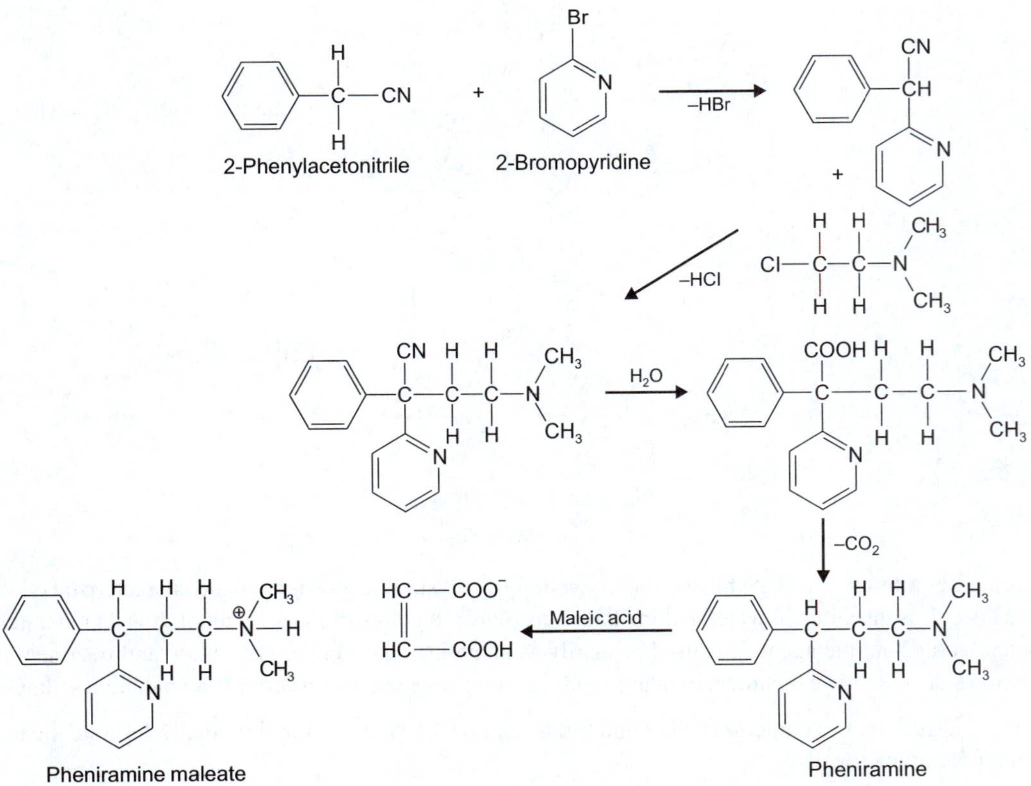

Route II. From: Picolinaldehyde

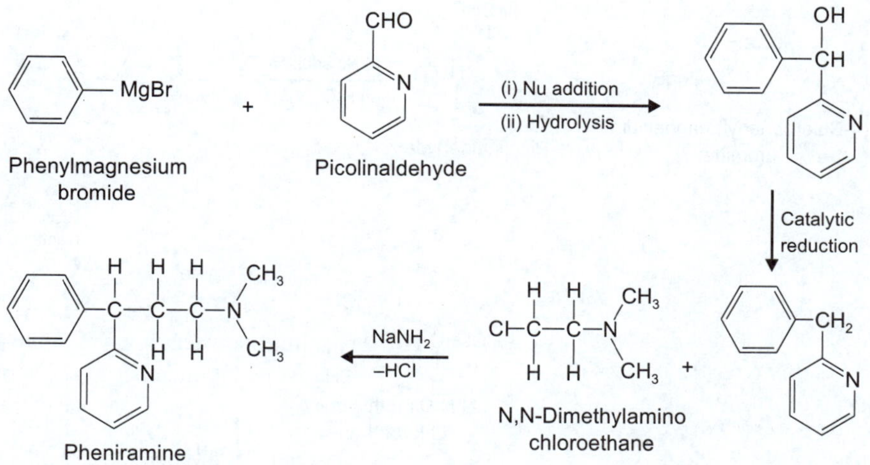

2. Chlorpheniramine HCl (Piriton, Alermine)

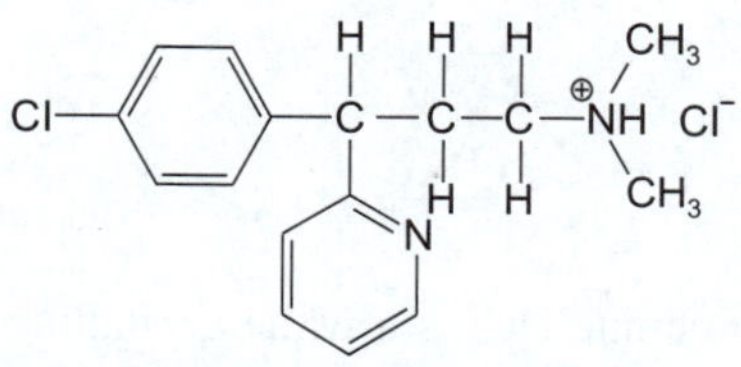

3-(4-Chlorophenyl)-N,N-dimethyl-3-(pyridin-2-yl)propan-1-amine

Synthesis

Route I. From: 2-(4-Chlorophenyl) acetonitrile

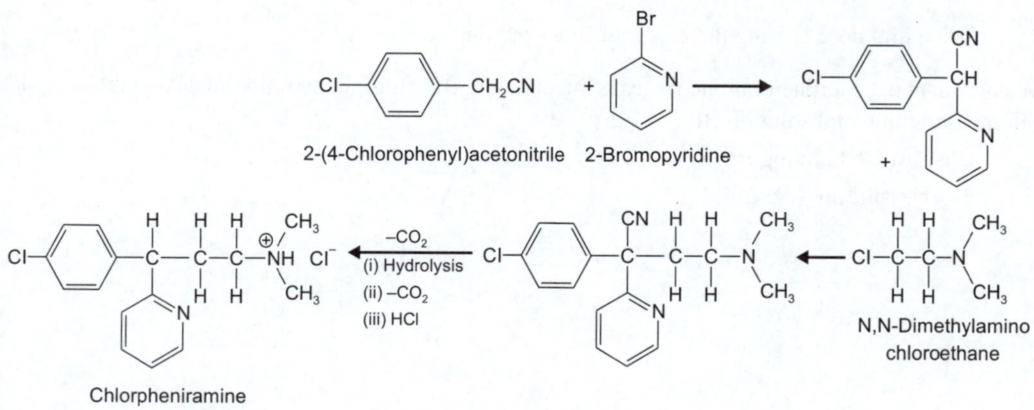

Route-II. From: Picolinaldehyde

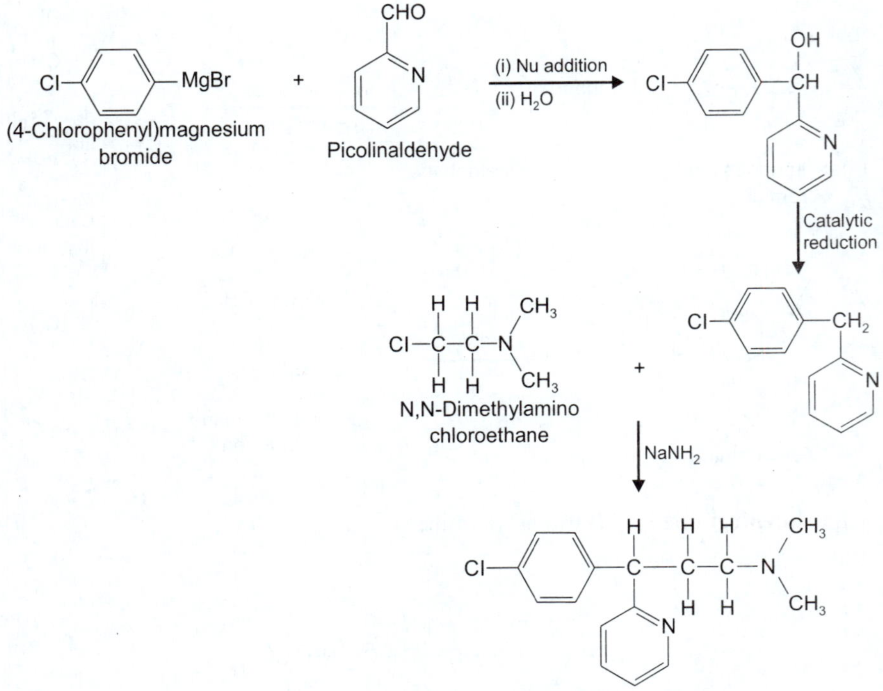

Chlorpheniramine

Properties and uses: Chlorpheniramine HCl is a white crystalline powder, soluble in water and in ethanol. Chlorination of pheniramine in the *para* position of the phenyl ring increases potency by almost 10-fold, with no appreciable change in toxicity. Most of the antihistaminic activity resides with the dextro isomer.

Assay: Dissolve the sample in anhydrous acetic acid and titrate against 0.1 M perchloric acid. Determine the end point potentiometrically.

Dose: Usual oral dose is 5 mg three or four times per day.

Dosage forms: Chlorpheniramine maleate injection IP, BP, chlorpheniramine maleate tablets IP, BP, chlorpheniramine oral solution BP.

ii. Unsaturated analogues

1. Triprolidine (Actidil)

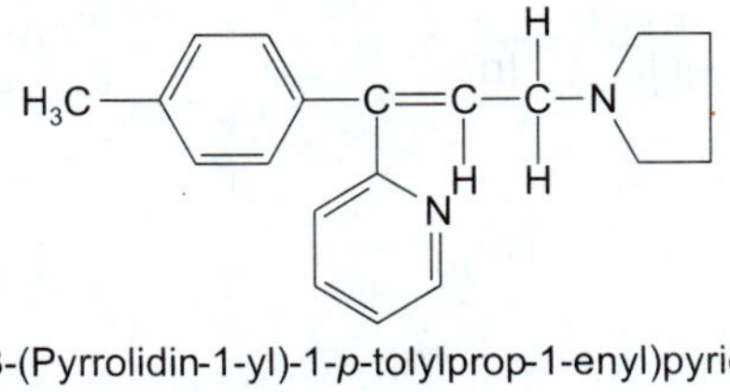

2-(3-(Pyrrolidin-1-yl)-1-*p*-tolylprop-1-enyl)pyridine

Synthesis

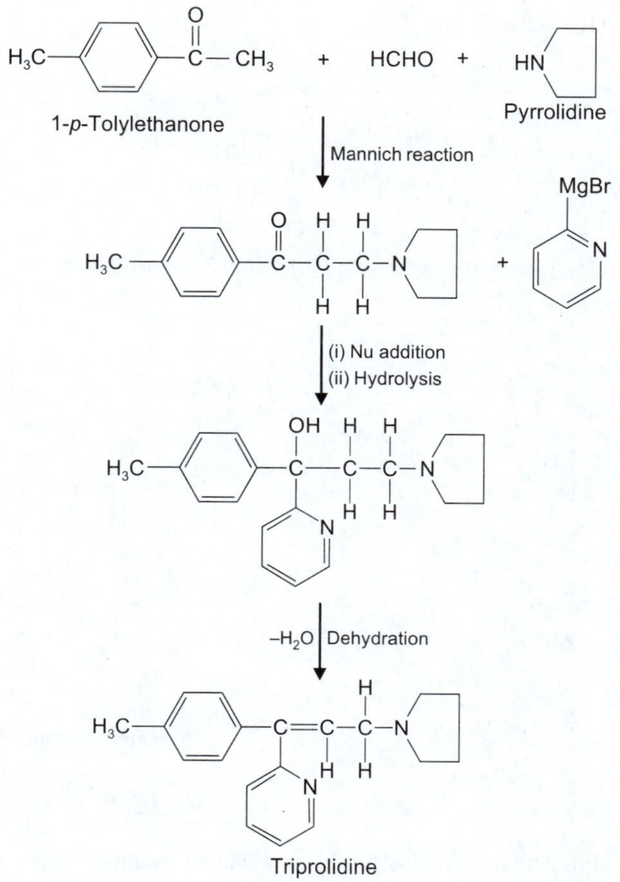

Properties and uses: Triprolidine hydrochloride is a white crystalline powder, practically insoluble in ether, soluble in water and in ethanol. The activity is mainly confined to the geometric isomer in which the pyrrolidino-methyl group is trans to the 2-pyridyl group. Pharmacological studies confirm the high activity of triprolidine and the superiority of (E) over corresponding (Z) isomers as H_1-antagonists. In guinea pig ileum sites, the affinity of triprolidine (E) for H_1-receptors was more than 1000 times the affinity of its (Z) partner.

Assay: Dissolve the sample in a mixture of anhydrous acetic acid and acetic anhydride and titrate against 0.1 M perchloric acid using crystal violet solution as indicator.

Dose: Usual dose is 5–7.5 mg per day.

Dosage forms: Triprolidine HCl tablets IP, triprolidine tablets BP.

e. Tricyclic ring system or phenothiazines

1. Promethazine HCl (Phenargen)

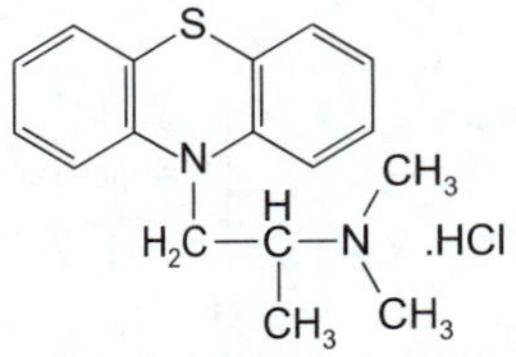

N,N-Dimethyl-1-(phenothiazin-10-yl)propan-2-amine hydrochloride

Synthesis

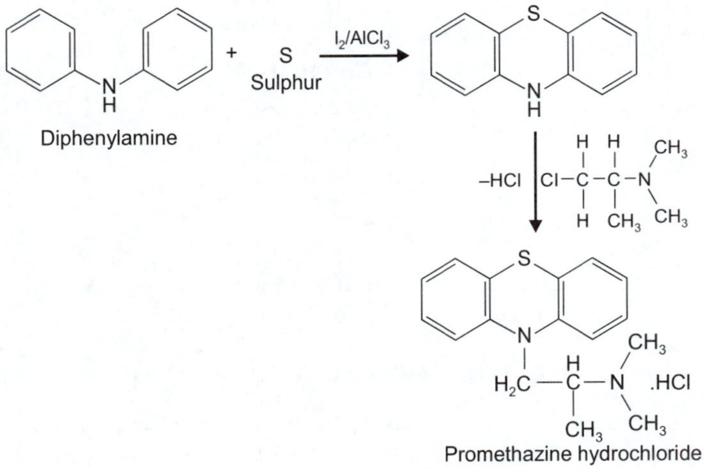

Properties and uses: Promethazine hydrochloride is a white or faintly yellowish crystalline powder, highly soluble in water, soluble in alcohol and in methylene chloride. It may be used effectively in perennial and seasonal allergic rhinitis, vasomotor rhinitis, allergic conjunctivitis due to inhalant allergens and foods, and certain milder type of skin manifestations of urticaria. It also possesses some anticholinergic, antiserotonergic, and marked local anaesthetic properties.

Assay: Dissolve the sample in a mixture of 0.01 M hydrochloric acid and alcohol and titrate against 0.1 M sodium hydroxide. Determine end point potentiometrically.

Dose: Usual dose is 20–50 mg per day.

Dosage forms: Promethazine hydrochloride injection IP, promethazine hydrochloride tablets IP, BP, promethazine hydrochloride syrup IP, promethazine injection BP, promethazine oral solution BP.

2. Trimeprazine (Temaril)

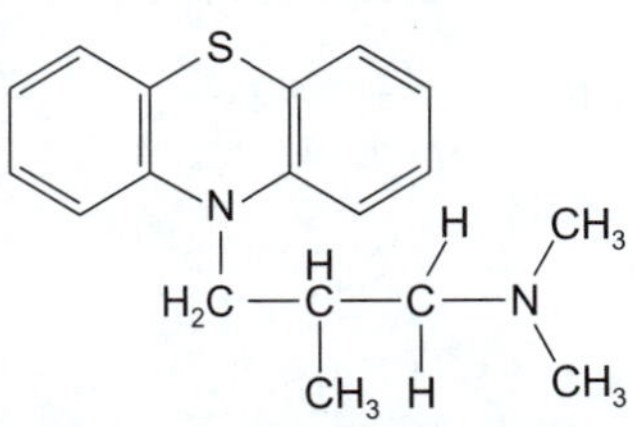

N,N,2-Trimethyl-3-(phenothiazin-10-yl)propan-1-amine

Synthesis

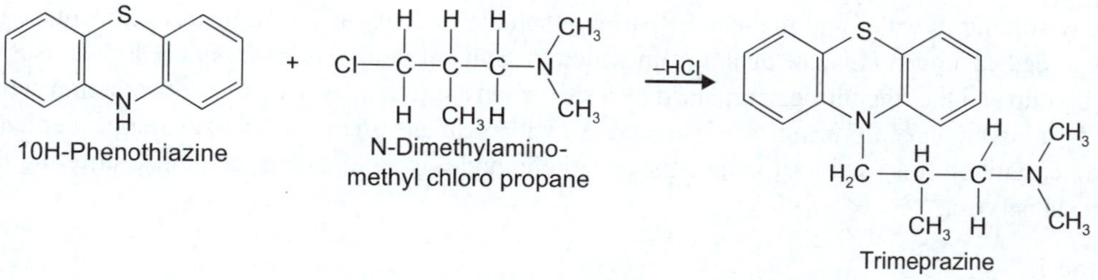

Properties and uses: It is a white crystalline powder, soluble in water. It is used as histamine H_1-receptor antagonist.

Dose: Usual dose for adults is 10–40 mg per day orally.

3. Methdilazine (Tacaryl HCl)

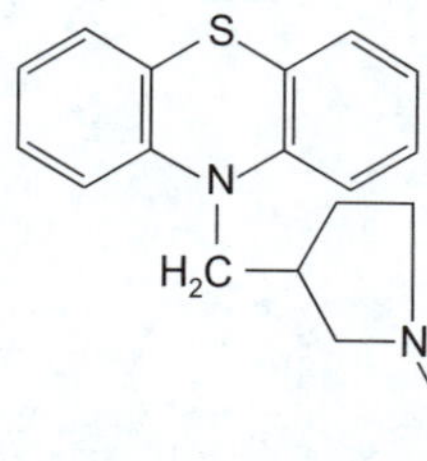

10-((1-Methylpyrrolidin-3-yl)methyl) phenothiazine

Synthesis

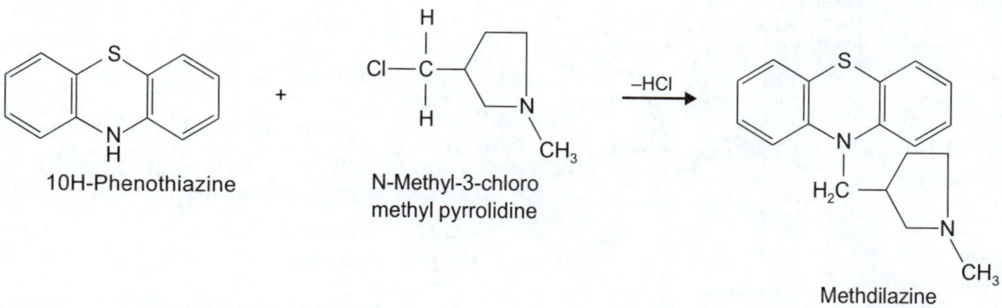

Properties and uses: It may be used for the symptomatic relief of urticaria. It has also been used successfully for the treatment of migraine headache.

Dose: Usual dose for adults is 8 mg taken orally two to four times a day.

f. Dibenzocycloheptene derivatives

1. Cyproheptadine (Periacetin)

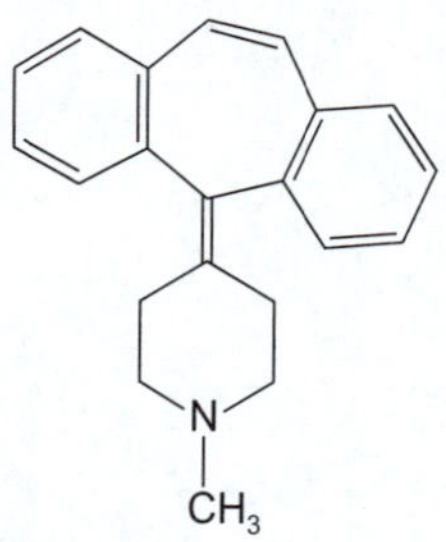

4-Dibenzo(a,(d) cyclohepten-5-ylidene)-1-methyl piperidine

Properties and uses: Cyproheptadine hydrochloride is a white or slightly yellow crystalline powder, slightly soluble in water and methanol, sparingly soluble in alcohol. This dibenzocycloheptene may be regarded as a phenothiazine analogue in which the sulphur atom has been replaced by an isosteric vinyl group and the ring nitrogen replaced by a sp^2 carbon atom. It also possesses antiserotonin activity and is used as an antipruritic agent associated with skin disorders (urticaria, allergic dermatitis, neurodermatitis). It is used to stimulate the appetite in under-weight patients and those suffering from anorexia nervosa.

Synthesis

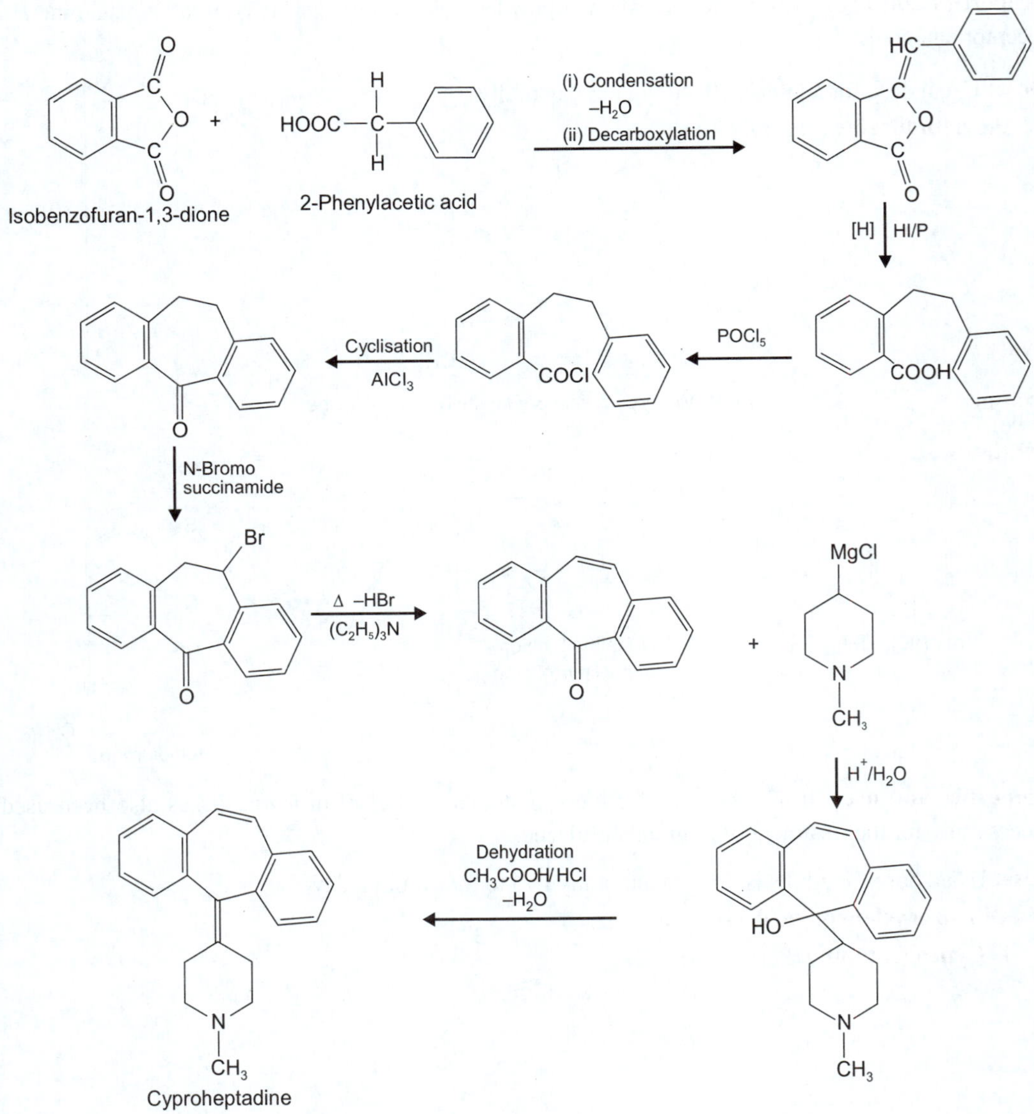

Assay: Dissolve the sample in a mixture of 0.01 M hydrochloric acid and alcohol and titrate against 0.1 M sodium hydroxide. Determine end point potentiometrically.

Dose: Usually, the dose is 4 mg taken orally three times a day.

Dosage forms: Cyproheptadine HCl syrup IP, cyproheptadine HCl tablets IP, cyproheptadine tablets BP.

2. Azatadine

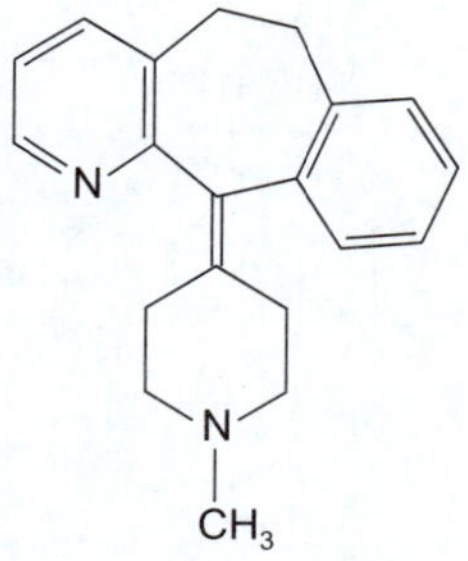

6,11-Dihydro-11-(1-methyl-4-piperidylidene)-5*H*-benzo-[5,6]-cyclohepta-9-[1,2-6]pyridine

Synthesis

Route I. From: 2-Chloro-3-phenethylpyridine

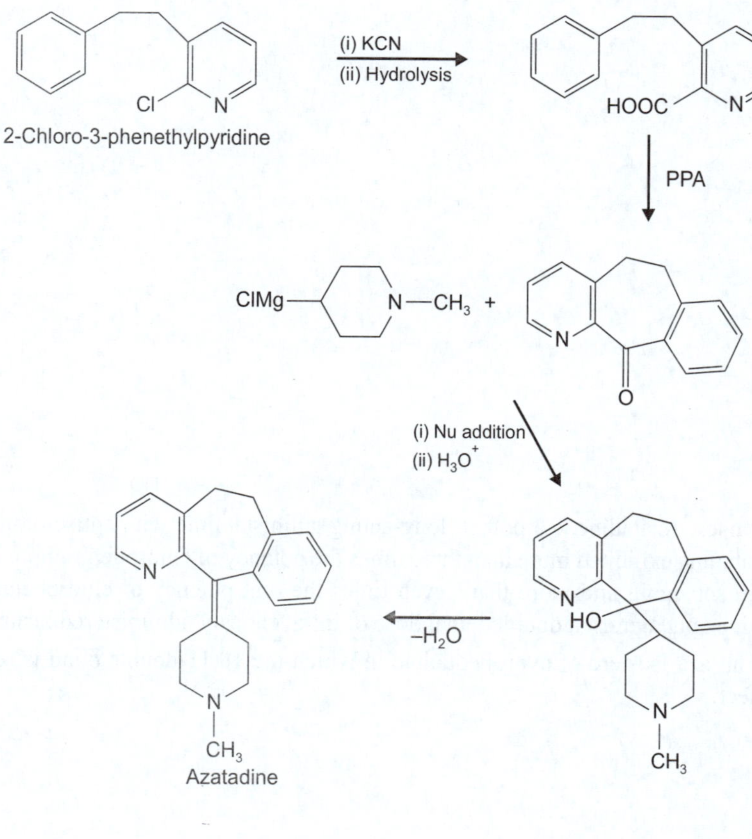

Route II. From: Phenylacetonitrile

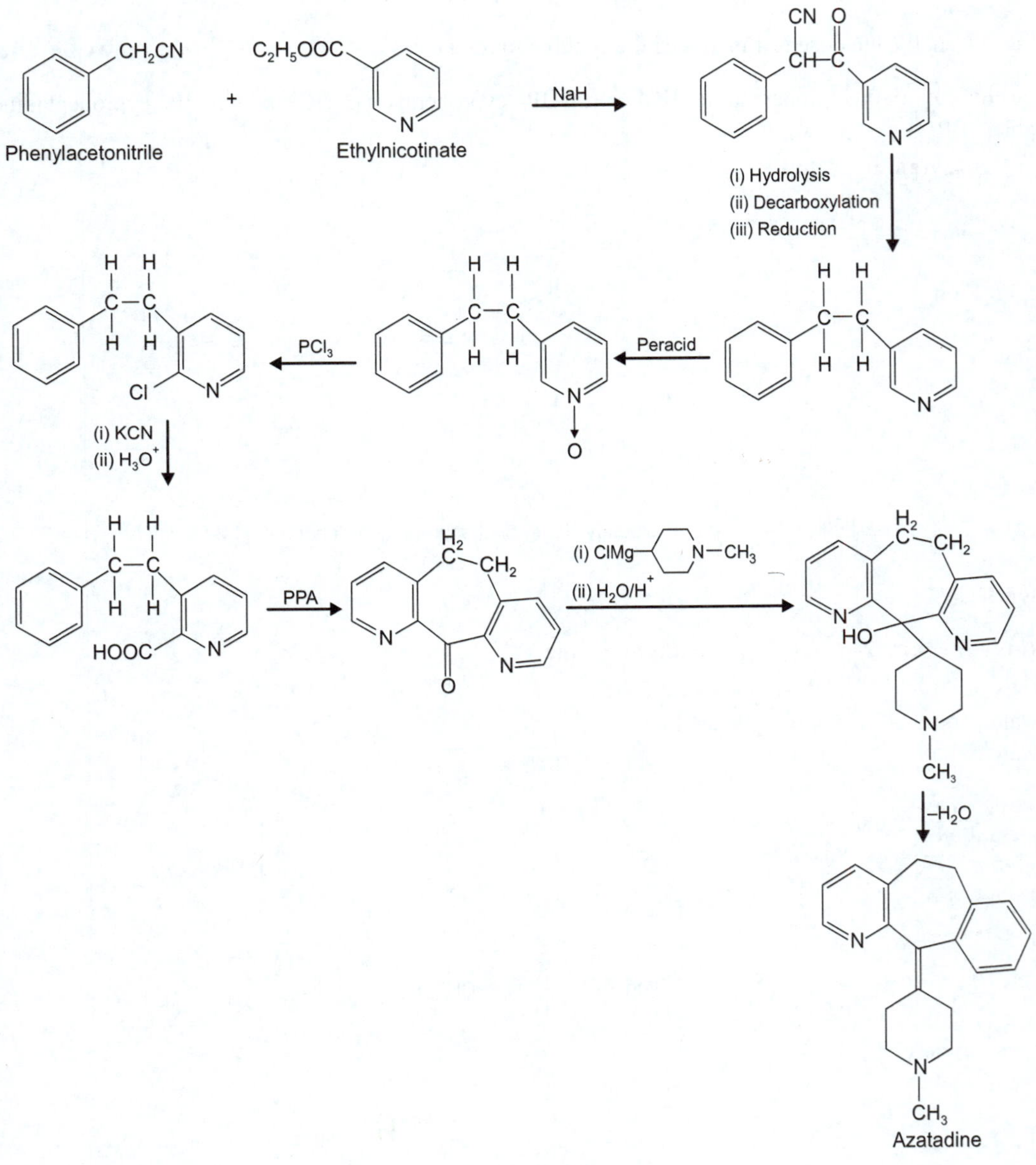

Properties and uses: Azatadine is a potent, long-acting antihistaminic with antiserotonin activity. In early testing, azatadine exhibited more than three times the potency of chlorpheniramine in the isolated guinea pig ileum screening and more than seven times the oral potency of chlorpheniramine in the protection of guinea pig against a double lethal dose of intravenously administered histamine.

Azatadine is an aza isostere of cyproheptadine in which the 10,11-double bond is reduced. It has low sedative effect.

g. Miscellaneous

1. Antazoline (Antistine)

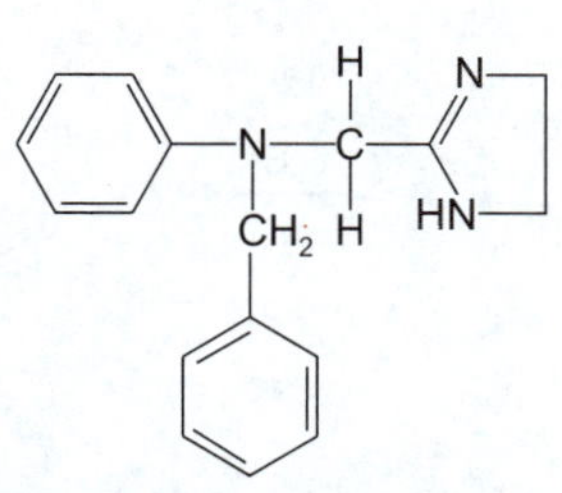

N-Benzyl-N-((4,5-dihydro-1*H*-imidazol-2-yl)methyl)benzenamine

Synthesis

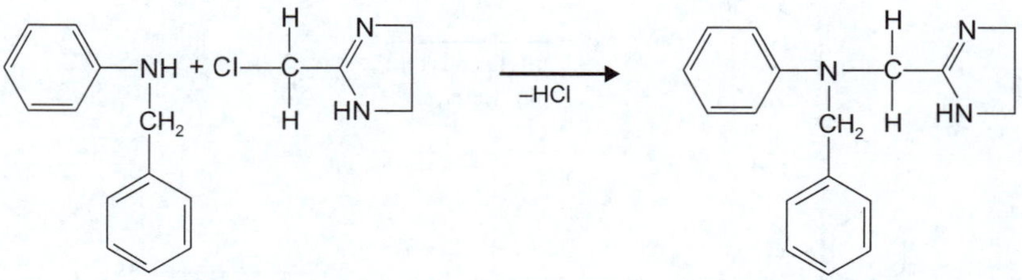

Properties and uses: Antazoline hydrochloride is a white crystalline powder, sparingly soluble in water, soluble in alcohol, and slightly soluble in methylene chloride. The phosphate salt is soluble in water, bitter taste. It is used for the treatment of rhinitis and conjunctivitis.

Assay: Dissolve the sample in alcohol and titrate against 0.1 M alcoholic potassium hydroxide using phenolphthalein as indicator.

Dose: Usual dose is 50–100 mg per day.

h. Newer agents

1. Ketotifen fumarate (Zaditen)

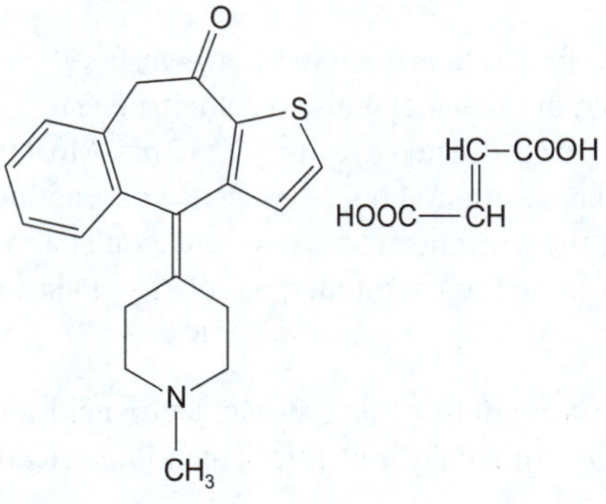

4-(1-Methyl-4-piperidylidene)-4H-benzo[4,5]cyclohepta[1,2-b]thiophen-10(9H)-one fumarate

Synthesis

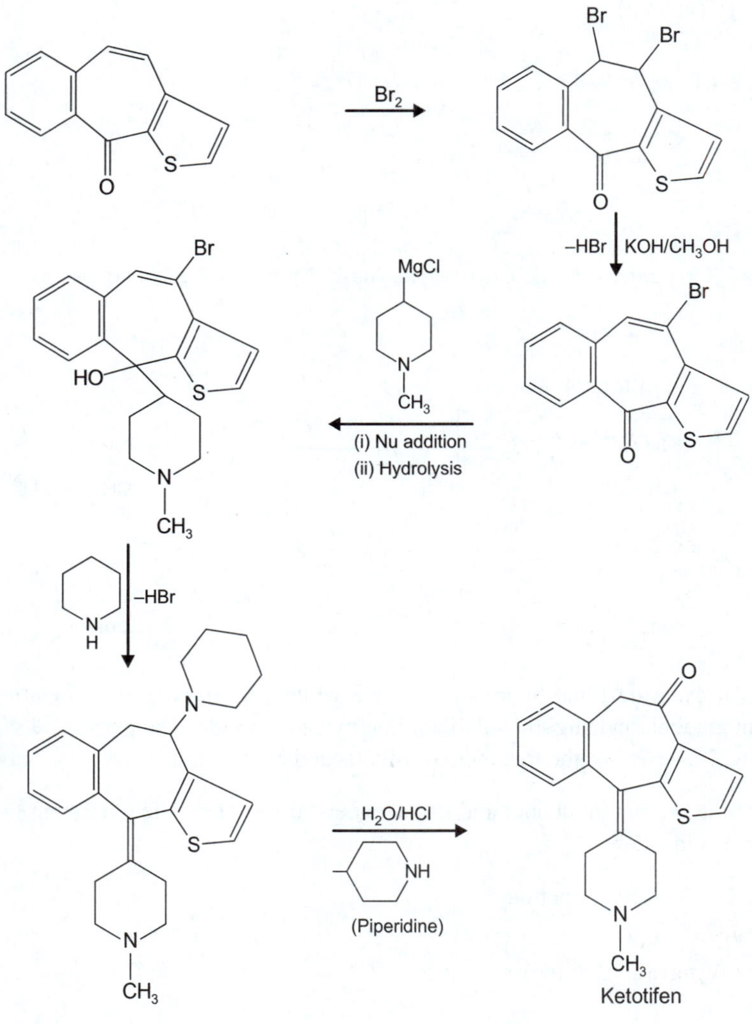

Properties and uses: Ketotifen fumarate is a white to brownish-yellow crystalline powder, sparingly soluble in water, slightly soluble in methanol and in acetonitrile. The recommended dose of ketotifen solution is one drop instilled into each affected eye every 8–12 hrs. Most frequently used for conjunctival infection, and rhinitis. Ketotifen solution should be used with caution during pregnancy or during nursing. This is an analogue of the tricyclic H_1-receptor antagonist and serotonin receptor antagonist. It has only minor anticholinergic and antiserotonergic activity. It has been used in the prophylactic treatment of asthma.

Assay: Dissolve the sample in a mixture of anhydrous acetic acid and acetic anhydride and titrate against 0.1 M perchloric acid. Determine the end point potentiometrically.

Dose: Usually, the dose is 1 mg orally two times a day.

II. H_1-Antagonists with Non-classical Structure

1. **Astemizole** (Histalong)

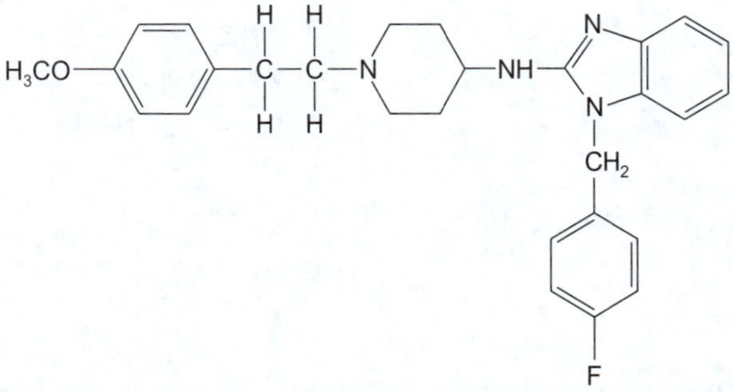

1-(4-Fluorobenzyl)-N-(1-(4-methoxyphenethyl)piperidin-4-yl)-1*H*-benzo[*d*]imidazol-2-amine

Synthesis

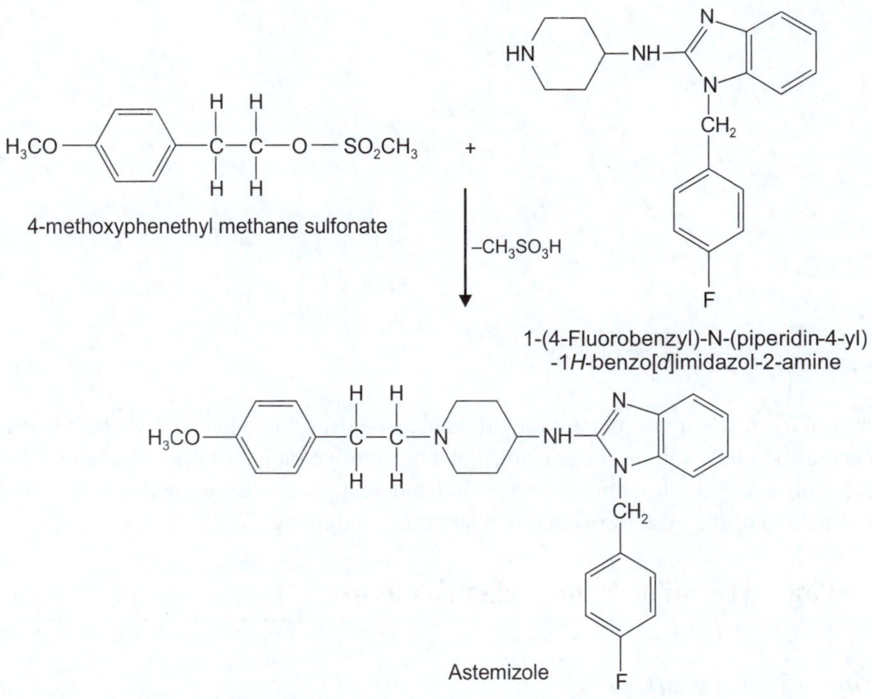

Properties and uses: Astemizole is a white powder, practically insoluble in water, soluble in methylene chloride, methanol, and alcohol. The drug is found to be more potent and possesses longer duration of action than the terfenadine. It has a slow onset, is long acting, and non-sedating piperidine antihistaminic having practically little anticholinergic activity. It is indicated for seasonal allergic rhinitis and chronic urticaria. It is an effective antiallergic agent giving protection against asthma, hay fever, and chronic urticaria. It does not exhibit any noticeable CNS activity.

Assay: Dissolve the sample in a mixture of anhydrous acetic acid and methyl ethyl ketone, and titrate against 0.1 M perchloric acid using naphtholbenzein solution as an indicator.

Dose: Usual dose is 10 mg (oral) increased, if required, to 30 mg per day for up to 7 days 1 hr before meals. It is not recommended for children below 6 years.

2. Tazifylline

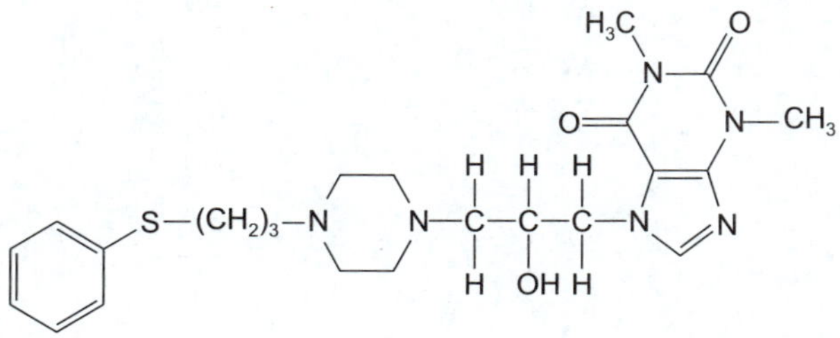

Properties and uses: Tazifylline is proved for its successful antiallergic activity, with no significant occurrence of side effects (dryness of mouth and sedation) and long duration of action.

3. Azelastine

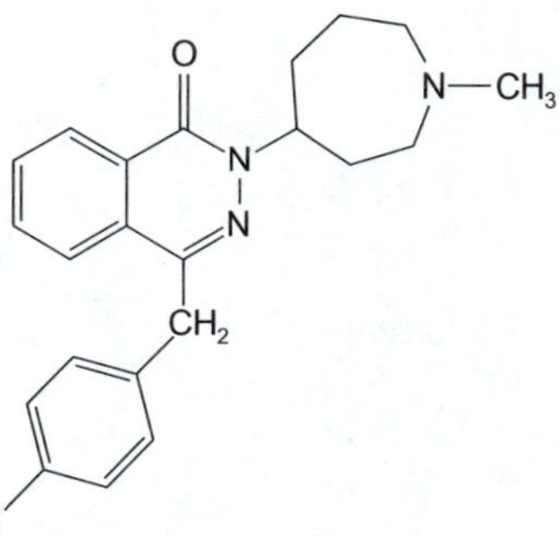

Properties and uses: It is a racemic mixture of white crystals, soluble in water, methanol or propylene glycol, but only slightly soluble in ethanol, octanol, or glycerine. It combines potent H_1-receptor antagonism with a negligible anticholinergic and moderate serotonergic activity. It is used in the treatment of itching of the eyes associated with allergic conditions.

III. Non-sedative H_1-antihistamines (H_1-antagonists)

1. Cetirizine (Zirtin, Cetin, Cetzine)

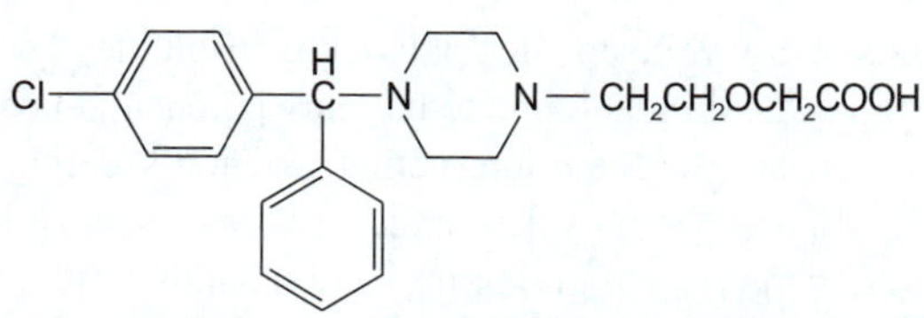

2-(2-(4-((4-Chlorophenyl)(phenyl)methyl)piperazin-1-yl) ethoxy)acetic acid

Synthesis

Route I. From: 1-[4-chlorophenyl (1-phenylmethyl)]-piperazine

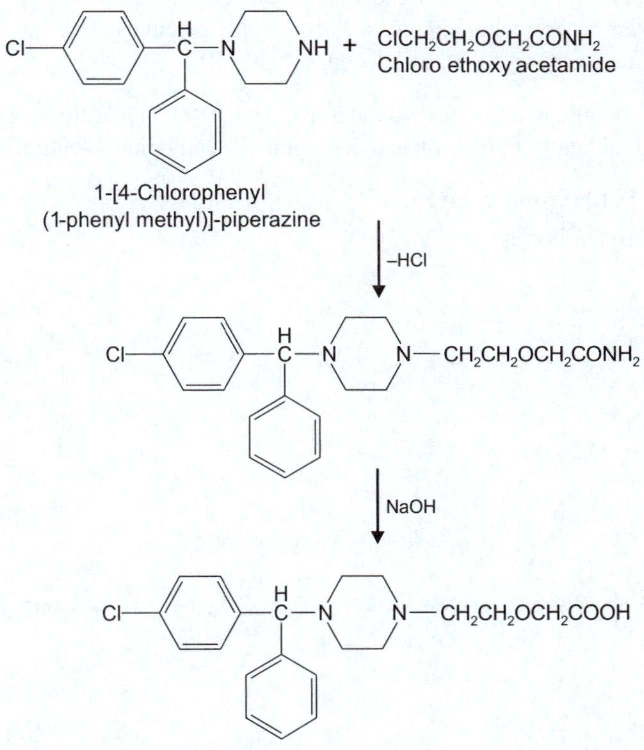

Cetirizine

Route II. From: Hydroxyzine

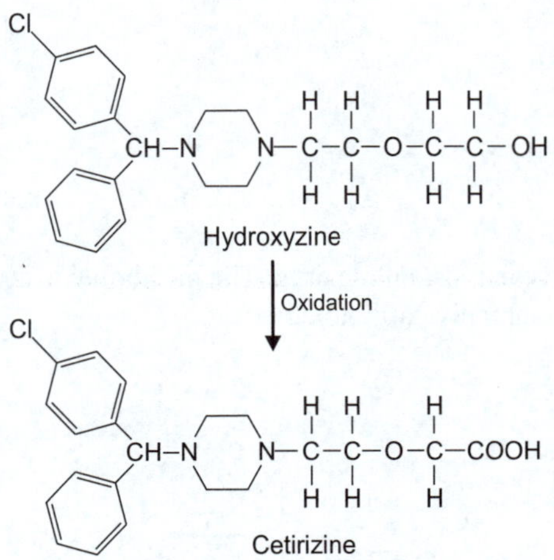

Cetirizine

Cetirizine is an acid metabolite formed by the oxidation of primary alcohol of antihistamine hydroxyzine.

Properties and uses: Cetirizine hydrochloride is a white powder, soluble in water, practically insoluble in acetone and methylene chloride. This is the principal metabolic product of hydroxyzine, the polar acid group prevents its penetration into the CNS. It is used as an antihistamine to treat various allergic conditions. Cetirizine is one of the most widely prescribed H_1-antihistamines. It is highly selective in its interaction with various hormonal binding sites and highly potent as well. Other effects of this drug include fatigue, dry mouth, pharyngitis, and dizziness.

Assay: Dissolve the sample in a mixture of water and acetone (1:7) and titrate against 0.1 M sodium hydroxide to the second point of inflexion and determine the end point potentiometrically.

Dose: Usual dose is 5–10 mg thrice/day.

2. **Loratadine** (Alaspan, Lorfast)

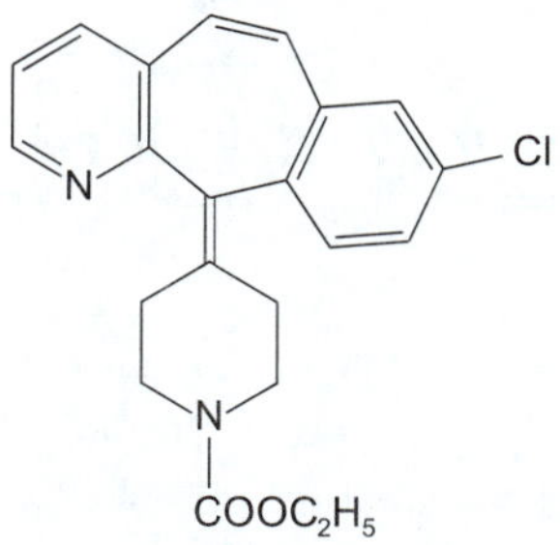

4-(8-Chlor-5,6-dihydro-benzocycloheptapyridin-11-ylidene)-1-piperidine carboxylic acid ethyl ester

Synthesis

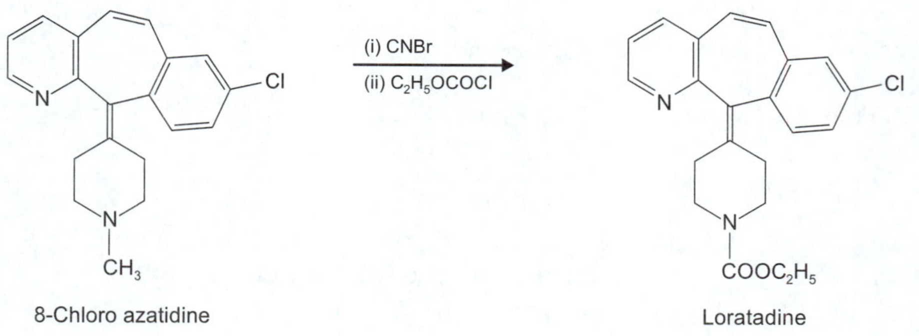

Metabolism: It is a non-sedative antihistaminic drug. The metabolite is desloratidine (descarboethoxy loratidine) is associated with potentially cardiotoxic effect.

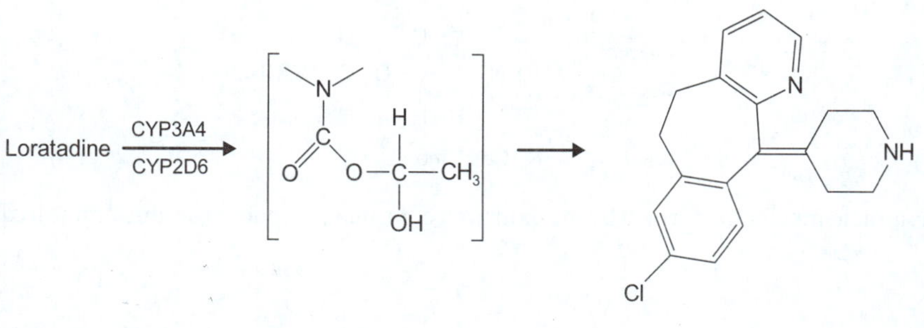

The metabolic conversion of loratidine to descarboethoxy loratidine occurs via oxidative process and not via hydrolysis, and both CYP2D6 and CYP3A4 are to be the isoenzymes catalysing this oxidative metabolism.

Properties and uses: Loratadine is a white crystalline powder, practically insoluble in water, soluble in acetone and methanol. Loratadine is an azo isomer of cyproheptadine. The replacement of methyl group of azatadine (piperidine nitrogen) by corresponding carbonate and introduction of 8-chloro substitution preserves the antihistaminic action and reduces the CNS effect. The potency of loratidine is comparable with that of astemizole and greater than of terfenadine.

Assay: Dissolve the sample in glacial acetic acid and titrate against 0.1 M perchloric acid. Determine the end point potentiometrically.

3. **Epinastine**

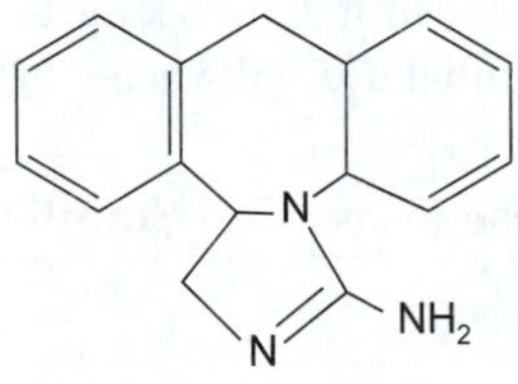

Properties and uses: This is structurally related to the antidepressant and non-sedative H_1-receptor antagonist mianserin. Introduction of an amidine moiety preserves the antihistamine action and reduces the CNS effect (sedation).

4. **Rocastine**

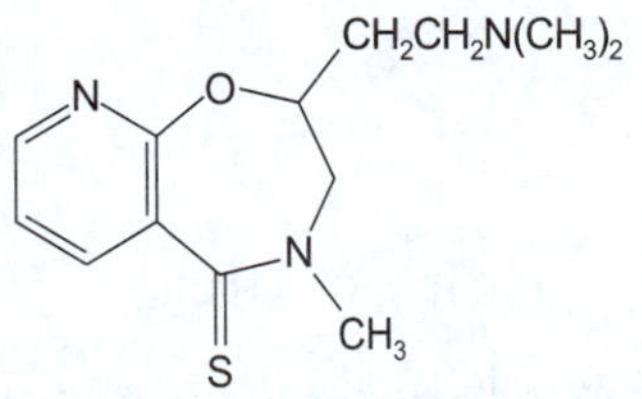

2-(2-(Dimethylamino)ethyl)-4-methyl-3,4-dihydropyrido[3,2-*f*][1,4]oxazepine-5(2*H*)-thione

Properties and uses: It is a rapid acting, non-sedating H_1-antagonist. The R-enantiomer was at least 300 times more potent than S-enantiomer.

5. **Olopatadine hydrochloride** (Patanase)

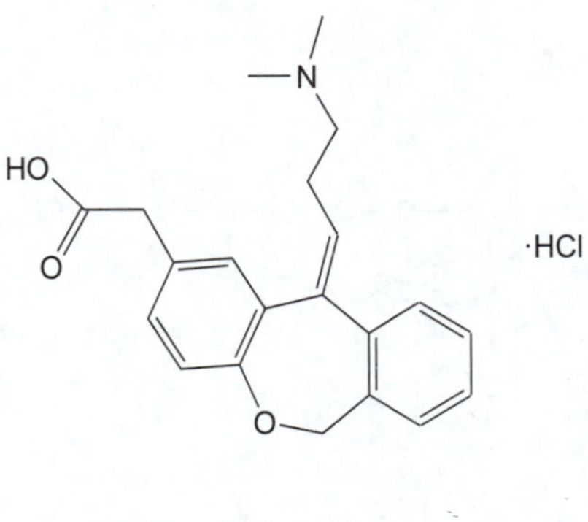

Mode of action: Olopatadine hydrochloride is an antihistamine with selective H_1-receptor antagonist activity. Its principal effects are mediated via inhibition of H_1-receptors. These drugs selectively bind to but do not activate histamine H_1-receptors, thereby blocking the actions of endogenous histamine. It inhibits the release of mast cell inflammatory mediators, i.e. histamine, tryptase, prostaglandin D_2 and TNFα. It is also an inhibitor of proinflammatory cytokine secretion from human conjunctival epithelial cells. Olopatadine acts as inhibitor of proinflammatory signal released from mast cells in response to allergic reactions or tissue damage from bronchi, capillaries, and other smooth muscles.

Properties and uses: Olopatadine hydrochloride is used for the relief of the symptoms of seasonal allergic rhinitis in patients 12 years of age and older. Adverse reactions associated with the use of olopatadine hydrochloride may include bitter taste, headache, epistaxis, pharyngolaryngeal pain, postnasal drip, cough, and urinary tract infection.

Dose: Olopatadine hydrochloride is supplied as a metered-dose manual spray pump designed for intranasal administration. The recommended initial dose of the drug is two sprays per nostril twice daily. Patanase must be primed before initial use and when it has not been used for more than 7 days.

IV. Inhibition of Histamine Release (Mast Cell Stabilizer)

i. Cromolyn sodium

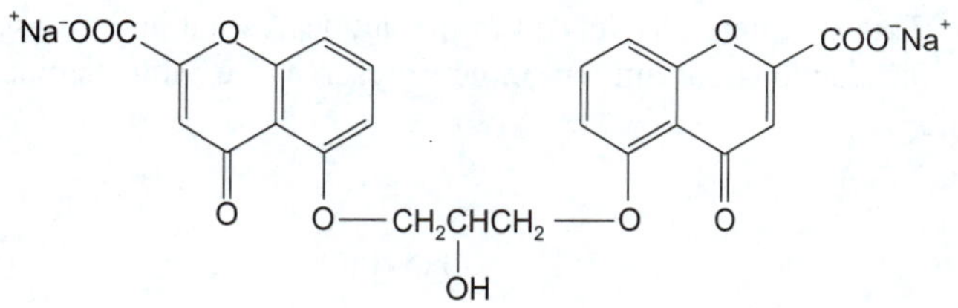

ii. Nedocromil sodium

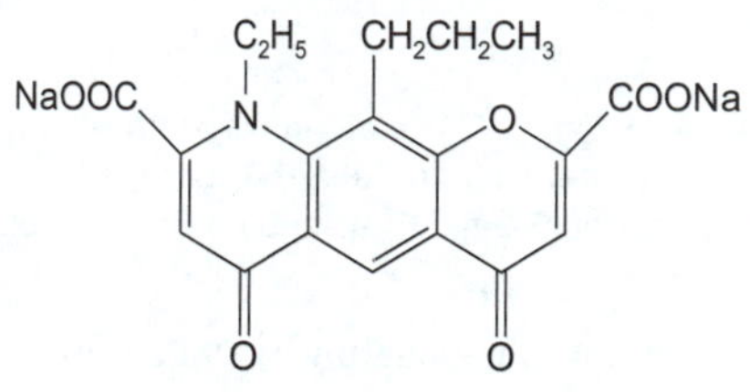

CLASSIFICATION BASED ON PCI SYLLABUS

Diphenhydramine hydrochloride

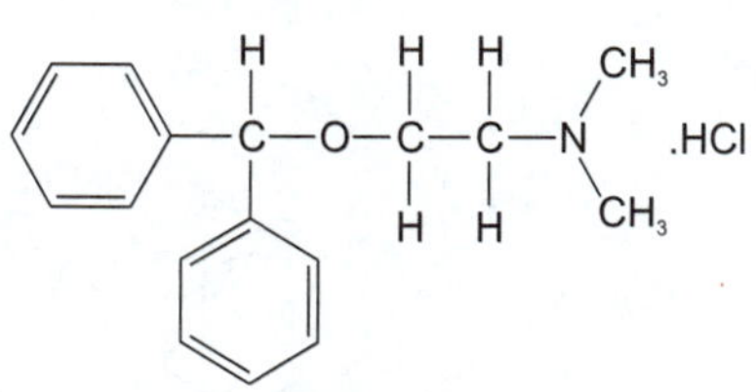

Dimenhydrinate [Diphenhydramine + 8-chlorotheophylline]

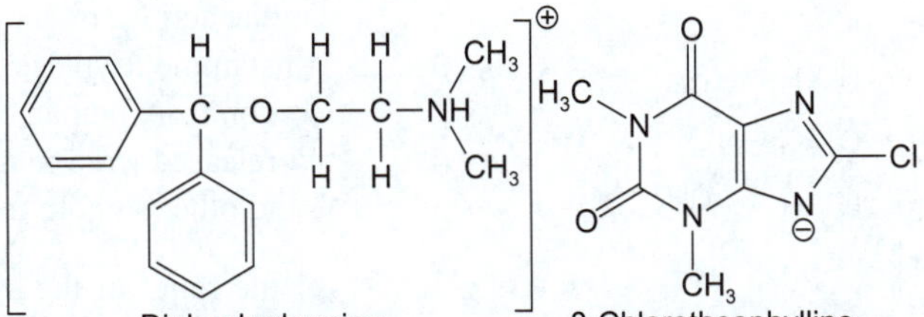

Diphenhydramine 8-Chlorotheophylline

Doxylamine succinate

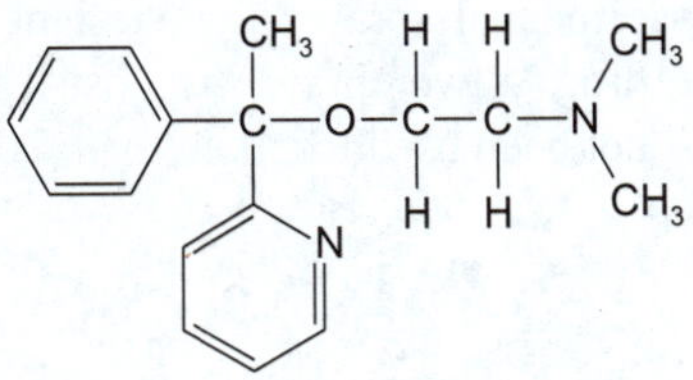

Clemastine fumarate

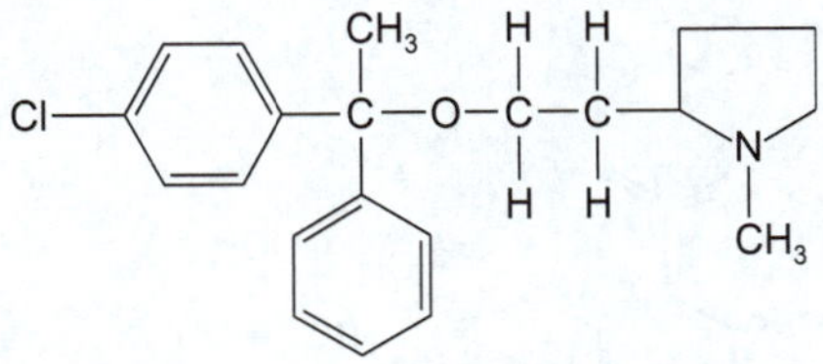

Diphenylphyraline hydrochloride

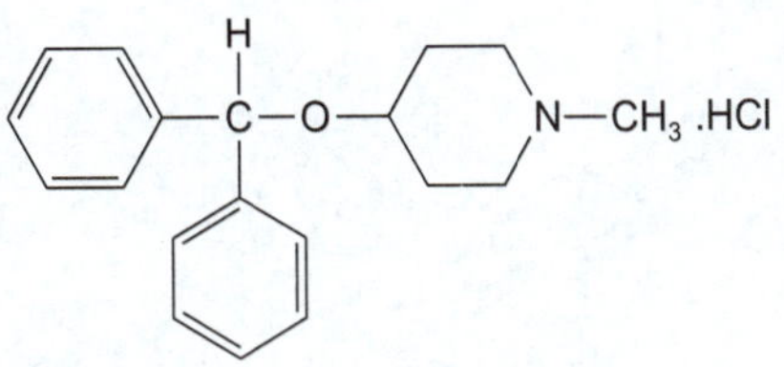

Tripelenamine hydrochloride

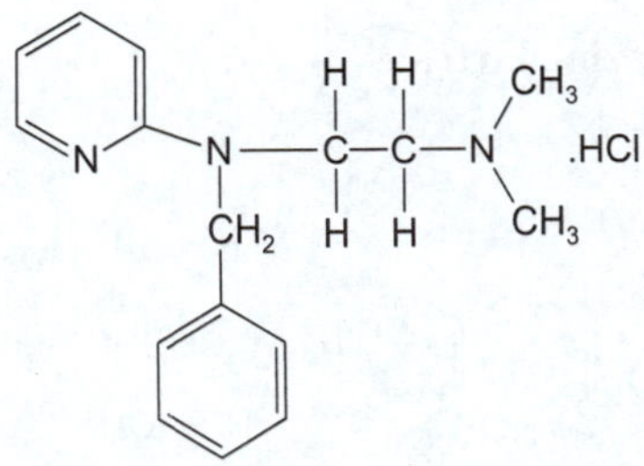

Chlorcyclizine hydrochloride

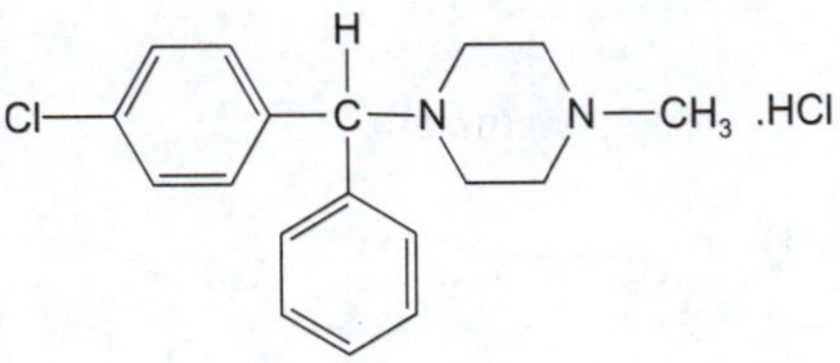

Meclizine hydrochloride

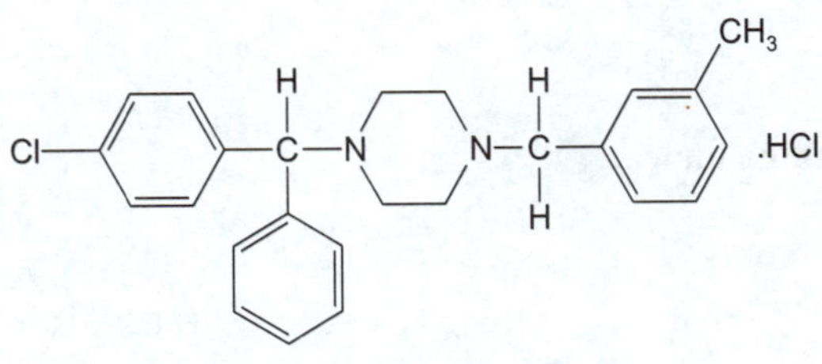

Buclizine hydrochloride

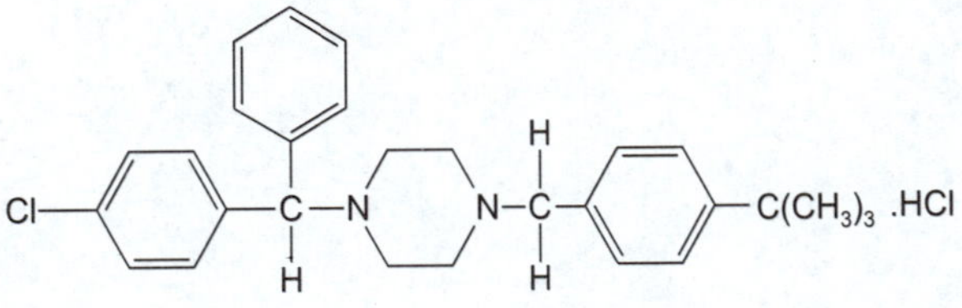

Chlorpheniramine maleate

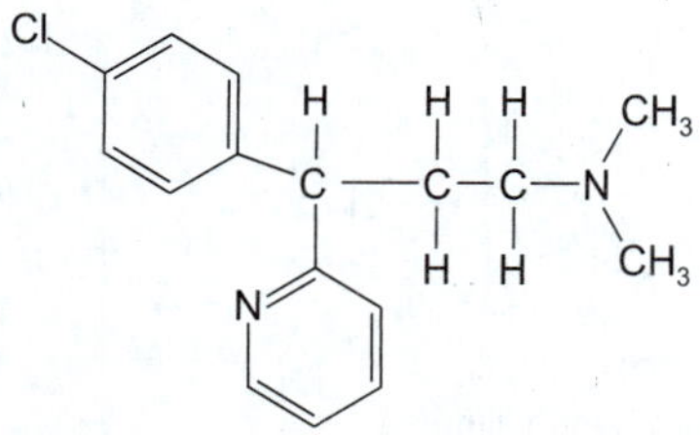

Triprolidine hydrochloride

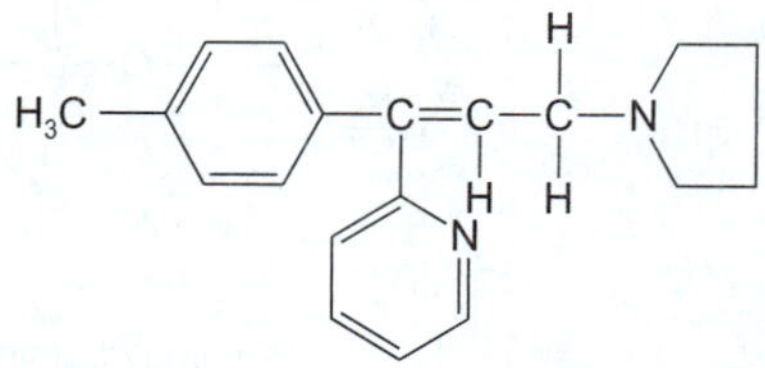

Phenindamine tartrate

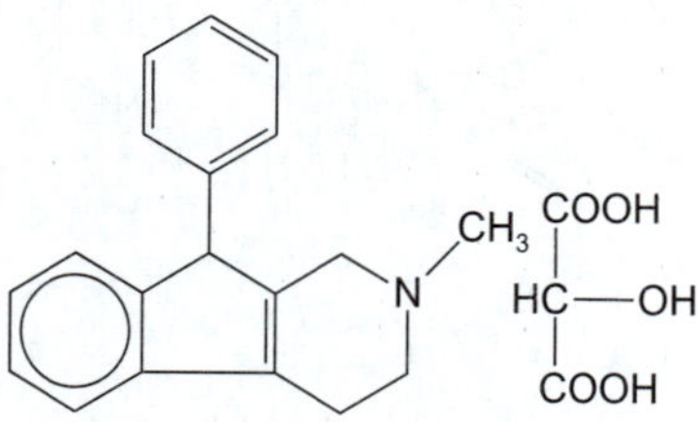

Promethazine hydrochloride

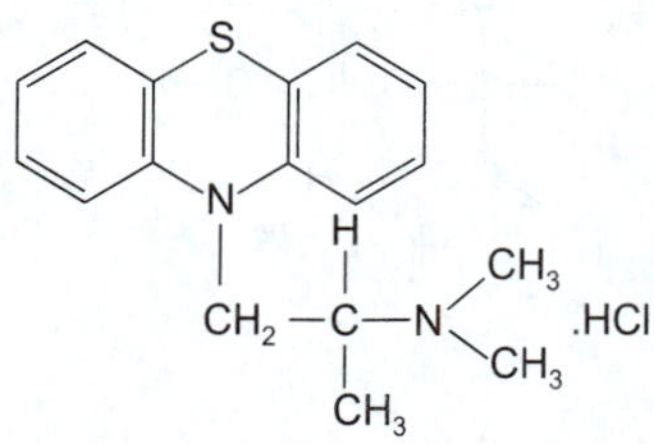

Trimeprazine tartrate

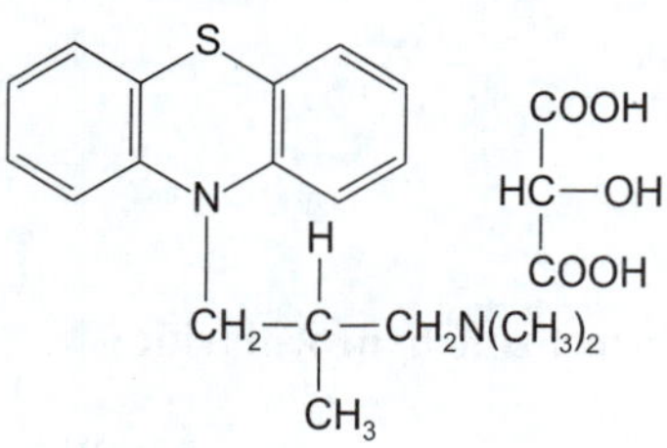

Cyproheptadine hydrochloride

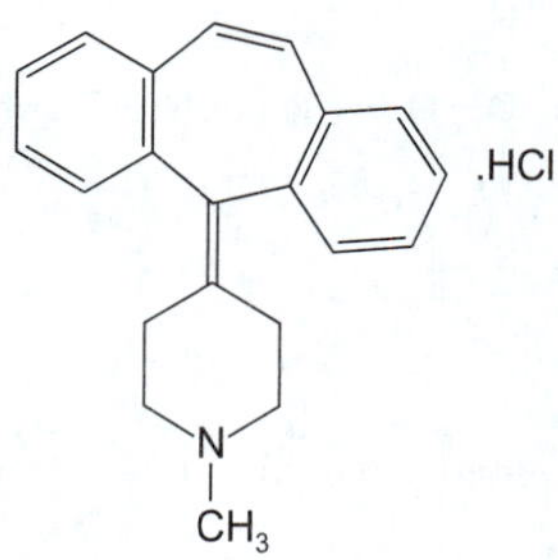

Azatidine maleate

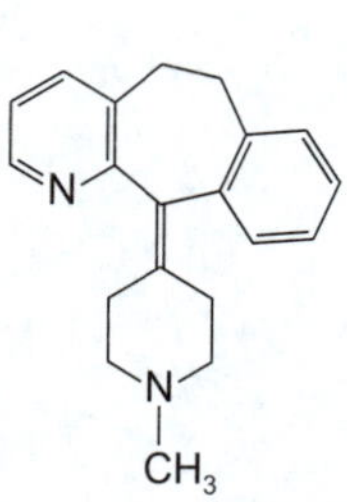

Astemizole

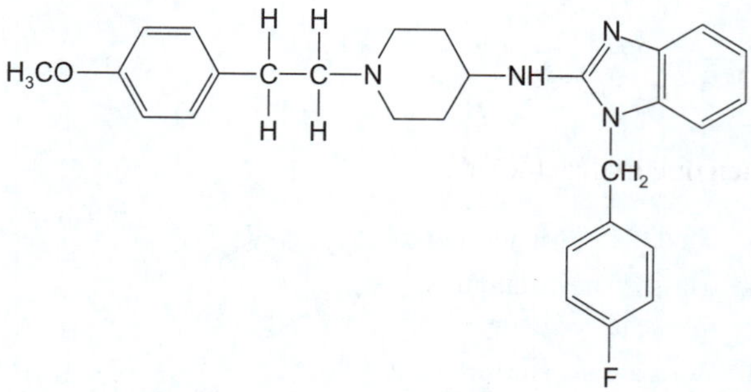

Loratadine

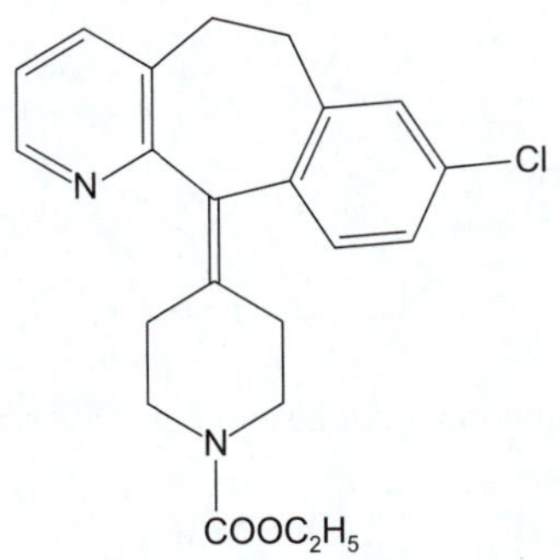

Cetirizine

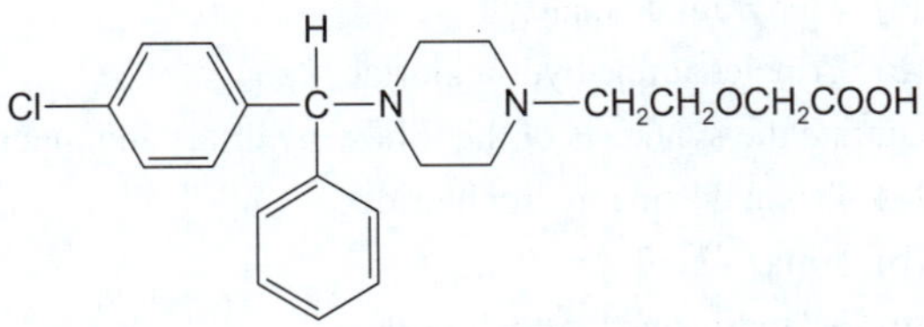

Levocetrizine

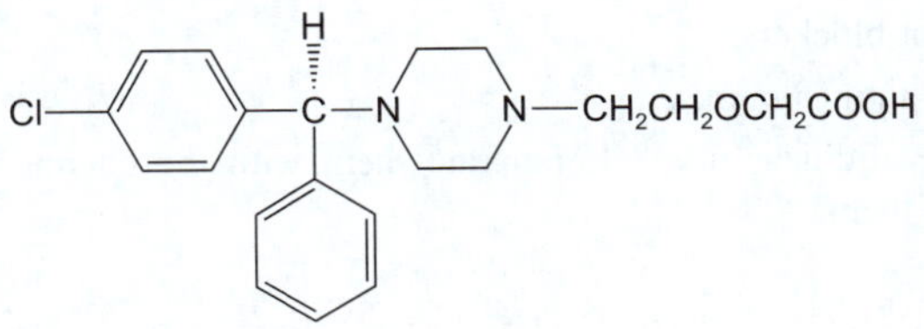

Cromolyn sodium

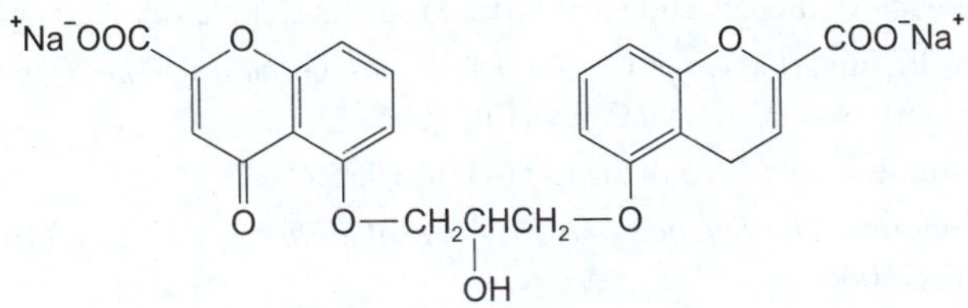

Phenindamine tartrate: This is closely related to cyproheptadine. It is an anticholinergic and antihistaminic agent. It is used to treat allergies and common cold such as itching, sneezing, hives and rashes.

PROBABLE QUESTIONS

1. What is histamine? What are its biological effects? Mention the different histamine receptors.
2. What are allergens? What is the importance of antihistamines in combating various types of allergic conditions? Mention suitable examples to support your answer.
3. Classify the histamine H_1-receptor antagonists. Write the structure, chemical name, and uses of one drug from each category.
4. What are the side effects of classical antihistamines?
5. Outline the synthesis of the following: Diphenhydramine, chlorpheniramine maleate, and triprolidine.
6. Name any three ethylene diamines being used as antihistamines. Outline the synthesis of any one of them.

7. Write the chemical structure, chemical name, and uses of the following and describe the synthesis of any one drug.
   (a) Mepyramine maleate
   (b) Tripelenamine hydrochloride
8. Outline the synthesis of the following drugs and mention their uses:
   (a) Promethazine hydrochloride
   (b) Antazoline
   (c) Methdilazine hydrochloride
9. Phenindamine tartrate and chlorpheniramine maleate are two important antihistamines. Describe the synthesis of any one drug in detail.
10. Write a brief account of the following:
    (a) Drugs used in the prevention of histamine release
    (b) Newer antihistamines
11. Write a comprehensive account of the following:
    (a) SAR of H_1-receptor blockers
    (b) Mode of action of antihistamines
12. What are non-sedative antihistamines? Enumerate them with the chemical structure and write the synthesis of any one of them.

SUGGESTED READINGS

1. Abraham DJ (ed). *Burger's Medicinal Chemistry and Drug Discovery* (6th edn). New Jersey: John Wiley, 2007.
2. *British Pharmacopoeia*. Medicines and Healthcare Products Regulatory Agency. London, 2008.
3. Bruntan LL, Lazo JS, and Parker KL. *Goodman and Gilman's: The Pharmacological Basis of Therapeutics* (11th edn). New York: McGraw Hill, 2006.
4. Burn JH. 'Antihistamines'. *Br Med J* 4(1): 1357–359, 1955.
5. Gennaro AR. *Remington's:The Science and Practice of Pharmacy* (21st edn). NewYork: Lippincott Williams and Wilkins, 2006.
6. Idson B. 'Antihistamine drugs'. *Chem Rev* 47: 307–527, 1950.
7. *Indian Pharmacopoeia*. Ministry of Health and Family Welfare. New Delhi, 1996.
8. Hunter RB and Dunlop DM. 'A review of antihistamine drugs'. *Q J Med* 25: 271–290, 1948.
9. Landsteiner K. The *Specificity of Serological Reactions*. New York: Dover Publications,1962.
10. Lemke TL and William DA. *Foye's Principle of Medicinal Chemistry* (6th edn). New York: Lippincott Williams and Wilkins, 2008.
11. Lednicer D and Mitscher LA. *The Organic Chemistry of Drug Synthesis*. New York: John Wiley, 1995.
12. Orange RP, Kaliner MA, and Austen KF. In *Biochemistry of the Acute Allergic Reaction*, Austen KF and Becker EL (eds). Oxford: Blackwell, 1971.

CHAPTER 2

Prostaglandins

INTRODUCTION

Prostaglandins (PGs) occur virtually in all mammalian tissues and possess numerous and diverse pharmacological actions. They are comprised of a large number of unsaturated hydroxy lipids like acids containing 20 carbon atoms. Since they were extracted from prostate gland and seminal vesicles of several animal species, including that of human semen, the term prostaglandin was used for them. It is isolated and purified as hydroxy fatty acid fraction from lipid extracts of seminal vesicles and from it the two biologically active substances, that is, PG E and F, were isolated. Some active compounds were derived from oxygenation of arachidonic acid, a precursor released from membrane phospholipids. The anti-inflammatory and analgesic effects of aspirin and the related non-steroidal anti-inflammatory drugs (NSAIDs) are due to their inhibitory effects on PG formation.

They are also reported to be present in significant quantities in the reproductive tissues, developing foetus and deciduals, umbilical cord, amniotic fluid, endometrium, menstrual fluid, epidermis, thymus, thyroid, and nerves. Further, in most of the organs, except for genital tissue, the PG is present as prostaglandin E (PGE) and prostaglandin F_2 (PGF_2). Therapeutic potential of PGs are in the treatment of blood pressure, bronchial functions, atherosclerosis, heart attack, inhibition of blood clot formation, childbirth, abortions, stomach ulcers, and other related syndromes.

FUNCTIONS OF PGs

There are varieties of physiological effects including the following:

1. Blood clots are formed when a blood vessel is damaged. A type of PGs called thromboxane (TXA_2) stimulates constriction and clotting of platelets. Conversely, PGI_2 have the opposite effect on the walls of blood vessels.
2. Certain PGs are involved in the induction of labour and other reproductive processes. PGE_2 causes uterine contractions and has been used to induce labour.

NOMENCLATURE

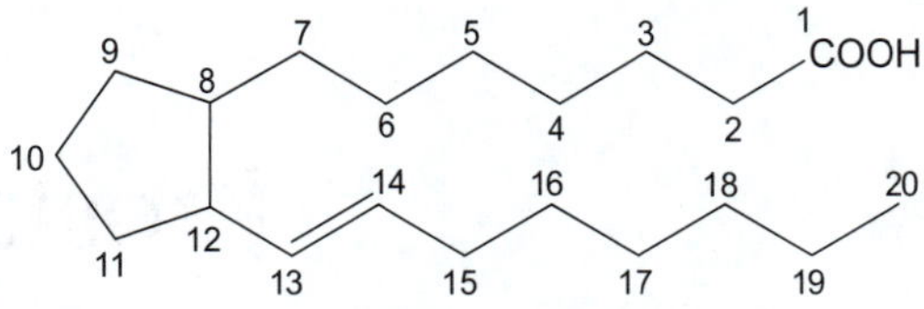

Prostanoic acid

PGs are considered as analogues of polyunsaturated fatty acids. It is a 20-carbon carboxylic acid containing a five-member ring. The PGs (Table 2.1) are classified according to the nature of:

A. Cyclopentane ring.

B. Two side chains.

C. Configuration of newly introduced functional group.

Table 2.1: Various types of PGs

Type	Structure	Function
A-type PGA	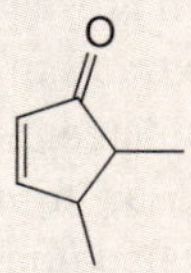	10,11-Unsaturated-9-keto function
B-type PGB	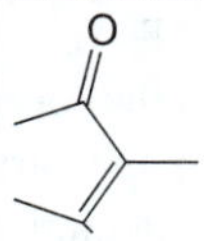	8,12-Unsaturated-9-keto function
C-type PGC	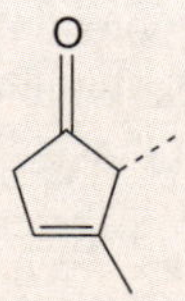	11,12-Unsaturated-9-keto function
D-type PGD	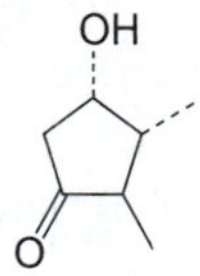	11-Keto-9-hydroxy function
E-type PGE	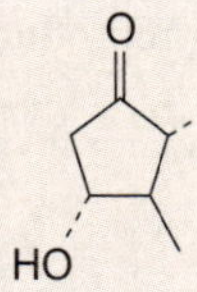	β-Hydroxyl ketone with keto moiety at C-9 and α-OH at C-11
F-type PGF	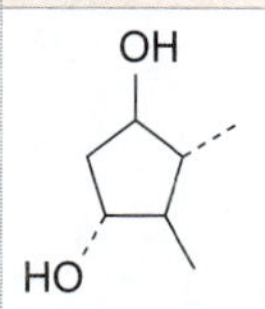	1,3-Diols

The main classes are further subdivided according to the number of double bonds in the side chain. This is indicated by the subscripts 1, 2, or 3 and refers to the fatty acid precursor in most instances. Examples: PGE_2 and $PGF_2\alpha$.

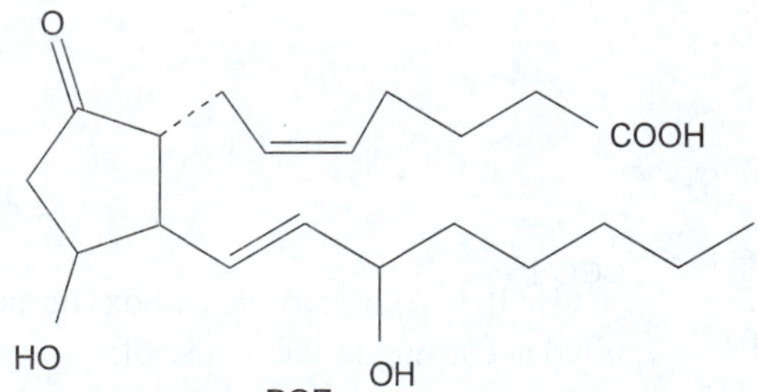

PGE_2

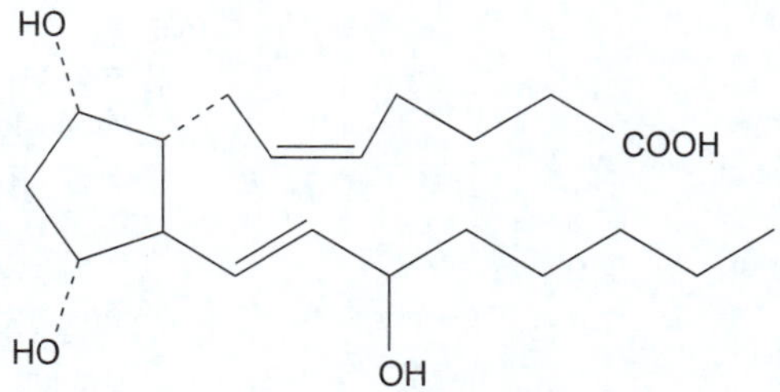

$PGF_2\alpha$

Two side chains are attached to the cyclopentane ring at C-8 and C-12. The upper chain, having a carboxylic acid group at the terminal, is α-side chain and the lower chain, having OH group at C-15 position, is a β-side chain. The α- and β-chains are in *trans* configuration in the prostanoic acid. The chiral centre C-15 is a δ nature (PGE). The OH group at C-11 in the E series has the configuration, however, in unnatural configurations the 11-OH is called 11-epi PGs, having arms fused C to each other and are named as isoprostaglandins.

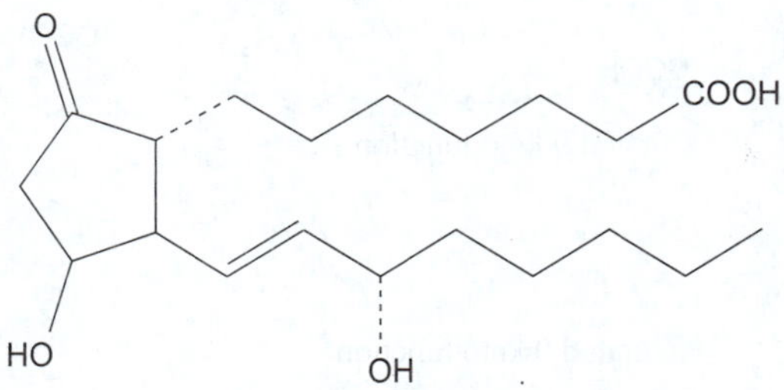

11-epi PGE_1

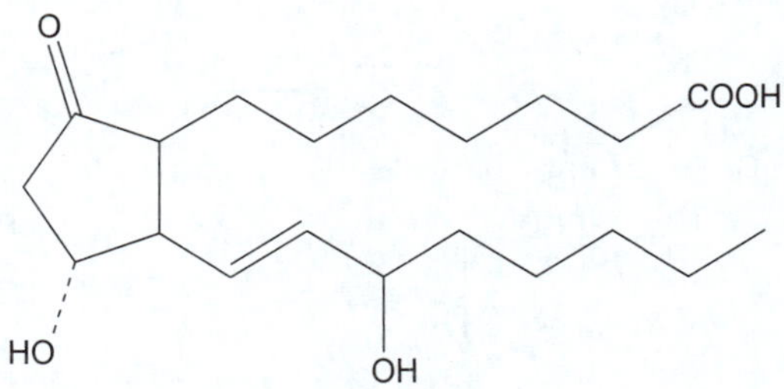

8-Isoprostaglandin

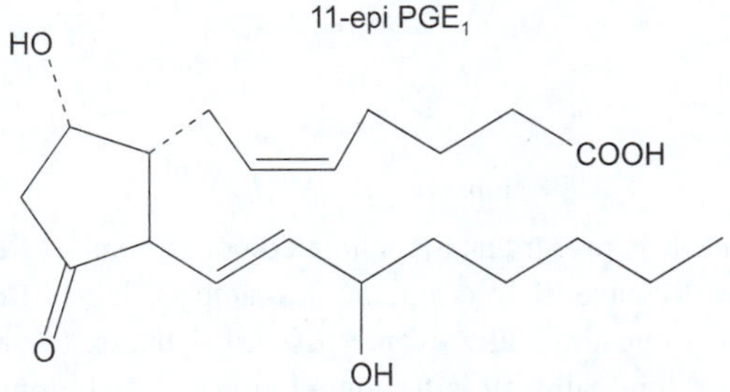

PGD_2

BIOSYNTHESIS

PGs are found virtually in all the tissues and organs. They are autocrine and paracrine lipid mediators that act on platelet endothelium, uterine tissues, and mast cells among others. The biosynthesis of PGE and PGF has been thoroughly established and both of them are derived from arachidonic acid. Two types of pathways have been proposed and are designated as follows:

1. Cyclooxygenase pathway
2. Lipoxygenase pathway

Cyclooxygenase Pathway

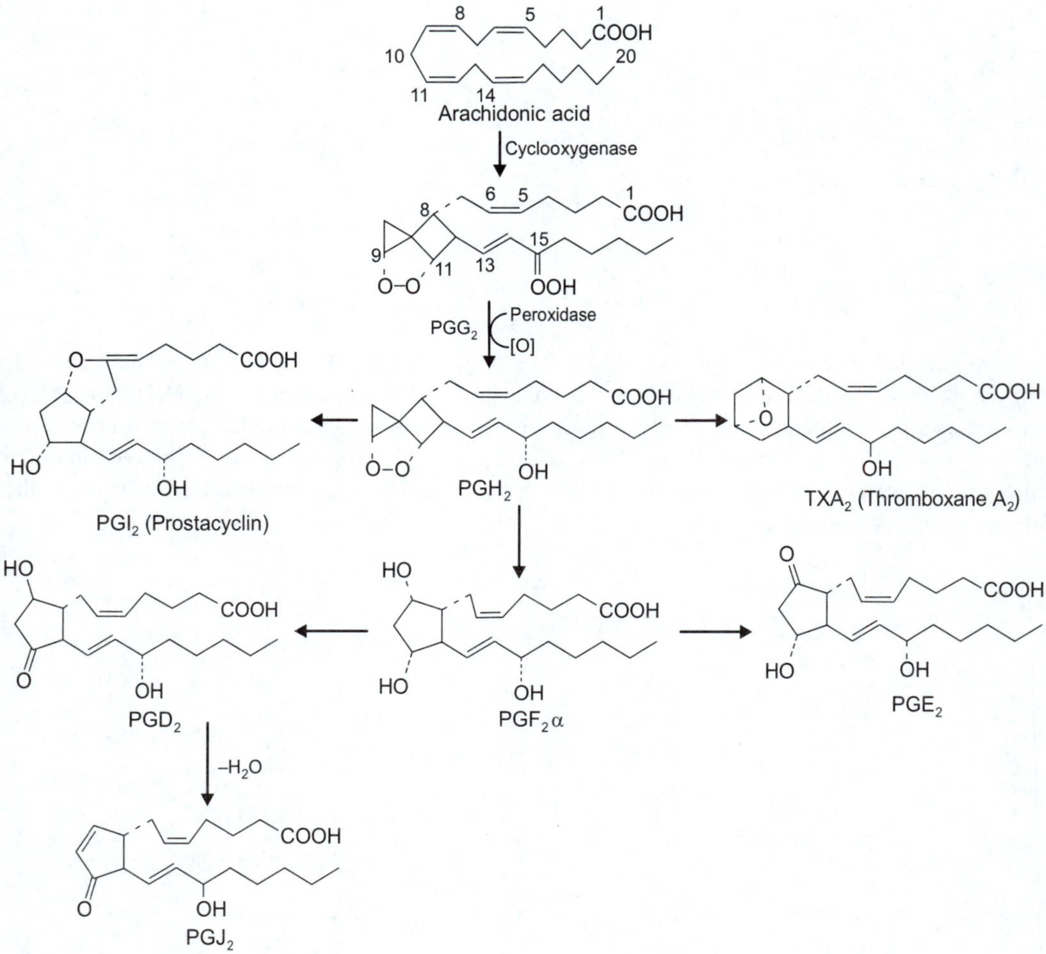

Arachidonic acid is derived from dietary linoleic acid. It is present as a conjugated component of the phospholipid matrix of the most cellular membrane. Release of free arachidonic acid is due to the stimulation of phospholipase enzyme in response to some traumatic events (tissues damage, toxin, exposure, and hormonal stimulation). The first step in this pathway is the interaction of arachidonic acid with PGH synthase, a haemoprotein, that catalyses both the addition of oxygen and subsequent reduction (peroxide activity) of the 15th position of hydroperoxide to 15(s) configuration alcohol prostaglandin H_2 (PGH_2). PGH synthase is also called cyclooxygenase I (COX-1) or cyclooxygenase II (COX-2). NSAIDs inhibit PGs synthesis; leading to relief of the pain, fever, and inflammation.

PGH_2 serves as a substrate for specific enzymes, leading to the production of various PGs, TXA_2, and PGI_2. While PGE_2 is formed by the action of endoperoxide isomerase on PGH_2 and PGD_2 by the action of isomerase or glutathione-s-transferase on PGH_2. PGF_2 is formed from PGH_2 via endoperoxidase reductase. Thromboxane synthetase acts on PGH_2 to produce thromboxane A_2.

Lipoxygenase Pathway

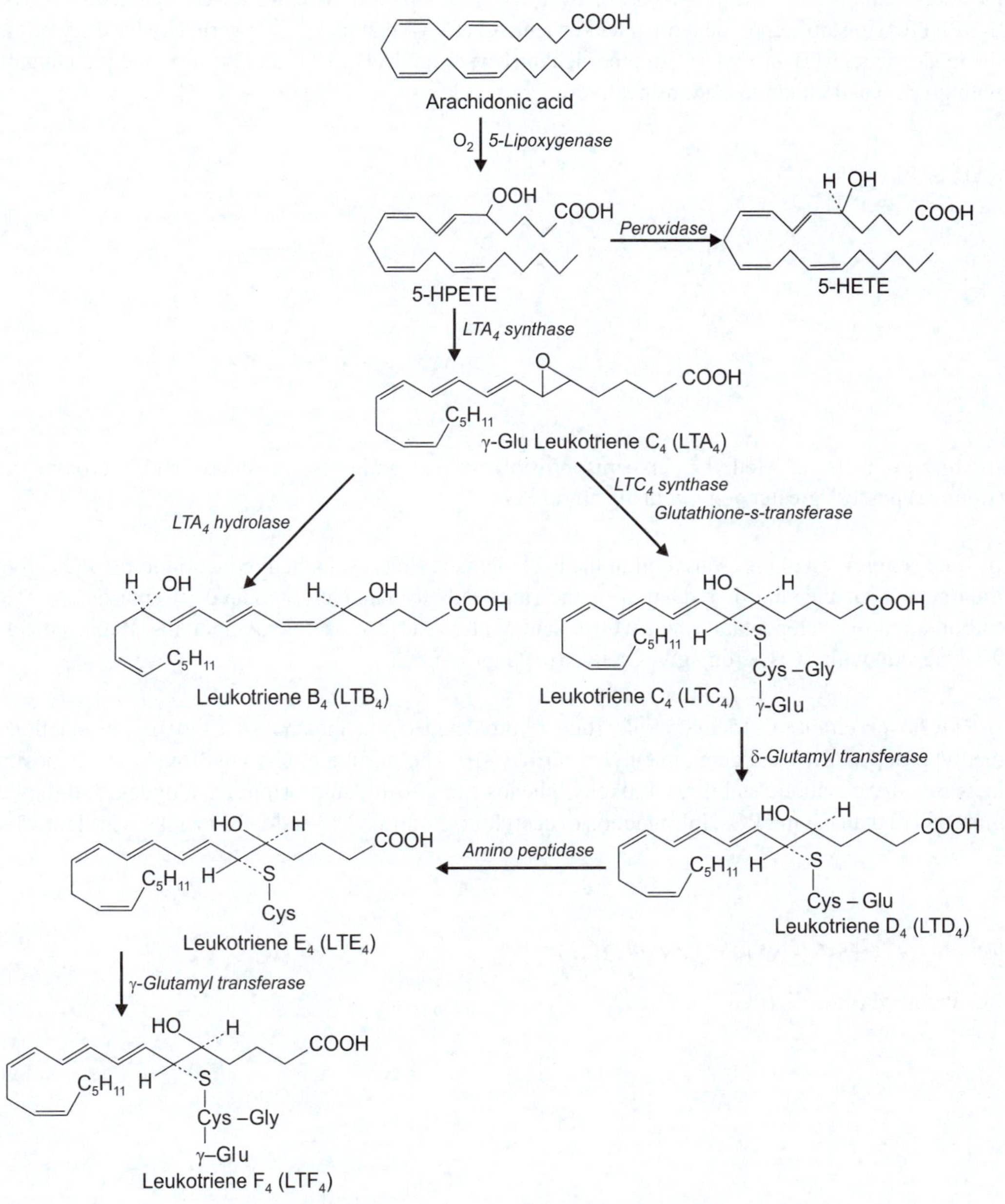

Lipoxygenase are a group of enzymes that oxidize polyunsaturated fatty acid possessing two *cis* double bonds separated by a methylene group to produce lipid peroxides. Arachidonic acid is metabolized to form a number of hydroperoxy eicosatetraenoic acid (HPETE) derivatives. These enzymes differ in the position at which they peroxidize arachidonic acid and in the tissues specificity. For example, platelets possess only 12-lipoxygenase, whereas leukocytes possess both 12-lipoxygenase and 5-lipoxygenase. Leukotriens are products of the 5-lipoxygenase pathways and are divided into major classes.

Hydroxylate eicosotetraenoic acid (LTs) is represented by lymphotoxin β_4 (LTB_4) and peptido leukotrienes (PLTs), such as leukotriene C4 (LTC_4), leukotriene D4 (LTD_4), and LTE_4. Lipoxygenase produces leukotrienase from 5-HPETE. Lysine epsilon-aminotransferase (LAT) synthetase converts 5-HPETE to unstable epoxide termed leukotriene A4 (LTA_4) that may be converted by the enzymes into the leukotriene, LTB_4 or by LTC_4 to other leukotrienes (e.g. LTD_4, LTE_4, and LTF_4), and reconjugation with glycine and glutamic acid, respectively.

SAR of PGs

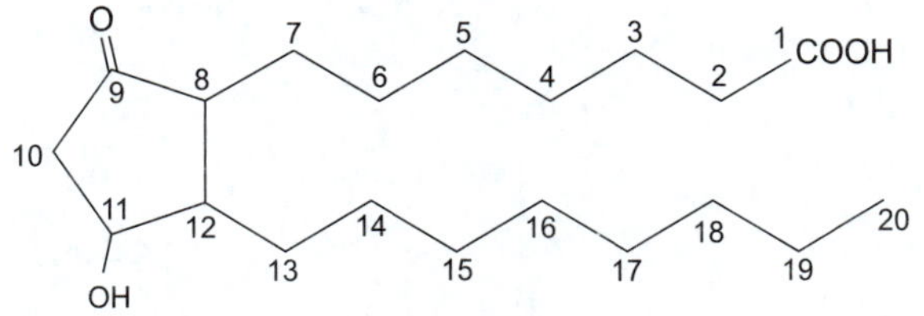

In the upper chain: Methyl esters (misoprostol), sulphonamide (sulprostone), and hydroxyl group (rioprost) possess greater activity than natural PGs.

In the cyclopentane ring: Variation in the cyclopentane ring results in a reduction in the PG activity. Enlargement of the ring or reduction of the ring leads to inactive compounds. Replacement of the carbon atom of cyclopentane ring by O, S, and N also leads to inactive compounds. Replacement of 9-keto group with $=CH_2$ group gives active (metenprost) PG.

In the lower chain: C-15 hydroxyl group is protected (from metabolism) by the introduction of methyl group at C-15 and gem dimethyl group at C-16. The shifting of C-15 hydroxyl to C-16 position increases the metabolic stability of alkoxy, phenoxy (enprostil, sulprostone) analogues, and they are more active than natural PGs. Introduction of acetylinic group at C-13 and C-14 increases the leuteolytic activity.

SYNTHESIS AND DRUG PROFILE

i. Prostaglandin E_1 (PGE_1)

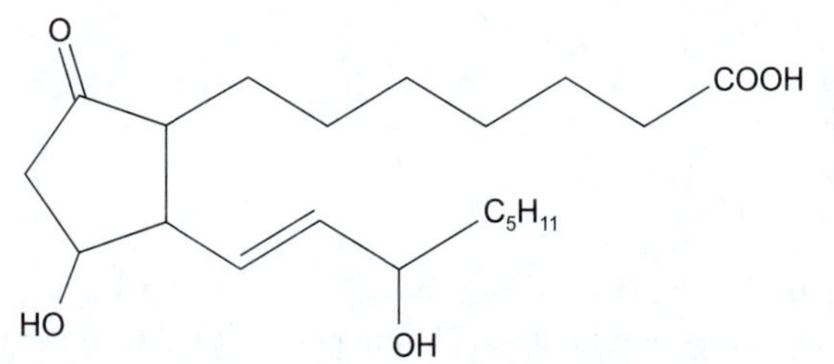

(E)-7-(3-hydroxy-2-(3-hydroxydec-1-enyl)-5-oxocyclopentyl)heptanoicacid

Synthesis

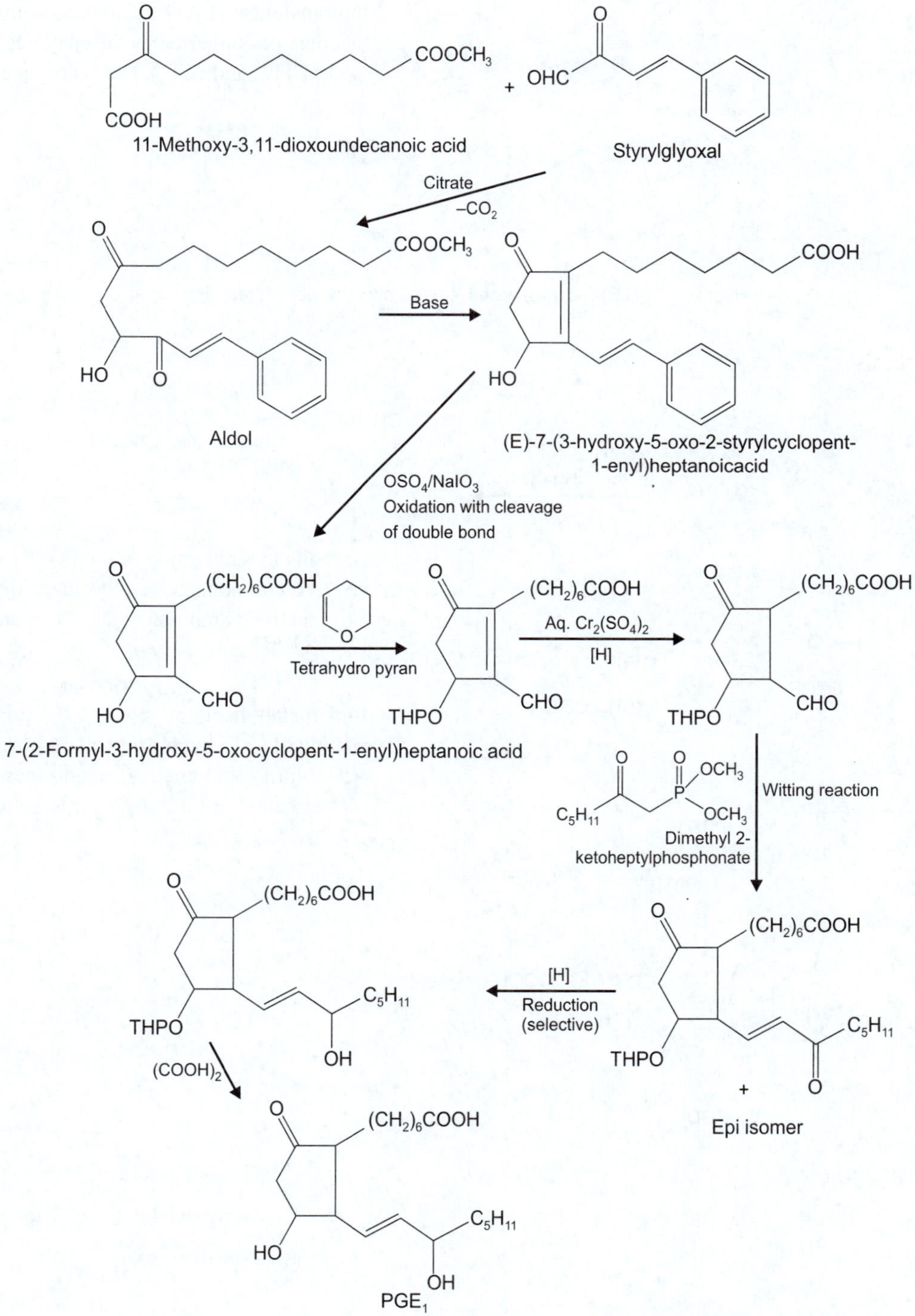

Dose: A dose of misoprostol, 200 µg three times a day for acute duodenal ulcer and comparable with cimetidine.

ii. Prostaglandin D_2 (PGD_2)

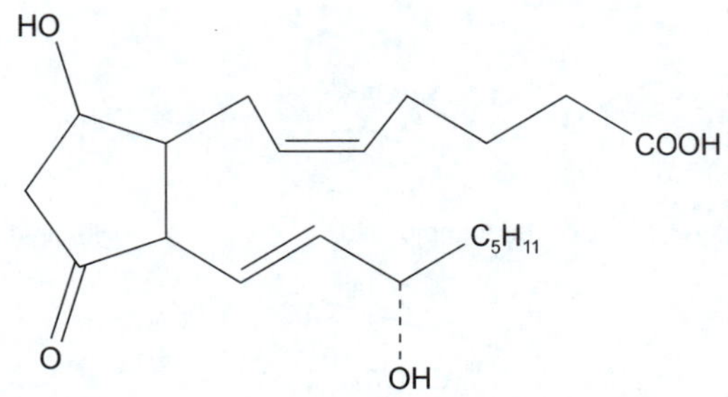

(Z)-7-(5-Hydroxy-2-((S,E)-3-hydroxyoct-1-enyl)-3-oxocyclopentyl)hept-5-enoic acid

Synthesis

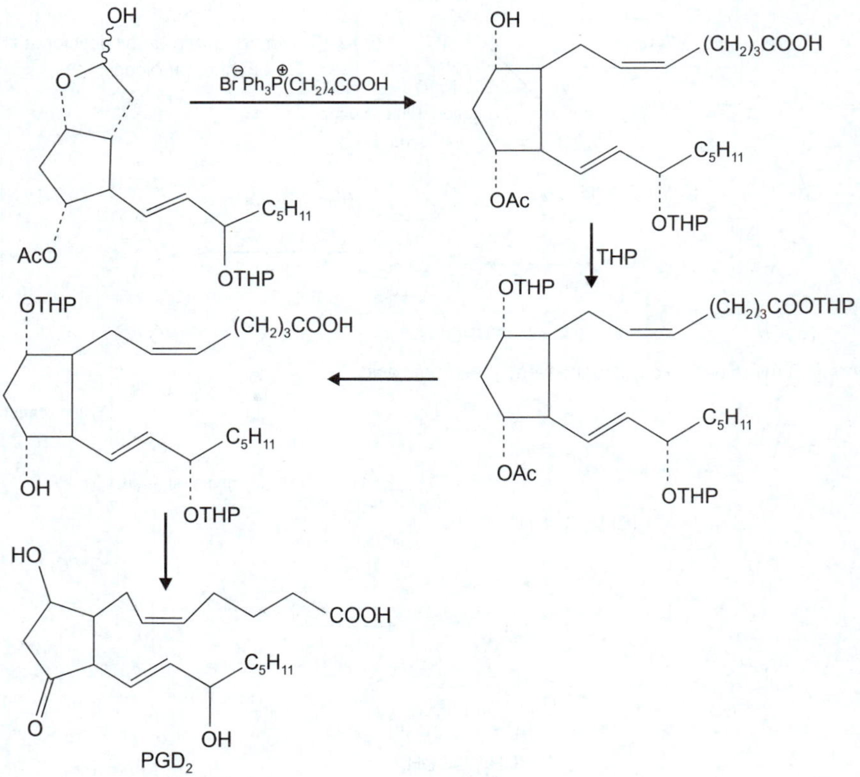

PGD_2

PGF$_2\alpha$

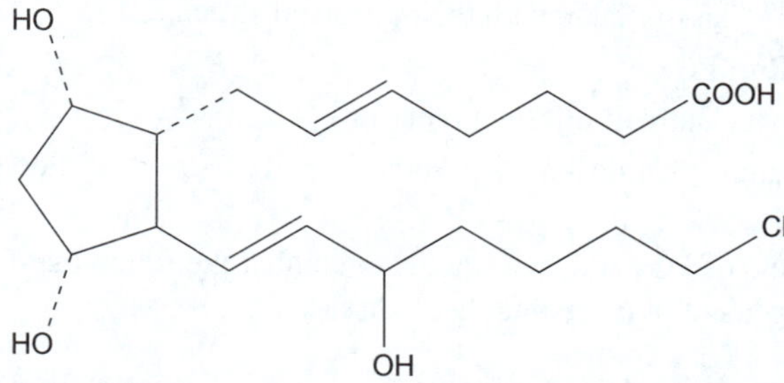

`(E)-7-((1R,3R,5S)-3,5-dihydroxy-2-((E)-3-hydroxyoct-1-enyl)cyclopentyl)hept-5-enoicacid

Synthesis

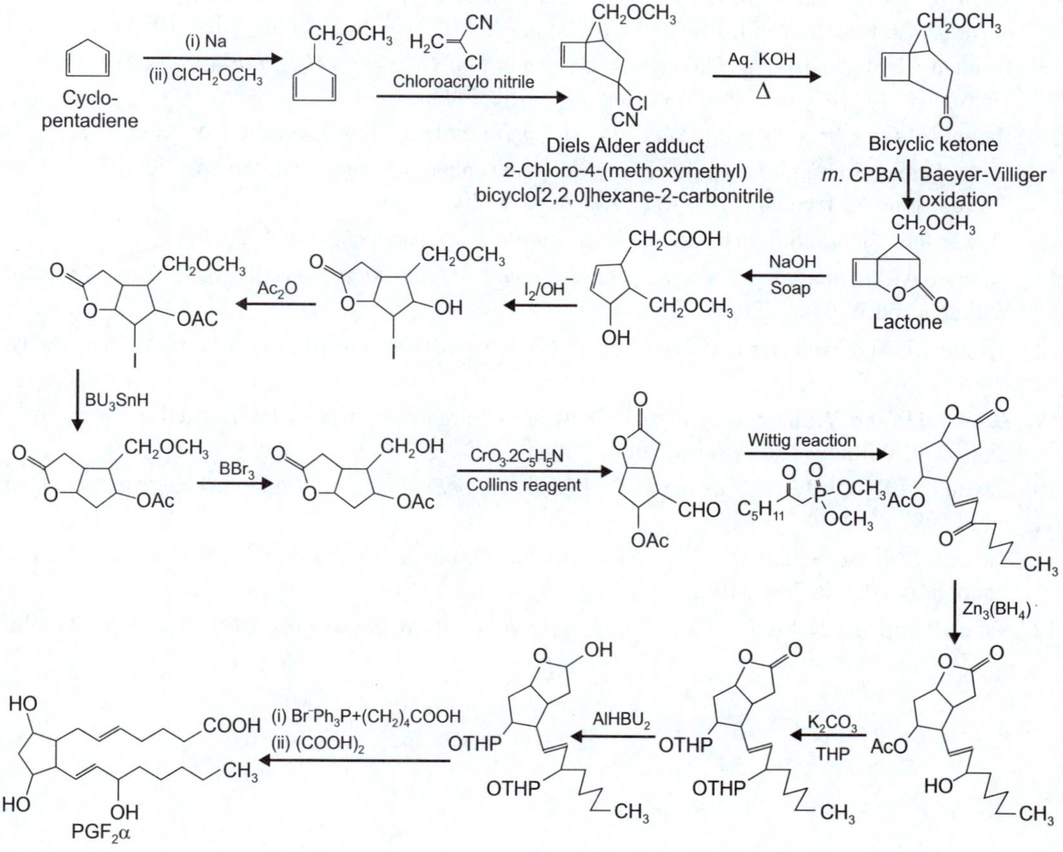

Metabolism: PGs are rapidly metabolized and inactivated by various oxidative and reductive pathways. The initial step involves rapid oxidation of the 15 α-OH group to the corresponding ketone by the PG-specific enzyme called PG 15 α-OH dehydrogenase. This is followed by a reduction of the C-13 and C-14 double bond by PG Δ^{13}-reductase to the corresponding dihydroketone, which represents the major metabolite in plasma. Subsequently, enzymes normally involved in 13 and ω-oxidation of fatty acids more slowly cleave the α-chain and oxidize the C-20 terminal methyl group to the carboxylic acid derivative, respectively.

PROBABLE QUESTIONS

1. What are PGs? Classify them with their chemical structure.
2. Write the SAR of PGs.
3. Write the nomenclature of different types of PGs.
4. Write the structure, chemical name, synthesis, and uses of the following compounds: (a) PGE_1 and (b) PGD_2.
5. Explain the role of PGs and eicosanoids to combat the following diseases: (a) Gastric ulceration and (b) management of congenital heart disease.

SUGGESTED READINGS

1. Abraham DJ (ed). *Burgers Medicinal Chemistry and Drug Discovery* (6th edn). New Jersey: John Wiley, 2007.
2. Axen U, Pike JE, and Schneider WP. 'The total synthesis of prostaglandins'. In: *The Total Synthesis of Natural Products*, Vol. I, J Apsimon (ed), pp. 81–142. New York: John Wiley, 1973.
3. Bruntan LL, Lazo JS, and Parker KL. *Goodman and Gilman's: The Pharmacological Basis of Therapeutics* (11th edn). New York: McGraw Hill, 2006.
4. Bailey JM (ed). *Prostaglandins, Leukotrienes and Lipoxins*. New York: Plenum Press, 1985.
5. Davis-Bruno KL and Halushka PV. 'Molecular pharmacology and therapeutic potential of thromboxane A2 receptor'. *Adv Drug Res* 25: 173–202, 1994.
6. Flower RJ. 'Eicosanoids: The nobel prize'. *Trends in Pharmacol Sci* 4: 1–2,1983.
7. Gennaro AR. *Remington's The Science and Practice of Pharmacy* (21st edn). New York: Lippincot Williams and Wilkins, 2006.
8. Lednicer D and Mitscher LA. *The Organic Chemistry of Drug Synthesis*. New York: John Wiley, 1995.
9. Lemke TL and William DA. *Foye's Principle of Medicinal Chemistry* (6th edn). New York: Lippincott Williams and Wilkins, 2008.
10. Reynolds EF (ed). *Martindale the Extra Pharmacopoeia* (31st edn). London: The Pharmaceutical Press,1997.
11. Roberts SM and Scheinmann F. *New Synthetic Routes to Prostaglandins and Thromboxanes*. London: Academic Press, 1982.
12. Vane JR and Grady J (eds). *Therapeutic Application of Prostaglandins*. Boston: Edward Arnold, 1993.

CHAPTER 3

Analgesics, Antipyretics and NSAIDs

INTRODUCTION

Non-steroidal anti-inflammatory drugs (NSAIDs) are used primarily to treat inflammation, mild-to-moderate pain, and fever. Specific uses include the treatment of headache, arthritis, sports injuries, and menstrual cramps. Aspirin is used to inhibit the clotting of blood and prevent strokes and heart attacks in individuals at high risk. NSAIDs are also included in many cold and allergic preparations.

NSAIDs are associated with a number of side effects. The frequency of side effects varies according to the drugs; the most common side effects are gastrointestinal tract (GIT) disturbances, such as nausea, diarrhoea, constipation, vomiting, decreased appetite, and peptic ulcer. NSAIDs may also cause fluid retention, leading to oedema; the most serious side effects are kidney failure, liver failure, ulcers, and prolonged bleeding after an injury of surgery. Some individuals are allergic to NSAIDs and may develop shortness of breath when NSAIDs are administered. People with asthma are at a higher risk for experiencing serious allergic reaction to NSAIDs. Use of aspirin in children and teenagers with chickenpox or influenza has been associated with the development of Reye's syndrome. Therefore, aspirin and salicylate should not be used in children and teenagers with suspected or confirmed chicken-pox or influenza.

Antipyretics are the drugs that reduce the elevated body temperature. Anti-inflammatory agents are used to cure or prevent inflammation caused by prostaglandin E_2 (PGE_2). These drugs are widely utilized for the alleviation of minor aches, pains, fever, and symptomatic treatment of rheumatic fever, rheumatoid arthritis, and osteoarthritis. The biosynthetic pathway of prostaglandins (PGs) is depicted in Figure 3.1.

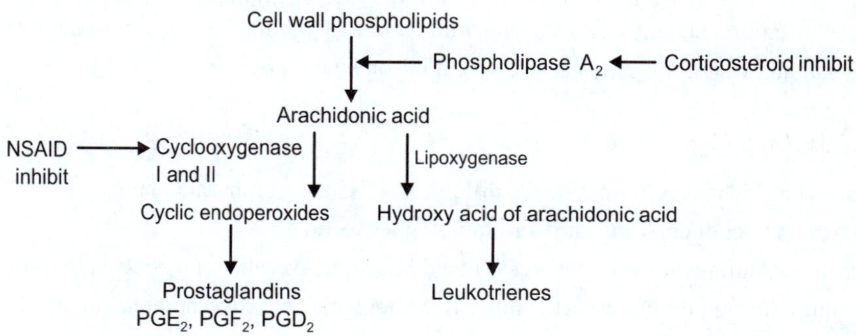

Figure 3.1: Biosynthetic pathway of PGs.

General Structure of PG

PG is a naturally occurring 20-carbon cyclopentano fatty acid derivative, derived from arachidonic acid.

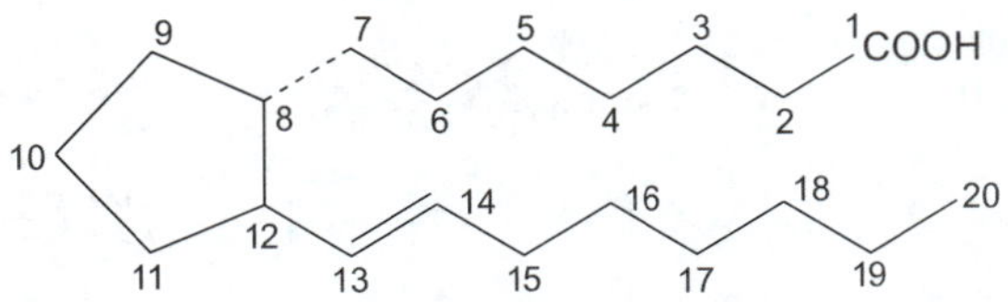

Mode of action: NSAIDs inhibit cycloxygenase (COX), the enzyme that catalyses the synthesis of cyclic endoperoxides, from the arachidonic acid to form PGs. The two COX isoenzymes are COX-1 and COX-2. The function of COX-1 is to produce PGs that are involved in normal cellular activity, (protection of gastric mucosa, maintenance of kidney function). While, COX-2 is responsible for the production of PGs at the inflammation sites, most NSAIDs inhibit both COX-1 and COX-2 with varying degree of selectivity. Selective COX-2 inhibitor may eliminate the side effects associated with NSAIDs due to COX-1 inhibition, such as gastric and renal effect.

Side Effects

In stomach: Biosynthesis of PGs, especially PGE_2 and PGI_2, serves as cytoprotective agents in gastric mucosa; these PGs inhibit acid secretion by the stomach, enhance mucosal blood flow, and promote the secretion of cytoprotective mucus in the GIT. Inhibition of the PGs synthesis may make the stomach more susceptible to damage and lead to gastric ulcer.

In platelets: Platelet's function get disturbed because NSAIDs prevent the formation of thromboxane A_2 (TXA_2) in platelets, as TXA_2 is a potent platelet-aggregating agent. This accounts for the tendency of these drugs to increase the bleeding time and this side effect has been exploited in the prophylactic treatment of thromboembolic disorder.

In uterus: NSAIDs prolong gestation because of the inhibition of PGF_2 in uterus. PGF_2 is a potent uterotropic agent and their biosynthesis by uterus increase dramatically in the hours before parturition. Accordingly, some anti-inflammatory drugs have been used as a colytic agent to inhibit preterm labour.

In kidney: NSAIDs decrease renal blood flow and the rate of glomerular filtration in patients with congestive heart failure, hepatic cirrhosis, and with chronic renal disease, in addition, they prolong the retention of salt and water, this may cause oedema in some patients.

CLASSIFICATION

I. Salicylic acid derivatives: Aspirin, diflunisal, salsalate, sulphasalazine.
II. *p*-Amino phenol derivatives: Paracetamol, phenacetin.
III. 3,5-Pyrazolidine dione derivatives: Phenyl butazone, oxyphenbutazone, sulphinpyrazone.
IV. Anthranilic acid derivatives (fonamates): Mefenamic acid, flufenamic acid, meclofenamate.

V. Aryl alkanoic acid derivative.
   a. Indole acetic acid: Indomethacin.
   b. Indene acetic acid: Sulindac.
   c. Pyrrole acetic acid: Tolmetin, zormipirac.
   d. Phenyl acetic (propionic) acid: Ibuprofen, diclofenac, naproxen, caprofen, fenoprofen, Ketoprofen, flurbiprofen, ketorolac, etodaolac.

VI. Oxicams: Piroxicam, meloxicam, tenoxicam.

VII. Selective COX-2 inhibitors: Celecoxib, rofecoxib, valdecoxib.

VIII. Gold compounds: Auronofin, aurothioglucose, aurothioglucamide, aurothiomalate sodium.

IX. Miscellaneous: Nabumetone, nimesulide, analgin.

X. Drug used in gout: Allopurinol, probenecid, sulphinpyrazone, febuxostat.

Salicylates

Salicylates not only possess antipyretic, analgesic, and anti-inflammatory properties, but also other actions that have been proven to be therapeutically beneficial because salicylates promote the excretion of uric acid and they are useful in the treatment of gouty arthritis. More attention has been given to the ability of salicylates (aspirin) to inhibit platelet aggregation, which may contribute to heart attack and strokes, and hence, aspirin reduces the risk of myocardial infarction. In addition, a recent study suggested that aspirin and other NSAIDs might be protective against colon cancer.

Structural–Activity Relationship (SAR) of Salicylates

- The active moiety of salicylates is salicylate anion, side effects of aspirin, particularly GIT effects appear to be associated with the carboxylic acid functional group.
- Reducing the acidity of the carboxy group results in a change in the potency of activity. Example, the corresponding amide (salicylamide) retain the analgesic action of salicylic acid, but is devoid of anti-inflammatory properties.
- Substitution on either the carboxyl or phenolic hydroxyl group may affect the potency and toxicity. Benzoic acid itself has only week activity.
- Placement of the phenolic hydroxyl group at meta or para to the carboxyl group abolishes the activity.
- Substitution of halogen atom on the aromatic ring enhances potency and toxicity.
- Substitution of aromatic ring at the 5th position of salicylic acid increases anti-inflammatory activity (diflunisal).

Metabolism of salicylic acid derivatives: The initial route of metabolism of these derivatives is their conversion to salicylic acid, which is excreted in urine as free acid (10%) or undergoes conjugation with either glycine to produce the major metabolites of salicylic acid (75%) or with glucuronic acid to form glucuronide (15%). In addition, small amount of metabolites resulting from microsomal aromatic hydroxylation leads to gentisic acid.

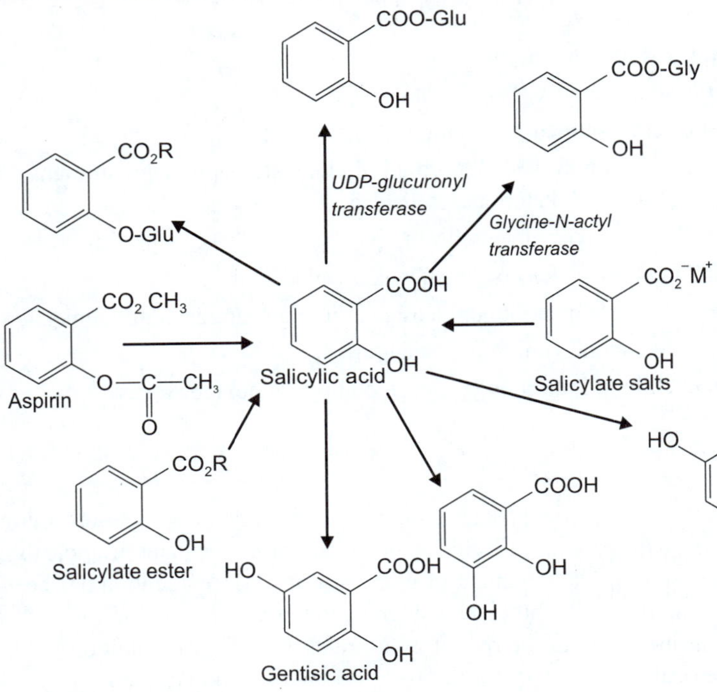

i. **Aspirin** (Emipirin, Bufferin)

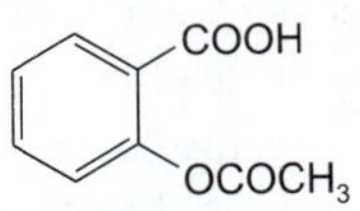

2-Acetoxybenzoic acid or Acetyl salicylate

Synthesis

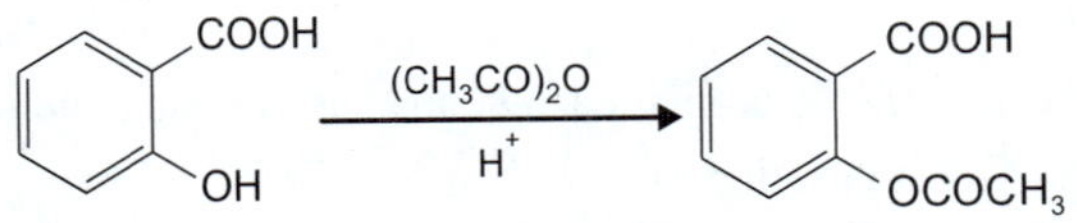

Properties and uses: Aspirin is a white crystalline powder, slightly soluble in water and soluble in alcohol, indicated for the relief of minor aches and mild-to-moderate pain in the conditions such as arthritis and related arthritic condition. Also used in myocardial infarction prophylaxis.

Assay: Dissolve the sample in alcohol and add 0.5 M sodium hydroxide. Allow to stand and titrate against 0.5 M hydrochloric acid using phenolphthalein as an indicator. Perform a blank titration.

Dose: Usual adult dose: 300 to 650 mg every 3 or 4 hrs orally or 650 mg to 1.3 g as the sustained-release tablet every 8 hrs; rectal, 200 mg to 1.3 g three or four times a day.

Dosage forms: Aspirin tablets IP, BP, dispersible aspirin tablets BP, effervescent soluble aspirin tablets BP, gastro-resistant aspirin tablets BP, aspirin and caffeine tablets BP, co-codaprin tablets BP, dispersible co-codaprin tablets BP.

ii. Sodium salicylate

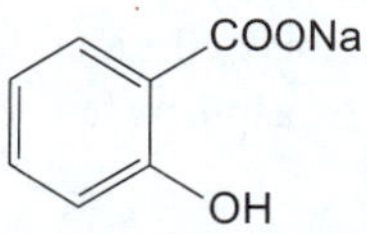

Sodium 2-hydroxybenzoate

Synthesis

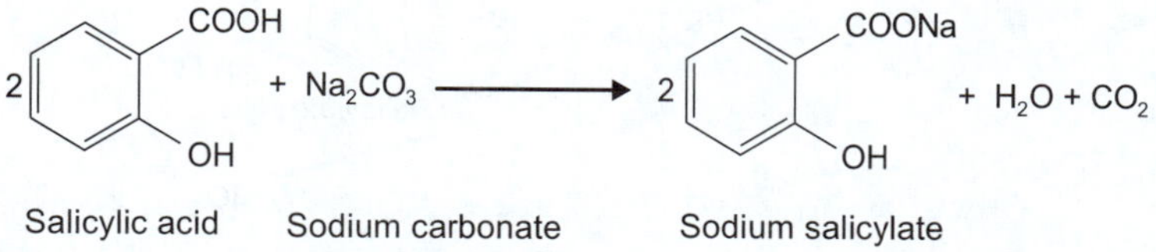

Properties and uses: Sodium salicylate is a white crystalline powder, soluble in water, sparingly soluble in alcohol. It is used for fever and for the relief of pain. It also possesses anti-inflammatory actions similar to aspirin and symptomatic therapy of gout.

Assay: Dissolve the sample in anhydrous acetic acid and titrate against 0.1 M per chloric acid. Determine the end point potentiometrically.

iii. Salsalate (Disalcid, Saloxium)

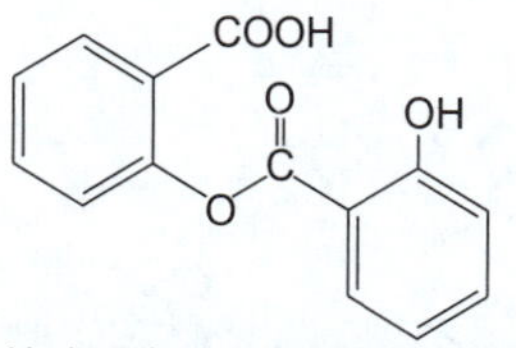

2-(2-Hydroxybenzoyloxy)benzoic acid

Synthesis

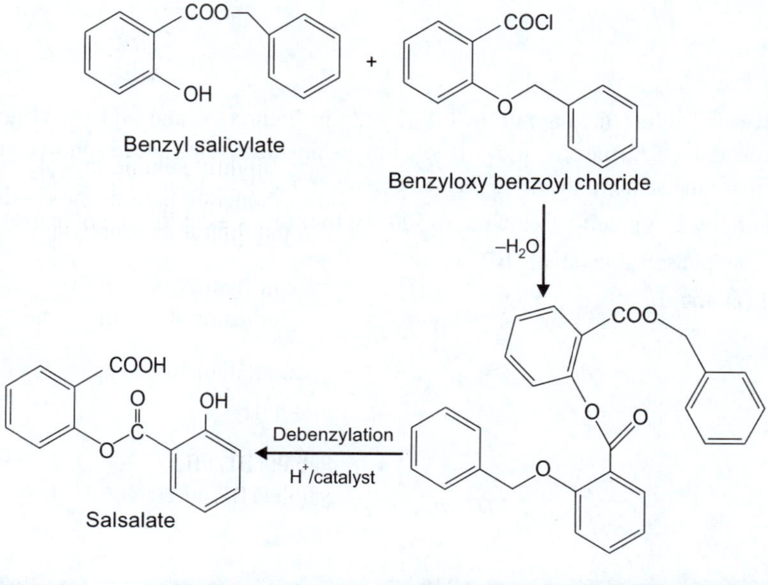

Properties and uses: Salsalate or salicylsalicylic acid is a dimer of salicylic acid. It is insoluble in gastric juice, but is soluble in the small intestine where it is partially hydrolyzed into two molecules of salicylic acid and absorbed. It does not cause GI blood loss. It has antipyretic, analgesic, and anti-inflammatory properties similar to those of aspirin. It is employed in the treatment of rheumatoid arthritis and other rheumatic disorders.

Dose: Usual adult dose is 325–1000 mg 2–3 times a day, orally.

iv. Sulphasalazine (Azultidine, Azaline)

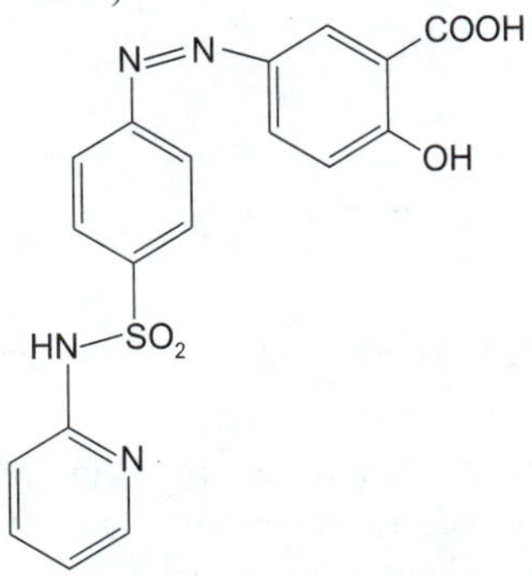

Properties and uses: Sulphasalazine is a bright yellow or brownish-yellow fine powder, practically insoluble in water and methylene chloride, very slightly soluble in alcohol, soluble in dilute solutions of alkali hydroxides. Sulphasalazine is a mutual prodrug. In large intestine, it is activated to liberate 5-aminosalicylic acid, which in turn inhibits PG synthesis and the sulphapyridine is useful for the treatment of infection. Hence, sulphasalazine is used in the treatment of ulcerative colitis.

Synthesis

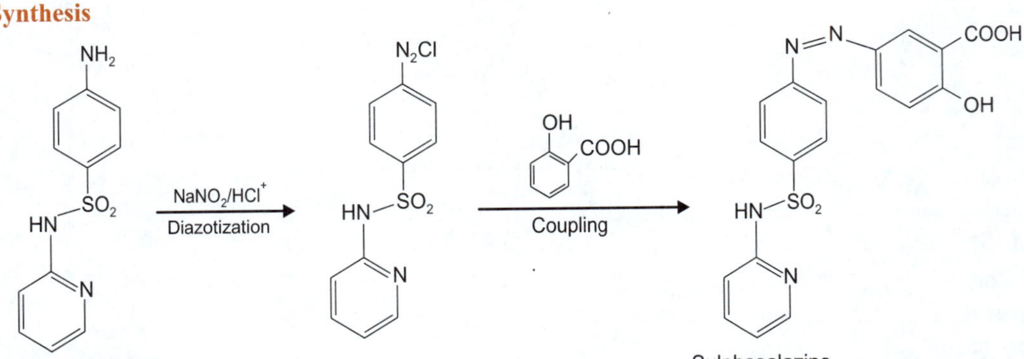

Assay: Dissolve and dilute the sample in 0.1 M sodium hydroxide and add 0.1 M acetic acid and measure the absorbance at the maxima of 359 nm using ultraviolet spectrophotometer. Prepare a standard solution at the same time and in the same manner, using sulphasalazine reference standard.

Dose: Orally initially 3–4 g daily, followed by 500 mg four times a day for maintenance.

Dosage forms: Sulphasalazine tablets BP.

v. Diflunisal (Dolobid)

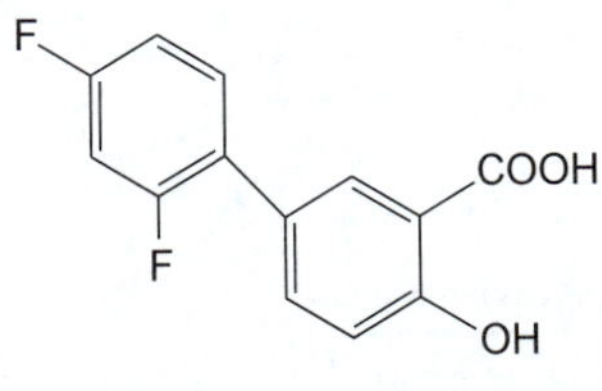

5-(2,4-Difluorophenyl) salicylic acid

Synthesis

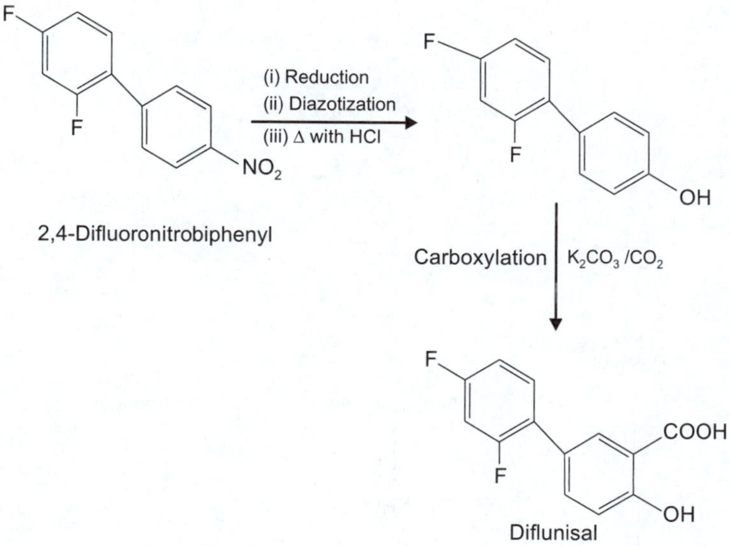

Properties and uses: Diflunisal is a white crystalline powder, practically insoluble in water, soluble in alcohol, and dilute solutions of alkali hydroxides. It is more potent than aspirin, but produces fewer side effects, and has a biological half-life 3–4 times greater than that of aspirin. It is a non-selective cyclooxygenase inhibitor used as antipyretic, analgesic, and anti-inflammatory.

Assay: Dissolve the sample in methanol, add water, and titrate against 0.1 M sodium hydroxide using phenol red as indicator, until the colour changes from yellow to reddish-violet.

p-Amino Phenol Derivatives

These derivatives possess analgesic and antipyretic action, but lack in anti-inflammatory effects. Acetanilide was introduced into the therapy in 1886 as an antipyretic–analgesic agent. However, it was subsequently found to be too toxic, having been associated with methemaglobinemia and jaundice.

Phenacetin was introduced in the following year and was widely used but was withdrawn recently because of its nephrotoxicity. Acetaminophen (paracetamol) was introduced in 1893 and it remains the only useful agent of this group used as an antipyretic and an analgesic.

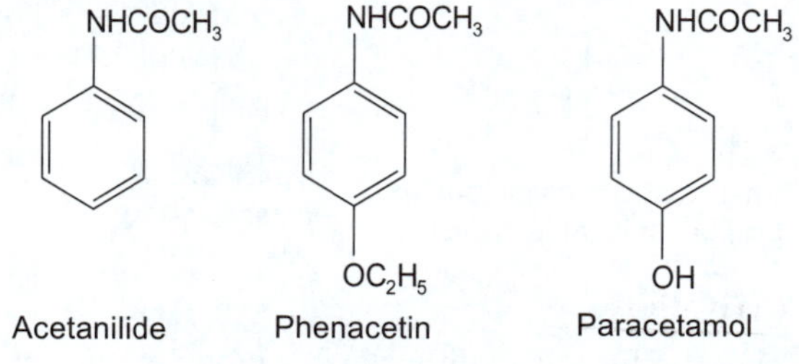

Metabolism of *para*-aminophenol derivatives: These drugs undergo hydrolysis to yield aniline derivatives that produce directly or through their conversion to hydroxylamine derivatives, such as acetaminophen that undergoes rapid first pass metabolism in the GIT to *o*-sulphate conjugate. The

N-hydroxylamine is then converted into a reactive toxic metabolite, acetiminoquinone, which produces toxicity to the kidney and liver in conjugation with hepatic glutathione to form mercapturic acid or cysteine conjugates.

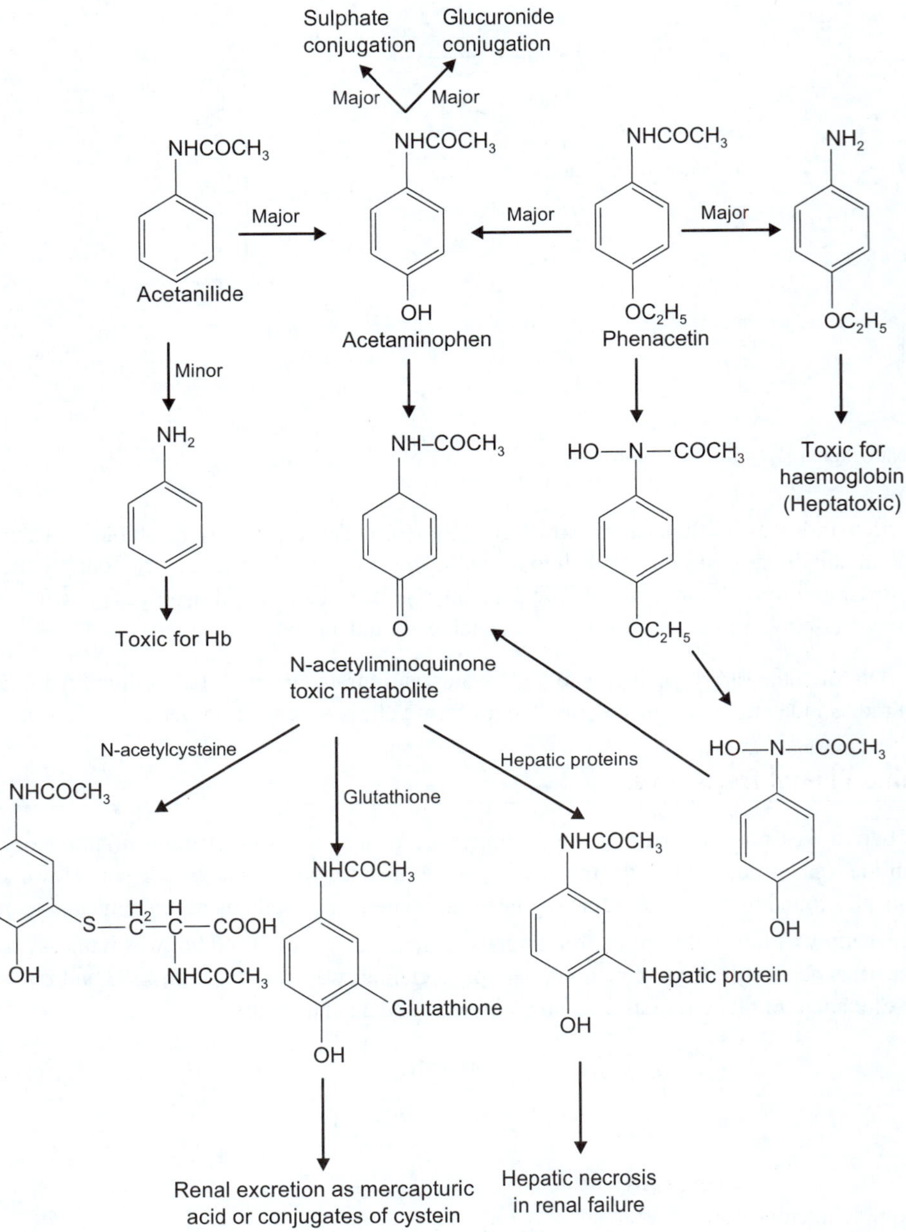

SAR of *p*-amino Phenol Derivatives

1. Etherification of the phenolic function with methyl or propyl groups produces derivatives with greater side effects than ethyl derivatives.
2. Substituents of the nitrogen atom, which reduce the basicity, also reduce activity unless the substituent is metabolically labile. Example, acetyl groups.
3. Amides derived from aromatic acid. Example, N-phenyl benzamides that are less active or inactive.

i. Phenacetin (Acetophenetidin)

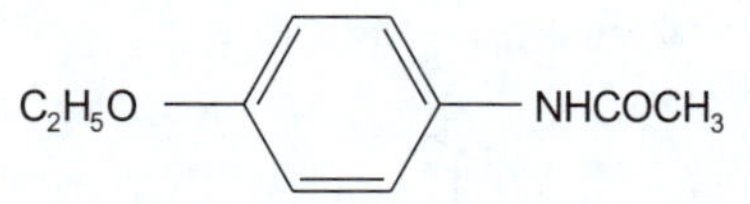

p-Ethoxy acetanilide

Synthesis

Route I. From: *p*-Nitrophenol

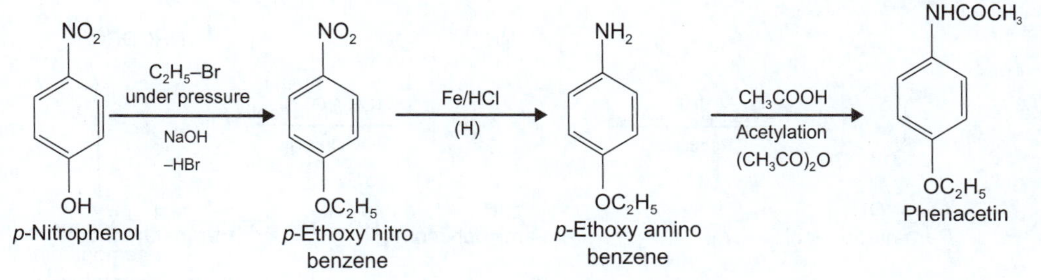

Route II. From: Aniline

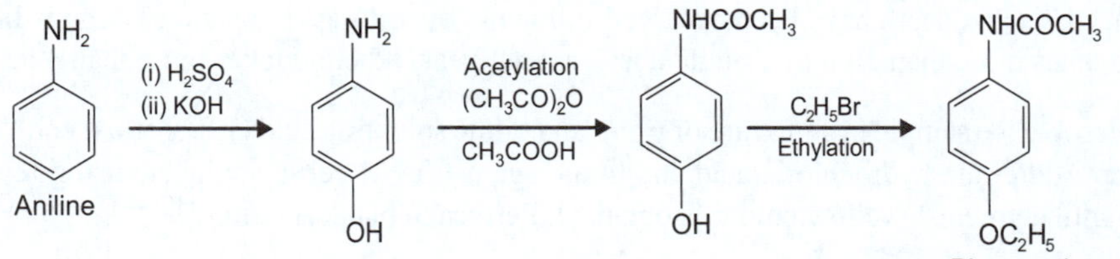

Route III. From: Chlorobenzene

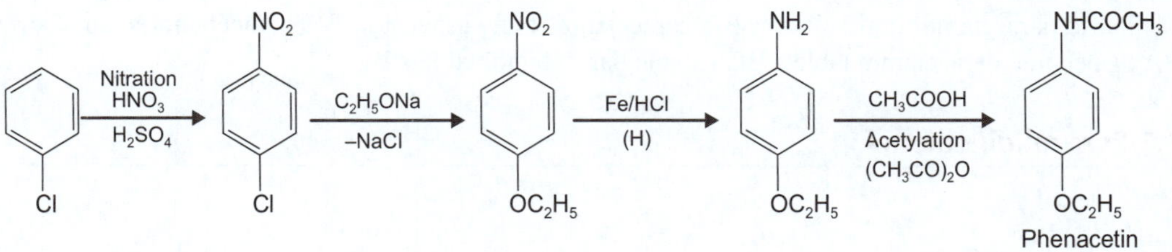

Properties and uses: It exists as a white glistering powder with a bitter taste, sparingly soluble in water and soluble in chloroform. It is an analgesic and an antipyretic with similar effectiveness as an aspirin. It has a greater potential for toxicity (hemolytic anaemia and methemoglobinaemia) than paracetamol.

Dose: Usual dose as oral for adults is 300 mg to 2 g per day.

ii. Paracetamol (Metacin, Tylenol, Tapar, Calpol)

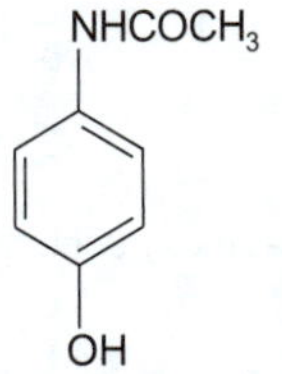

Para-acetaminophenol

Synthesis

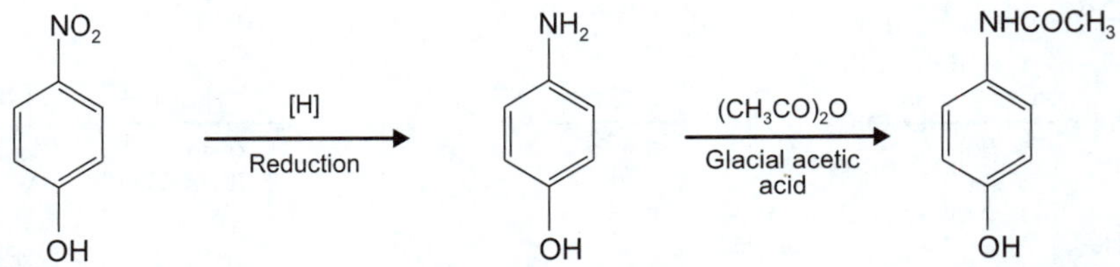

Para-nitrophenol *Para*-aminophenol Paracetamol

Properties and uses: Paracetamol exists as white crystalline powder, sparingly soluble in water, soluble in alcohol, and very slightly soluble in methylene chloride. Paracetamol produces antipyresis by acting on the hypothalamic heat-regulating centre and analgesia by elevating the pain threshold. Hepatic necrosis and death have been observed following over dosage; hepatic damage is likely in an adult who takes more than 10 g in a single dose or if a 2-year-old child takes more than 3 g.

Assay: Dissolve the sample in a mixture of water and dilute sulphuric acid (1:3), reflux, cool, and dilute with water. Add dilute hydrochloric acid and titrate against 0.1 M cerium sulphate using ferroin as an indicator until a greenish-yellow colour is obtained. Perform a blank titration.

Dose: Usual oral adult dose is 500 mg to 1 g for three or four times a day.

Dosage forms: Paracetamol tablets IP, BP, paracetamol syrup IP, co-codamol tablets BP, effervescent co-codamol tablets BP, co-dydramol tablets BP, co-proxamol tablets BP, paracetamol capsules BP, paediatric paracetamol oral solution BP, paracetamol oral suspension BP, paracetamol suppositories BP, dispersible paracetamol tablets BP, soluble paracetamol tablets BP.

3,5-Pyrazolidinediones

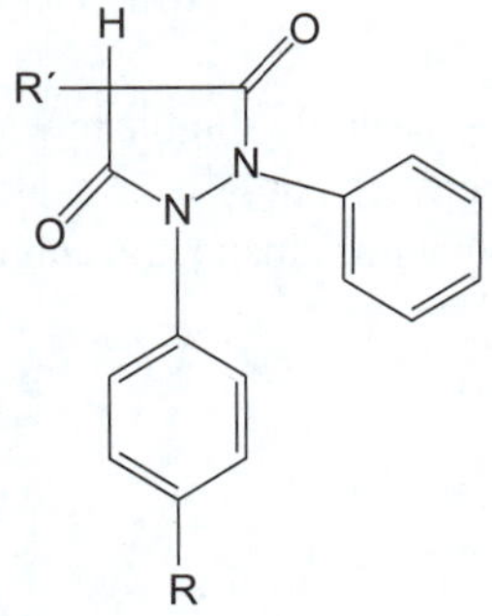

Name	*R*	*R′*
Phenyl butazone	–H	$-C_4H_9$
Oxyphenbutazone	–OH	$-C_4H_9$
Sulphin pyrazone	–H	$-(CH_2)_2SOC_6H_5$

SAR of 3,5-Pyrazolidinediones

- Replacement of one of the nitrogen atom in the pyrazolidinediones with an oxygen atom yields isoxazole analogues, which are as active as pyrazolidinedione derivatives.
- In 3,5-pyrazolidinedione derivatives, pharmacological activities are closely related to their acidity, the dicarbonyl function at the 3rd and 5th positions enhances the acidity of hydrogen atom at the 4th position.
- Presence of a keto group in the γ-position of the butyl side chain produces the active compound.
- Decreasing or eliminating acidity by removing the acidic proton at 4th position (e.g. 4,4-dialkyl derivatives) abolishes anti-inflammatory activity. Thus, if the hydrogen atom at the 4th position of phenylbutazone is replaced by substituents, such as a methyl group, anti-inflammation activity is abolished.
- If acidity is enhanced too much, anti-inflammatory and sodium-retaining activities decrease while other properties, such as the uricosuric effect increases.
- Introduction of polar function in these alkyl groups gives mixed results. The γ-hydroxy-*n*-butyl derivative possesses pronounced uricosuric activity, but give fewer anti-inflammatory effects.
- Substitution of 2-phenyl thio ethyl group at the 4th position produces antigout activity (sulphinpyrazone).
- Presence of both the phenyl groups is essential for neither anti-inflammatory nor analgesic activity.
- *m*-Substitution of aryl rings of the phenyl butazone gives uniformly inactive compounds. *p*-Substitution, such as methyl, chloro, nitro, or OH of one or both rings retains activity.

i. Phenylbutazone (Butazolidin, Busone)

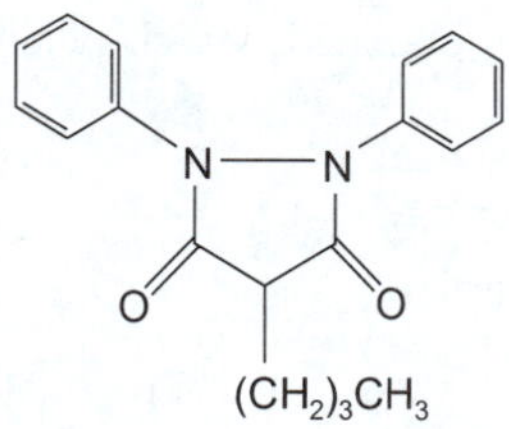

Synthesis

Route I. From: Diethylmalonate

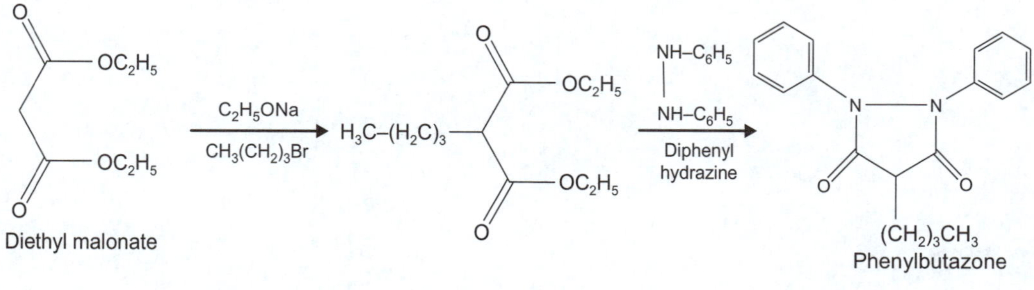

Route II. From: Diethyl butyl malonate or butyl malonylchloride

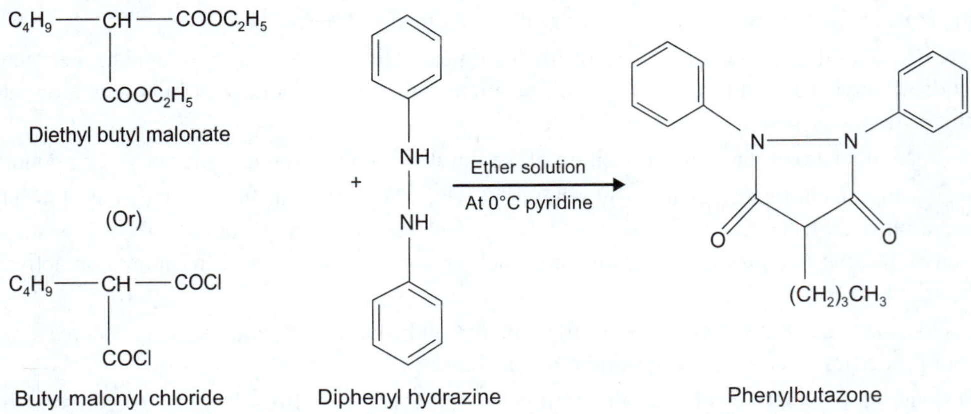

Properties and uses: Phenylbutazone is a white crystalline powder, practically insoluble in water, sparingly soluble in alcohol, and soluble in alkaline solutions. It is a pyrazole derivative that has antipyretic, analgesic, and anti-inflammatory actions, because of its toxicity it is not used as a general antipyretic or analgesic. It is a usual practice reserved for use in the treatment of osteoarthritis, ankylosing spondylitis, arthritis, acute superficial thrombophlebitis, painful shoulder, and Reiter's disease, where less toxic drugs have failed.

Assay: Dissolve the sample in acetone and titrate against 0.1 M sodium hydroxide using bromothymol blue as indicator until a blue colour is obtained, which persists for few seconds. Perform a blank titration.

Dose: The usual dose is 100–600 mg per day.

ii. **Oxyphenbutazone** (Tandearil, Oxaril)

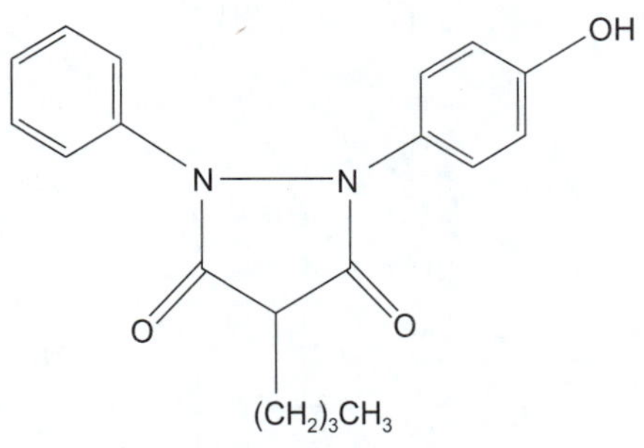

Synthesis

Route I. From: Aniline

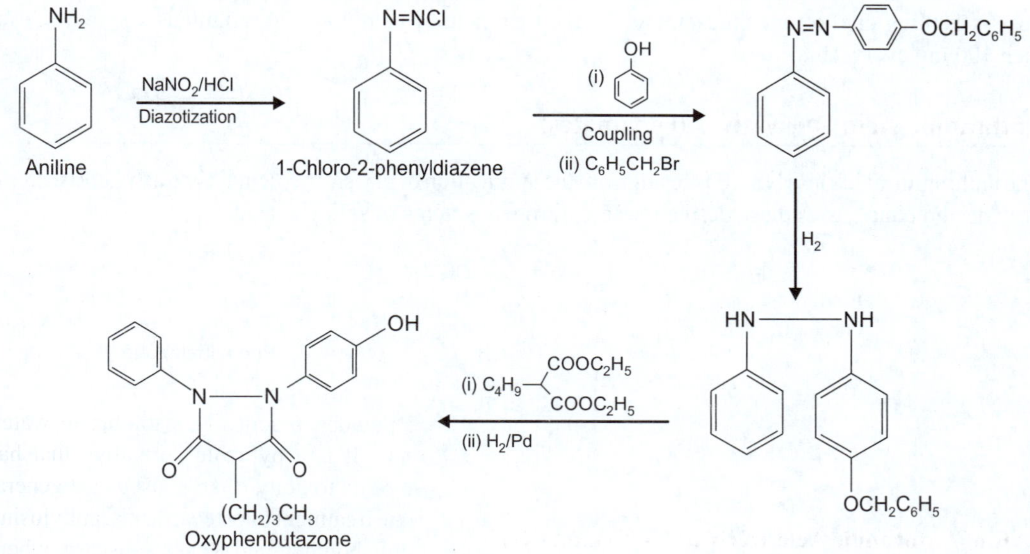

Route II. From: Diethyl butyl malonate

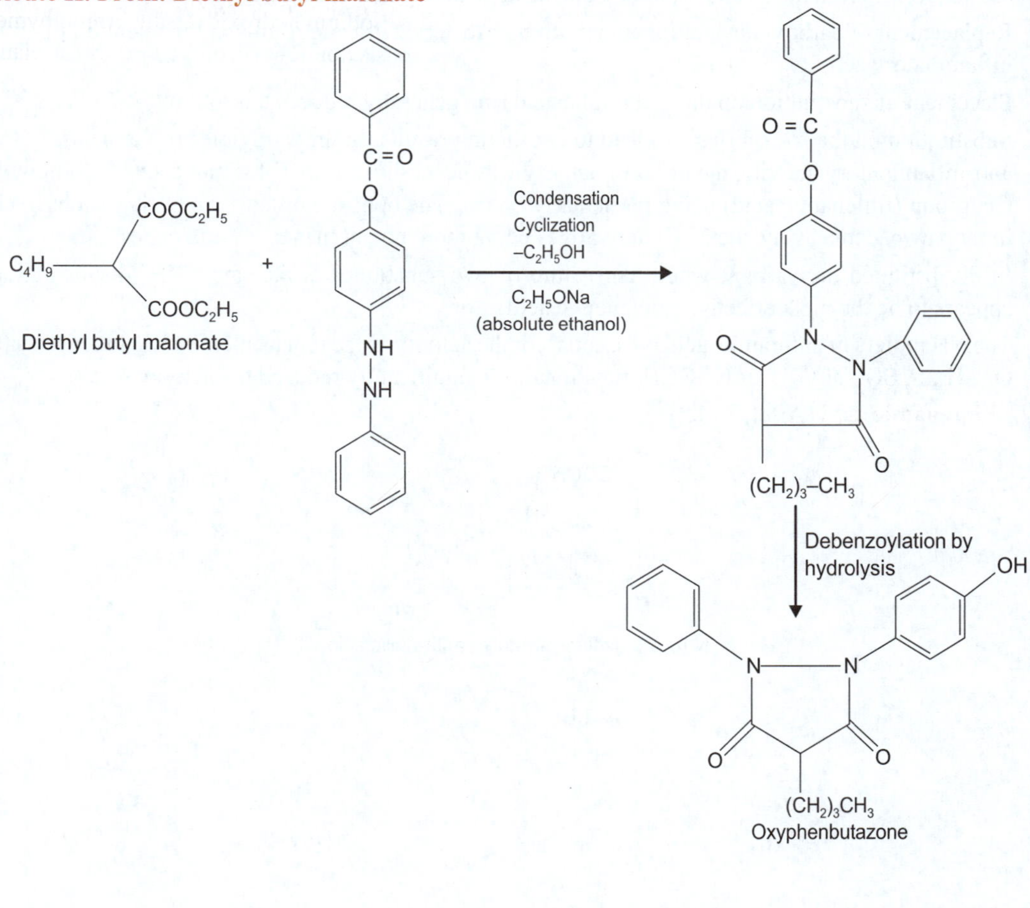

Properties and uses: It exists as a white to yellowish white, odourless, crystalline powder, soluble in water, alcohol, chloroform, and ether. Used as an analgesic and in arthritis.

Dose: Usual oral adult dose for antirheumatic is 100 or 200 mg three times daily; for maintenance the dose is 100 mg one to four times a day; for the treatment of gout 400 mg initially as a loading dose, then 100 mg every 4 hrs.

Anthranilic Acid Derivatives (Fenamates)

The anthranilic acid class NSAIDs result from the application of classic medicinal chemistry bioisosteric drug design concepts as these derivatives are nitrogen isoteres of salicylic acid.

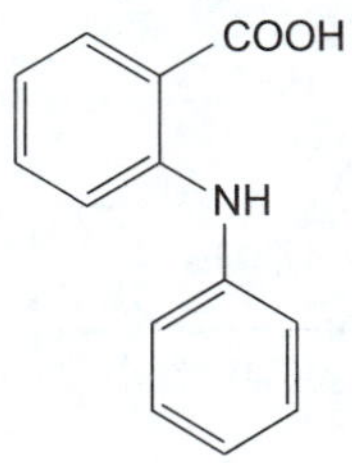

SAR of Anthranilic Acid Derivatives (Fenamates)

- The position of the carboxyl function is important for the activity of anthranilic acid derivatives that are active, whereas the 3- and 4-amino benzoic acid analogues are not active.
- Replacement of carboxylic acid function with the isosteric tetrazole results in the retention of anti-inflammatory activity.
- Placement of substitution on the anthranilic acid ring generally reduces the activity.
- Substitution on the N-aryl ring can lead to conflicting results. In the ultraviolet erythema assay for anti-inflammatory activity, the order of activity was generally 3′>2′>4′ for mono substitution with CF_3 group (flufenamic acid) being particularly potent. The opposite order of activity was observed in rat paw oedema assay, the 2′-Cl derivatives being more potent than 3′-Cl analogues.
- In disubstituted derivatives, where the nature of two substitutes is the same 2′,3′-disubstitution appears to be the most effective (mefenemic acid).
- The NH moiety of anthranilic acid is essential for the activity as the replacement of NH function with O, CH_2, S, SO_2, N-CH_3, or $NCOCH_3$ functionalities significantly reduced the activity.

i. **Flufenamic acid** (Arlef, Tarlef)

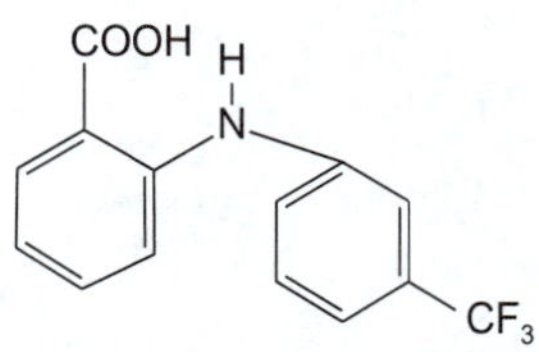

N-(α,α,α-Trifluoro-*m*-tolyl) anthranilic acid

Synthesis

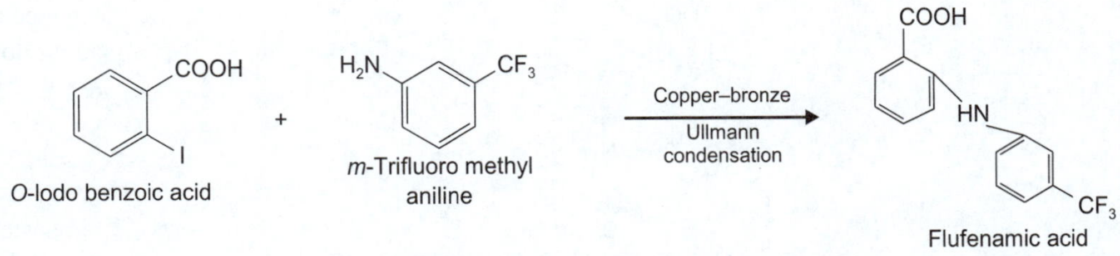

Properties and uses: Flufenamic acid is a pale yellow crystalline powder or needles. It has analgesic, anti-inflammatory, and antipyretic actions; it is employed in the treatment of rheumatic disorder and dysmenorrhoea.

Dose: 400–600 mg per day in divided doses.

ii. Mefenamic acid

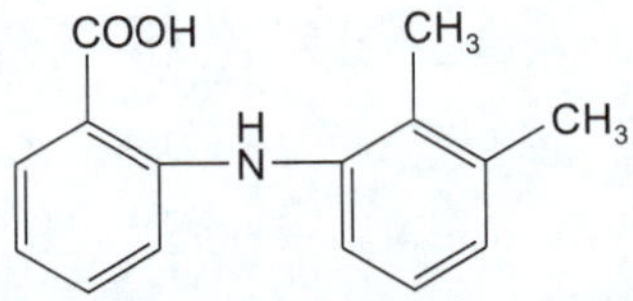

2-(2,3-Dimethylphenylamino)benzoic acid

Synthesis

An analogues approach by reaction of *o*-chlorobenzoic acid with 2,3-dimethyl aniline.

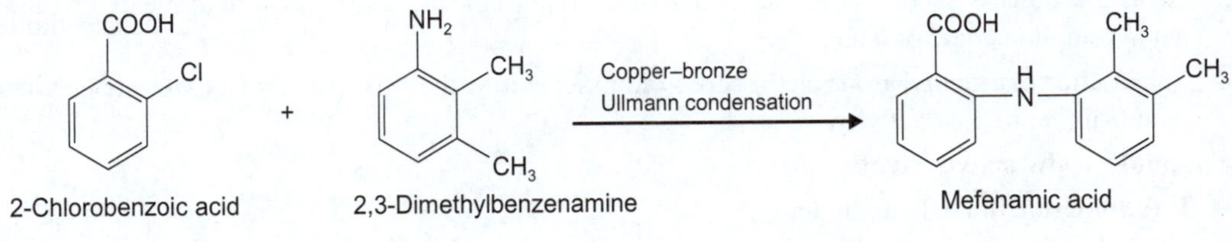

Metabolism: Its metabolism occurs through regioselective oxidation of 3-methyl group and glucuronidation of mephanamic acid. Majority of the 3-hydroxy methyl metabolite and dicarboxylic acid products are excreted.

Uses: Used as an analgesic and anti-inflammatory agent.

iii. Meclofenamate sodium

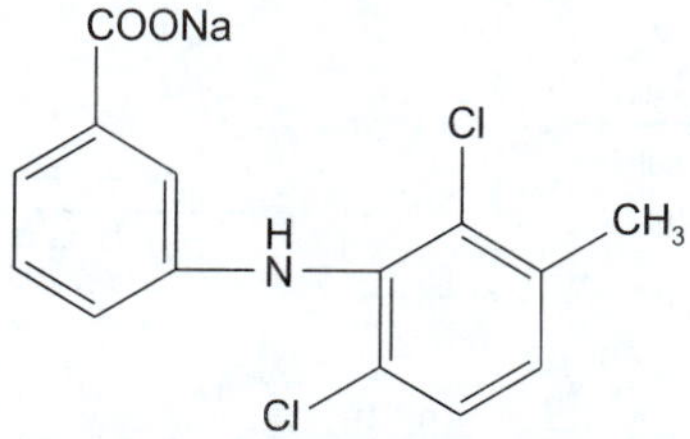

Sodium 3-(2,6-dichloro-3-methylphenylamino)benzoate

Synthesis: It is obtained by Ullmann condensation employing 2,6-dichloro-3-methyl aniline.

Aryl Alkanoic Acids

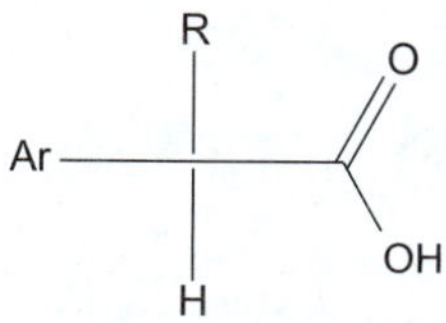

General structure

SAR of Aryl Alkanoic Acids

1. The centre of acidity is usually located one carbon atom adjacent to a flat surface represented by an aromatic or hetero-aromatic ring.
2. The distance between these centres is critical because increasing this distance to two or three carbons generally decreases activity.
3. All agents possess a centre of acidity, which can be represented by a carboxylic acid and hydroxamic acid, a sulphonamide or a terazole.
4. Substitution of a methyl group on the carbon atom separating the aromatic ring leads to enhancement of anti-inflammatory activity.

a. Indole acetic acid derivatives

i. Indomethacin (Indocin, Indocid)

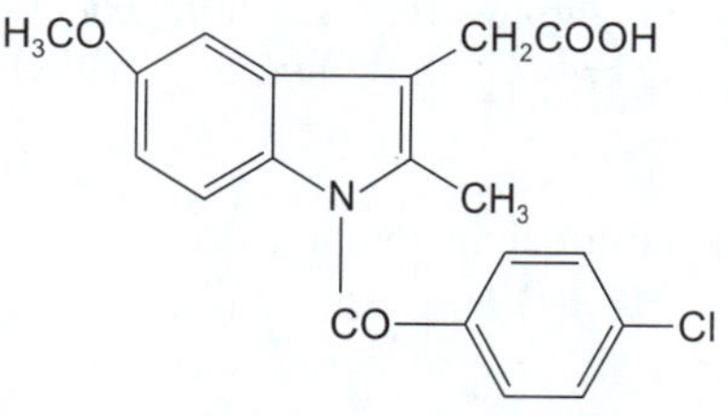

1-(*p*-Chlorobenzoyl)-5-methoxy-2 methylindole-3-acetic acid

Synthesis

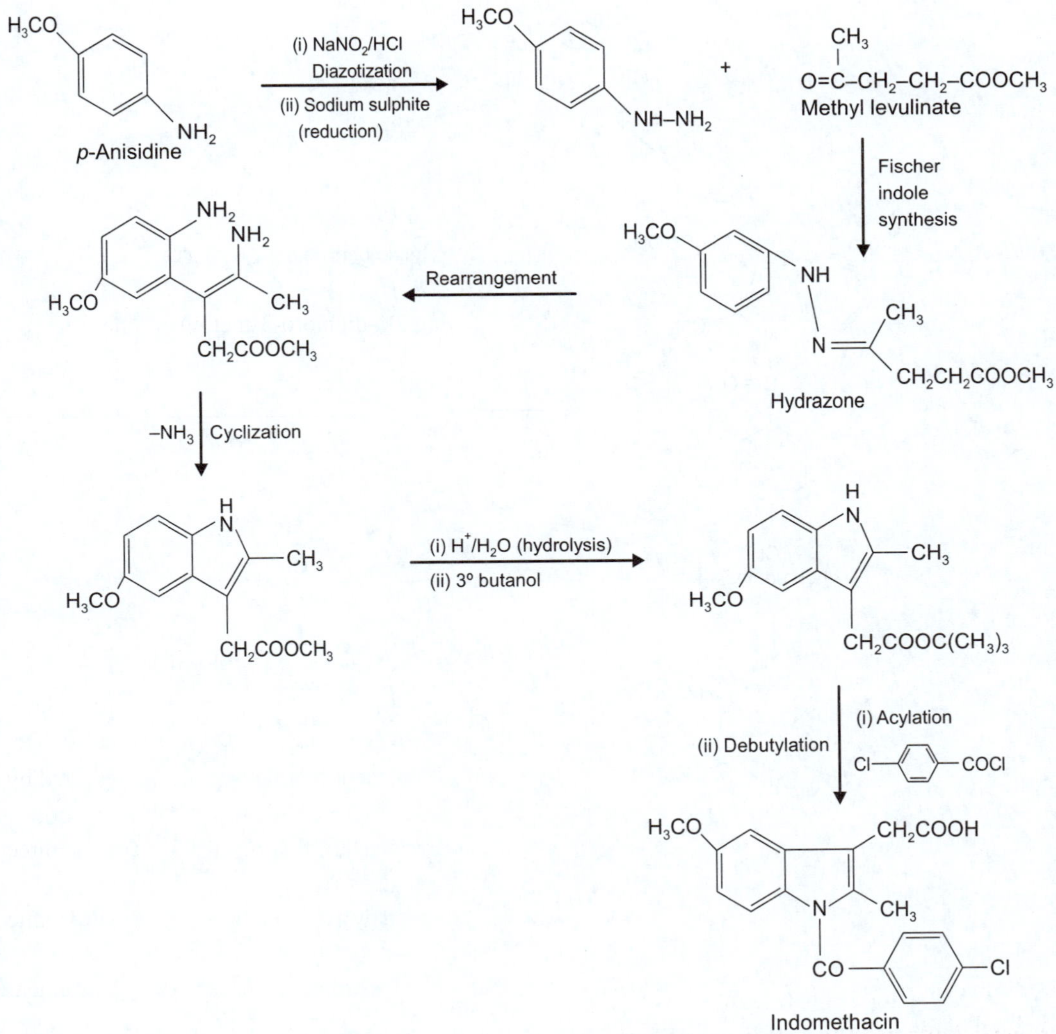

Metabolism: It is converted into inactive metabolites, that is, 50% of single dose is 5-*o*-demethylated and 10% conjugated with glucuronic acid. Non-hepatic enzymes hydrolyze indomethacin to N-deacetylated metabolite.

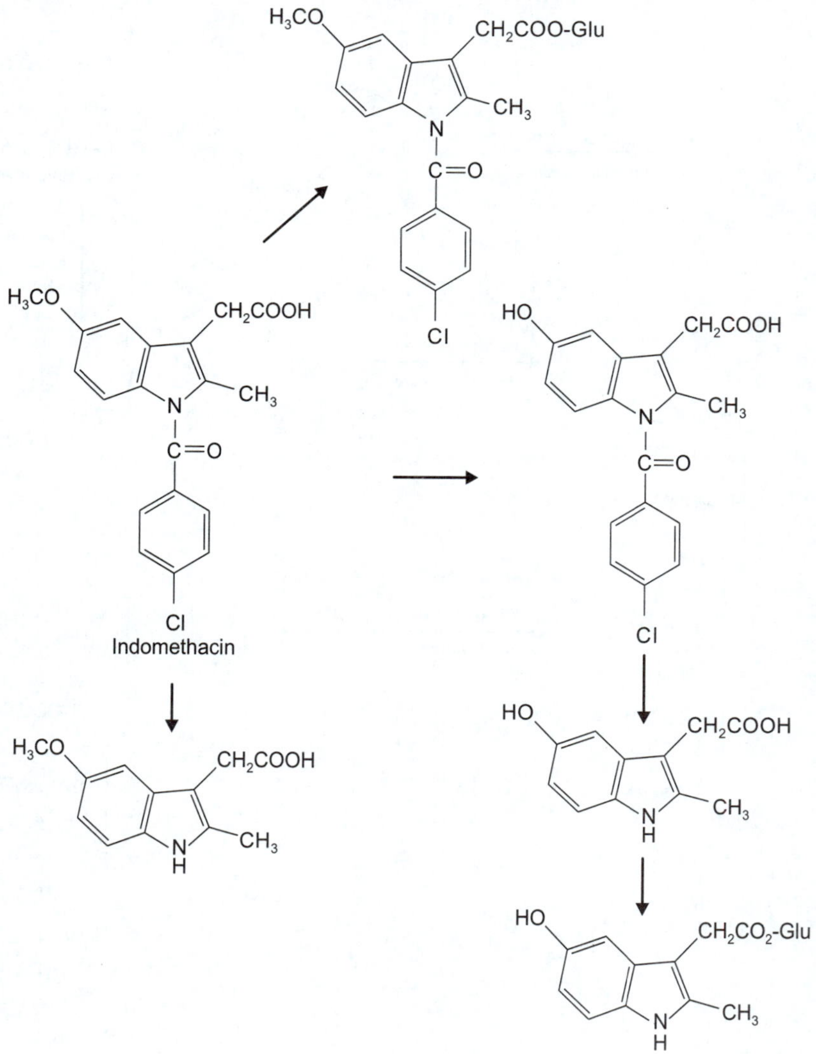

Properties and uses: It is a white or yellow crystalline powder, insoluble in water and sparingly soluble in alcohol. Indomethacin is more effective than aspirin. The most frequent side effects are gastric distress and headache. It also has been associated with peptic ulceration, blood disorders, and possible death (these side effects appear to be closely related and sometimes can be minimized by reducing the dose). It is not recommended for use in children because of possible interference with the resistance to infection. Used as anti-inflammatory and analgesic in rheumatic arthritis, spondylitis, and to lesser extent in gout.

Assay: Dissolve the sample in acetone and pass nitrogen for 15 min and titrate with 0.1 M sodium hydroxide using phenolphthalein as indicator.

Dose: In gout, usual adult dose orally is 100 mg initially, followed by 50 mg three times a day until pain is relieved. As an antirheumatic by oral route, the dose is 50 mg two or three times a day. And as an antipyretic, the dose is orally 25–50 mg three times a day.

Dosage forms: Indomethacin capsules IP, BP, indomethacin suppositories IP, BP.

b. Indeneacetic acid derivatives

i. Sulindac (Clinoril)

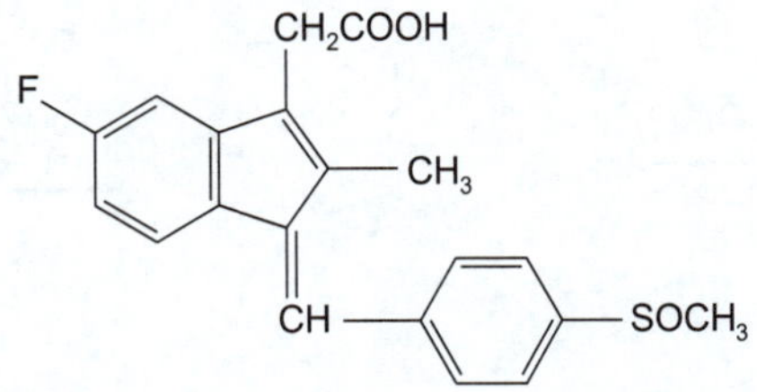

5-Fluoro-2-methyl-1[(4-methylsulphinyl) phenyl methylene] indene-3-acetic acid

Synthesis

Route I. From: 3-(4-Fluorophenyl)-2-methyl propanoic acid

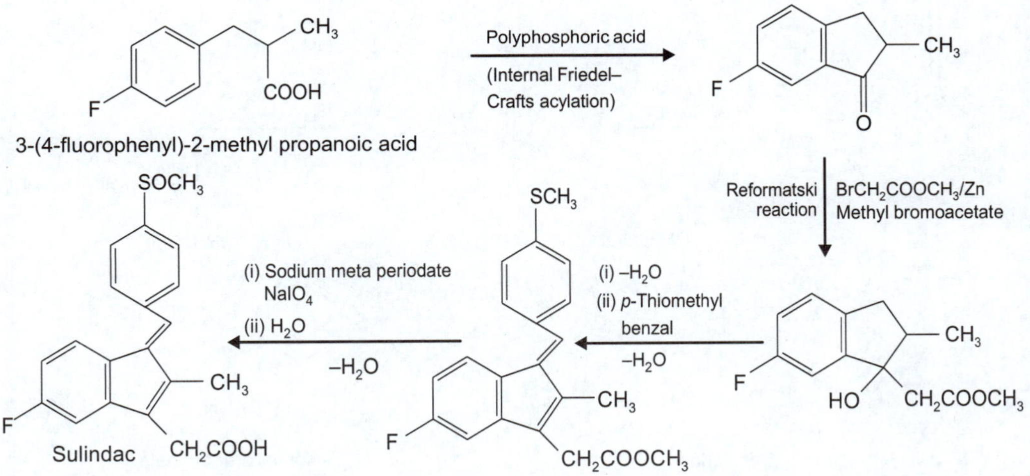

Synthesis

Route II. From: *p*-Fluorobenzaldehyde

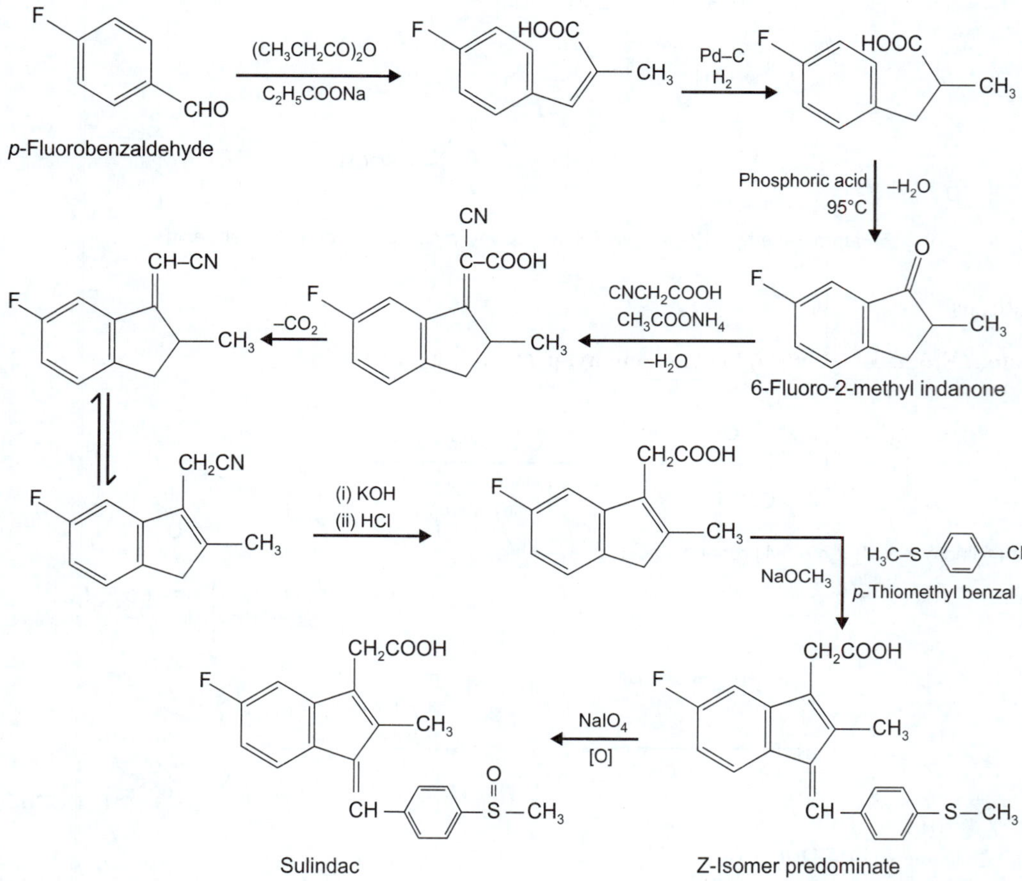

Metabolism: It is a prodrug to form active metabolites of sulphite. In addition to it, sulindac is oxidized to corresponding sulphone and other sulphone-glucuronide conjugates.

Properties and uses: Sulindac is a yellow crystalline powder, very slightly soluble in water, soluble in methylene chloride, and dilute solutions of alkali hydroxides, sparingly soluble in alcohol. The (Z)-isomer of sulindac showed much more potent anti-inflammatory activity than the corresponding (E)-isomer. The more polar and inactive sulphoxide is virtually the only form excreted. It has analgesic, antipyretic, and anti-inflammatory properties. It is usually employed in the treatment of rheumatic and muscular skeletal disorders, acute gouty arthritis, and osteoarthritis.

Assay: Dissolve the sample in methanol and titrate against 0.1 M sodium hydroxide. Determine the end point potentiometrically.

Dose: Usual adult oral dose is 150 mg twice a day with food.

Dosage forms: Sulindac tablets BP.

Metabolism of Sulindac

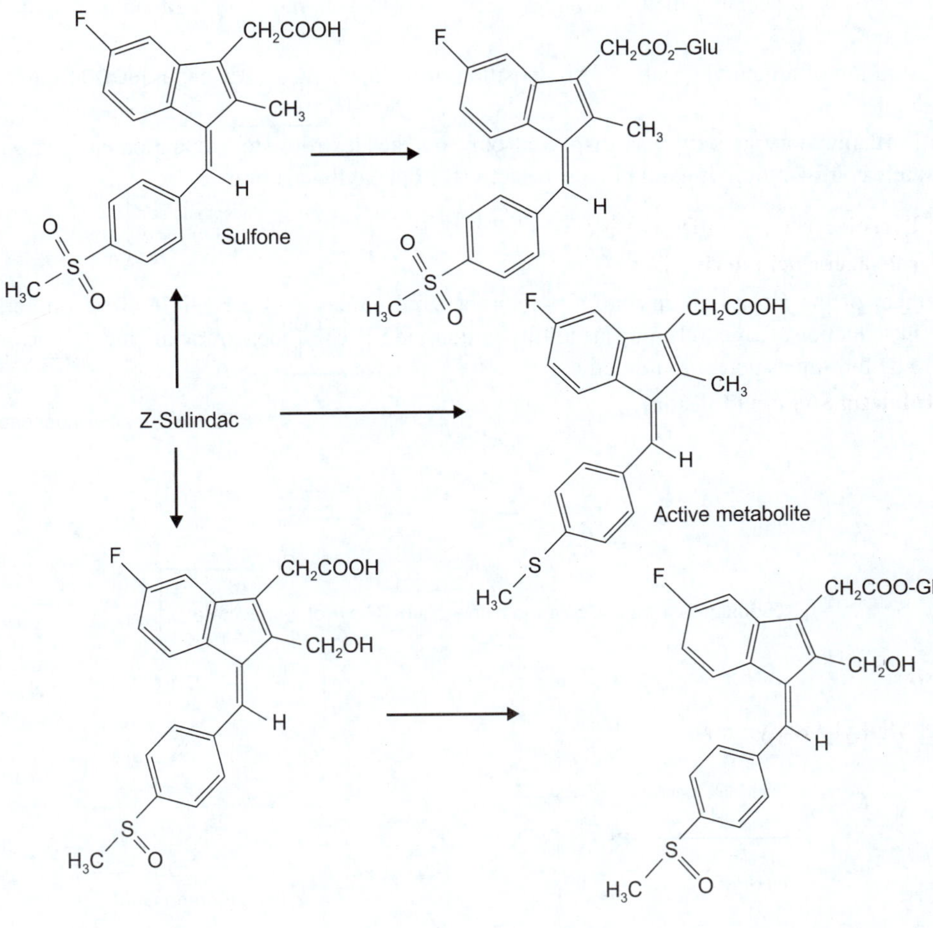

SAR of Indole Acetic Acid Derivatives

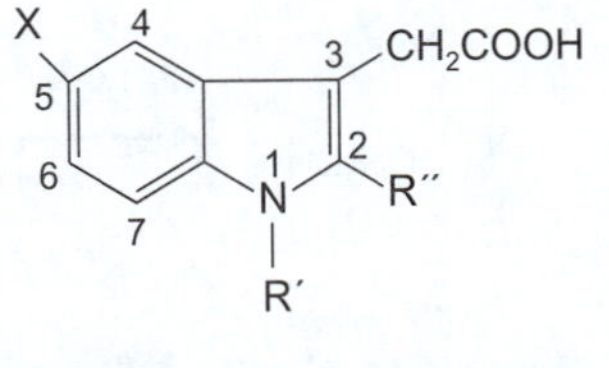

1. Placement of other acidic functionalities instead of the carboxyl group decreases activity and the amide derivatives are inactive.
2. Substituents of R′ useful for increasing anti-inflammatory activity are ranked as $C_6H_4CH_2$ > alkyl > H.
3. Acylation of the indole nitrogen with aryl/alkyl carboxylic acids results in the decrease of activity.
4. Presence of substituents on the N-benzoyl derivatives in the *p*-position with F, Cl, CF_3, or S-CH_3 groups provide greatest activity.
5. The order of potency of activity of x substituents is: 5-OCH_3 > N $(CH_3)_2$ > CH_3 > H.

6. The presence of indole ring nitrogen is not essential for activity because the corresponding 1-benzylidenylindene analogue (sulindac) is also active.
7. Alkyl groups, especially, methyl group at second position is much active than aryl substituted analogues.
8. Substitution of a methyl group at the α-position of the acetic acid side chain leads to equiactive analogues.
9. Anti-inflammatory activity was displayed only by the dextrorotatory enantiomer with similar absolute configuration; it has 25 times the activity of phenylbutazone.

SAR of Pyrrole Acetic Acid Derivative

c. Pyrrole acetic acid derivatives

Replacement of the *p*-tolyl group with a *p*-chlorobenzoyl moiety produced little effect on activity, whereas introduction of a methyl group in the 4th position and 5-*p*-chlorobenzoyl analogues (zomeapirac) proved to be four times potent as tolmetin.

i. Tolmetin Sodium (Tolectin)

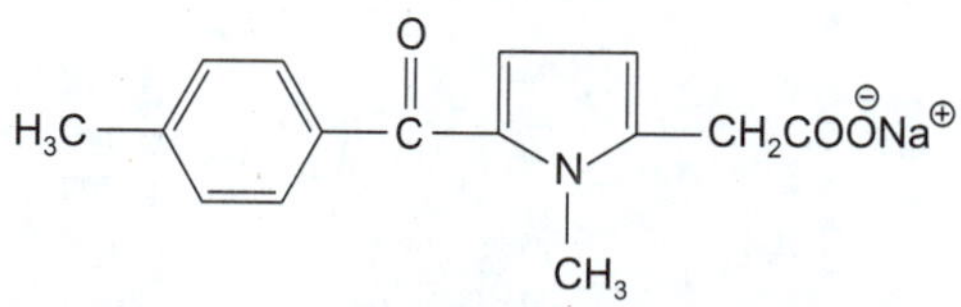

Sodium 2-(1-methyl-5-(4-methylbenzoyl)-1*H*-pyrrol-2-yl)acetate

Synthesis

From: 1-Methyl-1H-pyrrole

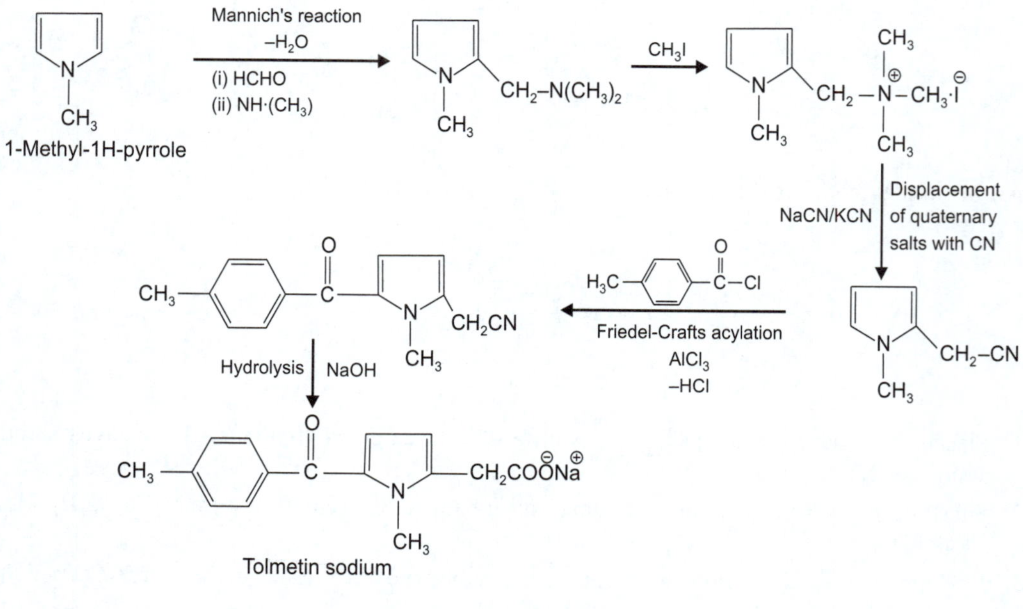

Metabolism: It is metabolized extensively first pass, involving hydroxylation of *p*-methyl group to primary alcohol, which is subsequently oxidized to dicarboxylic acid.

Properties and uses: It is a light yellow, crystalline powder, soluble in water, slightly soluble in alcohol. It has antipyretic, analgesic, and anti-inflammatory actions. It is employed in the treatment of rheumatic and musculoskeletal disorders. The drug is, however, comparable to indomethacin and aspirin in the control and management of disease activity.

Dose: Adult oral dose initially is 400 mg three times a day, subsequently adjusted as per patient's response.

ii. Zomepirac (Zomax)

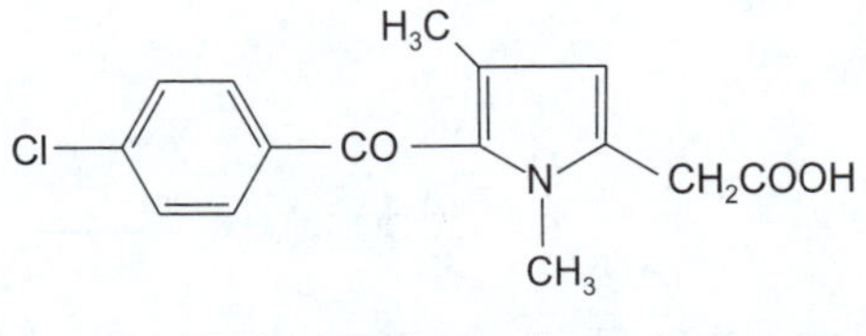

1,4-Dimethyl-5-(*p*-chlorobenzoyl) pyrrole-2-acetic acid

Synthesis

Route I. From: Chloroacetone

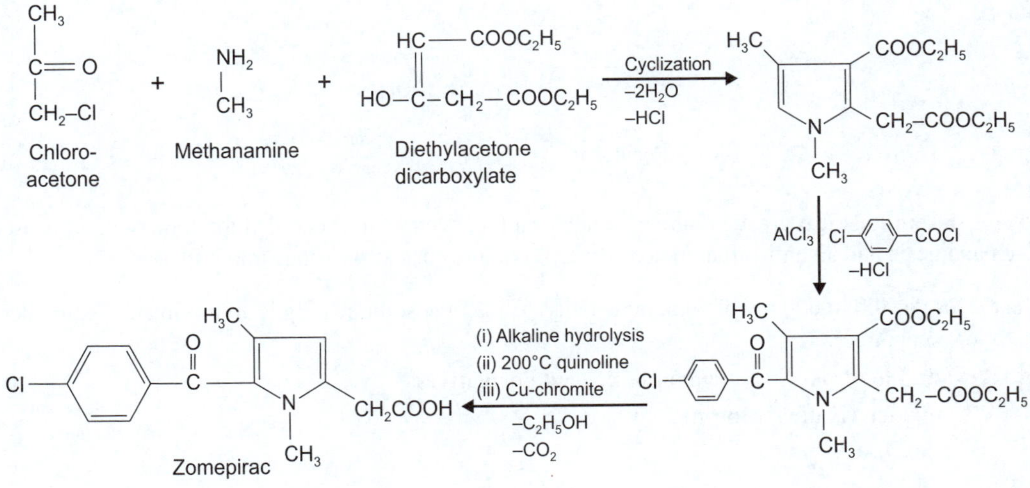

Route II. From: Enol of ethyl acetone dicarboxylate

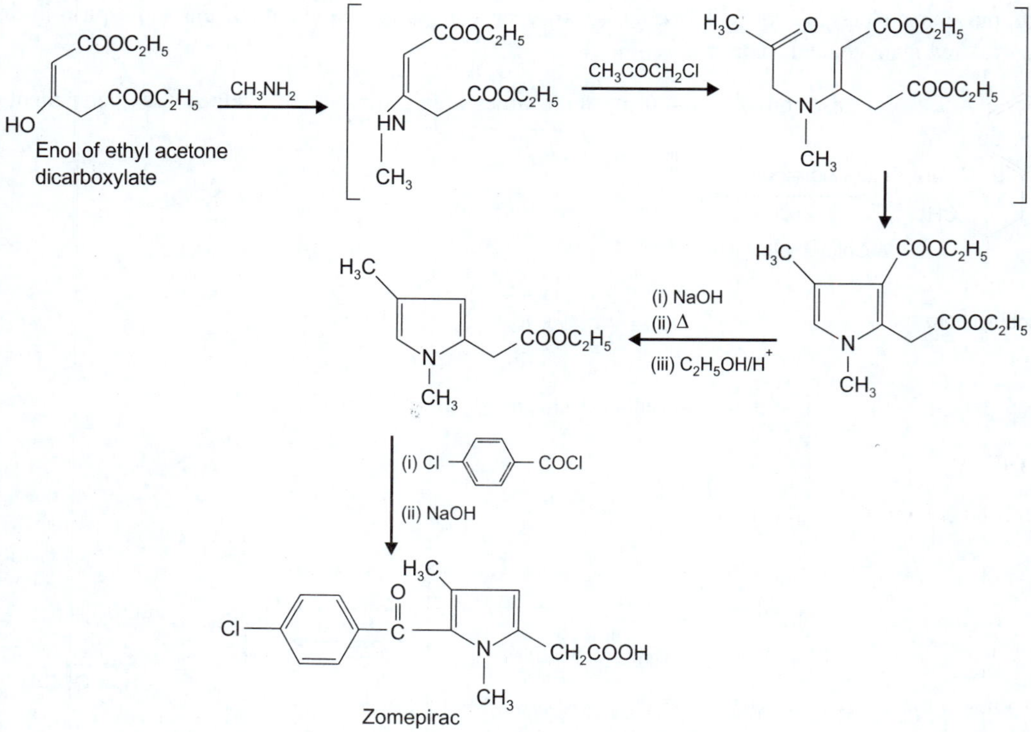

Properties and uses: A greater degree of analgesia for severe pain is claimed for zomepirac. It is used as an analgesic and an anti-inflammatory drug. It is four times as potent as tolmetin.

Dose: Dose is 400 to 600 mg of zomepirac daily (zomepirac sodium 1.2 g is approximately equivalent to 1 g of zomepirac).

d. Aryl and heteroaryl acetic/propionic acid derivatives

i. Ibuprofen (Brufen, Motrin)

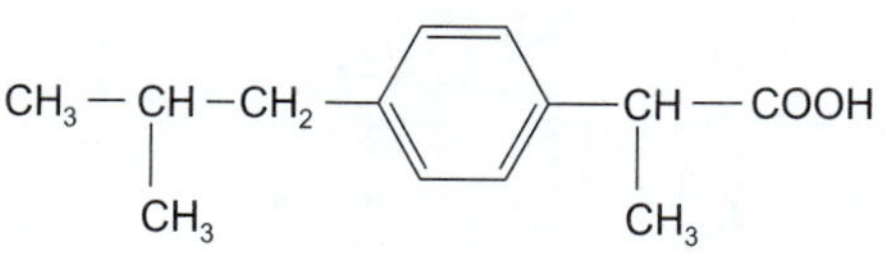

2-(4-Isobutyl phenyl) propionic acid

Synthesis

Route I. From: Isobutyl benzene

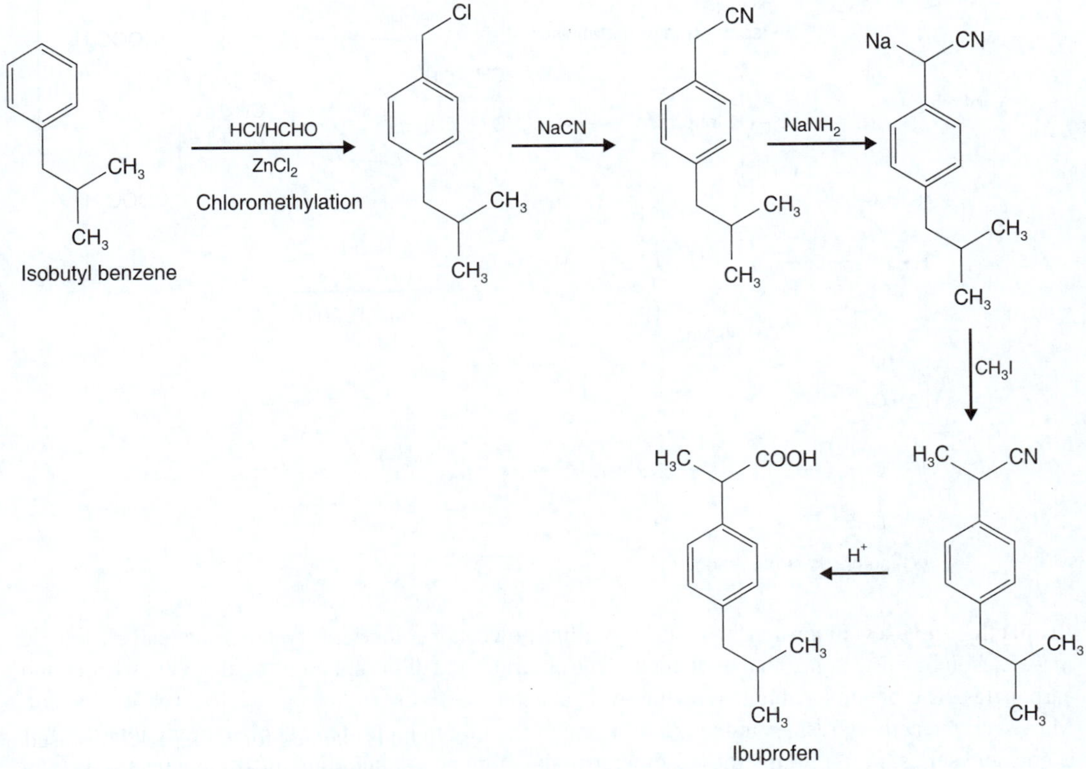

Route II. From: Isobutyl benzene

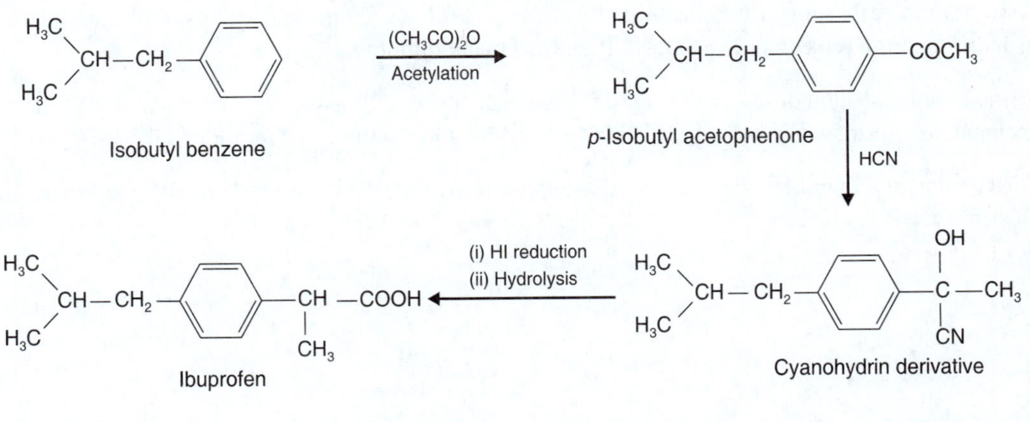

Metabolism: Oxidative metabolite of ibuprofen and unchanged drugs are excreted in urine. Oxidation involves ω, ω_1, and ω_2 oxidation of the *para*-isobutyl side chain, followed by alcohol oxidation, resulting from ω-oxidation to corresponding carboxylic acid.

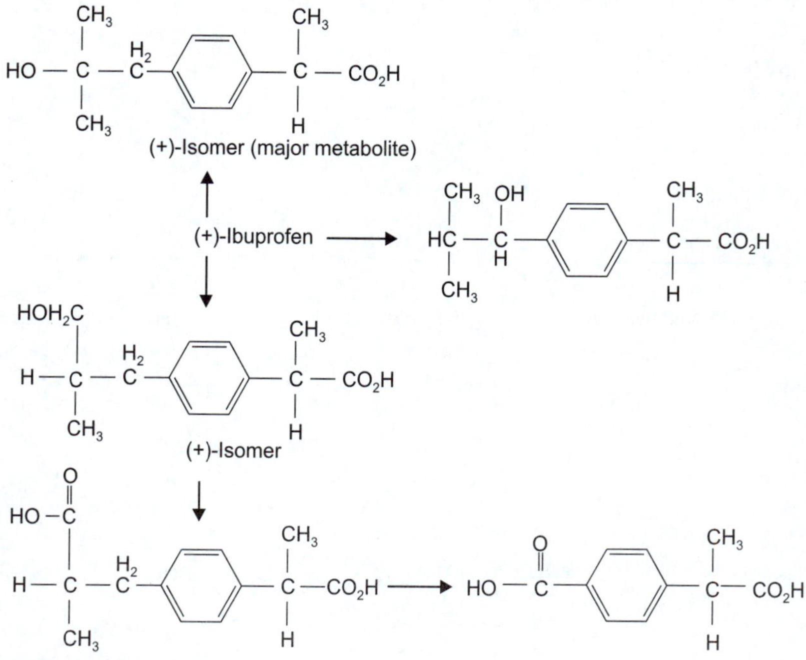

(+)-Isomer (major metabolite)

Properties and uses: Ibuprofen is a white crystalline powder or colourless crystals, practically insoluble in water, soluble in acetone, methanol, methylene chloride, and dilute solutions of alkali hydroxides and carbonates. The precursor ibufenac, which was abandoned owing to hepatotoxicity, was less potent. Moreover, the activity resides in the (s)-(+) isomer, not only in ibuprofen but also throughout the aryl acetic acid series. Furthermore, these isomers are the more potent inhibitors of PG synthetase. It is an anti-inflammatory drug that possesses antipyretic and analgesic action and is used for the treatment of rheumatoid arthritis and osteoarthritis.

Assay: Dissolve the sample in methanol and titrate against 0.1 M sodium hydroxide using phenolphthalein as indicator, until red colour is obtained. Perform a blank titration.

Dose: Usual oral adult dose as an analgesic (dysmenorrhoea) is 200–400 mg four to six times a day; in rheumatoid arthritis and osteoarthritis. The dose is 300–400 mg three or four times a day.

Dosage forms: Ibuprofen tablets IP, BP, ibuprofen cream BP, ibuprofen gel BP, ibuprofen oral suspension BP.

ii. Ibufenac

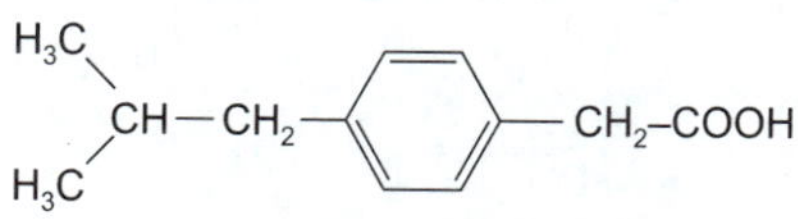

2-(*p*-Isobutyl-phenyl) acetic acid

Synthesis

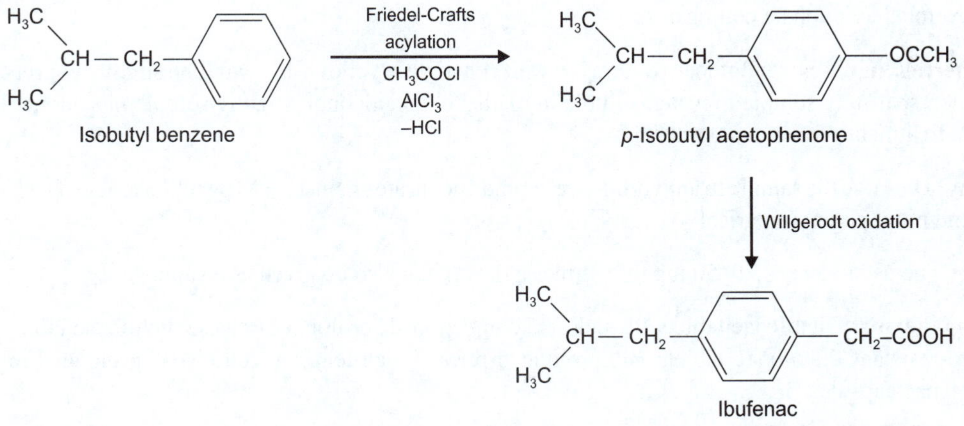

Properties and uses: It was formerly employed in the rheumatic conditions, but was found to cause hepatotoxicity. It has analgesic, antipyretic, and anti-inflammatory actions.

iii. Diclofenac (Voltaren, Voveran)

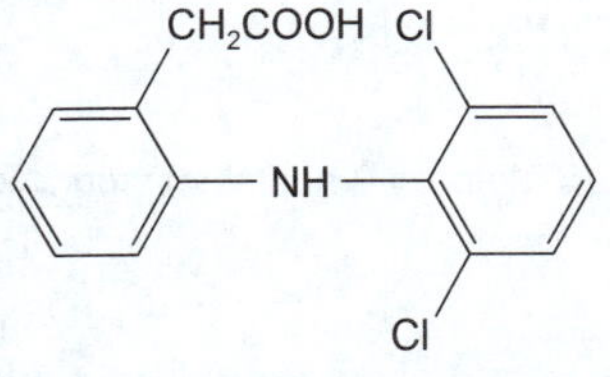

o-(2,6-Dichloro anilino) phenyl acetic acid

Synthesis

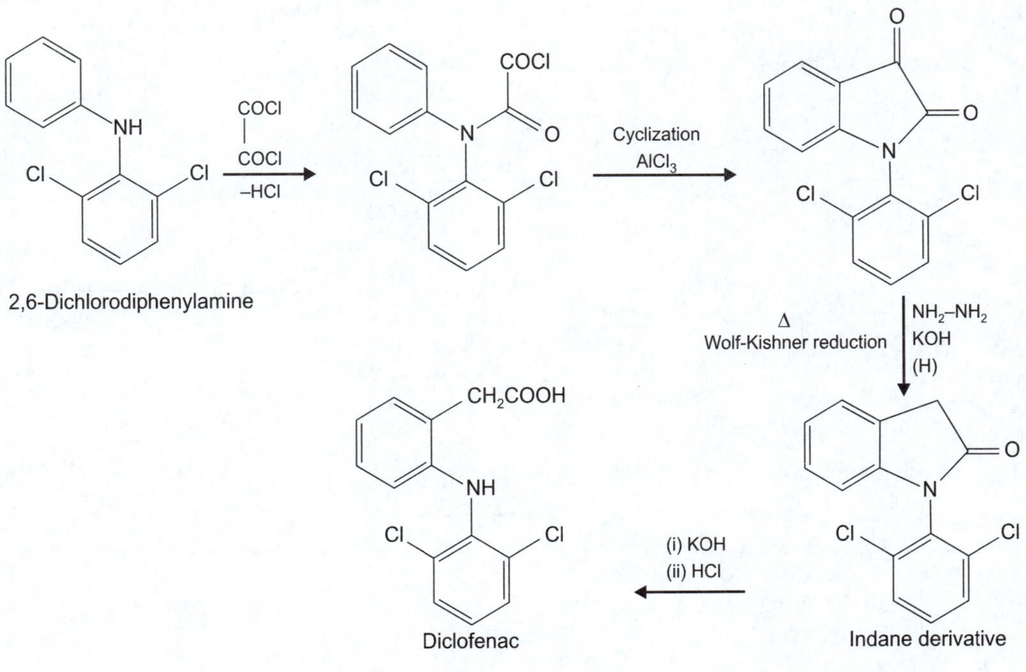

Metabolism: There are four major metabolites that are produced by aromatic hydroxylation, that is, 4-hydroxy derivative, 5-hydroxy, 3-hydroxy and 4,5-dihydroxy metabolites. Remaining metabolites are excreted as sulphate conjugates.

Properties and uses: Diclofenac sodium is a white or slightly yellowish crystalline slightly hygroscopic powder, sparingly soluble in water, soluble in methanol and alcohol, slightly soluble in acetone. Used in the treatment of rheumatic arthritis.

Assay: Dissolve the sample in anhydrous acetic acid and titrate against 0.1 M per chloric acid. Determine the end point potentiometrically.

Dose: The usual dose is 20–50 mg three times a day. It can also be given as a suppository.

Dosage forms: Diclofenac tablets IP, diclofenac injection IP, prolonged-release diclofenac tablets BP, gastro-resistant diclofenac tablets BP, prolonged-release diclofenac injection BP, prolonged-release diclofenac capsules BP.

iv. Naproxen (Naprosyn)

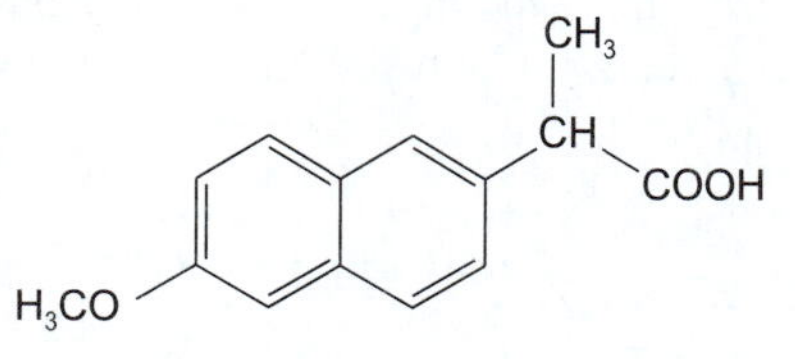

(±)2-(6-Methoxy-2-naphthyl) propionic acid

Synthesis

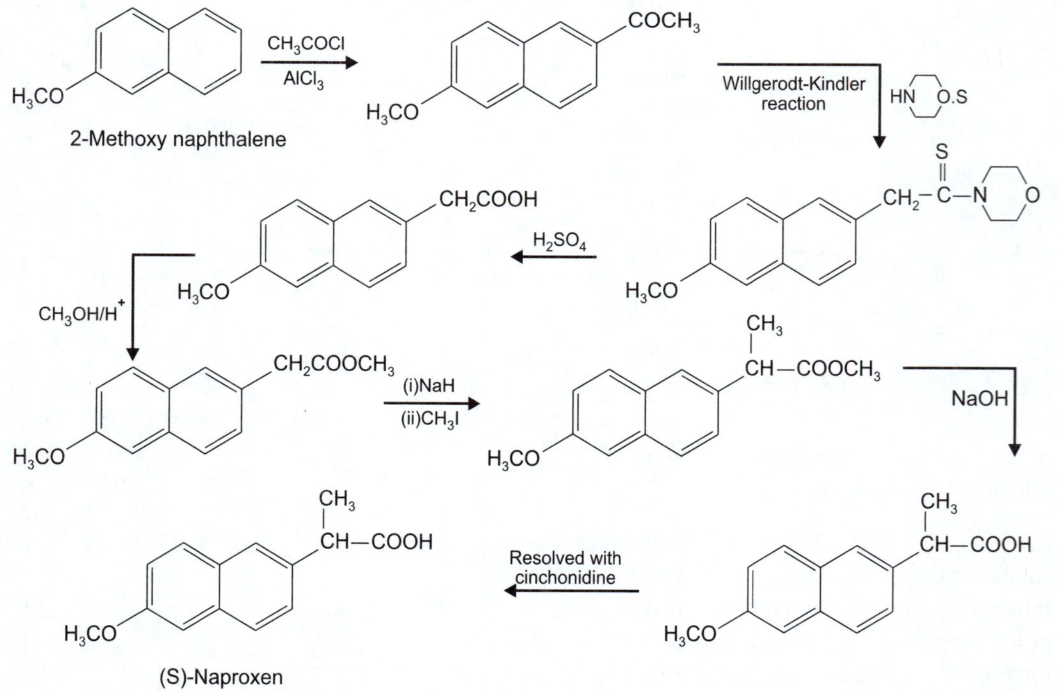

Metabolism: It is converted to 6-*o*-desmethyl metabolite and then to glucuronide conjugate.

Properties and uses: Naproxen is a white crystalline powder, practically insoluble in water, soluble in ethanol and in methanol. The drug is fairly comparable to aspirin both in the management and control of disease symptoms. Nevertheless, it has relatively lesser frequency and severity of nervous system together with milder GI-effects. It possesses analgesic, anti-inflammatory, and antipyretic actions, and it is used in the treatment of rheumatic arthritis, dysmenorrhea, and acute gout.

Assay: Dissolve the sample in a mixture of water and methanol (1:3) and titrate against 0.1 M sodium hydroxide, using 1 ml of phenolphthalein solution as indicator.

Dose: For adult in rheumatoid arthritis, 250–375 mg as initial dose two times a day; in acute gout, 750 mg as loading dose followed by 250 mg three times a day until relieved.

Dosage forms: Naproxen oral suspension BP, naproxen suppositories BP, naproxen tablets BP, gastro-resistant naproxen tablets BP.

v. **Fenoprofen** (Nalton)

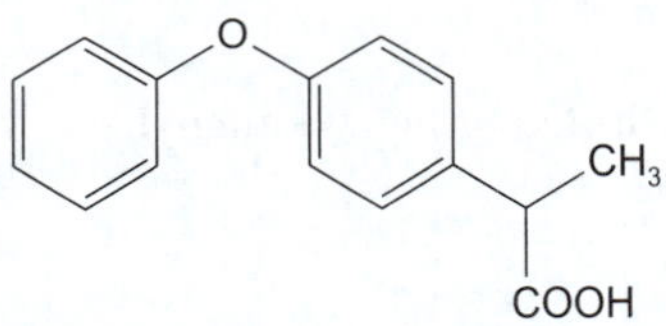

2-(3-Phenoxyphenyl) propionic acid

Synthesis

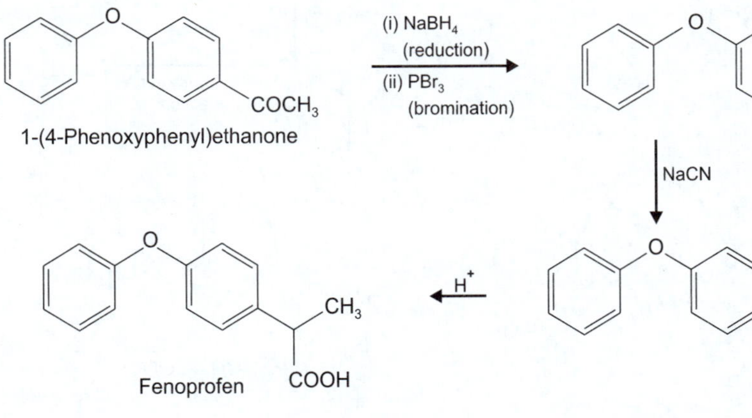

Metabolism: It is metabolized through glucuronide conjugation with a parent drug and CYP2C9 to 4-hydroxy metabolites.

Properties and uses: Fenoprofen calcium is a white crystalline powder, slightly soluble in water and soluble in ethanol. Fenoprofen calcium has anti-inflammatory (antiarthritic) and analgesic properties. It has been shown to inhibit PG synthetase. It is known to reduce joint-swelling, decrease the duration of morning stiffness, and relieve pain. It is also indicated for acute flares and exacerbations and in the long-term management of osteoarthritis and rheumatoid arhrtitis.

Assay: Dissolve the sample in anhydrous acetic acid and titrate against 0.1 M perchloric acid. Determine the end point potentiometrically. Perform a blank titration.

Dose: Dose is 50–100 mg twice daily with food.

Dosage forms: Fenoprofen tablets BP.

vi. **Ketoprofen** (Orudis)

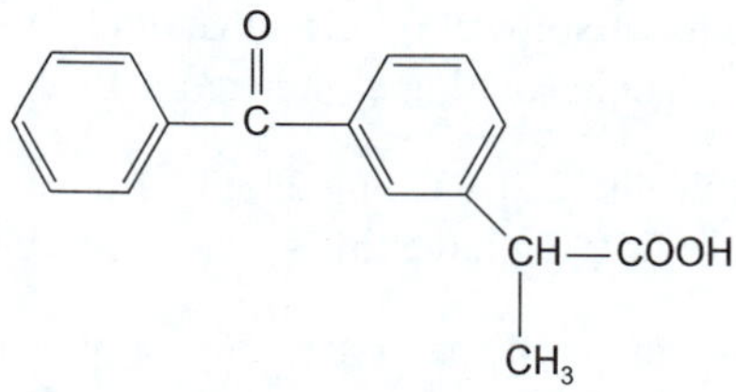

2-(3-Benzoyl phenyl) propionic acid

Synthesis

Route I. From: α-Methylene substituted *m*-benzyl phenyl acetic acid

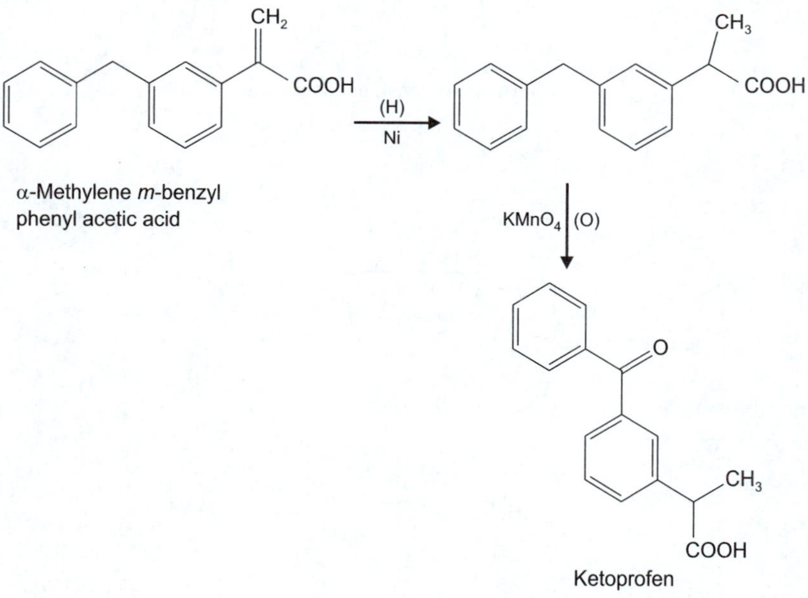

Route II. From: 2-(4-Aminophenyl)propanoic acid

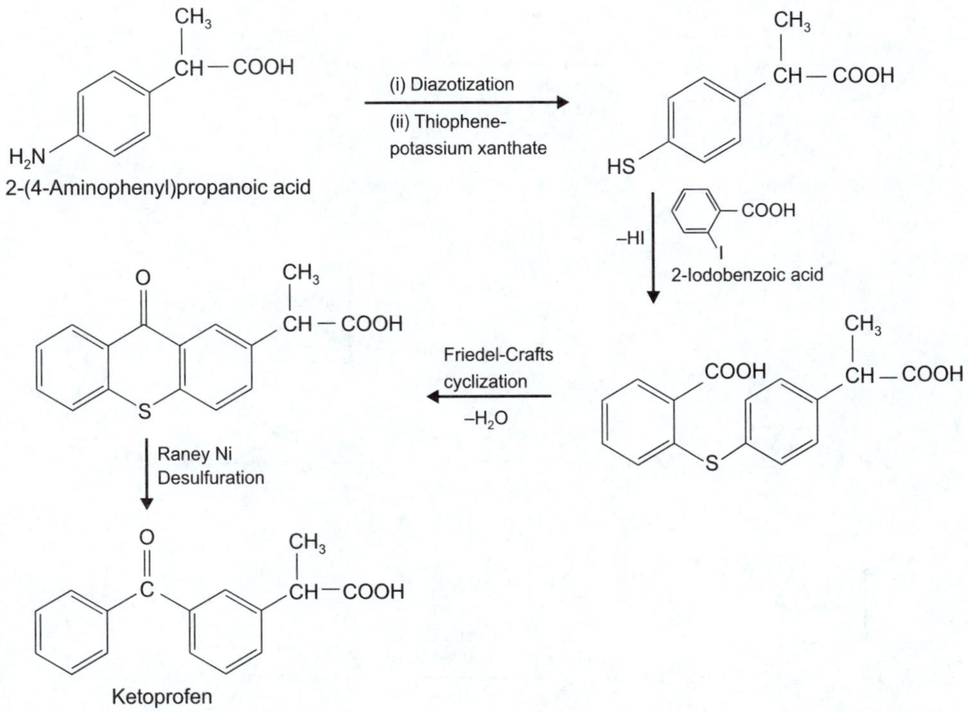

Metabolism: It is metabolized by glucuronidation of carboxylic acid, CYP3A4, and CYP2C9 hydroxylation of benzoyl ring and reduction of keto function.

Properties and uses: Ketoprofen is a white crystalline powder, practically insoluble in water, soluble in acetone, in ethanol, and in methylene chloride. It is closely related to fenoprofen in structure, properties, and indications and has a low incidence of side effects and has been approved for counter sale. It is used in the treatment of rheumatoid arthritis and osteoarthritis.

Assay: Dissolve the sample in ethanol and dilute with water and titrate against 0.1 M sodium hydroxide. Determine the end point potentiometrically.

Dose: Usual adult oral dose for rheumatoid arthritis is 600 mg four times daily; for osteoarthritis the dose is 300–600 mg four times a day.

Dosage forms: Ketoprofen capsules IP, BP, ketoprofen gel BP.

vii. **Flurbiprofen** (Ansaid)

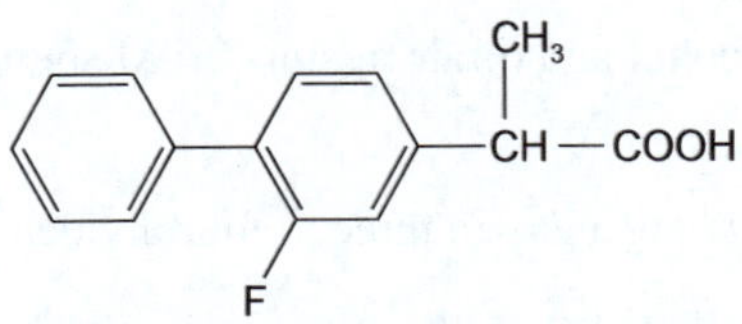

(±)-2-(2-Fluoro-4-biphenyl)-propionic acid

Synthesis

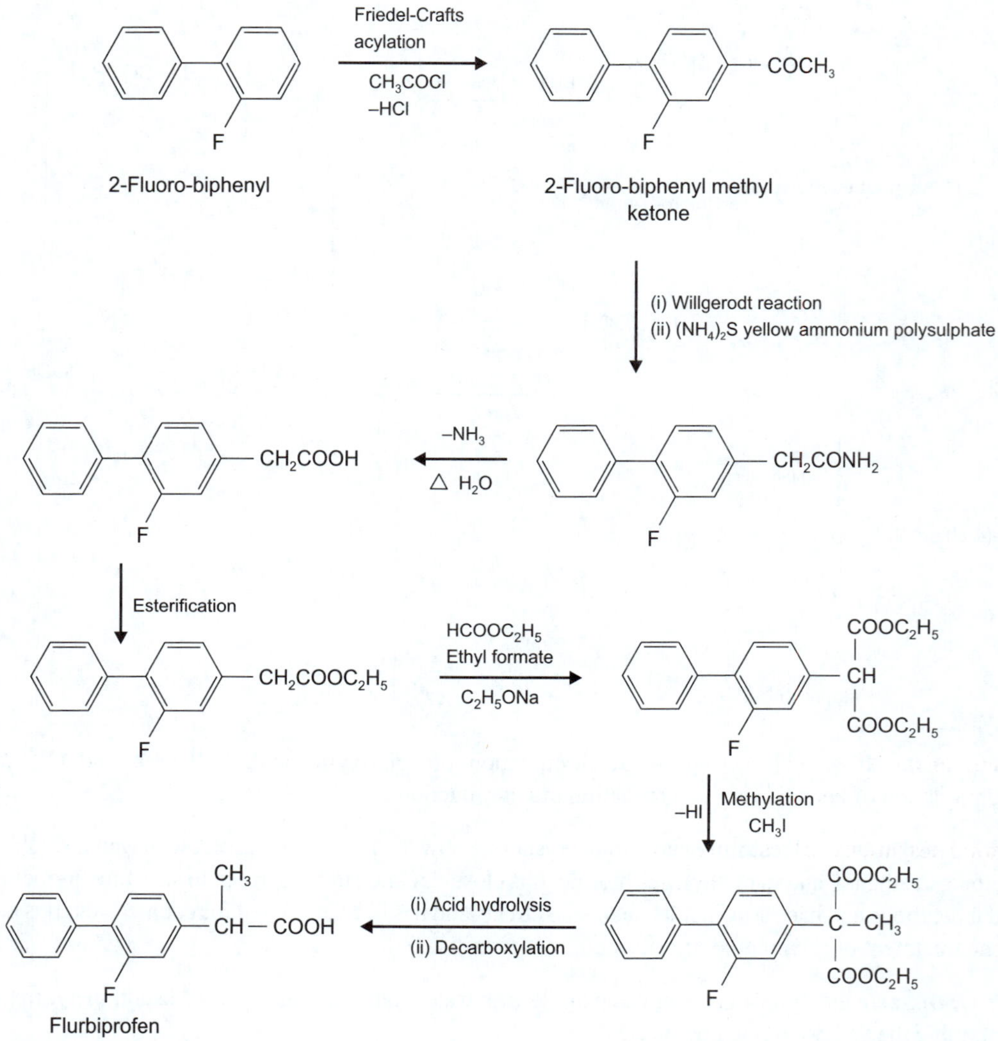

Properties and uses: Flurbiprofen is a white crystalline powder, practically insoluble in water, soluble in alcohol, in methylene chloride, and aqueous solutions of alkali hydroxides and carbonates. The drug is structurally and pharmacologically related to fenoprofen, ibuprofen, and ketoprofen. Another hydrotropic acid analogue that is used in the acute or long-term management of rheumatoid arthritis and osteoarthritis, it posses analgesic, anti-inflammatory, and antipyretic activities.

Assay: Dissolve the sample in alcohol and titrate against 0.1 M sodium hydroxide. Determine the end point potentiometrically.

Dose: Usual adult dose is 150–200 mg a day in three to four divided doses.

Dosage forms: Flurbiprofen tablets IP, BP, flurbiprofen suppositories BP.

viii. Caprofen

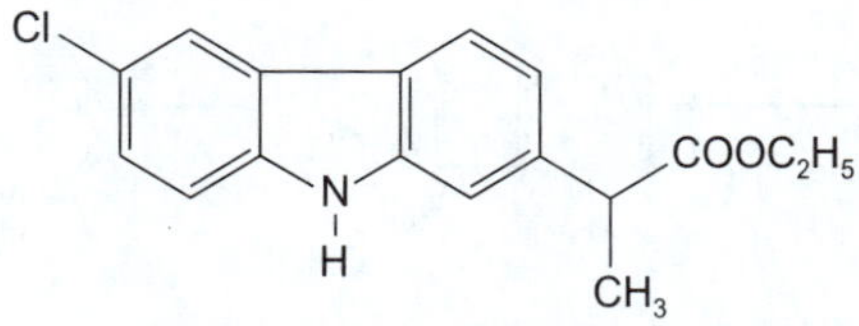

6-Chloro-α-methylcarbazole-2-acetic acid ethyl ester

Synthesis

From: 1-(4-chlorophenyl) hydrazine

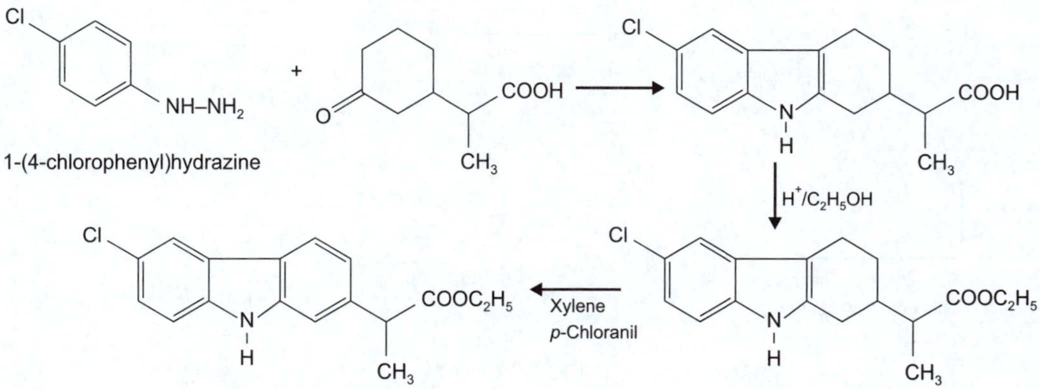

Uses: Used as an analgesic and anti-inflammatory agent.

ix. Ketorolac (Acular, Ketodrops, Ketlur)

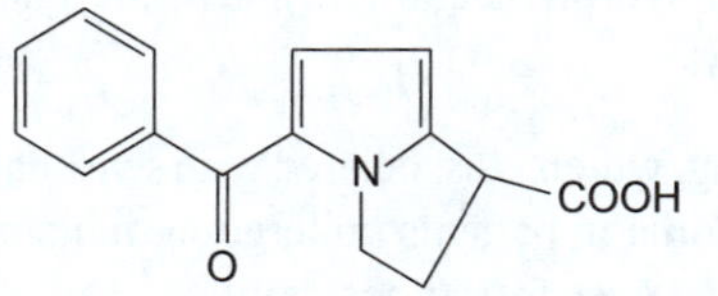

5-Benzoyl-2,3-dihydro-1H-pyrrolizine-1-carboxylic acid

Synthesis

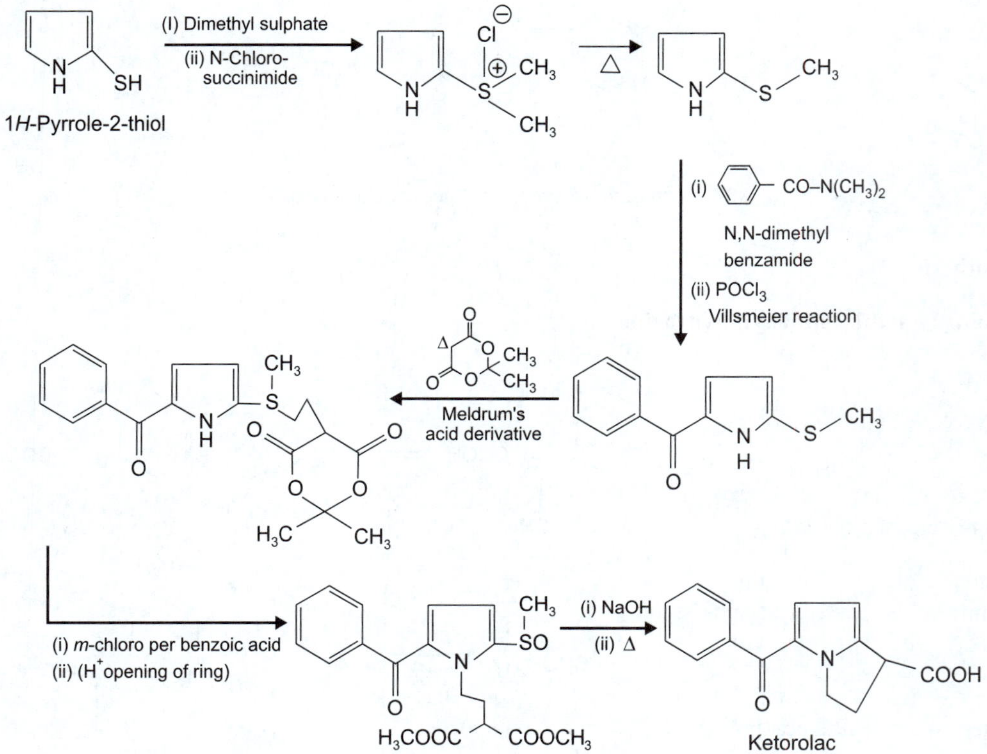

Properties and uses: Ketorolac is a white crystalline powder, soluble in water and in methanol, slightly soluble in ethanol, practically insoluble in methylene chloride. Ketorolac is a potent analgesic used for the treatment of moderately severe and acute pain.

Assay: Dissolve the sample in anhydrous acetic acid and titrate against 0.1 M per chloric acid. Determine the end point potentiometrically.

Dose: The dose for ocular itching, which is associated with seasonal allergic conjunctivitis, for reduction of ocular pain, and for photophobia in patients undergoing incisional refractive sugery, instil one drop of 0.5% solution into the affected eyes four times daily.

x. Etodolac

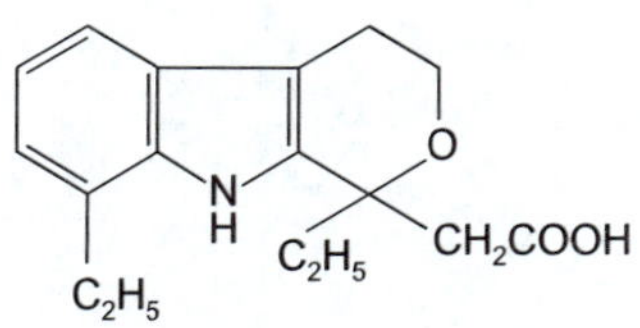

Synthesis

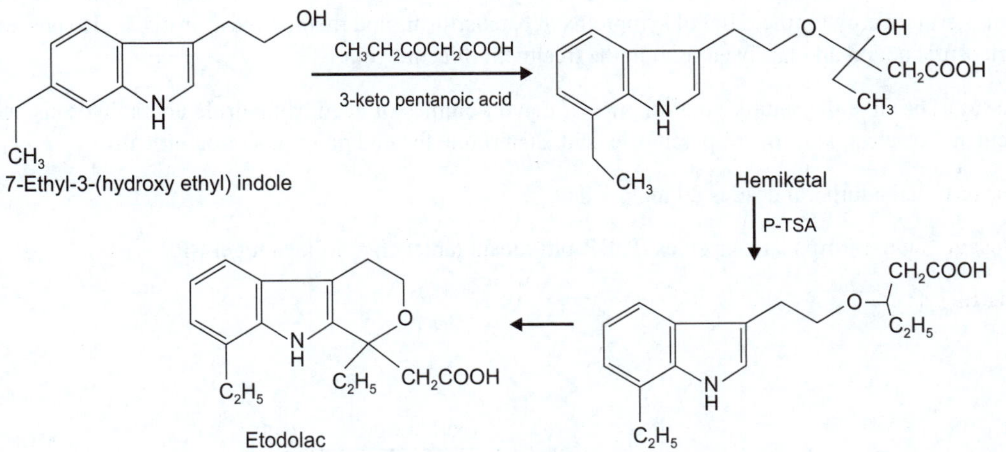

Metabolism: It is metabolized to 3-hydroxylated metabolite and to glucuronide conjugates.

Properties and uses: Etodolac is a white crystalline powder, practically insoluble in water, soluble in acetone and in ethanol. It has anti-inflammatory activity and inhibits cyclooxygenase. It is used in the treatment of osteoarthritis and rheumatoid arthritis. Gastrointestinal irritation and ulceration is less with this drug than with other drugs.

Assay: Dissolve the sample in methanol and titrate against 0.1 M tetrabutylammonium hydroxide. Determine the end point potentiometrically. Perform a blank titration.

Dosage forms: Etodolac capsules BP, etodolac tablets BP.

Oxicams

The term oxicam described the relatively new enolic acid class of 4-hydroxyl-1,2-benzothiazine carboxamide with anti-inflammatory and analgesic properties.

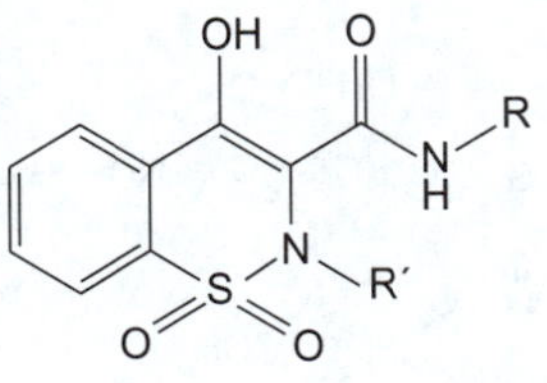

i. Piroxicam

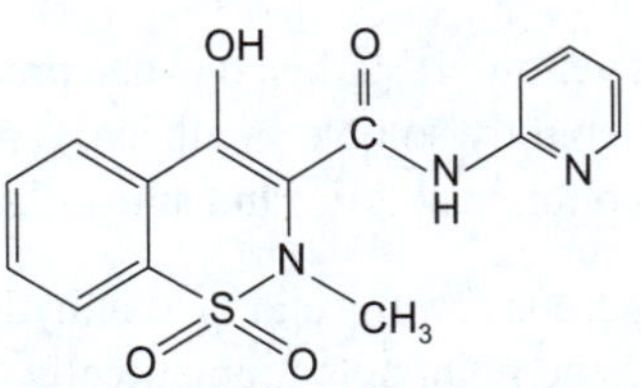

4-Hydroxy-2-methyl-N-2 pyridinyl-1,2 benzothiazine-3 carboxamide-1,1-dioxide

Properties and uses: Piroxicam is a white or slightly yellow crystalline powder, practically insoluble in water, soluble in methylene chloride, and slightly soluble in ethanol. It is employed for acute and long-term therapy for the relief of symptoms of osteoarthritis and rheumatoid arthritis. It also possesses uricosuric action and has been used in the treatment of acute gout.

Assay: Dissolve the sample in a mixture of equal volumes of acetic anhydride and anhydrous acetic acid and titrate against 0.1 M perchloric acid. Determine the end point potentiometrically.

Dose: Usual adult oral dose is 20 mg per day.

Dosage forms: Piroxicam capsules IP, BP, piroxicam tablets IP, piroxicam gel BP.

Synthesis

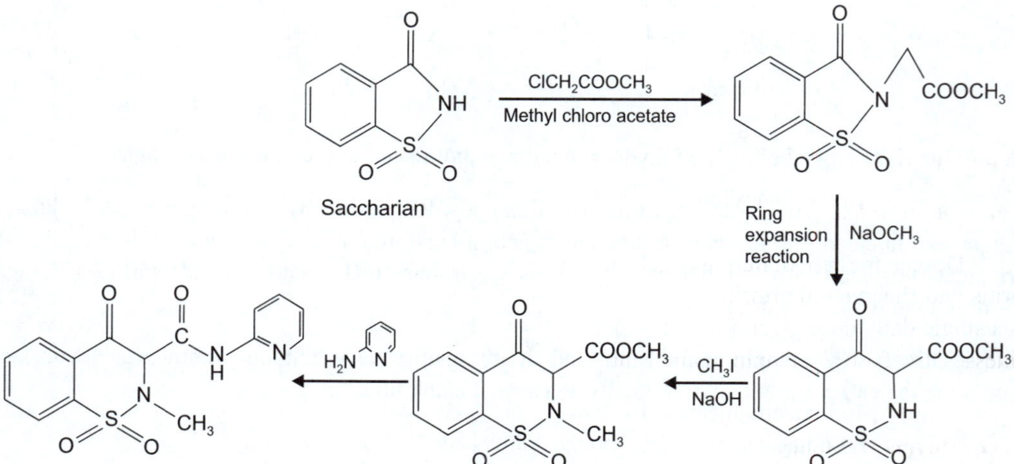

The two more closely related analogues are obtained by varying the heterocyclic amine used in the last step. 2-Amino thiazole thus leads to sudoxicam, while 3-amino-5-methylisoxazole affords isoxicam.

ii. Tenoxicam (Tobitil)

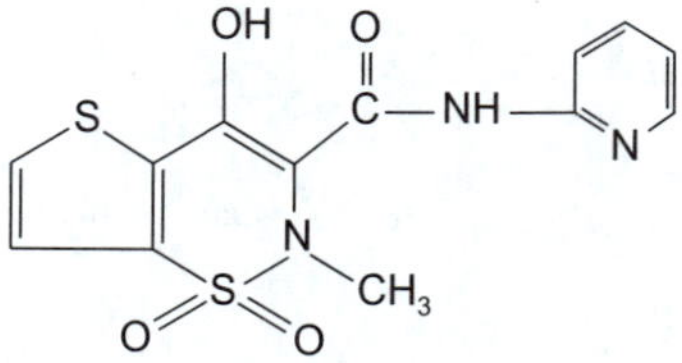

4-hydroxy-2-methyl-1,1-dioxo-pyridin-2-yl thieno [2,3-e] thiazine-3-carboxamide

Properties and uses: Tenoxicam is a yellow crystalline powder, practically insoluble in water, sparingly soluble in methylene chloride, very slightly soluble in ethanol, and soluble in solutions of acids and alkalis. Used as cyclooxygenase inhibitor, analgesic, and anti-inflammatory agent.

Assay: Dissolve the sample in anhydrous formic acid, add anhydrous acetic acid, and titrate against 0.1 M perchloric acid. Determine the end point potentiometrically.

Synthesis

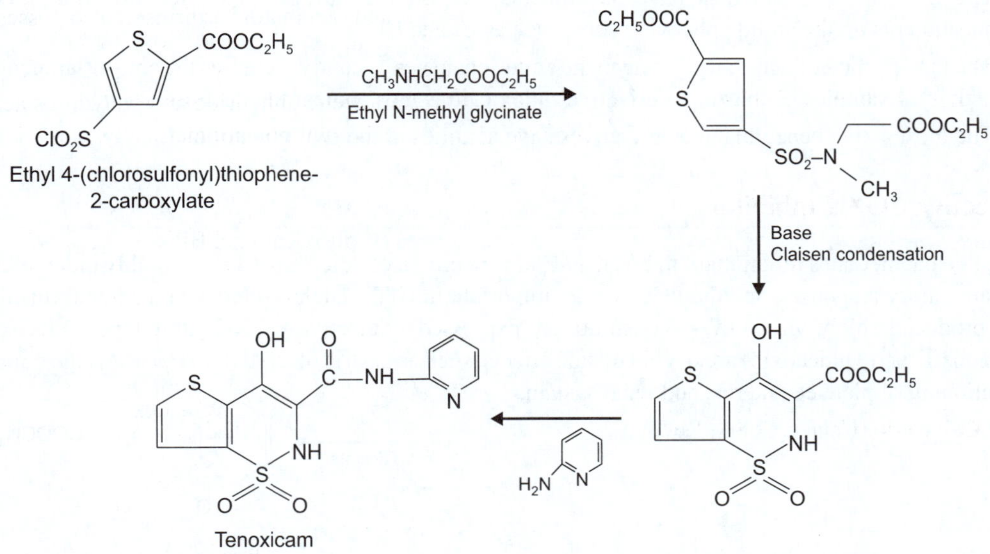

Dose: Dose in the case of musculoskeletal and joint disorders—such as ankylosing spondylitis, osteoarthritis and rheumatoid arthritis—and short-term management of soft tissue injury for adult is 20 mg as a single daily dose given for 7 days in acute cases. For musculoskeletal disorders and other related illnesses, the dose is a maximum of 4 mg a day up to 14 days in severe cases (short-term use).

Dosage forms: Tenoxicam injection BP, tenoxicam tablets BP.

iii. Meloxicam (Mobic)

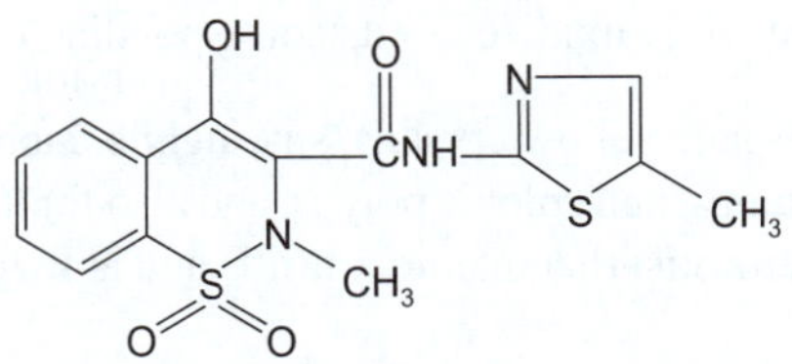

4-Hydroxy-2-methyl-N-(5-methyl-2-thiazolyl)-2*H*-1,2-benzothiazine-3-carboxamide-1,1-dioxide

Metabolism: This category of drugs undergoes aromatic hydroxylation at several positions of aromatic benzothiazine ring. Sudoxicam undergoes primary hydroxylation of thiazole ring, followed by ring-opening, whereas isoxicam undergoes primary cleavage reaction of benzothiazine ring.

Properties and uses: Meloxicam is a pale yellow powder, practically insoluble in water, slightly soluble in acetone, soluble in dimethylformamide, very slightly soluble in ethanol and in methanol. Used as cyclooxygenase inhibitor, analgesic, and anti-inflammatory.

Assay: Dissolve the sample in a mixture of anhydrous acetic acid and anhydrous formic acid (10:1) and titrate against 0.1 M perchloric acid. Determine the end point potentiometrically.

Dosage forms: Meloxicam tablets BP.

SAR of Oxicams

- The most active analogues have substituents CH_3 on the nitrogen and electron withdrawing substituents on the anilide phenyl groups, such as Cl and CF_3.
- The introduction of heterocyclic ring in the amide chain significantly increases the anti-inflammatory activity. Example—2-thiazolyl derivative sudoxicam is more potent than indomethacin.
- The most active benzothiazine derivatives have acidities in the pK_a range of 6–8.

Selective COX-2 Inhibitor

The PG that mediates inflammation, fever, and pain are produced solely via COX-2 (highly inducible by inflammatory response), and the PGs that are important in GIT, platelets, uterus, and adrenal function are produced solely via COX-1 (constitutively expressed). Selective COX-2 inhibitors (Celecoxib, Rofecoxib, and Valdecoxib) are devoid of side effects, such as gastric ulcer. It does not affect the normal functioning of platelets, uterus, and renal system.

i. **Celecoxib** (Celact, Cobix, Revibra)

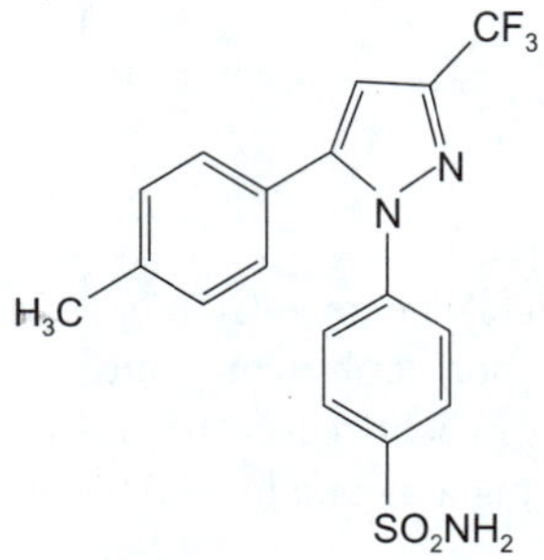

4-[5-(4-Methyl phenyl)-3-(trifluoro)-1*H*-pyrazo-lyl]-benzene sulphonamide

Metabolism: Metabolism of celecoxib occurs in the liver, involves hydroxylation of 4-methyl group to primary alcohol, which is subsequently oxidized to its corresponding carboxylic acid.

Properties and uses: It exists as pale yellow crystals, sparingly soluble in water. Celecoxib is used to treat arthritis, pain, menstrual cramps, and colonic polyps, and also for the relief of pain, fever, swelling, and tenderness caused by osteoarthritis, rheumatoid arthritis and ankylosing spondylitis.

Synthesis

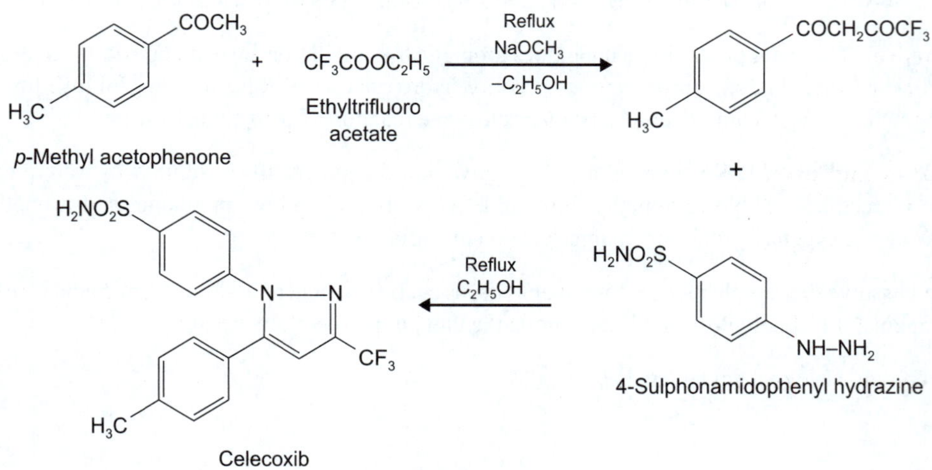

Dose: For osteoarthritis, the adult dose is 200 mg as a single dose or in two divided doses that may be increased to 200 mg two times a day, if necessary. For rheumatoid arthritis, the adult dose is 100–200 mg two times a day. For elderly people the dose is 100 mg two times a day. For dysmenorrhoea, initially the dose is 400 mg by 200 mg, if necessary, on the 1st day and maintenance dosage is 200 mg two times a day.

ii. **Rofecoxib** (Vioxx)

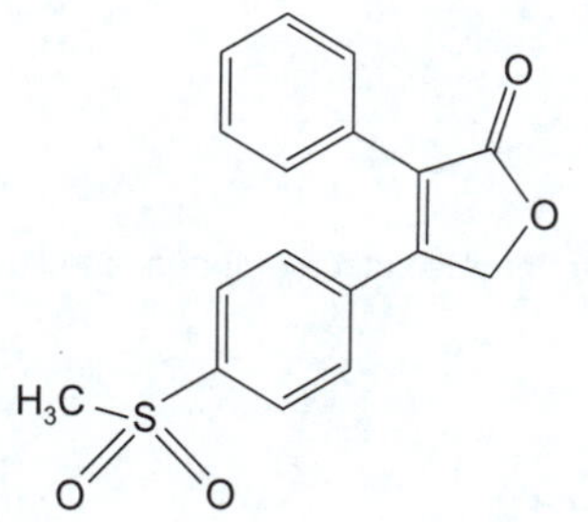

4-[4-(Methyl sulphinyl) phenyl]-3-phenyl-2-furanone

Synthesis

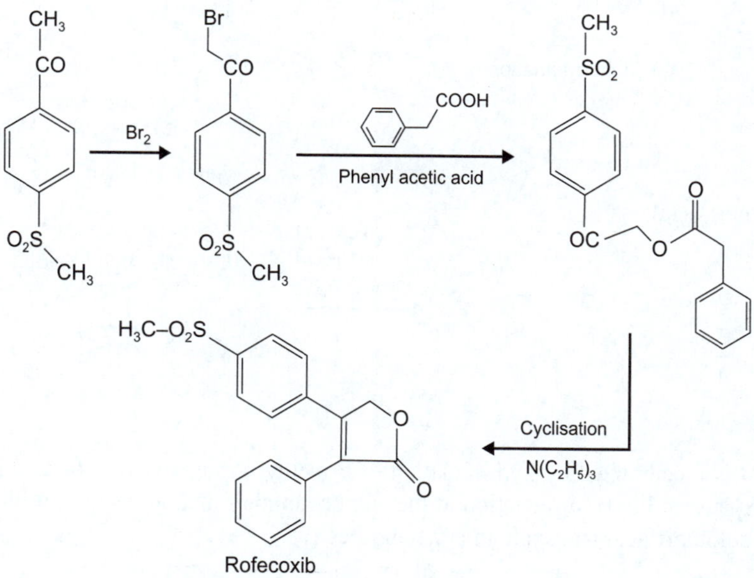

Metabolism: The metabolic route of rofecoxib appears to follow the reduction of dihydrofuranone ring system by cystolic enzyme to *cis* and *trans* hydroxy derivatives.

Properties and uses: It exists as white to light yellow powder, sparingly soluble in acetone, methanol, very slightly soluble in 1-octanol. It is a COX-2 inhibitor with greater potency and a longer half-life than celecoxib. Rofecoxib is used to relieve the pain, tenderness, inflammation (swelling), and stiffness caused by arthritis, and to treat painful menstrual periods and pain from other causes.

iii. Valdecoxib (Bextra)

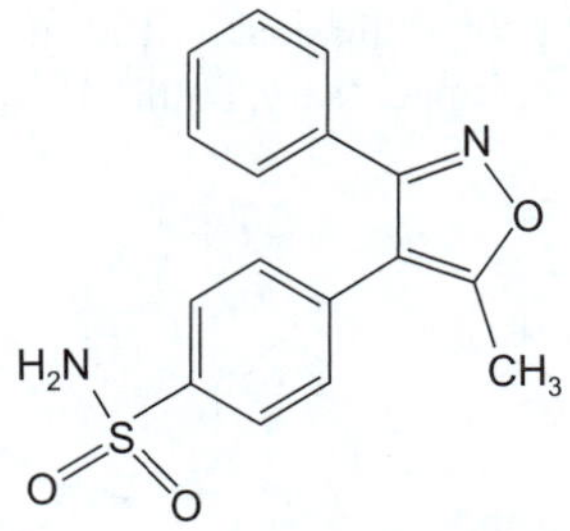

4-[5-Methyl-3-phenyl isoxazol-4-yl]-benzene sulphonamide

Synthesis

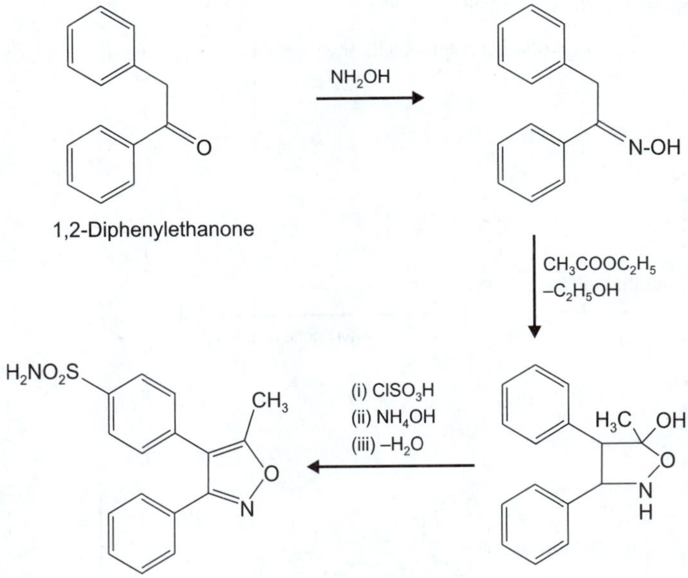

Metabolism: It is metabolized by hydroxylation of 5-methyl group and it is further metabolized to inactive carboxylate and *N*-Hydroxylation at the sulphonamide function, leading to the formation of corresponding sulphinic acid and suphomic metabolites.

Properties and uses: It is soluble in most organic solvents, insoluble in water. It is a NSAID drug that exhibits anti-inflammatory, analgesic, and antipyretic activities.

Dose: For dysmenorrhoea, the dose is 20 mg twice a day. For osteoarthritis and rheumatoid arthritis, the dose is 10 mg once daily.

Miscellaneous

i. Nabumetone (Nabuflam, Niltis)

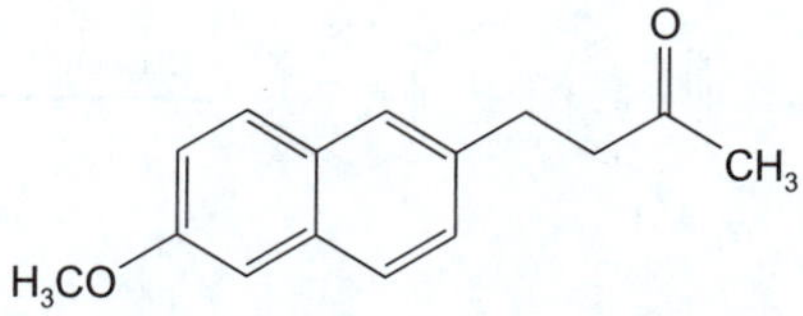

4-(6-Methoxy-2-naphthyl)-2 butanone

Properties and uses: Nabumetone is a white crystalline powder, practically insoluble in water, freely soluble in acetone, and slightly soluble in methanol. It is a non-acidic compound and because of this nature, it produces minimum gastrointestinal side effect. It is indicated in the treatment of acute and chronic treatment of osteoarthritis and rheumatoid arthritis.

Synthesis

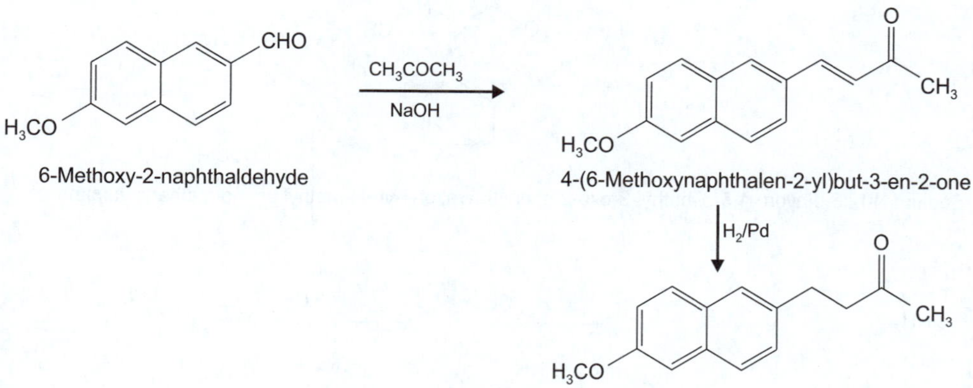

Dose: For pain and inflammation associated with osteoarthritis and rheumatoid arthritis adult dose is 1 g as a single dose in the evening followed by 0.5–1 g in the morning.

Dosage forms: Nabumetone oral suspension BP, nabumetone tablets BP.

Assay: It is assayed by adopting liquid chromatography technique.

ii. Nimesulide (Auronim)

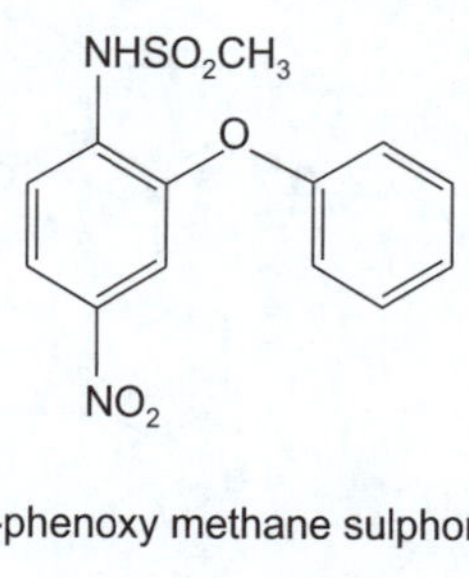

4-Nitro-2-phenoxy methane sulphonamide

Synthesis

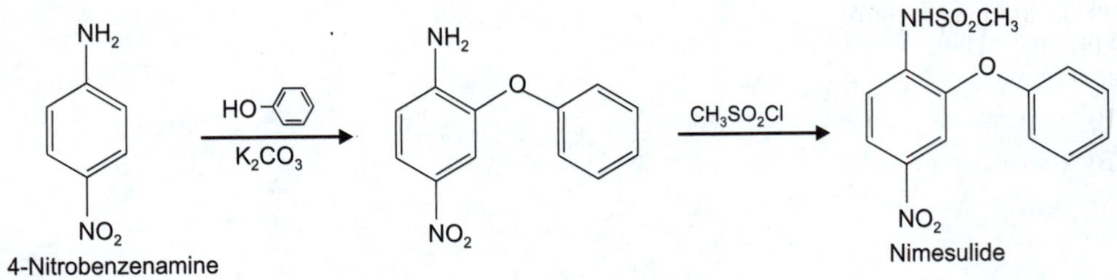

Properties and uses: Nimesulide is a yellowish crystalline powder, practically insoluble in water, soluble in acetone, and slightly soluble in anhydrous ethanol. It contains a sulphonamide moiety as an acidic group rather than a carbonic acid. It shows moderate incidence of gastric side effects because it exhibits significant selectivity towards COX-2, used as analgesic and anti-inflammatory agent.

iii. Analgin

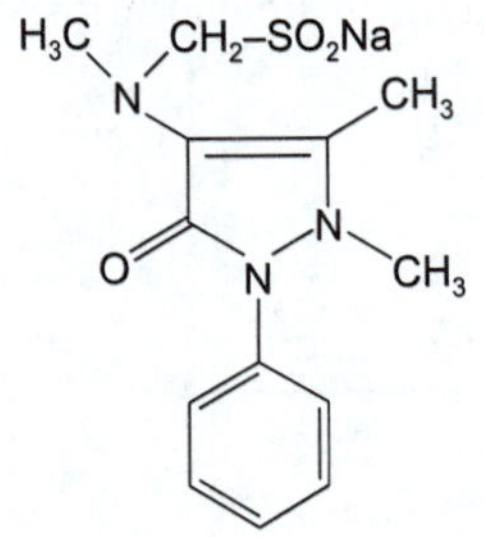

Sodium N-(2,3-dihydro-1,5-dimethyl-3-oxo-2 phenyl-pyrazol-4-yl)-N-methyl amino methane sulphonate

Synthesis

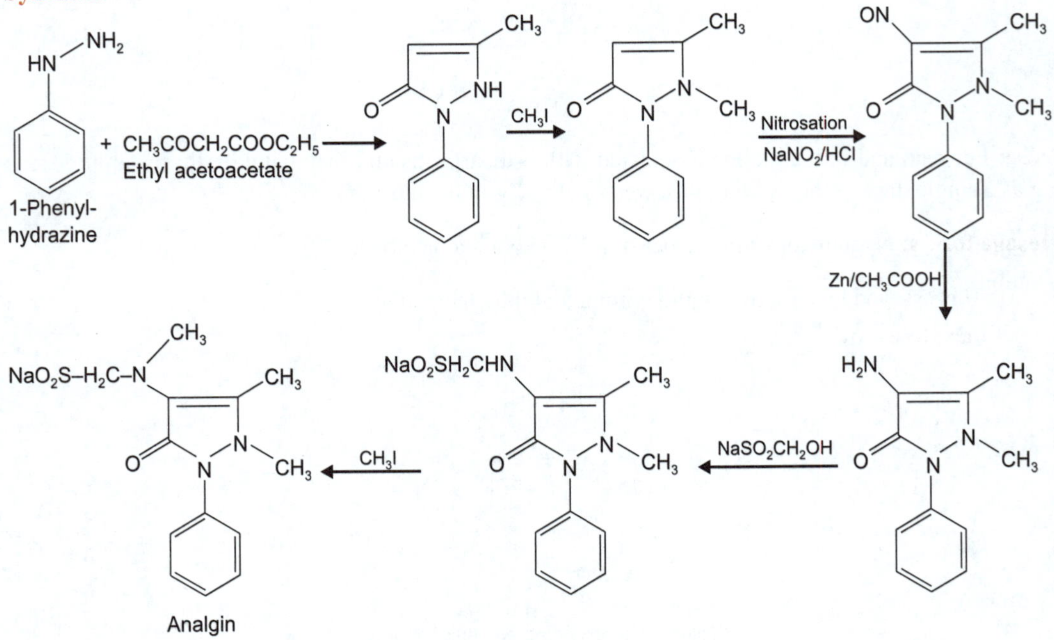

Uses: Used as an analgesic and anti-inflammatory agent.

Drugs Used in the Treatment of Gout

An acute attack of gout occurs as a result of anti-inflammatory reaction to crystals of sodium ureate (the end product of purine metabolism in human beings) that is deposited in the joint tissues. Drugs used to treat gout may act in the following ways:

- By inhibiting uric acid synthesis: Allopurinol.
- By increasing uric acid excretion: Probenecid, sulphinpyrazone.
- Miscellaneous: Colchicines (alkaloid obtained from *Colchicum autumnale*).

i. **Allopurinol** (Zyloprim)

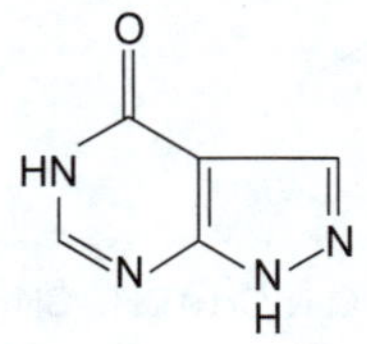

Pyrazolo pyrimidine-4-one

Synthesis

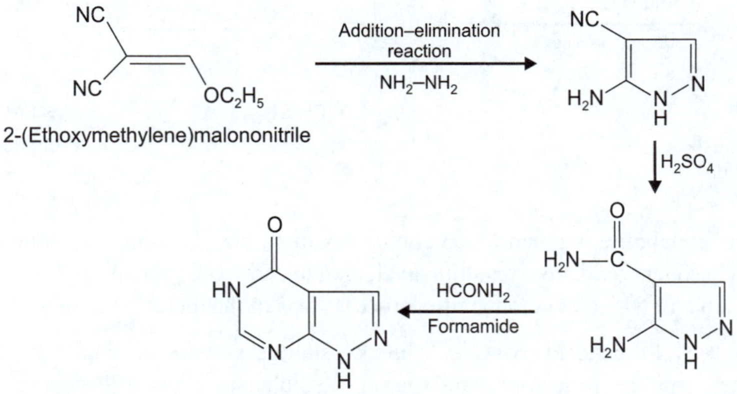

Mode of action: In human beings, uric acid is formed primarily by the xanthine oxidase-catalyzed oxidation of hypoxanthine and xanthine. At low concentrations, allopurinol is a substrate and competitive inhibitor of the enzyme at high concentrations; it is a non-competitive inhibitor.

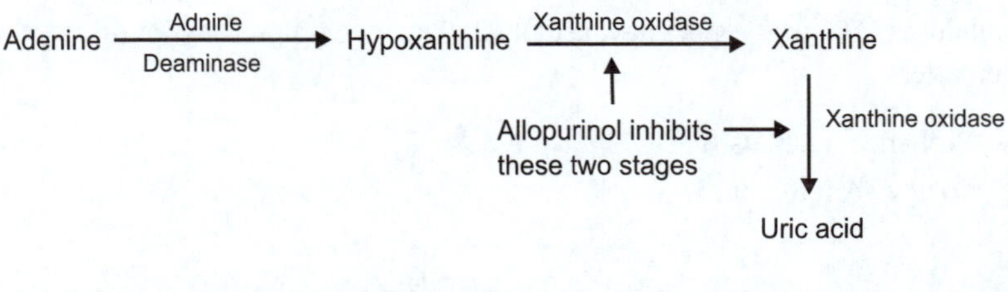

Metabolism: It is rapidly metabolized via oxidation and numerous ribonucleoside derivatives are formed. The major metabolites are alloxanthine or oxypurinol.

Properties and uses: Allopurinol is a white powder, very slightly soluble in water, in alcohol and in dilute solutions of alkali hydroxides. It is used in the treatment of gout and prevention of urate deposition in patients with leukaemia receiving anticancer drugs, which cause increasing serum uric acid levels.

Assay: It is assayed by adopting liquid chromatography technique.

Dose: Usual adult oral dose for gout is 100–200 mg two or three times a day.

Dosage forms: Allopurinol tablets IP, BP.

ii. **Probenecid** (Benemid)

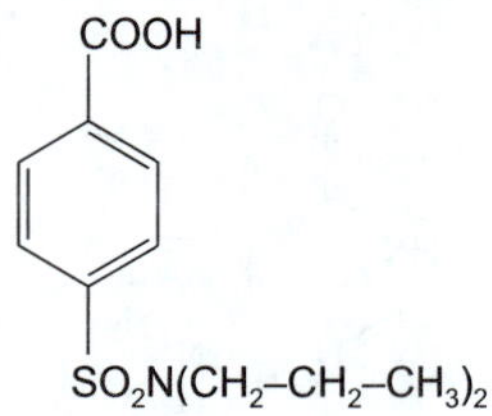

Synthesis

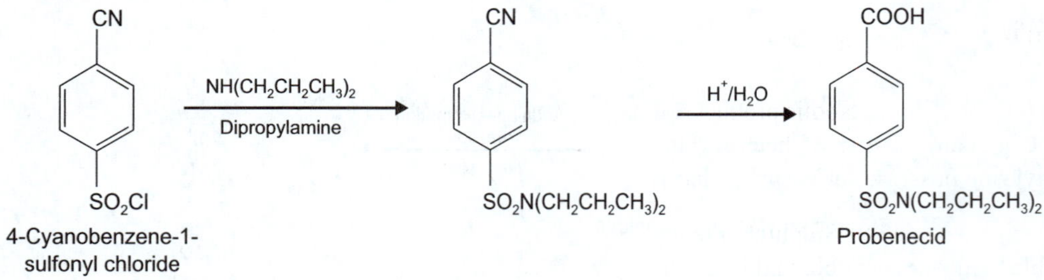

Metabolism: The metabolite is glucuronide conjugates of carboxylic acid, ω-oxidation of N-propyl side chain, and subsequent oxidation, resulting in alcohol to carboxylic acid derivative. ω-Oxidation of N-propyl side chain and N-dealkylation are the process steps in the metabolism of probenecid.

Properties and uses: Probenecid exists as white crystalline powder or small crystals, practically insoluble in water, soluble in acetone, and sparingly soluble in ethanol. Probenecid is uricosuric agent that increases the rate of excretion of uric acid and used in the treatment of chronic gout. The oral administration of probenecid in conjugation with penicillin G results in higher and prolonged concentration of the antibiotic in the plasma than when penicillin is given alone.

Assay: Dissolve the sample in alcohol, shaking and heating slightly, if necessary, and titrate against 0.1 M sodium hydroxide. Determine the end point potentiometrically.

Dose: Adult oral dose is 500 mg–2 g per day; usually 250 mg two times a day for one week, then 500 mg twice a day thereafter.

Dosage forms: Probenecid tablets IP, BP.

iii. **Sulphinpyrazone** (Anuturane)

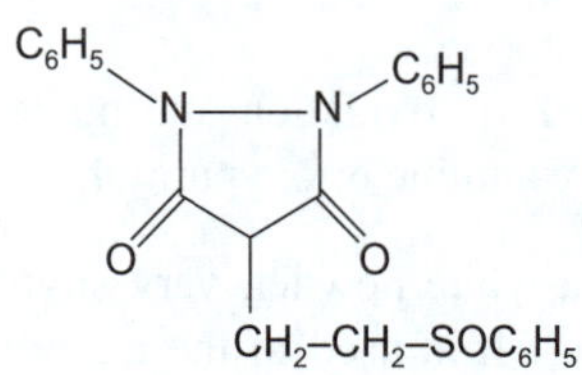

Synthesis

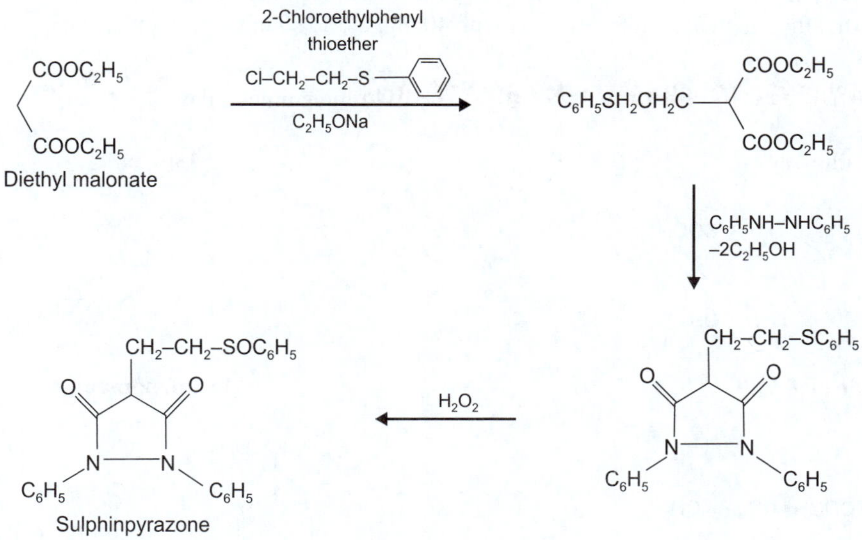

Metabolism: The metabolic product results from sulphoxide reduction, sulphur, and aromatic oxidation and C-glucuronidation of heterocyclic ring. The metabolite resulting from *para*-hydroxylation of phenyl ring possesses uricosuric effect.

Properties and uses: Sulphinpyrazone is a white powder, very slightly soluble in water, sparingly soluble in alcohol, soluble in dilute solutions of alkali hydroxides and used as uricosuric agent.

Assay: Dissolve the sample in acetone and titrate against 0.1 M sodium hydroxide using bromothymol blue as an indicator, until the colour changes from yellow to blue.

Dose: Initial oral dose is 100–200 mg per day, taken with meals or milk.

Dosage forms: Sulphinpyrazone tablets BP.

iv. Febuxostat (Uloric)

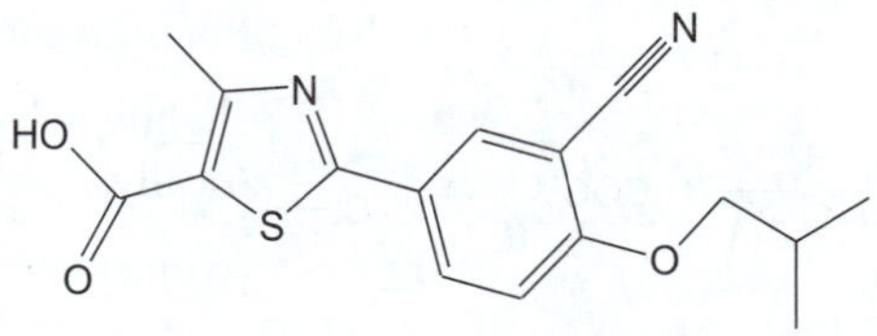

Mode of action: Febuxostat is a xanthine oxidase (XO) inhibitor. It achieves its therapeutic effect by decreasing serum uric acid. It is a non-purine selective XO inhibitor. Febuxostat inhibits both oxidized and reduced types of XO. It is not expected to inhibit other enzymes involved in synthesis and metabolism of purine and pyrimidine at therapeutic concentrations.

Properties and uses: Febuxostat is specifically used for the chronic management of hyperuricaemia in patients with gout. Adverse events associated with the use of febuxostat are liver function abnormalities, nausea, arthralgia, and rash.

Dose: Febuxostat is supplied as a 40 mg tablet designed for oral administration. The recommended initial dose of the drug is 40 mg once daily. For patients who do not achieve a serumuric acid less than 6 mg per dL after the treatment for 2 weeks with 40 mg, uloric 80 mg is recommended.

CLASSIFICATION BASED ON PCI SYLLABUS

Sodium salicylate

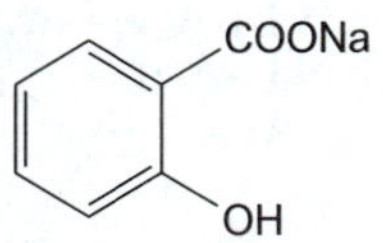

Aspirin

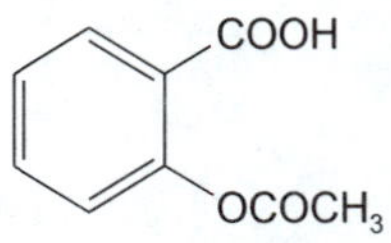

Mefenamic acid

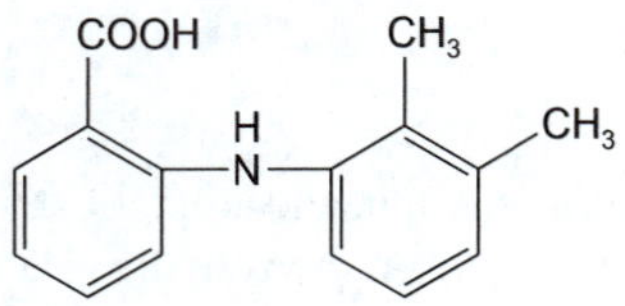

Meclofenamate

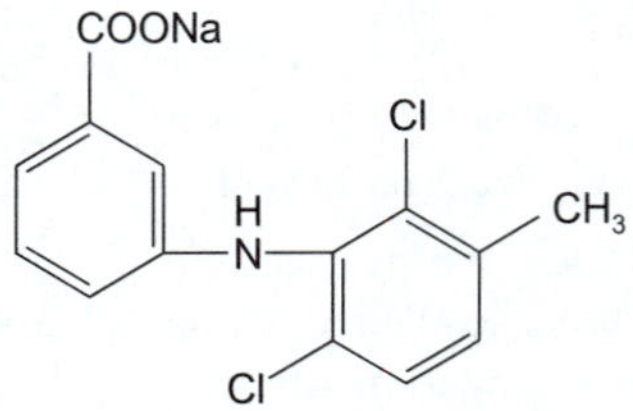

Indomethacin

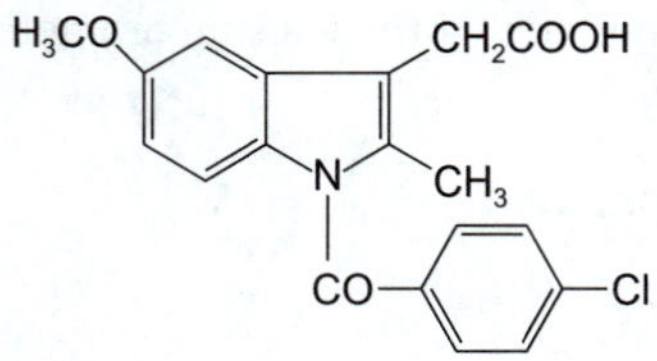

Sulindac

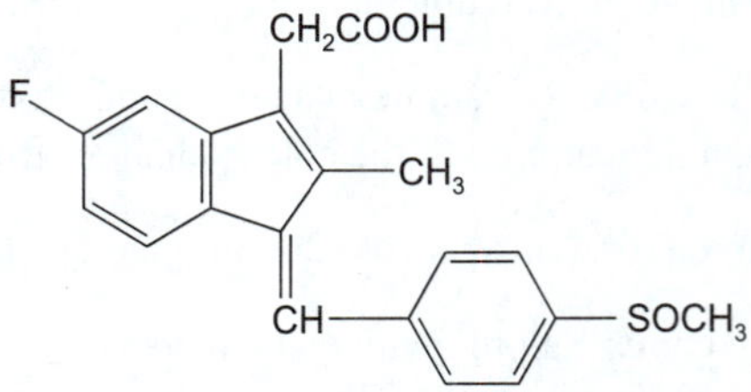

Tolmetin

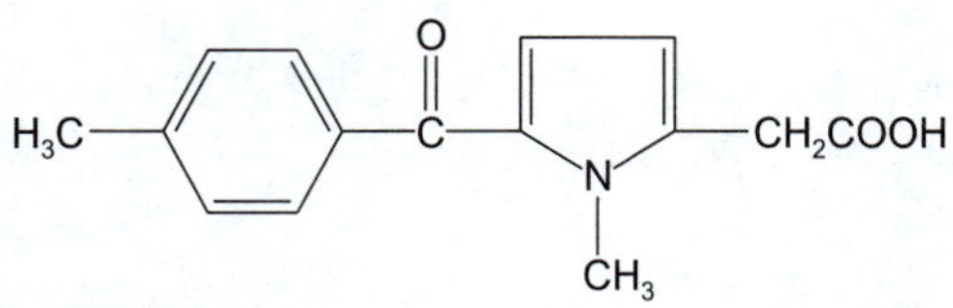

Zomepirac

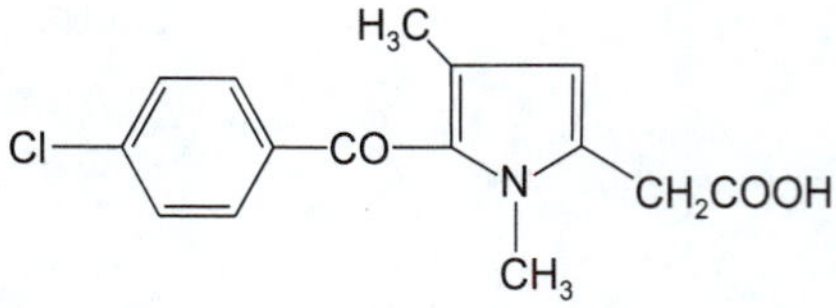

Diclofenac

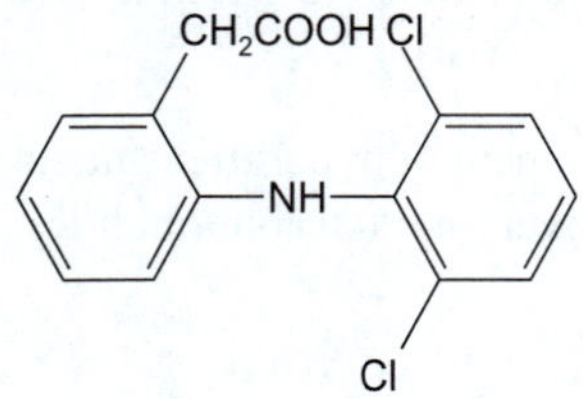

Ketorolac

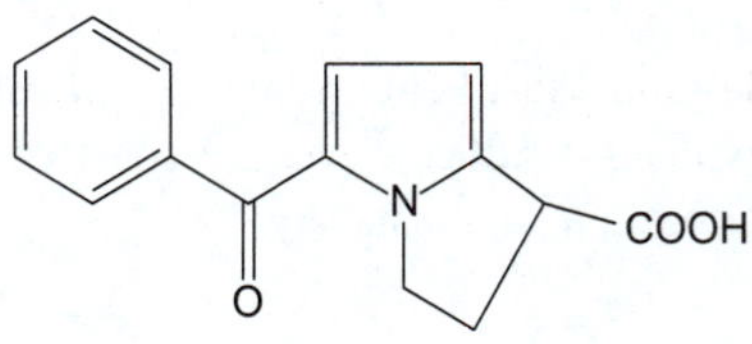

Ibuprofen

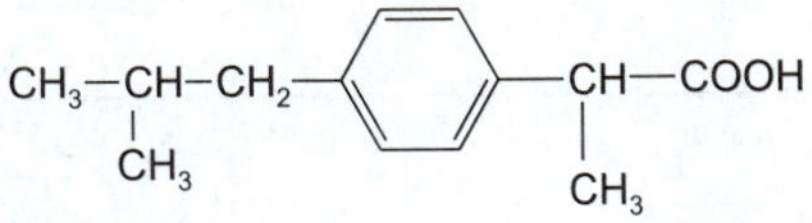

Naproxen

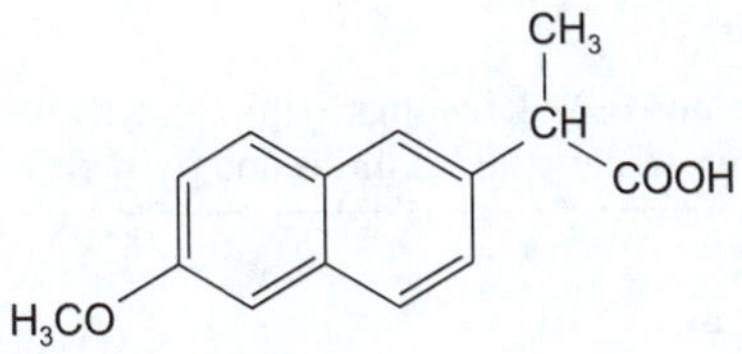

Piroxicam

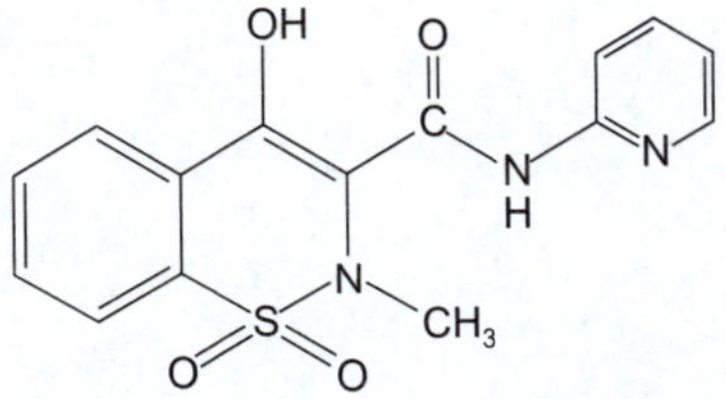

Phenacetin

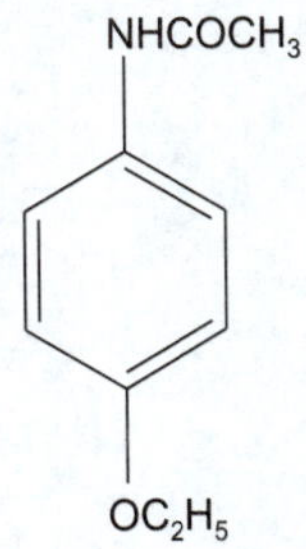

Acetaminophen

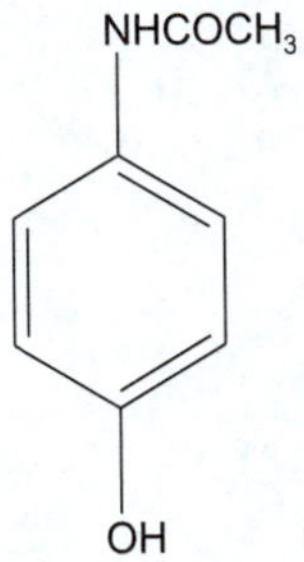

Antipyrine

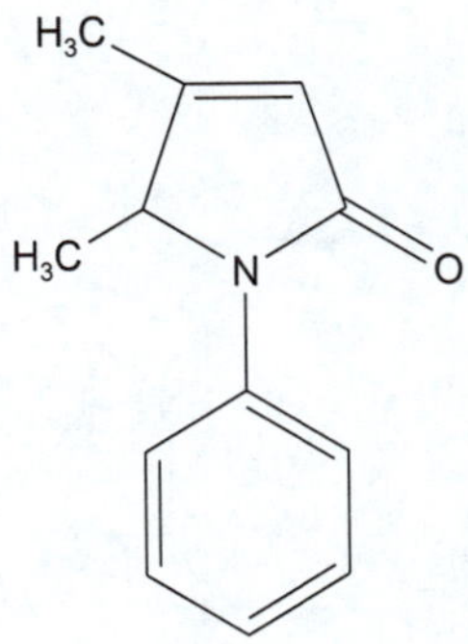

Phenylbutazone

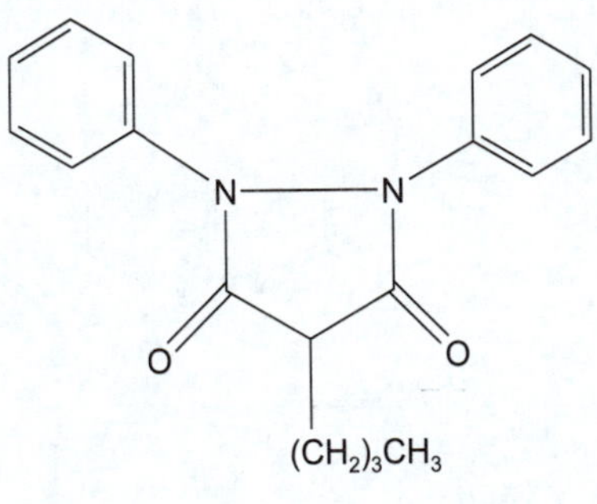

Meclofenamate

Properties and uses: It belongs to the category of anthranilic acid derivatives. It is a COX-inhibitor and used to treat joint and muscular pains, arthritis and dysmenorrhea.

Rimegepant

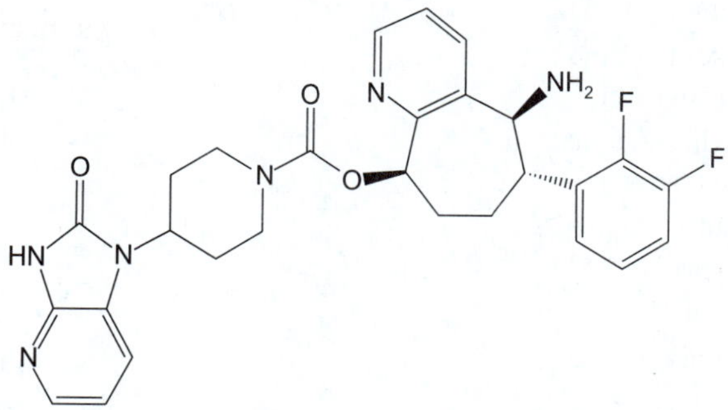

Uses: It is used to treat migraine.

Ubrogepant

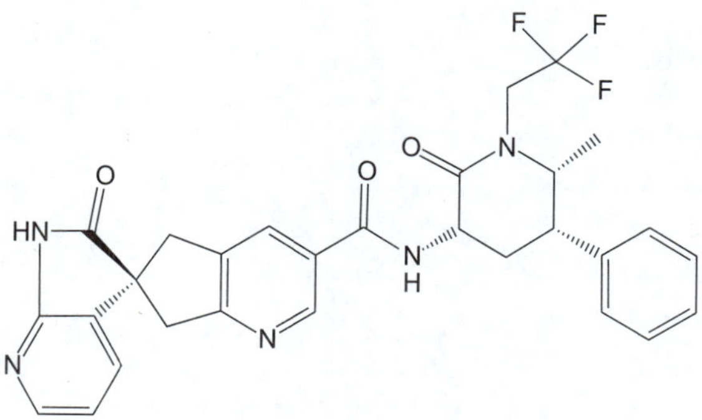

Uses: It is used for the treatment of acute (immediate) treatment of migraine.

Lasmiditan

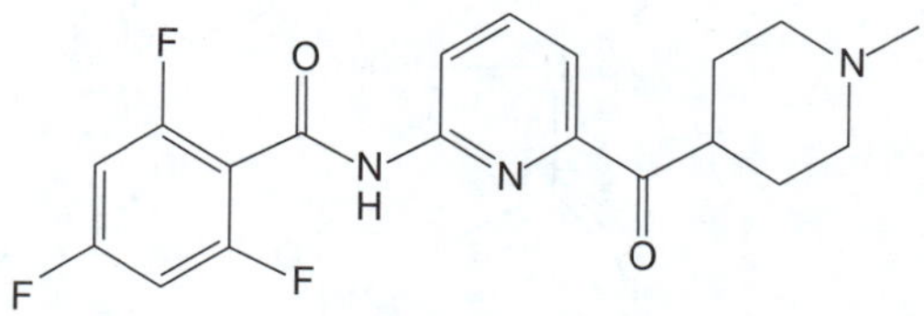

Uses: It is used for the treatment of migraine.

PROBABLE QUESTIONS

1. Explain schematically, the biosynthetic pathway of PGs and describe how does the NSAIDs act as antipyretics and analgesics?
2. Outline the synthesis of the following NSAIDs: Paracetamol, phenylbutazone, and indomethacin.
3. Classify the NSAIDs and write the structure, chemical name, and uses of at least one compound from each category.
4. Write the names of three drugs belonging to the category of aniline and *para*-aminophenol analogues. Outline the synthesis of one of them.
5. What is cyclooxygenase II? Name the drugs that selectively inhibit the cyclooxygenase II along with the synthesis of any one of them.
6. Explain how the salicylic acid analogues act as potent antipyretics and analgesics. Mention suitable examples to support your answer.
7. Write the metabolism of *para*-amino phenol derivatives with their chemical structure and indicate the metabolic product responsible for hepatotoxic.
8. The metabolite of phenylbutazone is a more effective drug. Outline its synthesis and the important uses.
9. Name a sulphur-containing pyrazolidine drug used as an antipyretic and analgesic, and write its synthesis.
10. Structural analogues of N-aryl anthranilic acid yielded some potent antipyretics, analgesics, and anti-inflammatory compounds. Justify the statement with two examples and write their synthesis.
11. Outline the synthesis of the following NSAIDs: Ibuprofen, diclofenac, and nabumetone.
12. Explain the mode of action of antipyretics and analgesics by citing the examples of some typical drugs, which you have studied.
13. Write in detail about antipyretics and analgesics.
14. What are salicylates? Enumerate the derivatives of salicylic acid used as NSAIDs with their chemical structure. Describe the SAR and metabolism of salicylates.
15. Outline the synthesis and uses of the following NSAIDs: Piroxicam, sulindac, and zomepirac sodium.
16. Write a brief note on aryl acetic acid derived from NSAIDs.
17. What are the major side effects of NSAIDs? Explain how the GIT disturbances can be corrected.
18. Explain the mode of action of antigout drugs and outline the synthesis, metabolism, and uses of any two of them.

SUGGESTED READINGS

1. Abraham DJ (ed). *Burger's Medicinal Chemistry and Drug Discovery* (6th edn). New Jersey: John Wiley, 2007.
2. *British Pharmacopoeia*. Medicines and Healthcare Products Regulatory Agency, London, 2008.
3. Bruntan LL, Lazo JS, and Parker KL. *Goodman and Gilman's: The Pharmacologica Basis of Therapeutics* (11th edn). New York: McGraw Hill, 2006.
4. *Indian Pharmacopoeia*. Ministry of Health and Family Welfare. New Delhi, 1996.
5. Lednicer D and Mitscher LA. *The Organic Chemistry of Drug Synthesis*. New York: John Wiley, 1995.
6. Lemke TL and William DA. *Foye's Principle of Medicinal Chemistry* (6th edn). New York: Lippincott Williams and Wilkins, 2008.
7. Gennaro AR. *Remington's: The Science and Practice of Pharmacy* (21st edn). New York: Lippincot Williams and Wilkins, 2006.
8. Reynolds EF (ed). *Martindale the Extra Pharmacopoeia* (31st edn). London: The Pharmaceutical Press, 1997.

SECTION II

Drugs Acting on Respiratory System

CHAPTER 4

Expectorants and Antitussives

INTRODUCTION OF RESPIRATORY SYSTEM

There are many drugs acting on respiratory system, that is, antitussives, antiasthmatics, expectorants, and mucolytics. There are some drugs that act centrally for suppression of cough through the inhibition of mechano or chemoreceptors. Normally, cough is beneficial for expelling all the dust particles that enter into the respiratory tract. However, when the cough becomes severe due to any inflammation in the respiratory tract or in the lungs, it is necessary to treat with some drugs, such as mucolytics, antiasthmatics, or any expectorants.

The drugs that are used for bronchial asthma are β_2-adrenergic agonists because it is caused due to the irregulation of autonomic control towards these receptors in the lungs and respiratory tract, which produces constriction. Therefore, the difficulty in breathing persists and can be treated, especially, with β_2 adrenergic agonists. For example, salmeterol, terbutaline, formeterol, and some methyl xanthines (caffeine, theophylline) as well as anticholinergics (ipratropium bromide, tiotropium bromide). The inflammation persisting may be treated better with corticosteroids. Bronchial asthma may also be due to the hypersensitive reactions, due to the release of histamine and acetylcholine in the tracheo-bronchial regions. These can be treated by using some mast cell stabilizers called sodium chromoglycate and leukotriene antagonists, that is, montelukast and zafirlukast.

Antitussives are the drugs that act in the central nervous system (CNS) to raise the threshold of cough centre or act peripherally in the respiratory tract to reduce tussal impulse, for example, opioids and non-opioids.

Mucolytics are the drugs that depolymerize the mucopolysaccharides and they break the network of tenacious sputum. These events mark the expulsion of sputum with the help of ciliary movement. Examples: bromhexine, adathoda vasika.

Expectorants are the drugs that increase the bronchial secretion and reduce the viscosity of sputum for removal by coughing. Sodium and potassium citrate and ammonium chloride are used as expectorants.

EXPECTORANTS AND ANTITUSSIVES

Antitussives are drugs that reduce coughing. Coughing may be diminished by reducing respiratory secretion, eliminating a source of irritation, or decreasing the sensitivity of irritant receptors within the respiratory tract. Antitussives can act either by raising the threshold of the cough centre or by reducing the number of impulses transmitted to the centre from the peripheral receptors. The antitussives are divided into two main classes:

1. Centrally-acting antitussives that affect the cough centre in the medulla.

2. Peripherally, active antitussives that act at the receptor level in the respiratory tract.

Pharyngeal demulcents sooth the throat and reduce the afferent impulse from the inflammed/irritated mucosa. Expectorants are drugs that increase the secretion of bronchus and reduce the viscosity, thereby removing cough and sputum. The drugs usually used as expectorants are salts of sodium, potassium, and ammonium compounds. Guaiphenesin, vasaka, and balsam of tolu are plant products. These also enhance the mucociliary movement. Ammonium salts are nauseating and reflexly increase the respiratory secretion. Antitussives act centrally and relieve the cough. They act on the cough centre in the medulla oblongata and increase the threshold to cough. These drugs control the cough rather than eliminate it. The drugs that are used as antitussives are codeine, an opium alkaloid, and selective drugs are also there for the action on the cough centre, but it may produce respiratory depression at higher dosage. In non-opioids, noscapine and dextromethorphan are usually used. Noscapine is an opium alkaloid of benzoisoquinoline series. It depresses cough, but has no narcotic, analgesic, or dependence effects. Dextromethorphan is a synthetic compound and it is a α-isomer and used as antitussives.

CLASSIFICATION

I. Centrally-acting Antitussive Agents

i. Dextromethorphan HBr

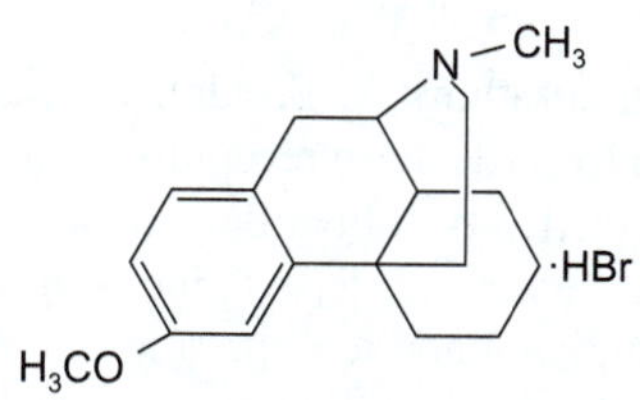

ii. Levopropoxyphene napsylate

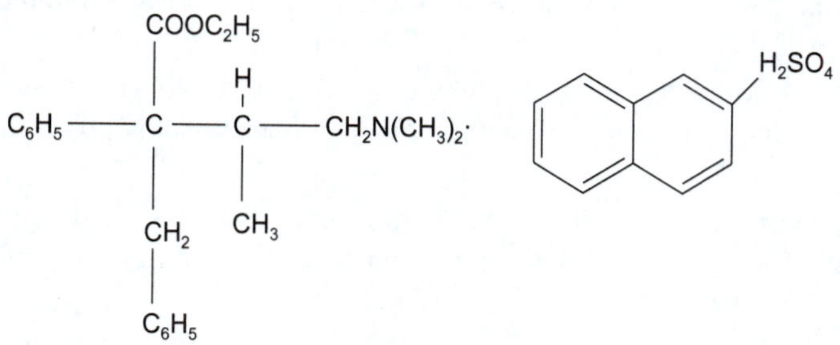

iii. Noscapine

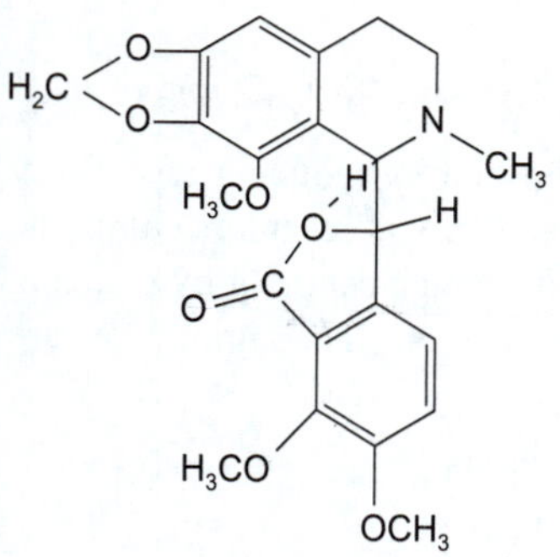

iv. Pholcodine

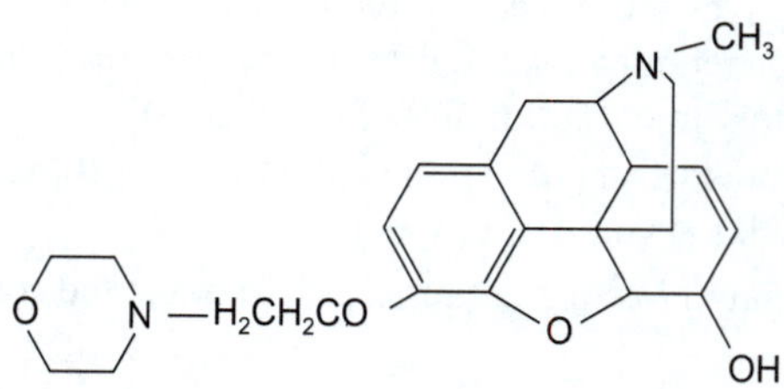

v. Codeine phosphate

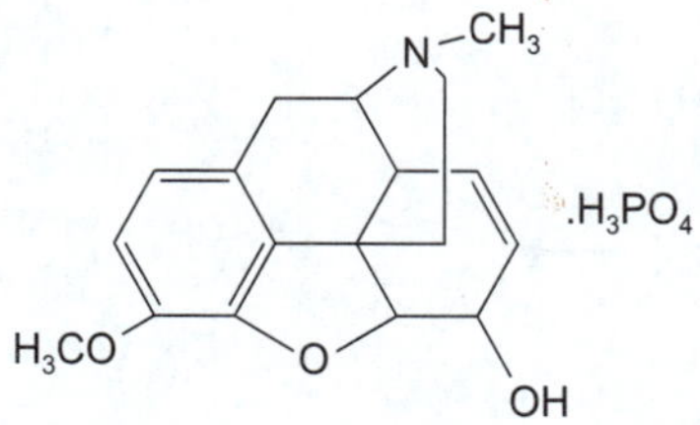

II. Peripherally-acting Antitussives

i. Benzonatate

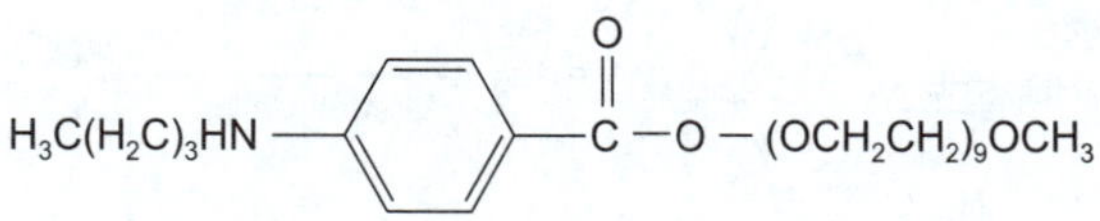

ii. Carbetapentane

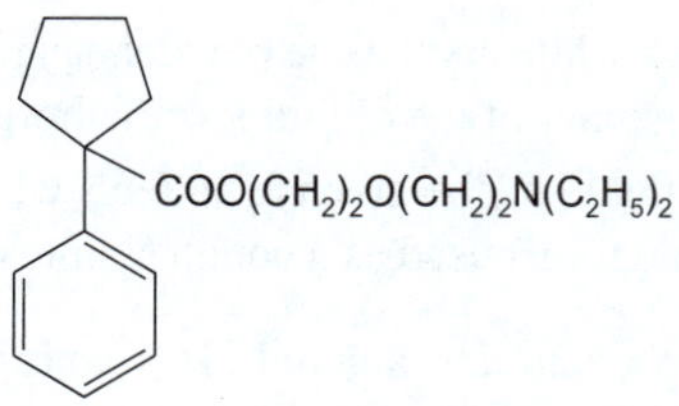

iii. Caramiphen

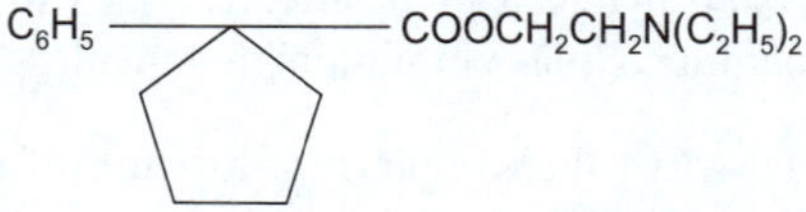

iv. Chlophedianol hydrochloride

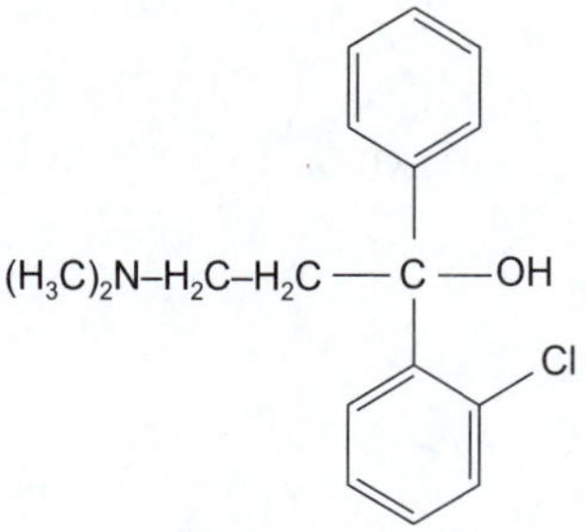

v. Isoaminile

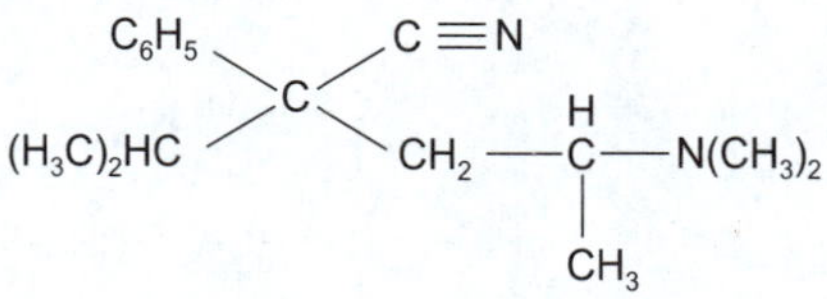

SYNTHESIS AND DRUG PROFILE

I. Centrally-acting Antitussive Agents

i. Dextromethorphan HBr

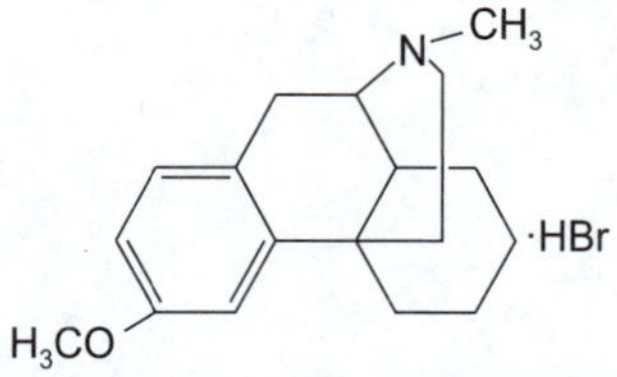

3-Methoxy-17-methyl-9α,13α,14α,-morphinan hydrobromide

Synthesis

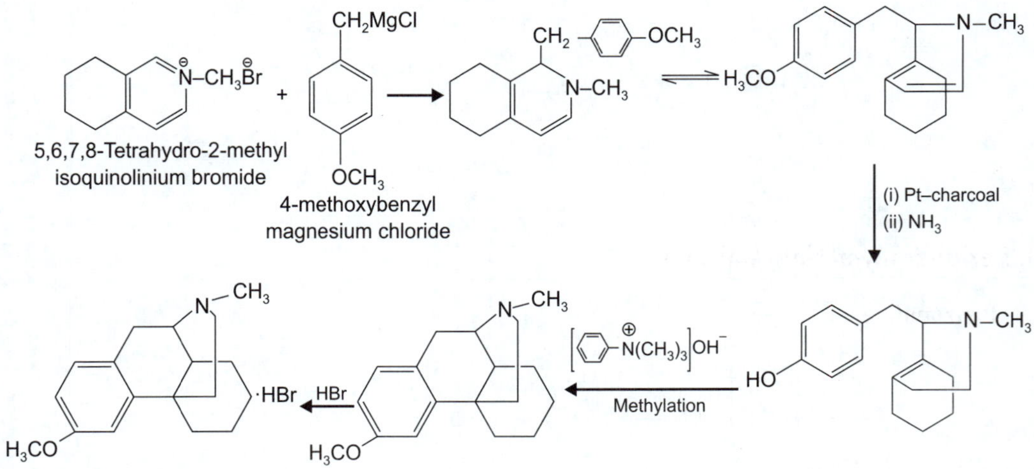

Dextromethorphan hydrobromide

Properties and uses: Dextromethorphan hydrobromide (HBr) is a white crystalline powder, sparingly soluble in water, and soluble in alcohol. It is a substituted dextro isomer of the opioid levomethorphan.

It is not an analgesic or an addictive. Dextromethorphan HBr should not be given to patients who are on monoamine oxidase inhibitors therapy. It is an opioid receptor agonist used as a cough suppressant.

Assay: Dissolve the sample in a mixture of 0.01 M hydrochloric acid and alcohol (1:4) and titrate against 0.1 M sodium hydroxide. Determine the end point potentiometrically. Read the volume added between the two points of inflexion.

ii. **Levo proproxyphene napsylate** (Novrad)

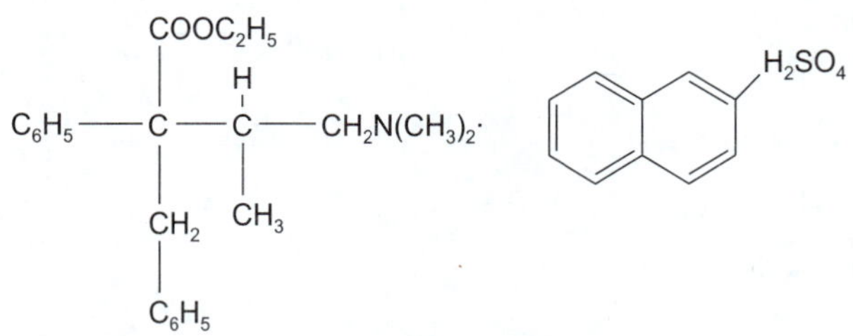

(–)-α-[(2-Dimethylamino)-1-methyl ethyl]-α-phenyl phenylethyl propionate(1:1)monohydrate-2-naphthalene sulphonic acid salt

Properties and uses: It is a white, bitter, crystalline powder, odourless, soluble in water, alcohol, or chloroform. It has little or no analgesic activity. It has been found to be relatively less potent than codeine in the treatment of cough reflexes. The (–)-isomer of the drug showed greater antitussive activity in comparison to either the (+)-isomer or the racemic mixture.

Dose: Usually, 50–100 mg after every 4 hrs.

Synthesis

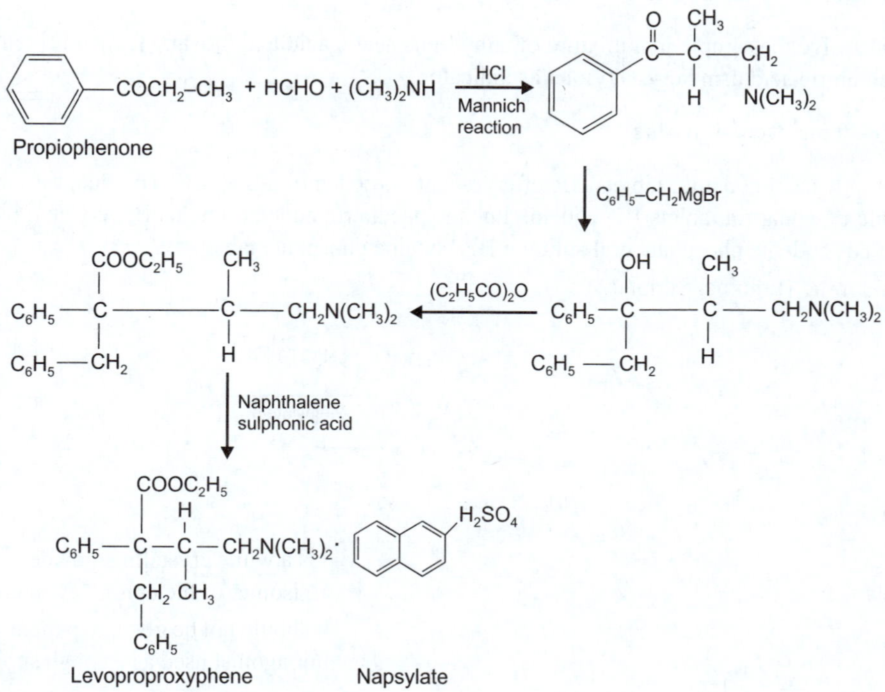

iii. Codeine phosphate (Zenodyl)

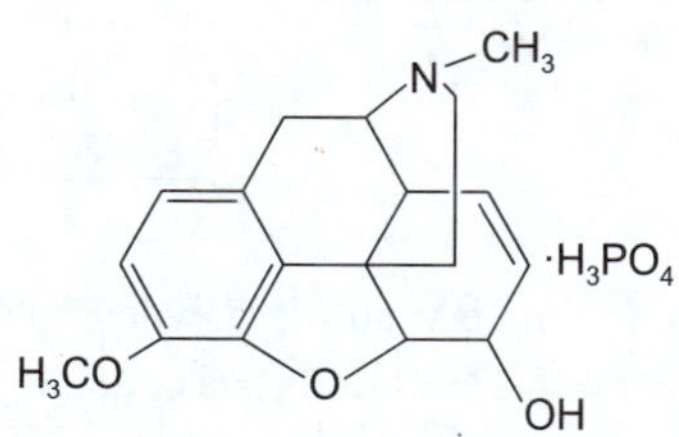

Synthesis

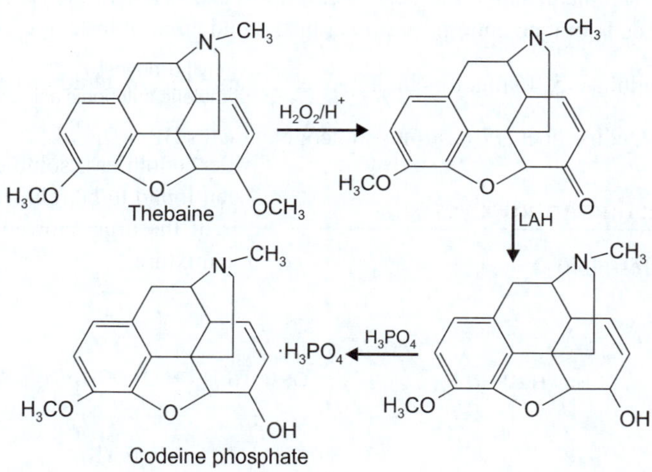

Properties and uses: Codeine phosphate is a white crystalline powder, soluble in water, and slightly soluble in ethanol. This drug acts by suppression of the cough centre in the brain stem.

Assay: Dissolve the sample in a mixture of anhydrous acetic acid and dioxan (1:2) and titrate against 0.1 M perchloric acid using crystal violet as indicator.

Dose: 10–20 mg every 4 to 6 hrs.

Dosage forms: Co-codamol tablets BP, effervescent co-codamol tablets BP, co-codaprin tablets BP, dispersible co-codaprin tablets BP, codeine linctus, paediatric codeine linctus BP, codeine phosphate injection BP, codeine phosphate oral solution BP, codeine phosphate tablets BP.

iv. **Pholcodine** (Ethnine, Simplex)

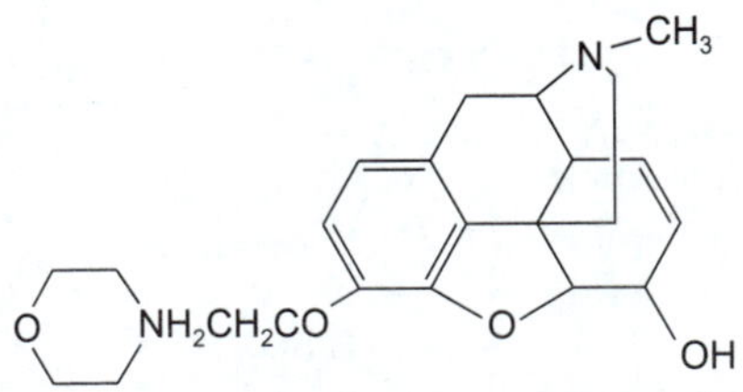

Synthesis

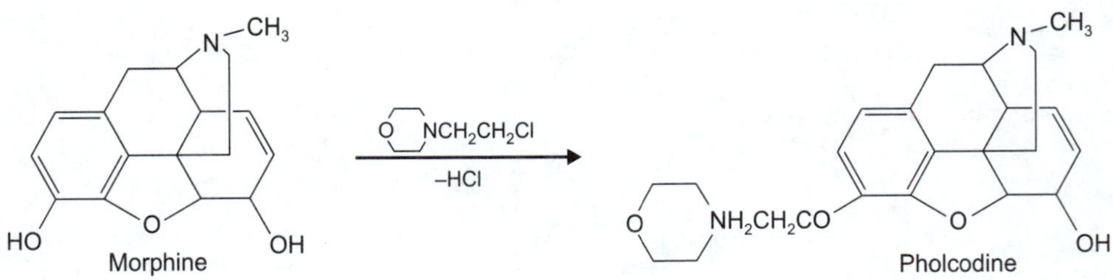

Properties and uses: Pholcodine is a white crystalline powder, sparingly soluble in water, soluble in acetone, alcohol, and dilute mineral acid. It is as effective as codeine. It is a cough suppressant with mild sedative, but practically negligible analgesic action. It is employed for the relief of unproductive cough.

Assay: Dissolve the sample in anhydrous acetic acid, warm gently and titrate against 0.1 M perchloric acid. Determine the end point potentiometrically at the second point of inflexion.

Dose: The dose for adults is 5–15 mg, for children over 2 years 5 mg, for children below 2 years 2.5 mg.

Dosage forms: Pholcodine linctus BP, strong pholcodine linctus BP.

II. Peripherally-acting Antitussives

i. **Benzonatate** (Tessalon)

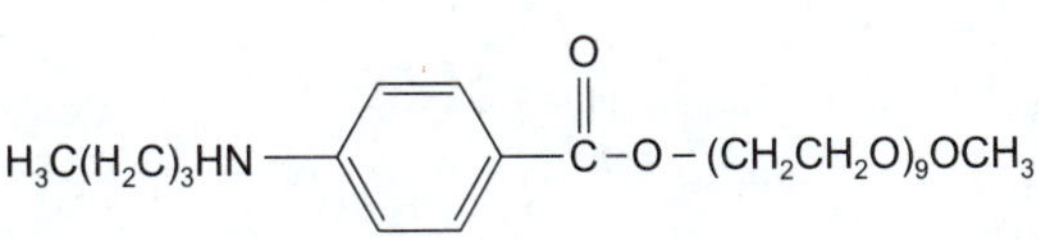

Synthesis

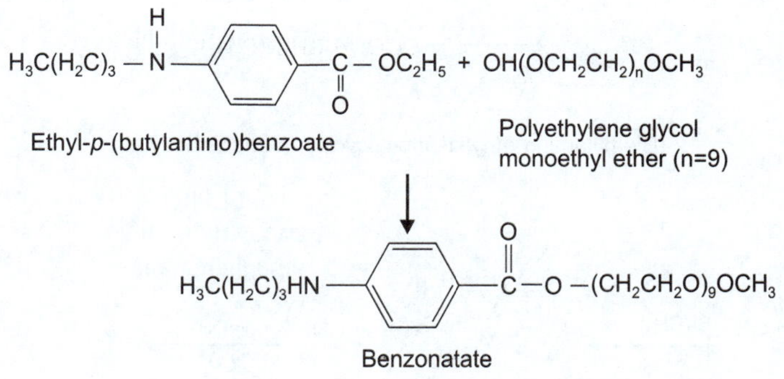

Properties and uses: It is a long-chain polyglycol derivative chemically related to tetracaine and benzocaine. It is a potent antitussive agent. It usually acts by inhibiting the transmission of impulses of the cough reflex in the vagal nuclei of the medulla and predominately depresses polysynaptic spinal reflexes. It is regarded as a cough suppressant acting both centrally and peripherally.

Dose: The usual dose is 100 mg three times daily.

ii. Carbetapentane (Toclase)

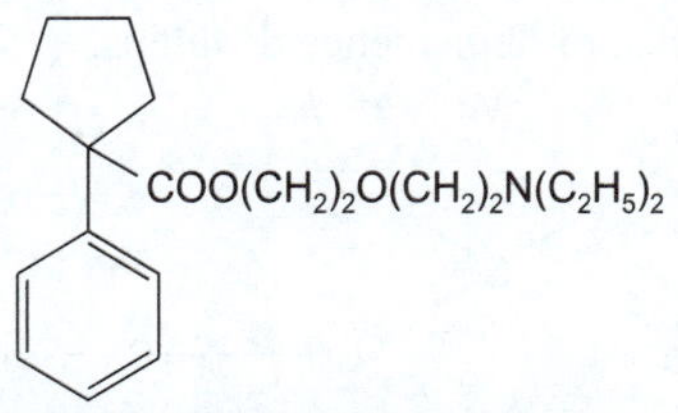

2-(2-(Diethylamino)ethoxy)ethyl-1-phenylcyclopentanecarboxylate

Synthesis

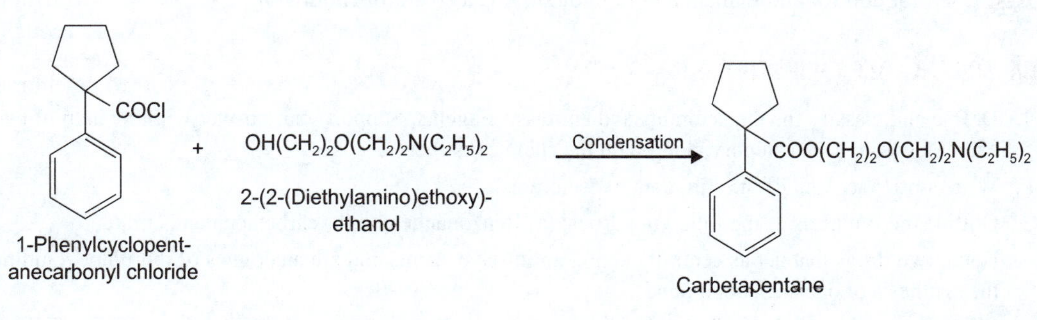

Properties and uses: It is a cough suppressant and is reported to reduce bronchial secretions. It is found to be effective in acute coughs associated with common upper respiratory infections.

Dose: The usual dose is 25–150 mg per day in divided doses.

iii. Caramiphen

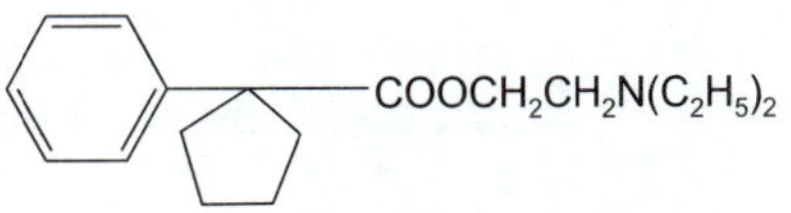

2-(Diethylamino)ethyl-1-phenylcyclopentanecarboxylate

Synthesis

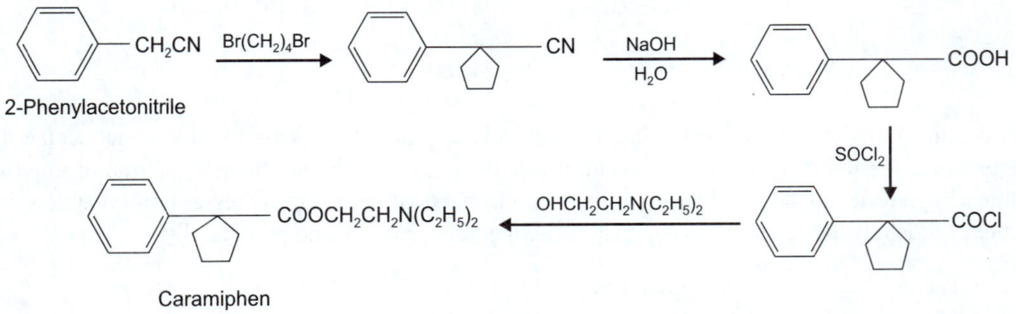

Uses: It is a cough suppressant, less active than codeine, but with longer duration of action. It has little effect on respiration and no tolerance of dependence develops.

iv. Isoaminile

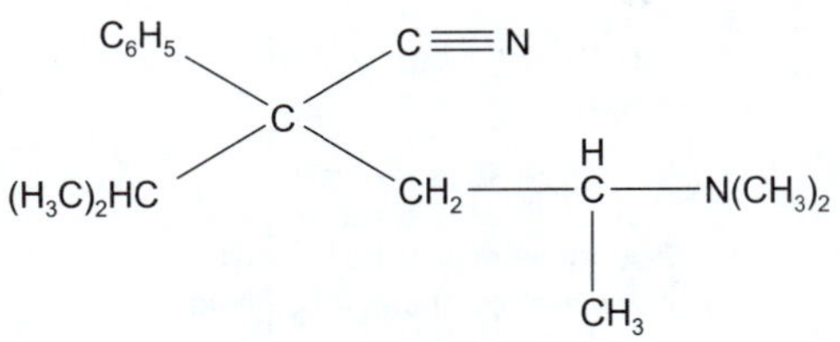

Uses: Used for control and management of cough, it is also a bronchodilator.

PROBABLE QUESTIONS

1. Define and classify the expectorants and antitussive agents. Support your answer with the help of two examples from each category along with the chemical structure.
2. Write a brief account of the stimulant expectorants.
3. Outline the synthesis of the following drugs: (a) Benzonatate and (b) carbetapentane citrate.
4. Name two drugs that act as centrally acting antitussive agents and are analogues of morphine. Outline the synthesis of one such compound.
5. Mannich reaction of propiophenone yields levopropoxphene napsylate. Describe the synthetic route to yield the final product.
6. Write the structure and chemical name of the five important drugs that are used abundantly in suppressing cough.
7. What are sedative expectorants? Classify them and give the structure, chemical names and uses of one compound from each group.
8. Centrally-acting antitussive agents act by depressing medullary cough centre in the CNS to suppress cough reflexes. Justify the statement by citing at least three potent drugs.

SUGGESTED READINGS

1. Abraham DJ (ed). *Burger's Medicinal Chemistry and Drug Discovery* (6th edn). New Jersey: John Wiley, 2007.
2. Boyd EM. 'Expectorants and respiratory tract fluids'. *Pharmacol Rev* 6(4): 521–42, 1954.
3. Bruntan LL, Lazo JS, and Parker KL. *Goodman and Gilman's: The Pharmacological Basis of Therapeutics* (11th edn). New York: McGraw Hill, 2006.
4. Lemke TL and William DA. *Foye's Principle of Medicinal Chemistry* (6th edn). New York: Lippincott Williams and Wilkins, 2008.
5. Lednicer D and Mitscher LA. *The Organic Chemistry of Drug Synthesis*. New York: John Wiley, 1995.
6. Gennaro AR. *Remington's The Science and Practice of Pharmacy* (21st edn). New York: Lippincot Williams and Wilkins, 2006.

SECTION III

Drugs Acting on Digestive System

CHAPTER 5

Antiulcer Agents

INTRODUCTION

Antiulcer agents are drugs that are used in the treatment of peptic and gastric ulcers. These are classified on the basis of mechanism of action.

CLASSIFICATION

I. Reduction of gastric acid secretion
   a. H_2-antihistamines: Cimetidine, ranitidine, and famotidine.
   b. Proton pump inhibitors: Omeprazole, lansoprazole, and pantoprazole.
   c. Anticholinergics: Pirenzepine, propantheline, and oxyphenonium.
   d. Prostaglandin analogues: Misoprostol.

II. Neutralization of gastric acid (antacids)
   a. Systemic: $NaHCO_3$ and sodium citrate.
   b. Nonsystemic: $Mg(OH)_2$, $CaCO_3$, aluminium hydroxide gel, and magnesium trisilicate.

III. Ulcer protectives: Sucralfate, colloidal bismuth subcitrate (CBS).

IV. Anti-*Helicobacter pylori* drugs: Amoxicillin, clarithromycin, metronidazole, tinidazole, and tetracycline.

CHEMICAL STRUCTURES OF GASTRIC ACID SECRETION INHIBITORS

I. a. H_2-Antihistamines

i. Nizatidine

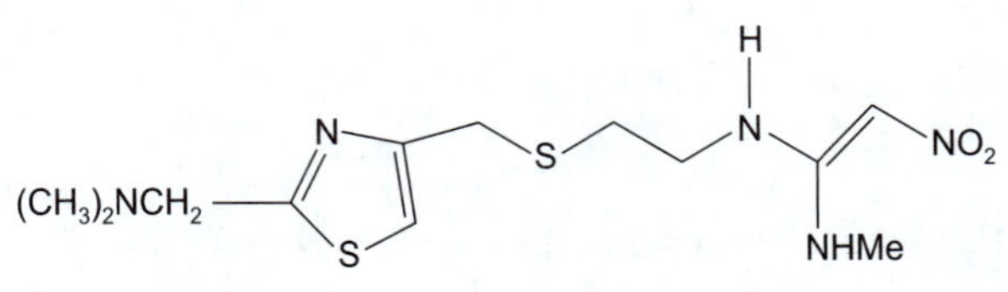

ii. **Cimetidine**

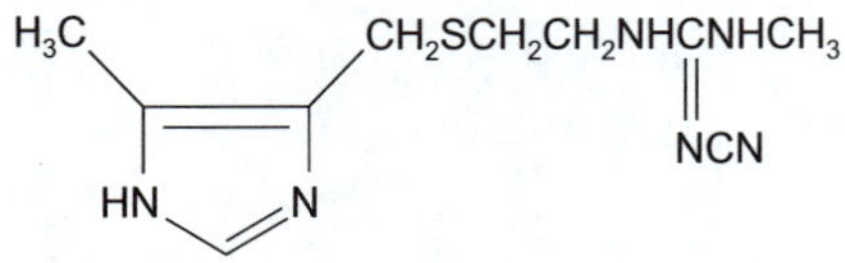

iii. **Roxatidine**

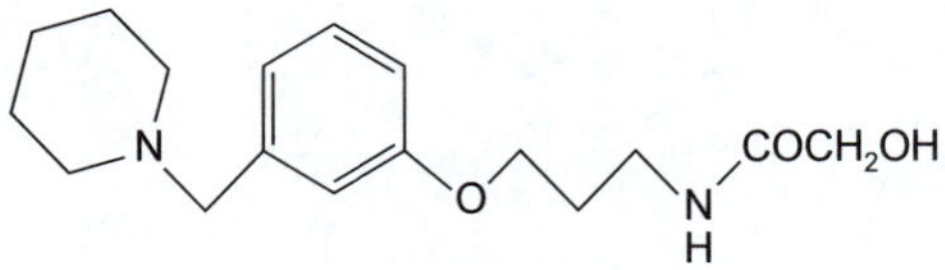

iv. **Famotidine**

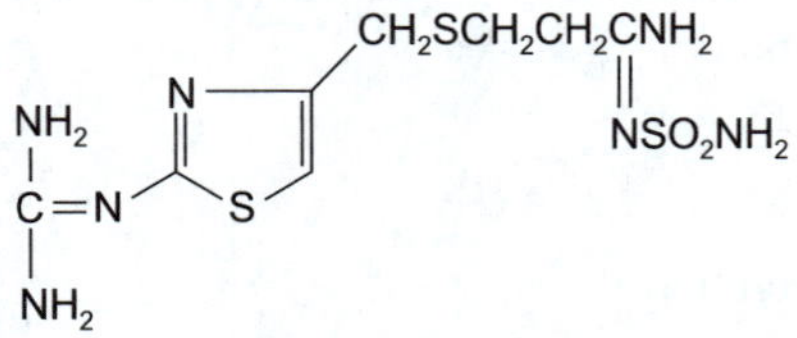

v. **Ranitidine**

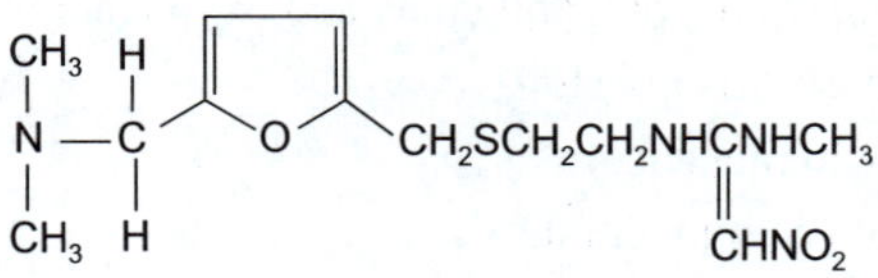

vi. **Oxmetidine**

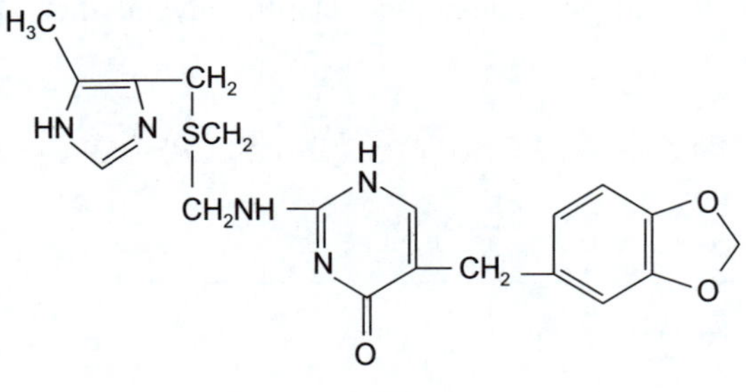

vii. **Etintidine**

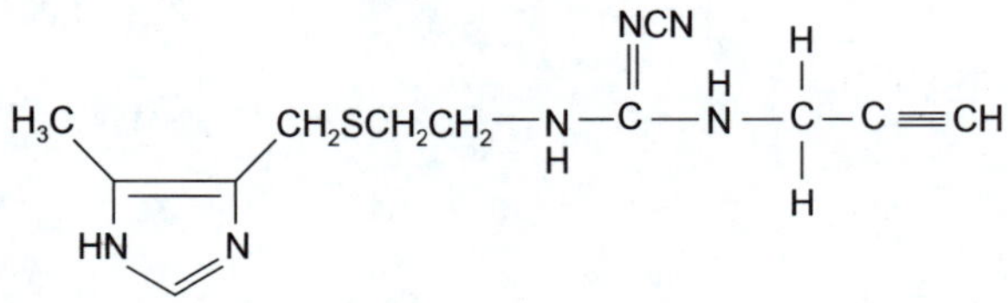

viii. Lupitidine

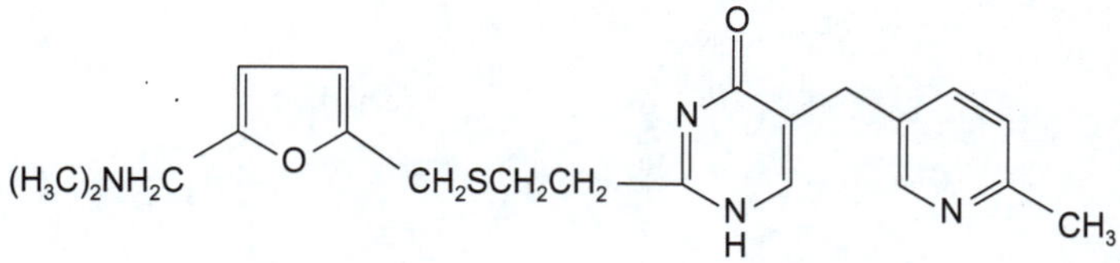

ix. Tiotidine

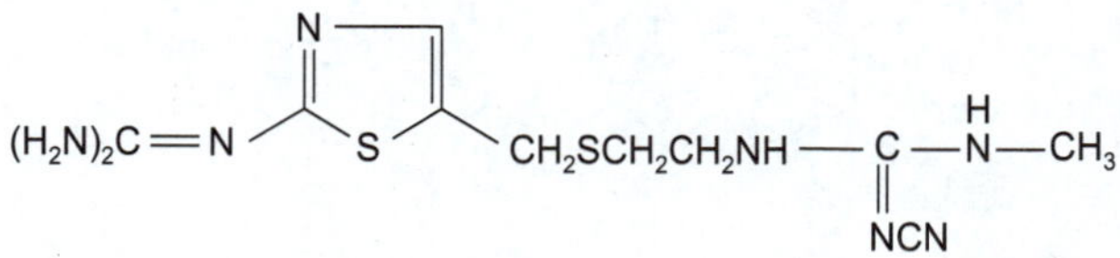

Lamitidine analogues

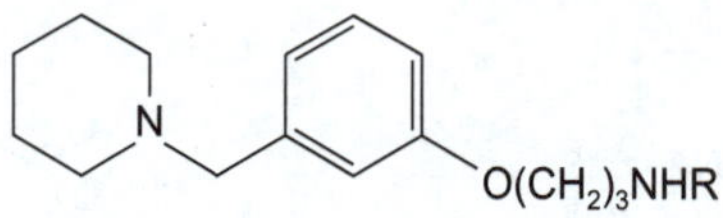

Name	*R*
Lamitidine	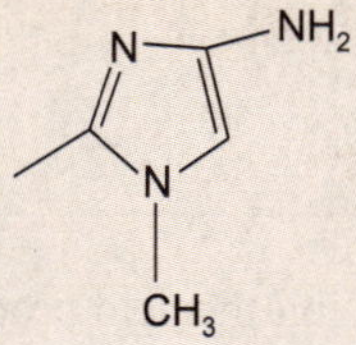
Pifatidine	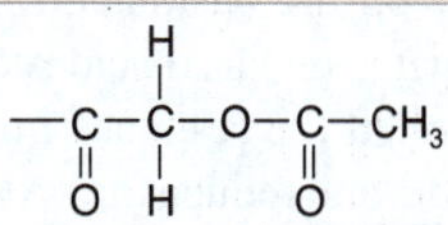
Loxtidine	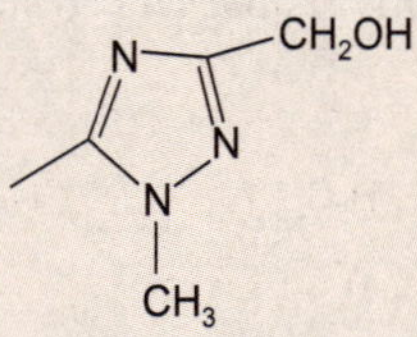

I. b. Proton Pump Inhibitors

i. Omeprazole

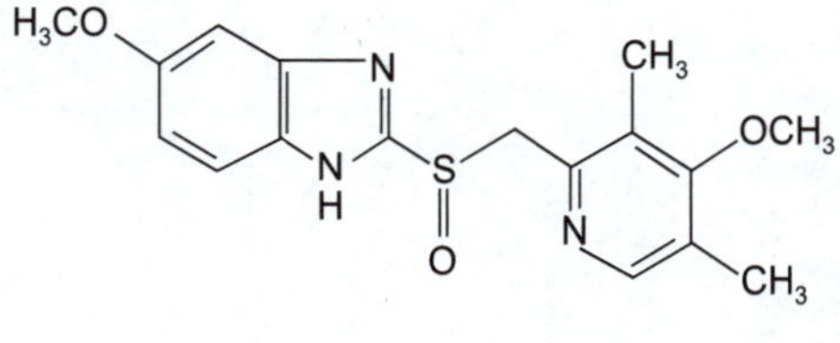

ii. Lansoprazole

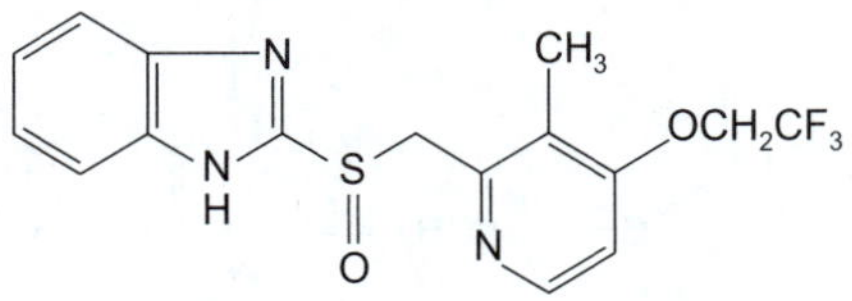

iii. Pantoprazole

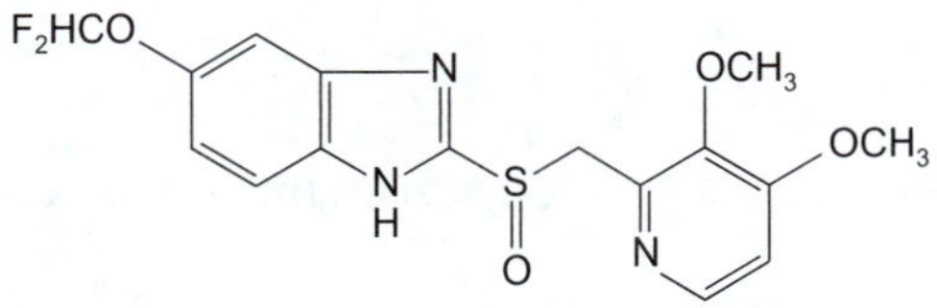

iv. Rabeprazole

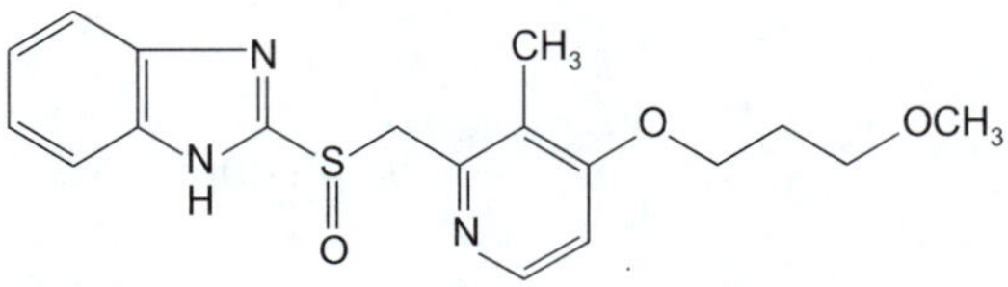

SYNTHESIS AND DRUG PROFILE

I. a. H_2-receptor Antagonists

Mode of action: These drugs inhibit the acid production by reversibly competing with histamine for the binding with H_2-receptor on the basolateral membrane of parietal cells. The most predominant effect of H_2-receptor antagonist is on basal acid secretion. Histamine on H_2-receptors produces cAMP-dependent protein kinase to elicit the response in the gastrointestinal tract (GIT). The H_2-antagonists reversibly bind the H_2-receptors and reduce the cAMP formation, which is responsible for the activation of proton pump and subsequently reduces the gastric acid formation in the GIT.

i. Cimetidine (Tagamet)

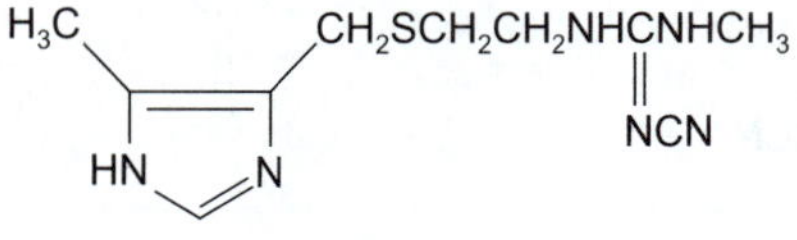

Synthesis

Route I. From: Ethyl-5-methyl-imidazole-4-carboxylate

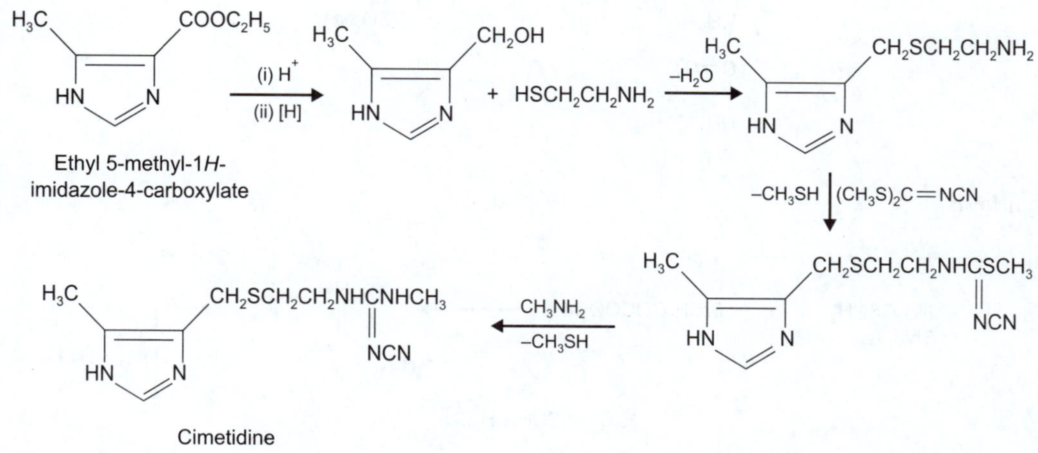

Route II: From: Ethyl-2-chloro acetoacetate

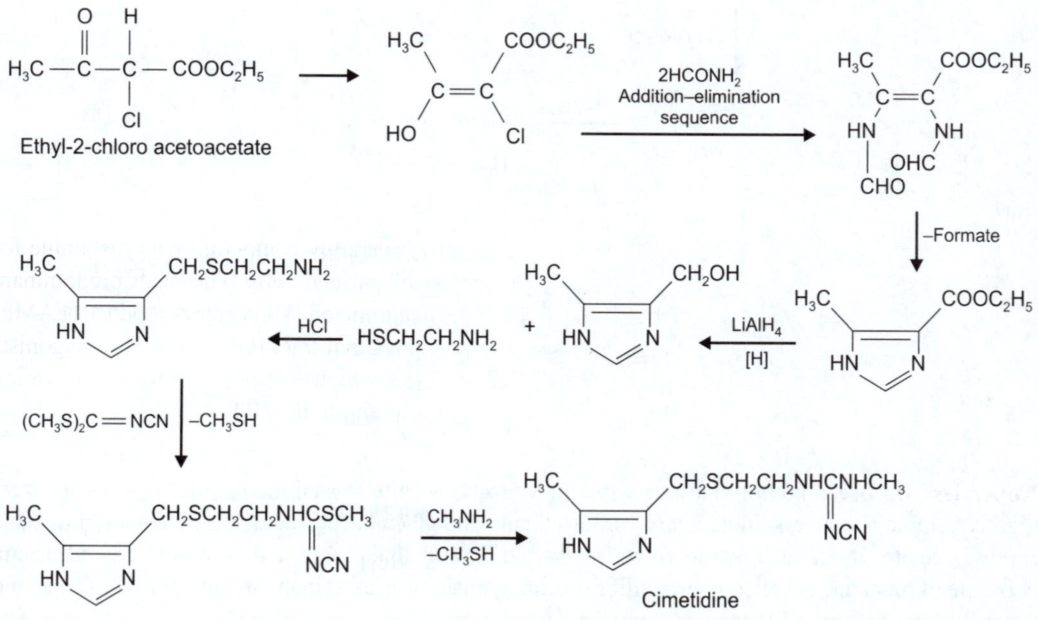

Properties and uses: Cimetidine hydrochloride is a white crystalline powder, soluble in water, and sparingly soluble in ethanol. It is a H_2-receptor antagonist that not only inhibits gastric acid secretion, but also prevents other actions of histamine mediated by H_2-receptors. It is used in the treatment of peptic ulceration. Cimetidine has a weak antiandrogenic effect. Gynaecomastia may occur in patients treated for a month or more.

Assay: Dissolve the substance in a mixture of 0.01 M HCl and alcohol (1:10) and titrate against 0.1 M sodium hydroxide. Determine the end point potentiometrically.

Dose: Oral dose is 200 mg thrice a day with meals and 400 mg at night.

ii. Famotidine (Famocid, Famtac)

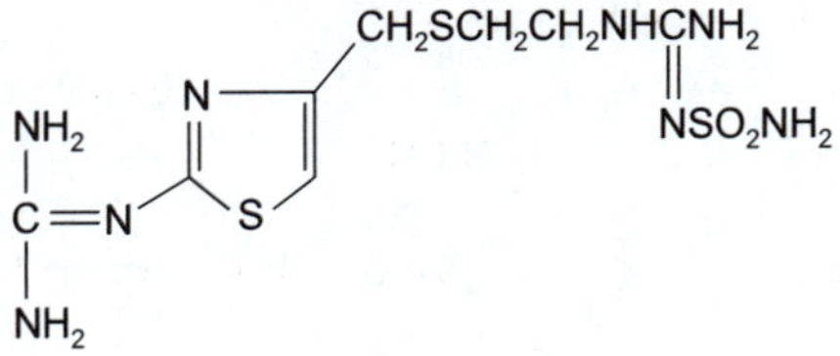

Synthesis

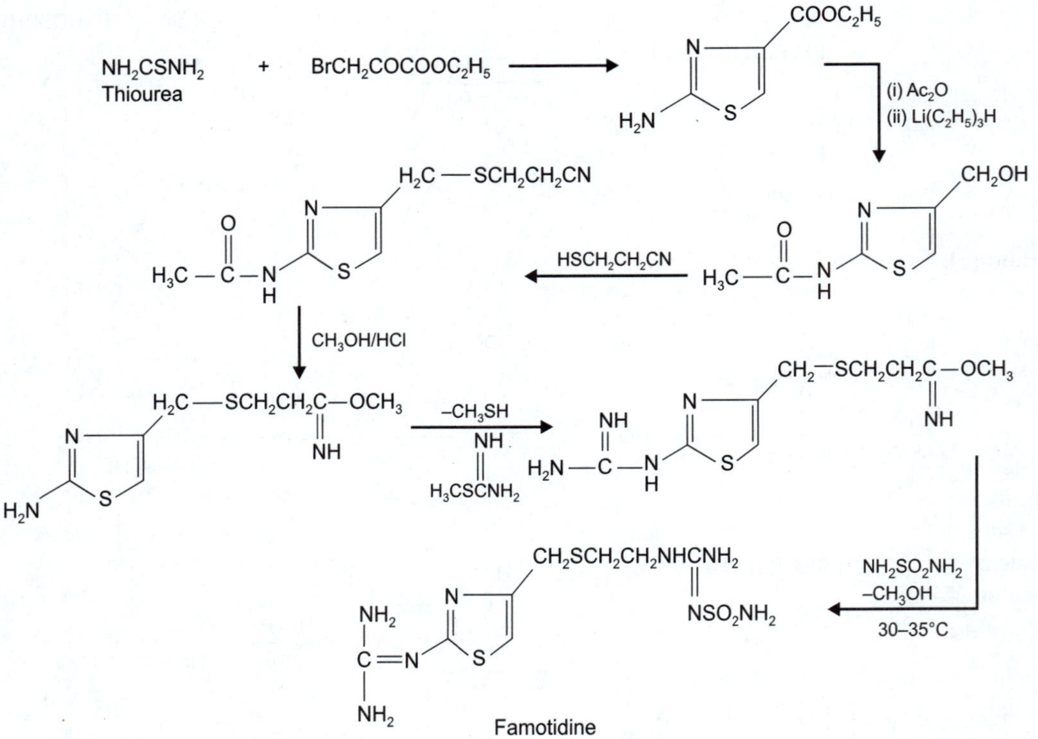

Properties and uses: Famotidine is a white or yellowish-white crystalline powder or crystals, very slightly soluble in water, soluble in anhydrous ethanol and glacial acetic acid, but practically insoluble in ethyl acetate. It acts as a competitive, reversible H_2-antagonist with a slow onset of equilibrium. This type of blockade is called non-equilibrium antagonism. It is used in the treatment of duodenal and gastric ulcers, Zollinger-Ellison syndrome, and heart burn.

Assay: Dissolve the sample in anhydrous acetic acid and titrate against 0.1 M perchloric acid. Determine the end point potentiometrically.

Dose: The dose for gastric or duodenal ulcer is 40 mg at night for 4–8 weeks. The dose for prophylaxis or relapse is 20 mg at night. Not recommended for usage in children.

Dosage forms: Famotidine tablets BP.

iii. Ranitidine (Zantac)

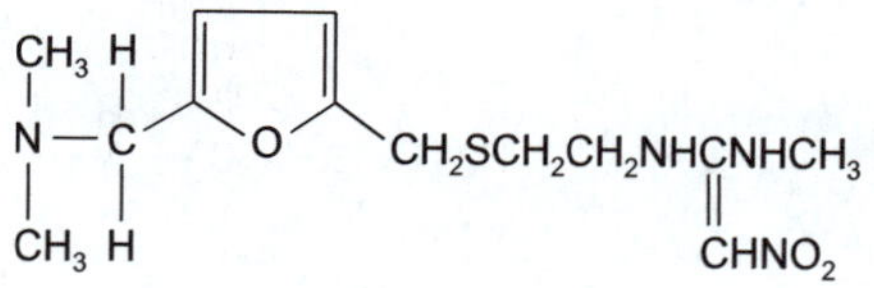

Synthesis

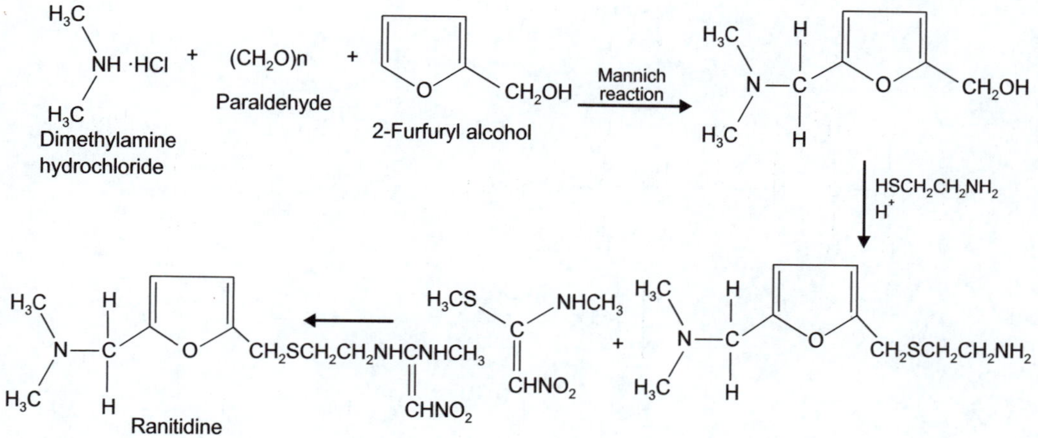

Properties and uses: Ranitidine hydrochloride is a white or pale yellow crystalline powder, soluble in water, slightly soluble in anhydrous ethanol and methylene chloride. In Ranitidine, the imidazole ring of cimitidine was replaced by furan in conjugation with some rearrangement of the terminal functionality; the substituted guanidine group has been isosterically modified by utilizing a nitromethenyl moiety to basicity. It is used in the treatment of duodenal ulcer, gastric ulcer, and pathological hypersecretory conditions.

Metabolism of cimetidine, ranitidine, and famotidine: Hydroxylation of the imidazole C-4 methyl group of cimitidine occurs. Ranitidine is excreted largely unchanged, but minor metabolic pathways include N-demethylation as well as N- and S-oxidation. The metabolites are thought not as contributing to the therapeutic properties of parent drugs, with the exception of nizanidine, from which the N-demethyl metabolites retains H_2-antihistamine activity.

Assay: Dissolve the sample in water and titrate against 0.1 M sodium hydroxide. Determine the end point potentiometrically.

Dose: The dose is 150 mg (as the hydrochloride) two times a day.

Dosage forms: Ranitidine HCl injection IP, ranitidine HCl tablets IP, ranitidine injection BP, ranitidine oral solution BP, ranitidine tablets BP.

iv. Etintidine

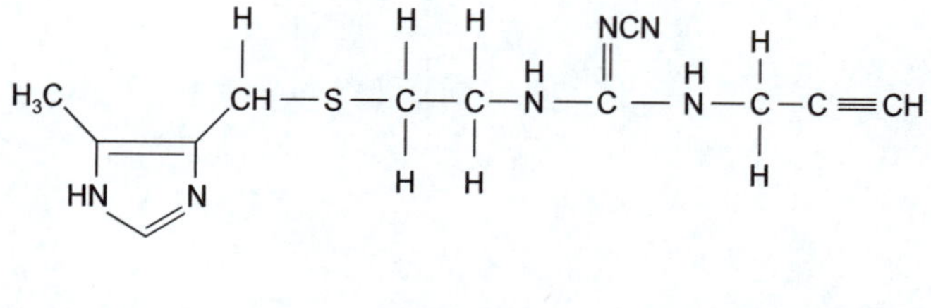

Synthesis

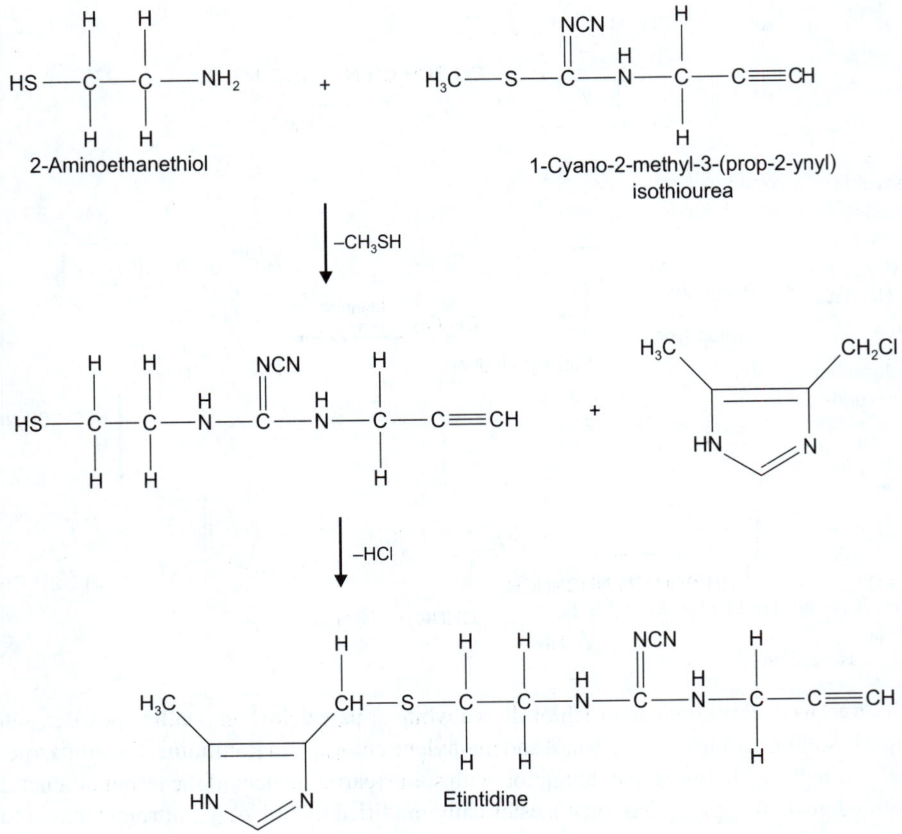

Uses: Used as antiulcer and it is twice as active as cimetidine.

v. Oxmetidine

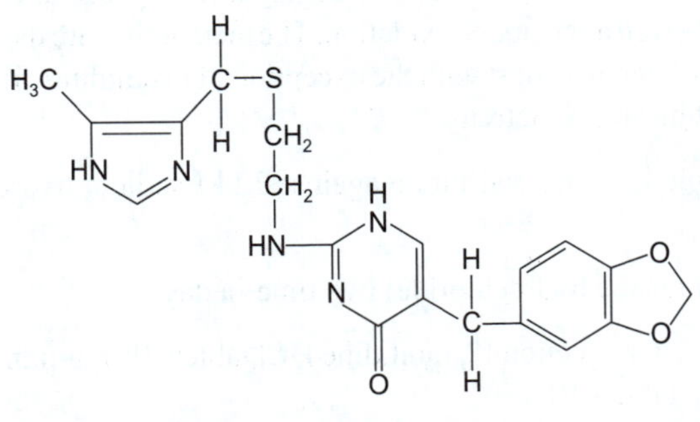

5-(Benzo[d][1,3]dioxol-5-yl methyl)-2-(2-((5-methyl-1*H*-imidazol-4-yl) methylthio)ethylamino)pyrimidin-4(1*H*)-one

Synthesis

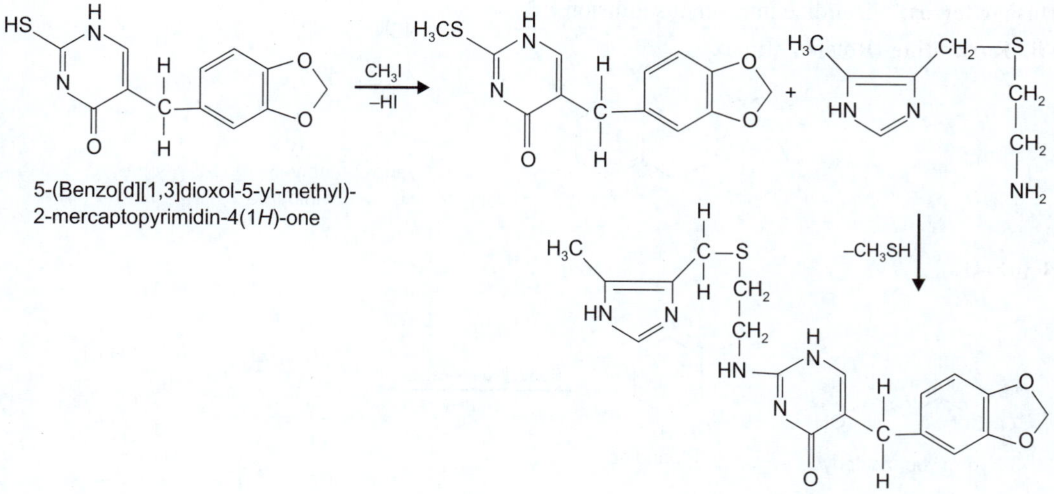

5-(Benzo[d][1,3]dioxol-5-yl-methyl)-2-mercaptopyrimidin-4(1*H*)-one

Oxmetidine

Properties and uses: It shows a time-dependent and slow onset of action, which differentiates it from ranitidine. It is reported to have histamine H_2-receptor blocking activity.

vi. Nizatidine

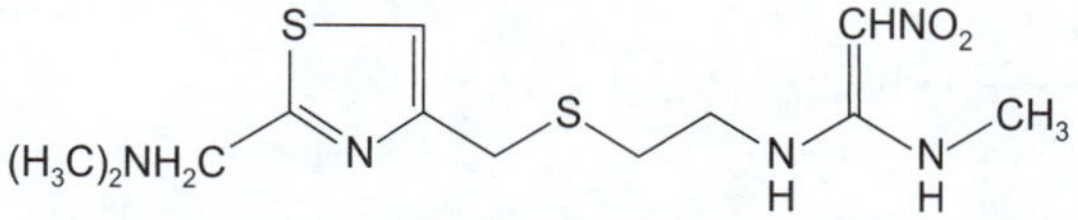

N,N-Dimethyl-4-((2-(1-(methylamino)-2-nitrovinylamino) ethylthio)methyl)thiazol-2-methyl amine

Synthesis

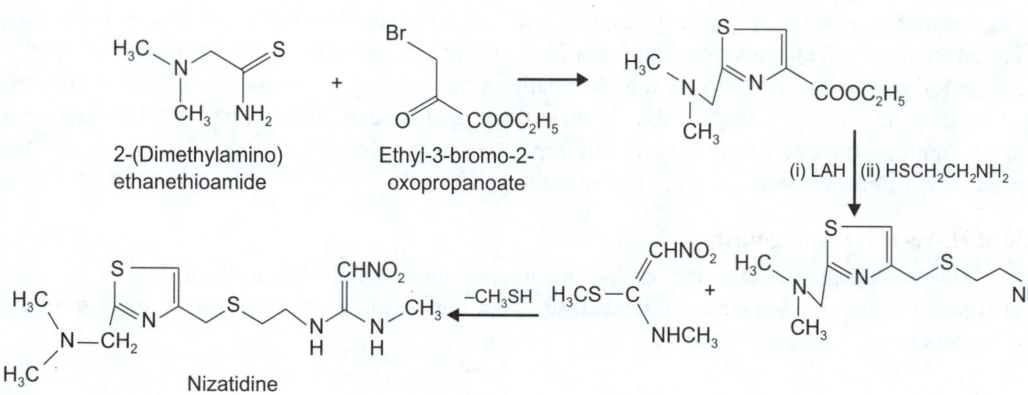

2-(Dimethylamino) ethanethioamide

Ethyl-3-bromo-2-oxopropanoate

Nizatidine

Properties and uses: Nizatidine is a white or slightly brownish crystalline powder, sparingly soluble in water, and soluble in methanol. It is used as histamine H_2-receptor antagonist in the treatment of peptic ulcer.

Assay: It is assayed by adopting liquid chromatography techniques.

Dosage forms: Nizatidine intravenous infusion BP.

vii. Roxatidine (Rotane, Zorpex)

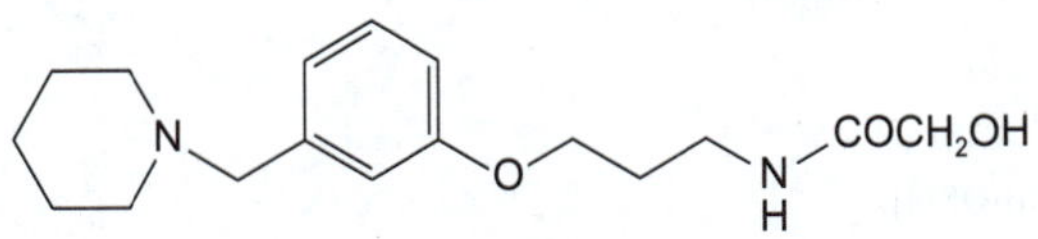

Synthesis

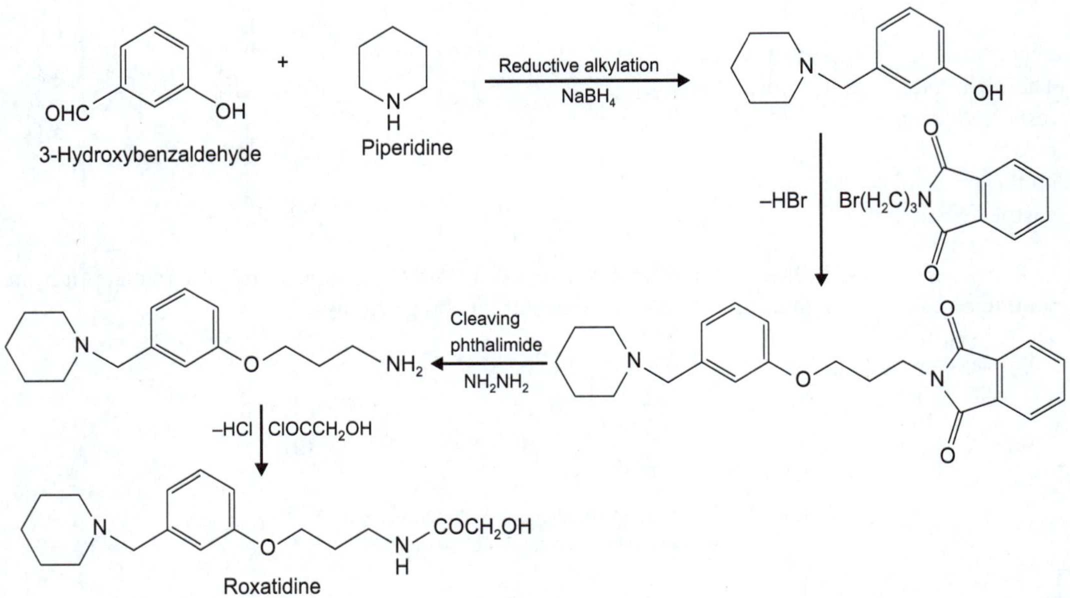

Dose and uses: Oral dose for peptic ulcer for adults is 150 mg at bedtime or 75 mg twice a day for 4–6 weeks; maintenance dose is 75 mg at bedtime. Dose for gastroesophageal reflux disease/oesophagitis, including erosions and ulcerations for adults is 75 mg twice a day or 150 mg at bedtime for 6–8 weeks. The dose for gastritis for adults is 75 mg once daily in the evening. For Zollinger-Ellison syndrome, the dose for adult is 75 mg twice a day. In anaesthetic premedication for adults, the dose is 75 mg in the evening on the day before surgery and repeated every 2 hrs before induction of anaesthesia, alternatively, 150 mg once on the night before surgery.

SAR of H_2-receptor Antagonists

The H_2-receptor antagonists were the result of the international modification of the histamine structure and deliberate search for a chemically-related substance that would act as competitive inhibitor of the H_2-receptors.

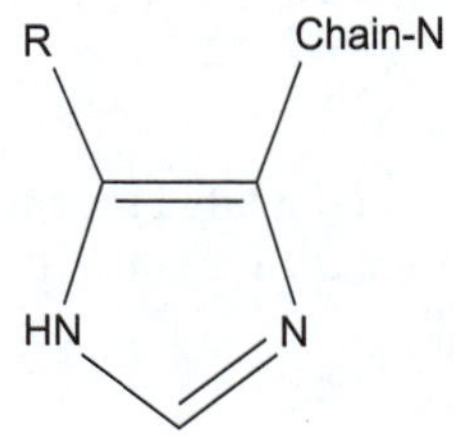

- Imidazole ring is not the only required ring for competitive antagonism of histamine H_2-receptors. Other heterocyclic rings (furan, thiophene, thiazole, etc.) that enhance the potency and selectivity of H_2-receptor antagonism can be used.
- The ring and terminal nitrogen should be separated by four carbon atoms for optimum antagonistic activity. The isosteric thioether link is also present in certain drugs.
- The terminal nitrogen group should be polar, non-basic substituents for maximal antagonist activity. In general, antagonistic activity varies inversely with the hydrophilic character of the nitrogen group (exception ranitidine and nizatidine).

I. b. Proton Pump Inhibitors

Mode of action: These drugs suppress gastric acid secretion through H^+-K^+- ATPase pump, the two major signalling pathways that are present with the parietal cells, that is, cAMP-dependent and Ca^{2+}. The respective receptors for the actions are M_3 and H_2. These receptors are modulated through the respective ionic mechanism and elicited by the acetylcholine from M_3 and histamine from H_2 receptor for release of the gastric acid mediated through H^+-K^+-ATPase pump. The proton pump inhibitors act on these receptors and inhibit H^+-K^+-ATPase, and reduce the activation of parietal cells to release the gastric acid.

i. **Omeprazole** (Ocid, Omez, Omicap)

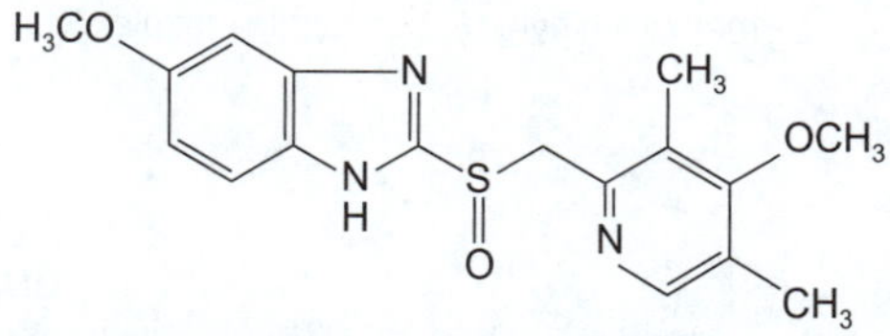

5-Methoxy-2-((4-methoxy-3,5-dimethylpyridin-2-yl)
methylsulfinyl) benzimidazole

Synthesis

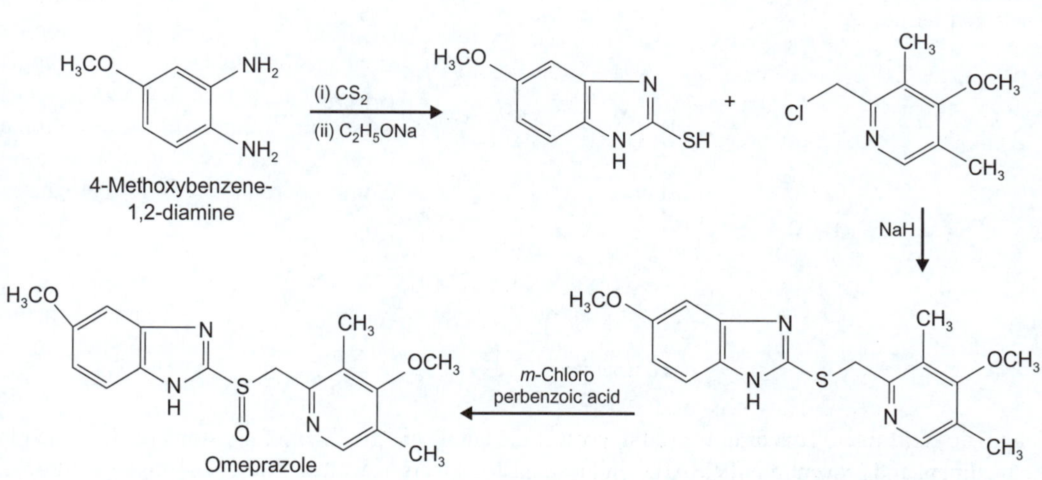

Properties and uses: Omeprazole sodium is a white hygroscopic powder, soluble in water, alcohol, and propylene glycol, very slightly soluble in methylene chloride. It is used in the treatment of duodenal ulcer, gastric ulcer, and pathological hypersecretory conditions.

Assay: Dissolve the sample in water and titrate against 0.1 M HCl. Determine the endpoint potentiometrically.

Dose: The oral dose for NSAID-associated duodenal or gastric ulcer, gastroduodenal erosions, and prophylaxis in patients with history of gastroduodenal lesions for adult is 20 mg daily. For prophylaxis of acid aspiration during anaesthesia, the dose for adults, initially, is 40 mg given in the evening before surgery and another dose is 40 mg 2–6 hrs before the procedure. For acid-related dyspepsia, the dose for adults is 10 or 20 mg daily for 2–4 weeks. For peptic ulcer, the dose for adult is 20 mg daily as a single dose or 40 mg daily in severe cases. Duration of treatment for duodenal ulcers is 4 weeks; gastric ulcers is 8 weeks. Maintenance dose is 10–20 mg once daily. Capsule/tablet should be swallowed whole, do not crush or chew. Eradication of *H. pylori* infection: Dose for this treatment for adults varies with regimen, that is, 20 mg once daily or 40 mg a day as single or in two divided doses, and requires combination therapy with antibiotics.

ii. Lansoprazole (Lancid, Lancus, Lansec)

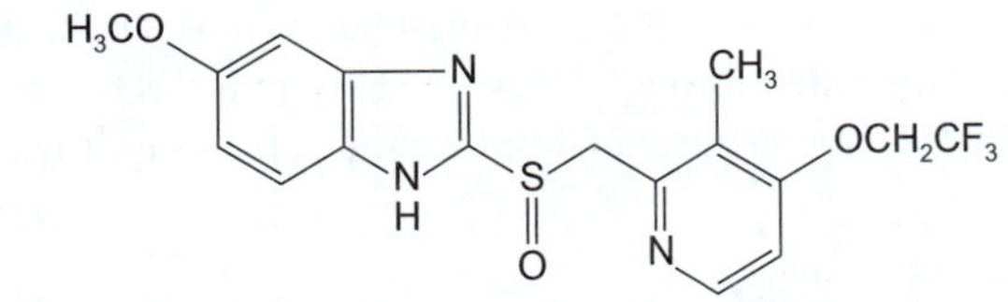

5-Methoxy-2-((3-methyl-4-(2,2,2-trifluoroethoxy)pyridin-2-yl) methylsulfinyl)-1*H*-benzo[d]imidazole

Synthesis

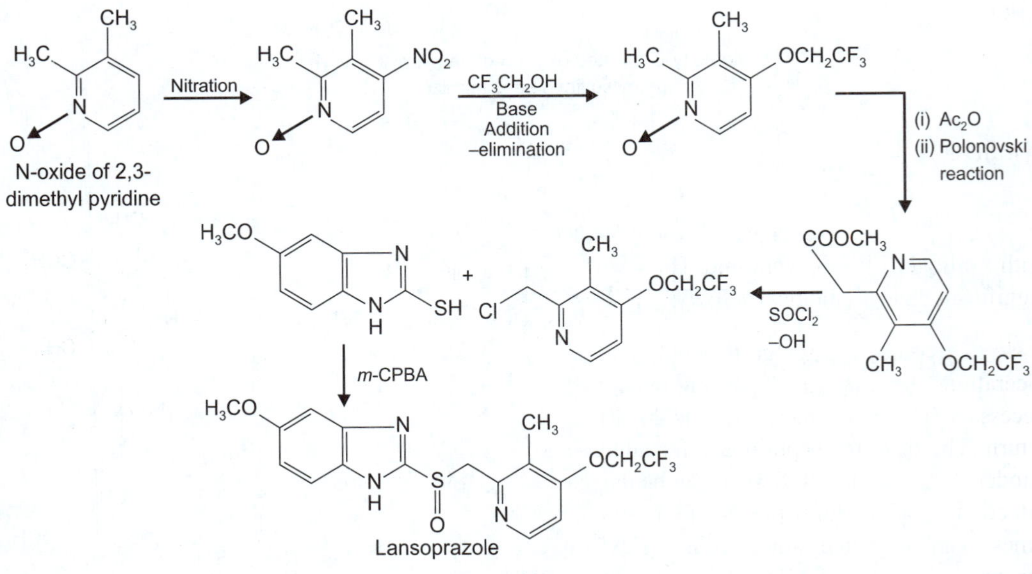

Properties and uses: This drug is used to protect the acidic environment in the stomach. It is used in the treatment and prevention of NSAIDs-induced gastric ulcers as well as Zollinger-Ellison syndrome.

Dose: The oral dose for pathological hypersecretory conditions for example, Zollinger-Ellison syndrome, for adults initially is 60 mg daily and adjusted as required, daily doses greater than 120 mg should be given in two divided doses. For acid-related dyspepsia for adults, the dose is 15–30 mg once daily in the morning for 2–4 weeks. For peptic ulcer, the dose for adults is 30 mg once daily in the morning, given for 4 weeks (duodenal ulcer) or for 8 weeks (gastric ulcer). For NSAID-associated ulceration and prevention of NSAID-induced ulcers, the dose for adults is 15–30 mg daily for 4–8 weeks. For the eradication of *H. pylori* infection, the dose for adults is 1-week triple therapy, that is, 30 mg two times a day combined with clarithromycin 500 mg two times a day and either amoxicillin 1 g two times a day or metronidazole 400 mg two times aday.

iii. Pantoprazole (Pantop, Pantodac, Pantocid)

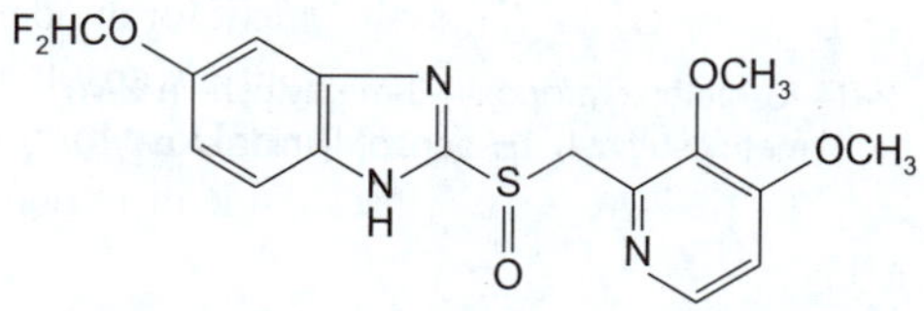

5-(Difluoromethoxy)-2-((3,4-dimethoxypyridin-2-yl)methylsulfinyl)-1*H*-benzo[d]imidazole

Synthesis

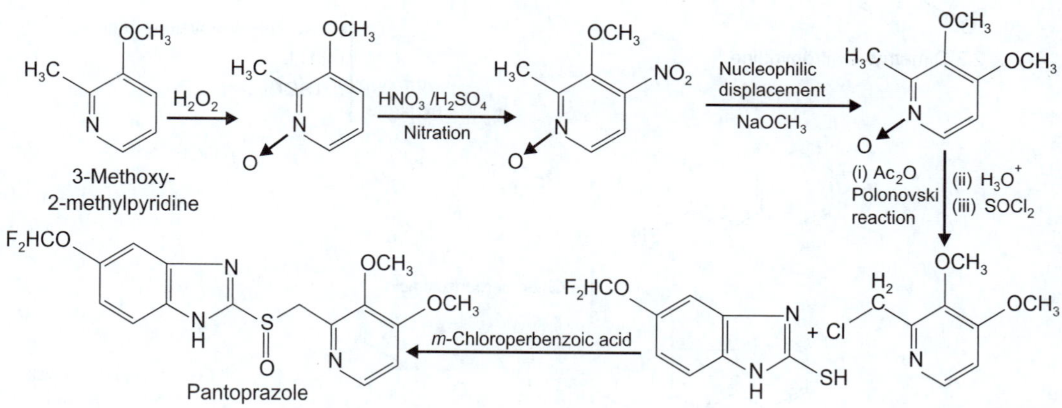

Properties and uses: It is used in the treatment of pathological hypersecretory conditions associated with Zollinger-Ellison syndrome. There is no evidence that any of the pantoprazole metabolites have significant pharmacological activity.

Dose: The oral dose for gastroesophageal reflux disease and oesophagitis, including erosions and ulcerations, for adults is 20–40 mg once daily in the morning for 4 weeks, increased to 8 weeks, if necessary. The maintenance dose is 20–40 mg daily increased to 40 mg each morning, if symptoms return. The dose for peptic ulcer for adults is 40 mg once daily in the morning for 2–4 weeks for duodenal ulceration or 4–8 weeks for benign gastric ulceration. The dose for the eradication of *H. Pylori* infection for adults for triple therapy is 40 mg twice a day combined with clarithromycin 500 mg two times a day and either amoxicillin 1 g twice a day or metronidazole 400 mg twice a day. The dose for prophylaxis of NSAIDs-associated peptic ulcer for adults is 20 mg daily. For Zollinger-Ellison syndrome and other hypersecretory states, the adult dose initially is 80 mg daily, adjusted to individual requirements. Maximum daily dose is 240 mg daily. Daily doses greater than 80 mg should be given in two divided doses.

- **Intravenous:** The intravenous dose for Zollinger–Ellison syndrome and other hypersecretory states for adults is 80 mg (as the Na salt) daily over 2–15 min. Maximum doses are 240 mg daily in divided doses, if rapid control is required. In the cases of peptic ulcer, gastroesophageal reflux disease, oesophagitis, including erosions and ulcerations the adult dose is 40 mg (as the Na salt) daily (over 2–15 min) until the patient can be resumed.

iv. Rabeprazole (Rabeloc, Rabifast, Rabitop)

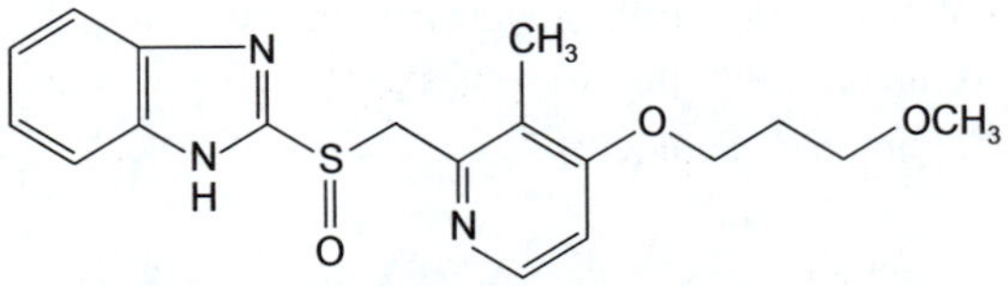

2-((4-(3-Methoxypropoxy)-3-methylpyridin-2-yl) methylsulfinyl)-1*H*-benzo[d]imidazole

Synthesis

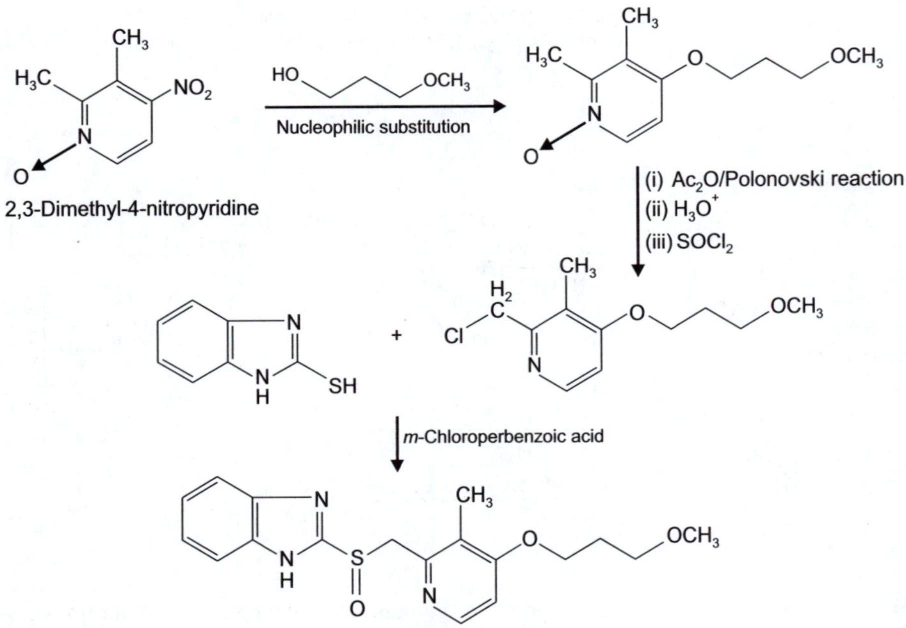

Rabeprazole

Uses: It is used in gastric hypersecretory disorders.

Dose: The dose for pathological hypersecretory conditions, for example, Zollinger-Ellison syndrome, for adults initially is 60 mg daily, adjusted according to response. Maximum dose is 120 mg daily. For active peptic ulcer diseases for adults is 20 mg daily given for 4–8 weeks for duodenal ulcer and 6–12 weeks for gastric ulcer. In the case of eradication of *H. Pylori* infection the dose for adults as a combination with antibacterials is 20 mg twice a day combined with clarithromycin 500 mg twice a day and either amoxicillin 1 g twice a day or metronidazole 400 mg twice a day to be taken for a week.

Metabolism of proton pump inhibitors: Metabolism of omeprazole and other proton pump inhibitors occurs primarily in the liver. The sulphonated, hydroxylated, and *o*-demethylated metabolites have been reported as products. The oxidative metabolism of omeprazole is catalyzed principally by CYP2C19 (primarily 5'-hydroxylation and to a lesser extent, benzimidazole *o*-demethylation).

Different proton pump inhibitors depend differently on CYP2C19 for the oxidative metabolism, and the enantiomer show variation of independence on CYP2C19 and other pathways. Pantaprazole and lansoprazole show greater metabolism via CYP2C19. The enantiomer being affected differently than rabeprazole, which is metabolized only to a small extent by oxidative CYP450 enzyme.

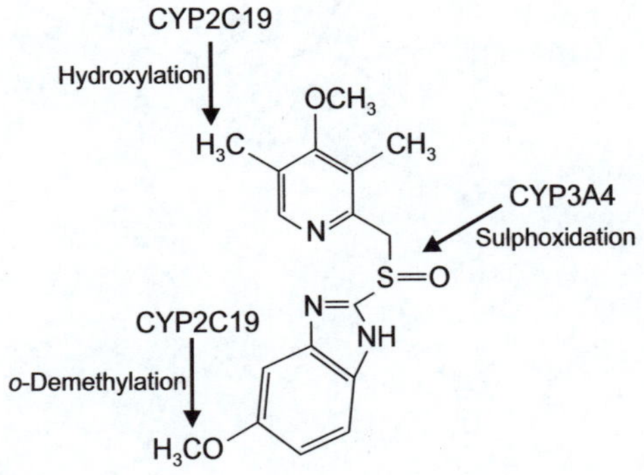

CLASSIFICATION BASED ON PCI SYLLABUS

Cimetidine

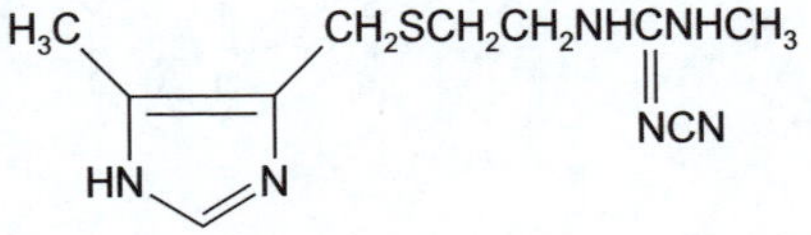

Famotidine

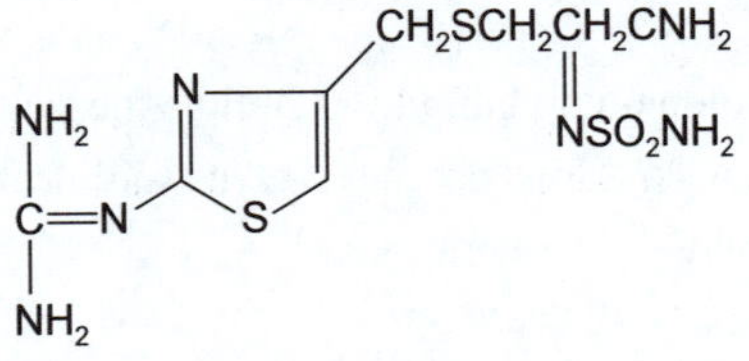

Ranitidine

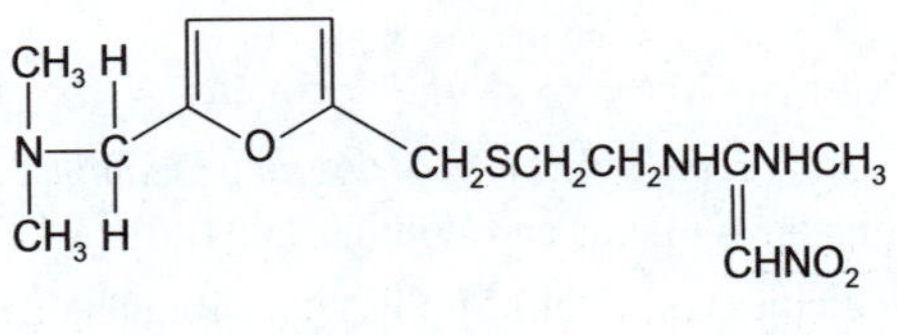

GASTRIC PROTON PUMP INHIBITORS

Omeprazole

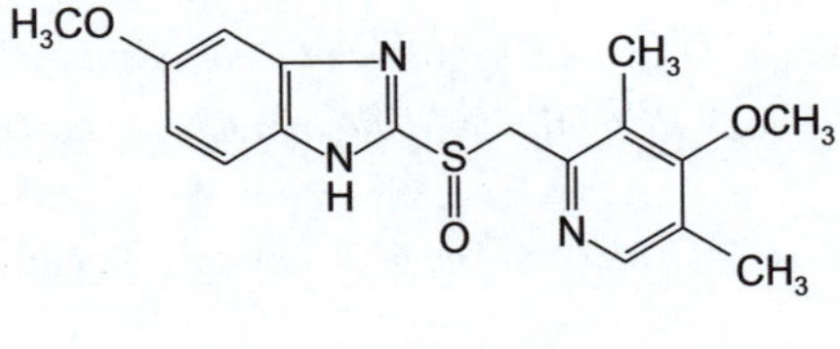

Lansoprazole

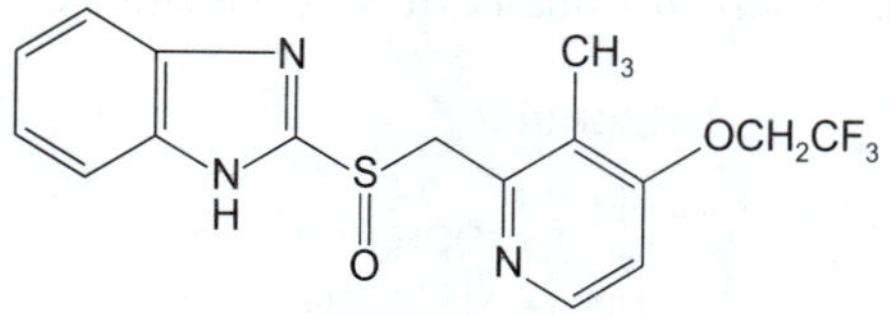

Rabeprazole

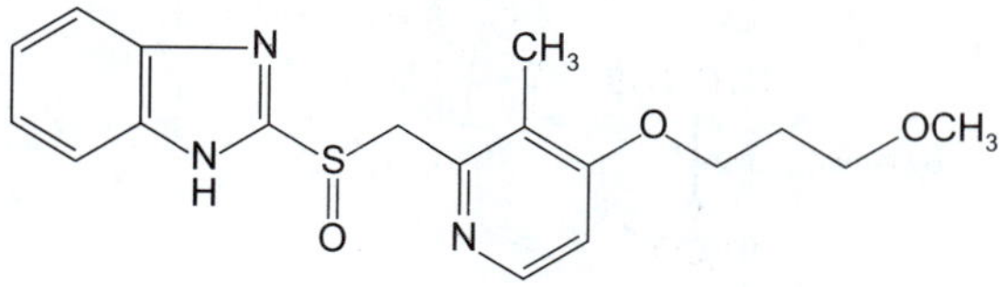

Pantoprazole

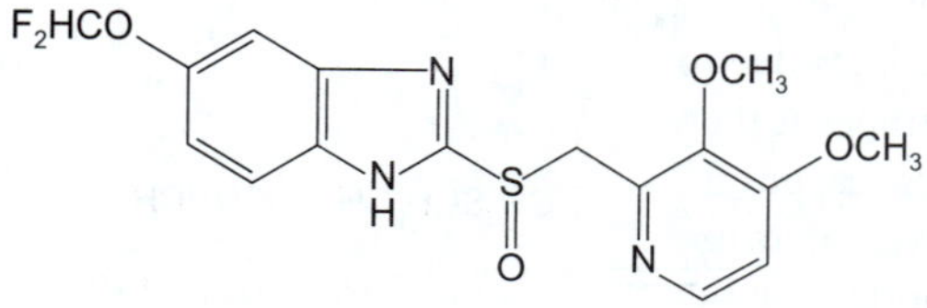

PROBABLE QUESTIONS

1. Define and classify antiulcer agents with one example in each category and write the synthesis and uses of one of them.
2. Write the mode of action of proton pump inhibitors. Outline the synthesis and uses of lansoprazole.
3. What are H_2-receptor antagonists? How do they act as antiulcer agents? Describe the synthesis, metabolism, and uses of ranitidine.
4. Write a short note on anti-*H. pylori* drugs.
5. Name the thiazole and imidazole containing H_2-blockers and write the synthesis, metabolism, and uses of one of them.

SUGGESTED READINGS

1. Block JH and Beale JM. *Wilson Gisvold's Textbook of Organic Medicinal and Pharmaceutical Chemistry* (11th edn). New York: Lippincott Williams and Wilkins, 2004.
2. *British Pharmacopoeia*. Medicines and Healthcare Products Regulatory Agency. London, 2008.
3. Bruntan LL, Lazo JS, and Parker KL. *Goodman and Gilman's: The Pharmacological Basis of Therapeutics* (11th edn). New York: McGraw Hill, 2006.
4. Gennaro AR. *Remington: The Science and practice of Pharmacy* (21st edn). New York: Lippincot Williams and Wilkins, 2006.
5. *Indian Pharmacopoeia*. Ministry of Health and Family Welfare. New Delhi, 1996.
6. Lednicer D and Mitscher LA. *The Organic Chemistry of Drug Synthesis*. New York: John Wiley, 1995.
7. Lemke TL and William DA. *Foye's Principle of Medicinal Chemistry* (6th edn). New York: Lippincott Williams and Wilkins, 2008.
8. Wolff ME. *Burger's Medicinal Chemistry and Drug Discovery* (5th edn). New York: John Wiley, 1995.

CHAPTER 6

Antidiarrhoeals

INTRODUCTION

Diarrhoea means loose bowel movements resulting into the frequent passage of watery, uniformed stools with or without mucous and blood. This condition may arise due to the change in the nature of the diet and routine or sometimes due to bacterial infection. The former type of diarrhoea is the mild form while the infective diarrhoea is more powerful and persistent. Organism escapes from gastric acid and other digestive processes reaches the bowel. Their metabolic products irritate the nerve ending of intestinal wall leading to severe diarrhoea. In this condition, to compensate the loss of body fluids, a mixture of salt (sodium chloride or sodium bicarbonate) and water is to be given frequently. The simple type of diarrhoea may be controlled just by using intestinal adsorbents while infected diarrhoea needs the use of intestinal antiseptics.

ADSORBENTS

These substances have the power of adsorbing gases, bacteria, and toxins without undergoing any chemical reaction. They also posses the protective property apart from their adsorbent action. They form a coating over the intestinal mucosa to reduce its irritation, examples of this category are kaolin, calcium carbonate, magnesium trisilicate, and aluminium hydroxide, pectin, bismuth subsalicylate and polycarbophill and various psyllium seed derivatives.

1. **Diphenoxylate HCl** (Lemotil)

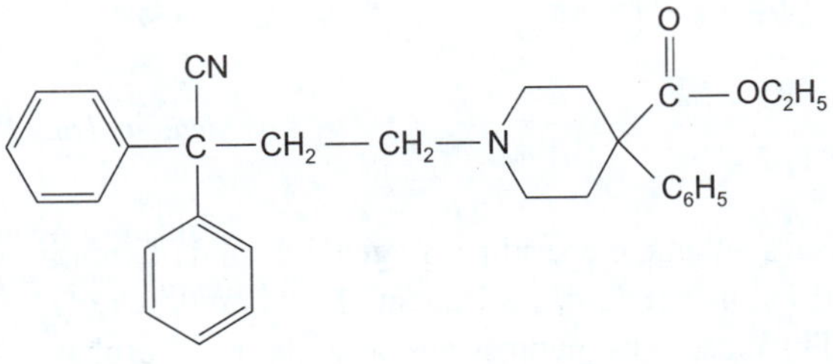

Synthesis

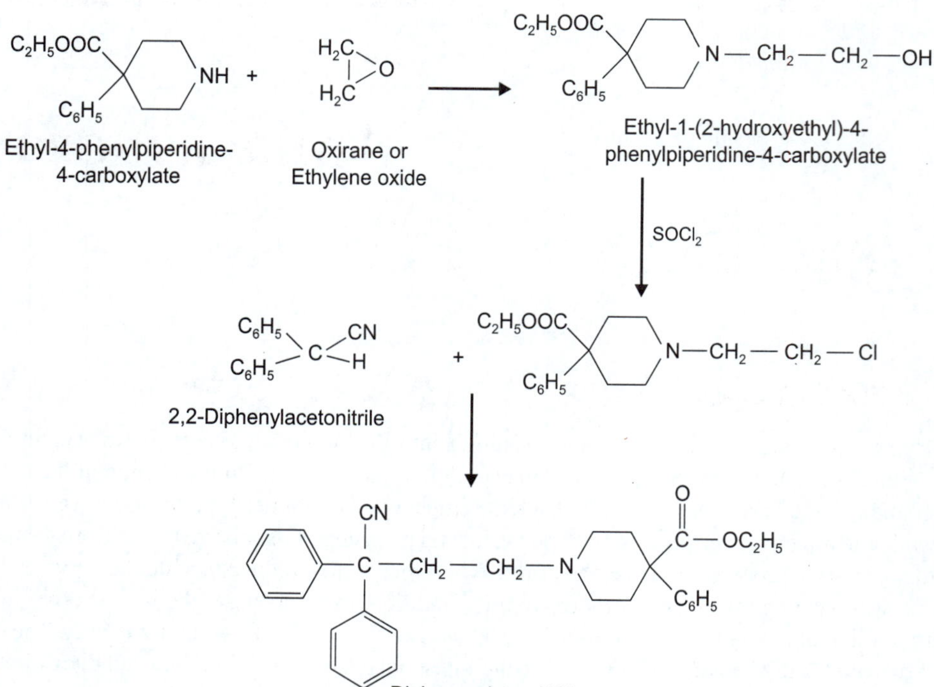

Diphenoxylate . HCl

Properties and uses: It is a weak meperidine congener lacking analgesic activity. It is used for the symptomatic activity of diarrhoea in patients with mild chronic inflammatory bowel disease and for infectious gastroenteritis.

Dose: The usual adult dose orally is 5 mg four times a day.

2. Loperamide

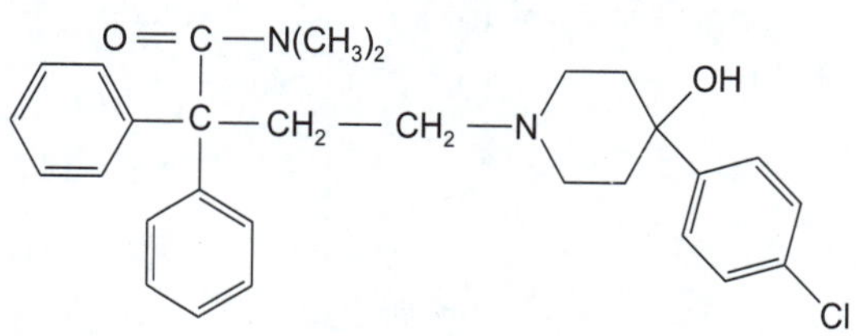

Properties and uses: It is a synthetic meperidine congener devoid of sedative or respiratory depressant actions. It is orally used as an antidiarrhoeal agent. Loperamide exerts spasmolytic effect on the gastrointestinal tract (GIT) muscle by depressing slow cholinergic phase and rapid prostaglandin-mediated phase of smooth muscle contraction. It may act on the intestinal nerve endings or on the ganglia.

INTESTINAL ANTISEPTICS

These agents are used to treat severe diarrhoeal forms, which are due to microbial infection. They mainly comprise of certain members of the sulphonamides and antibiotics that are poorly absorbable in the GIT, and thus, reach in high concentrations to the small and large bowels. Examples are sulphasalazine, sulphaguanidine, phthalyl sulphathiazole, succinyl sulphathiazole. Various combinations of sulphonamides and antibiotics along with kaolin are available either in the form of cream or suspension. Streptomycin, neomycin, chloramphenicol, tetracyclines and nystatin are the examples of such antibiotics used for this purpose.

1. Antisecretory drugs

i. Sulphasalazine (salicylazosulphapyridine)

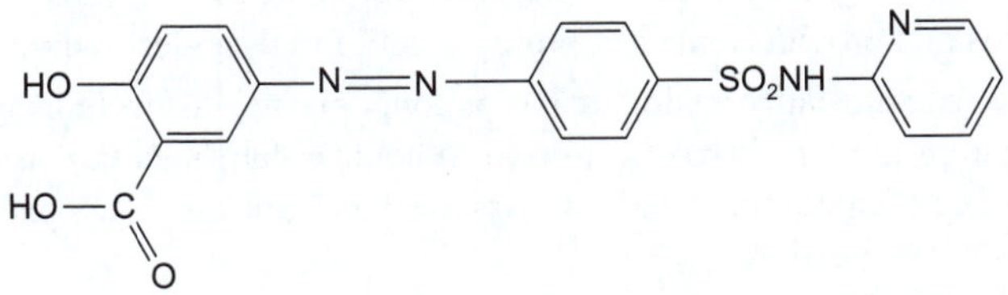

Synthesis

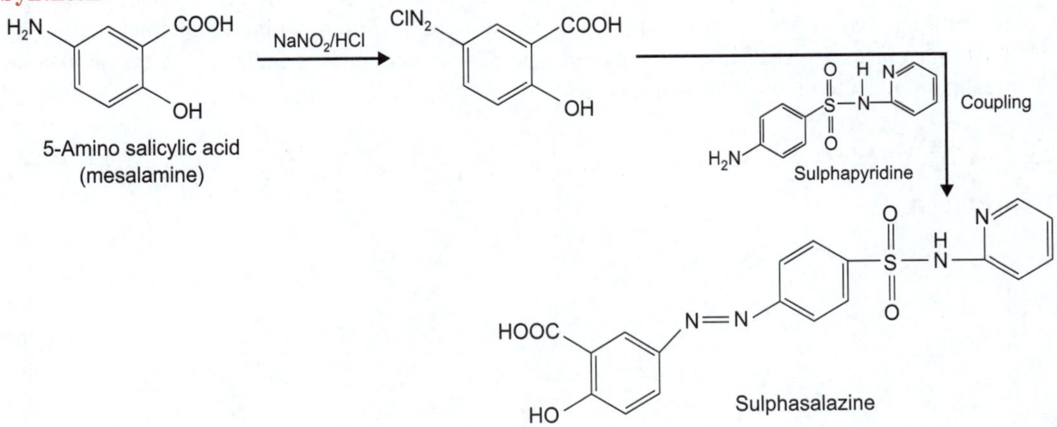

Metabolism: It undergoes reductive metabolism by gut bacteria, converting the drug into sulphapyridine and 5-amino salicylic acid, which are the active components.

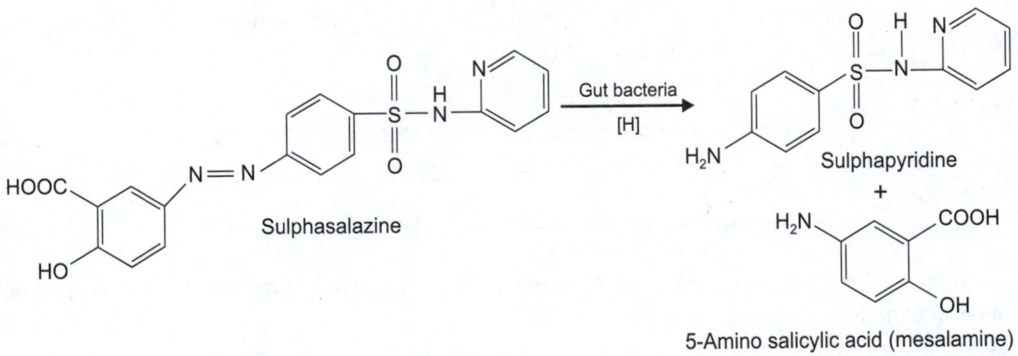

Properties and uses: Sulphasalazine is a bright yellow or brownish-yellow fine powder, practically insoluble in water and methylene chloride and sparingly soluble in alcohol. It dissolves in dilute solutions of alkali hydroxides and used in the treatment of inflammatory bowel diseases such as ulcerative colitis.

Assay: Dissolve and dilute the sample in 0.1 M sodium hydroxide and add 0.1 M acetic acid and measure the absorbance at the maxima of 359 nm using ultraviolet spectrophotometer.

Dosage forms:

i. Sulphasalazine tablets BP.

ii. **Bismuth subsalicylate:** It acts by decreasing prostaglandin synthesis in the intestinal mucosa, thereby reducing Cl^- secretion. It has some prophylatic value in traveller's diarrhoea (probably due to weak antibacterial action also), but it is rather inconvenient to carry and take.

iii. **Atropine:** Atropinic drugs can reduce bowel motility and secretion, but have poor efficacy in secretory diarrhoeas. They may benefit nervous/drug-(neostigmine, metaclopramide, reserpine) induced diarrhoeas and provide some symptomatic relief in dysenteries diverticulitis.

iv. **Octreotide:** This somatostatin analogue has a long plasma as well as potent antisecretory/antimotility action on the gut. It has been used to control diarrhoea in carcinoid and vasoactive intestinal peptide secreting tumours and for refractory diarrhoea in AIDS patients, but needs to be given by subcutaneous injections.

v. **Racecadotril:** This recently introduced prodrug is rapidly converted to thiorphan, an enkephalinase inhibitor. It prevents the degradation of endogenous enkephalins, which are mainly δ-opioid receptor agonists. Racecadotril decreases intestinal hypersecretion, without affecting motility by lowering mucosal cAMP due to enhanced enkephalins action. It is indicated in the short-term treatment of acute secretory diarrhoeas.

NEWER AGENTS

Telotristat ethyl

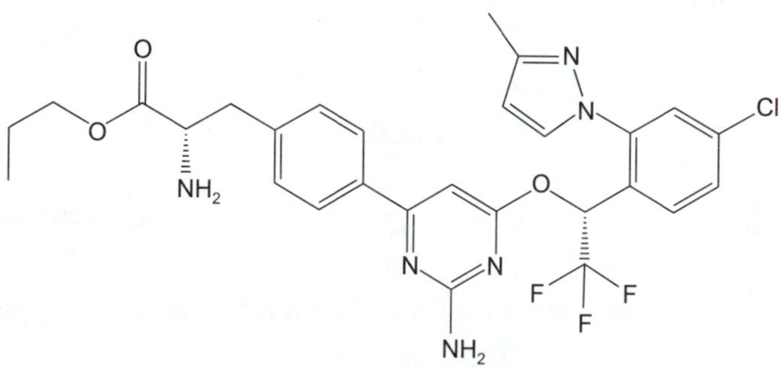

Uses: It is a prodrug of telotristat and used as combination therapy with somatastatin for the treatment of diarrhoea associated with carcinoid syndrome.

Plecanatide

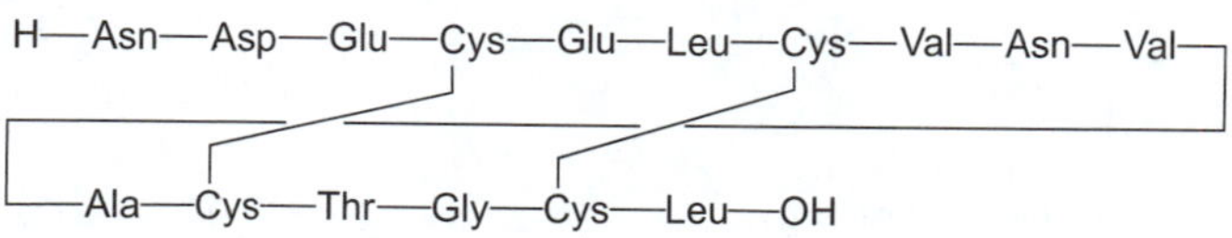

Uses: It is used for the treatment of chronic idiopathic constipation (CIC) and irritable bowel syndrome with constipation.

PROBABLE QUESTIONS

1. Define and classify antidiarrhoeal agents with suitable examples. Write the synthesis and uses of any two of them.
2. Write short notes on antisecretary drugs used in diarrhoea.
3. Write the synthesis of loperamide and diphenoxylate.

SECTION IV

Drugs Acting on Blood and Blood-Forming Organs

CHAPTER 7

Coagulants and Anticoagulants

INTRODUCTION

Haemostasis is the cessation of blood loss from damaged vessels. Platelets first adhere to macromolecules in the subendothelial regions of injured blood vessels; they aggregate to form the primary haemostatic plug. Platelets stimulate the local activation of plasma coagulation factors, leading to generation of a fibrin clot that reinforces the platelet aggregate. Later, as wound healing occurs, the platelet aggregates and fibrin clots are degraded. Thrombosis is a pathological process in which a platelet aggregates and a fibrin clot occludes blood vessels. Arterial thrombosis may result in ischaemic necrosis of tissues supplied by the artery (e.g. myocardial infarction due to thrombosis of coronary artery). Venous thrombosis may cause tissue drain by the vein to become edematous and inflamed.

Coagulation of blood comprises the formation of fibrin by a series of interactions among a large number of protein factors and other substances. Blood coagulation process requires coagulation factors, calcium, and phospholipids.

- The coagulation factors (proteins) are manufactured by the liver.
- Ionized calcium (Ca^{2+}) is available in the blood and forms intracellular sources.
- Phospholipids are prominent components of the cellular and platelet membranes. They provide a surface on which the chemical reactions of coagulation can take place. The coagulation factors are numbered in the order of their discovery.

  Factor I—fibrinogen

  Factor II—prothrombin

  Factor III—tissue thromboplastin (tissue factor)

  Factor IV—ionized calcium (Ca^{2+})

  Factor V—labile factor or proaccelerin

  Factor VI—unassigned

  Factor VII—stable factor or proconvertin

  Factor VIII—antihaemophilic factor

  Factor IX—plasma thromboplastin component, Christmas factor

  Factor X—Stuart-Prower factor

  Factor XI—plasma thromboplastin antecedent

  Factor XII—Hageman factor

  Factor XIII—fibrin stabilizing factor

MECHANISM OF BLOOD CLOTTING

Coagulation can be initiated by either of the two distinct pathways (Figure 7.1):

1. The intrinsic pathway can be initiated by events that take place within the lumen of blood vessels. This requires only elements (clotting factors, Ca^{2+} platelet surface, etc.) found within or intrinsic to the vascular system.
2. The extrinsic pathway is the other route to coagulation. It requires tissue factor (tissue thromboplastin), a substance that is extrinsic to or not normally cumulating in the vessel. Tissue factor is released when the vessel wall is ruptured.

1. **Calcium salts:** Calcium salts, especially Ca^{2+} intravenous injections, are very popular, but it does not help much unless there is deficiency of Ca^{2+} in the blood.

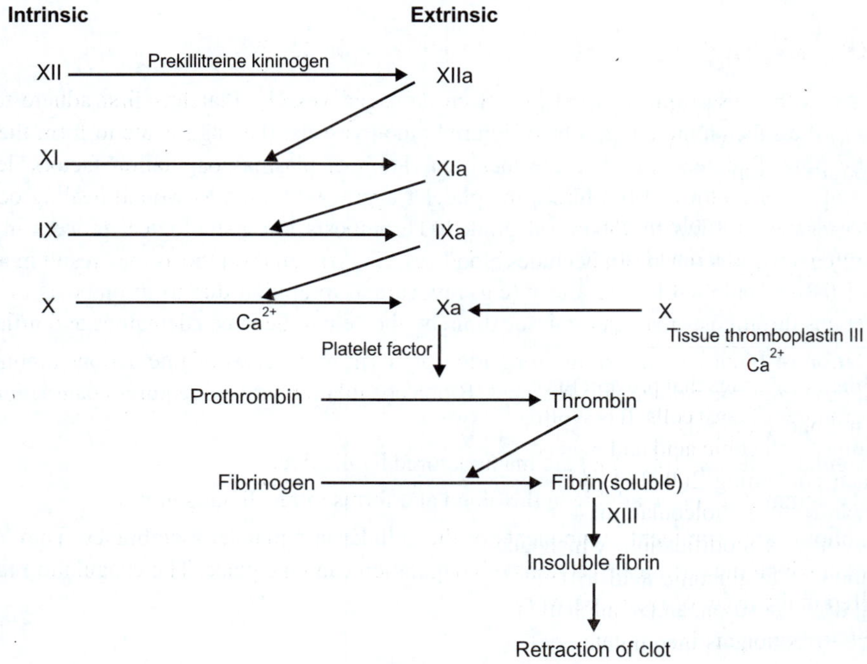

Figure 7.1: Mechanism of blood clotting.

2. **Vitamin K** (Synonym: Vitamin K_1—phytomenadione)

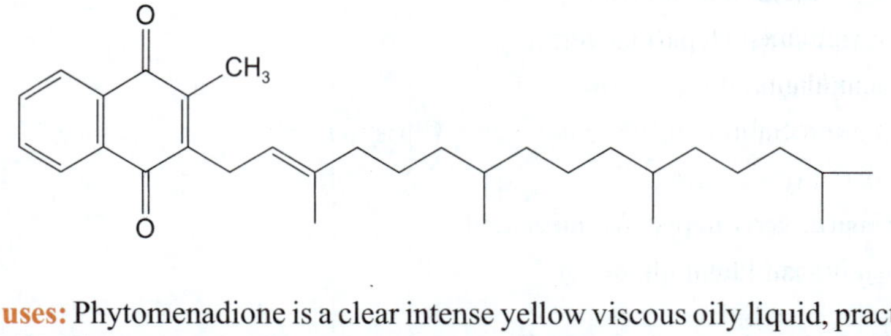

Properties and uses: Phytomenadione is a clear intense yellow viscous oily liquid, practically insoluble in water, sparingly soluble in ethanol, and miscible with fatty oils. Vitamin K is essential to keep up the prothrombin level in blood by forming prothrombin in the liver. Hence, it is used orally and intramuscular (IM), now water-soluble vitamin K is available for intravenous (IV) administration. This is called methyl naphthaquinone and is very useful in emergency.

Assay: It is assayed by adopting liquid chromatography technique.

Dosage forms: Phytomenadione injection BP, phytomenadione tablets BP.

3. **Vitamin K_3** (Menadione)

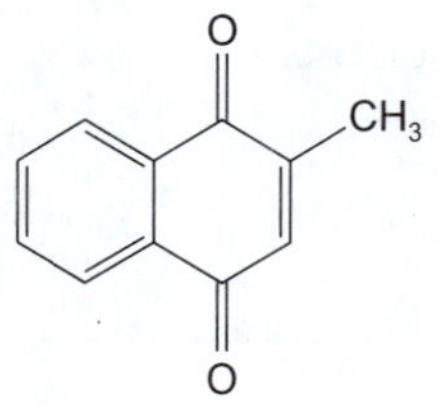

Properties and uses: Menadione is a pale-yellow crystalline powder, practically insoluble in water, soluble in toluene, sparingly soluble in alcohol and methanol. Used as source of vitamin K and has prothrombogenic property.

Assay: Dissolve the sample in glacial acetic acid and add dilute hydrochloric acid and zinc powder. Allow the mixture to stand and titrate against 0.1 M ammonium cerric nitrate using ferroin as indicator.

Anticoagulants

Anticoagulants are drugs that prevent the clotting of blood. Heparin is a glucosaminoglycan found in the secretory granules of mast cells. It is synthesized from uridine diphosphate sugar precursor as a polymer of alternating D-gluconic acid and *N*-acetyl-*D*-glucosamine residue. About 10–15 glucosaminoglycan chains, each containing 200–300 monosaccharide units, are attached to a core protein and yield a proteoglycan with a molecular mass of 750,000–1,000,000 daltons. The glucosaminoglycan then undergoes a series modification, which includes *n*-acetylation and *n*-sulphonation of glucosamine, epimerization of D-gluconic acid to L-iduronic acid, *o*-sulphation of iduronic and glucoronic acid residues at the C_2 position, and *o*-sulphation of glucosamine residue at C_3 and C_6 position. Each of these modification reactions is incomplete, yielding variety of oligosaccharide structures. After the heparin proteoglycan has been transported to the mast cell granule, an endo-β-D-glucuronidase degrades the glycosamionoglycan chains to 5000–30,000 dalton fragments over a period of hours.

CLASSIFICATION

Anticoagulants are classified as follows:

I. *In vitro* anticoagulants: Heparin, sodium oxalate, and sodium citrate

II. *In vivo* anticoagulants
   1. Heparin—injectable
   2. Oral
      a. Coumarin derivatives: Warfarin, bishydroxycoumarin
      b. Indandiones: Phenindione, diphenadion

I. *In vitro* Anticoagulants

Heparin, sodium citrate, sodium oxalate.

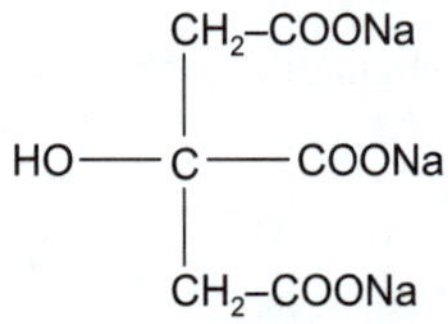
Sodium citrate

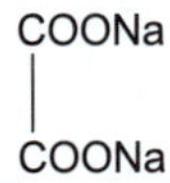
Sodium oxalate

II. *In vivo* Anticoagulants

a. Coumarin derivatives

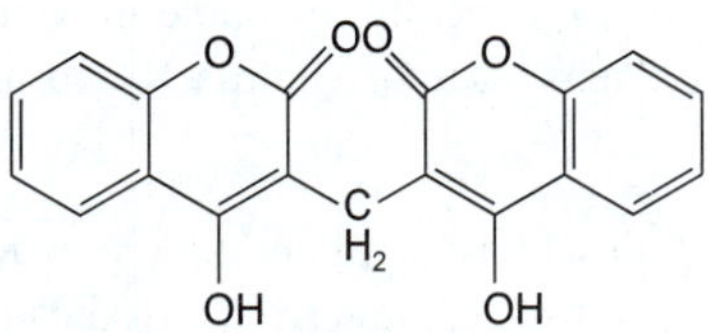
Dicoumarol

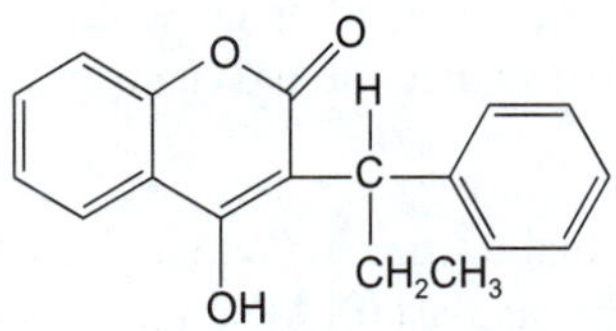
Phenprocoumon

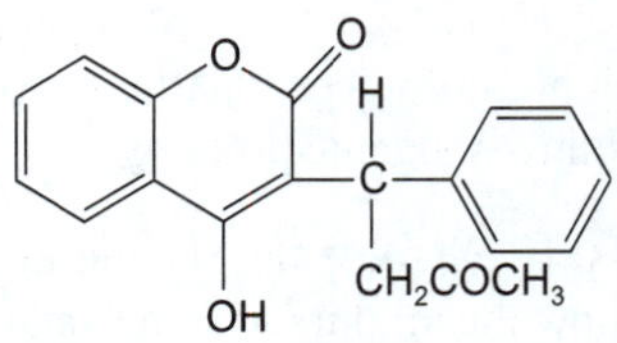
Warfarin

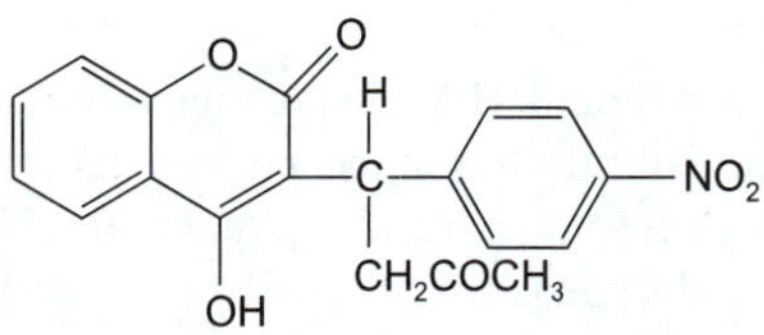
Acenocoumarol

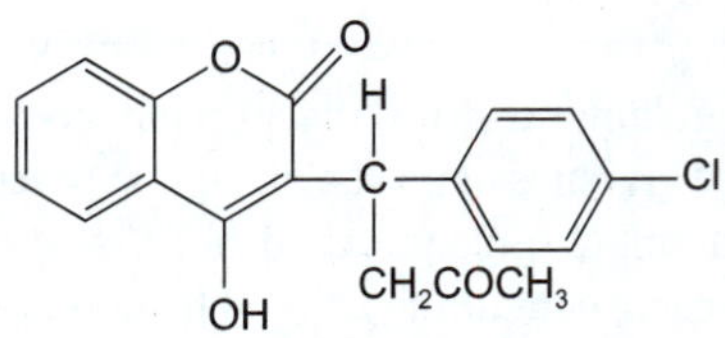
Coumachlor

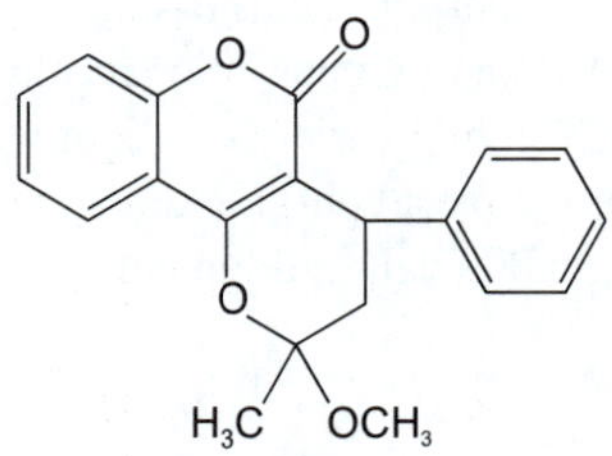
Cyclocoumarol

b. Indandione derivatives

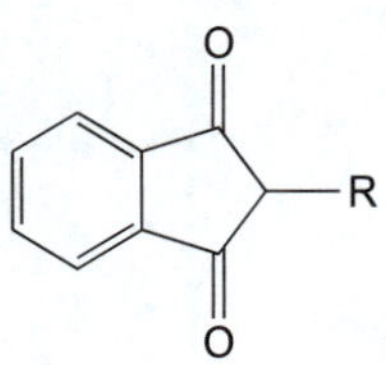

Name	*R_1*
Phenindione	$-C_6H_5$
Anisindione	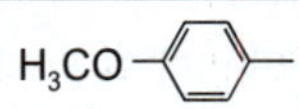
Bromindione	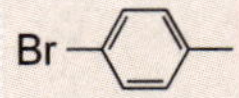
Diphenadione	$-COCH(C_6H_5)_2$

SYNTHESIS AND DRUG PROFILE

I. *In vitro* Anticoagulants

i. Sodium citrate

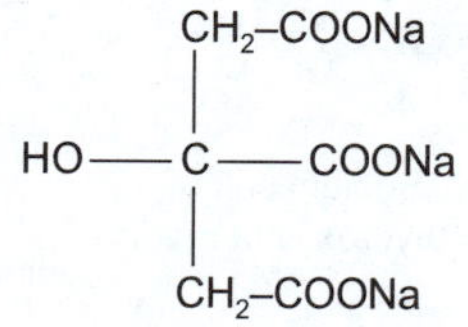

Synthesis

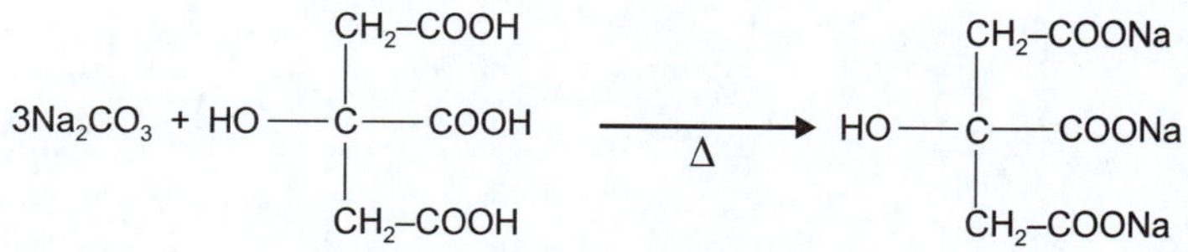

Citric acid Sodium citrate

Properties and uses: Sodium citrate exists as white crystalline powder or granular crystals, soluble in water, but insoluble in alcohol and used as systemic alkalinizing substance.

Assay: Dissolve the sample in anhydrous acetic acid. Heat it, allow to cool and titrate against 0.1 M perchloric acid using naphtholbenzein as indicator until a green colour is obtained.

Dosage forms: Sodium citrate eyedrops BP, sodium citrate irrigation solution BP.

ii. Sodium oxalate

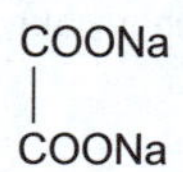

Synthesis

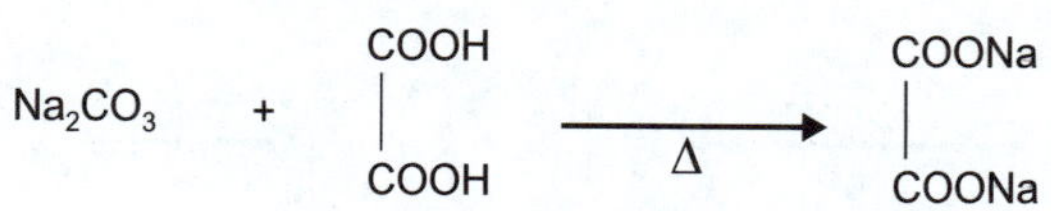

Oxalic acid Sodium oxalate

II. a. *In vivo* Anticoagulants or Coumarin Derivatives

i. Bishydroxycoumarin (Dicoumarol)

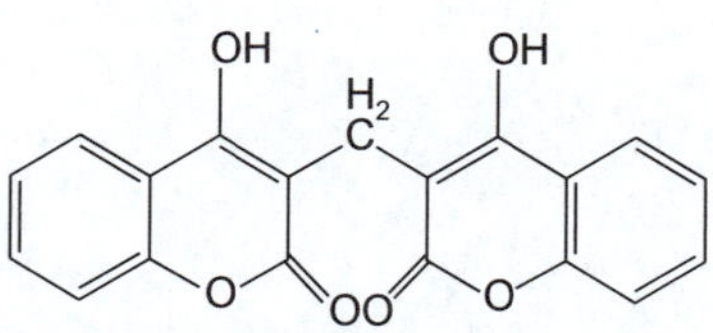

4-Hydroxy-3-((4-hydroxy-2-oxochroman-3-yl)methyl)-2*H*-chromen-2-one

Synthesis

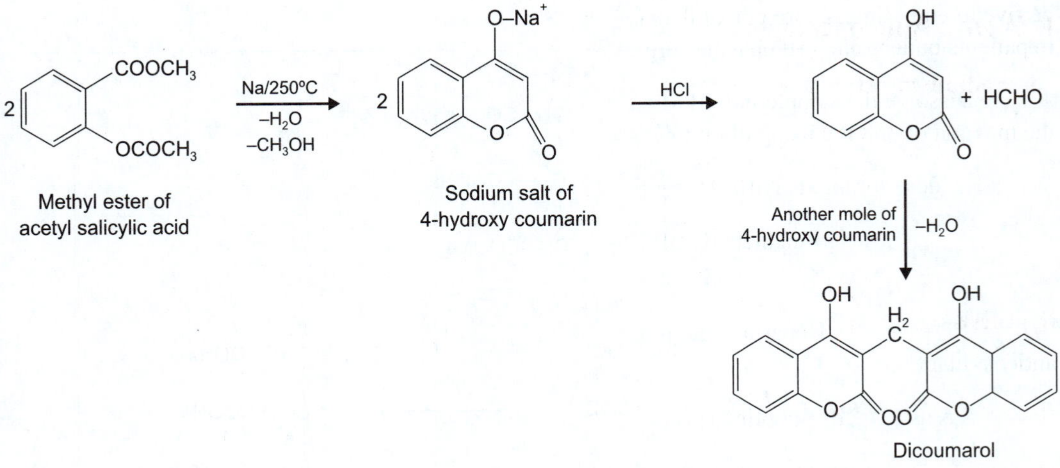

Properties and uses: It is used in postoperative thrombophlebitis, pulmonary embolus, acute embolic, and thrombolic occlusion of peripheral arteries.

ii. **Warfarin** (Coumarin, Coumadia)

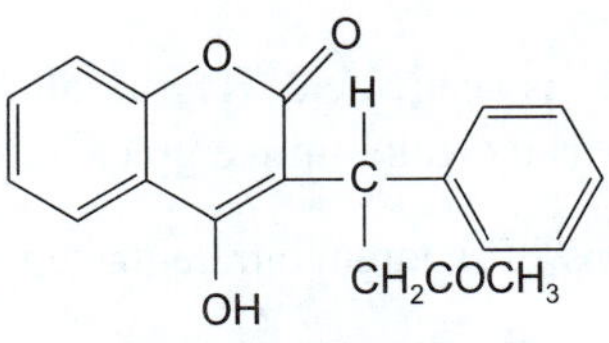

4-Hydroxy-3-(3-oxo-1-phenylbutyl)-2*H*-chromen-2-one

Synthesis

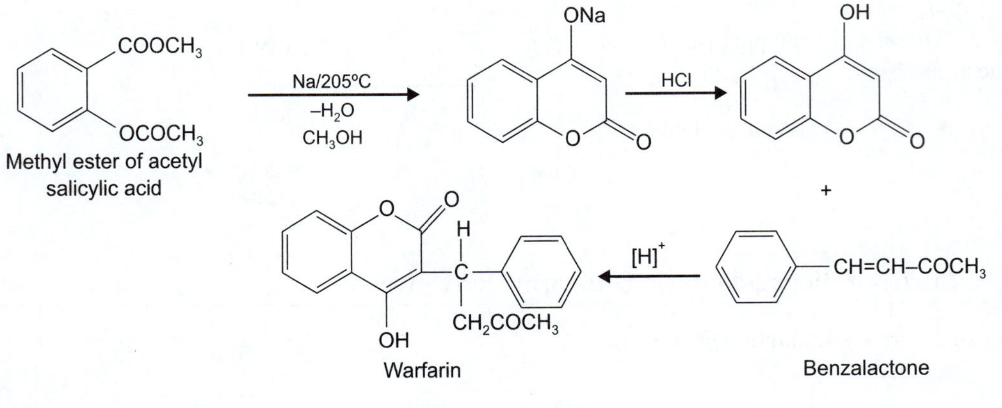

Properties and uses: Warfarin sodium is a white hygroscopic powder, soluble in water, alcohol, and acetone, very slightly soluble in methylene chloride. The (–)-(S)-isomer of warfarin has shown itself to be five to eight times more potent than (+)-(R)-enantiomer. Warfarin is a synthetic anticoagulant used in patients undergoing orthopaedic surgery.

Assay: Dissolve the sample in 0.01 M sodium hydroxide and measure the absorbance after dilution at the maxima of 308 nm using ultraviolet spectrophotometer.

Dose: The dose for adults is 10–15 mg per day for 2 to 4 days.

Dosage forms: Warfarin tablets IP, BP.

iii. Heparin

Properties and uses: Heparin sodium is a white hygroscopic powder, soluble in water and used as an anticoagulant.

Assay: It is assayed by adopting spectrophotometric method.

Dosage forms: Heparin injection BP.

iv. Ethyl biscoumacetate

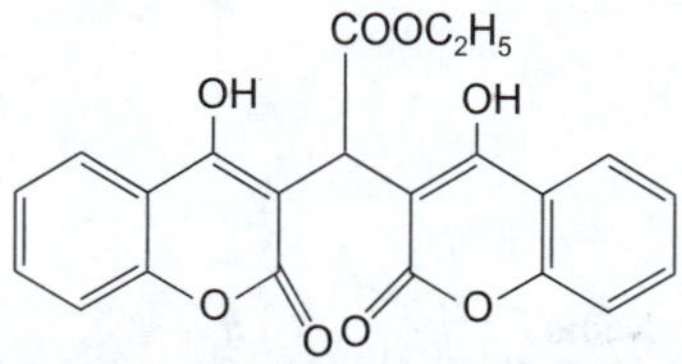

Ethyl-2,2-bis(4-hydroxy-2-oxo-2*H*-chromen-3-yl)acetate

v. Acenocoumarol

Properties and uses: Acenocoumarol is a white to buff-coloured powder, practically insoluble in water and ether, slightly soluble in ethanol. It dissolves in aqueous solutions of the alkali hydroxides. Used as vitamin K epoxide reductase inhibitor and as oral anticoagulant.

Assay: Dissolve the sample in acetone and titrate against 0.1 M sodium hydroxide using bromothymol blue as indicator.

Dosage forms: Acenocoumarol tablets BP.

II. b. Indandione Derivatives: General Method of Preparation

Synthesis of Phenindione, Anisindione, and Bromindione

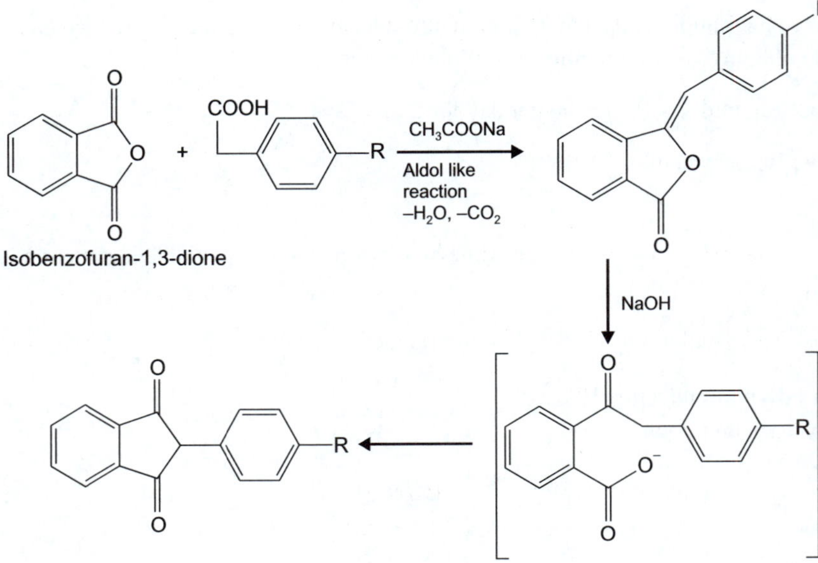

Name	*R*
Phenindione	–H
Anisindione	$-OCH_3$
Bromindione	–Br

These 1,3-indandiones have been recognized for their anticoagulant activity.

i. **Phenindione**

Properties and uses: Phenindione exists as white crystalline powder, very slightly soluble in water, slightly soluble in ethanol and ether. Used as oral anticoagulant.

Assay: To the sample, add ethanol and warm it, cool to room temperature, add 10% v/v solution of bromine in ethanol, and allow standing with occasional shaking. Add 2-naphthol and shake until the colour of the bromine is discharged. Add water, and dilute potassium iodide solution and titrate the liberated iodine against 0.1 M sodium thiosulphate using starch mucilage as indicator.

Dosage forms: Phenindione tablets IP, BP.

ii. **Thrombolytics** (Fibrinolytics)

Fibrinolytics are drugs used to lyse thrombi and to recanalize occluded blood vessels mainly coronary artery. Anticoagulants are designed to prevent thrombus formation. A proteolytic enzyme, known as plasmin, which is released by its precursor protein plasminogen causes the destruction or dissolution of a thrombus. Plasminogen activators (e.g. streptokinase, urokinase) bring about this conversion (Figure 7.2).

Certain other compounds have been found to promote the synthesis of various plasminogen activators. For example, anabolic steroids, act indirectly as fibrinolytic agents. All these agents are useful in the treatment of pulmonary embolic and acute coronary thrombosis. Streptokinase and urokinase are commonly used fibrinolytic agents in the treatment of acute thromboembolic diseases.

a. **Streptokinase:** Streptokinase is obtained from group-C beta-haemolytic streptococci. It is inactive; therefore, to be active it must be converted to plasminogen, which causes proteolysis of plasmin. It is typically used in myocardial infarctions and arterial thrombosis.

b. **Urokinase:** It is isolated from the human urine, now prepared from the cultures of human renal cells. It is non-antigenic and is a glycosylate serine protease containing 41 amino acid residues. It is a substrate for plasminogen, which is activated to plasmin.

c. **Anistrepalse:** It is a streptokinase–plasminogen complex in which plasminogen is isolated and acts as a slow released form of plasminogen activator. Coupling of the streptokinase–plasminogen complex to *p*-amidinophenyl-*p*-anisate blocks the catalytic centre of the complex, but allows it to bind to fibrin. As the anisoyl group is slowly hydrolyzed *in vivo*, the complex is allowed to bind to fibrin prior to activation. It is used in the management of acute myocardial infarction.

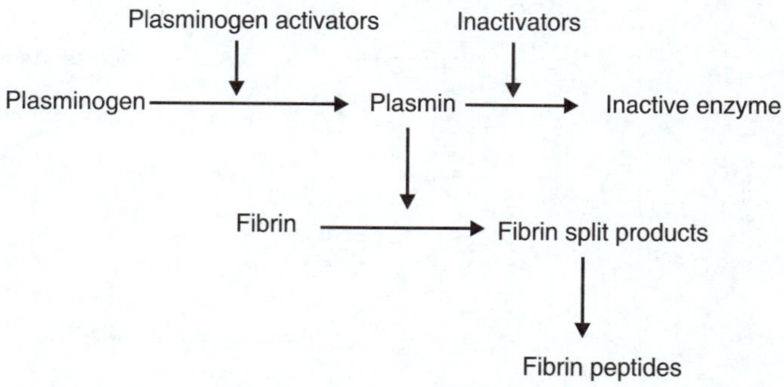

Figure 7.2: Dissolution of thrombus

d. **Aspirin:** Synthesis and drug profile is discussed in Section I, Chapter 3: Analgesics, Antipyretics and NSAIDs.

Antiplatelet drugs (Antithrombocytic drugs)

Platelets provide the initial haemostatic plug at the sites of vascular injury. Platelet aggregation is implicated in thrombus formation in arterial systems and pathogenesis of atherosclerosis. Thus, agents that inhibit platelet aggregation should be able to modify or prevent atherosclerotic disease and thrombosis.

Drugs interfering with platelet functions are as follows:

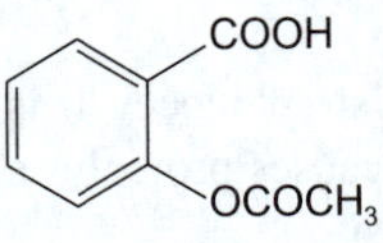

Aspirin

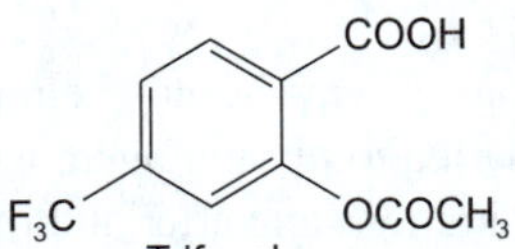

Trifusal

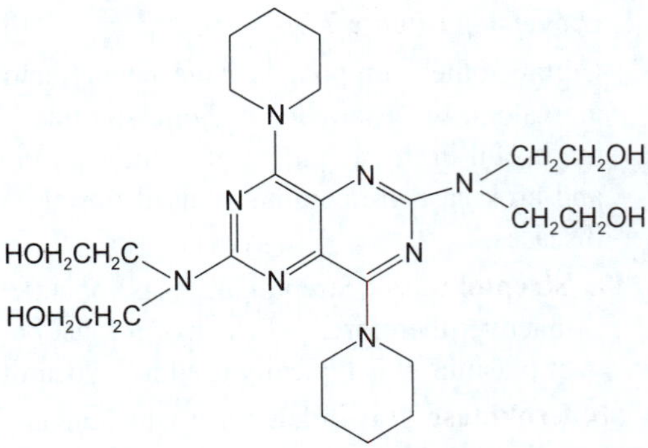

Dipyridamole

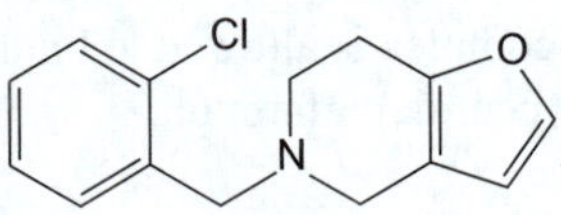

Ticlopidine

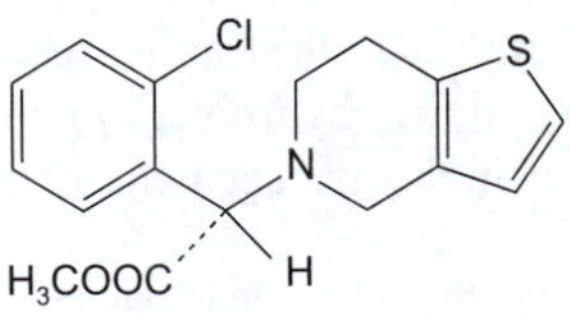

Clopidogrel

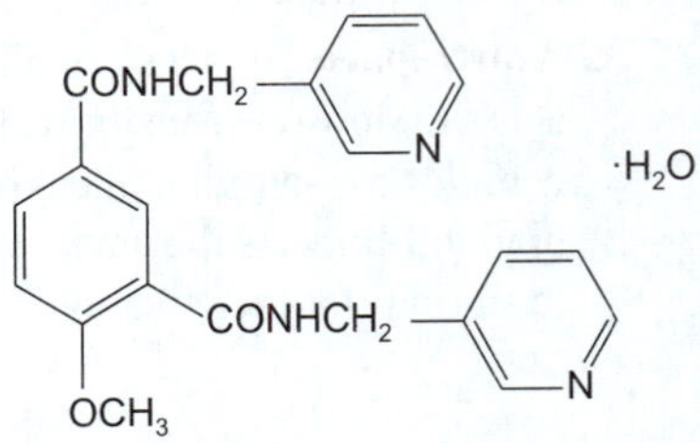

Picotamide monohydrate

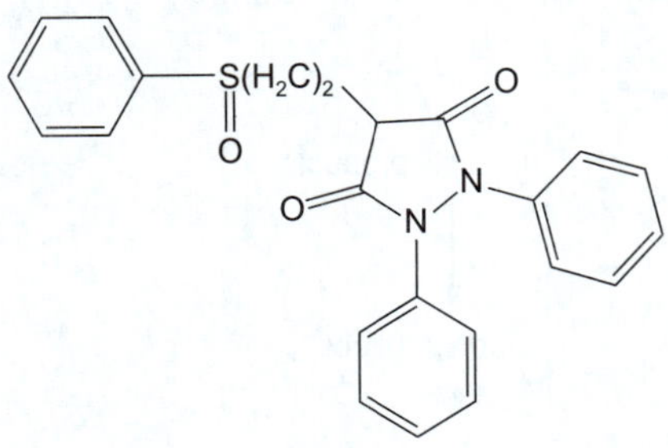

Sulphinapyrazone

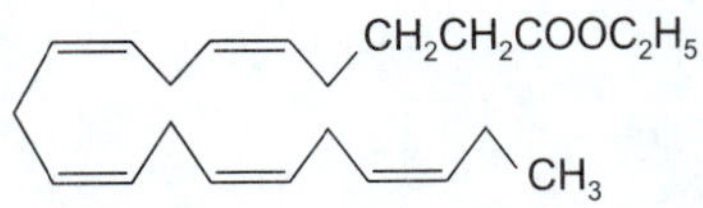

Ethyl icosapentate

SYNTHESIS AND DRUG PROFILE

i. Aspirin

Mode of action: Aspirin inhibits the enzyme cycloxygenase and thromboxane synthetase (TxA_2) by binding irreversibly and interfering with the platelet aggregation.

Synthesis and drug profile of aspirin is discussed under Section I, in Chapter 3. Analgesics, Antipyratics and NSAIDs.

ii. Dipyridamole (Persantine, Cardiwell)

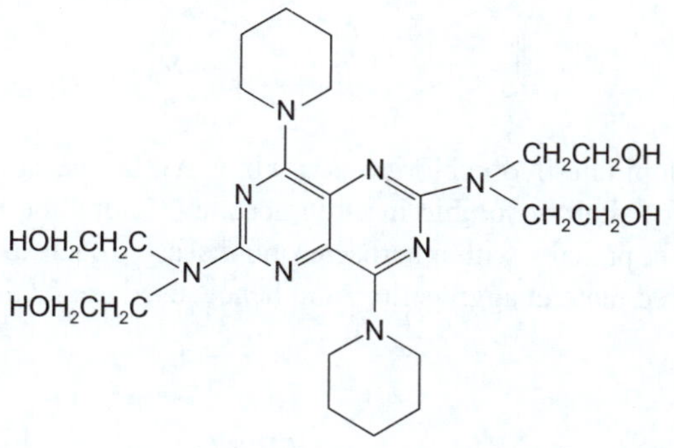

Synthesis

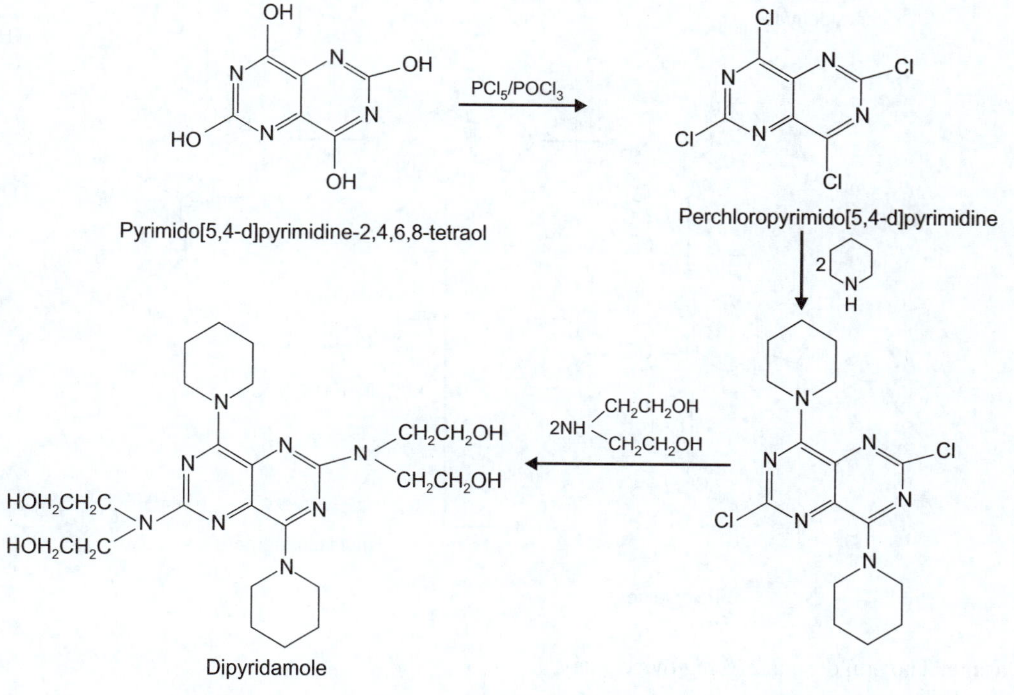

Properties and uses: Dipyridamole is a bright yellow crystalline powder, practically insoluble in water, soluble in acetone, ethanol, and dilute solutions of mineral acids. It is an adenosine reuptake inhibitor, inhibitor of platelet aggregation, and useful in transient ischaemic attacks and secondary prevention of myocardial infarction.

Assay: Dissolve the sample in methanol and titrate against 0.1 M perchloric acid. Determine the end point potentiometrically.

Dose: 50–75 mg 8 hourly in combination with aspirin.

Dosage forms: Dipyridamole tablets BP.

iii. Ticlopidine HCl (Tyklid, Ticlid)

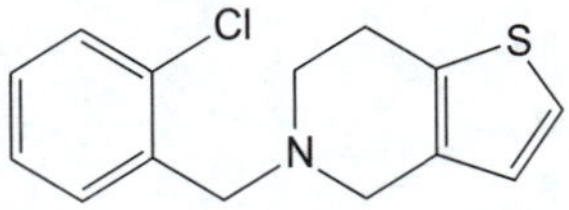

Properties and uses: Ticlopidine hydrochloride is a white crystalline powder, sparingly soluble in water and ethanol, and very slightly soluble in ethyl acetate. Ticlopidine is a thieno pyridines used for thrombosis prevention in patients with atherosclerotic disease. It acts as an inhibitor of adenosine diphosphate (ADP)-mediated platelet aggregation, and hence, used as an antiplatelet drug.

Synthesis

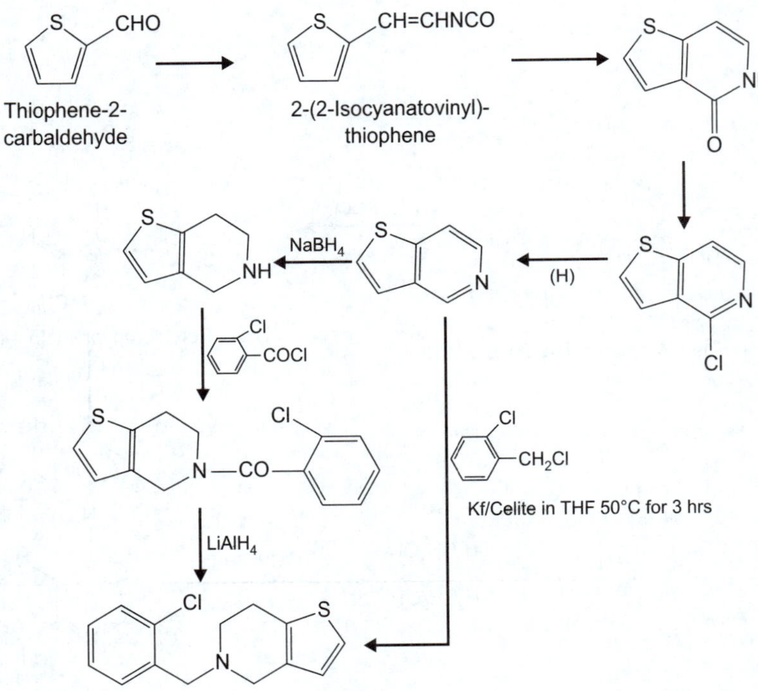

Ticlopidine

Dosage: The oral dose is 250 mg twice a day.

Assay: Dissolve the sample in anhydrous acetic acid and add acetic anhydride. Titrate against 0.1 M perchloric acid and determine the end point potentiometrically.

iv. Sulphinpyrazone (Anturane)

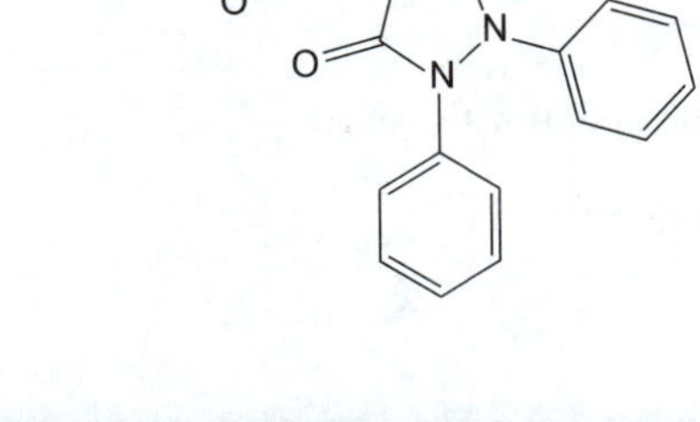

Properties and uses: Sulphinpyrazone is a white powder, very slightly soluble in water, sparingly soluble in alcohol, but soluble in dilute solutions of alkali hydroxides. It has antiplatelet and potent uricosuric effects, and hence, used in the treatment of gout.

Synthesis

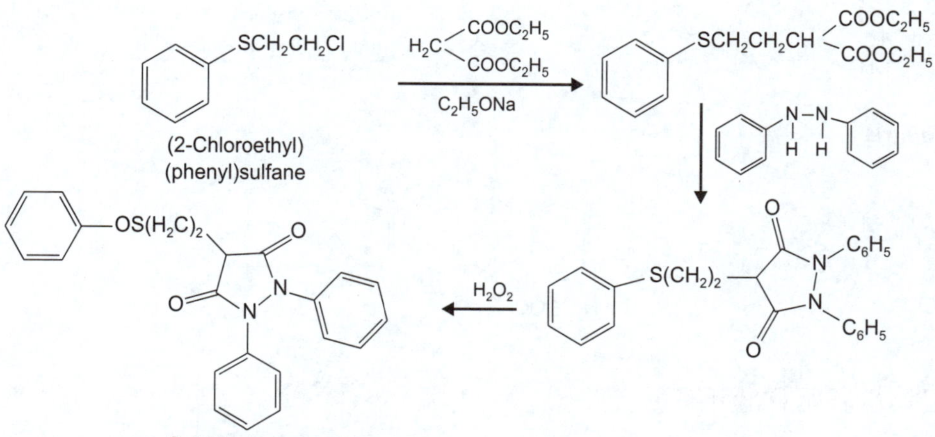

Assay: Dissolve the sample in acetone and titrate against 0.1 M sodium hydroxide using bromothymol blue as indicator until the colour changes from yellow to blue.

Dose: The dose is 300 mg four times a day.

Dosage forms: Sulphinpyrazone tablets BP.

v. **Picotamide monohydrate**

Properties and uses: Picotamide monohydrate is a white crystalline powder, slightly soluble in water, soluble in ethanol, methylene chloride, and dilute mineral acids. It acts as thromboxane synthetase inhibitor and thromboxane receptor antagonist; used as antiplatelet agent.

Assay: Dissolve the sample in a mixture of anhydrous acetic acid and acetic anhydride (1:1) and titrate against 0.1 M perchloric acid. Determine the end point potentiometrically.

CLASSIFICATION BASED ON PCI SYLLABUS

Menadione

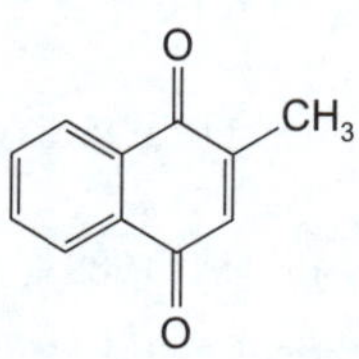

Acetomenadione

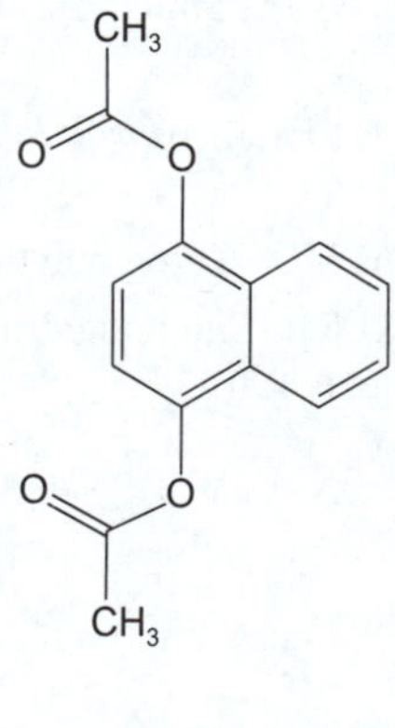

Warfarin

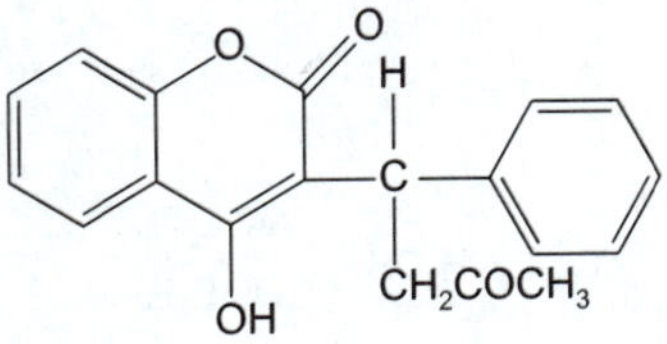

Anisindione

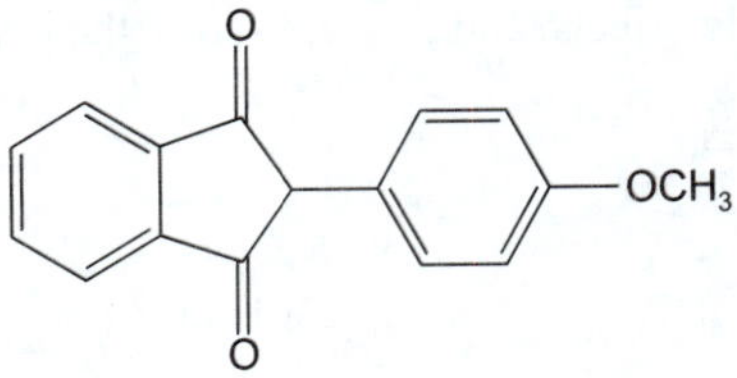

Clopidogrel

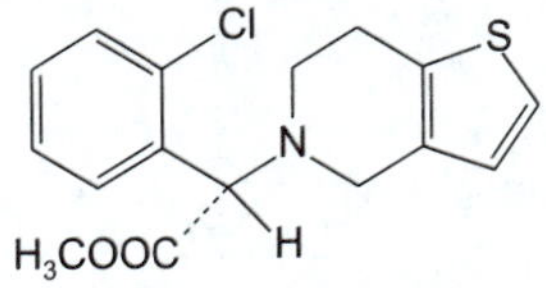

PROBABLE QUESTIONS

1. Classify anticoagulants with suitable examples and write the synthesis of any two of them.
2. Enumerate the coumarin-derived anticoagulants and write the synthesis of one of them.
3. Write a short note on *in vivo* anticoagulants.
4. Write a note on indandione derivatives.
5. Describe in detail about antithrombocytic and fibrinolytic agents.

SUGGESTED READINGS

1. *British Pharmacopoeia*. Medicines and Healthcare products regulatory agency. London, 2008.
2. Bruntan LL, Lazo JS, and Parker KL. *Goodman and Gilman's: The Pharmacological Basis of Therapeutics* (11th edn). New York: McGraw Hill, 2006.
3. Colmon RW, Hirsch J, Marder VJ, and Salzman EW. *Hemostasis and Thrombosis* (2nd edn). Philadelphia: JB Lippincott, 1987.
4. Coller BS. 'Platelets and thrombolytic therapy'. *N Engl J Med* 322: 33, 1990.
5. Gennaro AR. Remington: *The Science and Practice of Pharmacy* (21st edn). New York: Lippincot Williams and Wilkins, 2006.
6. Ito M, Smith A, and Lee M. '*Ticlopidine hydrochloride*'. Clin Pharm 11: 603–17, 1992.
7. *Indian Pharmacopoeia*. Ministry of Health and Family Welfare. New Delhi, 1996.
8. Jakabowski JA, Smith GF, and Sail DJ. 'Future antithrombatic therapy'. *Ann Rept Med Chem* 27: 99–108, 1992.
9. Reynolds EF (ed). *Martindale the Extra Pharmacopoeia* (31st edn). London: The Pharmaceutical Press, 1997.
10. Simmons ML. 'Thrombolytic therapy in acute mycocardial infarction'. *Ann Rev Med* 40: 181, 1989.
11. Shebuski RJ. 'Emerging drug discovery targets in thrombosis and coagulation'. *Ann Rept Med Chem* 26: 93–101, 1997.

CHAPTER 8

Plasma Expanders

INTRODUCTION

A haemorrhagic shock may result from the loss of blood during burns, wounds, or surgery. Mild shock results when there is a loss of 15 to 20% in the total blood volume. Further loss of blood, up to 40% of total blood volume may lead to severe shock during which the cardiovascular functioning is severely affected. To restore this functioning, saline should be administered as an initial emergency measure. Plasma expanders can also be used to overcome the initial losses.

There are of two types of plasma expanders: (i) Natural products and (ii) synthetic products.

Natural products: These include transfusion of whole blood or the preparations of plasma proteins. Blood products containing plasma proteins are human albumin (albumisol) and plasma protein fraction (PPF). Both of these preparations are usually given by intravenous infusion.

Synthetic products: Dextran, hetastarch, perfluorochemicals, polyvinylpyrrolidone, and gelatin are some of the synthetic plasma expanders, out of which dextran has been used extensively.

i. Dextran

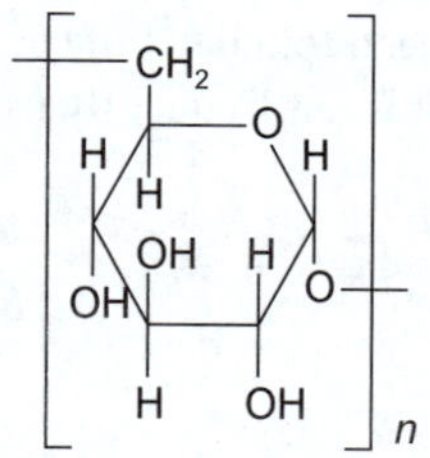

Dextran could be considered as being almost close to ideal plasma expanders. Dextrans are colloidal glucose polymers that are obtained from sucrose by the action of bacteria, *Leuconostoc mesenteroides*. The dextran molecule consists mainly of 1:6 glucoside linkages with relatively few 1:4 linkages and has an average molecular weight of 40 millions. This form is not clinically suitable. Hence, it is partially hydrolyzed *in vitro* to give dextran with average molecular weight of 40,000, 70,000, 11,000, and 15,000 daltons. They are known as dextran-40, dextran-70, dextran-110, and dextran-150, respectively. Of these, dextran-40 and dextran-70 are of clinical importance. Solutions of dextran in isotonic sodium chloride is used to increase the circulating blood volume and to maintain the venous pressure, right arterial pressure, stroke volume, and cardiac output.

Only dextran solutions are used in the treatment of hypoproteinaemia, nephrosis, and toxaemia of late pregnancy. Dextran does not posses oxygen-carrying capacity.

The dextran solution is pharmacologically inactive and has been reported as having no significant deleterious effect on renal, hepatic, or any other vital functions. Occasionally, sensitization reaction may occur in some patients. The bleeding time, fibrin polymerization on platelet function may be impaired *in vivo*. Dextrans are contraindicated in patients with anaemia, severe thrombocytopenia, and low plasma fibrinogen level.

ii. **Human albumin**

It is obtained from pooled human plasma; 100 ml of 20% human albumin solution is the osmotic equivalent of about 400 ml of fresh frozen plasma or 800 ml of whole blood. It can be used without regard to the patient's blood group and does not interfere with coagulation. Unlike whole blood or plasma, it is free of risk of transmitting serum hepatitis because the preparation is heat-treated. There is also no risk of sensitization with repeated infusions. It has been used in acute hypoproteinaemia, acute liver failure, and dialysis.

iii. **Degraded gelatin polymer** (polygeline)

It is a polypeptide with an average MW 30,000, which exerts osmotic pressure similar to albumin, and is not antigenic and hypersensitivity reactions are rare. It does not interfere with the grouping and cross-matching of blood and remains stable for 3 years. It can be used for the priming of heart–lung dialysis machines.

iv. **Hydroxyethyl starch** (HES, hetastarch)

It is a complex mixture of ethoxylated amylopectin of various molecular sizes, average MW 4.5 lakh (range 10,000–1,000,000). The colloidal properties of 6% HES approximate those of human albumin. Plasma volume expands slightly in excess of the volume infused. It has been used to improve harvesting of granulocytes because it accelerates erythrocyte sedimentation. Adverse effects are vomiting, mild fever, itching, chills, flu-like symptoms, swelling of salivary glands, urticaria, perorbital oedema, and bronchospasm are the anaphylactoid reactions.

v. **Polyvinylpyrrolidone** (PVP)

It is a synthetic polymer (average MW 40,000) used as a 3.5% solution. It interferes with the blood grouping and cross-matching. It has been found to bind penicillin and insulin in circulation, so that the same is not available for action. It is not frequently used as a plasma expander.

PROBABLE QUESTIONS

1. What are plasma expanders? Write their uses and describe briefly about any two of the products used as plasma expanders.
2. Write a brief note on dextran.

SECTION V

Drugs Acting on Endocrine System

CHAPTER 9

Oral Hypogylcaemic Drugs

INTRODUCTION

Diabetes mellitus is a metabolic disorder characterized by hyperglycaemia, glycosuria, hyperlipidemia, negative nitrogen balance, and ketonaemia. Most patients can be classified, clinically, as having either type I diabetes mellitus (insulin-dependent diabetes mellitus (IDDM) or type II non-insulin-dependent diabetes mellitus (NIDDM). The incidence of each type of diabetes varies widely throughout the world. In the United States, about 5 to 10% of the diabetic patients have type I diabetes mellitus, with an incidence of 17 per 100,000 found in United Kingdom. The vast majority of diabetic patients have type II diabetes mellitus.

Type I diabetes is also called juvenile onset diabetes mellitus. There is β-cell destruction in the pancreatic islets of langerhans. Majority of the cases are due to autoimmune (type I A) antibodies that destroy β cells, are detectable in blood, but some are idiopathic (type I B) no β (beta)-cell antibody is found. In all type I cases, circulating insulin levels are low or very low and ketosis may occur. Genetic predisposition is also a cause for this condition.

Type II diabetes is also called maturity onset diabetes mellitus. There is no loss or moderate reduction in the β-cell mass, insulin in circulation levels is low and generally has a late onset of disease after middle age. This may be due to an abnormality in the glucoreceptors of β-cells, therefore, they respond at higher glucose concentrations or at relative β-cell deficiency. The reduced sensitivity of peripheral tissues to insulin and reduction in the number of insulin receptors are a consequence for producing diabetes. When glucagons exceed a normal amount, it produces hypoglycaemia. The insulin is secreted by the β-cells of Langerhans, synthesized by a single chain precursor of 110 amino acid preproinsulin. After translocation through the membrane of rough endoplasmic reticulum, the 24 amino acid N-terminal peptide of preproinsulin is rapidly cleared off to form proinsulin. Here, the molecules folds and the disulphide bonds are formed. In the conversion of proinsulin to insulin in the Golgi complex, four basic amino acids and the remaining connector or C peptide are removed by proteolysis. This gives rise to two peptide chains (A and B) of insulin molecules, which contains one intrasubunit and two intersubunits disulphide bonds. The A chain consists of 21 amino acids and B with 30 amino acids and molecular mass is about 5734 daltons.

The regulatory factors of insulin secretion are chemical, hormonal, and neural. Chemical regulation depends upon the glucose entry in to the β-cells by glucose transport. Once, after the entry of glucose and its phosphorylation by glucokinase, glucoreceptor activation indirectly inhibits the adenosine triphosphate (ATP) sensitive potassium channels and increases intracellular calcium, which triggers the exocytic release of insulin. Hormonal change in corticosteroids modify the release of insulin. Insulin inhibits glucagon secretion and glucagons increase the insulin secretion.

The neural control is mediated by α_2-and β_2-receptors. Stimulation of α_2-receptor decreases the insulin release and stimulation of β_2-receptors increases insulin release. Cholinergic stimulation increases the insulin secretion.

Hypoglycaemic drugs are agents, which decrease the blood sugar level. Oral hypoglycaemic agents must be distinguished from more hypoglycaemic drugs, such as salicylates, which are too toxic for clinical use in doses that effectively lower the blood sugar. An ideal antidiabetic drug should be non-toxic and correct the basic metabolic defects in diabetics, in addition to lowering the blood sugar.

CLASSIFICATION

I. Sulphonylureas

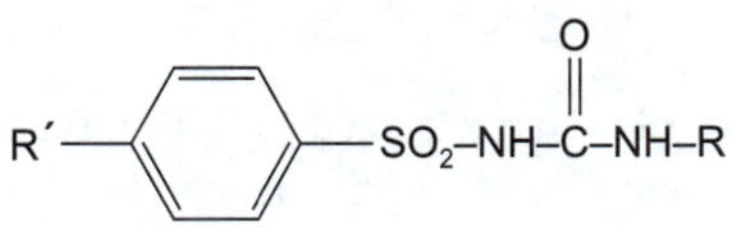

a. First-generation drugs

Name	*R*	*R'*
Carbutamide	$-^{n}C_4H_9$	$-NH_2$
Tolbutamide	$-^{n}C_4H_9$	$-CH_3$
Chloropropamide	$-^{n}C_3H_7$	–Cl
Tolazamide	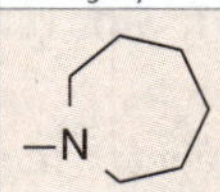	$-CH_3$
Acetohexamide	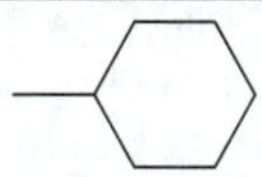	$-COCH_3$

b. Second-generation drugs

Name	*R*	*R'*
Glibenclamide (glyburide)	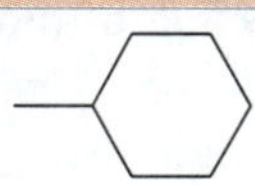	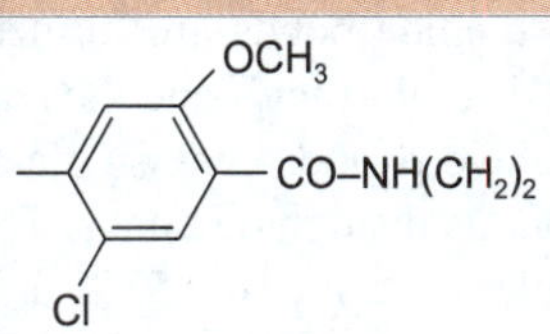
Glipizide	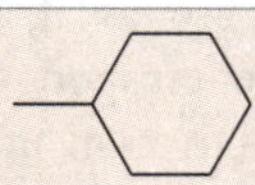	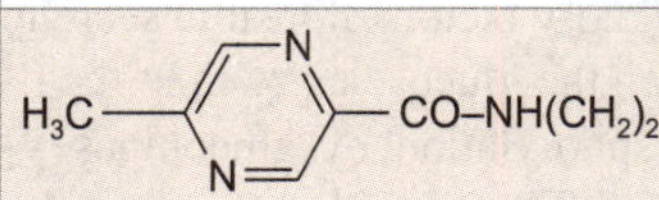
Gliclazide	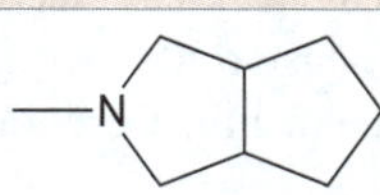	$-CH_3$

Name	R	R′
Glibornuride	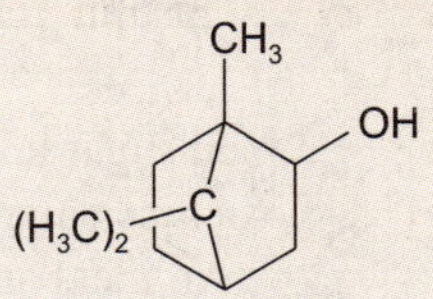	$-CH_3$

II. Biguanides

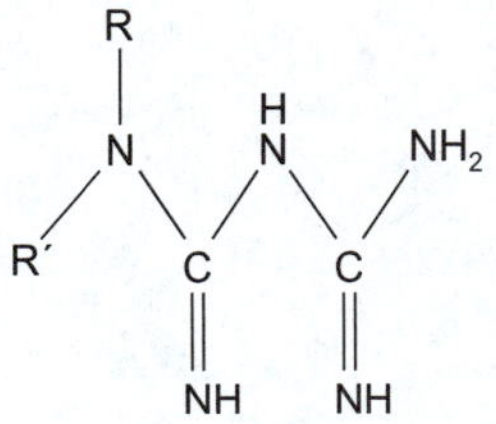

Name	R	R′
Phenformin	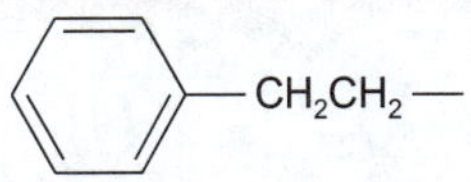	–H
Metformin	$-CH_3$	$-CH_3$
Buformin	$-CH_2CH_2CH_2CH_3$	–H

III. Substituted Benzoic Acid Derivatives (Meglitinides)

i. Meglitinide

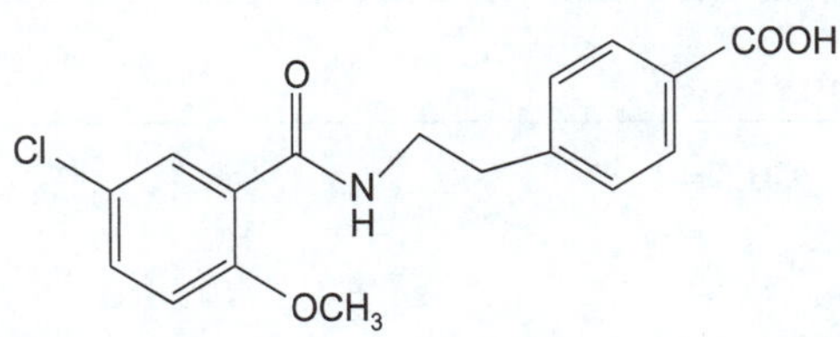

ii. Repaglinide

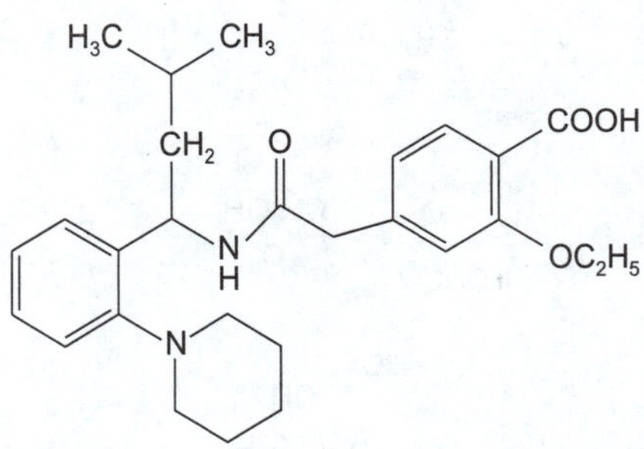

iii. Nateglinide

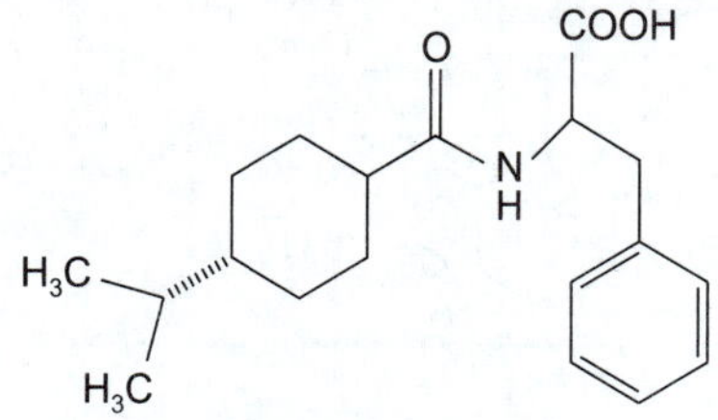

IV. Thiazolidinediones (Glitazones)

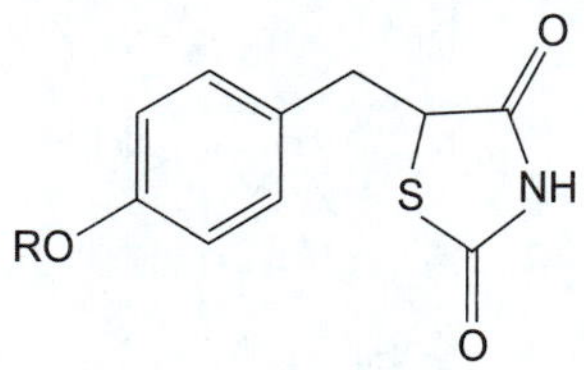

Name	*R*
Pioglitazone	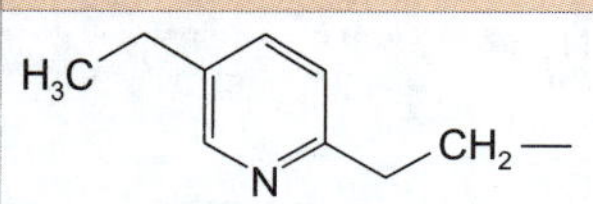
Ciglitazone	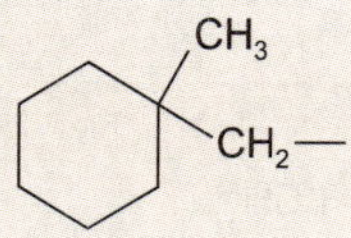
Rosiglitazone	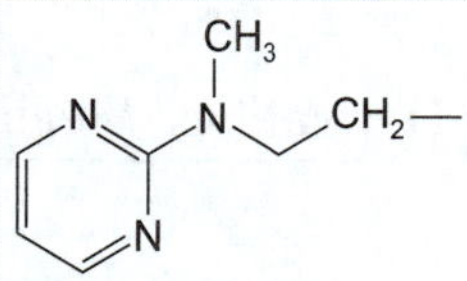

V. α-Glucosidase Inhibitors

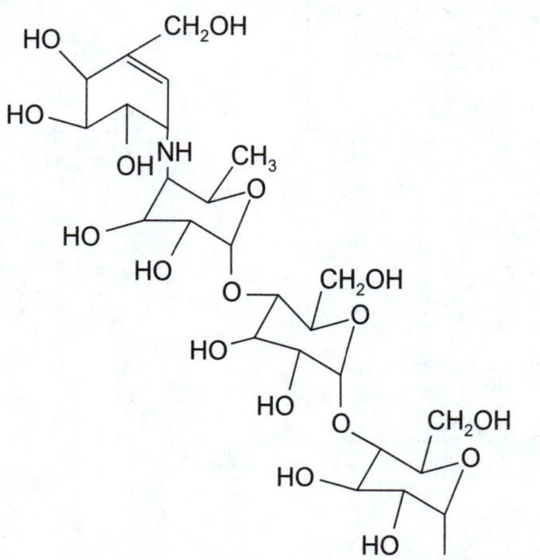

Acarbose

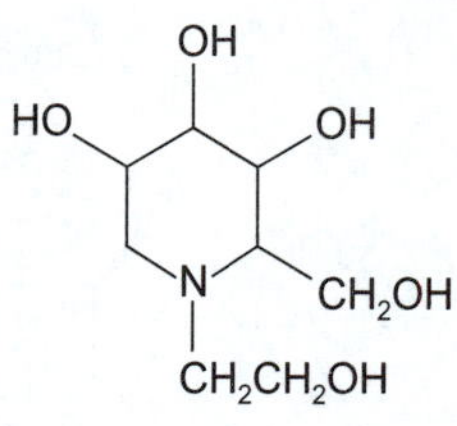

Miglitol

VI. Aldose Reductase Inhibitors

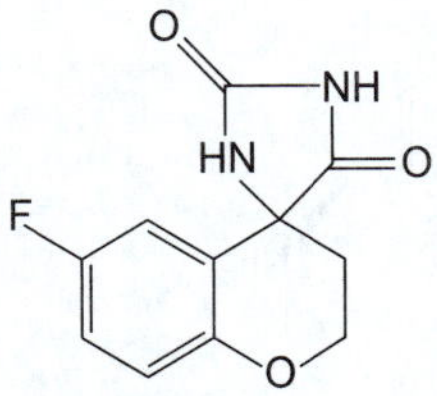

Sorbinil

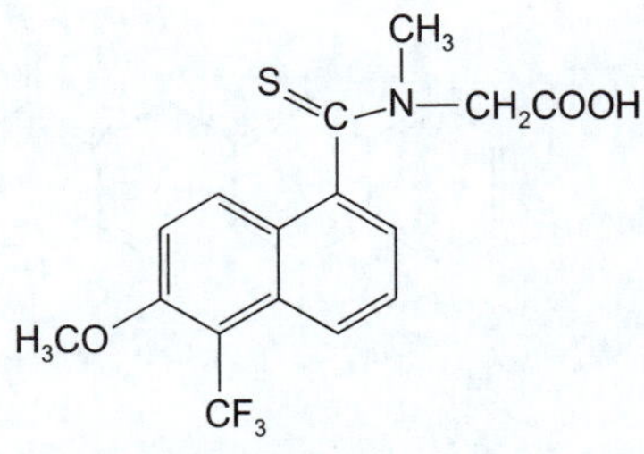

Tolrestat

VII. Miscellaneous

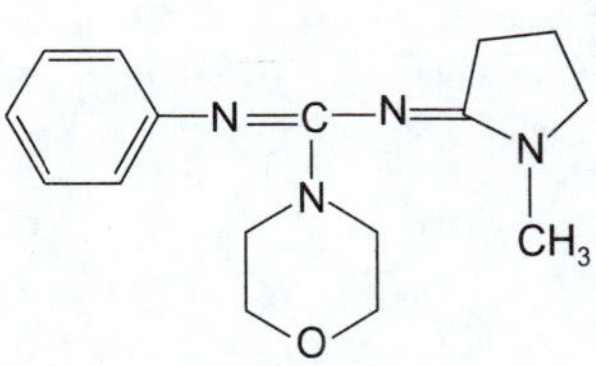

Linogliride

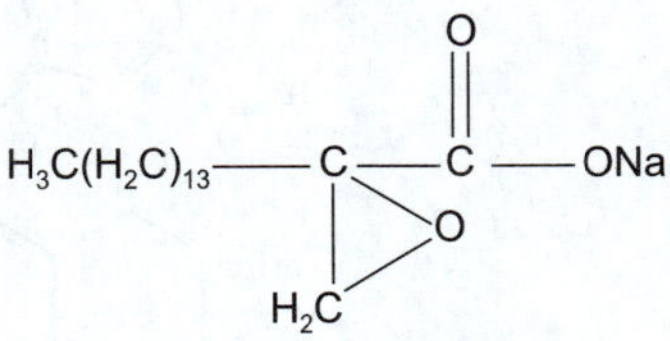

Palmoxirate sodium

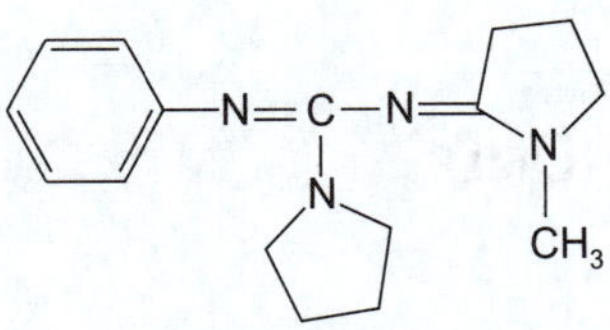

Pirogliride

Newer Drugs

Saxagliptin (Onglyza)

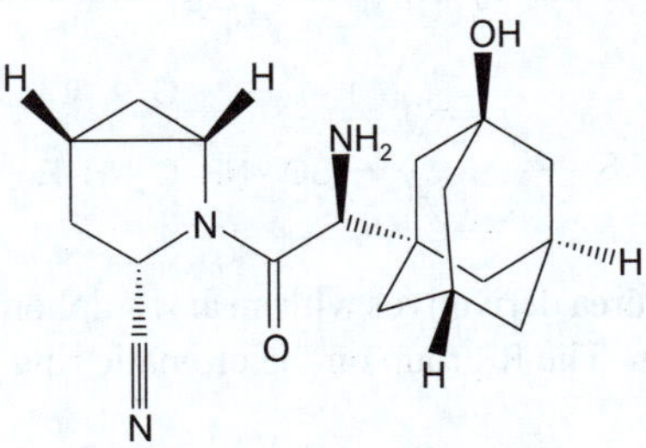

Linagliptin (Tradjenta)

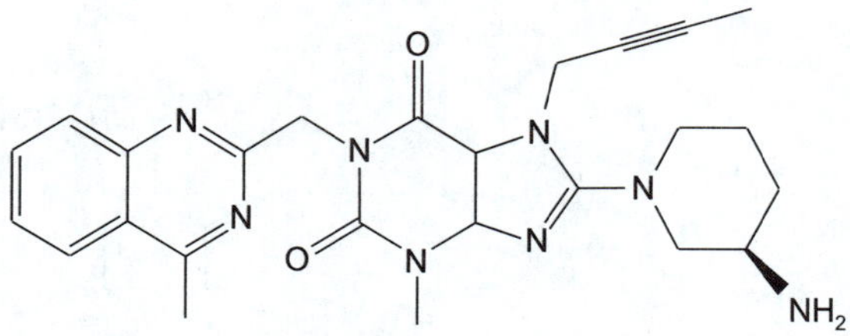

Mifepristone

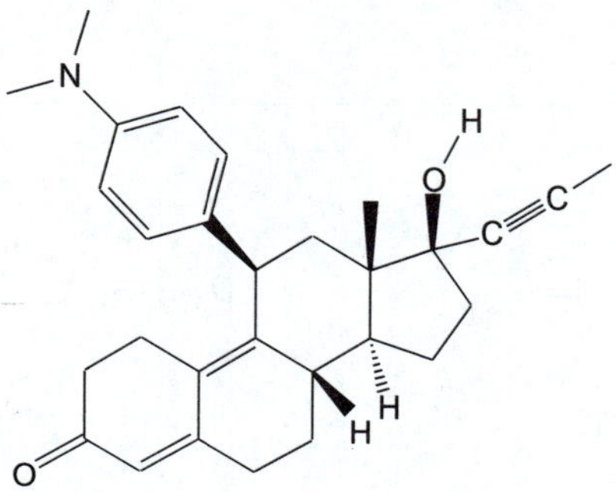

Liraglutide (Victoza) $C_{172}H_{265}N_{43}O_{51}$

SYNTHESIS AND DRUG PROFILE

I. Sulphonylurea Derivatives

a. First-generation drugs

Mode of action: They target on the specific receptors in the β-cells of islets of Langerhans called sulphonylurea receptors, and cause depolarization by reducing the conductance of ATP sensitive K^+ channels. This enhances the Ca^{2+} influx and produces degranulation, leading to the secretion of insulin. The sulphonylureas may be represented by the following general structure.

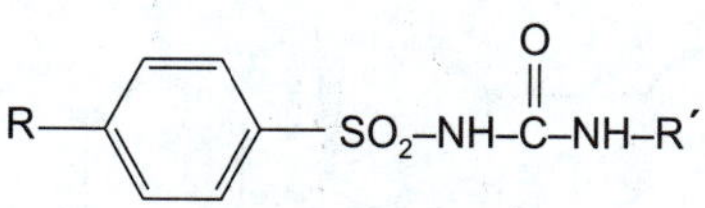

All members of this group are urea derivatives with an aryl sulphonyl group in the 1st position and an aliphatic group at the 3rd position. The R group on the aromatic ring primarily influences the duration of action of the compound.

i. Tolbutamide (Orinase)

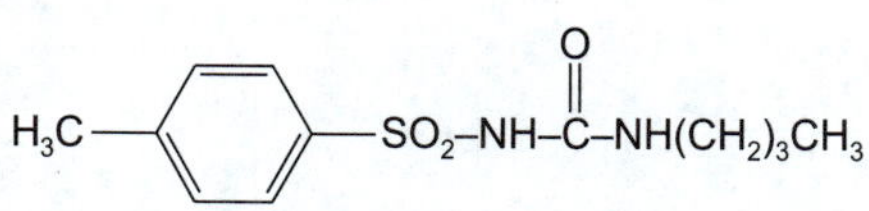

1-Butyl-3-(*p*-tolylsulphonyl) urea

Properties and uses: Tolbutamide is a white crystalline powder, practically insoluble in water, soluble in acetone, alcohol, and dilute solutions of alkali hydroxides. It is useful in the treatment of selected cases of diabetes mellitus, namely, mild and uncomplicated, stable diabetes of adult.

Assay: Dissolve the sample in a mixture of water and alcohol (1 : 2) and titrate against 0.1 M sodium hydroxide using phenolphthalein as indicator.

Synthesis

Route I. From: 4-Methylbenzene sulphonamide

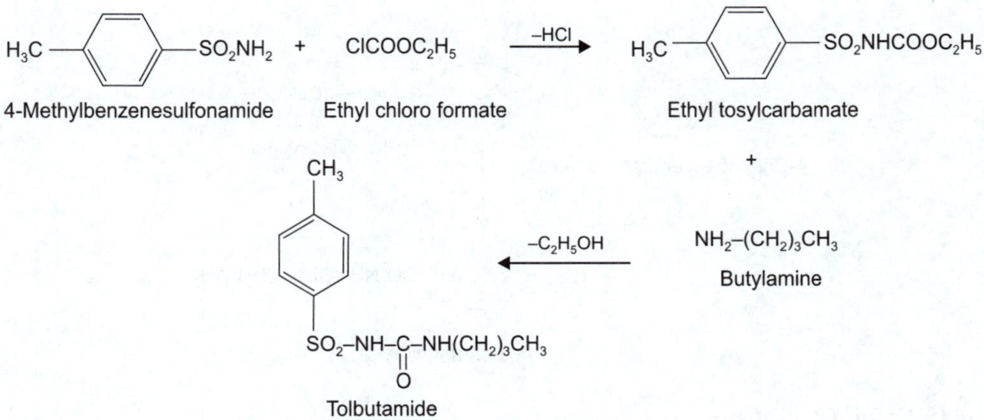

Route II. From: Toluene

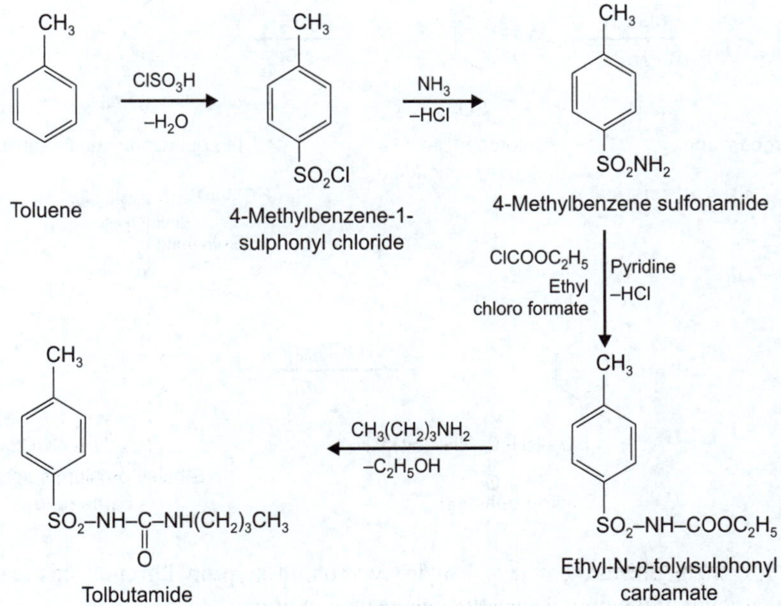

Dose: The usual dosage is 250 and 500 mg with an initial dose of 500 mg.

Dosage forms: Tolbutamide tablets BP.

ii. Chloropropamide (Diabenese)

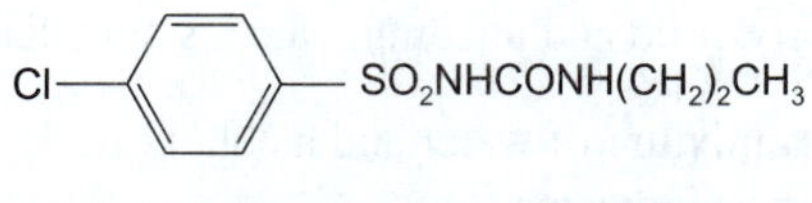

1-[(*p*-Chlorophenyl sulphonyl)]-3-propyl urea

Synthesis

Route I. From: 4-Chlorobenzenesulphonamide

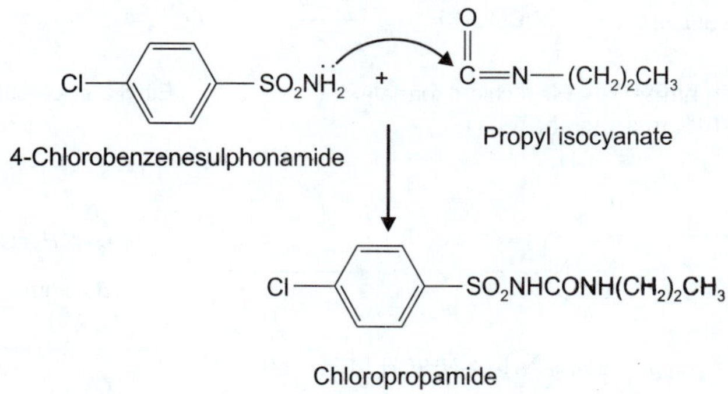

Route II. From: Chlorobenzene

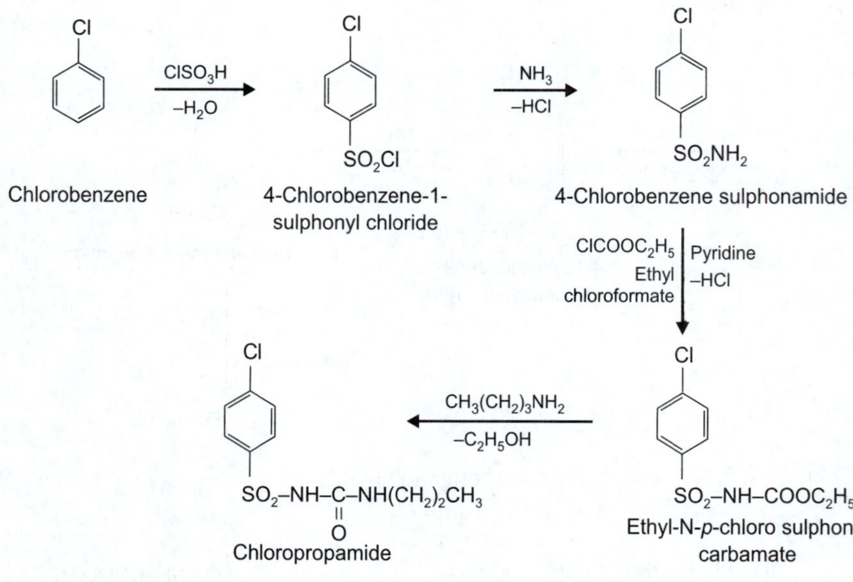

Metabolism: It is metabolized by ω or ω-1 hydroxylation of the propyl group. This reaction is slow and significant amount of the drug is excreted unchanged in urine.

Properties and uses: Chloropropamide is a white crystalline powder, practically insoluble in water, soluble in acetone, methylene chloride, alcohol, and dilute solutions of alkali hydroxides. Used in the treatment of diabetes mellitus.

Assay: Dissolve the sample in alcohol and add water. Titrate against 0.1 M sodium hydroxide using phenolphthalein as indicator until a pink colour is obtained.

Dose: The usual dose is 100–250 mg per day.

iii. Tolazamide (Tolamide, Tolinase)

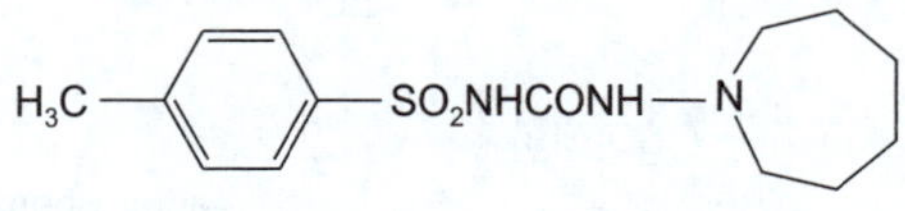

1-(Hexahydro-azepine-1-yl)-3-(*p*-tolylsulphonyl)urea

Metabolism of tolbutamide and tolazamide: They undergo a more rapid benzylic oxidation, leading to an inactive benzoic acid derivative. An alternative hydroxylation of the aliphatic ring of tolazamide becomes active and results in a metabolite of prolonged duration of action.

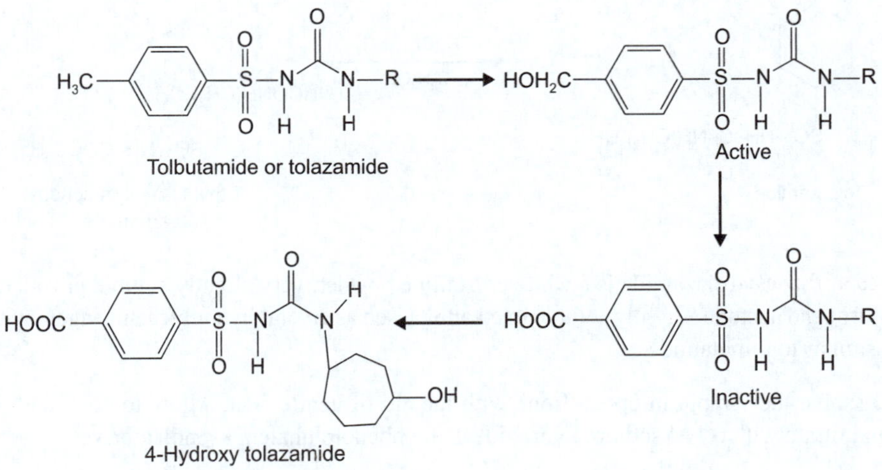

Synthesis

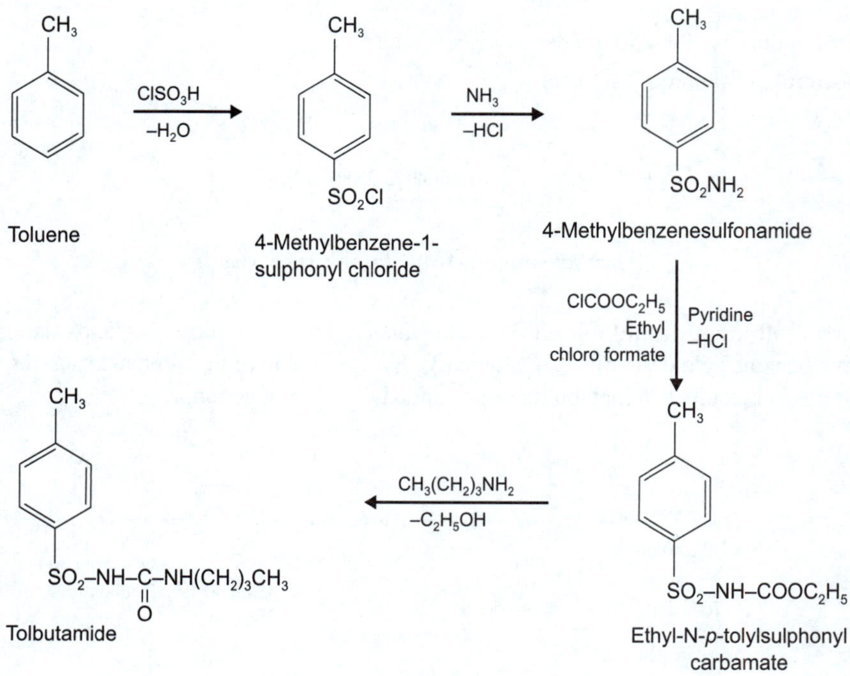

Properties and uses: Tolazamide is a white crystalline powder, very slightly soluble in water, soluble in chloroform and acetone, slightly soluble in ethanol. Used as an oral hypoglycaemic agent with action and uses similar to tolbutamide.

Assay: Dissolve the sample in butan-2-one with the aid of gentle heat. Allow to cool, add 30 ml of ethanol and titrate with 0.1 M sodium hydroxide using phenolphthalein as indicator.

Dose: The dose is 100–250 mg daily.

Dosage forms: Tolazamide tablets BP.

iv. Acetohexamide

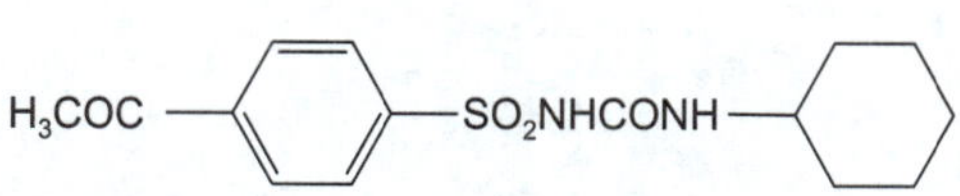

1-[(4-Acetylphenyl) sulphonyl]-3-cyclohexyl urea

Synthesis

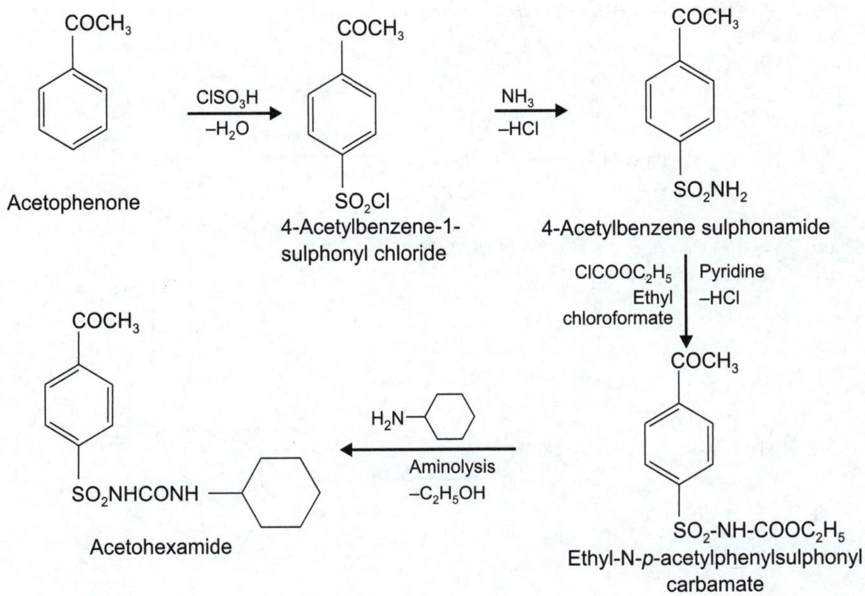

Metabolism: The major metabolite of acetohexamide is a reduced product of the keto group, forming an alcohol. The hydroxy metabolite exhibits 2.5 times the hypoglycaemic activity of the parent molecule.

Properties and uses: It is a white, odourless crystalline powder, soluble in alcohol and chloroform, but insoluble in water or ether. It is an orally active hypoglycaemic drug.

b. Second-generation drugs

i. Glibenclamide (Glyburide)

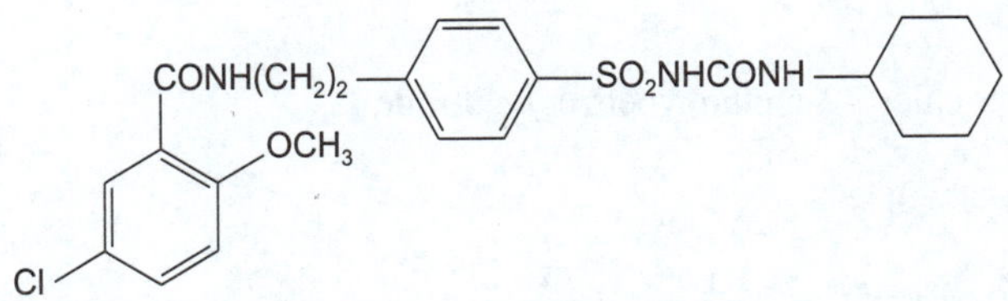

5-Chloro-N-[2-4[[[(cyclohexylamino) carbonylamino] sulphonyl] phenyl] ethyl]-2-methoxy benzamide

Synthesis

Route I. From: 5-Chloro-2-methoxybenzoylchloride

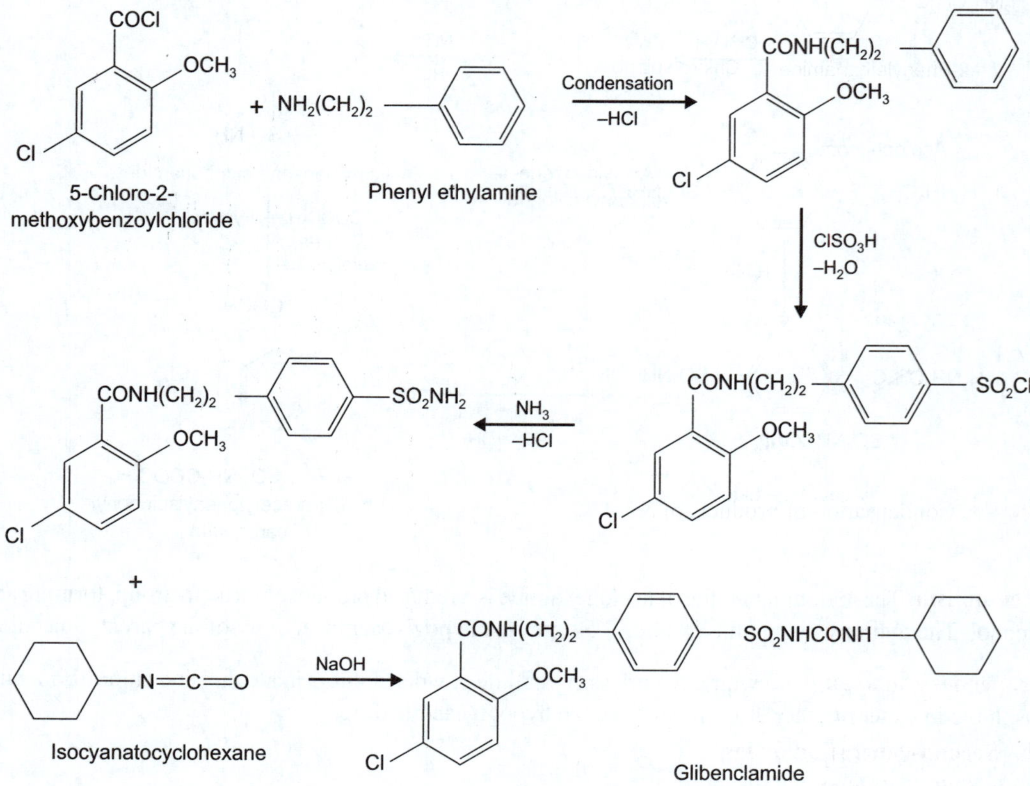

Route II.

Step I: Synthesis of 5-chloro-2-methoxybenzoyl chloride

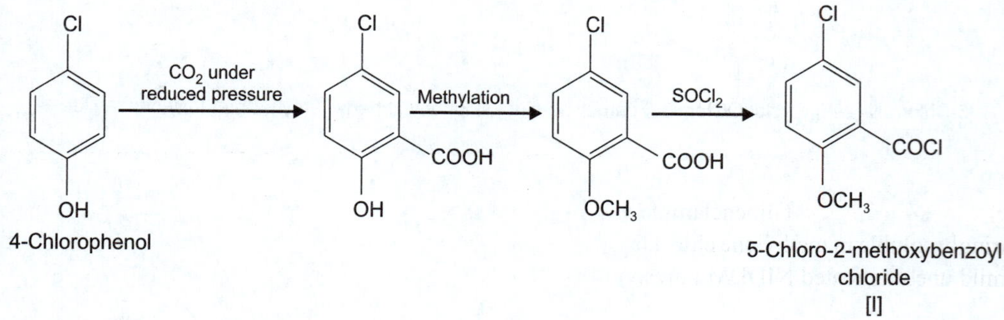

Step II: Synthesis of 4-(aminoethyl)-1-cyclohexylamino carbonyl benzene sulphonamide

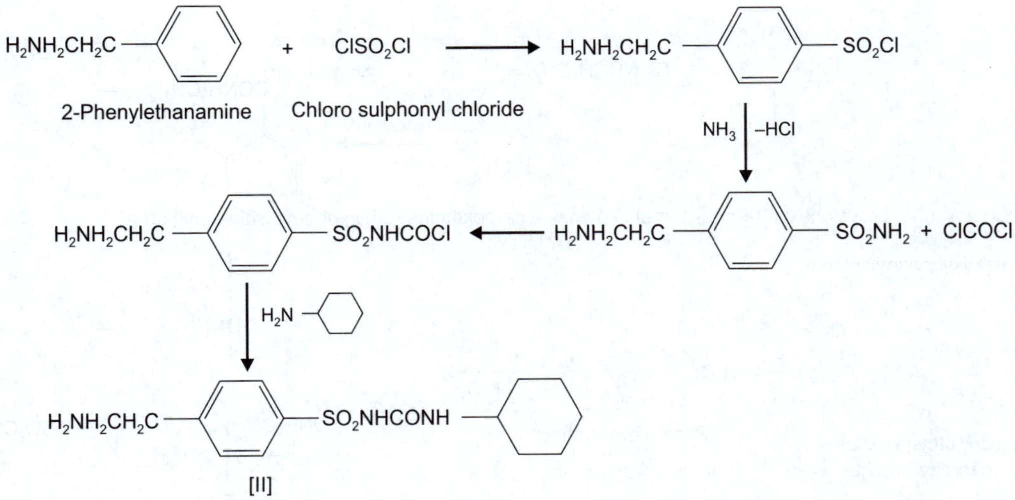

Step III: Condensation of products of *Steps I* and *II.*

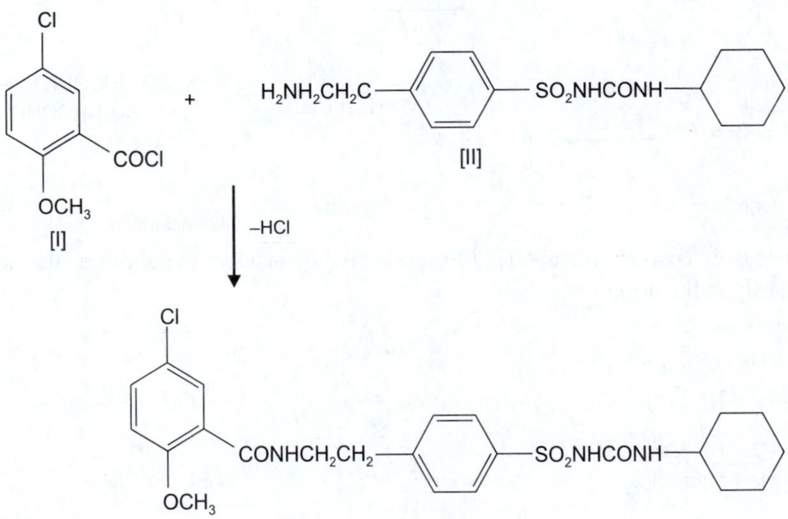

Glibenclamide

Properties and uses: Glibenclamide is a white crystalline powder, practically insoluble in water, sparingly soluble in methylene chloride, slightly soluble in alcohol and methanol. Used in the treatment of mild uncomplicated NIDDM unresponsive to diet alone.

Assay: Dissolve the sample in alcohol by heating and titrate against 0.1 M sodium hydroxide, using phenolphthalein as indicator, until a pink colour is obtained.

Dose: The dose is 2.5–5 mg per day to be taken with breakfast.

Dosage forms: Glibenclamide tablets BP.

ii. Glipizide (Dibizide, Glucolip, Glynase)

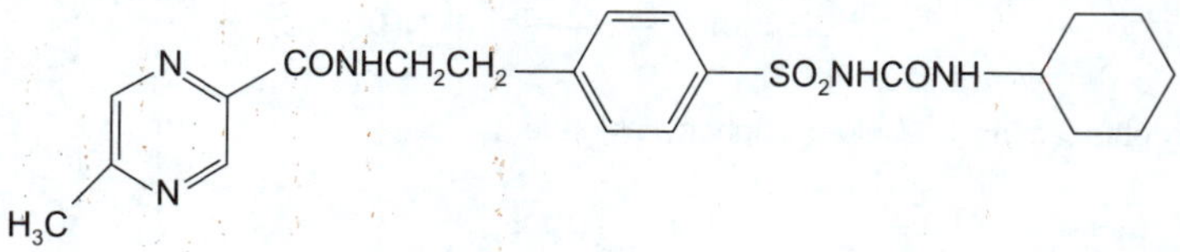

1-Cyclohexyl-3-[[*p*-[2-(5-methylpyrazine carboxamide) ethyl] phenyl] sulphonyl] urea

Synthesis

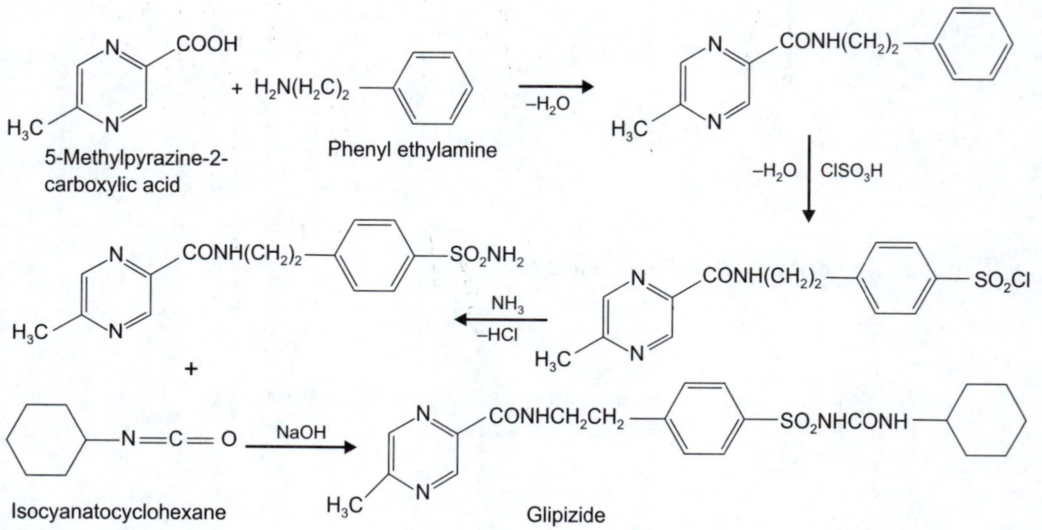

Metabolism: It is extensively metabolized to less active or inactive metabolites. Its metabolites are excreted primarily in the urine.

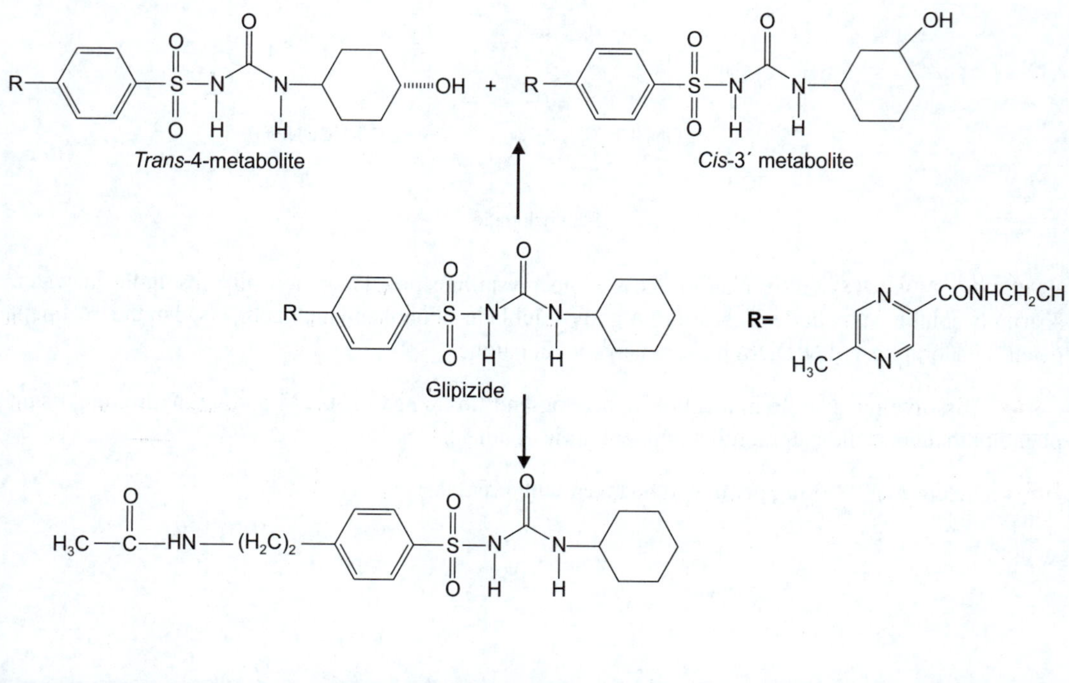

Properties and uses: Glipizide is a white crystalline powder, practically insoluble in water and ethanol, very slightly soluble in methylene chloride and acetone, soluble in dilute solutions of alkali hydroxides. It is an orally active hypoglycaemic drug.

Assay: Dissolve the sample in dimethylformamide and titrate against 0.1 M lithium methoxide add quinaldine red as indicator, until the colour changes from red to colourless.

Dose: The dosage is 25–50 mg once a day or in divided doses.

Dosage forms: Glipizide tablets BP.

iii. Gliclazide

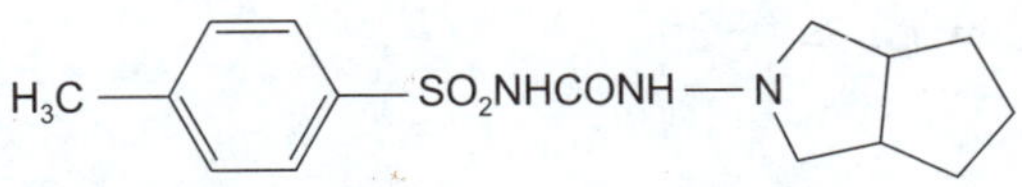

1-(3-Azabicyclo-oct-3-3-yl)-3-(*p*-tolylsulphonyl)urea

Properties and uses: Gliclazide is a white powder, practically insoluble in water, soluble in methylene chloride, sparingly soluble in acetone, and slightly soluble in alcohol. It is an orally active hypoglycaemic drug.

Assay: Dissolve the sample in anhydrous acetic acid and titrate against 0.1 M perchloric acid. Determine the end point potentiometrically.

Dosage forms: Gliclazide tablets BP.

SAR of Sulphonylureas

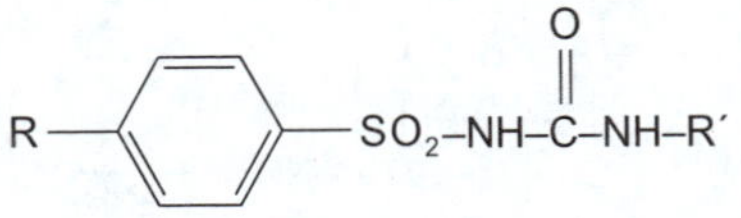

1. The benzene ring should contain a substitutent preferably in the *para* position. The substituents, such as methyl, acetyl, amino, chloro, bromo, trifluoro methyl, and dithiomethyl were found to enhance the antihyperglycaemic activity.
2. When the *para* position of benzene is substituted with aryl carboxamidoalkyl group (second-generation sulphonylureas, such as glibenclamide) the activity was found to be enhanced further.
3. The size of the group attached to the terminal nitrogen is crucial for activity. The group should also impart lipophilicity to the compound *N*-methyl and ethyl substituents that show no activity, whereas N-propyl and higher homologues were found to be active and the activity is lost when the N-substituent contains 12 or more carbons.

II. Biguanides

Mode of action: Biguanides do not have direct action on increasing or decreasing the glucose level. This reduces glucose levels primarily by decreasing hepatic gluconeogenisis by increasing the insulin action on muscles and fat. It also reduces the absorption of glucose from intestine.

i. Phenformin

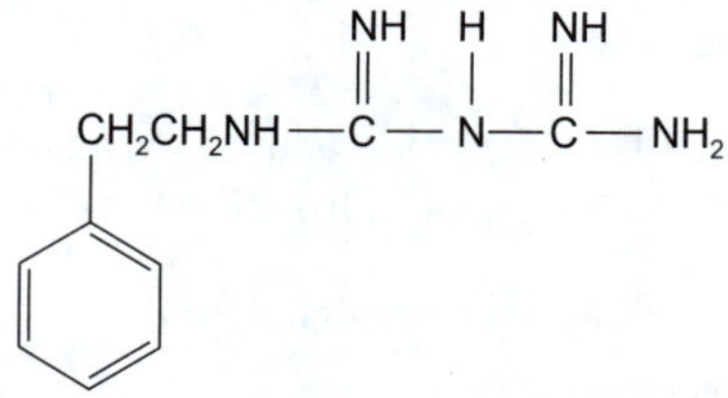

Synthesis

Route I. From: 2-Phenylethylamine

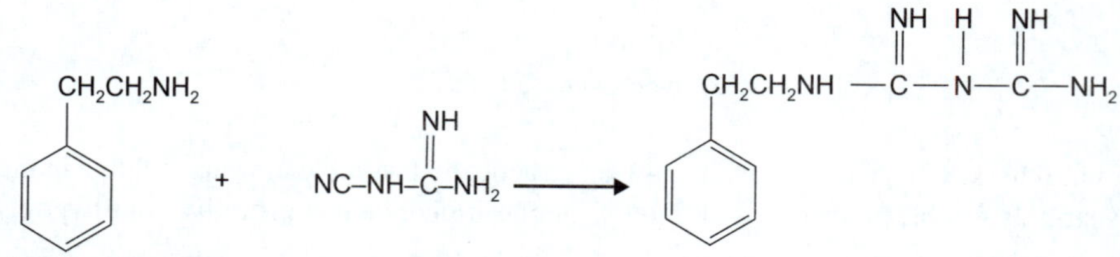

Route II. From: 1-(2-Chloroethyl) benzene

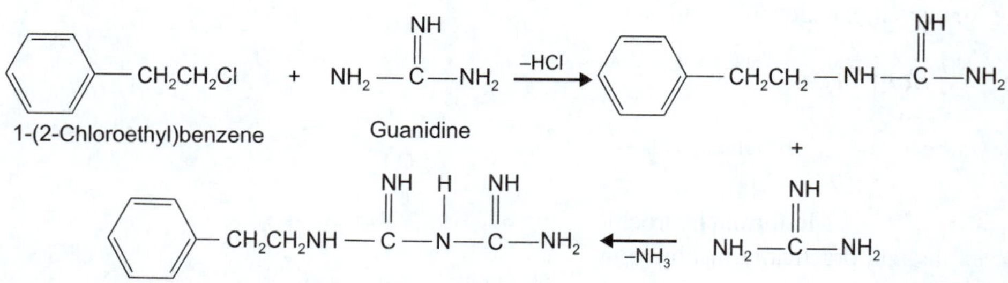

Properties and uses: Used only in stable type II diabetics, it may be used alone or in conjunction with another oral hypoglycaemic agents, such as sulphonylureas or with insulin.

Dose: The normal dose is 25 mg tablets 1–4 times a day, usually 50–150 mg daily with breakfast.

ii. Metformin (Diamet, Diaphage Glyciphage, Glycomet)

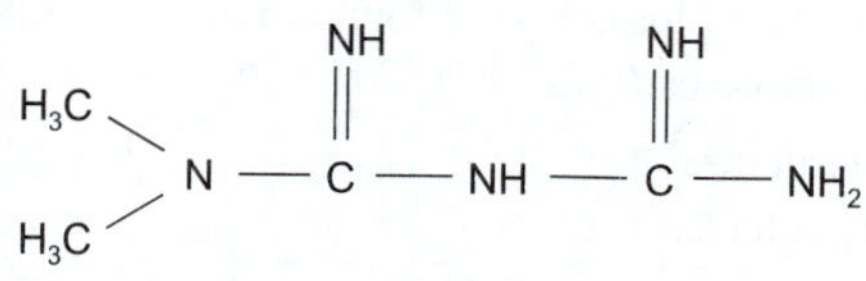

1,1-dimethyl biguanide

Synthesis

Route I. From: Dimethylamine

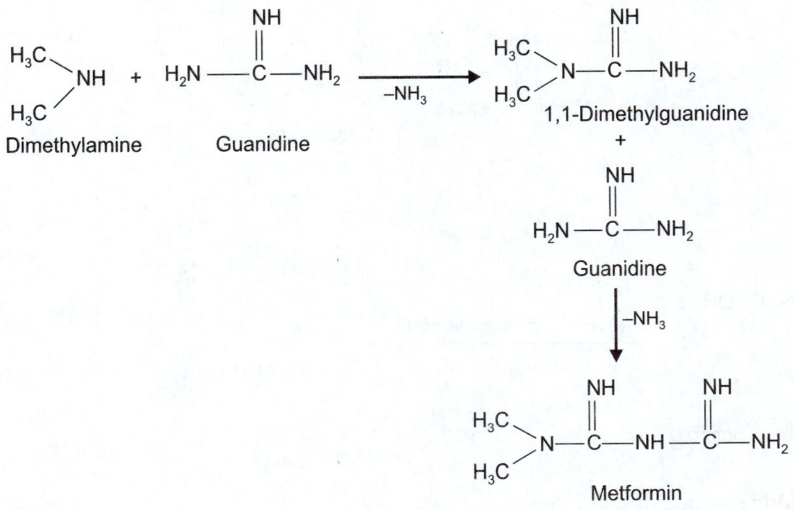

Route II. From: Dimethylamine

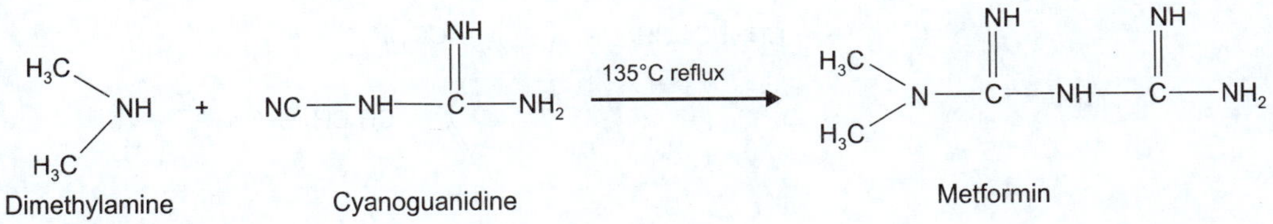

Properties and uses: Metformin hydrochloride exists as white crystals, freely soluble in water, slightly soluble in alcohol, practically insoluble in acetone and methylene chloride. It is usually given along with sulphonylureas.

Assay: Dissolve the sample in anhydrous formic acid, add acetonitrile, and titrate against 0.1 M perchloric acid. Determine the end point potentiometrically.

Dose: Initial dose is 500 mg thrice daily or 850 mg twice daily with meals.

Dosage forms: Metformin tablets BP.

III. Substituted Benzoic Acid Derivatives (Meglitinides)

The meglitinides are similar in structure to sulphonylureas. The sulphonylurea and meglitinide classes of oral hypoglycaemic drugs are referred to as endogenous insulin secretagogues because they induce the pancreatic release of endogenous insulin.

Mode of action: Even though, these are not sulphonylureas they act on sulphonylurea receptors as well as the other variant receptors and closes the ATP dependent K^+ channels, leading to insulin secretion by depolarization.

i. Meglitinide

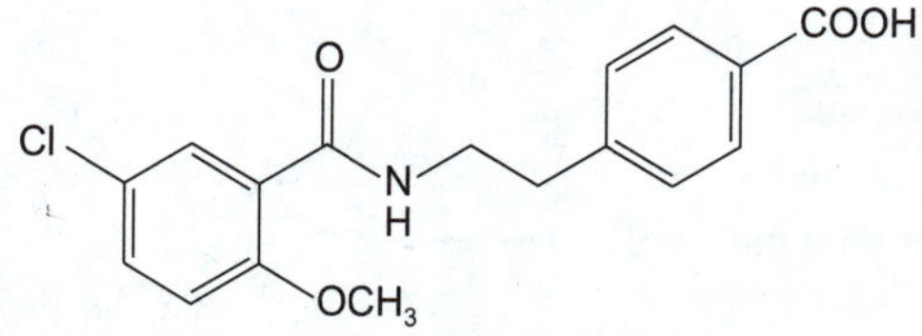

Synthesis

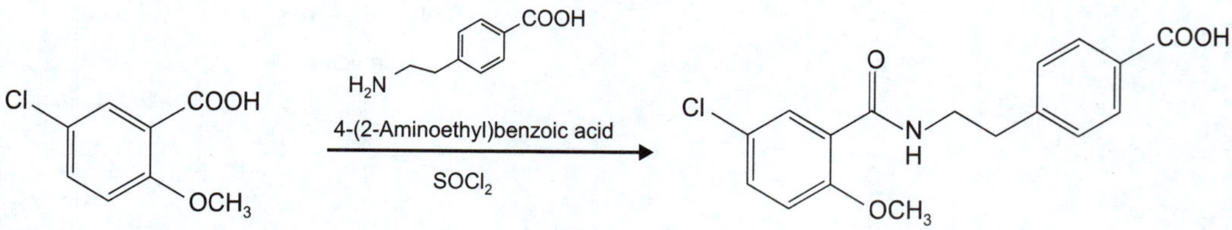

5-Chloro-2-methoxybenzoic acid

Meglitinide

ii. Repaglinide (Repide, Repa, Eurepa)

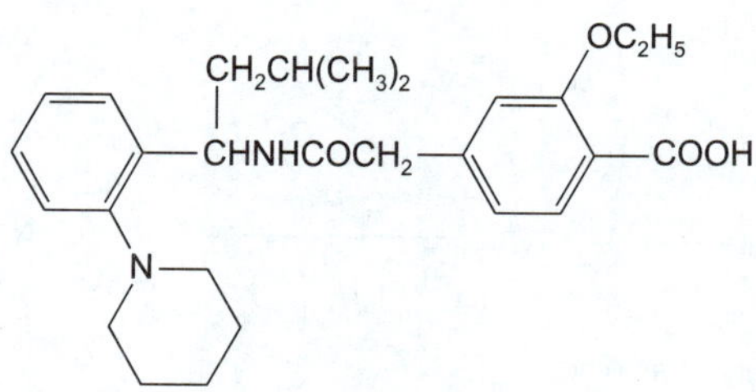

Synthesis

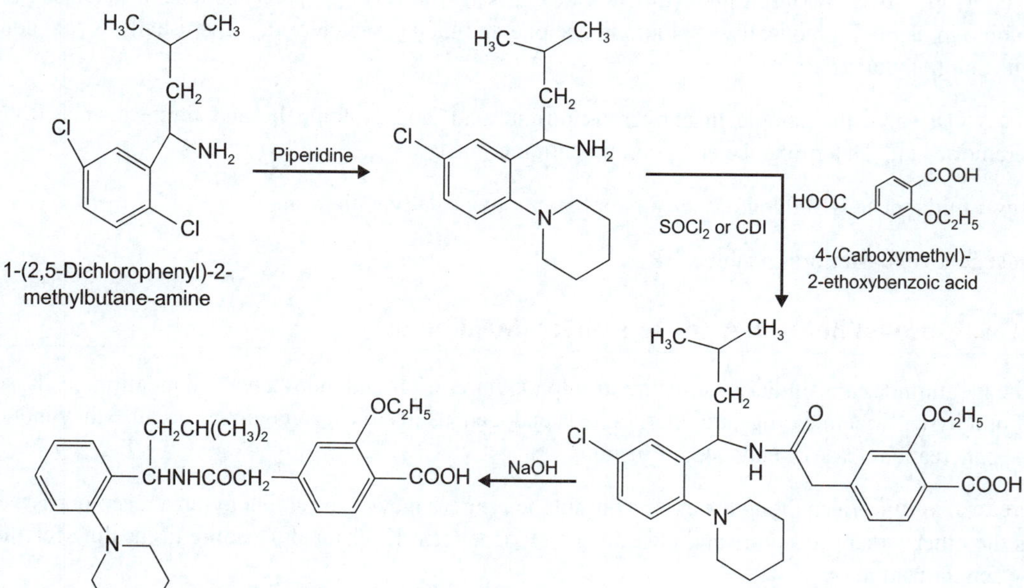

Repaglinide

Properties and uses: Repaglinide is a white powder, practically insoluble in water, soluble in methanol, and methylene chloride. It stimulates insulin release and is used in the treatment of diabetes mellitus.

Assay: Dissolve the sample in methanol and add anhydrous acetic acid and titrate against 0.1 M perchloric acid. Determine the end point potentiometrically.

Dose: The usual initial dose for adults is 0.5 mg, taken within 30 min of main meals. Initial doses of 1 or 2 mg may be used in patients who have had previous hypoglycaemic treatment. Dose may be adjusted at intervals of 1–2 week up to 4 mg before meals; maximum dose is 16 mg daily.

iii. Nateglinide

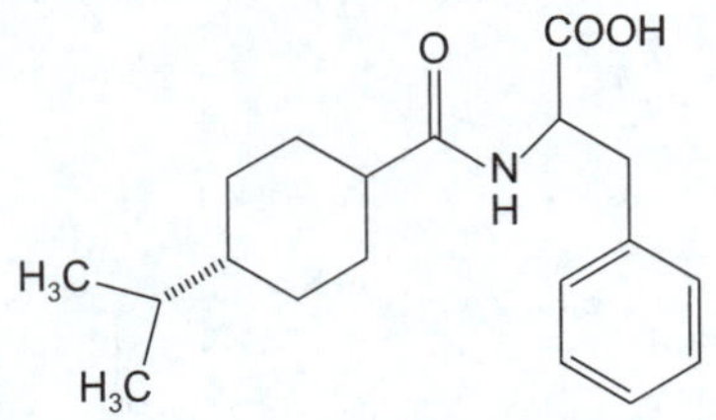

Metabolism: It is metabolized in the liver and 16% is excreted in the urine unchanged. The major metabolites are hydroxyl derivative (CYP2C9 70%, CYP3A4 30%) that are further conjugated to the glucuronide derivative (Figure 9.1).

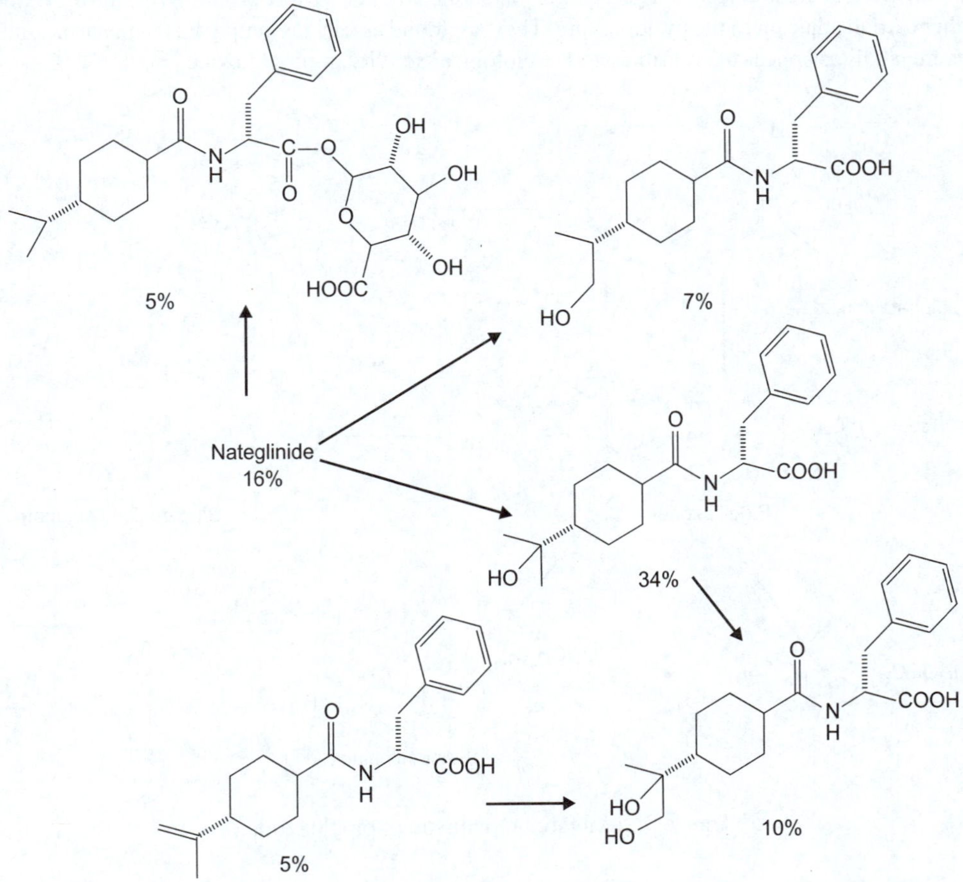

Fig. 9.1: Metabolic pathway of nateglinide

Uses: It is used as an oral hypoglycaemic agent in type II diabetic mellitus.

IV. Thiazolidinediones (Glitazones)

Thiazolidinediones are a new class of oral antidiabetic agents (commercially known as glitazones) that enhance insulin sensitivity in peripheral tissues. It is relatively safe in patients with impaired renal function because they are highly metabolized by the liver and excreted in the faeces.

Mode of action: These drugs produce gene-mediated transcription for the release of insulin by forming new proteins. They act on the nuclear peroxisome proliferator-activated receptor γ (*ppar* γ) and elicit the genes. It also inhibits the resistance to insulin by activating glucose transporters (Glut and Glut 1) in the plasma membrane.

i. Pioglitazone

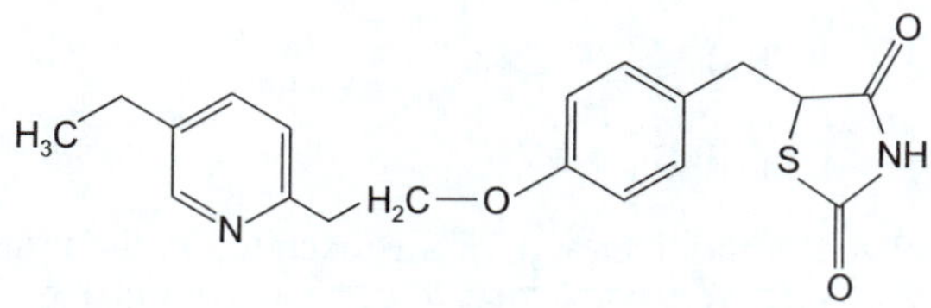

Metabolism: It is metabolized and gives eight metabolic products. These products result from oxidation at either carbon adjacent to the pyridine ring. They are found as various conjugates in the urine and bile. Three metabolites appear to contribute to the biological activity of pioglitazone (Figure 9.2).

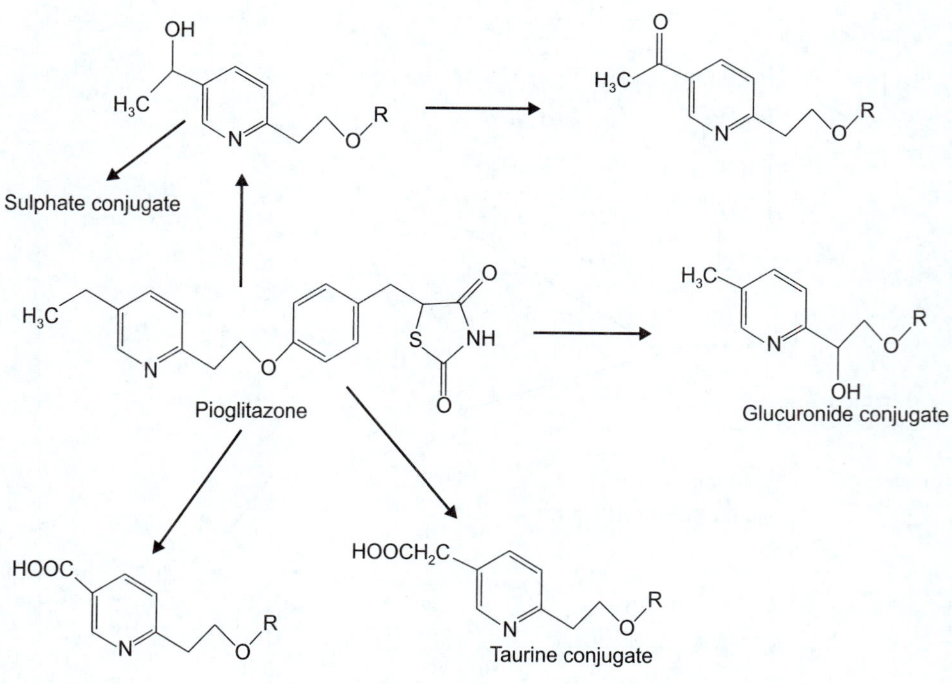

Figure 9.2: Metabolic pathway of pioglitazone.

ii. Ciglitazone

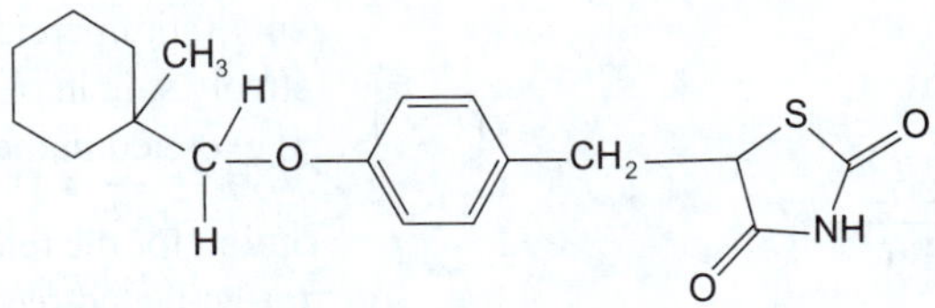

Synthesis

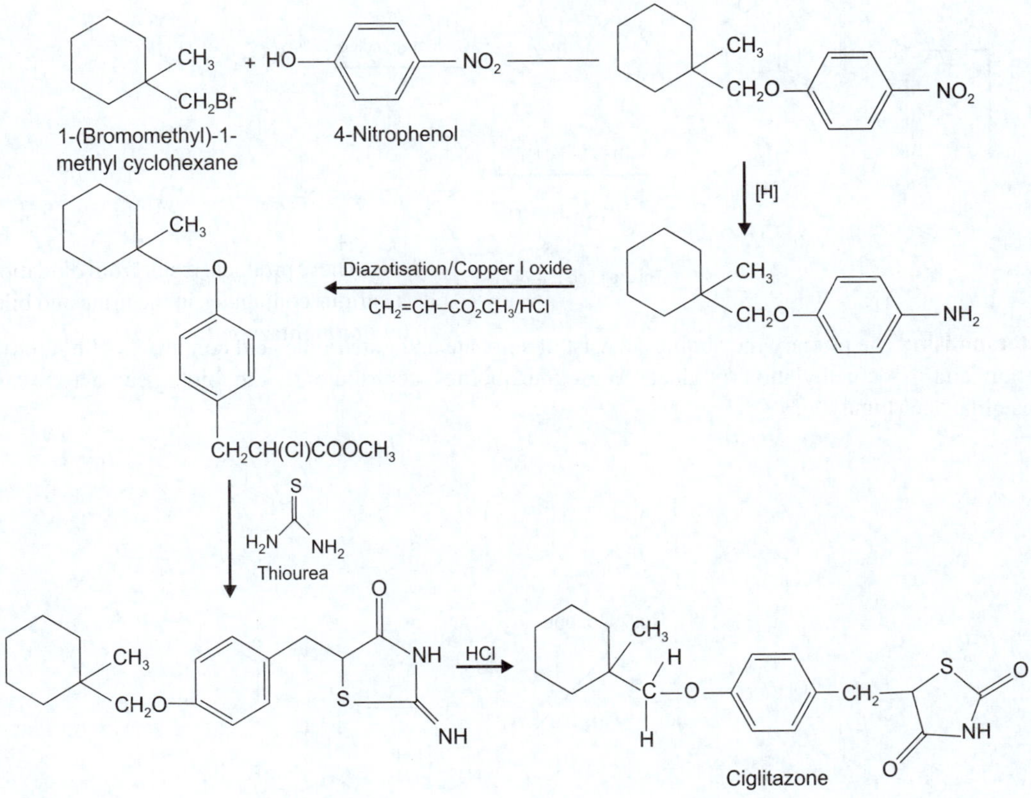

Use: It is used in the treatment of NIDDM.

iii. Rosiglitazone (Rosicon, Reglit, Rosinorm)

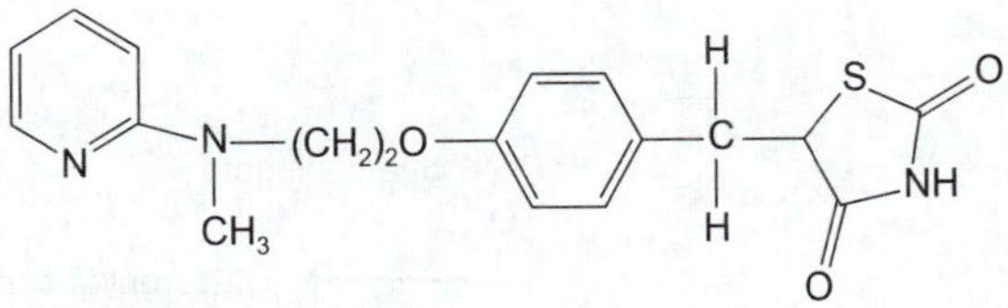

(±)-5-[[4-[2-Methyl-2-pyridinylamino]ethoxy]phenyl methyl]-2,4-thiazolidinedione

Synthesis

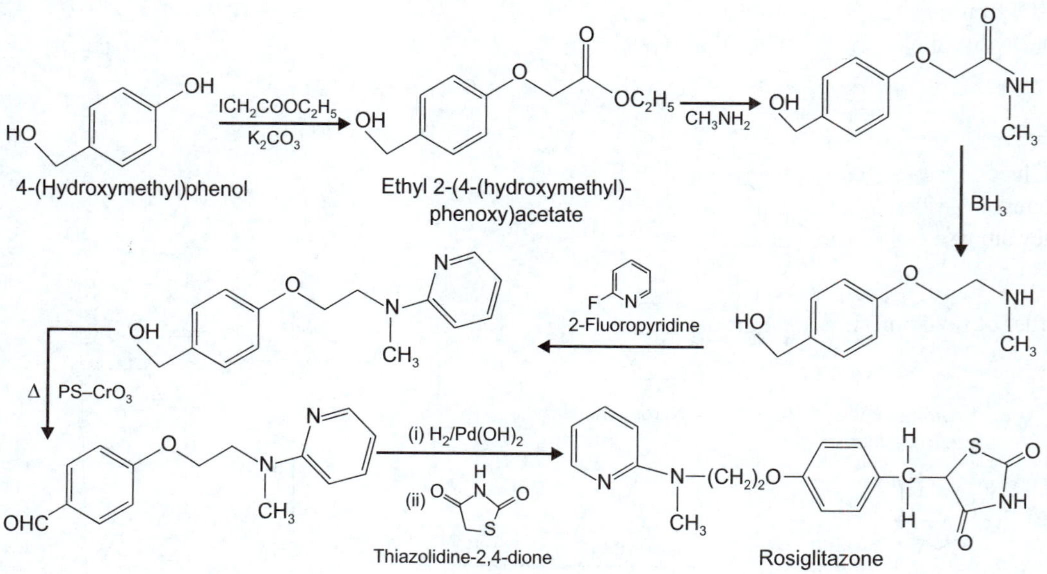

Metabolism: The primary metabolites consist of sulphate and glucuronic acid conjugates of hydroxylation and N-demethylation product. These metabolites contribute to the biological activity of rosiglitazone (Figure 9.3).

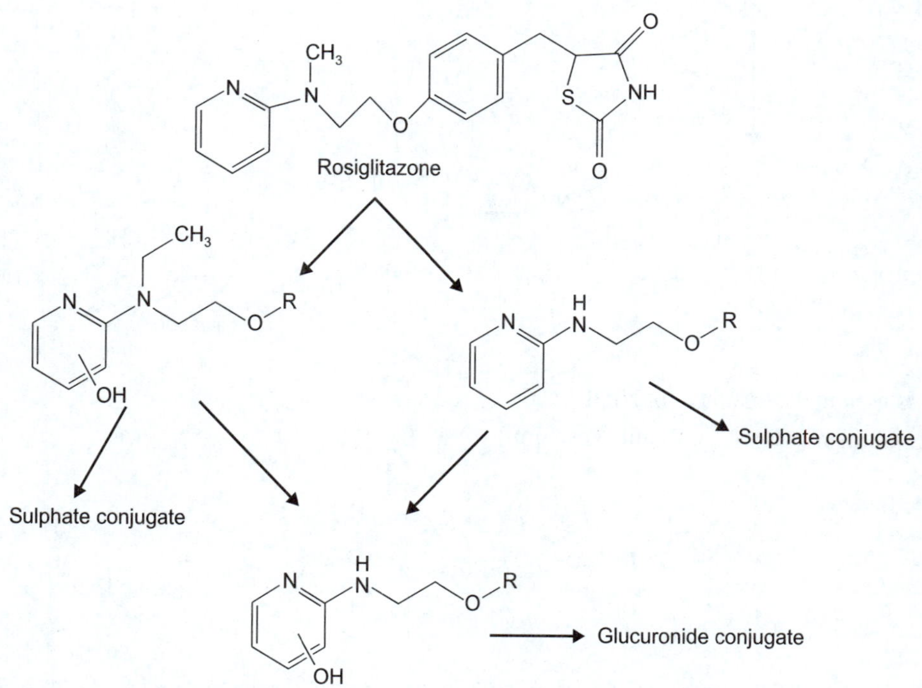

Figure 9.3: Metabolic pathway of rosiglitazone.

Uses: It is used in the treatment of NIDDM.

Dose: The dosage for type II diabetes mellitus for adult is 4 mg daily, which may be increased after 8–12 week of therapy, according to response and the maximum dosage is 8 mg daily.

V. α-Glucosidase Inhibitors

α-Glucosidase enzyme is responsible for breaking down the complex polysaccharides and sucrose to monosaccharides, which are then absorbed; α-glucosidase inhibitors decrease the rate of breakdown. They are also called starch blockers.

Mode of action: These acts on the final enzymes in the digestion of carbohydrates present in the brush border of small intestine and transport of polysaccharides and sucrose.

i. Acarbose

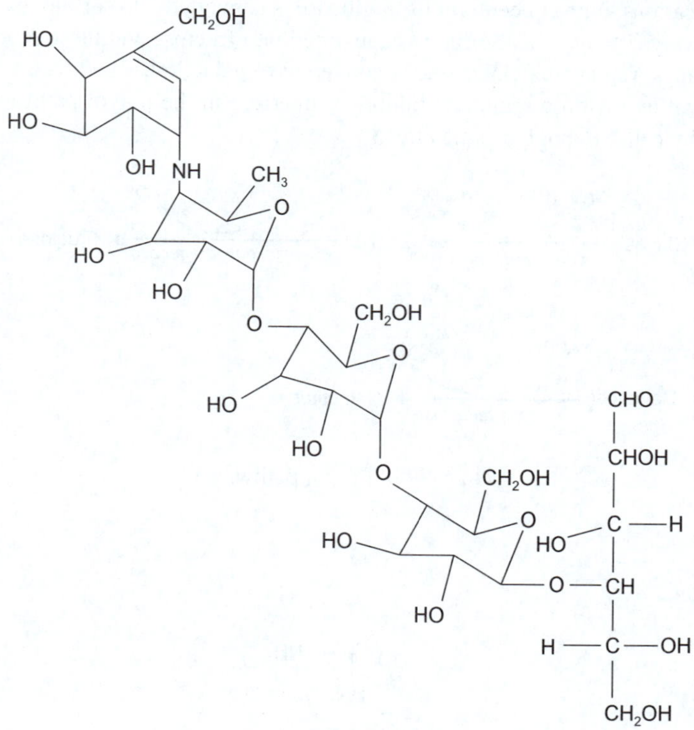

Properties and uses: Acarbose is a white or yellowish amorphous hygroscopic powder, very soluble in water, soluble in methanol, and practically insoluble in methylene chloride. It is an alpha-glucosidase inhibitor and used in the treatment of diabetes mellitus.

Assay: It is assayed by adopting liquid chromatography technique.

ii. Miglitol

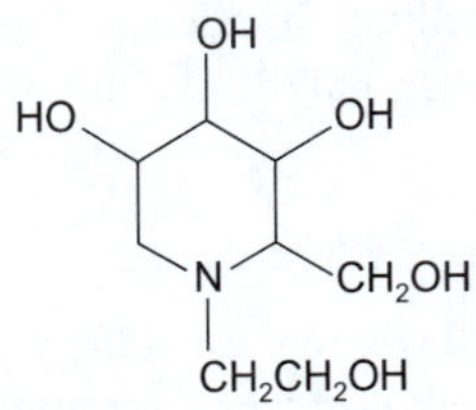

Properties and uses: It is a crystalline substance, soluble in water. It is a α-glucosidase inhibitor and used as an antidiabetic agent.

VI. Aldose Reductase Inhibitors

In diabetic complications, high concentrations of glucose is converted into sorbitol by aldose reductase by the polyol pathway (Figure 9.4). Sorbitol is converted into fructose and these products accumulate in the nerves, kidneys, retina, etc. Galactone is converted to galactitol, which is not metabolized and causes osmotic swelling. Aldose reductase inhibitors interfere in the polyol pathway of sorbitol and fructose and thereby cause hypoglycaemic effects.

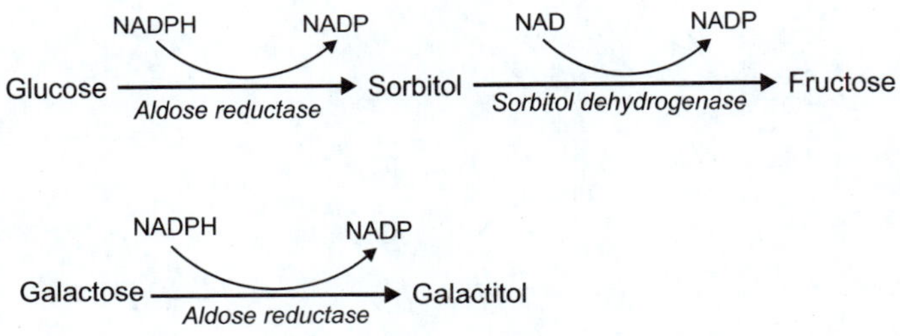

Figure 9.4: Polyol pathway

i. Sorbinil

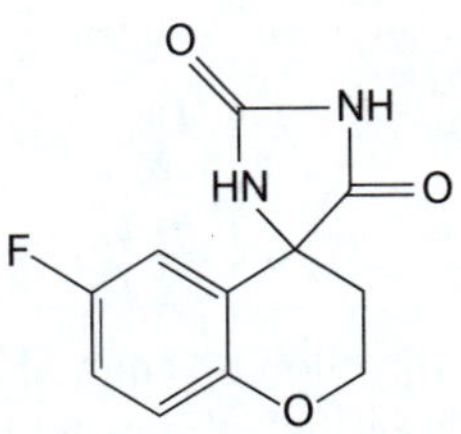

Uses: It is used in the treatment of diabetic neuropathy.

ii. Tolrestat

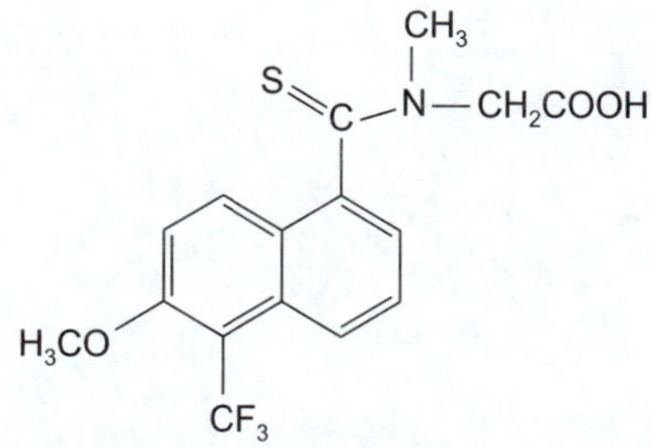

N-[6-Methoxy-5-trifluoromethyl-1-naphthyl(thiocarbonyl)]-N-methylglycine

Uses: It is useful in the prophylaxis of diabetic neuropathy and cataracts.

VII. Miscellaneous

Linogliride

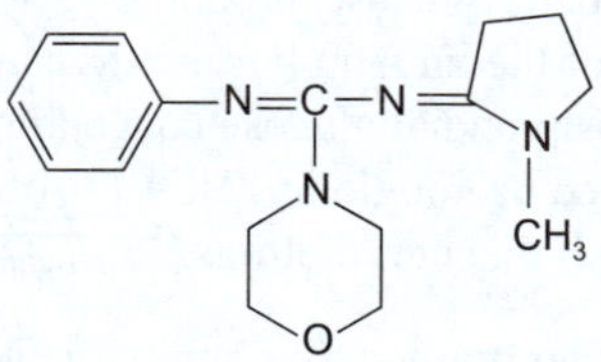

Synthesis

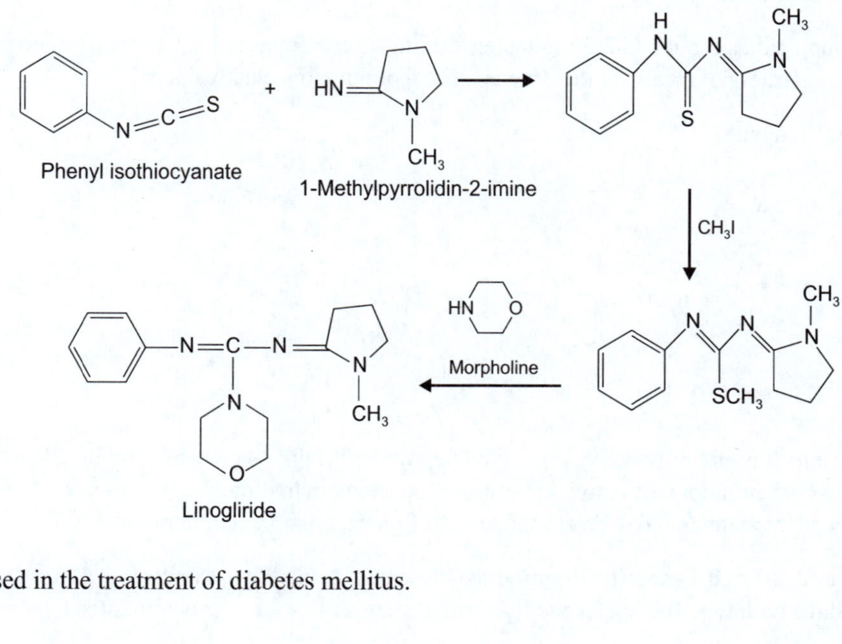

Linogliride

Uses: Used in the treatment of diabetes mellitus.

NEWER DRUGS

Saxagliptin (Onglyza)

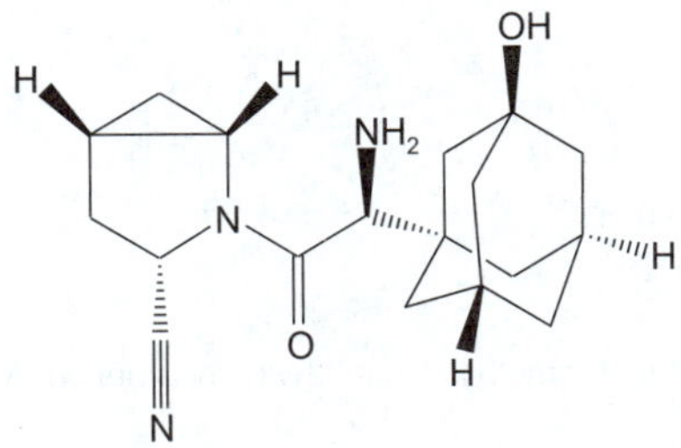

Mode of action: It is an orally-active DPP4 enzyme inhibitor, which acts by affecting the action of natural hormones known as incretins. From small intestine after meals, more amount of incretin hormones such as glucagon-like peptide-1 (GLP-1) and glucose-dependent insulinotropic polypeptide (GIP) are released into bloodstream, which cause insulin release in a glucose-dependent manner from the beta cells of pancreas, but DPP4 enzyme inactivates them within minutes. GLP-1 also lowers glucagon secretion for reducing hepatic glucose production. This drug acts as competitive DPP4 inhibitor that slows the inactivation of the incretin hormones, hence their bloodstream concentrations increased and reduces fasting and postprandial glucose concentration in a glucose-dependent manner. It produces reductions in (glycosylated haemoglobin) HbA (1c) and increases in the rate of achieving target HbA (1c) in patients with type II diabetes mellitus.

Properties and uses: Saxagliptin is an orally-active inhibitor of the DPP4 enzyme. It is used as an adjunct to diet and exercise to improve glycemic control in adults with type II diabetes mellitus. Adverse events associated with the use of onglyza may include, upper respiratory tract infection, urinary tract infection, headache, nasopharyngitis.

Dose: It is supplied as 5 mg and 2.5 mg tablet formulated for oral administration. The recommended initial dose, regardless of meals, of the drug is 2.5 mg or 5 mg once daily taken.

Linagliptin (Tradjenta)

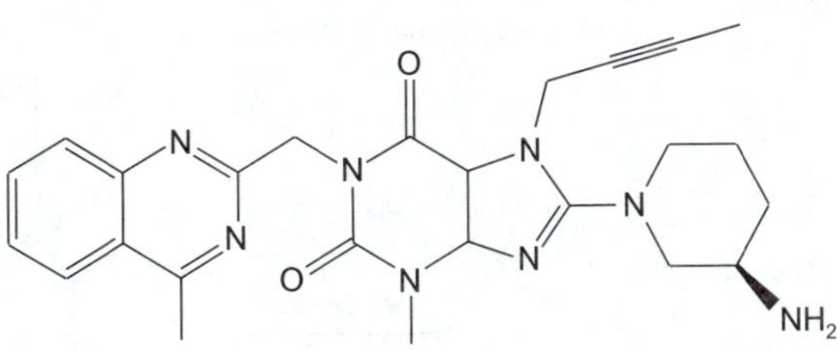

Mode of action: It is an orally-active dipeptidyl peptidase-4 (DPP-4) enzyme inhibitor, Thus, the drug increases the concentrations of active incretin hormones, which stimulate the release of insulin in a glucose-dependent manner and decrease the levels of glucagon in the circulation.

Properties and uses: It is specifically used as an adjunct to diet and exercise to improve glycemic control in adults with type II diabetes mellitus. Adverse reactions are nasopharyngitis, hypoglycaemia, pancreatitis.

Dose: The recommended dose is 5 mg once daily with or without food.

Mifepristone (Korlym)

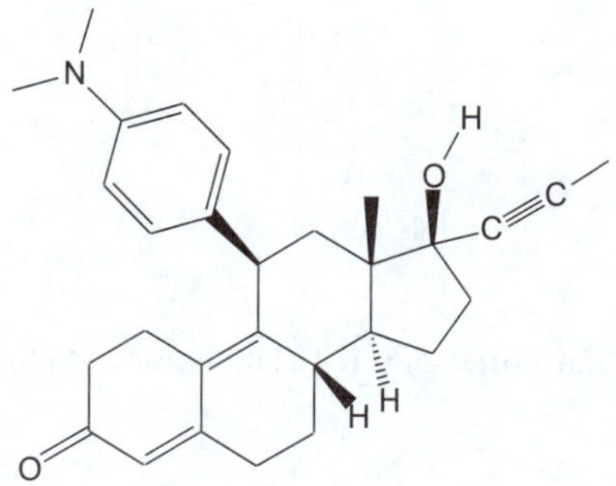

Properties and uses: Mifepristone is a small-molecule progesterone and glucocorticoid antagonist. It blocks the binding of cortisol to its receptor. It does not decrease cortisol production but reduces the effects of excess cortisol, such as high blood sugar levels. Used to control hyperglycemia secondary to hypercortisolism in adults with endogenous Cushing's syndrome who have type II diabetes mellitus or glucose intolerance and have failed surgery or are not candidates for surgery. Adverse events are, nausea, headache, decreased blood potassium, fatigue, hypertension, arthralgia, vomiting, peripheral edema, dizziness.

Dose: Initial dose is a single dose of 300 mg orally once daily. The daily dose of the drug may be increased in 300 mg increments. The dose may be increased to a maximum of 1200 mg once daily but should not exceed 20 mg/kg per day. Increases in dose should not occur more frequently than once every 2–4 weeks.

Mode of action: It is a small-molecule progesterone and glucocorticoid antagonist. It is a selective antagonist of the progesterone receptor at low doses and blocks the glucocorticoid receptor (GR-II) at higher doses. It has high affinity for the GR-II receptor but little affinity for the GR-I (MR, mineralocorticoid) receptor.

Liraglutide (Victoza)

$$C_{172}H_{265}N_{43}O_{51}$$

Properties and uses: Liraglutide an analog of human GLP-1 and acts as a GLP-1 receptor agonist, specifically used as an adjunct to diet and exercise to improve glycemic control in adults with type II diabetes mellitus. Adverse events associated with the use of liraglutide may include, nausea, vomiting, diarrhea, constipation, headache.

Dose: At any time of day it can be administered once daily, independent of meals. It can be injected subcutaneously in the abdomen, thigh, or upper arm. Initial dose is 0.6 mg per day for one week. After one week at 0.6 mg per day, it should be increased to 1.2 mg. The dose can be increased to 1.8 mg, if the 1.2 mg dose does not yield acceptable glycaemic control.

Mode of action: It increases intracellular cyclic AMP (cAMP), which results in insulin release in the presence of elevated glucose concentrations. As blood glucose concentrations decrease and approach euglycaemia, this insulin secretion subsides. It also reduces glucagon secretion in a glucose-dependent manner. Blood glucose lowering also involves a day in gastric emptying.

Steglatro

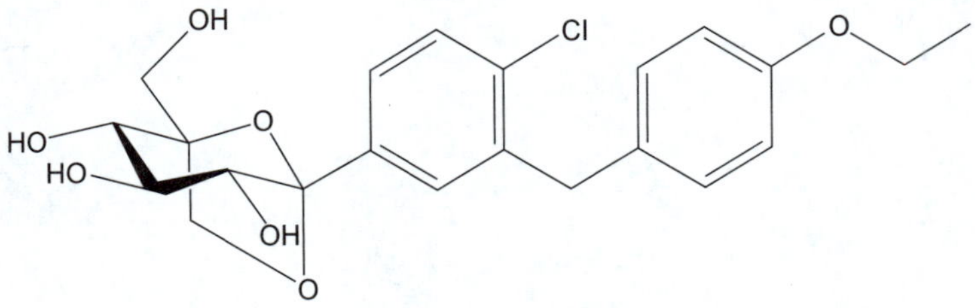

Uses: It is a sodium glucose co-transporter 2 (SGLT2) inhibitor and improves glycemic control in adults with type II diabetes mellitus.

CLASSIFICATION BASED ON PCI SYLLABUS

Sulfonyl Ureas

Tolbutamide

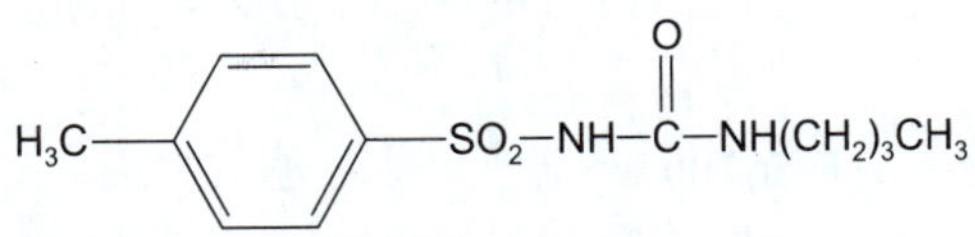

Chlorpropamide

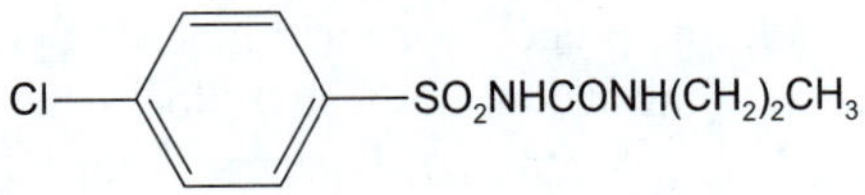

Glipizide

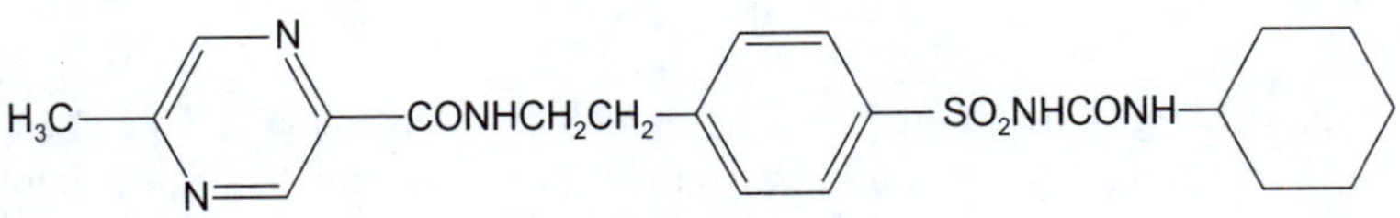

Glimepiride

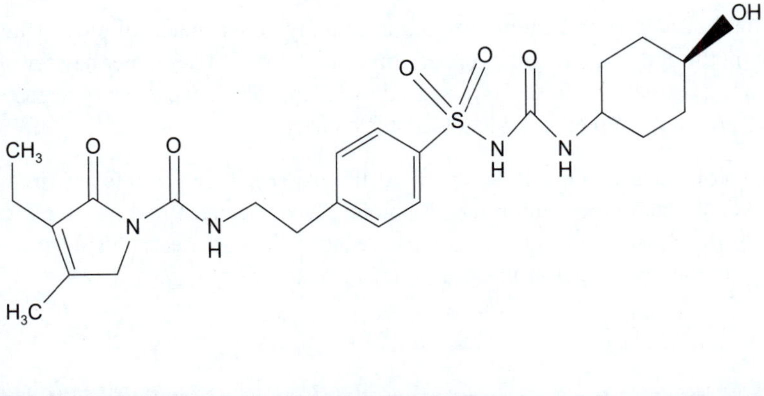

Biguanides

Metformin

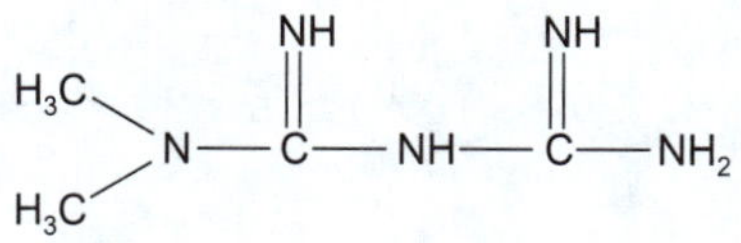

Thiazolidinediones

Pioglitazone

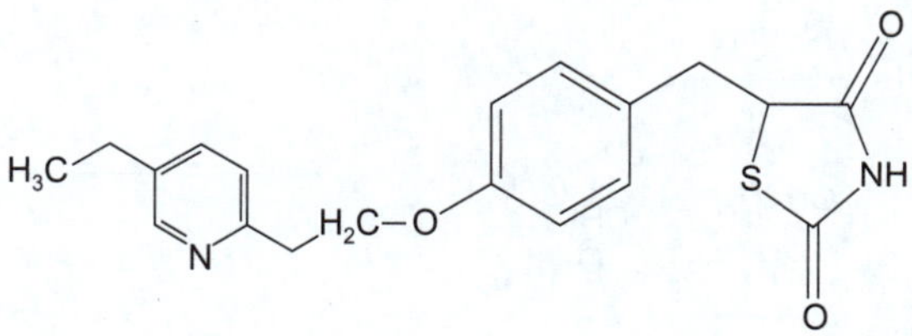

Rosiglitazone

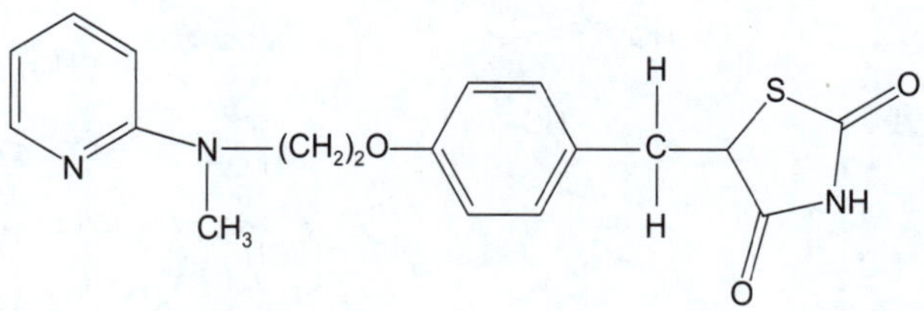

Meglitinides

Repaglinide

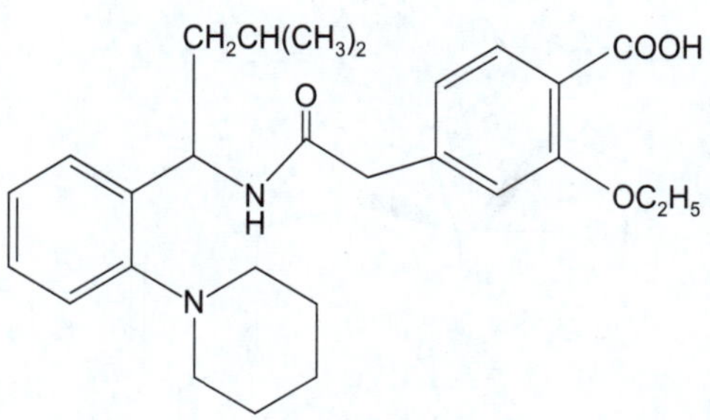

Nateglinide

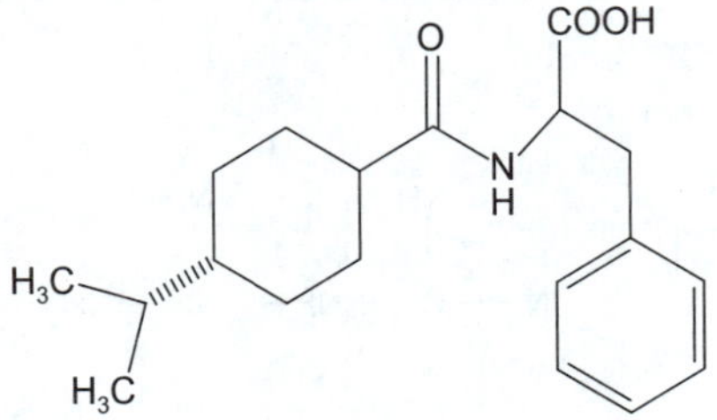

Glucosidase Inhibitors

Acarbose

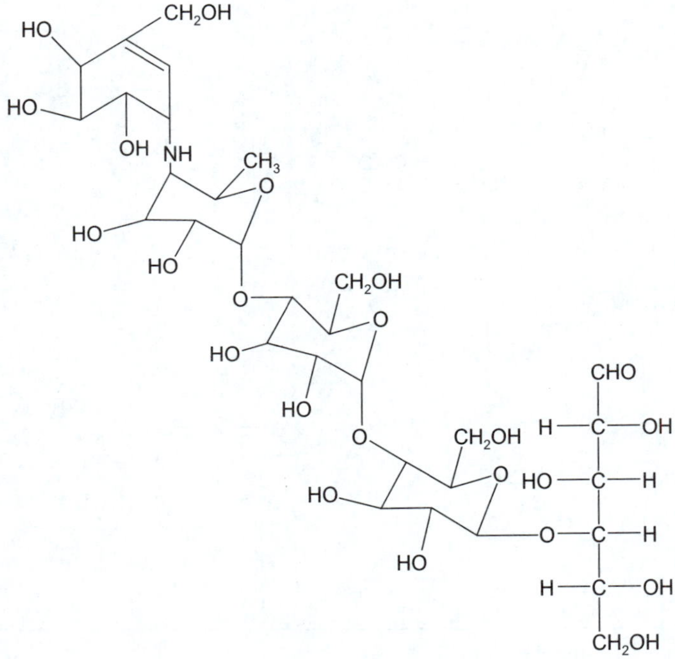

Voglibose

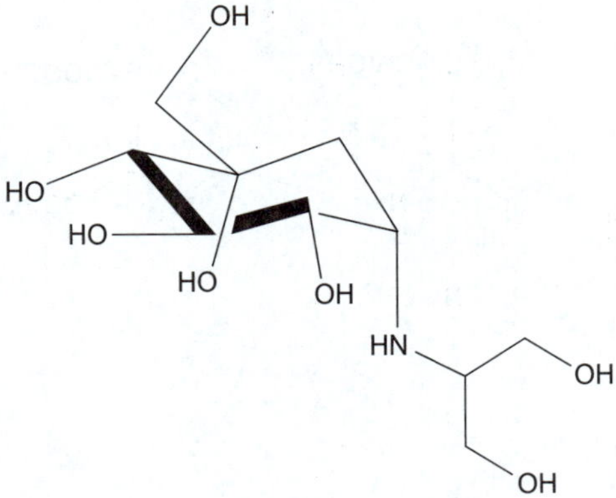

Properties and uses: It is an α-glucosidase inhibitor which delays the absorption of glucose. It is used to treat diabetic.

INSULIN AND ITS PREPARATIONS

Insulin is a hormone secreted by the β-cells of islets of Langerhans and regulates the blood glucose level in the body. It facilitates the transport of glucose to skeletal muscles and adipose tissue by increasing the number of glucose transporters such as GLUT-1 and GLUT-4. It regulates metabolism of carbohydrates, fats and proteins and controls the sugar level in the blood. The β-cells synthesize insulin from a single-chain precursor of 110 amino acids termed preproinsulin. Insulin promotes the synthesis of glycogen, triacylglycerols and proteins and hence it is considered as anabolic hormone.

Structure of Insulin

It was discovered by Banting and Best. It contains 51 amino acids and two peptide chains, i.e. Chain A and Chain B, which are connected via two disulphide bridges (Fig. 9.4). C–P or connecting peptide is responsible for immunogenic reactions. The amino acids present in insulin are glycine, alanine, valine, leucine, iso-leucine, proline, phenylalanine, tyrosine, serine, threonine, lysine, glutamic acid, glutamine, asparagine, arginine, histidine.

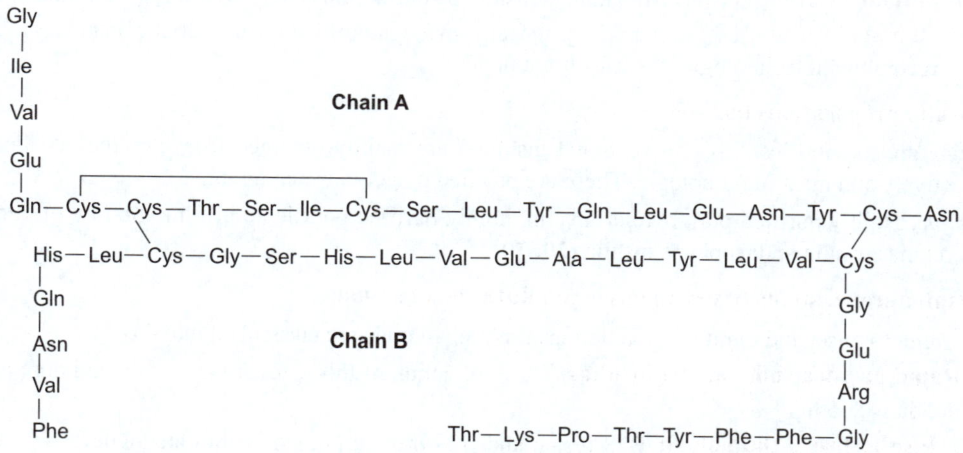

Fig 9.4: Structure of human insluin

Structure of chain A: The chain A of insulin is found to contain 21 amino acids and is acidic in nature.

Structure of chain B: The chain B contains 30 amino acid residues and is basic in nature.

Mode of Action

Insulin binds with the specific insulin receptors such as 2α and 2β receptors. The 2β receptor is tyrosine kinase receptor. Insulin binds with 2α receptor and activates the tyrosine kinase activity of β-subunits which increases the glucose entry to the cell via phosphorylation.

Functions of insulin: The various functions of insulin are:

1. Regulates glucose metabolism
2. Stimulates lipogenesis
3. Diminishes lipolysis
4. Increases amino acid transport into cells
5. Modulates transcription
6. Alters the cell content of numerous mRNAs

7. Stimulates growth
8. DNA synthesis
9. Cell replication

Insulin Preparations

They are classified into different ways as follows.

1. Insulin preparations based on source.
2. Insulin preparations based on purity.
3. Insulin preparations based on onset and duration of action.

Let us discuss in detail.

1. Insulin preparations based on source:

a. **Bovine insulin:** It differs from human insulin by 3 amino acid residues and more immunogenic to humans.

b. **Porcine insulin:** It differs from human insulin by one amino acid residue and less immunogenic.

c. **Human insulin:** It is prepared by the enzymatic modification of porcine insulin or DNA recombinant technology. It is least immunogenic.

2. Insulin preparations based on purity:

Porcine and bovine insulins (conventional insulins) are mainly obtained from porcine and bovine, respectively and most immunologic. These are purified by gel-chromatography.

Example: Highly purified pork regular insulin, highly purified pork lente insulin, mixture of purified pork regular insulin and isophane insulin (30:70).

3. Insulin preparations based on onset and duration of action:

According to onset and duration of action insulin preparations are classificed into 4 types:

i. **Rapid or ultra short-acting insulins:** Onset of action of this category is 15 min and duration of action is 2–6 hrs.

a. **Insulin lispro (humalog):** B28 lysine and B29 proline human insulin analogue in which the usual B28 proline and B29 lysine is reversed.

b. **Insulin aspirate (novolog):** It is similar to human insulin but the B28 proline is replaced by aspartic acid.

c. **Insulin glulisine:** It is also a human insulin analogue in which B3 asparagine is replaced by lysine and B29 lysine is replaced by glutamic acid.

ii. **Short-acting insulin preparations:** Regular soluble insulin (humulin/novolin). The onset of action is 0.5 to 1 min and the duration of action is 6–8 hrs. It is the only insulin approved to be administered via IV route. It is prepared from porcine, bovine or genetically engineered rDNA technology from some microorganisms such sa *E. coli*.

iii. **Intermediate-acting:** The onset of action is 1–2 hrs and duration of action is 18–24 hrs.

a. **Isophase or NPH (neutral protamine Hage dog):** It contains a sterile suspension of zinc insulin crystals and protamine sulphate.

b. **Lente (Insulin zinc suspension):** It is a sterile suspension of insulin modified by the addition of zinc chloride. The main advantage of this is, produces less allergic reactions when compared with NPH.

iv. **Long-acting:** The onset of action is 2 to 5 hrs and the duration of action is 20 to 24 hrs.

a. **Glargine (lantus):** It differs from human insulin wherein A21 asparagine is replaced by glycine and additional 30B-a-L-arginine and 30 b-b-L-arginine.

b. Ultra lente/extended insulin zinc suspension: It is a sterile suspension of insulin modified with addition of zinc chloride. Onset of action is 4–8 hrs and the duration of action is 36 hrs.

iii. Insulin detemir: It is a neutral soluble human insulin analogue in which the terminal amino acid B30 has been replaced by a 14-carbon chain fatty acid, myristic acid.

Insulin combinations

i. Novolin 70/30: It contains 70% NPH and 30% regular insulin.

ii. Humulin 50/50: It contains 50% NPH and 50% regular insulin.

PROBABLE QUESTIONS

1. Explain type I and type II diabetes with some typical examples.
2. How do you classify the oral hypoglycaemic agents? Write the structure, chemical names, and uses of at least two compounds.
3. Write the mode of action of tolbutamide and phenformin.
4. Write in detail about thiazolindiones with specific reference to the following drugs: Rosiglitazone, troglitazone.
5. Write a short note on the following oral hypoglycaemic agents: (a) Biguanides and (b) α-glucosidase inhibitors.
6. Write a brief account of the following with a few examples: (a) First-generation sulphonylureas and (b) second-generation sulphonylureas.
7. How will you synthesize the following drugs: (a) Chloropropamide, (b) tolbutamide, and (c) glipizide.
8. Explain about the meglitinides' specific mechanism of action. Write the structure, synthesis, metabolism, and uses of any one of them.

SUGGESTED READINGS

1. Boyd AE. 'Sulfonylurea receptors ion channels, and fruit flies'. *Diabetes* 37: 847–50, 1988.
2. *British Pharmacopoeia*. Medicines and Healthcare Products Regulatory Agency. London, 2008.
3. Bruntan LL, Lazo JS, and Parker KL. *Goodman and Gilman's: The Pharmacological Basis of Therapeutics* (11th edn). New York: McGraw Hill, 2006.
4. Cook NS. *Potassium Channels: Structure, Classifi cation, Function and Therapeutic Potential*. New York: John Wiley, 1990.
5. Datt N. 'Insulin pharmacotherapy'. *J Pharm Pract* 5: 260–70, 1992.
6. Ferner RE. 'Oral hypoglycemic agents'. *Med Clin North Am* 72: 1323–335, 1988.
7. Gennaro AR. *Remington: The Science and practice of Pharmacy* (21st edn). New York: Lippincot Williams and Wilkins, 2006.
8. Gerich JE. 'Oral hypoglycemic agents'. *N Engl J Med* 321: 1231, 1989.
9. *Indian Pharmacopoeia*. Ministry of Health and Family Welfare. New Delhi, 1996.
10. Lednicer D and Mitscher LA. *The Organic Chemistry of Drug Synthesis*. New York: John Wiley, 1995.
11. Lebovitz HE. 'Oral antidiabetic agents'. *Drugs* 44 (Suppl) 3: 21–28, 1992.
12. Miyahera RL. 'Pharmacotherapy of oral hypoglycaemic agents'. *J Pharm Pract* 5: 271–79, 1992.
13. Pandeya SN and Murthi KN. 'Recent developments in antidiabetics'. *Eastern Pharmacist* 35 (416): 69–76, 1992.
14. Pandey SK, Theberge JF, Bernier M, and Srivastava AK. *Biochemistry* 38: 14667–675, 1999.
15. Srivastava V and Pandeya SN. 'Recent trends in hypoglycemic research'. *J Sci Industr Res* 47: 706–21, 1988.

CHAPTER 10

Steroids

INTRODUCTION

Steroids are a unique class of chemical compounds that are found widely in the animal and plant kingdom, these are characterized by the presence of a 1,2-cyclopentanoperhydrophenanthrene nucleus in their structure. Steroids consist of four rings. Perhydrophenanthrene (rings A, B, and C) is a completely saturated derivative of phenanthrene, while D is a five-membered cyclopentane ring. The steroids include a wide variety of naturally occurring and synthetic substances, such as sterols including vitamin D, bile acids, adrenal cortical and sex hormones, various contraceptive drugs, cardiac-active lactones (cardiac glycosides), sapogenins, and certain alkaloids and antibiotics.

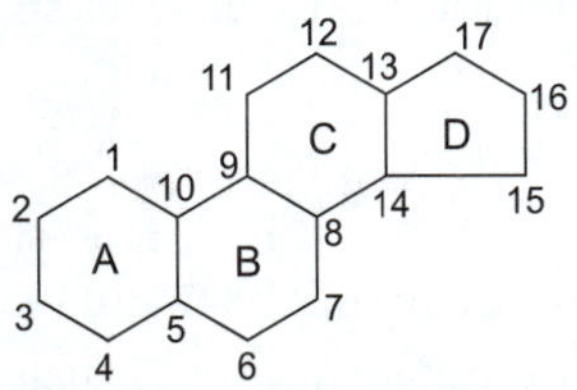

Steroid template

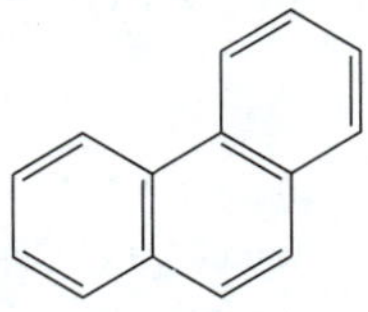

Phenanthrene

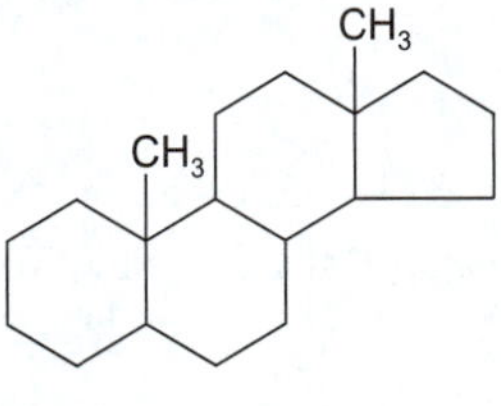

Steroid backbone

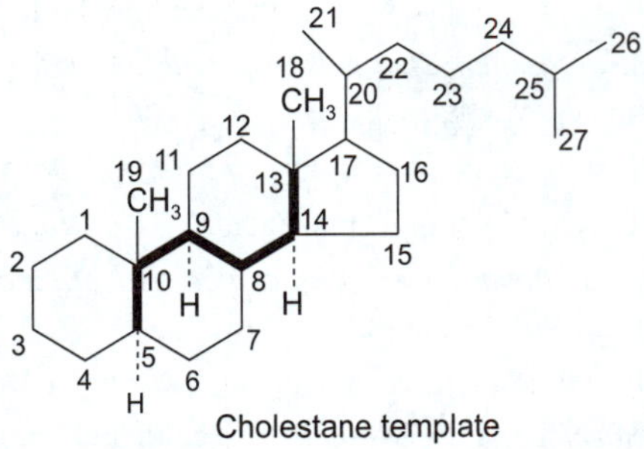

Cholestane template

The term *cholesterol* was derived from the Greek words *bile* (meaning 'chole') and *solid* (meaning 'sterols'). The modern era of steroid research began with steroid chemistry in the 1900s. Dr A O Windaus worked for over 20 years and received the Nobel Prize in 1928 for his research on the *constitution of sterols*.

Dr Heinrich and Dr Wieland engaged in natural products chemistry, including bile acids, were awarded the Nobel Prize in 1928.

Totally six Nobel Prizes were awarded to scientists working in the area of steroids; among the six, four were in steroid chemistry. The pioneer work of Adolf Windaus and Heinrich Wieland in structural elucidation of a number of important steroids lead to the many significant discoveries in the steroids.

The two interesting discoveries (mentioned in points a and b below) in the late 1940s and early 1950s had a dramatic effect not only on steroid research but also on the pharmacological applications of steroids, which led to an extensive research on the medicinal chemistry, pharmacology, and clinical studies of steroid agonists and antagonists.

a. The clinical report on the anti-inflammatory effect of cortisone in patients with rheumatoid arthritis.
b. The use of oestrogen and progestin preparations for contraception.

Steroids when dehydrogenated with selenium at 360°C yield Diels hydrocarbon. On the basis of this reaction, a steroid may be defined as any compound which yields Diel's hydrocarbon when distilled with selenium. However, if the steroids are distilled with selenium at 420°C, they yield mainly chrysene and a small amount of picene.

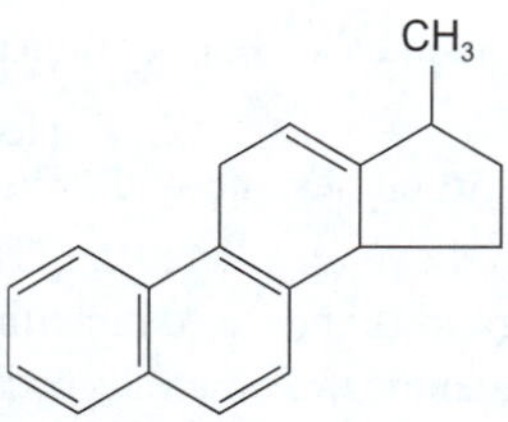

Diels hydrocarbon

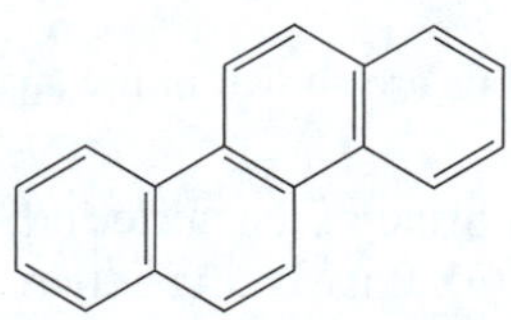

Chrysene

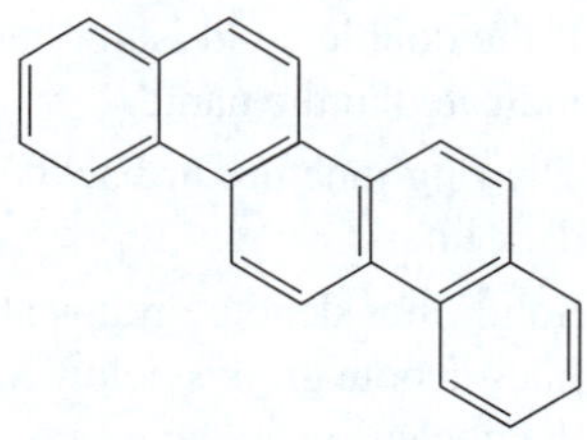

Picene

The overall class of steroids is found almost entirely as solids and the melting points for steroids range from approximately 100 to 250°C. Generally, steroids are insoluble in water, but they are reasonably soluble in organic solvents such as ethanol, acetone, chloroform and dioxane. Oestrogens with a phenolic hydroxyl group on the aromatic A ring are soluble in dilute sodium hydroxide.

NOMENCLATURE OF STEROIDS

1. Steroids consist of four fused rings (A, B, C, and D). Chemically, these hydrocarbons are cyclopentanoperhydrophenanthrenes. They contain a five-membered cyclopentane (D) ring and three rings of phenanthrene, i.e. perhydrophenanthrene (ring A, B, and C) is the completely saturated derivative of phenanthrene.

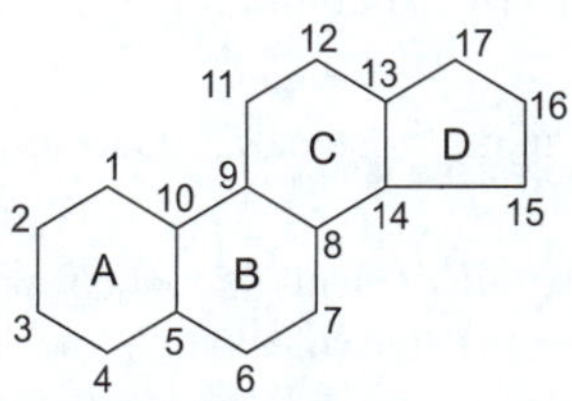

Steroid template

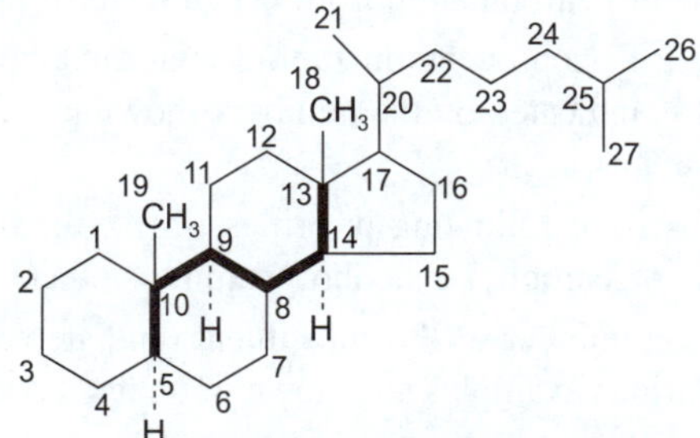

Cholestane template

2. Earlier, the various steroids were generally designated by their common or trivial names, such as cholesterol, progesterone, testosterone, and oestradiol. However, the developments in chemistry lead to discard these names and favour for the systematic names as per the International Union of Pure and Applied Chemistry (IUPAC) nomenclature.

3. The steroid scaffold contains 17 carbon atoms, and the numbering of the carbon atoms begins with the carbons of the phenanthrene and is then followed by numbering the remaining carbons of the cyclopentane ring. Additional carbon atoms on steroids including angular methyl groups attached to C10 and C13 and alkyl substituents on C17 are numbered.
4. The systematic names for steroids are based upon the stem name (Fig. 10.1), which in turn is based on the hydrocarbon system. Cholestane is the term used for steroids with 27 carbon atoms, pregnanes are steroids with 21 carbon atoms, androstanes have 19 carbon atoms, estranes have 18 carbon atoms, while gonanes have 17 carbon atoms.
5. If any unsaturation (double bond) is present in the steroid, the 'ane' ending of the stem name is replaced with 'ene' if it contains one double bond; 'diene' if it contains two double bonds; 'triene' if it contains three double bonds.
6. The symbol Δ is often used to designate a C=C bond in a steroid. If C=C is in between carbons 4 and 5, the compound is referred to as a Δ^4 steriod, and if the C=C bond is between positions 5 and 10, the compound is designated as $\Delta^{5(10)}$ steroid.
7. If the double bond is not between sequentially numbered carbons, in such cases both carbons are indicated in the name.
8. The ring juncture or backbone carbons are shown in the structure of 5α-cholestane with a heavy dark line.
9. Solid lines denote groups above the plane of the nucleus (β-configuration) and dotted or broken lines denote groups below the plane (α). If the configuration of substituent is unknown, its bond to the nucleus is drawn as a wavy line (ξ).
10. Circles were sometimes used to indicate α-hydrogens and dark dots to indicate β-hydrogens.
11. If the steroid contains a three-membered ring, it is indicated by the prefix 'cyclo', preceded by the number of positions concerned.
12. The configuration of the H at C-5 is always indicated in the name.
13. Compounds with 5α-cholestane belong to allo- series, while compounds derived from 5β-cholestane belong to the normal series.
14. If any contraction of the ring of a steroid occurs, it is indicated by the prefix *nor* and preceded by a small capital letter indicating the ring affected.
15. If there is any enlargement of the ring of a steroid, it is indicated by the prefix *homo* and preceded by a small capital letter indicating the ring affected.
16. When a methyl group is missing from the side chain this is again indicated by the prefix *nor* with the number of carbon atom from which it has disappeared.
17. If any ring fission occurs in steroid with the addition of a hydrogen atom to each new terminal group, it is indicated by the numbers showing the positions of the bond broken, followed by the prefix, *seco*.
18. On the basis of following priorities, suffix for the stem name is selected: Carboxylic acid (or derivative) > carbonyl > alcohol > amine > ether.
19. The carbon number of the substituent (and stereochemistry, if present) is placed in front of the suffix. Various examples are shown in Figure 10.1 to illustrate these rules.

Steroid skeleton (stem) name | **Steroidal skeleton containing compounds**

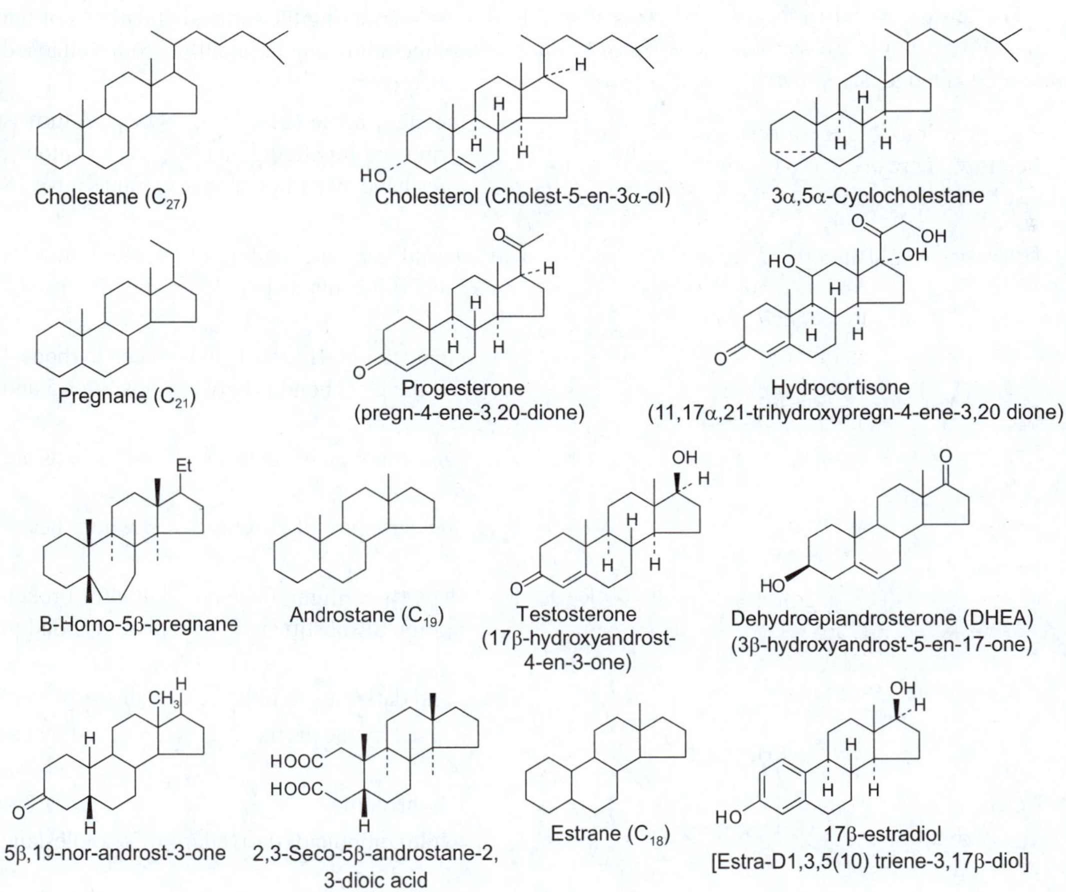

Figure 10.1: Steroid stem name and naming of their derivatives

Stereochemistry: The absolute stereochemistry of the molecule and any substituent is shown with solid (β) and dashed (α) bonds; the axial bond (a) is perpendicular to the plane of the molecule, while the equatorial bond (e) is horizontal to the plane of the molecule.

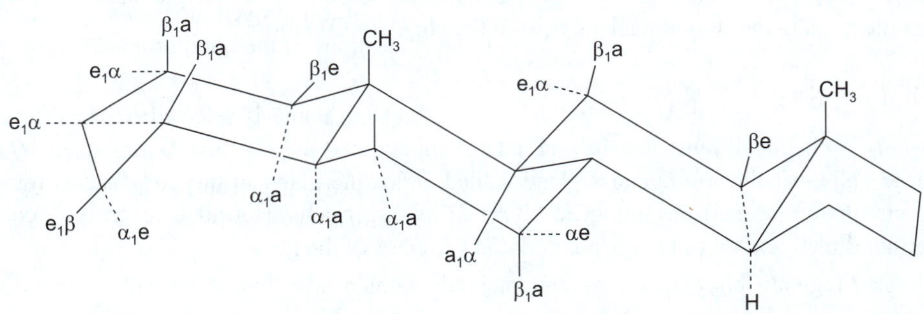

5α-Androstane

The aliphatic side chain at position is always assumed to be of β-configuration.

The terms *cis* and *trans* are used occasionally to indicate the backbone stereochemistry between rings. For example, 5α-steroids are A/B *trans* and 5 β-steroids are A/B *cis*. The terms 'syn' and 'anti' are used analogously to *trans* and *cis*.

Conformations: There are six asymmetric carbon atoms in the nucleus: 5, 8, 9, 10, 13, and 14. Therefore, there are $2^6 = 64$ optically active forms possible. Cholestane, androstane, and pregnane can exist in two conformations, that is chair form and boat form.

Cholestone A,B-*trans* form

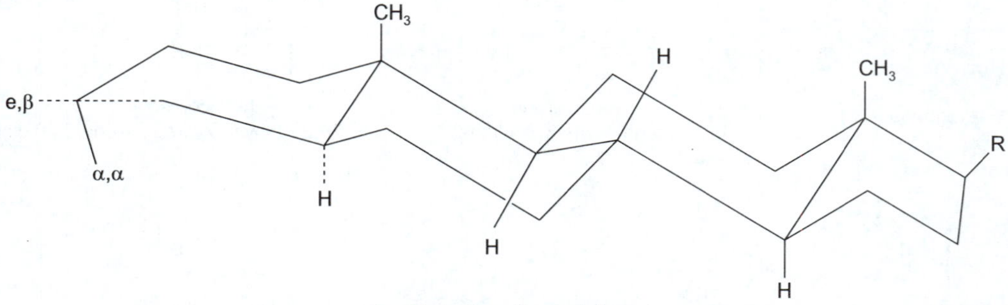

5α-Cholestane (in chair forms)

Coprostane A,B-*cis* form

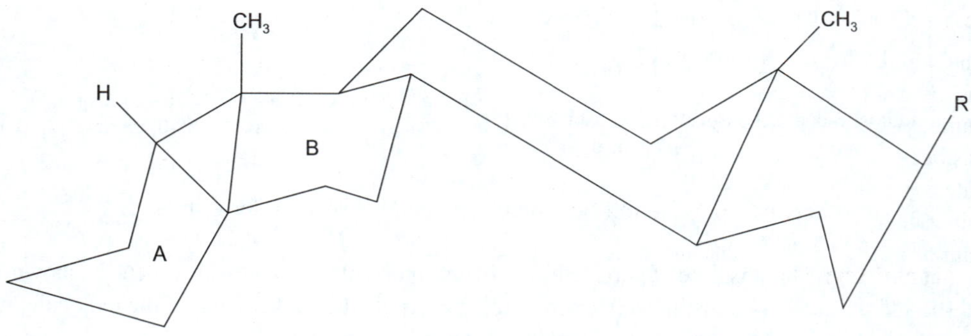

Chair confirmation is more stable than boat confirmation due to less angle strain, and hence all cyclohexane rings in the steriod nucleus exist in the chair confirmation.

HORMONES

Hormone is a chemical substance having intense biological activity that is produced by certain specialized cells usually in a ductless gland, called endocrine gland in the body and is transported through circulation to exert physiological effect on its target cells. Hormones exert their control by acting either directly or, more likely, indirectly on the DNA of the genes.

Hormones regulate body functions and maintain homeostasis in the variable external/internal environment. The deficiency of a hormone leads to a particular disease, which can be cured by the administration of the concerned hormone.

Some of the hormones and their body functions are given below:

Major regulator hormone	***Body function***
Aldosterone, antidiuretic hormone	Circulating volume
Glucocorticoids, adrenaline	Adoption to stress
Gonadotropins, androgens, oestrogens, progestins	Sex and reproduction
Insulin, glucagon	Availability of fuel
Thyroxine	Metabolic rate

Classification

Hormones are classified as follows:

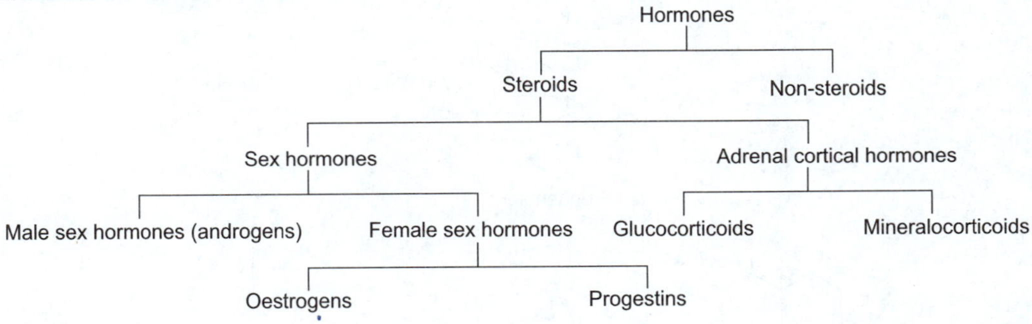

ADRENAL CORTICAL HORMONES (CORTICOSTEROIDS)

The adrenal glands located in superior part of kidney consist of two distinct parts: The medulla and the cortex. The medulla synthesizes catecholamines (adrenaline), while the cortex synthesizes a number of steroid hormones called corticosteroids. The production of these adrenocortical hormones has been controlled by the hormone ACTH (adrenocorticotrophic hormone) which is produced in the anterior lobe of the pituitary. The corticosteroids are classified into two types, i.e. glucocorticoids or mineralocorticoids. They are labelled as per the type of actions found among corticoids, which include natural glucocorticoids and mineralocorticoids and their synthetic analogues. Their main function is to maintain fluid-electrolyte, cardiovascular, and energy substrate homeostasis and functional status of skeletal muscles and nervous system.

Glucocorticoids: These steroids regulate the carbohydrates, proteins, and the fat metabolism and are intimately involved in the operation of the processes that enable the body to resist infections and stress. Example, hydrocortisone and cortisone.

Mineralocorticoids: These steroids mainly influence salt and water balance (and hence the control of blood volume and blood pressure) by maintaining proper electrolyte balance. Example, aldosterone and 11-deoxycorticosterone.

Biological Effects of Glucocorticoids

1. They act on carbohydrate and protein metabolism and promote glycogen deposition in liver.
2. Promote lipolysis due to glucagon, growth hormone, adrenaline, and thyroxine.
3. They inhibit intestinal absorption and enhance renal excretion of Ca^{2+}.
4. Glucocorticoids restrict capillary permeability, and maintain tone of arterioles and myocardial contractility.

5. Irrespective of the type of injury or insult, the attending inflammatory response is suppressed by glucocorticoids.

Biosynthesis of the adrenocorticoids from cholesterol

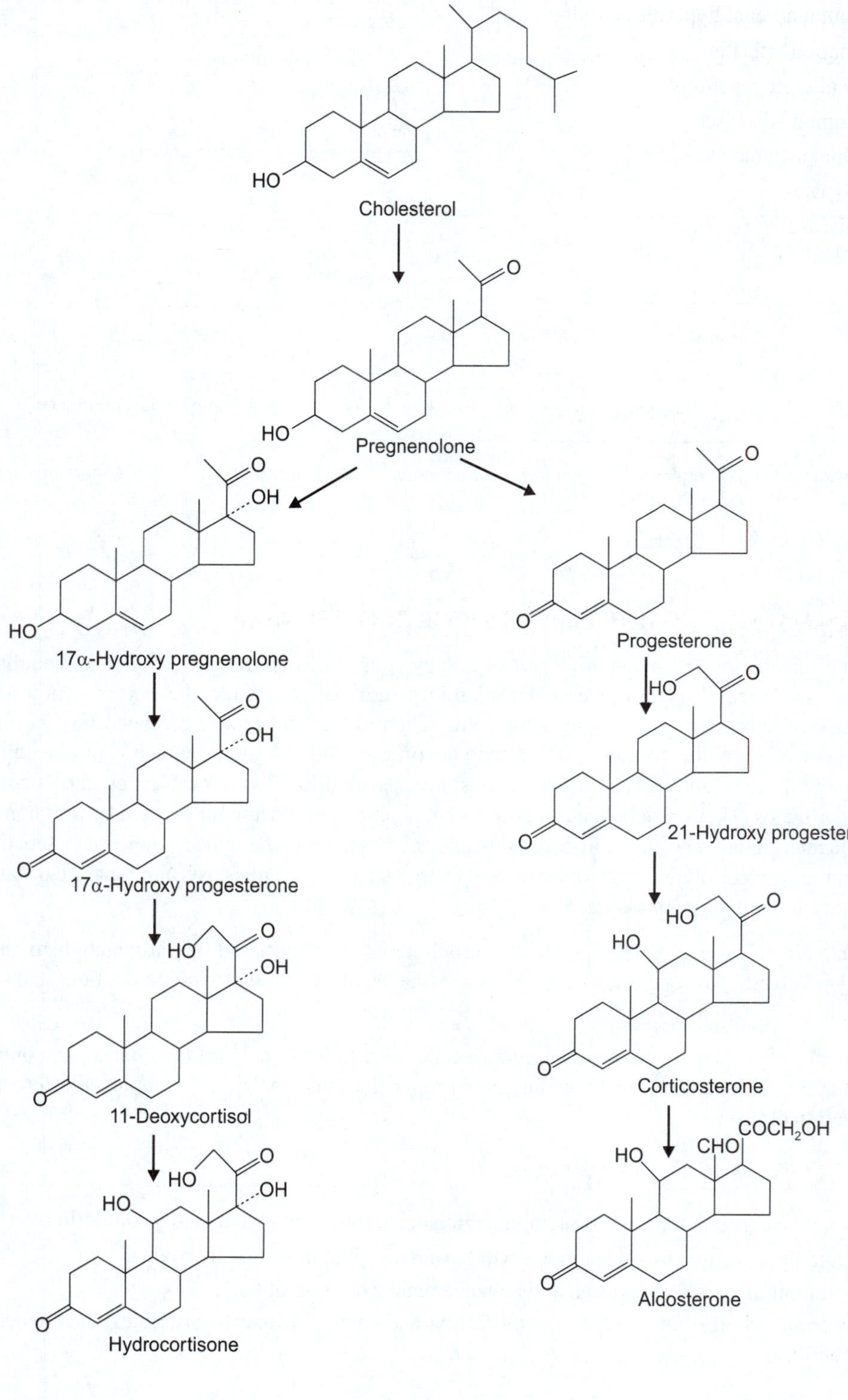

Therapeutic uses of glucocorticoids: Therapeutically, they are used in the following conditions:

- Acute adrenal insufficiency
- Chronic adrenal insufficiency (Addison's disease)
- Congenital adrenal hyperplasia (adrenogenital syndrome)
- Rheumatiod arthritis
- Severe allergic reactions
- Autoimmune diseases
- Bronchial asthma
- Eye diseases
- Skin diseases

Classification of Corticosteroids

1. **Mineralocorticoids with high salt retention**

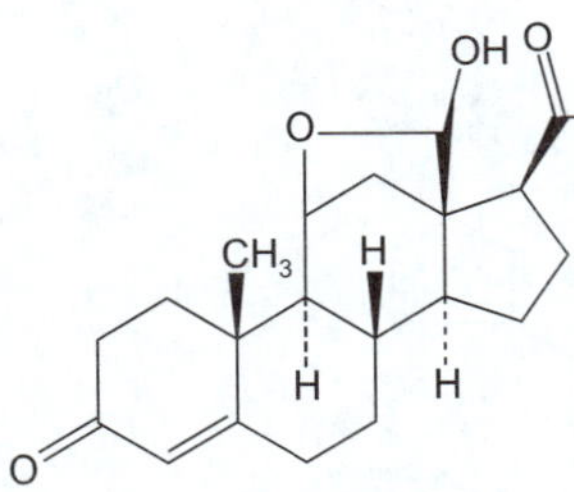

Aldosterone

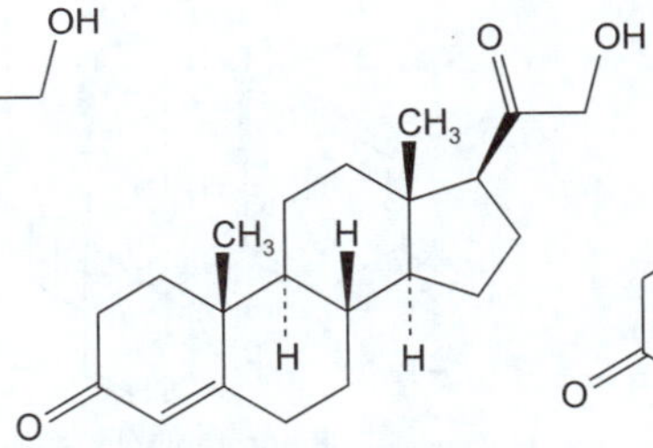

11-Deoxycorticosterone

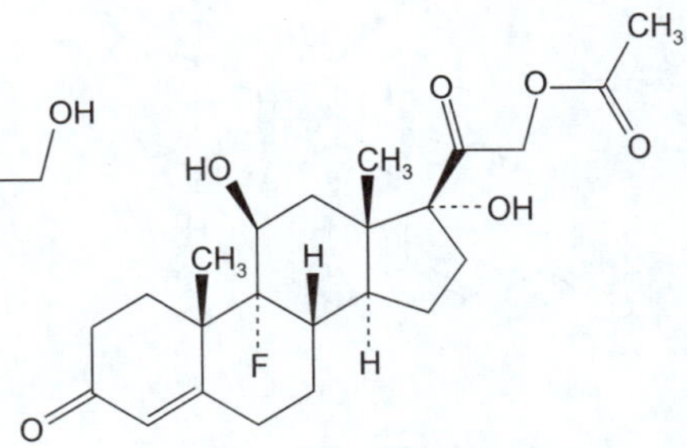

Fludrocortisone acetate

2. **Glucocorticoids with moderate-to-low salt retention**

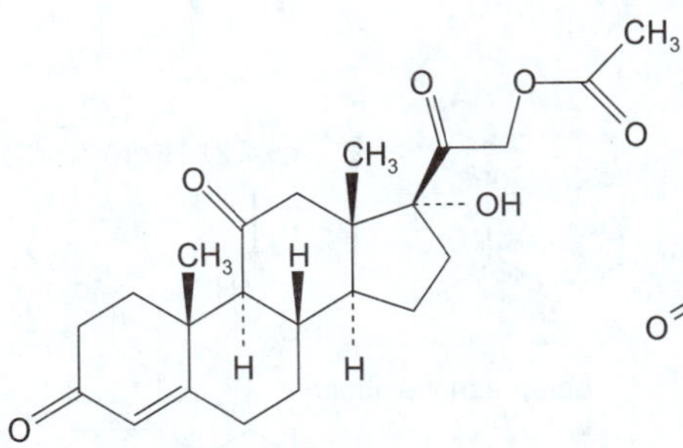

Cortisone acetate

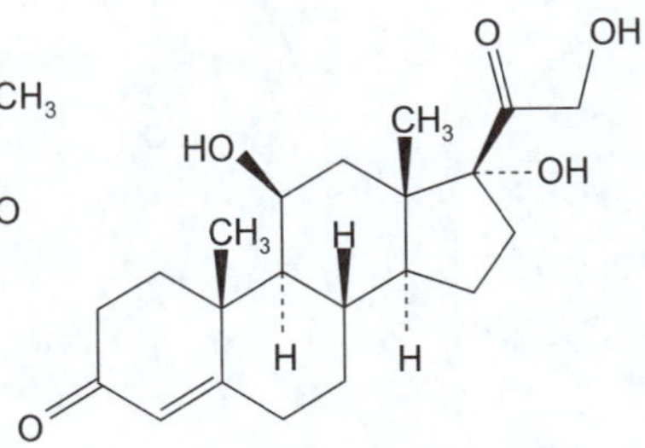

Hydrocortisone (cortisol)

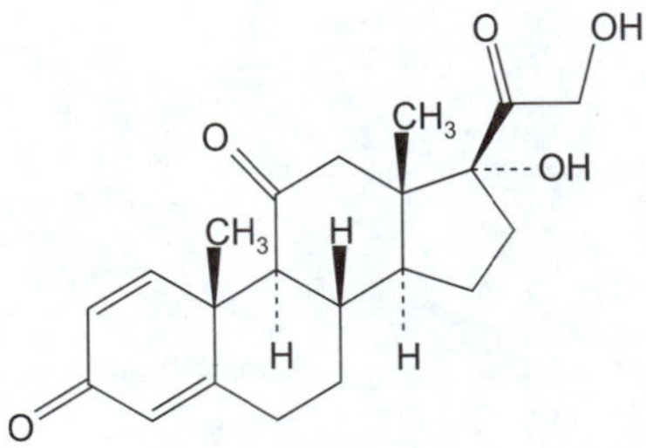

Prednisone

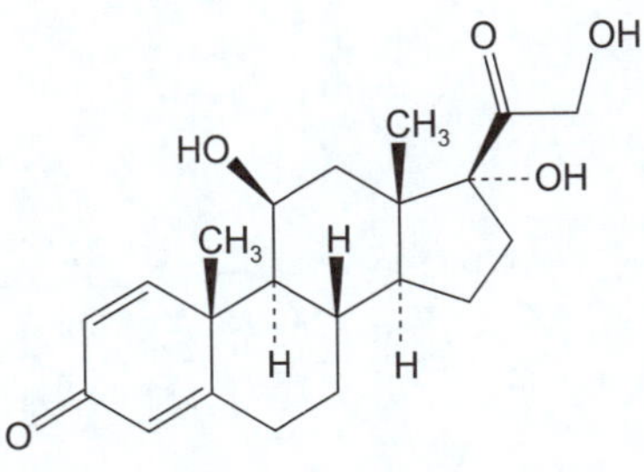

Prednisolone

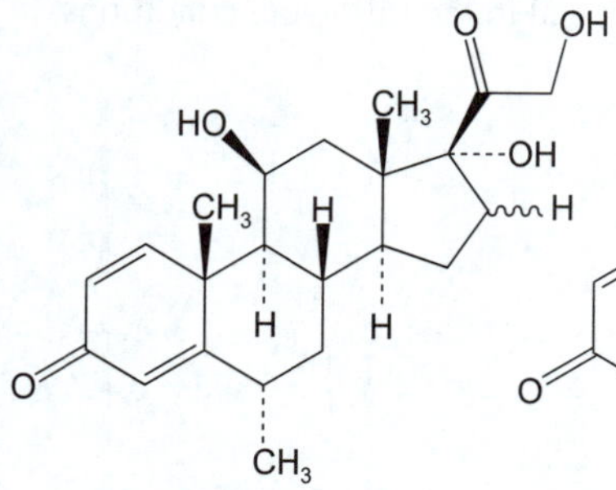

Methylprednisolone

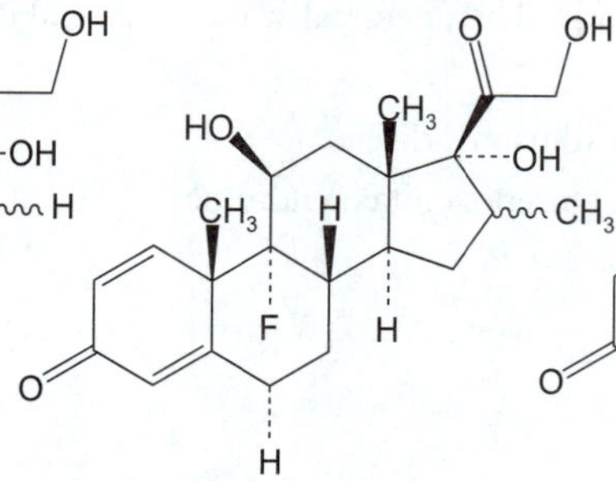

Betamethasone

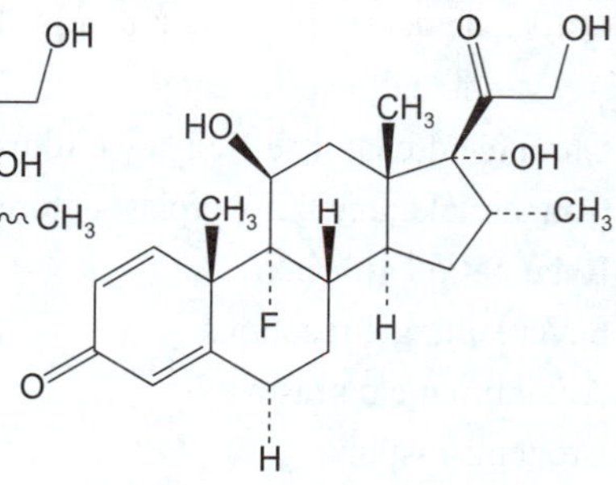

Dexamethasone

3. Ophthalmic glucocorticoids

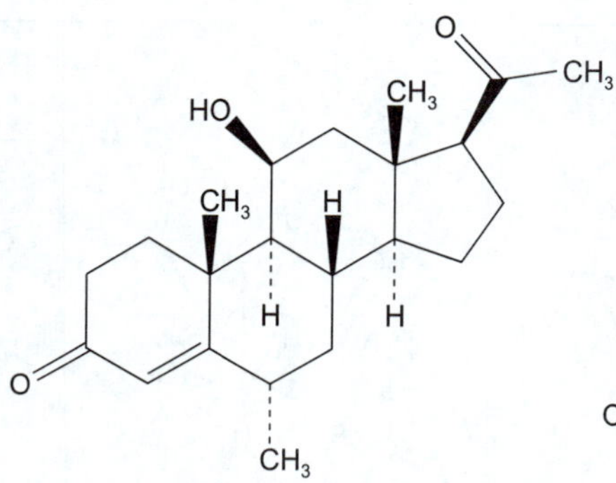

Medrysone

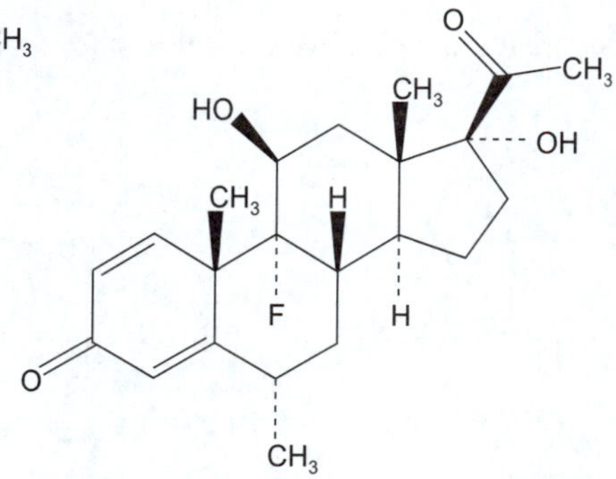

Fluorometholone

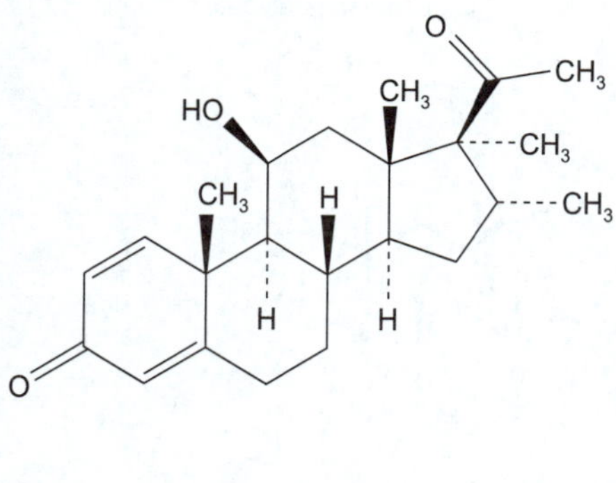

Rimexolone

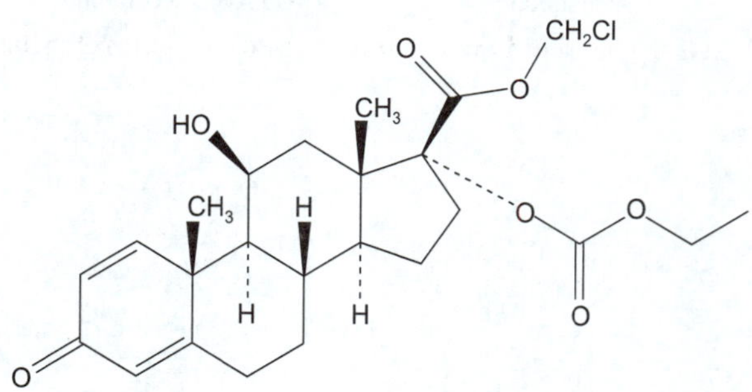

Loteprednol etabonate

4. Glucocorticoids used for the treatment of asthma and allergy

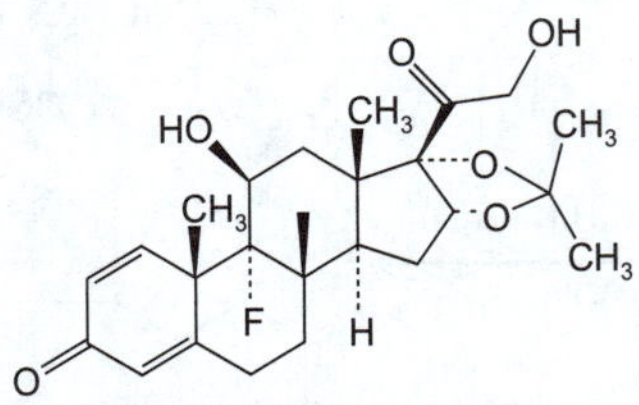

Triamcinolone acetate

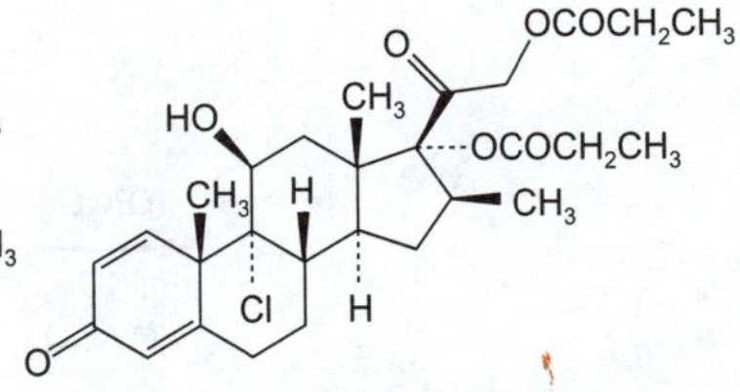

Beclomethasone dipropionate

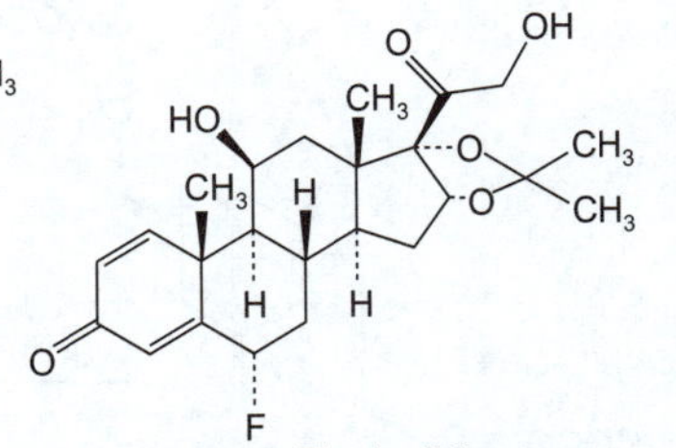

Flunisolide

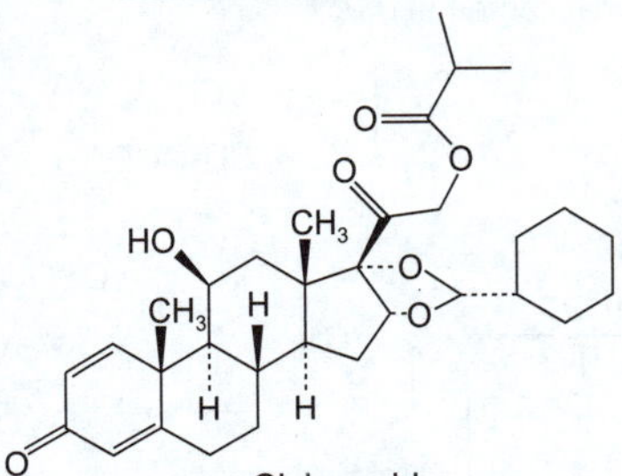

Ciclesonide

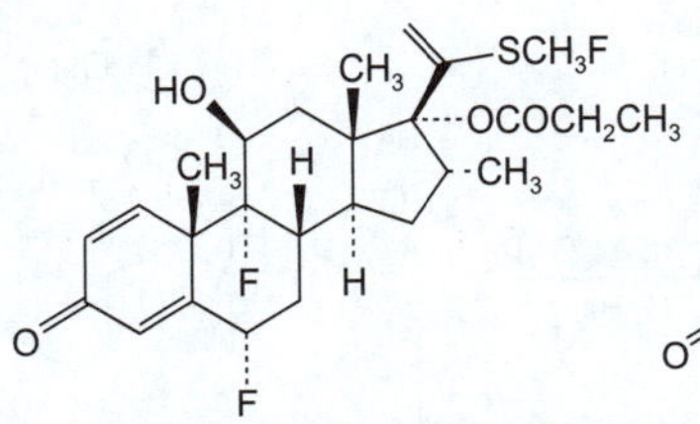

Fluticasone propionate

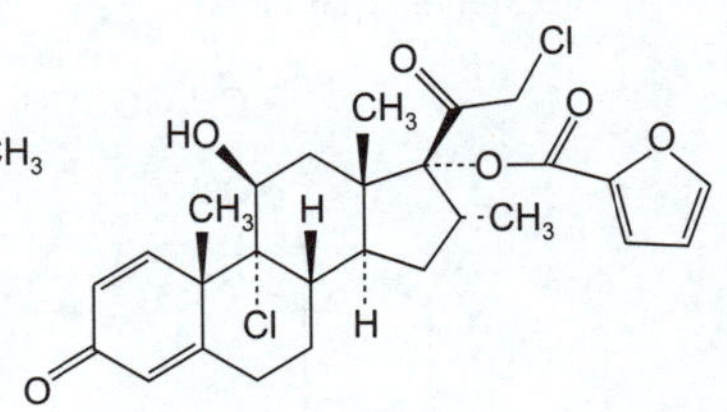

Mometasone furoate

Cortisone (Cortogen, Cortone)

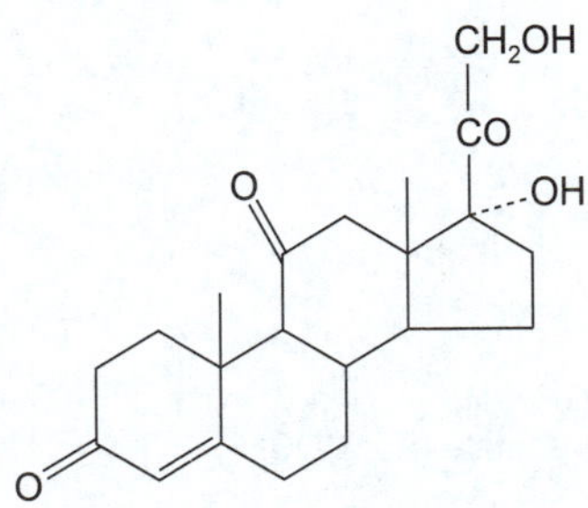

Synthesis

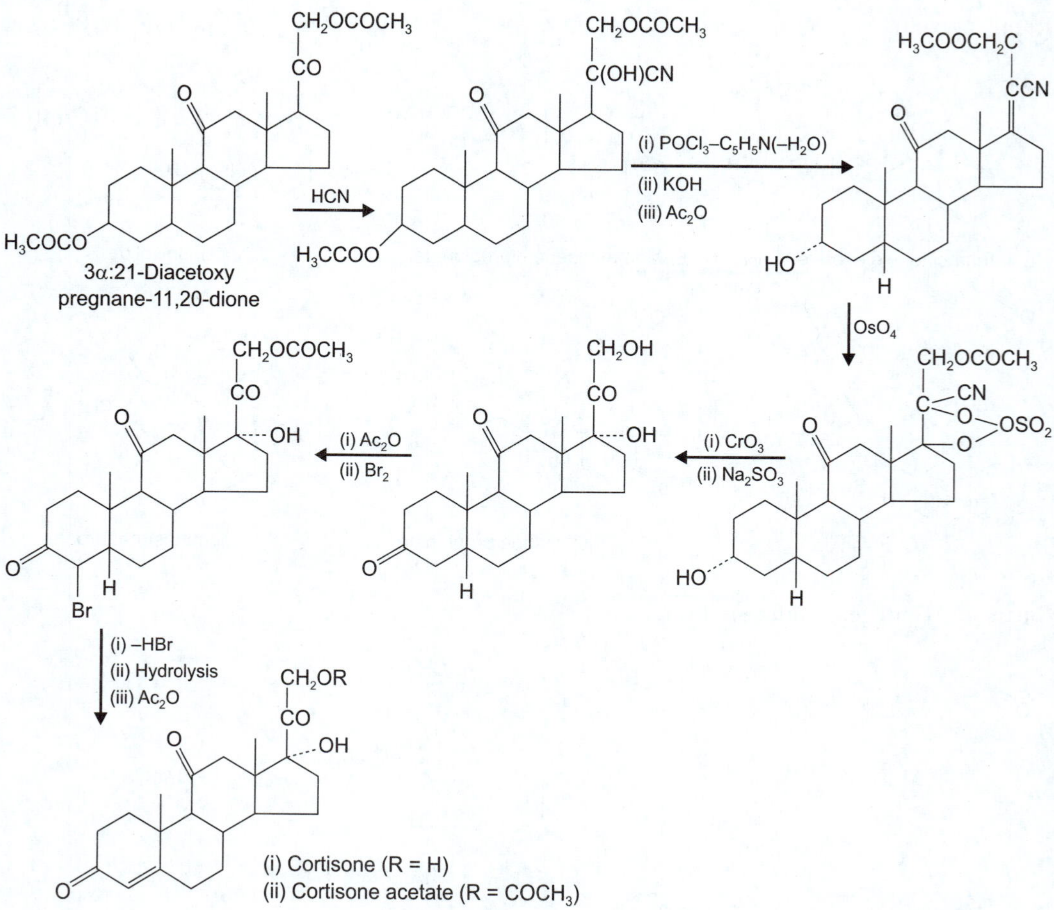

Properties and uses: It is a white crystalline powder, which is insoluble in water and soluble in alcohol. It is used in rheumatoid arthritis, severe shock, allergic conditions, and chronic lymphatic leukaemia.

Dose: The dosage for adults is 20–100 mg per day by oral or intramuscular (IM).

Hydrocortisone (Cortisol, Hydrocortone, Lortef)

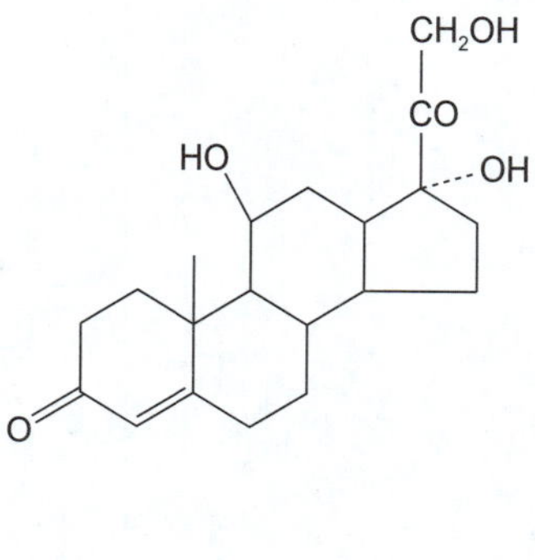

Synthesis

Route 1. From: Progesterone

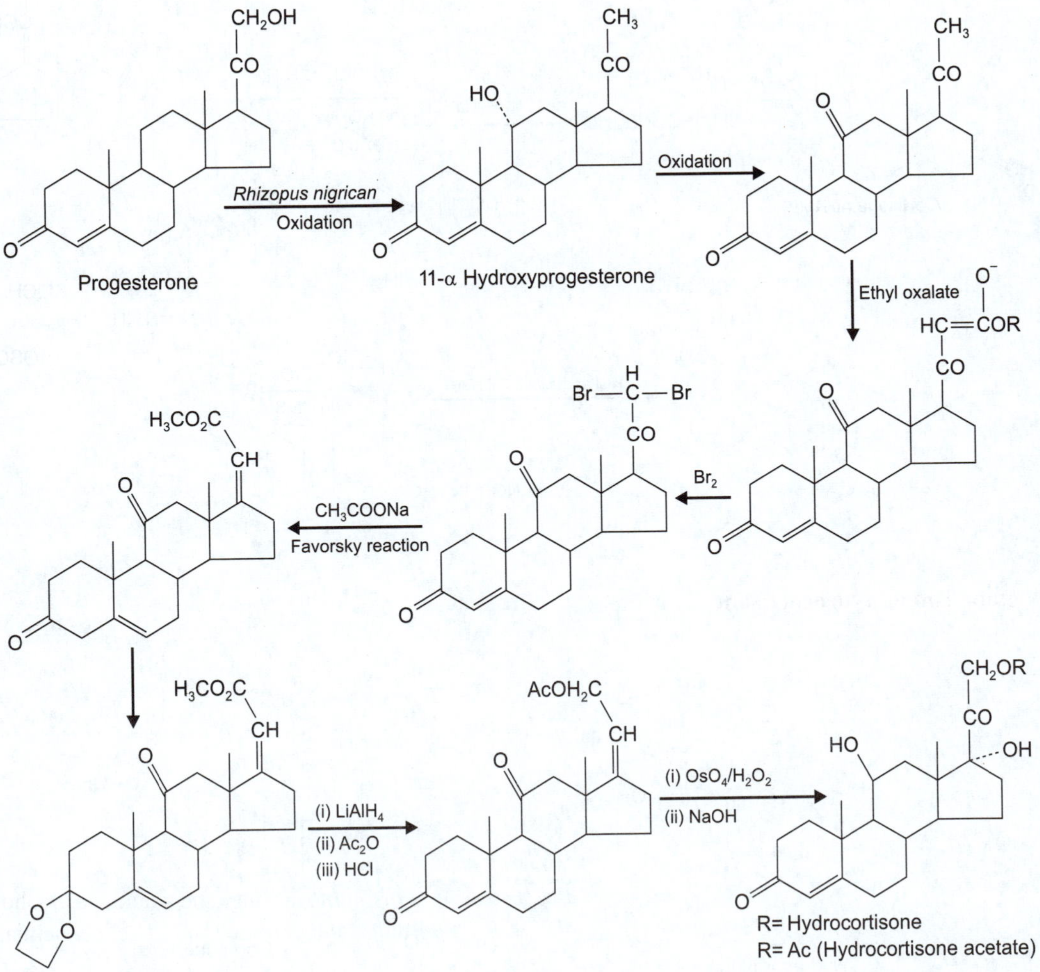

Route 2. From: Cortisone acetate

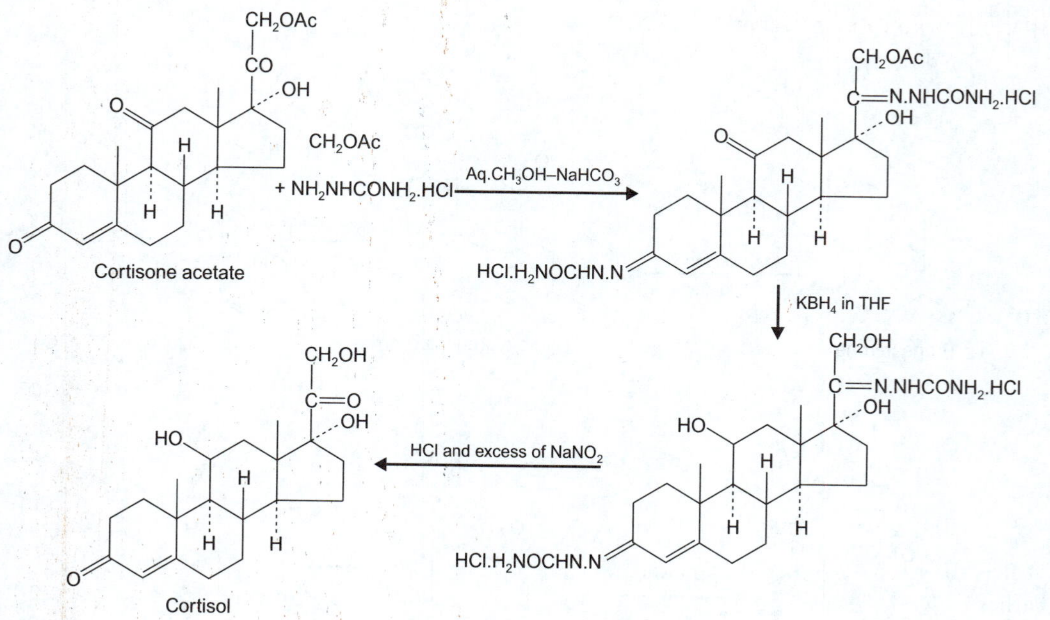

Metabolism of hydrocortisone

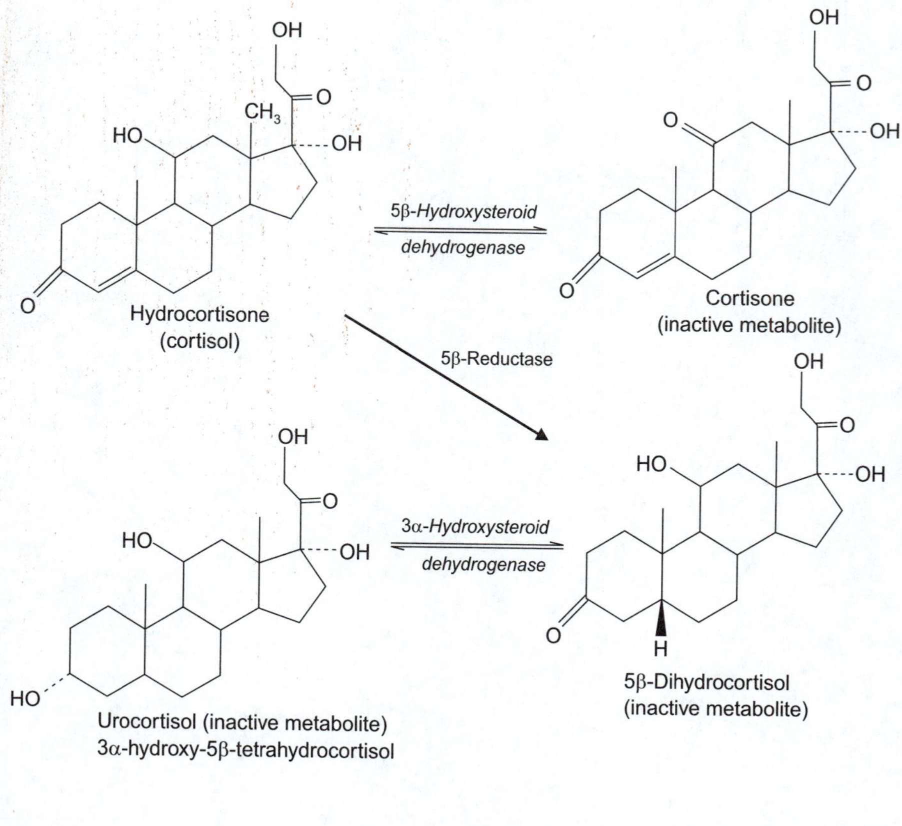

Properties and uses: It exists as white crystalline powder, which is soluble in water and alcohol. It is used as an anti-inflammatory agent.

Dose: The dose as injection is 100 mg IM and as topical cream 1–2.5% for skin, ear, and eye.

Aldosterone

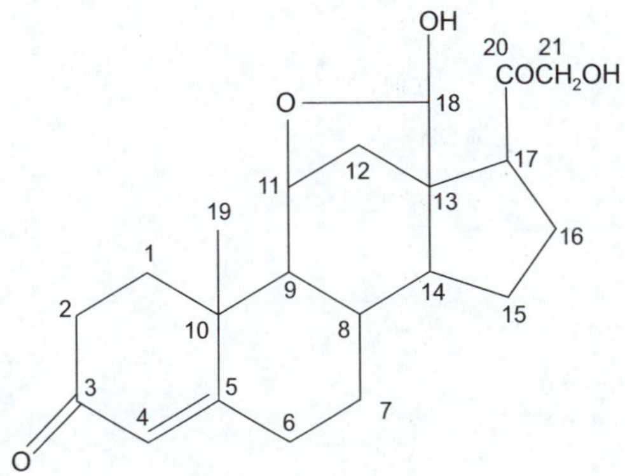

It is the mineralocorticoid that was first isolated in a crystalline form by Mason et al. in 1953. Earlier, it was named electrocortin but later was renamed to *aldosterone* because of its aldehydic and ketonic groups. Aldosterone in solution exists as an equilibrium mixture of the 18-aldehyde and 11, 18-hemiacetal forms.

Prednisolone (Prelone, Emsolone)

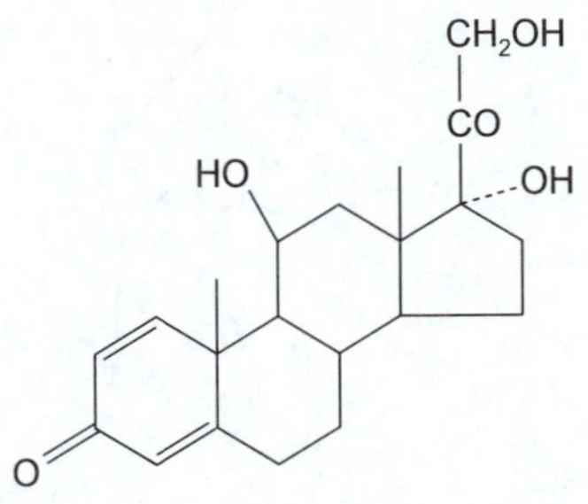

Synthesis

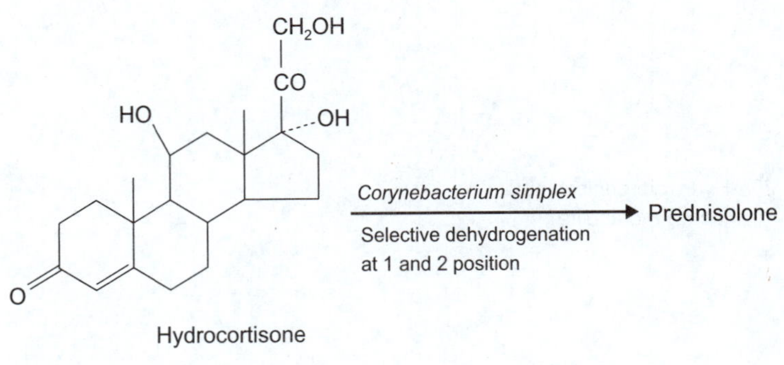

Properties and uses: It is a white crystalline powder, which is sparingly soluble in alcohol. It is four times as potent as hydrocortisone.

Dose: The oral dose for adult is 5–60 mg per day. As IM, intravenous (IV), and intra-articular (IA) injection, the dose is 10–40 mg, and for topical use (skin and eyes) the dose is 0.25%.

Metabolism for prednisolone:

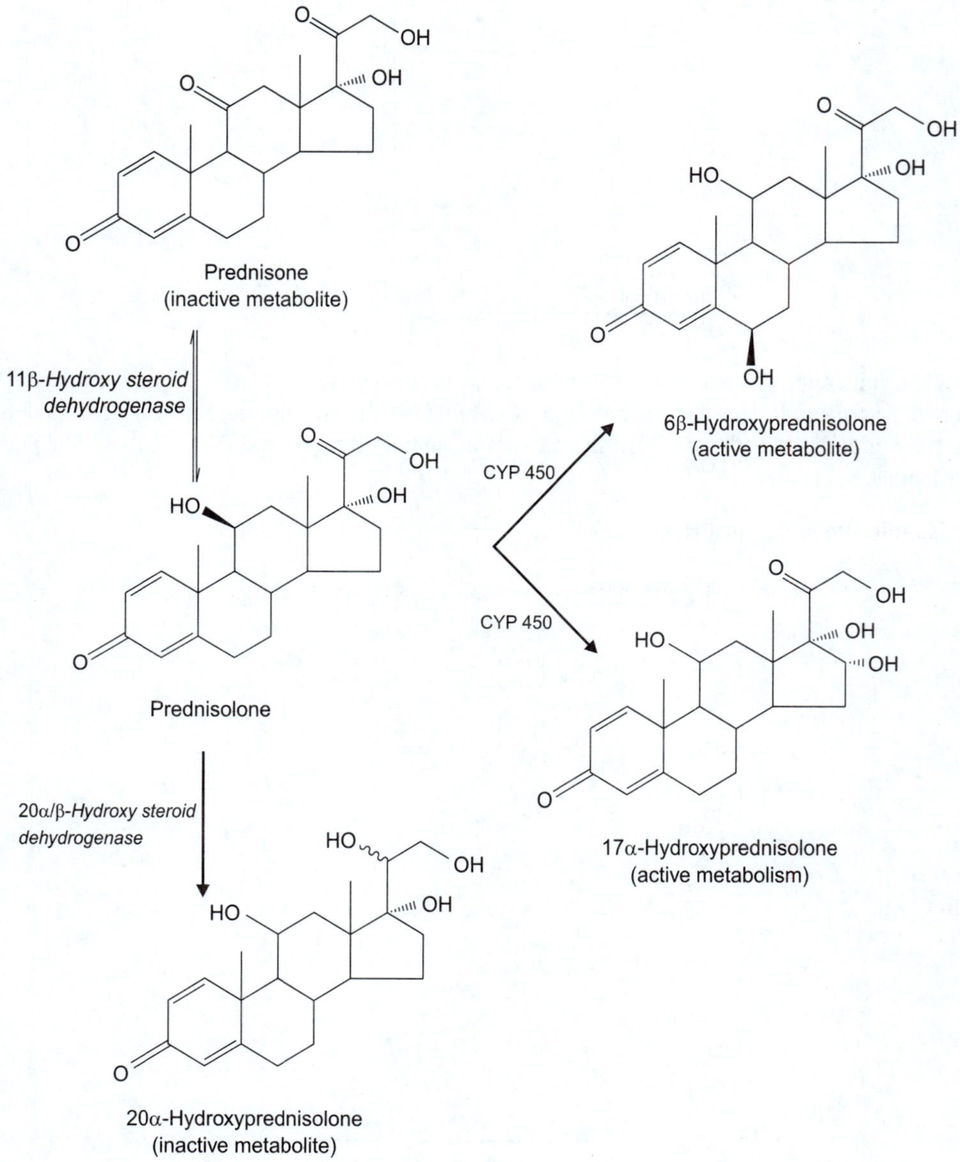

Dexamethasone (Dalalone)

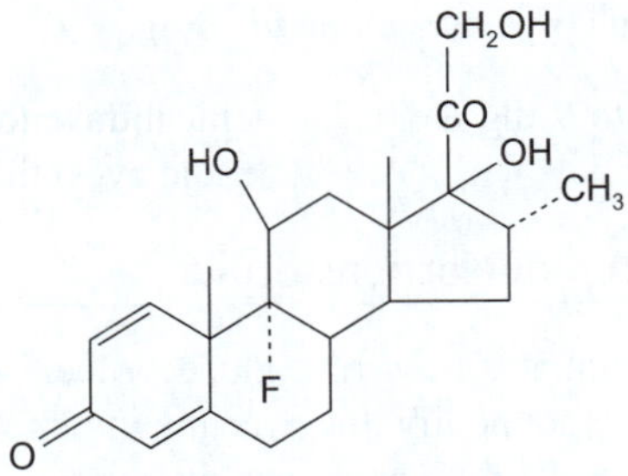

Synthesis

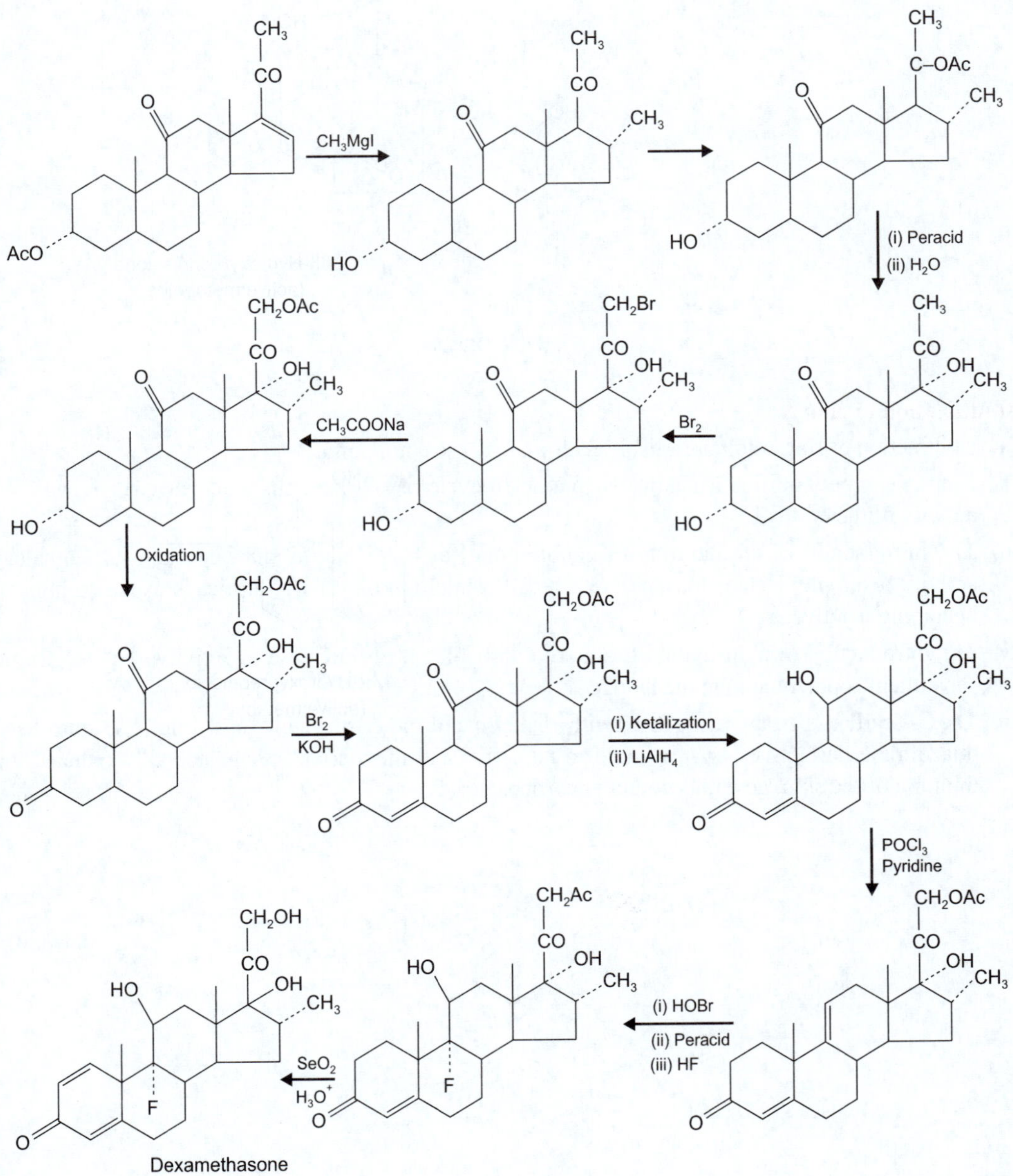

Properties and use: It exists as white crystalline powder, which is soluble in alcohol and insoluble in water. It is used as an anti-inflammatory and antiallergic drug.

Dose: Oral adult dose is 500 μg to 9 mg daily. The topical dose for conjunctiva is 1 drop of 0.1% suspension.

Structure–Activity Relationship of Corticosteroids

Hydrocortisone (cortisol) is the naturally occurring glucocorticoid with mineralocorticoid acitivity. The aim of the medicinal chemists is to modify this structure in increasing glucocorticoid potency and decreasing sodium retention capacity. The structure–activity relationship studies are described herein.

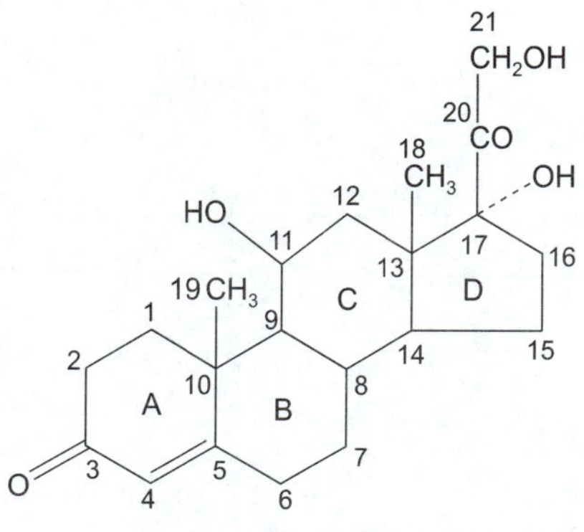

Hydrocortisone

Modification in ring A

i. Contraction of ring A to norcortisol yields an inactive compound.

ii. Ring A can be modified isosterically to a heterocycle like 2-oxacortisol acetate, which has 25% activity of the cortisol.

iii. The introduction of unsaturation (a double bond) at C-1 leads to enhanced anti-inflammatory activity (example: Betamethasone). Whereas the addition of –OH group leads to the compound becoming inactive.

iv. The introduction of a 2α-methyl group into cortisol leads to increase in activity, the C-2 bromo substituent is potent among the halogens.

v. The C-3 carbonyl group can be fused with a heterocyclic moiety to yield a 'soft drug'. C-3 spirofused thiazolidine derivative (1) was found to be active and this derivative considerably reduced the thinning of the skin, generally found in corticosteroids.

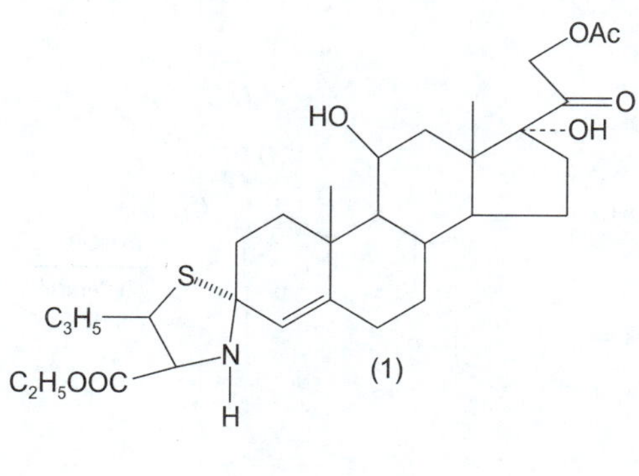

(1)

vi. The Δ^4 double bond is important but not essential for anti-inflammatory activity.
Example: 5 α- pregnane-3-one is more active than cortisone.

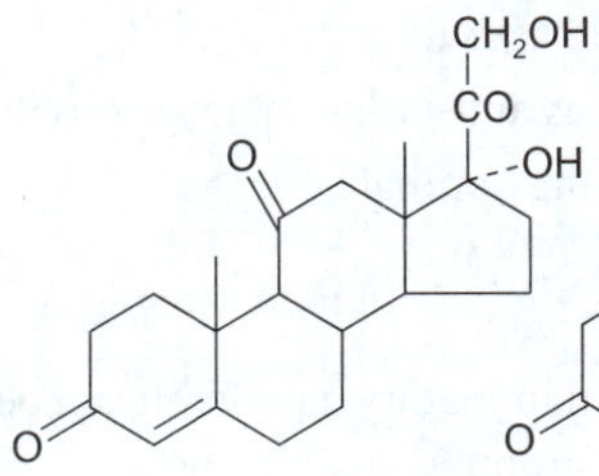

Cortisone

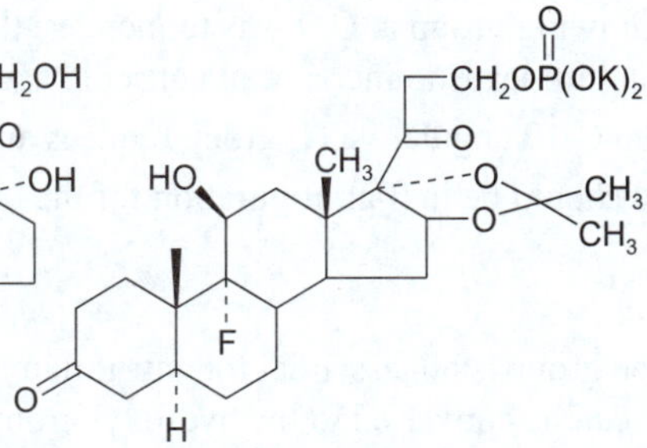

5α-Pregnane-3-one

vii. Ring A can be fused with a pyrazole ring. Compound (2) has 2000 times the potency of cortisol, but also lacks mineralocorticoid activity.

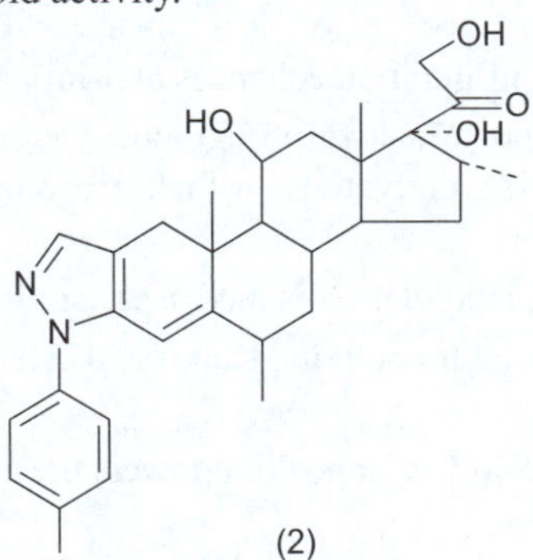

(2)

Modification in ring B

i. Substitution of 6α position with hydrophobic groups like alkyl or halogens (methyl, chloro, and fluoro) leads to increase in activity.
ii. Polar substituents such as –OH or =O at 6α position decreases the activity.
iii. 7α and 7β substituents decrease the anti-inflammatory activity. Thus, 7α- and 7β-methyl cortisol derivatives are less potent than cortisol.
iv. Introduction of –OH group at both 6α and 7α position leads to decrease in activity.
v. 6α- and 7α- difluoromethylene and 6β and 7β derivatives show enhanced activity.
vi. Introduction of 8(9) double bond in prednisolone affords compound with lower anti-inflammatory activity.

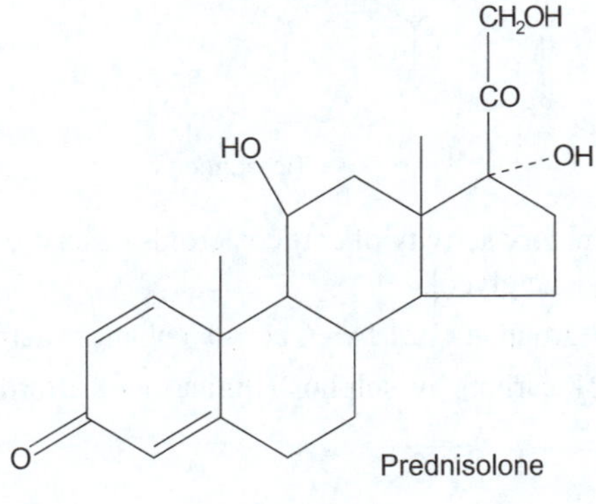

Prednisolone

vii. Anti-inflammatory potency of corticosteroids drastically influenced by the substituents at C-9 position. The groups added were –F, –Cl, –Br, –I, –OH, and $-CH_3$. The activity of the compounds increases with increasing hydrophobic bonding of the C-9α substituents. The function of the electron withdrawing group at C-9 was to increase the acidity of the neighbouring 11β-hydroxy group which in turn leads to increase in corticoid activity.

viii. Removal of the C-19 angular $-CH_3$ group reduces anti-inflammatory activity.

ix. The H at C-10 should be in β-configuration for the optimal activity.

Modification in ring C

i. The C-11 oxygen group is not essential for anti-inflammatory activity. It can be replaced by groups like –Cl, which can be converted to the hydroxyl group *in vivo*.

ii. Ester substituents at C-12 have showed anti-inflammatory activity and the potency is in the following order: Propionyl > butyl > isovaleryl.

Modification in ring D

i. Methyl group at C-15 with α configuration enhances anti-inflammatory activity.

ii. Placement of 16α-hydroxy and 17α-hydroxy groups yields potent compounds. These two groups may also form acetonide derivatives, which are more potent than the corresponding 16,17-dihydroxy derivatives.

iii. At C-16 introduction of chloro, methyl groups increases activity.

iv. The 17α-OH group is not essential for activity. Ketals and esters yield compounds with improved potency.

v. Introduction of –Cl, –Br, and –F at C-17α position lowers the activity.

Modification in the side chain at C-17

i. Acetonide derivatives across the 17,20-diol arrangement resulted in more potent analogues compared to free diols.

ii. Hydroxyethanone side chain attached at C-17 in the classical corticosteroid is not essential for activity. Tipredane, a 17-thioketal is a potent topical anti-inflammatory drug.

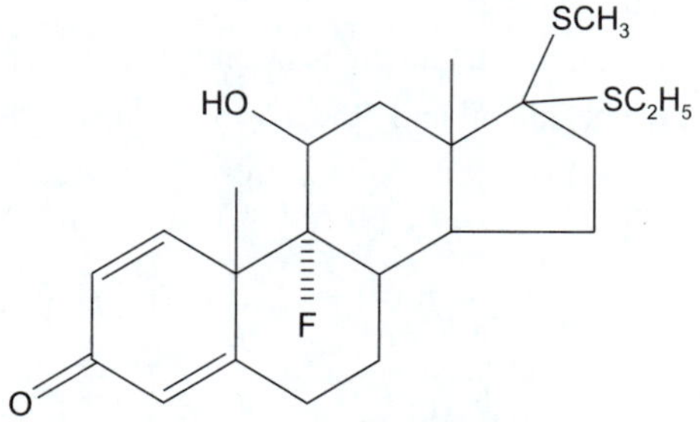

Tipredane

iii. Retaining of anti-inflammatory activity of corticosteroids observed upon ketalization of the C-20 carbonyl group with ethylene glycol.

iv. Replacement of the –OH group at C-21 by –Cl or –F enhances activity.

v. Replacement of the C-21 carbon by sulphur (fluticasone) afforded 21-thioesters, also useful clinically.

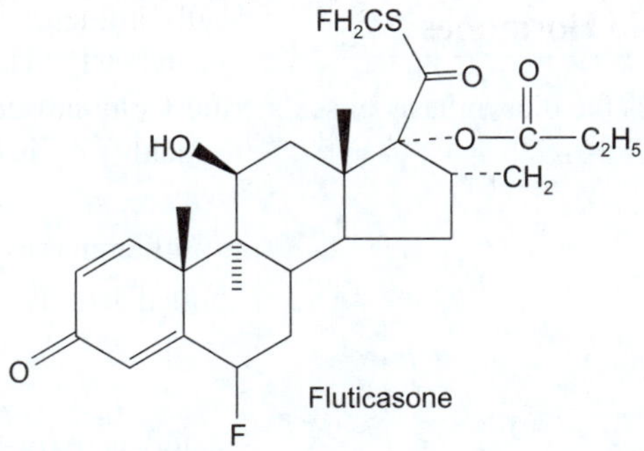

Fluticasone

vi. Replacement of $-CH_2OH$ group with an aldehyde (3) leads to compound with some systemic absorption.

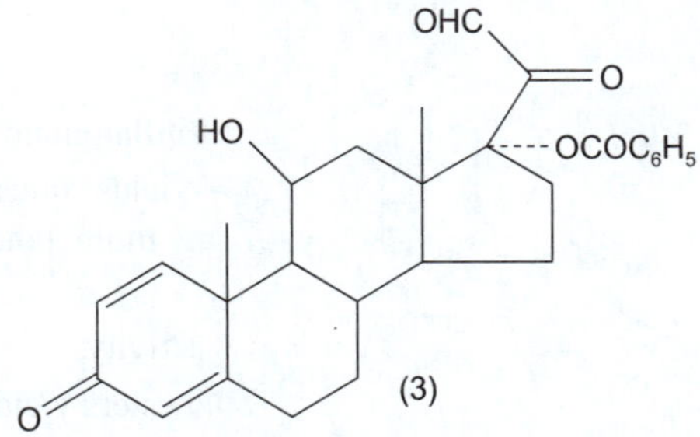

(3)

vii. The C-21 –OH group can be esterified to afford lipophilic compounds that are meant for repository use.

viii. Introduction of activating groups at C-21; conversion of $-CH_2OH$ group to a $-CH_3$ group (medrysone) yields clinically useful ophthalmic anti-inflammatory compound with relatively little effect on intraoccular pressure.

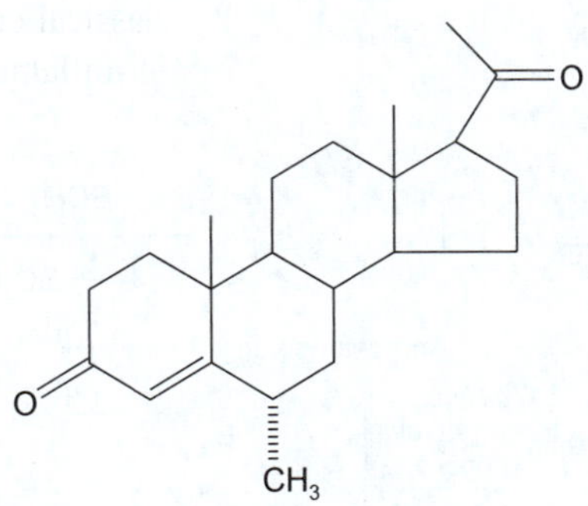

Medrysone

SEX HORMONES

These are a group of steroids biosynthesized in the testes, ovaries, adrenals, and placenta of pregnancy. The activity of these sex hormones is controlled by the hormones that are produced in the anterior lobe of the pituitary gland.

The sex hormones regulate reproductive functions and sexual processes and are responsible for the development of secondary male and female sex characteristics.

Biosynthesis of Sex Steroid Hormones

The following scheme outlines the biosynthesis of sex steroid hormones in the body.

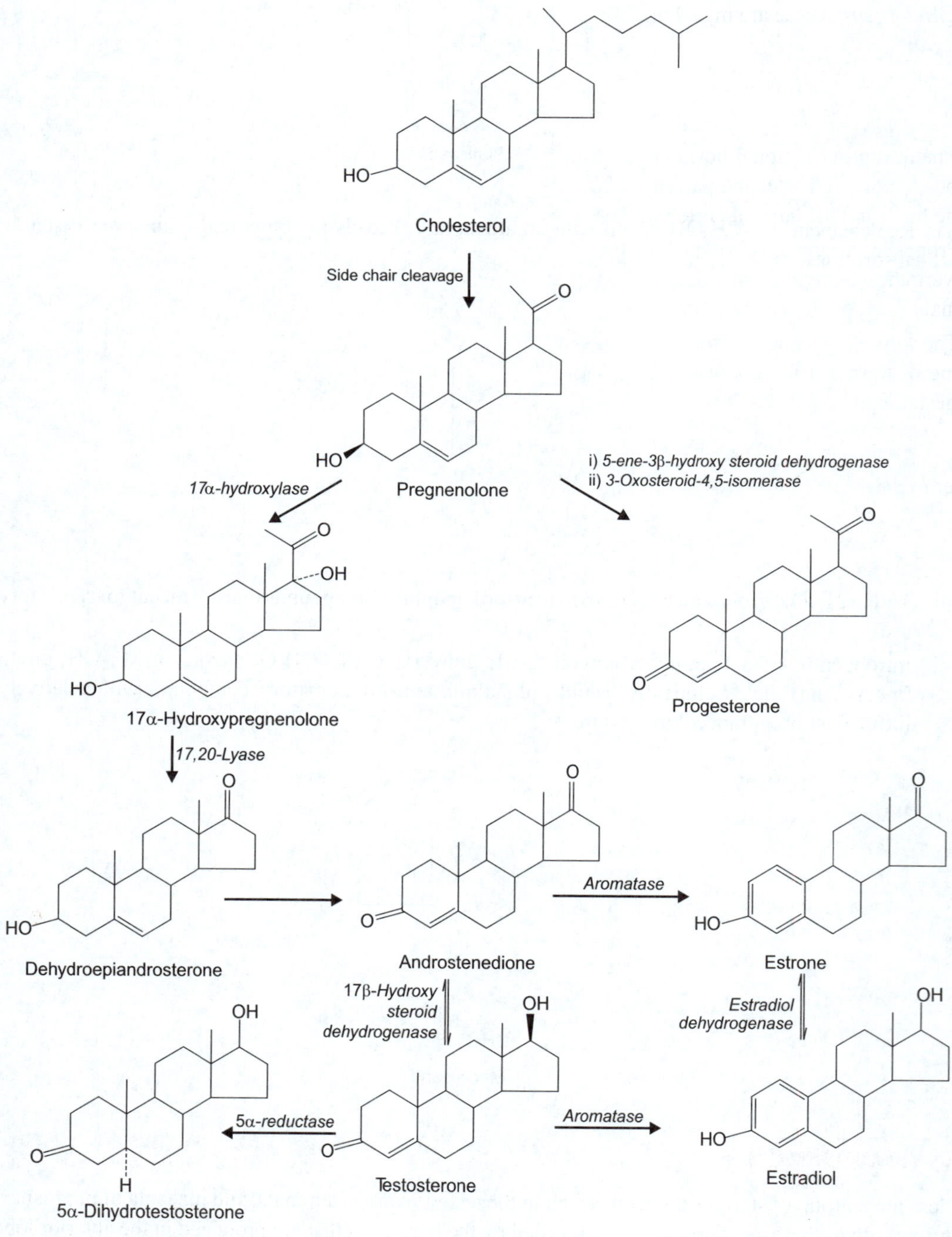

The sex hormones are classified into three types:

a. *Gestogens*: These are corpus luteum hormones.
b. *Oestrogens*: These are female or follicular hormones.
c. *Androgens*: These are male hormones.

PROGESTERONES OR GESTOGENS OR CORPUS LUTEUM HORMONES OR PROGESTINS

The natural progestational hormone or progestogen is progesterone, which is secreted mainly by the corpus luteum in the second part of the menstrual cycle. Small amounts are also secreted by the testes in the male and the adrenal cortex in both sexes, and large amounts are secreted by the placenta.

Progestin means favouring pregnancy. These are substances secreted in corpus luteum, which convert the oestrogen primed endometrium to secretory endometrium and maintain pregnancy in animals spayed after conception.

The key endogenous steroid hormone that acts at the progesterone receptors is progesterone. It is one of the most important members of gestogens. All other endogenous steroids lack significant progestational action.

Biosynthesis of progesterones

Refer to the section biosynthesis of sex steroid hormones.

Metabolism of progesterone

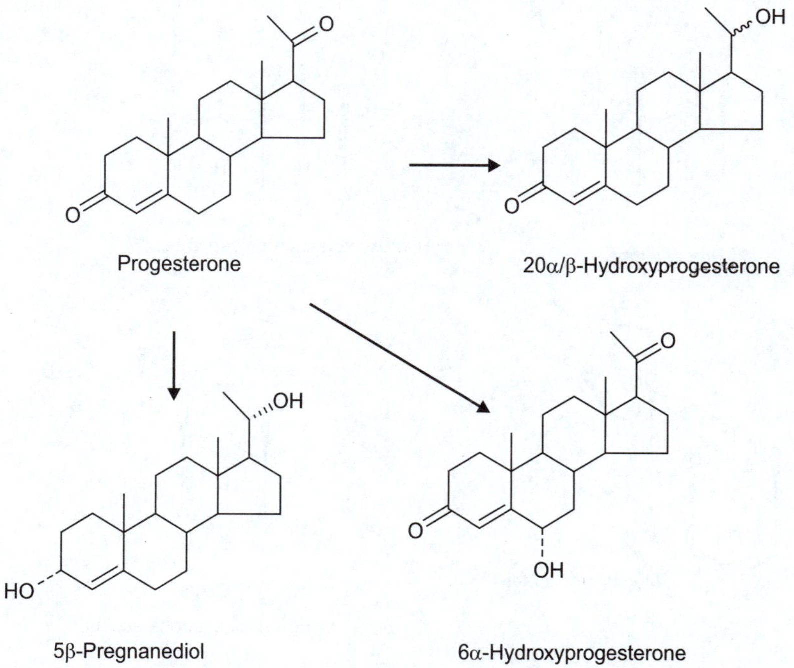

Biological activities of progestins

Progesterone has various pharmacological actions, with the main target tissues being the uterus, breast, and brain. Progesterone in the uterus helps in the development of secretory endometrium. It also acts to thicken cervical secretions and decreasing cervical penetration by sperm. Progesterone is important for the maintenance of pregnancy by suppressing menstruation and decreasing uterine contractility. In the breast, during pregnancy, progesterone acts in conjunction with oestrogens to prepare for lactation.

Therapeutic uses of progestins

Therapeutic uses of progestins are as follows:

- A significant use of the progestins, as of the oestrogens, is inhibition of ovulation.
- The combination of a progestin with oestrogens may significantly reduce the risk of endometrial cancer in women taking postmenopausal oestrogens.
- Progestins have been used very effectively to treat primary and secondary amenorrhoea, functional uterine bleeding, and related menstrual disorders caused by hormonal deficiency or imbalance.
- Progestins can be used for palliative treatment of advanced carcinoma of the breast or endometrium.

CLASSIFICATION OF PROGESTERONES

1. Derivatives of Progesterone

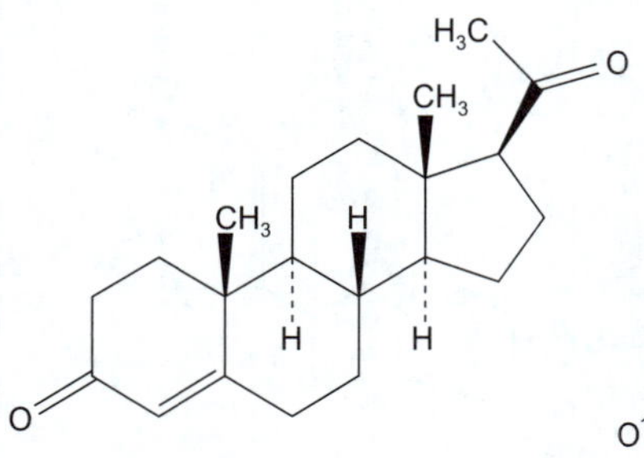

Progesterone

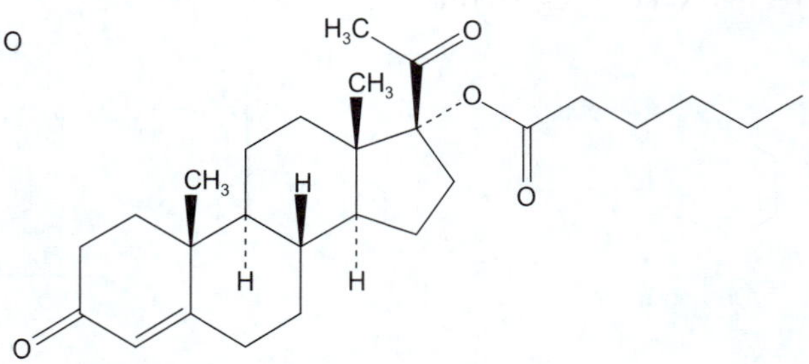

Hydroxyprogesterone caproate

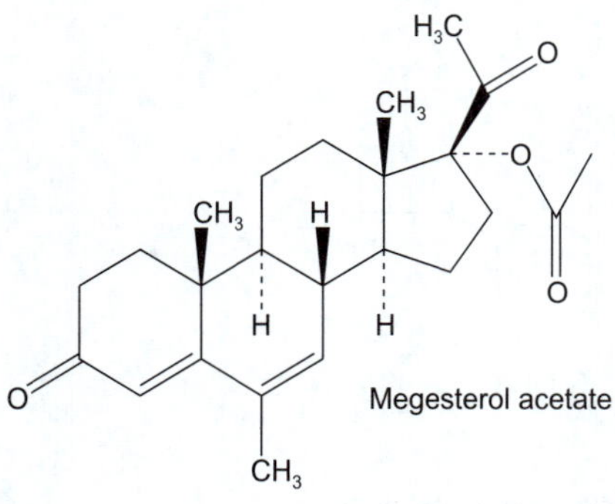

Megesterol acetate

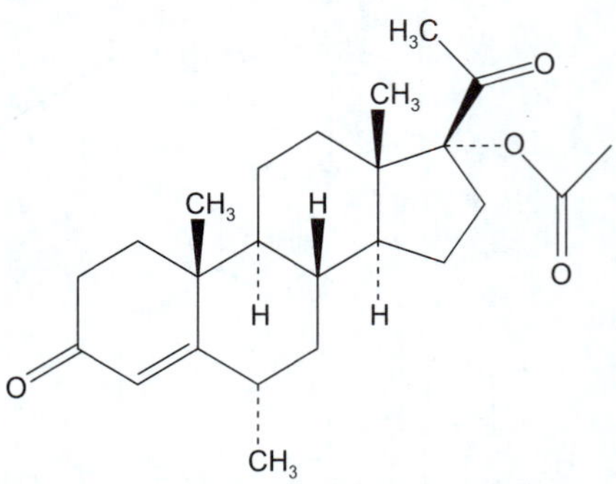

Medroxyprogesterone acetate

2. Synthetic Progesterones

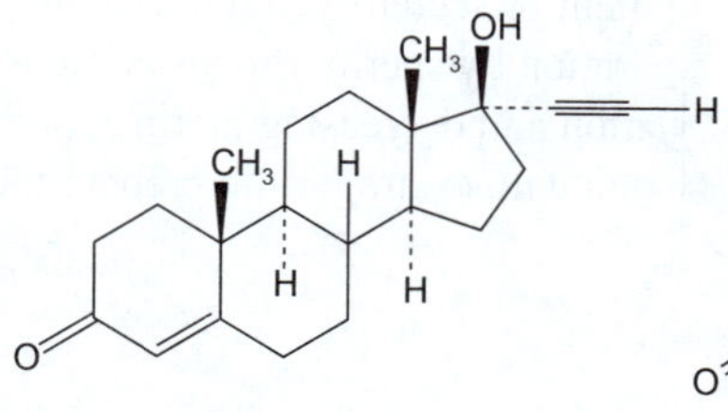

Ethisterone

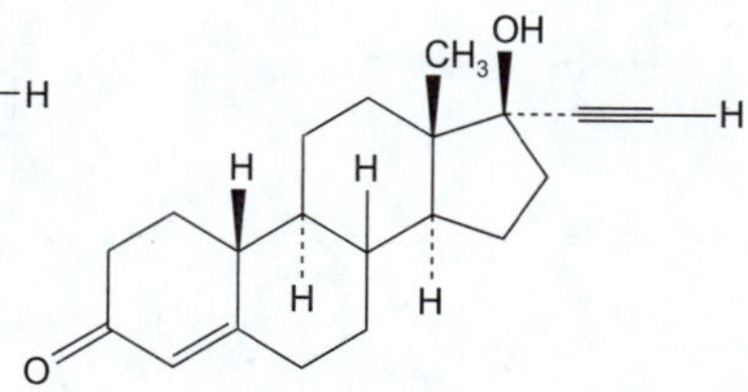

Norethindrone

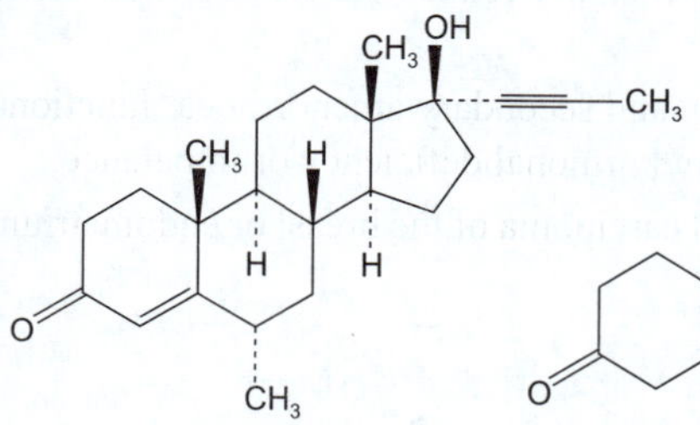

Dimethisterone

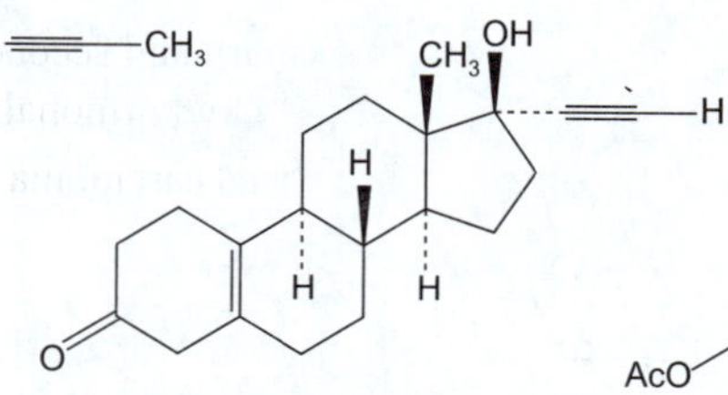

Norethynodrel

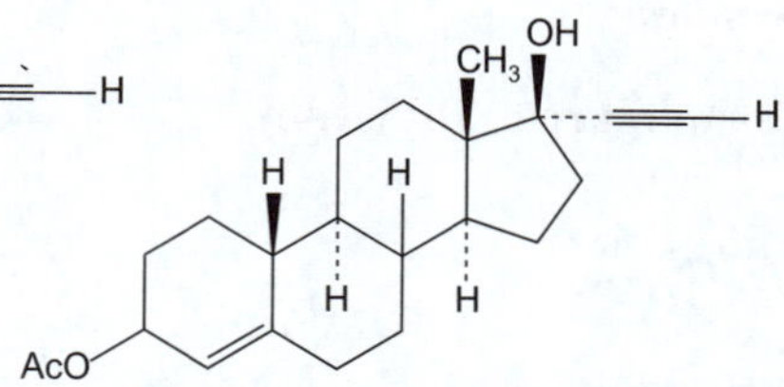

Ethynodiol diacetate

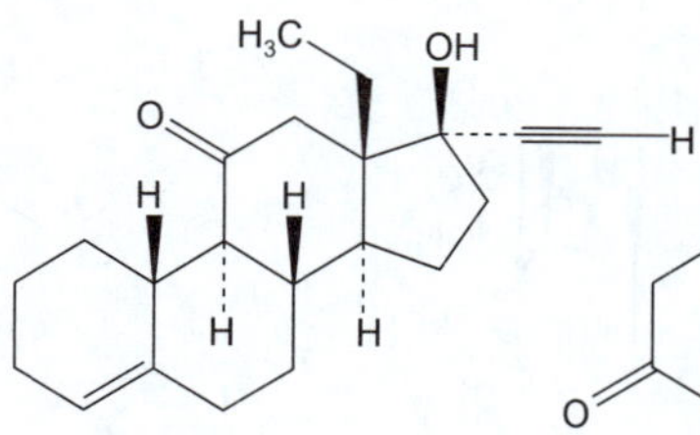

Desogestrel

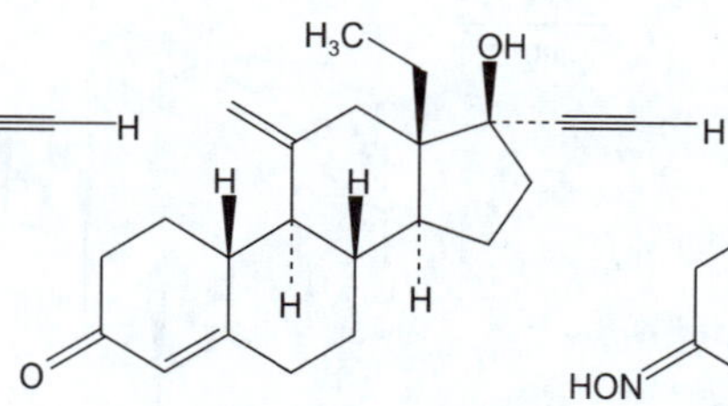

Etonogestrel

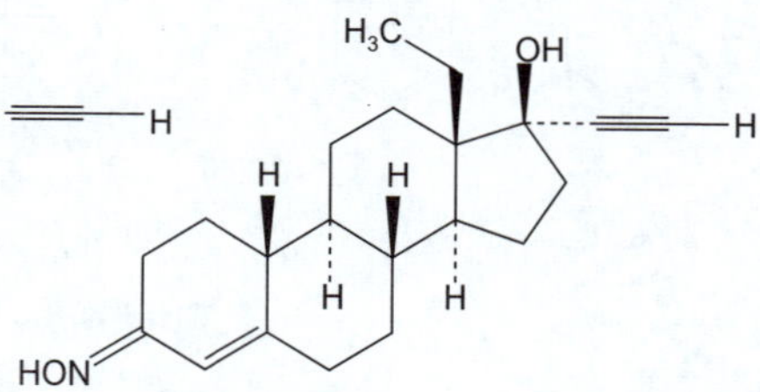

Norgestromin

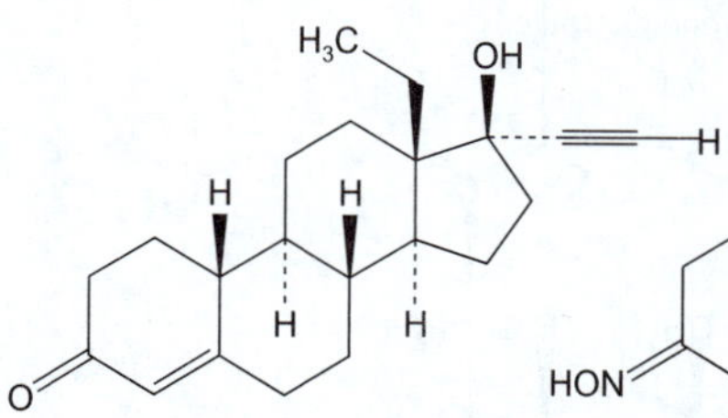

Norgestrel

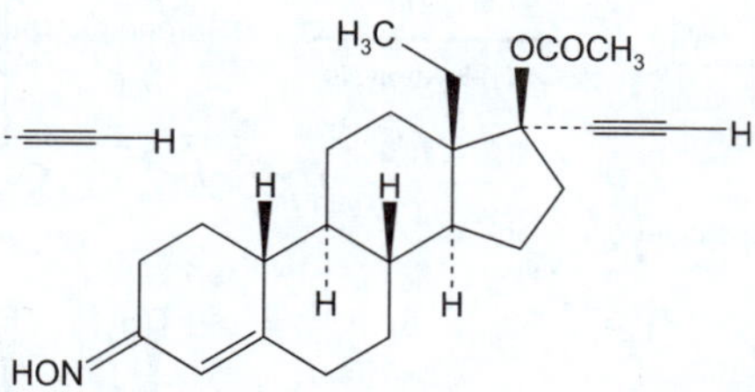

Norgestimate

Progesterone (Alza)

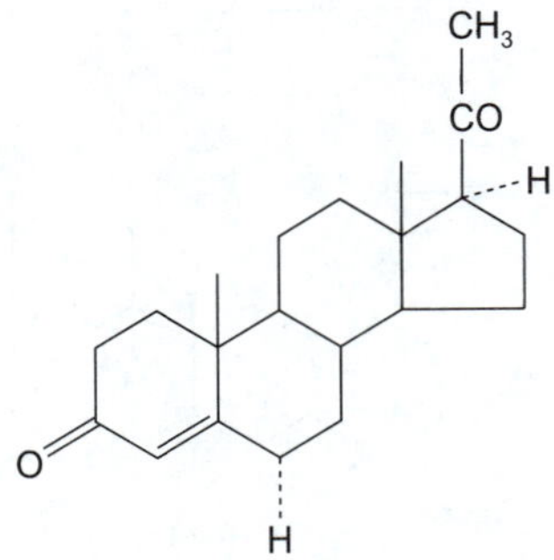

Synthesis

Route 1. From: Diosgenin

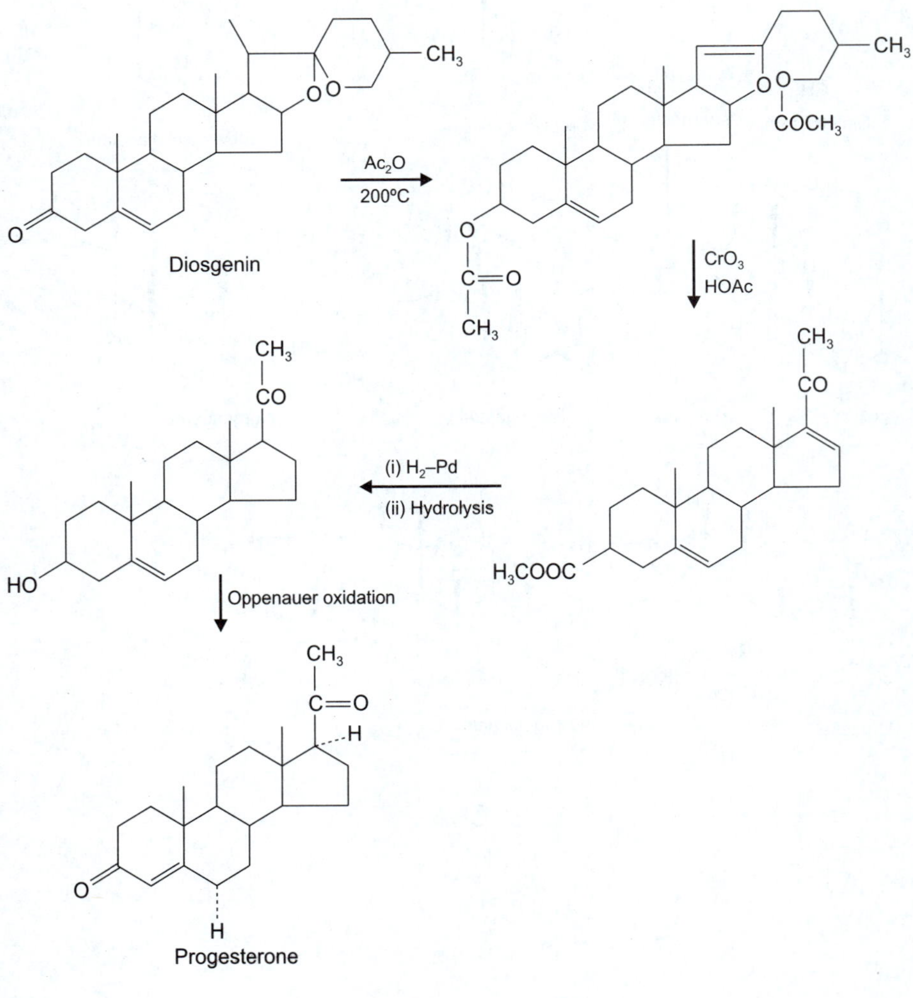

Route 2. From: Ergosterol

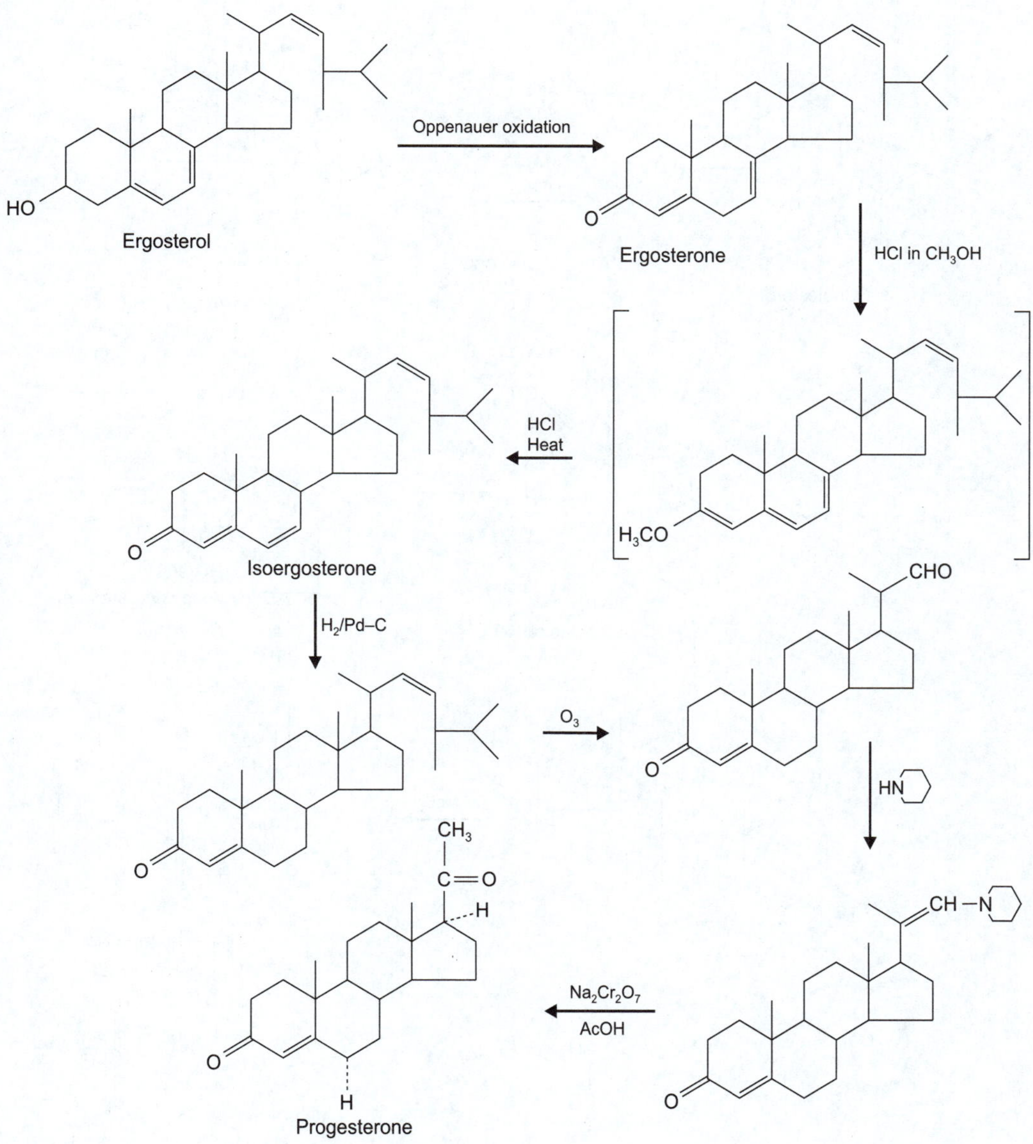

Route 3. From: Cholesterol

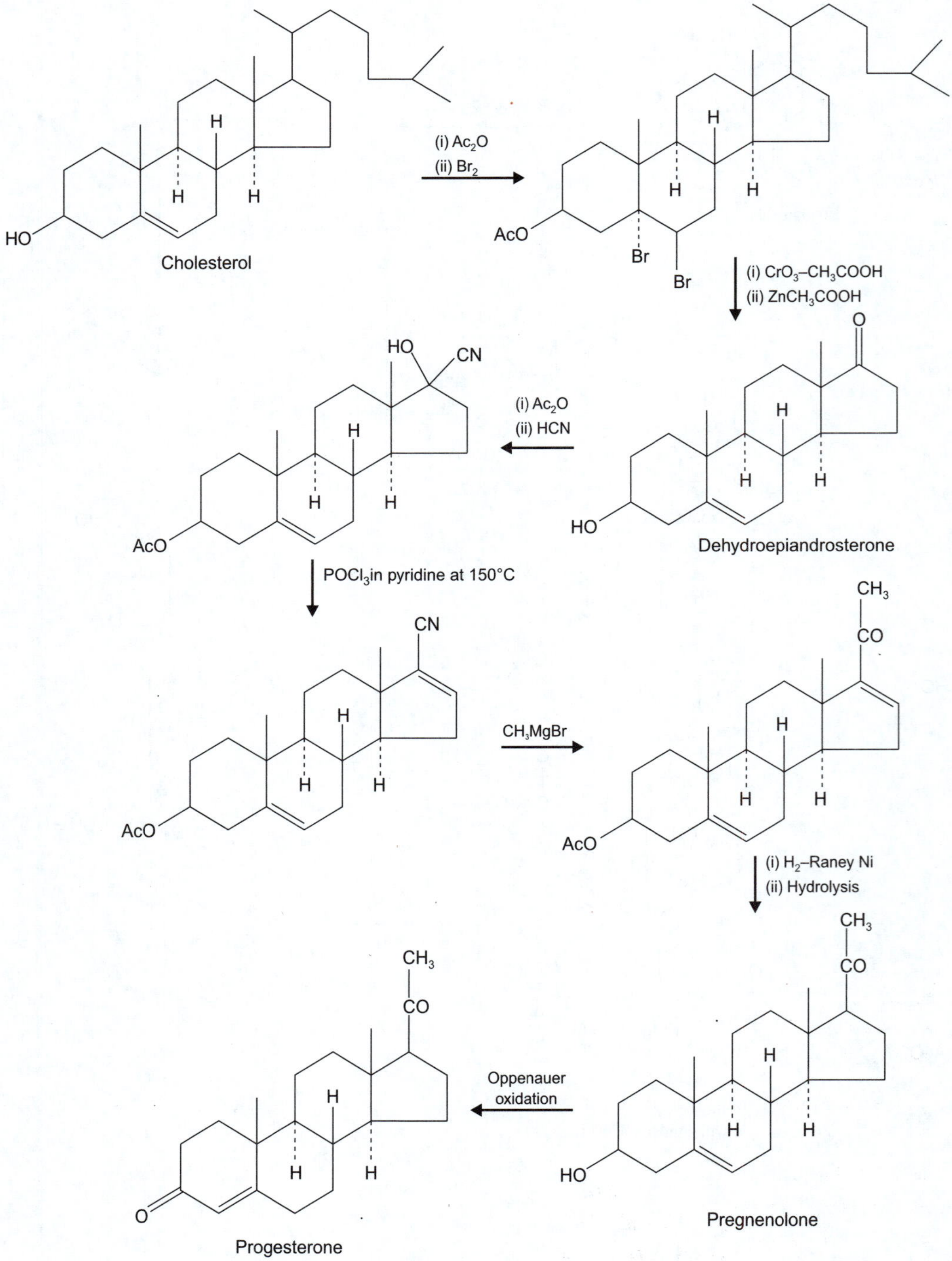

Properties: It exists as white crystalline powder, which is insoluble in water and alcohol.

Dose: The dose for uterine bleeding is 5–10 mg injected per day up to 5–10 days. For habitual abortion, the dosage is 5–20 mg twice or thrice a week by IM injection.

Hydroxyprogesterone caproate

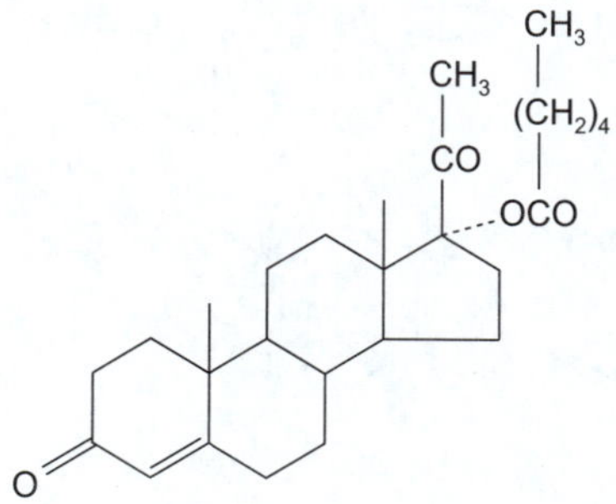

Synthesis

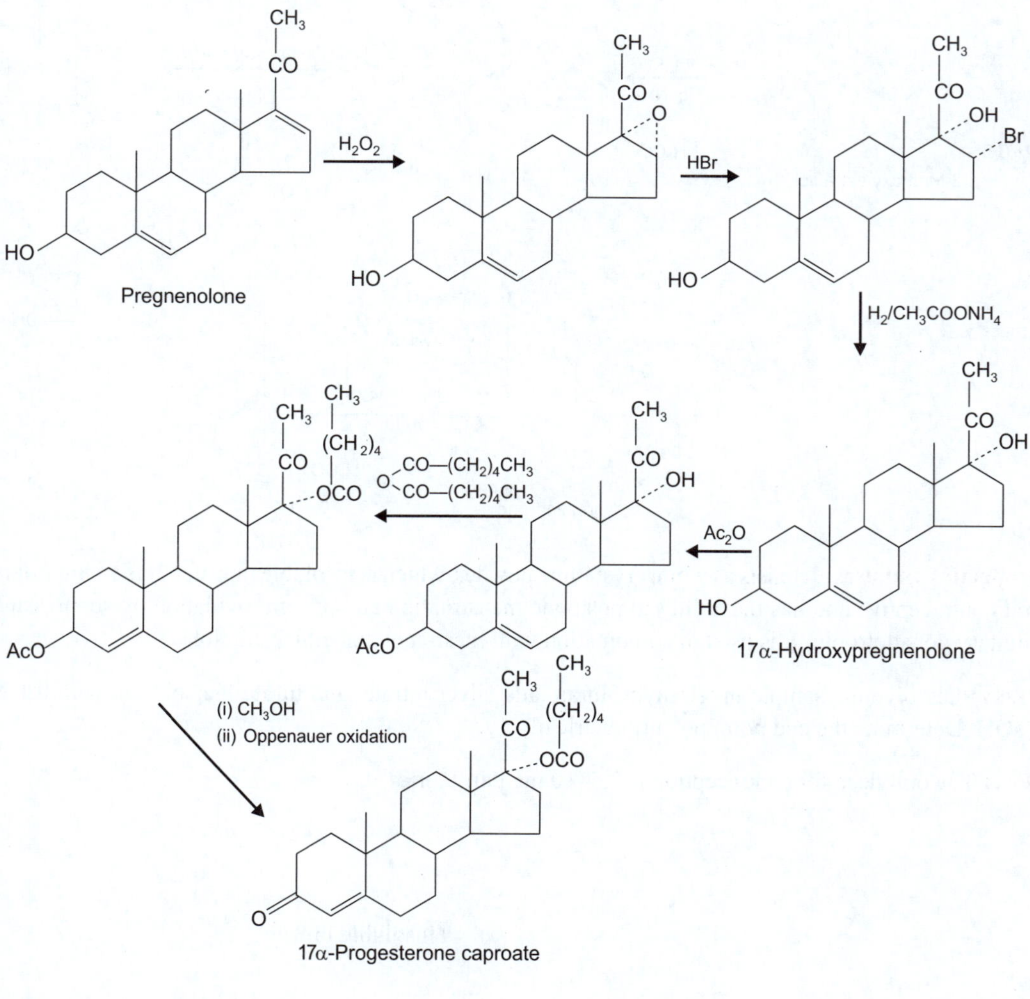

Properties and uses: It exists as white crystalline powder, which is insoluble in water. It is more potent than progesterone, and has longer duration with short onset of action.

Norethindrone (Norethiesterone, Micronor)

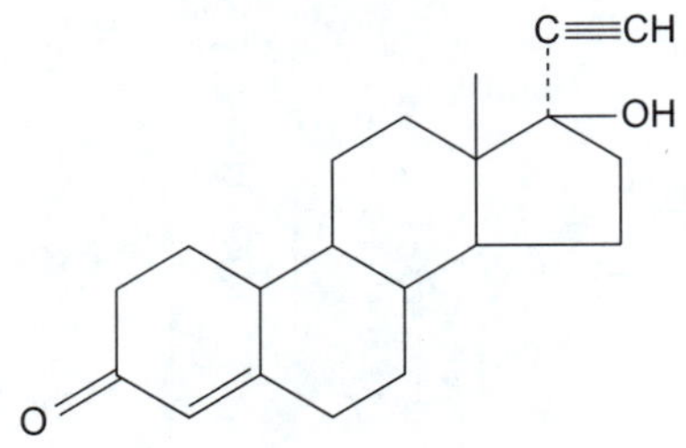

Synthesis

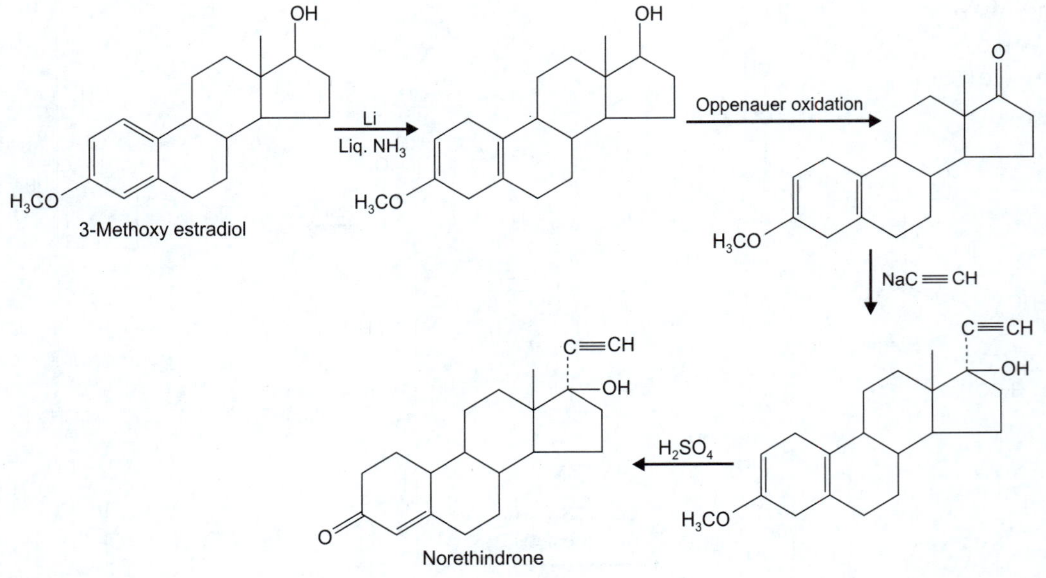

Properties and uses: It exists as white crystalline powder, which is insoluble in water. It is an important oral contraceptive and has the ability to postpone menstruation and prevent ovulation by suppressing pituitary gonadotropin. It is used in combination with mestranol and ethinestradiol.

Assay: Dissolve the sample in tetrahydrofuran, add silver nitrate, and titrate the solution with 0.1 N NaOH. Determine the end point potentiometrically.

Dose: The oral dose for contraception is 2.5–10 mg daily for 21 days.

Norgestrel (Ovrette, Ovval)

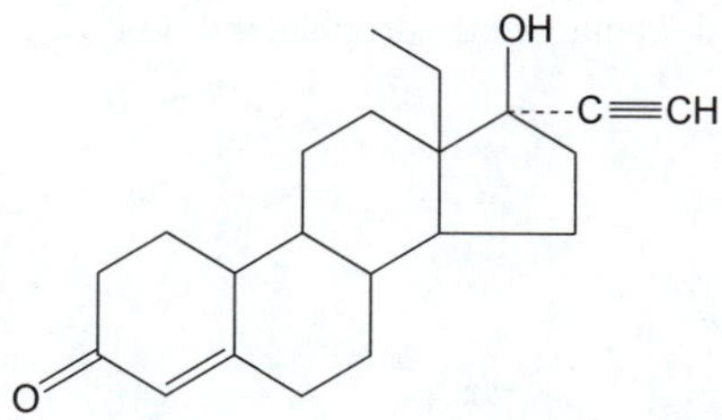

Synthesis

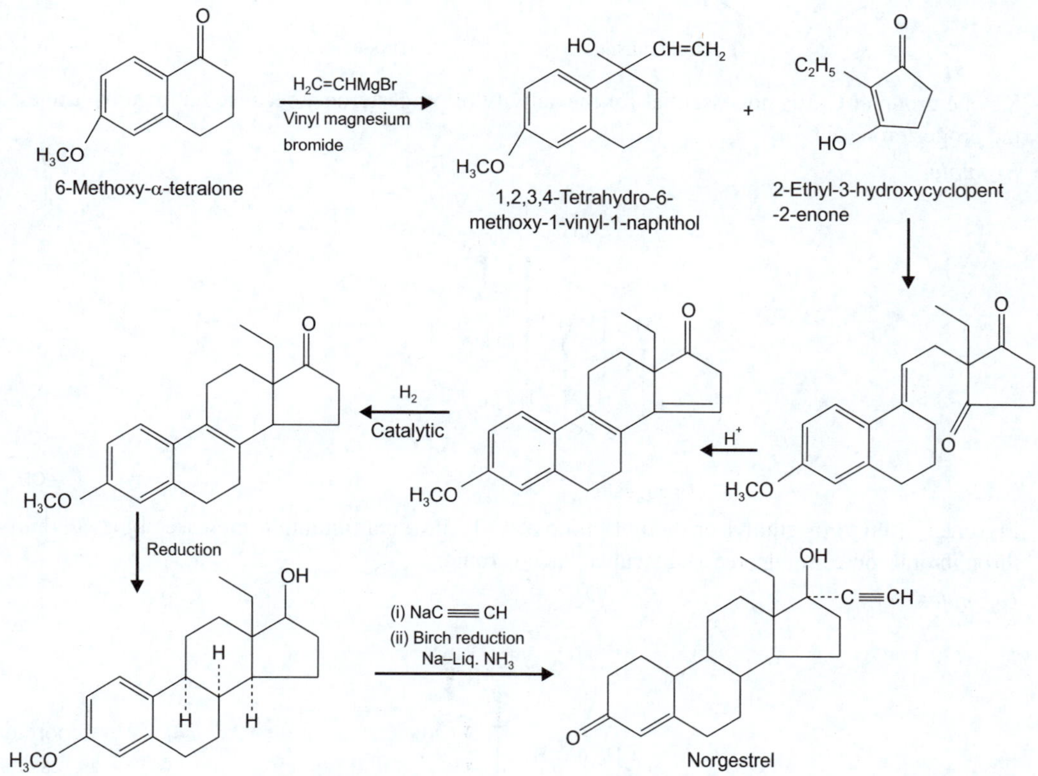

Properties and uses: It exists as white crystalline powder, which is insoluble in water and slightly soluble in alcohol. It is used as an oral contraceptive.

Dose: The oral dose as a single agent is 75 μg per day.

Structure–Activity Relationship of Progesterones

Presence of steroid nucleus (cyclopentanoperhydrophenanthrene ring) is compulsory for pharmacological activity of progestins.

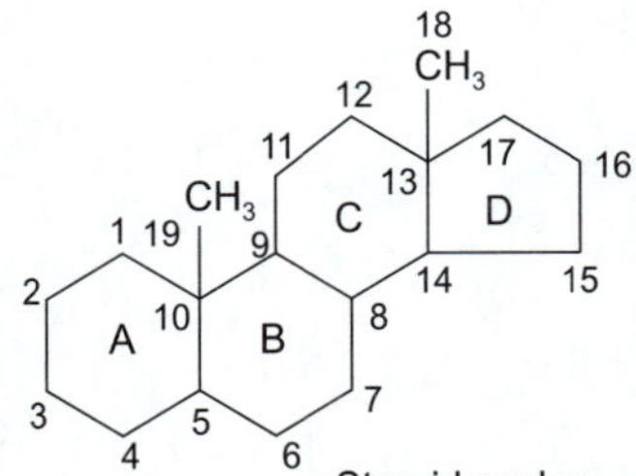

Steroid nucleus

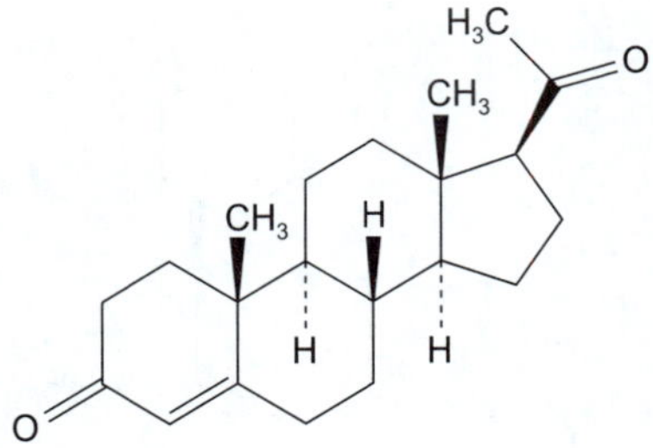

Progesterone

- Ketone group at C-3 is not essential for the activity of progesterone, because removal of it retains the progesterone activity.

  Example:

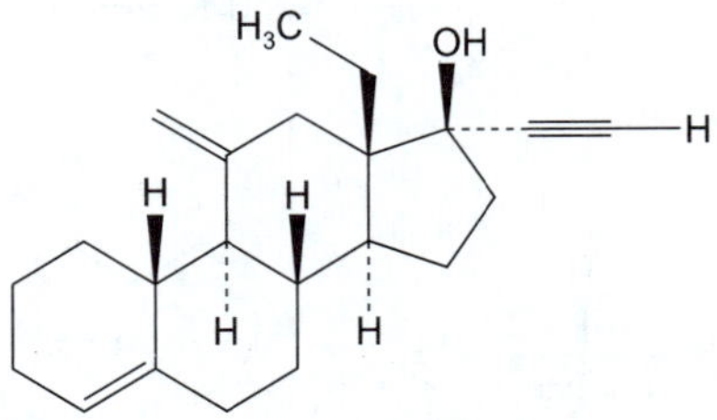

Desogestrel

- Presence of ethyl or ethinyl or diethyl group at C-17 in α-configuration increases bioavailability through oral route, but decreases by subcutaneous route.

  Example:

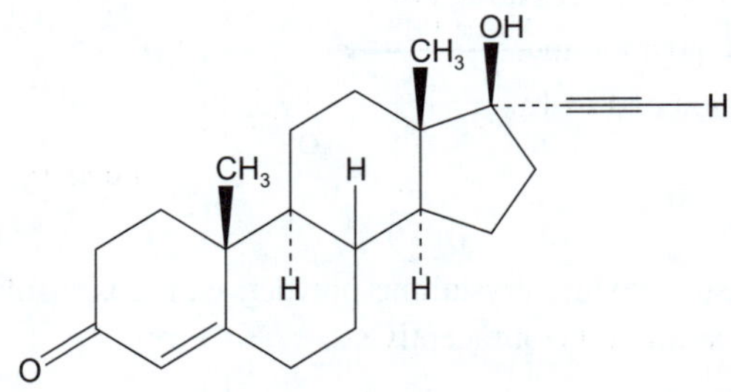

Ethisterone

- The L-enantiomer of the compound resulting from substitution of ethyl group at C-ring juncture is found to be active.
- Derivatives of the progestins like 3-oxime-17-ester decreases androgenic side effect, while retaining the progestin activity.

- Introduction of halogen or CH_3 at C-6 or C-7 atoms in α-configuration increases hormonal activity of progestins.

  Example:

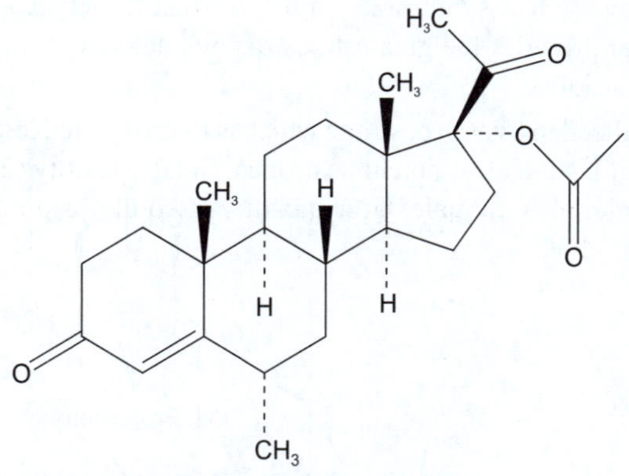

Medroxyprogesterone acetate

- Presence of methyl at C-19 is not essential for activity because its removal leads to formation of compound with increased activity.

  Example:

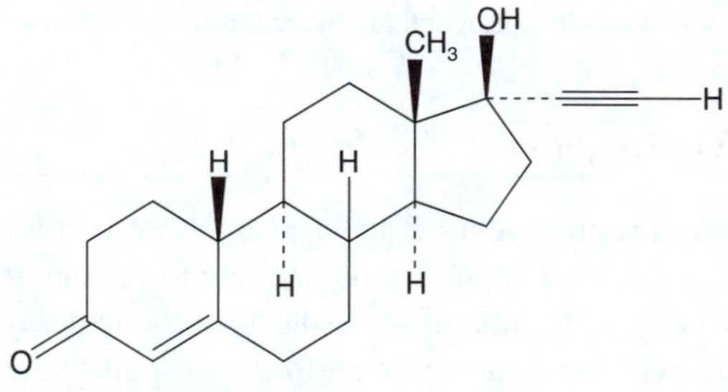

Norethindrone

- Addition of Cl or F at C-21 prevents metabolic hydroxylation, which also enhances oral effectiveness.
- Unsaturation at ring A and B enhances activity of 19-norethindrone. Example: Trimegestone.
- Addition of methyl at 18th position increases the activity.
- In ring D at C-17, acetylation of 17α-hydroxyl group increases the duration of action.

  Example:

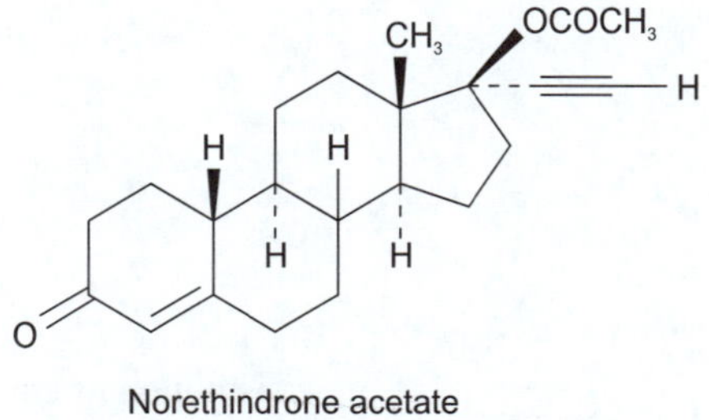

Norethindrone acetate

OESTROGENS

Oestrogens are classified as organic compounds that control the uterine cycle. Oestradiol is the major oestrogen secreted by the ovary. It is synthesized in the graffian follicle, corpus luteum, and placenta from cholesterol. Oestradiol provides the greatest oestrogenic activity, with less activity for oestrone and the least activity for oestriol.

Oestradiol is rapidly oxidized in liver to oestrone which is hydroxylated to form oestriol. All three are found in blood, but oestradiol is the most potent oestrogen. Small quantity (2–20 µg/day) of oestradiol is synthesized in human males also. In male, large quantity of equilin is produced which has one-fifth oestrogenic potency of oestradiol.

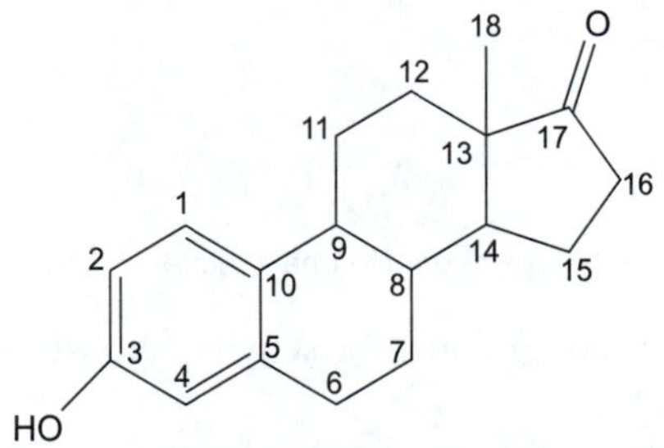

Estrogen or 3-hydroxy-13-methyl-7,8,9,11,12,13,15,16-octahydro-6*H*-cyclopenta[a]phenanthren-17(14*H*)-one

Biological Activities of Oestrogens

The oestrogens and, to a lesser extent, progesterone are largely responsible for the development of secondary sex characteristics in women at puberty, in addition to the important role in the menstrual cycle. The oestrogens also cause a proliferation of the breast ductile system, and progester one stimulates development of the alveolar system. The oestrogens stimulate the development of lipid and other tissues, which contribute to the breast shape and function. Fluid retention in the breasts during the later stages of the menstrual cycle is a common effect of the oestrogens.

Metabolism of oestrogens

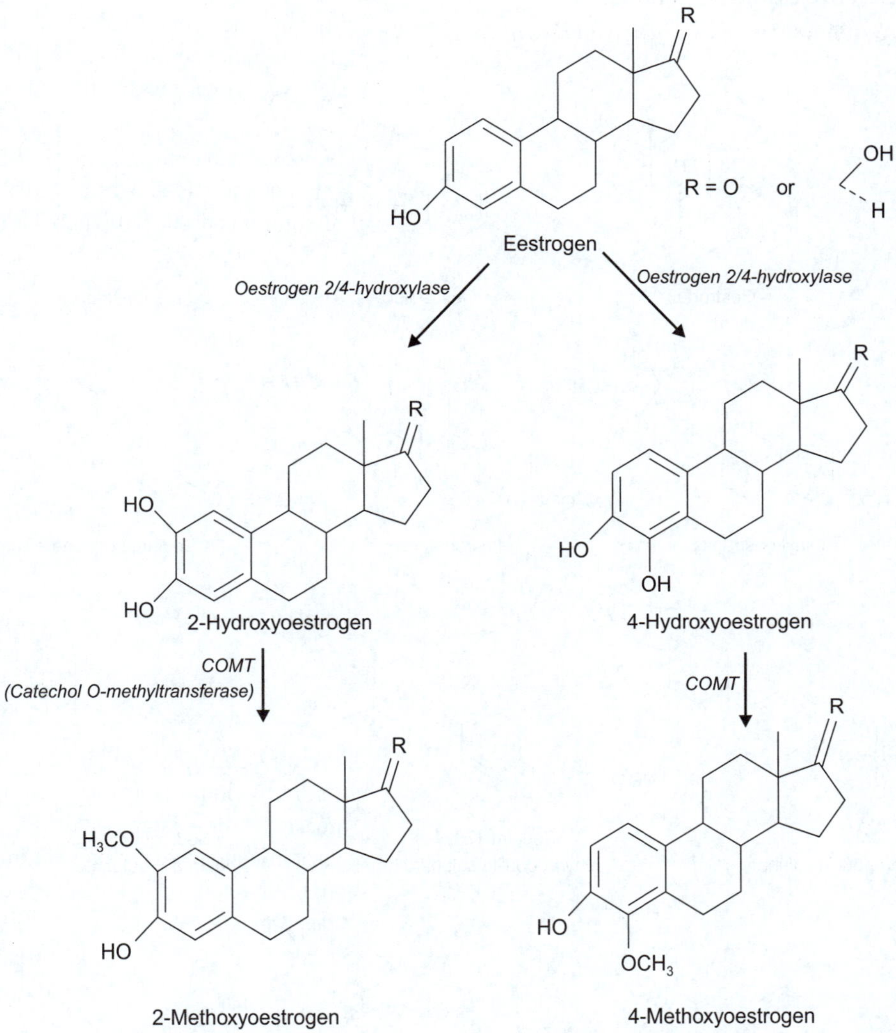

Therapeutic Uses of Oestrogens

Oestrogens are used therapeutically as follows:

- A major use of oestrogens is for inhibition of ovulation, in combination with progestins (birth control).
- Another major use of oestrogens is in hormone replacement therapy for postmenopausal women.
- Used in the treatment of advanced, inoperable breast cancer (in men and postmenopausal women) and prostate cancer (in men).

Classification of oestrogens

Oestrogens are classified as follows:

1. Steroidal oestrogens and their derivatives

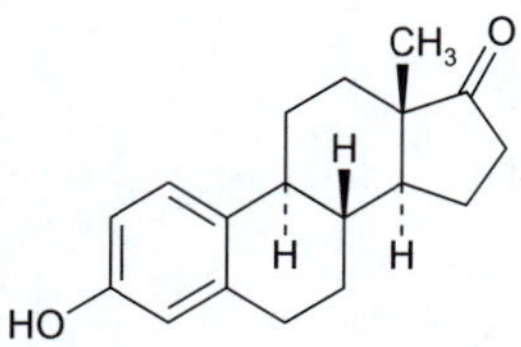

Oestrone

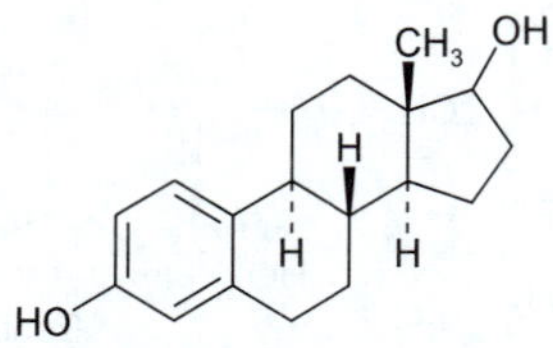

Oestradiol

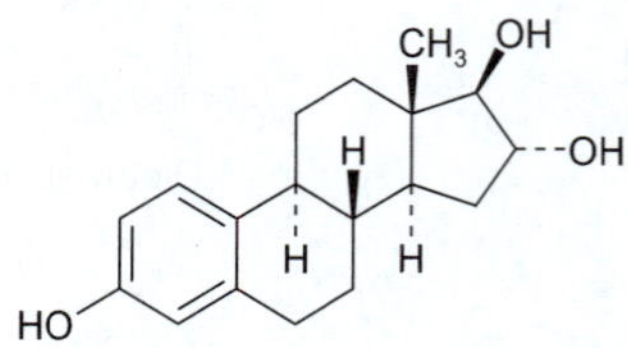

Oestriol

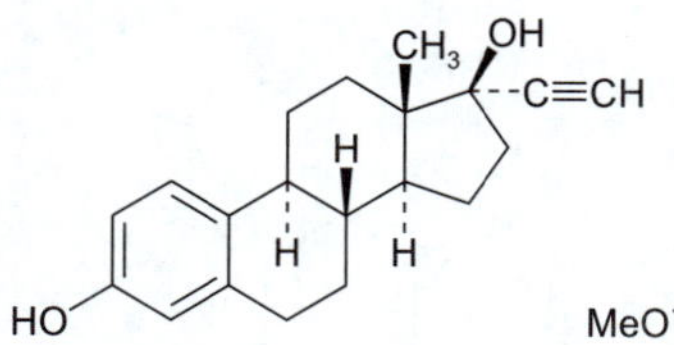

Ethinyl oestradiol

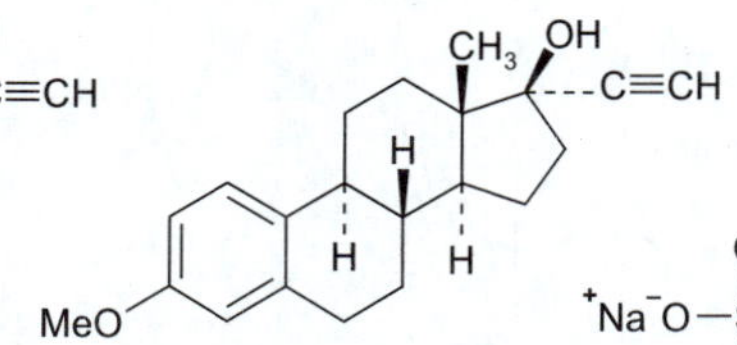

Mestranol

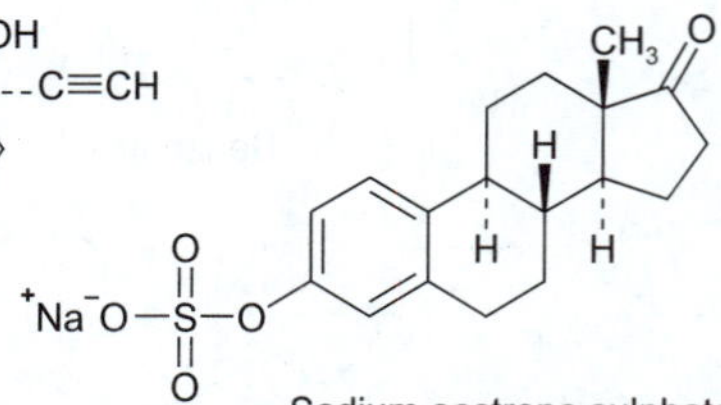

Sodium oestrone sulphate

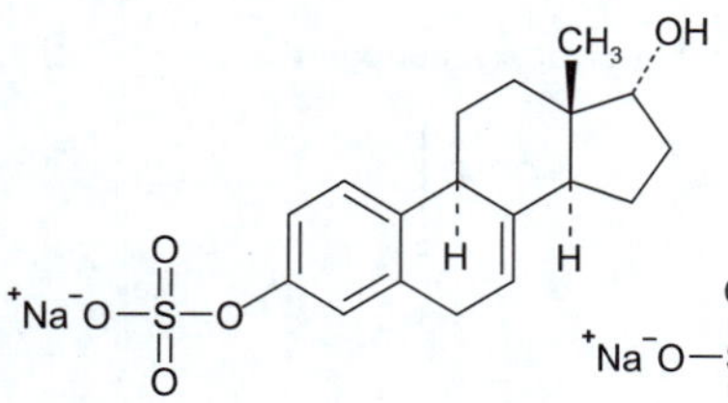

Sodium 17α-dihydroequilin sulphate

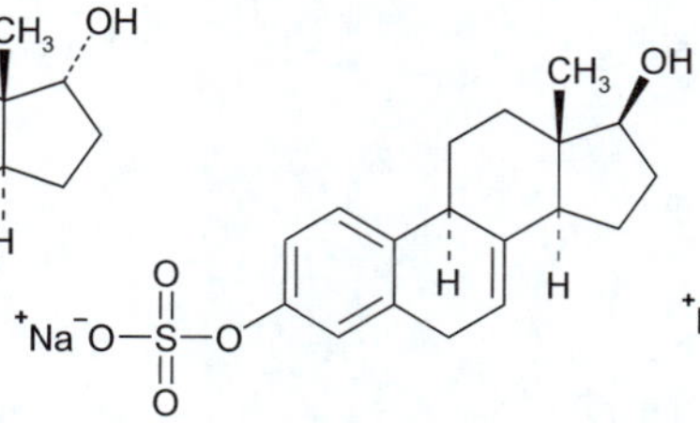

Sodium 17β-dihydroequilin sulphate

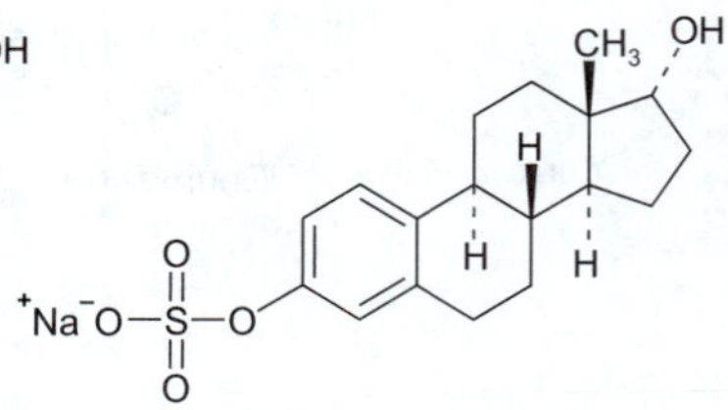

Sodium 17α-oestradiol sulphate

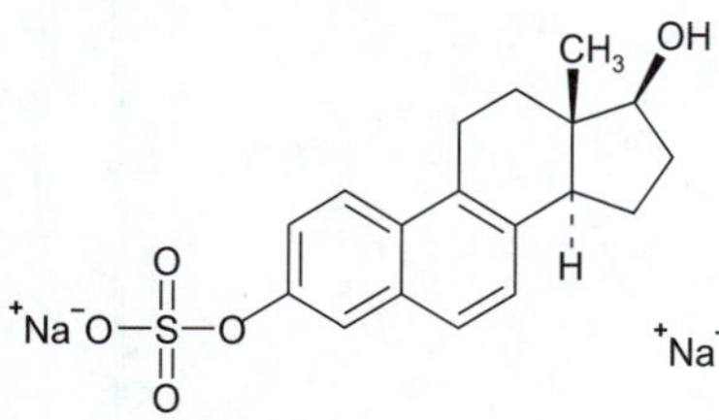

Sodium 17β-dihydroequilenin sulphate

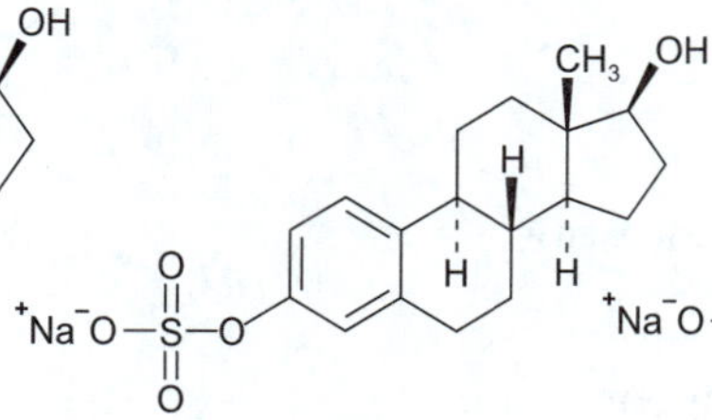

Sodium 17β-oestradiol sulphate

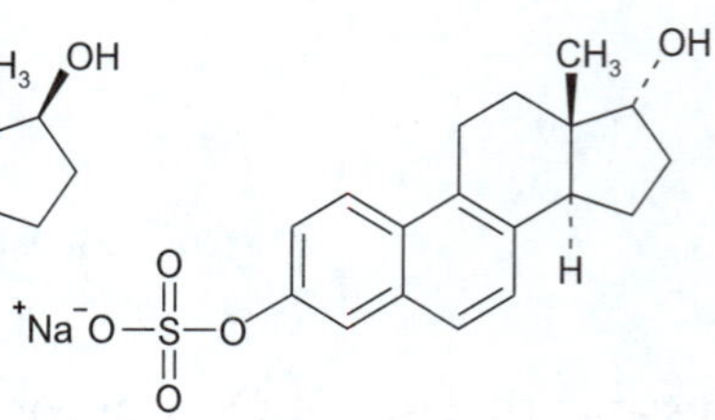

Sodium 17α-dihydroequilenin sulphate

2. Non-steroidal or synthetic oestrogens or artificial hormones

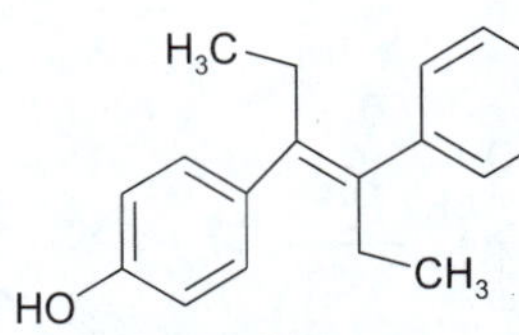

Diethylstilbestrol

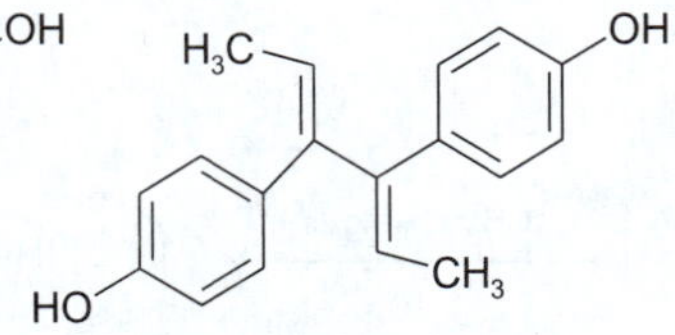

Dienestrol

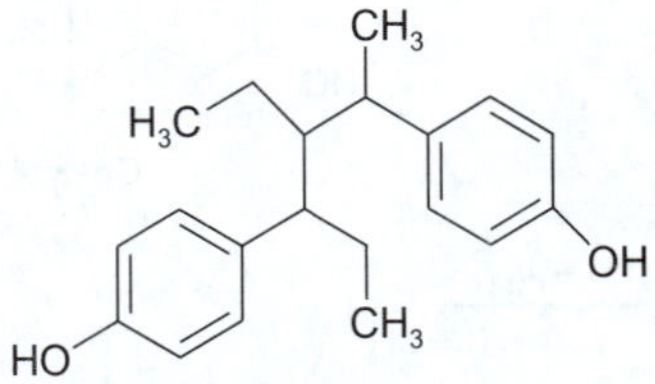

Benzestrol

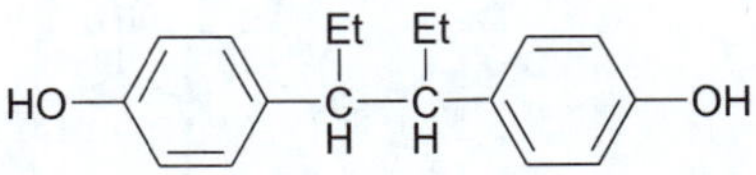

Hexoestrol

3. Oestrogens of plant origin

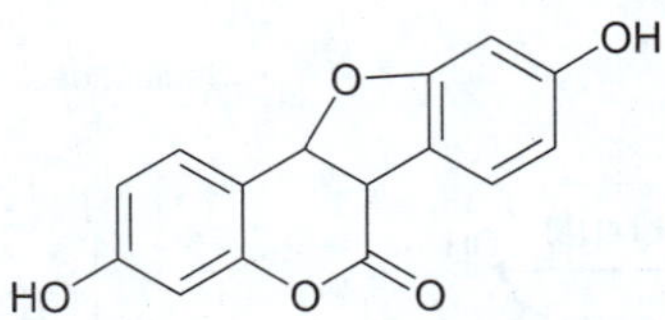

Coumestrol

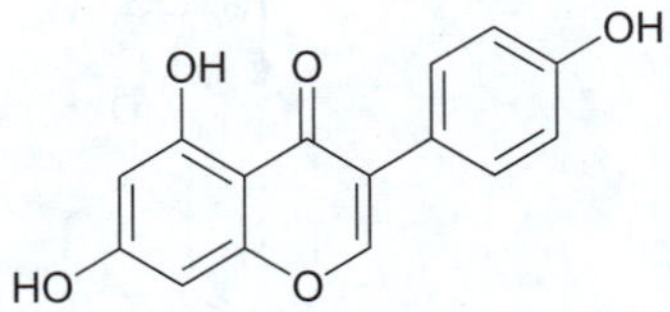

Genistein

Oestrone

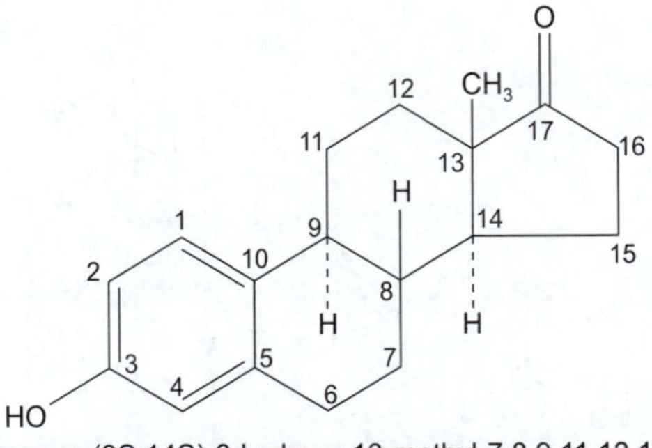

Oestrogen or (9S,14S)-3-hydroxy-13-methyl-7,8,9,11,12,13,15,16-octahydro-6*H*-cyclopenta[a]phenanthren-17(14*H*)-one

From the urine of pregnant women, it was isolated in the year 1929 by Butenandt and Doisy. It is the first known member of sex hormones. The main sources of oestrone are urine of pregnant or non-pregnant women, human placenta, and adrenal cortex. It is a stable, white substance existing in three crystal forms.

The main function of oestrone is to induce the state of heat in the female animals, and it thus acts in the control of uterine cycle. It also helps in the development of female secondary sex characteristics by which they become different from males.

Synthesis of oestrone

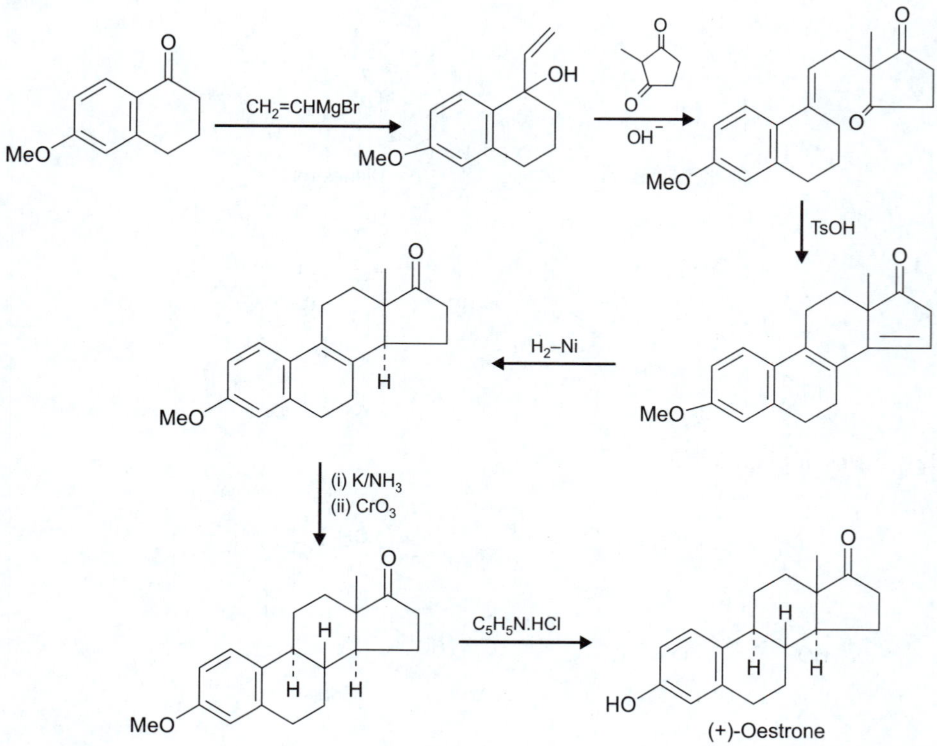

Oestriol

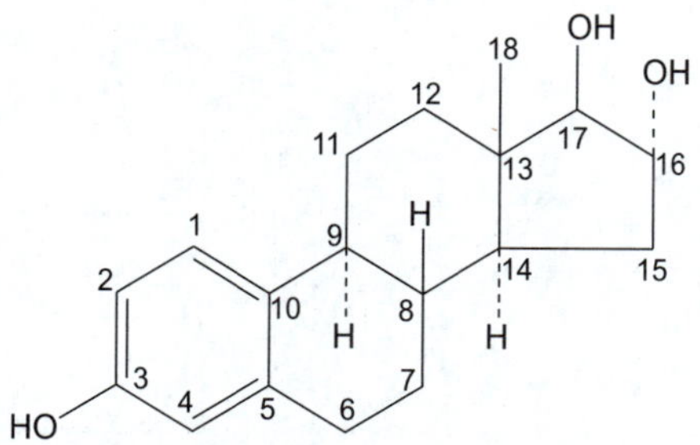

Oestrogen or (9S,14S,16R)-13-Methyl-7,8,9,11,12,13,14,15,16,17-decahydro-6*H*-cyclopenta[a]phenanthren-3,16,17-triol

It was isolated from human pregnancy urine by Marrian in the year 1950. It is useful in some cases of oestrogen deficiency, especially for the relief of menopausal symptoms and, in paediatrics, to combat gonorrhoeal vaginitis. It occurs mainly in human placenta and pregnant women. It is effective orally.

Synthesis of oestriol

Route 1.

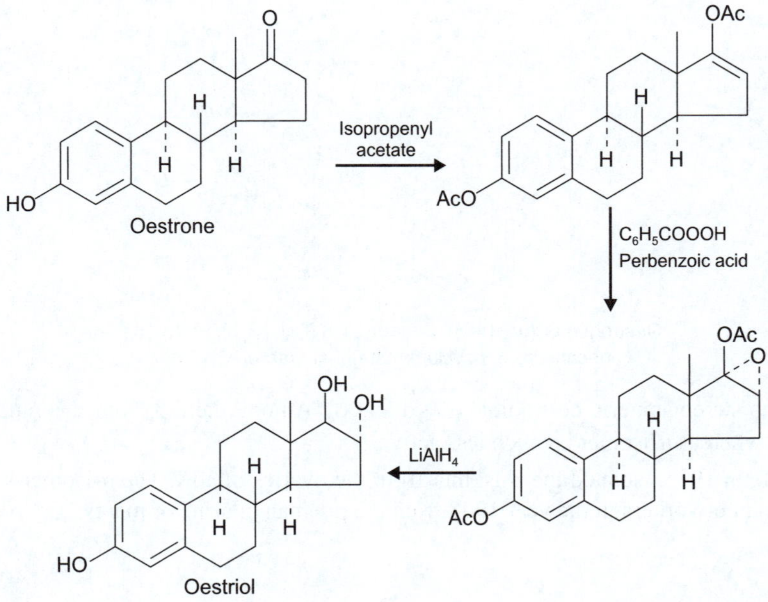

Route 2.

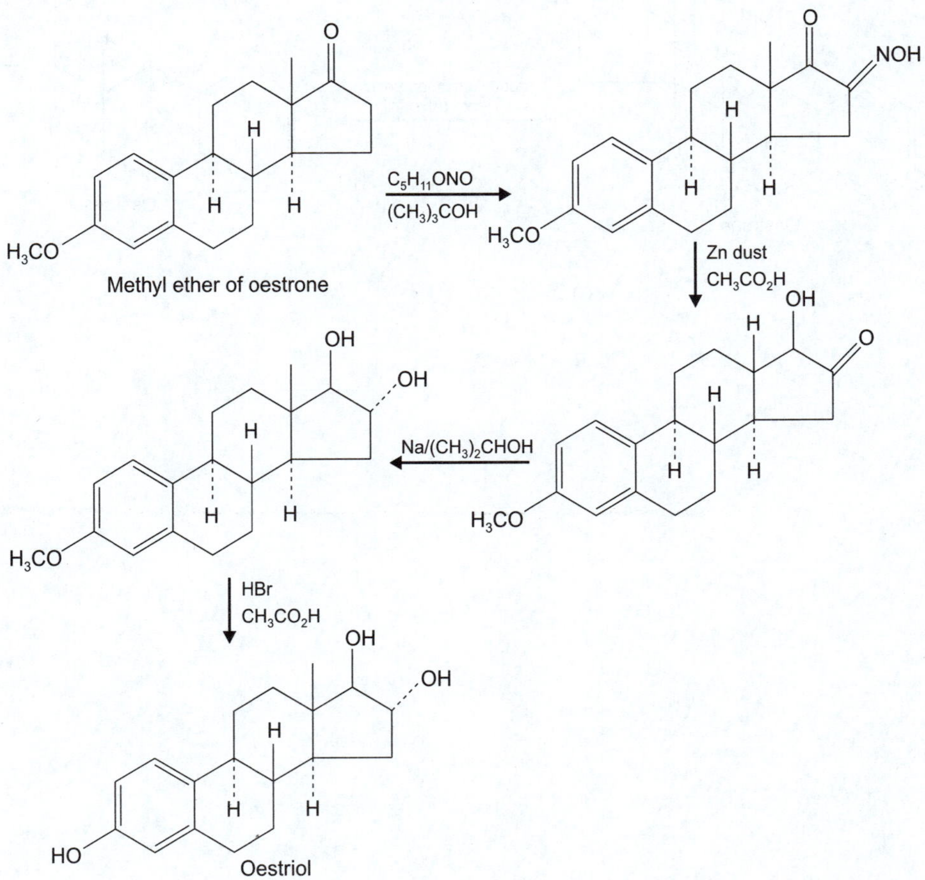

Oestradiol

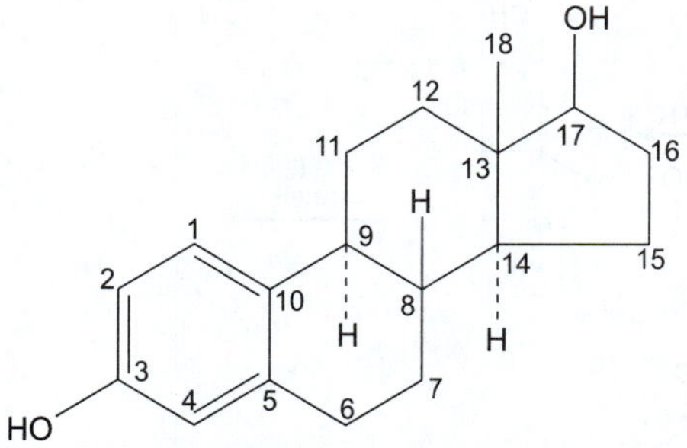

Oestrogen or (9S,14S)-13-methyl-7,8,9,11,12,13,14,15,16,17-decahydro-6*H*-cyclopenta[a]phenanthren-3,17-diol

It exists as two stereoisomeric oestradiols (i.e. α and β). Among them β-isomer is much more active than oestrone whereas α-isomer is much less active.

Doisy et al., in 1935, isolated the β-isomer from the ovaries of cow. The α-isomer was isolated by Winterstein and co-workers in the year 1938 from the pregnancy urine of mares.

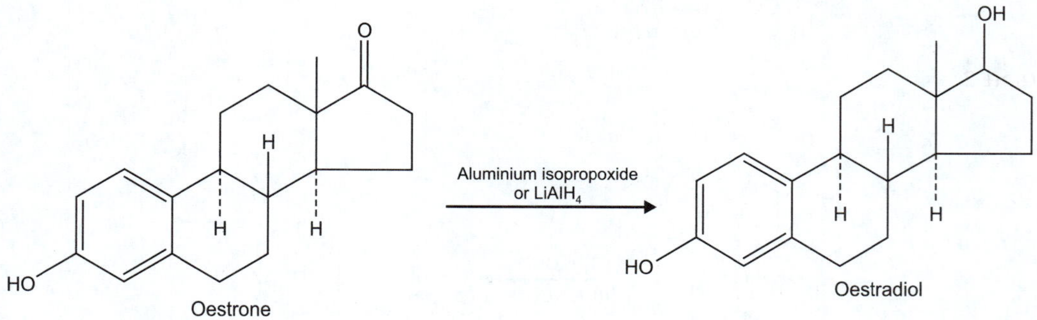

Synthesis of oestrogen derivatives

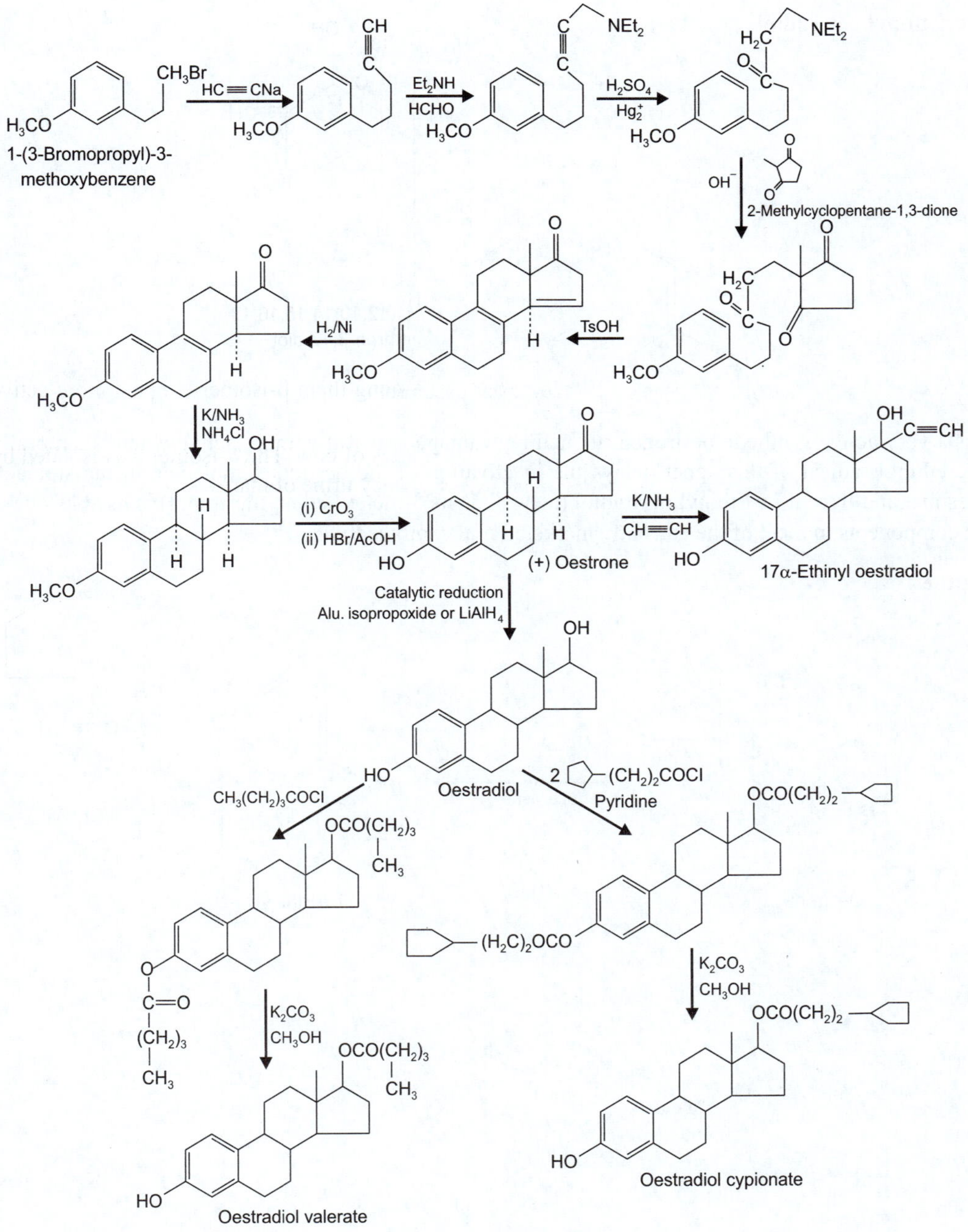

Synthetic Oestrogens

17α-Ethinyl oestradiol

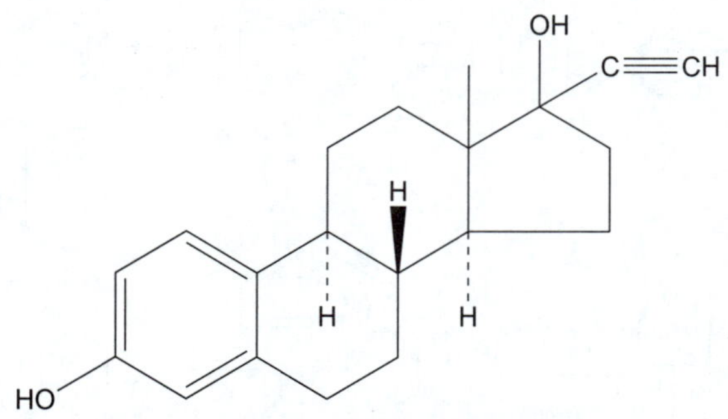

17α-Ethinyl oestradiol

It is a very active synthetic oestrogen. Its main advantage is that it is more active when taken orally. The ethinyl radical of this agent delays the inactivation of the oestradiol molecule in the stomach, intestine, and liver. 17α-Ethinyl oestradiol (as well as its 3-methyl ether, mestranol) is used as one of the components in most of the currently marketed oral contraceptive.

Synthesis

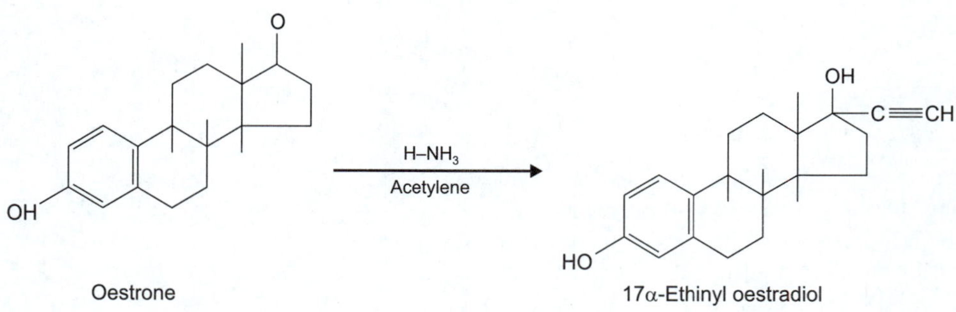

Conversion Among Oestrone, Oestriol, and Oestradiol

Interconversion taking place during metabolism is given below.

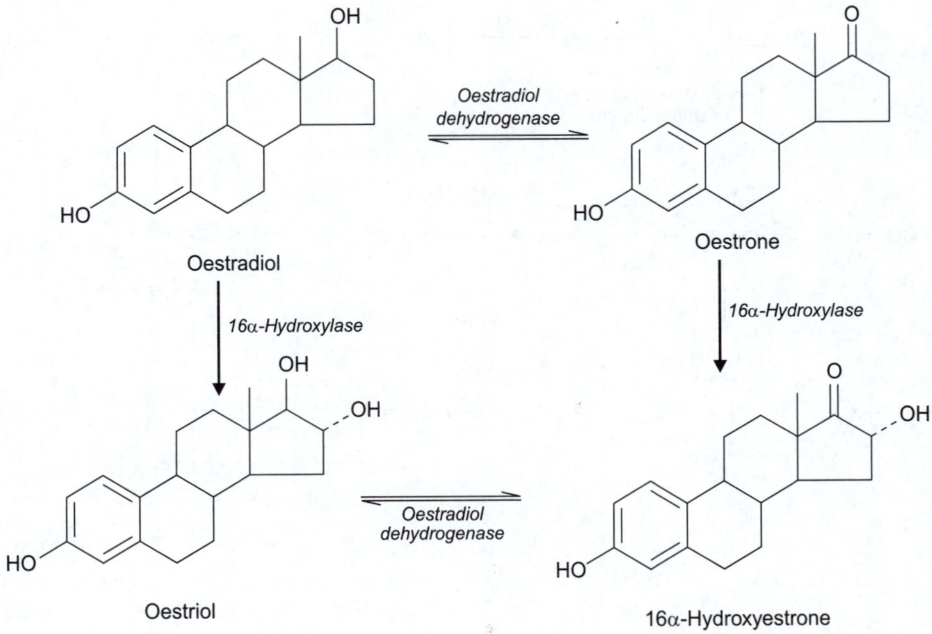

Non-steroidal Oestrogens or Artificial Hormones

A large number of synthetic oestrogens have been prepared which have oestrogenic activity without having steroid skeleton. Because of their relatively low cost and their efficiency when administered orally over oestrogens of natural origin, these agents are preferred.

1. **Stilbestrol** (Diethylstilbestrol, Stilbetin, Stilphostrol)

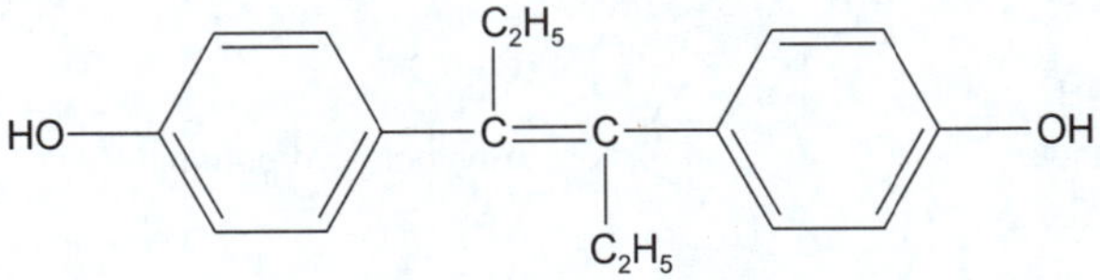

4,4-Dihydroxydiethylstilbene

Synthesis: It can be synthesized by the following routes.

Route 1. From: Anisaldehyde (Dodds method)

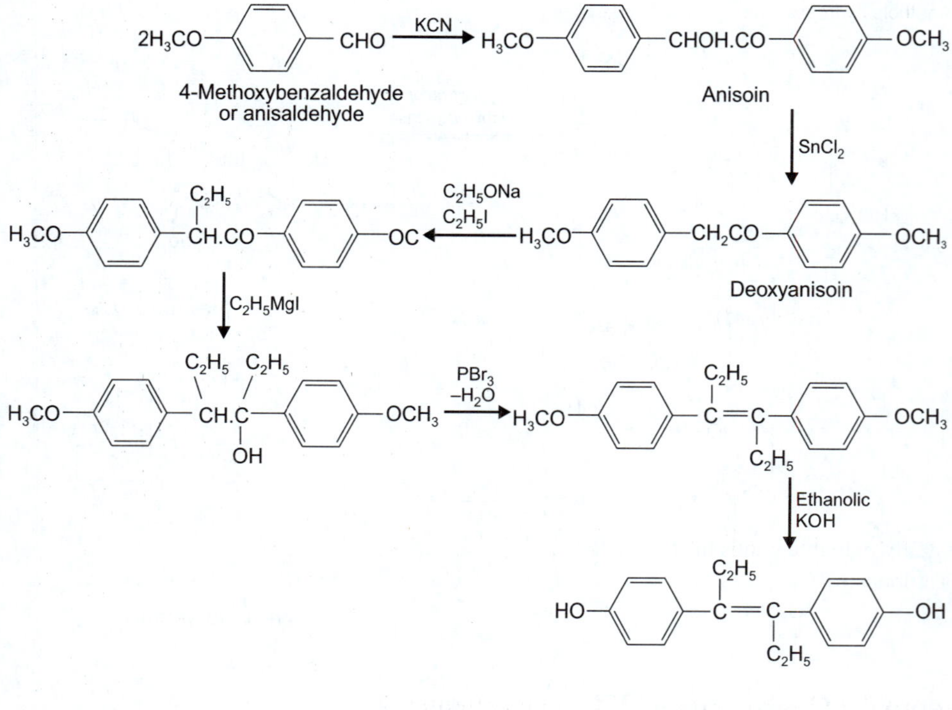

Diethylstilbestrol (*trans*)

Route 2. From: Anethole

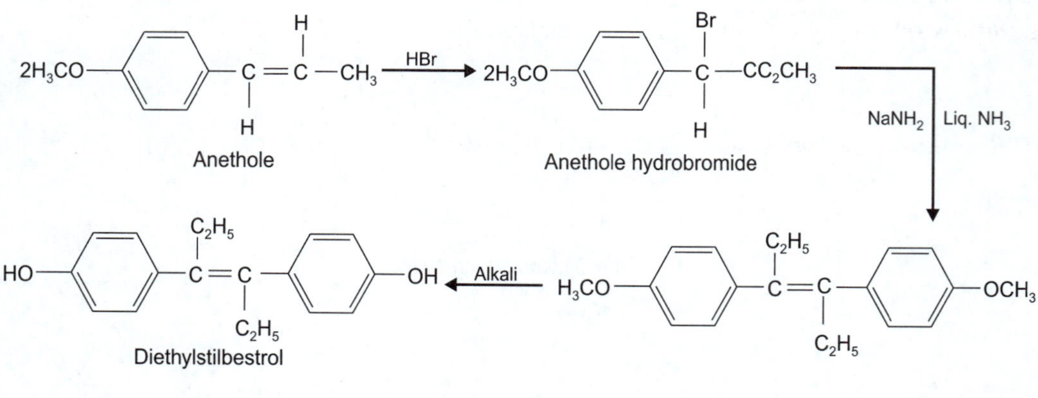

Properties: It is a white crystalline powder, which is insoluble in water and soluble in alcohol.

2. **Hexoestrol:** Hexoestrol contains two asymmetric carbon atoms, hence it exists in diastereomeric forms. The meso form is much more potent than the racemic form, and it is only the meso form which is of commercial importance. It is synthesized from anethole hydrobromide.

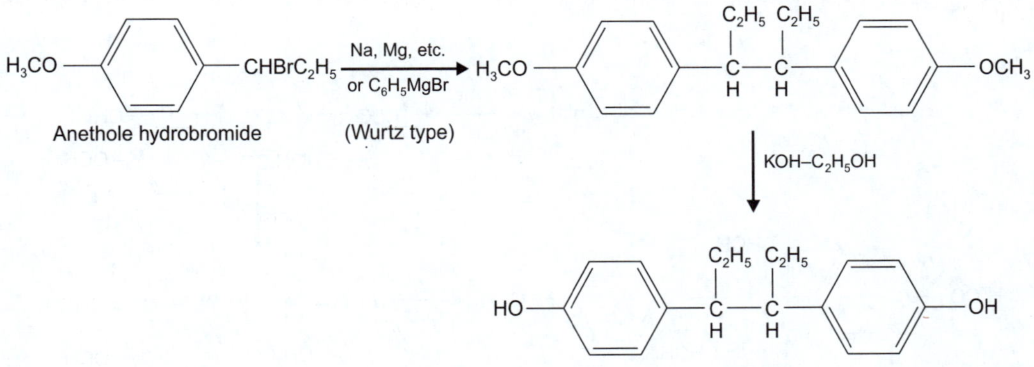

Hexoestrol

3. Dienoestrol (Estragard)

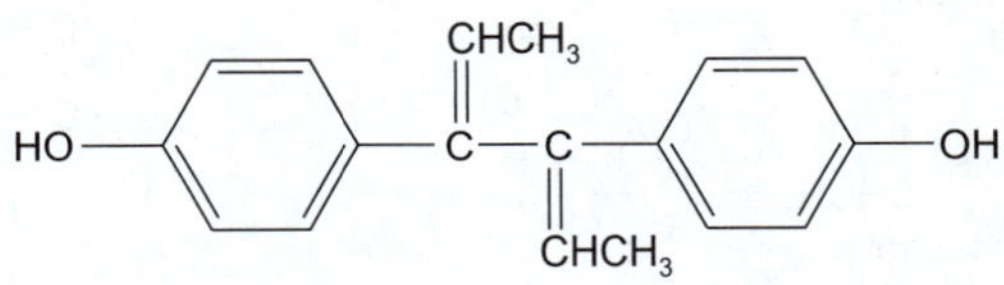

It has two double bonds in side chain as indicated in the name itself. It is about one-fourth as potent as stilboestrol.

Synthesis

Route 1.

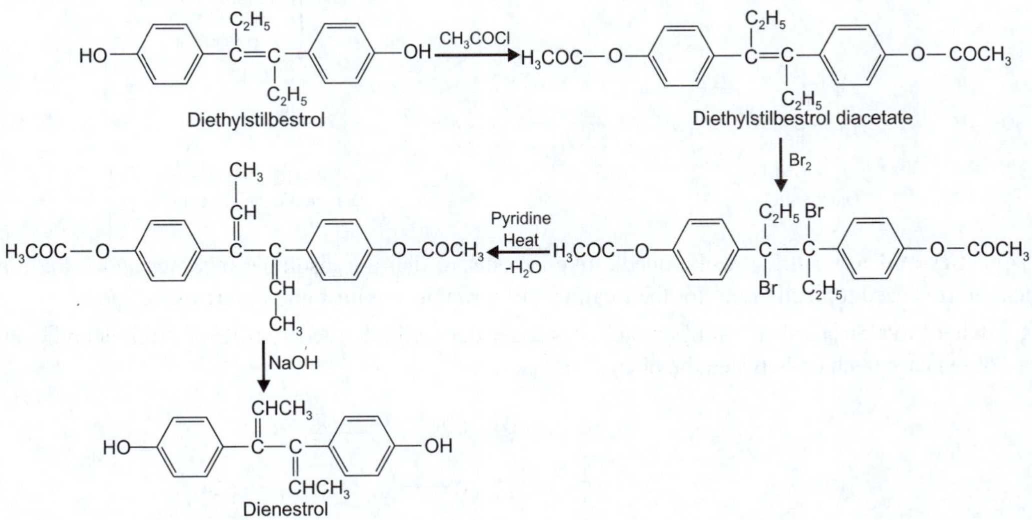

Route 2.

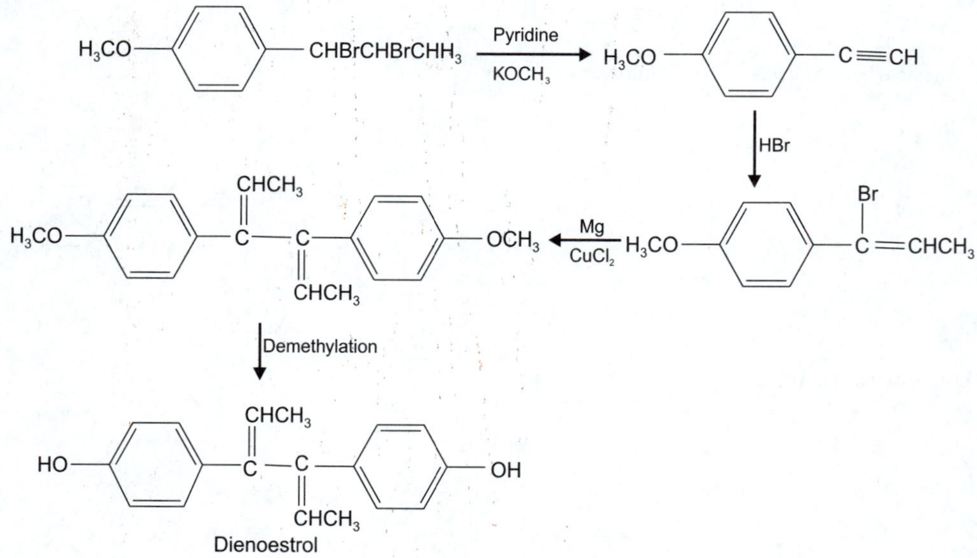

Route 3.

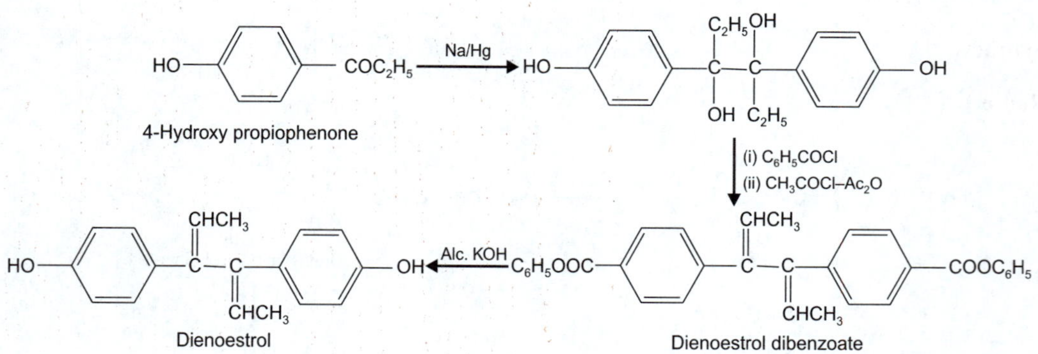

Properties and uses: It has white needle-like crystals, which are insoluble in water and soluble in alcohol. It is used topically only for the treatment of atrophic vaginitis and kraurosis vulvae.

4. **Benzoestrol:** It is an example of synthetic oestrogen that can be derived from hexoestrol by lengthening of the carbon chain between the phenyl groups.

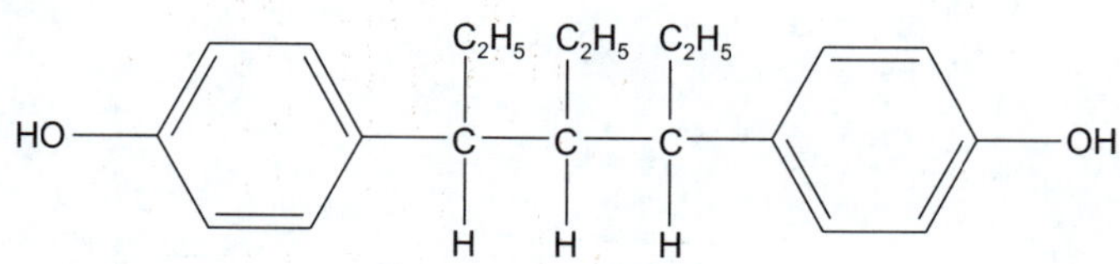

Benzoestrol

Synthesis

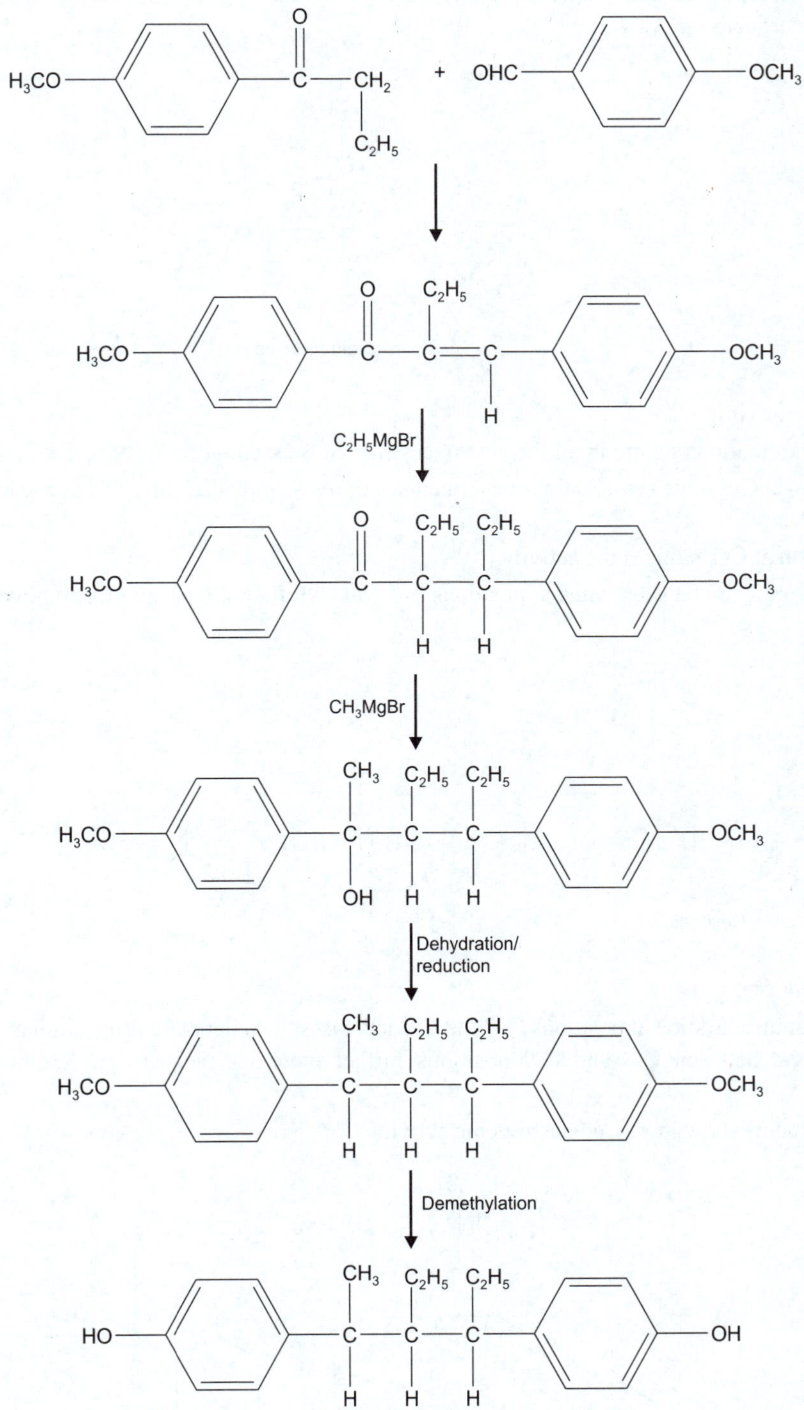

Benzoestrol

Structure–activity relationship of oestrogens

Presence of steroid nucleus (cyclopentanoperhydrophenanthrene ring) is essential for pharmacological activity of oestrogens.

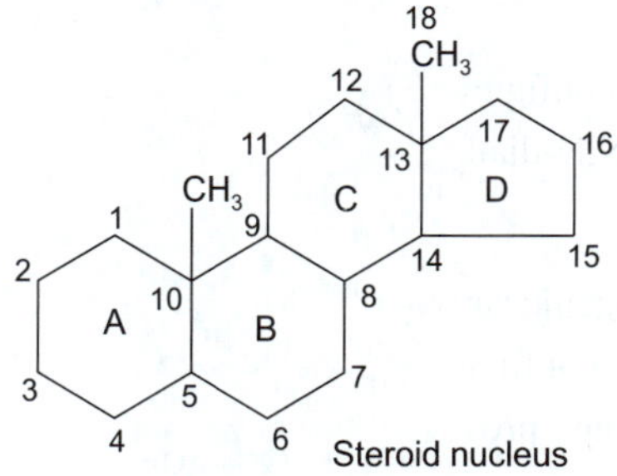

Steroid nucleus

Modification of ring A

- Ring A is aromatic in nature in all the oestrogens, which is essential for oestrogenic activity.
- –OH group at C-3 is also essential for oestrogenic activity. Removal of this –OH group leads to great loss of activity.
- Substitution at C-1 reduces the activity.
- Smaller groups can be substituted at positions C-2 and C-3. Example: 2-hydroxy ethinyl oestradiol.

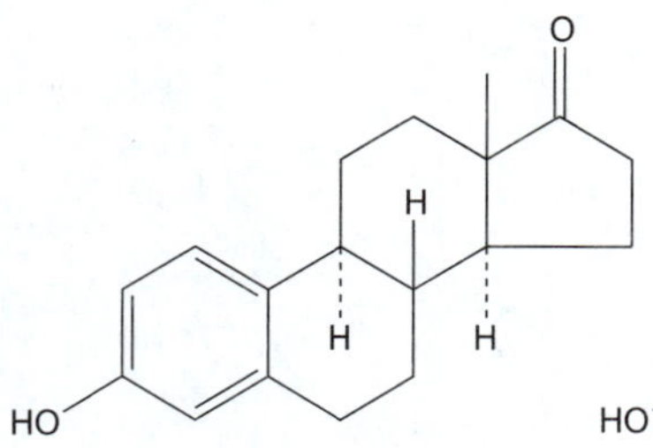

Oestrone

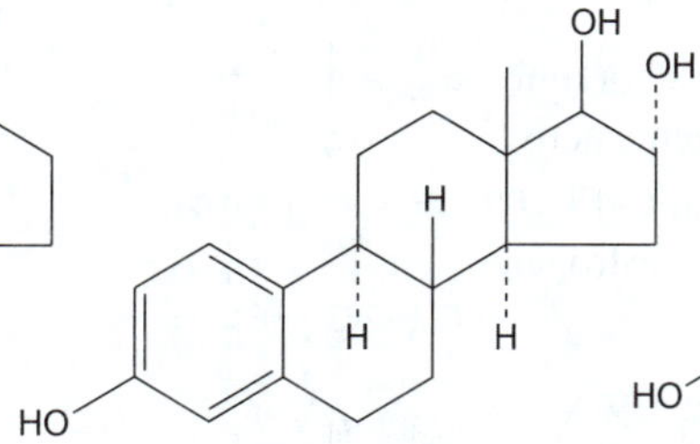

Oestriol

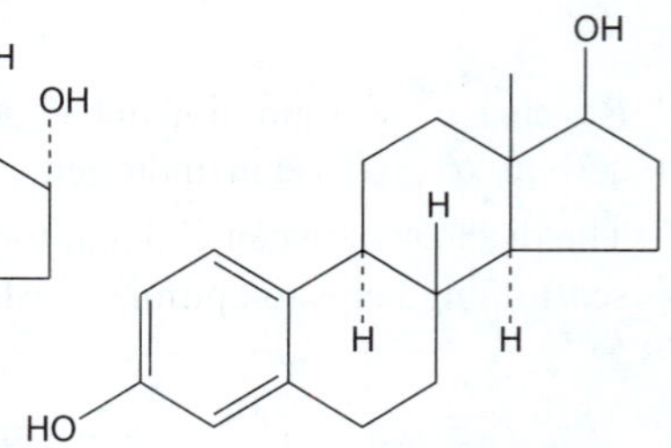

Oestradiol

Modification of ring B

- Presence of unsaturation at positions C-6 and C-7 increases the potency of drug, similarly additional double bond between C-8 and C-9 positions further increases the activity. Example: Equilin, equilenin.
- 7α-Substituents show increased oestrogenic activity.

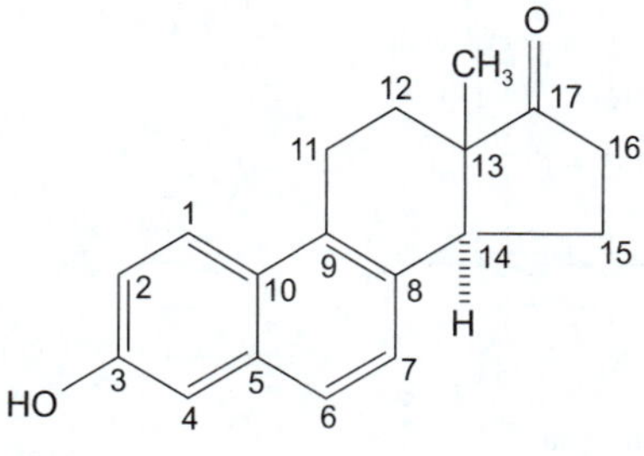

Equilenin

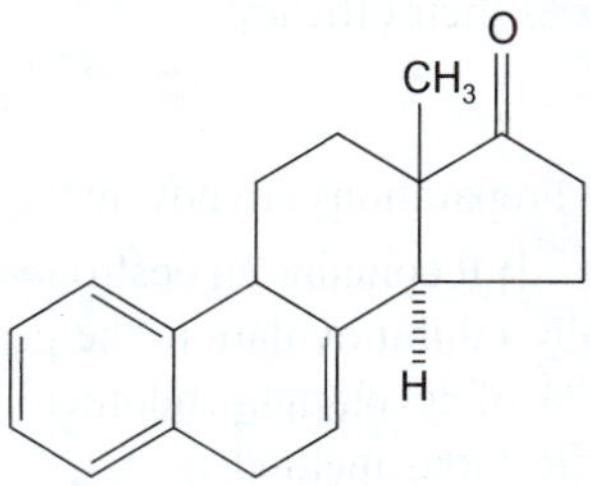

Equilin

Modification of ring C

- Substitution of –OH groups at C-6, C-7, and C-11 position reduces the activity.
- Substitution at C-11 β-position with alkyl group or alkoxy groups which has 17-ethinyl group greatly increases affinity for the oestrogenic receptor compared to oestradiol. Example: 11β-methoxy or 11β-ethyl oestradiol.
- $-CH_2Cl$ group at C-11 with β-configuration shows more potent activity.
- Larger substituents, example N,N-dialkyl undecylamides, show antagonistic activity.

Modification of ring D

- 17β-OH is essential for oestrogenic activity.
- Epimerization of 17β-OH to α-configuration results in the formation of less active analogues.
- 17α-Ethinyl or 17α-vinyl groups provide greatest activity due to increase in polarity. Example: Ethinyl oestradiol.

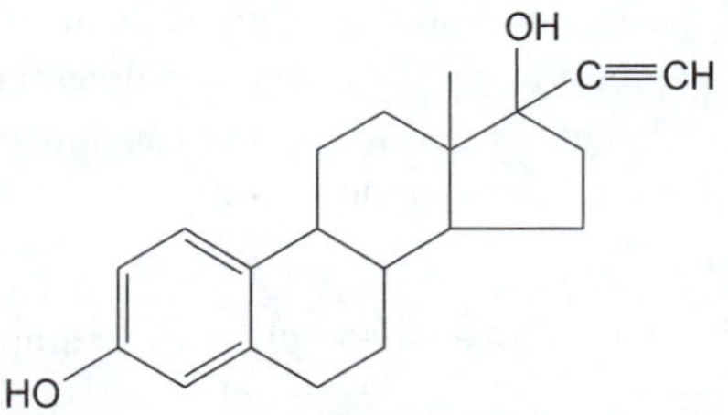

17α-Ethinyl oestradiol

- Reversal of configuration of C-2 or replacement of H for ethynyl in D ring leads to loss of oestrogenic activity or increase in androgenic activity.
- The distance between C-3 and C-17 –OH groups should be 10–12 Å, presence of this hydrophobic scaffolding helps to optimize oestrogenic activity. Example: All oestrogens and diethylstilbestrol.

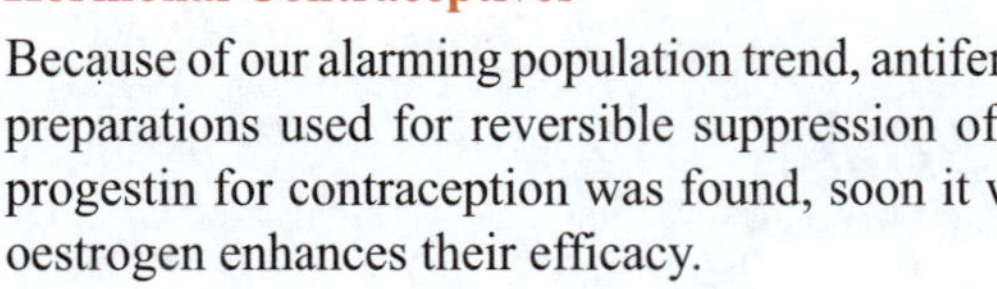

Diethylstilbestrol

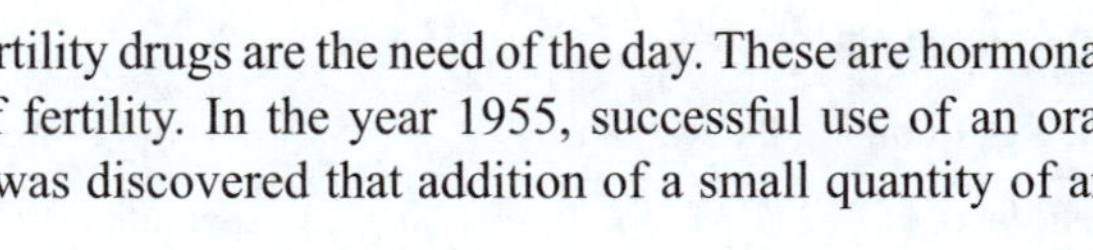

Benzoestrol

Hormonal Contraceptives

Because of our alarming population trend, antifertility drugs are the need of the day. These are hormonal preparations used for reversible suppression of fertility. In the year 1955, successful use of an oral progestin for contraception was found, soon it was discovered that addition of a small quantity of an oestrogen enhances their efficacy.

Oral Contraceptives

A variety of oral preparations are now available as per individual choices.

1. **Combined pill:** It contains an oestrogen and a progestin. Although both oestrogens and progestins synergistically inhibit ovulation, the progestin ensures prompt bleeding at the end of a cycle and blocks the risk of developing endometrial carcinoma due to the oestrogen. This is the most popular and most efficacious method.
2. **Phased regimens:** This is recommended for women over 35 years of age or when other risk factors are present. These have been introduced to reduce steroid dose without compromising efficacy. It

may be biphasic or triphasic. The oestrogen dose is kept constant while the amount of progestin is low in the first phase and progressively higher in the second and third phases.

3. **Minipill (progestin only pill):** A low-dose progestin only pill is taken daily continuously without any gap. It has been devised to eliminate the oestrogen, because of the many long-term risks.
4. **Postcoital (emergency) contraception:** Currently three regimens are available:
   - This regimen, called the *Yuzpe method*, has been the most popular. It is estimated to prevent 3 out of 4 possible pregnancies.
   - Levonorgestrel 0.5 mg + ethinyl oestradiol 0.1 mg (2 ovral tablets) taken as early as possible but within 72 hrs of unprotected intercourse and repeated after 12 hrs.
   - Emergency postcoital contraception should be used for unexpected or accidental exposure (rape, condom rupture) only, as it has higher failure rate and side effects than regular low-dose combined pill.

Side effects: The signs and symptoms are similar to those usually occurring during pregnancy. Women using the oral contraceptives experience undesirable side effects like nausea, vomiting, breast fullness, mastalgia, headache, dizziness, depression, apathy, fatigue, pelvic pain and chloasma, fluid retention, and weight gain are also observed. This is due to the mild increase in aldosterone secretion by the adrenals or to some anabolic activity inherent in the steroid.

Trade name	*Progestin (dose)*	*Oestrogen (dose)*
Combined pill		
Mala-D (21 tabs + 7 ferrous sulphate [60 mg] tabs)	Norgestrel (0.3 mg)	Ethinyl oestradiol (30 μg)
Ovral-G	Norgestrel (0.5 mg)	Ethinyl oestradiol (50 μg)
Ovral-L, Bandhan	Levonorgestrel (0.15 mg)	Ethinyl oestradiol (30 μg)
Novelon	Desogestrel (0.15 mg)	Ethinyl oestradiol (30 μg)
Femilon	Desogestrel (0.15 mg)	Ethinyl oestradiol (20 μg)
Phased pill		
Triquilar (6 + 5 + 10 tablets)	Levonorgestrel (50–75–125 μg)	Ethinyl oestradiol (30–40–30 μg)
Orthonovum (7 + 7 + 7 tabs)	Norethindrone (0.5–0.75–1.0 mg)	Ethinyl oestradiol (35–35–35 μg)
Postcoital pill		
Ovral, duoluton-L (2 + 2 tabs)	Levonorgestrel (0.25 mg)	Ethinyl oestradiol (50 μg)
Norlevo, ECEE2 (1 + 1 tab)	Levonorgestrel (0.75 mg)	Nil
Mini pill		
Micronor	Norethindrone (0.35 mg)	Nil

ANDROGENS (MALE SEX HORMONES)

Introduction: The testes produce mainly one androgen, 'testosterone'. It is excreted in the urine as such or mainly as metabolites like androsterone and dehydroepiandrosterone (DHEA). Testosterone and its more potent reduction product 5α-dihydrotestosterone (DHT) are produced in significantly greater amounts in males, in low amounts of these 'male' sex hormones females also produce. These androgens have two important activities, i.e. promoting male sex characteristics (androgenic activity) and muscle building activity (anabolic activity). Androsterone is the most potent, having approximately one-seventh of the activity of testosterone.

Urine contains approximately 1 mg of androsterone per litre of urine. In 1931, Butenandt isolated the first male sex hormone, namely androsterone. He had isolated 15 mg of the crystalline androsterone from 15,000 litres of urine.

Classification

1. **Androgenic or male sex characteristics promoting activity:** Compounds with androgenic activity are called androgens. It includes normal development, functioning, and maintenance of the male sex organs and sexual characteristics.
2. **Anabolic or muscle building activity:** Compounds with anabolic activity are called anabolic agents. It causes nitrogen retention by increasing the rate of protein synthesis, decreasing the rate of protein catabolism, and thus promotes laying down of new tissues. It also stimulates the thickness rise and linear growth of the bones to some extent. The distinction of anabolic therapy of such wasting conditions as cancer, trauma, osteoporosis, and effects of immobilizations are also treated by the anabolic agents.

Biological Activities of Androgens

Testosterone and DHT cause masculinizing effects, even in the male foetus. They induce the development of prostate, penis, and related sexual tissues at puberty. The secretion of testosterone by the testes increases greatly, leading to an increase in facial and body hair, deepening of the voice, increased protein anabolic activity and muscle mass, and increase in the size of sexual organs. Spermatogenesis begins, and the prostate and seminal vesicles increase their activity. The skin becomes thicker, and sebaceous glands increase in number leading to acne in many young people. The androgens also play important roles in male psychology and behaviour. Testosterone plays a role in libido, mood, muscle mass and strength, as well as bone density of women.

Therapeutic Uses of Anabolic–androgenic Steroids (AAS)

- Mainly used in androgen replacement therapy in men, either at maturity or in adolescence.
- Used in advanced or metastatic breast carcinoma of selected patients.
- Used to relieve bone pain associated with osteoporosis and to treat certain anaemias.

Following are the testosterone and its synthetic anabolic–androgenic steroids.

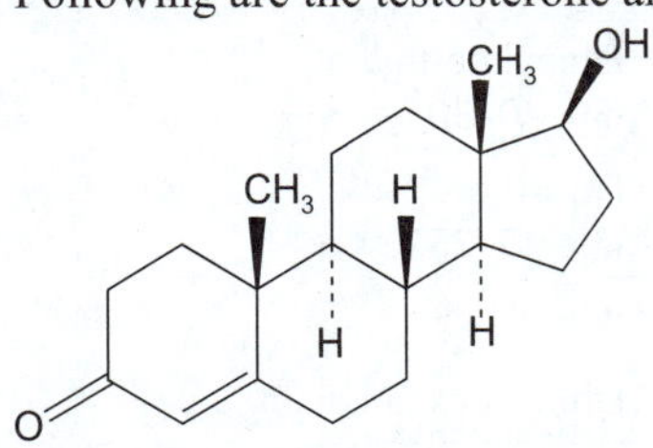

Testosterone

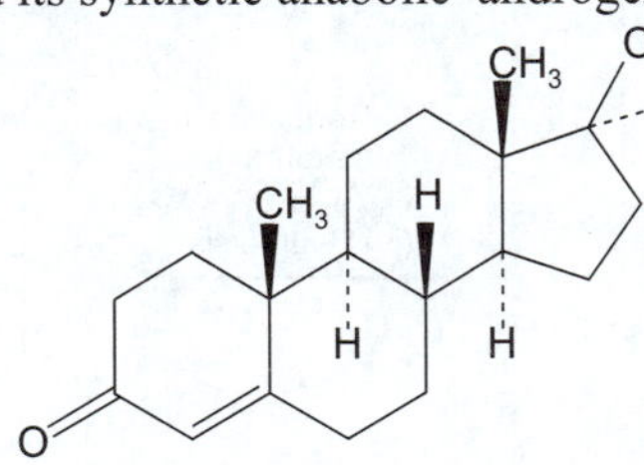

17α-Methyltestosterone

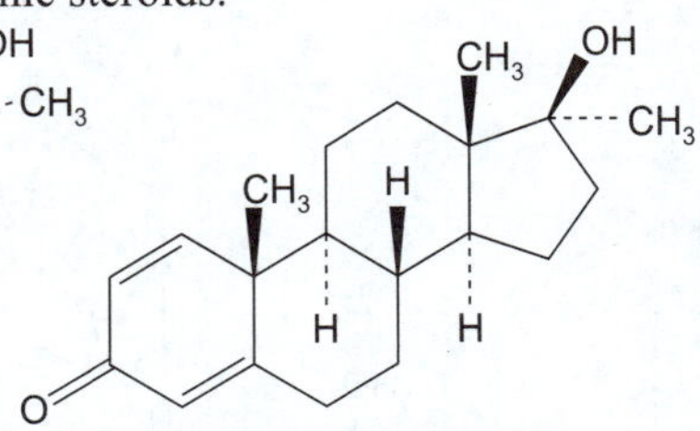

Methandrostenolone (dianabol)

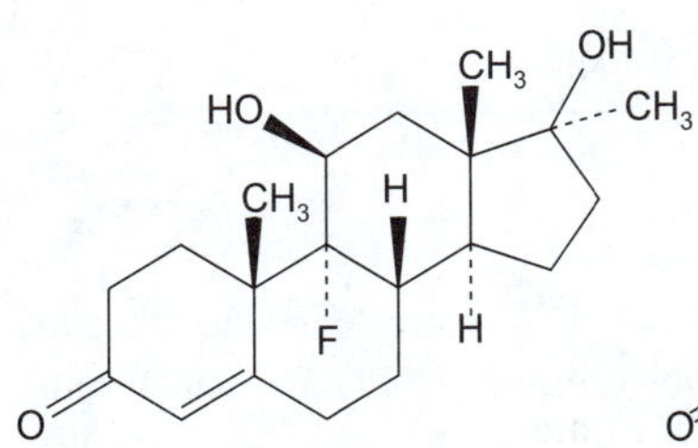

Fluoxymesterone

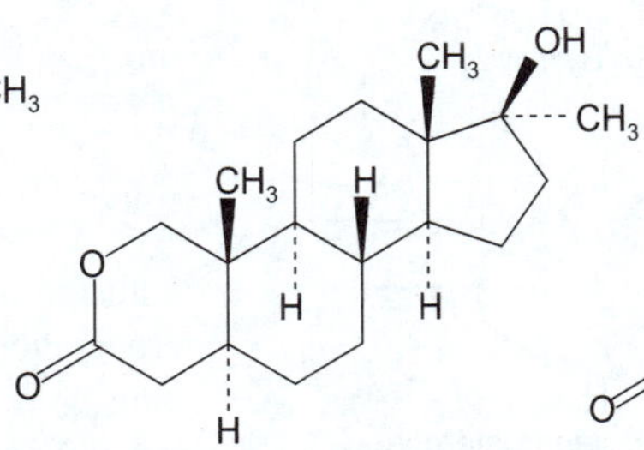

Oxandrolone (oxandrin)

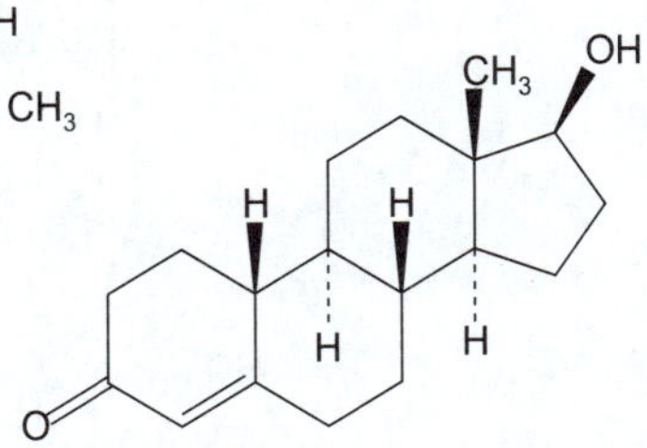

Nandrolone

ANDROSTERONE

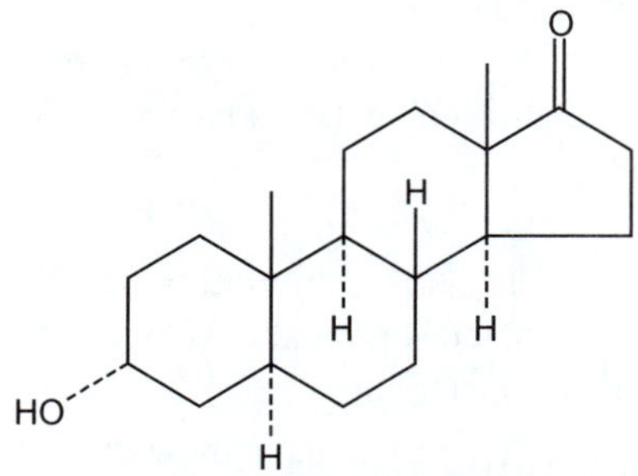

Androsterone

The androsterone occurs in urine as a conjugate with glucuronic acid of male and female animals and in the testicular extract. This also occurs in blood as sulphate. Small amounts in adrenal cortex, human sperm, and ovary are also available.

For the isolation of androsterone, urine is concentrated, hydrolysed with acid and extracted with chloroform. The chloroform layer containing hormone is treated with potassium hydroxide repeatedly to get rid of all the acidic and phenolic impurities. By steam distillation, the neutral fraction of the additional quantity of the inactive materials is removed. The steam distilled fraction is treated with Girard's reagent. The Girard derivative is extracted and hydrolysed to yield the androsterone.

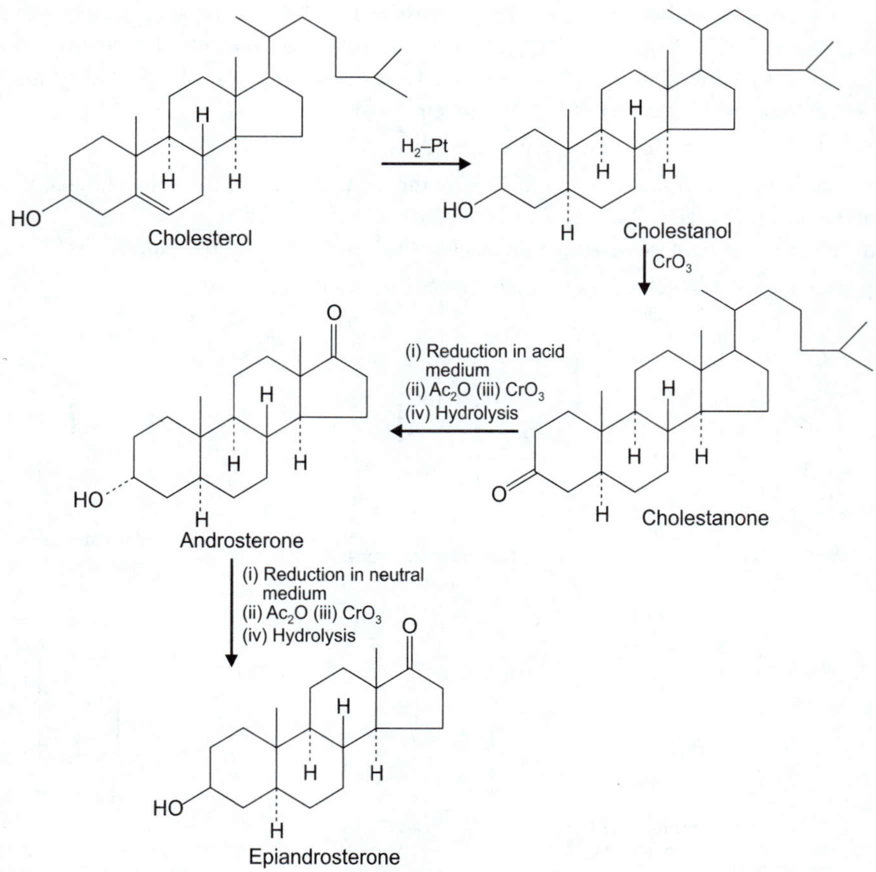

DEHYDROEPIANDROSTERONE (DHEA)

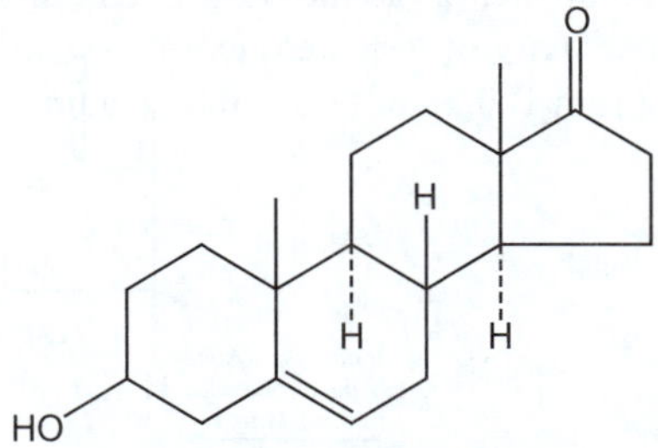

Dehydroepiandrosterone

In the year 1935, Butenandt isolated DHEA from urine. The activity of this hormone is from one-third to half that of androsterone. It is of interest to note that DHEA has also been obtained from the urine of pregnant and non-pregnant women. Its structure resembled quite markedly the structure of oestrone.

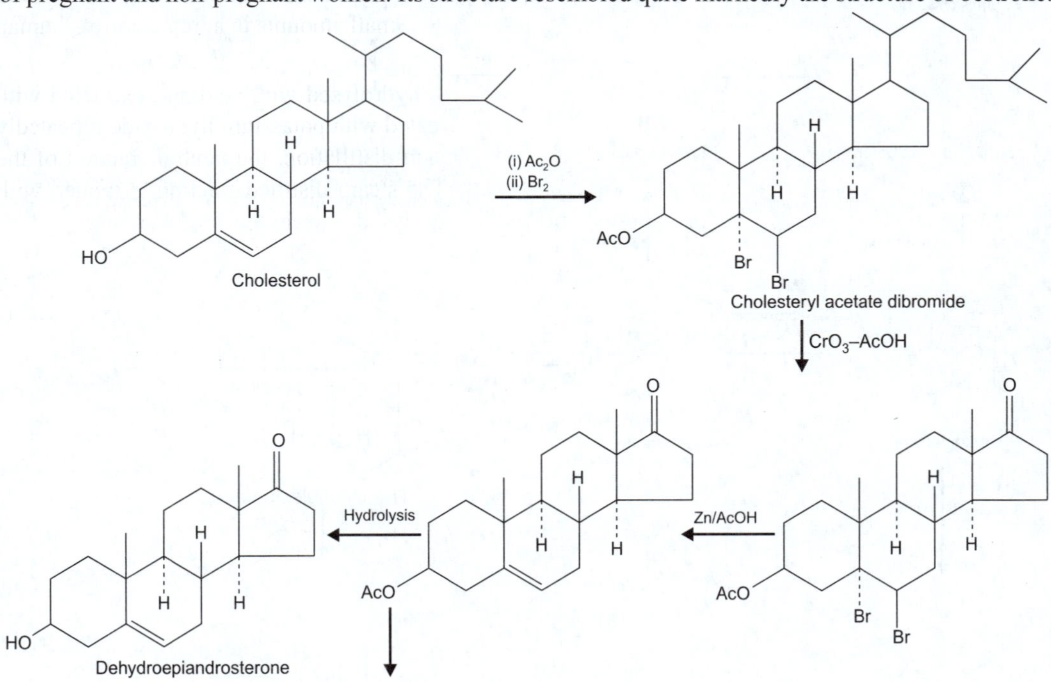

TESTOSTERONE (NUVIR, ANDRIOL, TESTOVIRON)

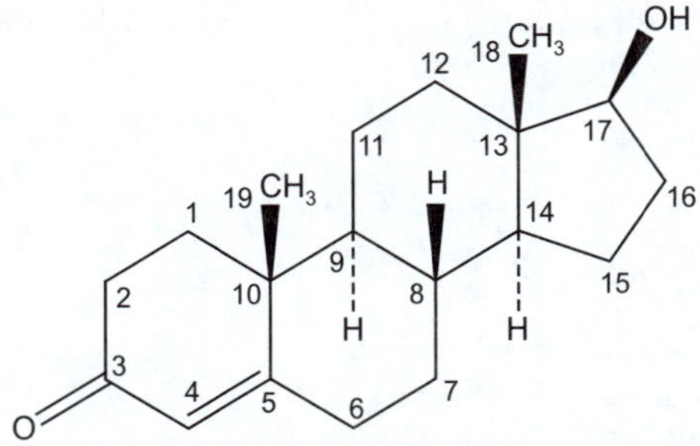

Testosterone or (8R,9S,10R,13S,14S,17S)-17-hydroxy-10,13-dimethyl-1,7,8,10,11,12,13,15,16,17-decahydro-2*H*-cyclopenta[a]phenanthren-3(6*H*,9*H*,14*H*)-one

All steroidal hormones that exhibit a typical androgenic activity are derivatives of androstane and the most potent one is testosterone. Androsterone is the most potent among the other androgens having approximately one-seventh of the activity of testosterone. In the year 1935, testosterone was isolated by E. Laqueru et al., from testes. From 100 kg of testes, they obtained 10 mg of testosterone.

Metabolism of Testosterone

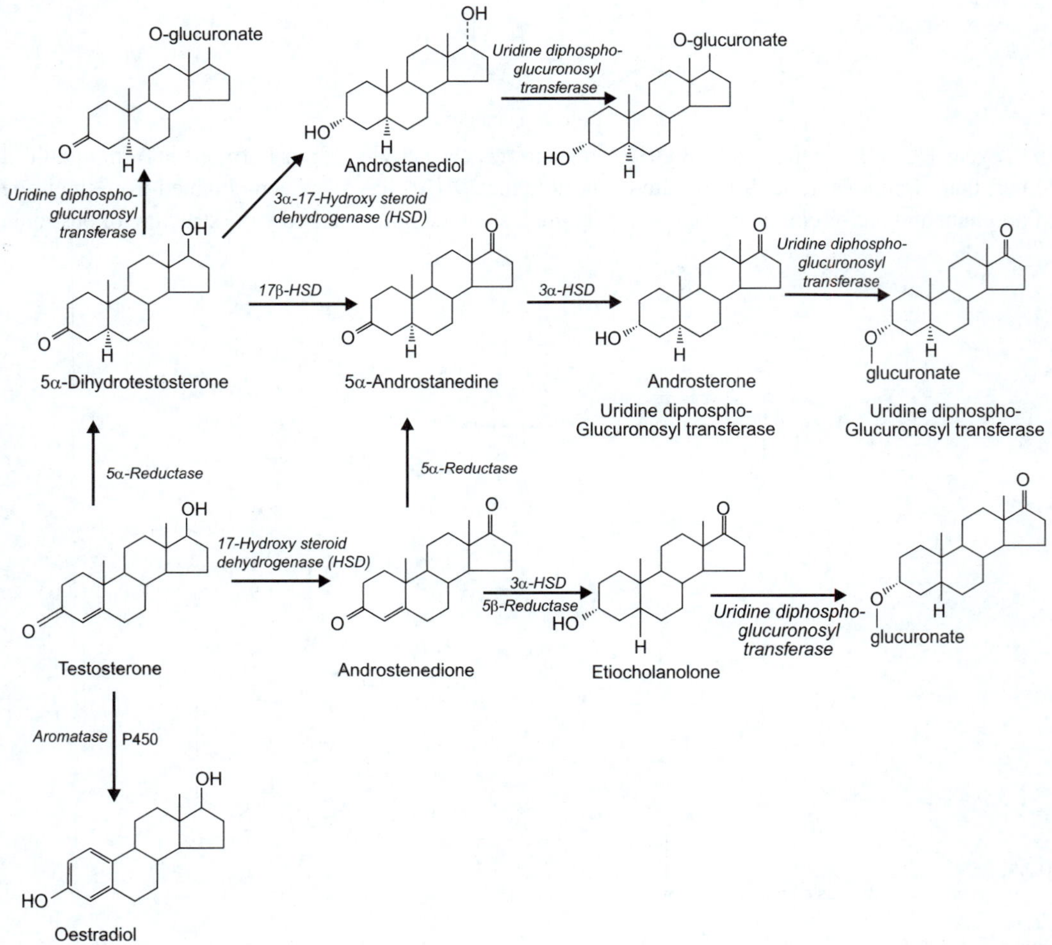

Synthesis

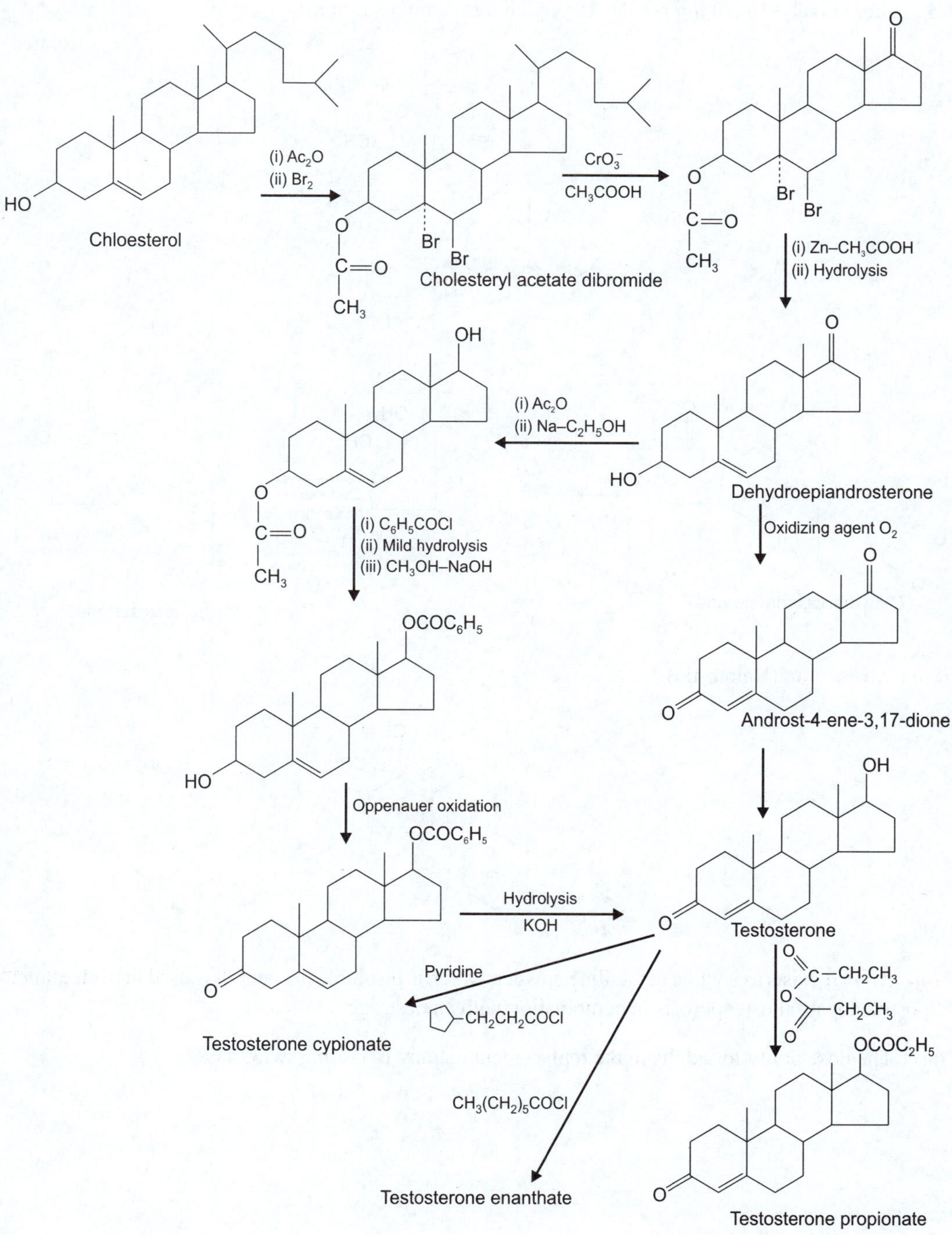

Properties and uses: It is a creamy white crystalline powder, which is insoluble in water and soluble in alcohol. It may be used for palliative treatment of breast carcinoma in postmenopausal women.

Assay: Dilute the sample in alcohol to 50 ml with ethyl alcohol. Measure the absorption at 241 nm using ethanol in the blank.

Dose: The dose for prolonged treatment subcutaneously is 600 mg. For breast cancer, the dose is up to 1.5 g; alternatively, 10–30 mg per day through buccal administration.

Methyl testosterone

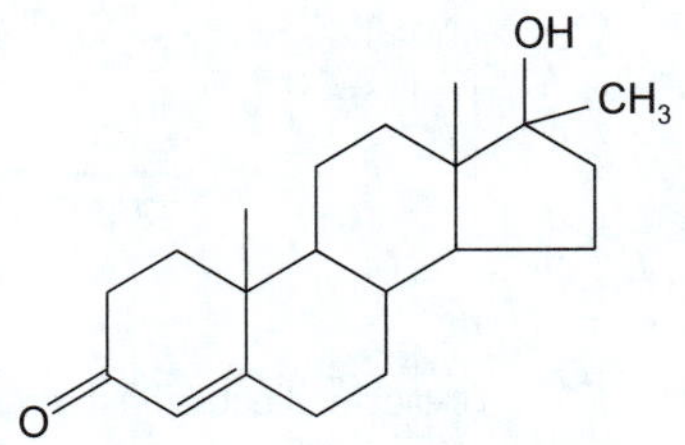

Synthesis

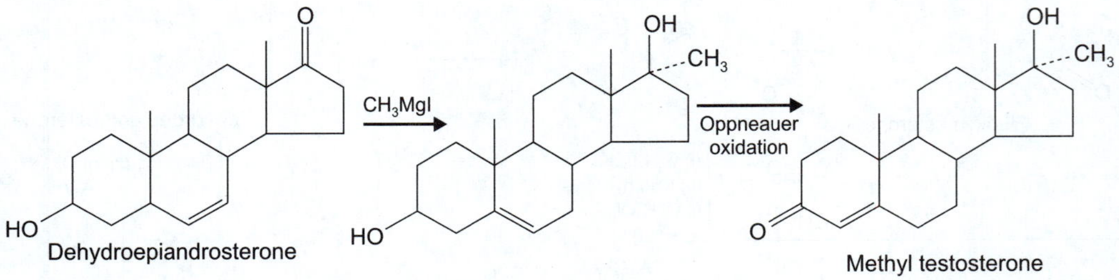

Fluoxymesterone (Halotestin)

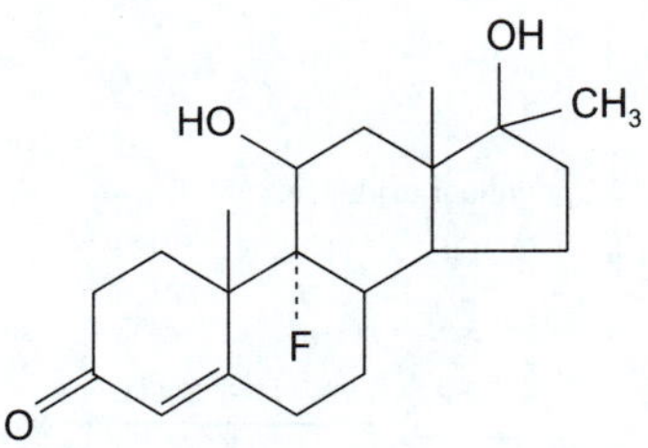

Properties: It exists as a white crystalline powder, which is insoluble in water. It is used in the treatment of postmenopausal osteoporosis in combination with an oestrogen.

Dose: The dose orally for adults in the replacement therapy is 1–3 mg twice a day.

Synthesis

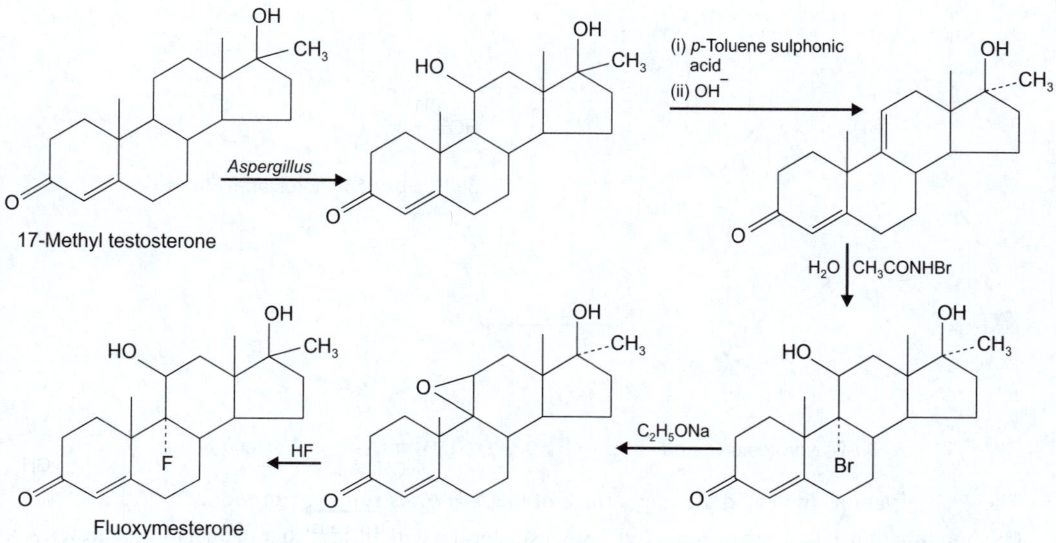

Structure–Activity Relationship of Androgens

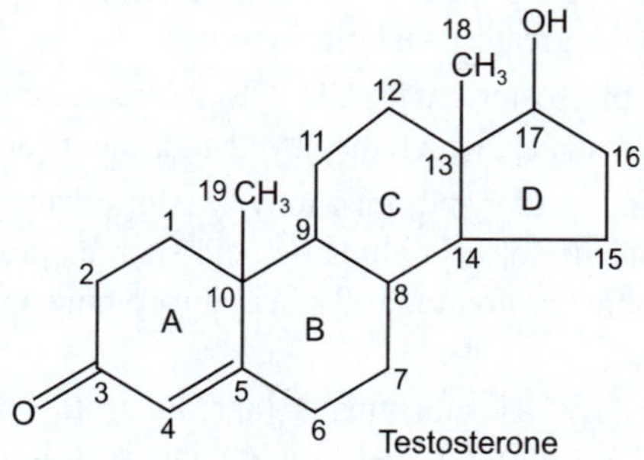

Conversion of testosterone to dihydrotestosterone (DHT) has little effect or may increase potency. Changing the A/B *trans* stereochemistry of known androgens such as androsterone and DHT to the A/B *cis*-derivative 3β-hydroxy-5β-androstane-17-one and 17β-hydroxy-5β-androstan-3-one, respectively, reduces both the anabolic and androgenic properties drastically.

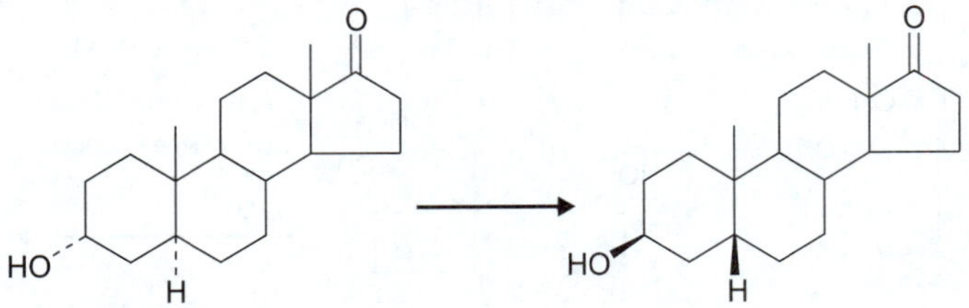

Androsterone → 3β-Hydroxy-5β-androstane-17-one

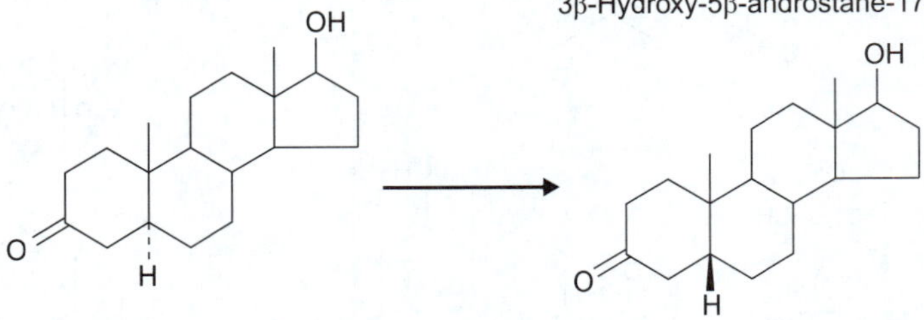

5α-Dihydrotestosterone → 17β-Hydroxy-5β-androstane-3-one

- These observations indicated the importance of the A/B *trans* ring juncture for activity.
- Oxygen function at C-3 can be removed from testosterone with little reduction in androgenic activity, removal of the –OH group from C-17 sharply reduced the androgenic activity.
- The position of the oxygen atom is important. The substitution of oxygen at C-2 affords the most active compound and the order of activity is 2 > 3 > 4.
- The relative androgenicity of the olefins of 3-deoxytestosterones is in the order of $\Delta^1 > \Delta^2 > \Delta^3 > \Delta^4$. But the Δ^2-isomer displayed the greatest anabolic activity.
- On the basis that sulphur is bioisosteric with CH=CH Wolff and co-workers have synthesized the thia, seleno, and tellurio androstanes, which displayed androgenic activity.
- Esterification of testosterone prolonged the activity significantly when it was administered parenterally. Long-chain aliphatic or aryl aliphatic acid such as propionic, heptanoic (enanthoic), decanoic, cyclopentylpropionic (cypionic), or β-phenylprorpionic acid are used for esterification of testosterone.
- Placement of a 9α and an 11β-OH substituents (analogous to synthetic glucocorticoids) gives fluoxymesterone (9α-F-11β,17β-dihydroxy-17α-methylandrost-4-en-3-one), which is an orally active androgen showing approximately four times the oral activity than that of 17α-methyl testosterone.

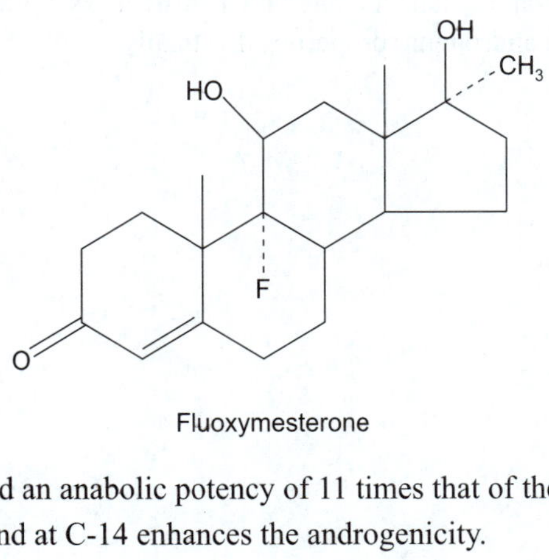

Fluoxymesterone

- Fluoxymesterone indicated an anabolic potency of 11 times that of the unhalogenated derivative.
- Introduction of double bond at C-14 enhances the androgenicity.

- The17β-hydroxyl group is essential for androgenic and anabolic activity. Esterification of the 17β-hydroxyl group not only enhanced but also prolonged the anabolic and androgenic properties in some cases.
- C-17α methylation conferred oral activity on testosterone, whereas increasing the chain length beyond methyl invariably led to a decrease in activity.

CLASSIFICATION BASED ON PCI SYLLABUS

Sex Hormones

Testosterone

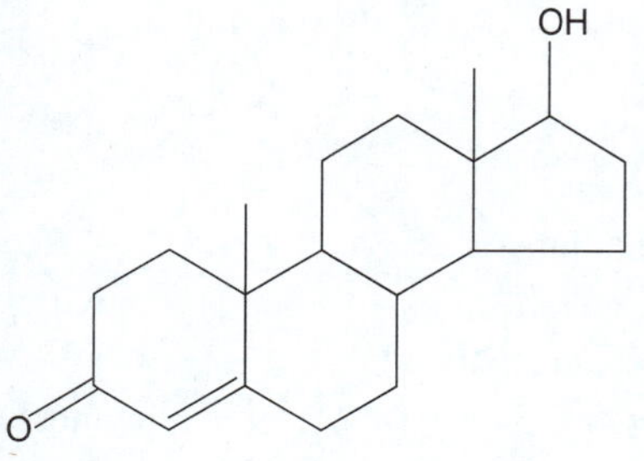

Nandralone

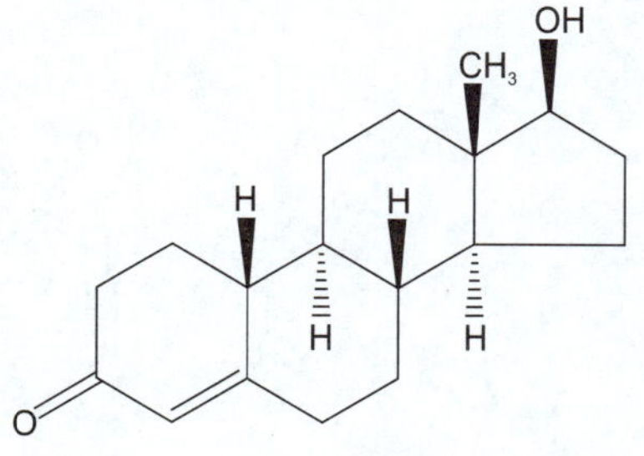

Progestrones

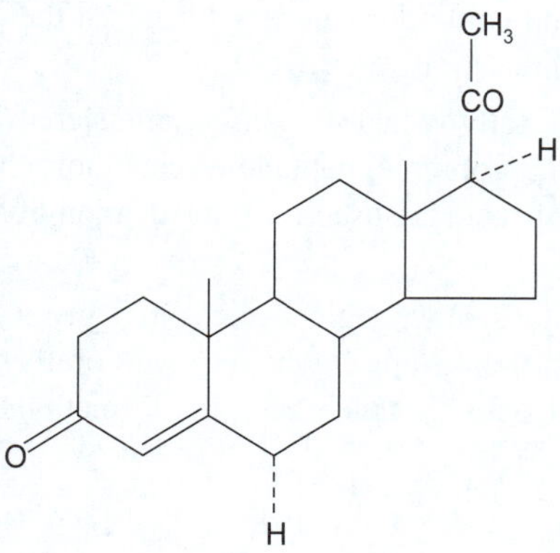

Oestriol

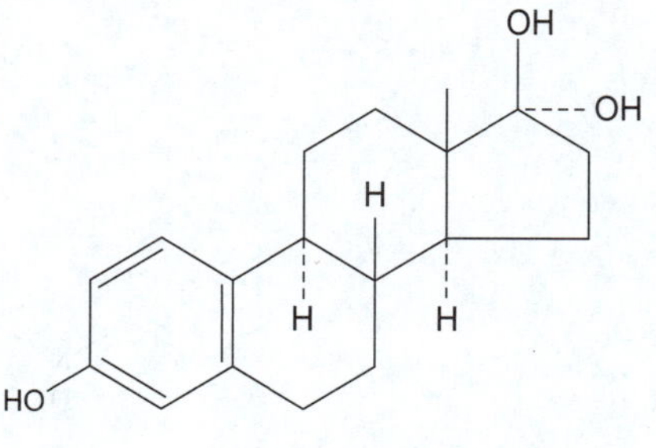

Oestradiol

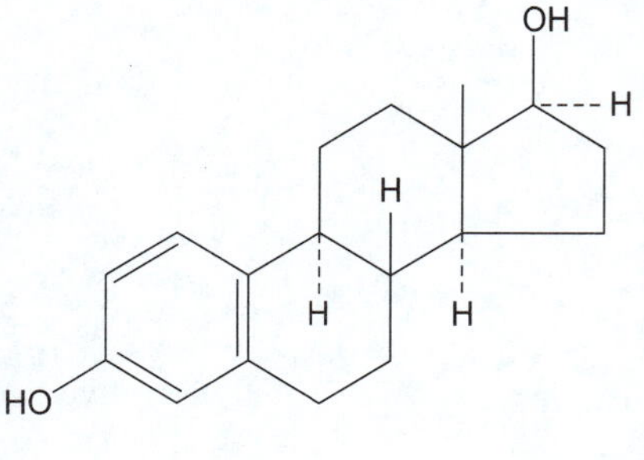

Oestrione

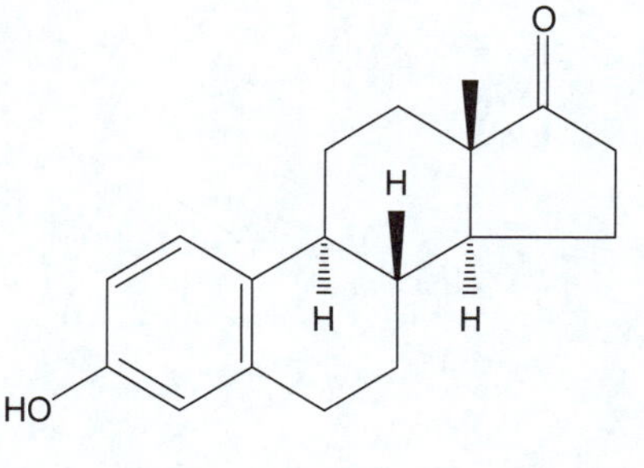

Diethylstilbestrol

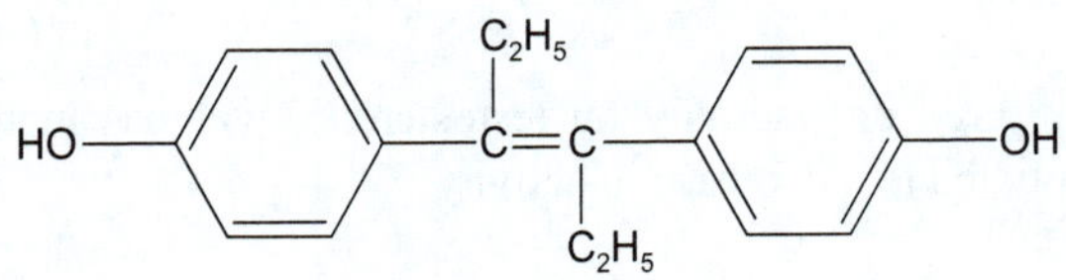

Drugs for Erectile Dysfunction

Sildenafil

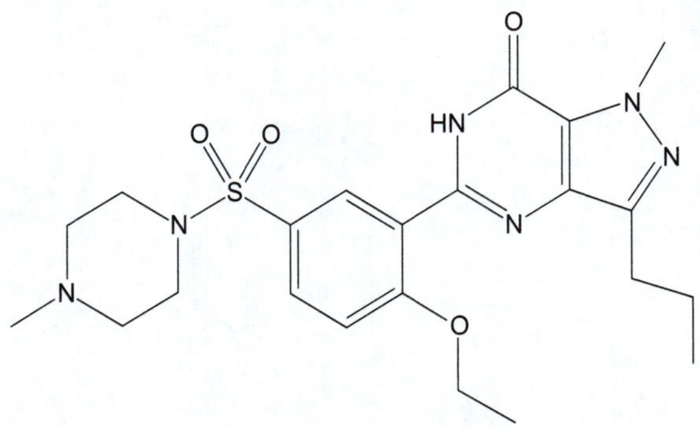

Tadalafil

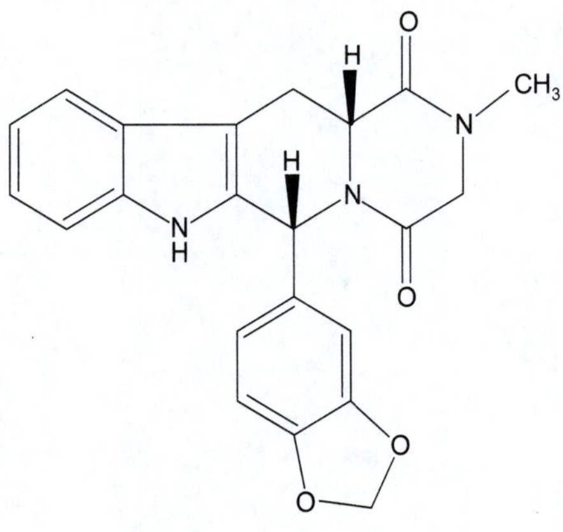

Oral Contraceptives

Mifepristone

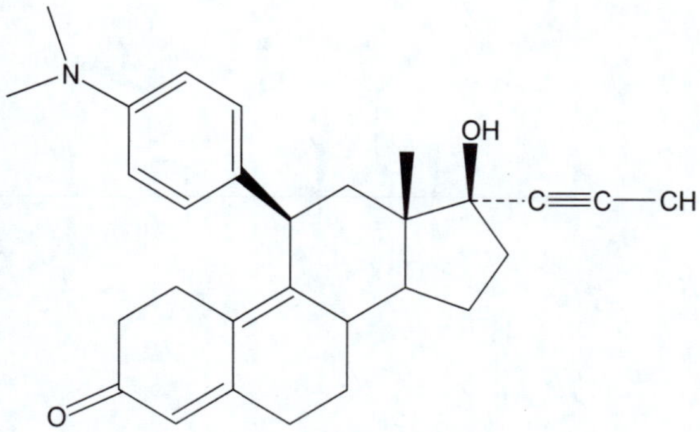

Norgestrel

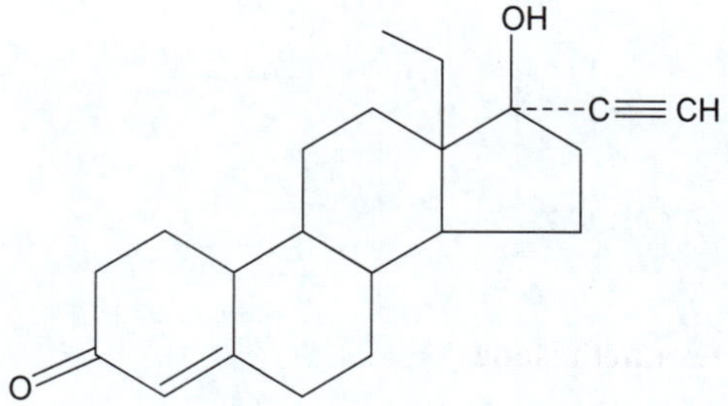

Levonorgestrol

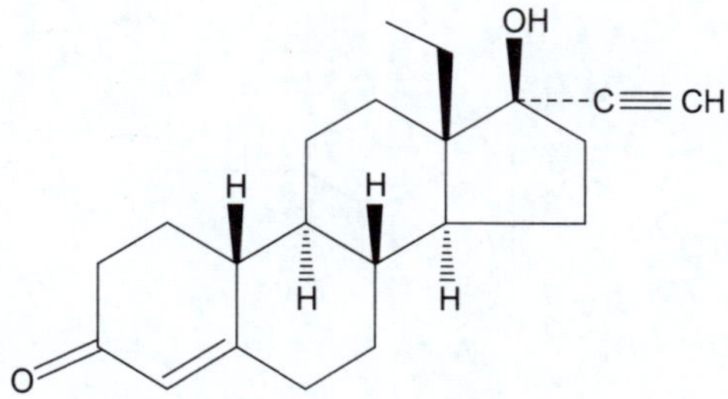

Corticosteroids

Cortisone

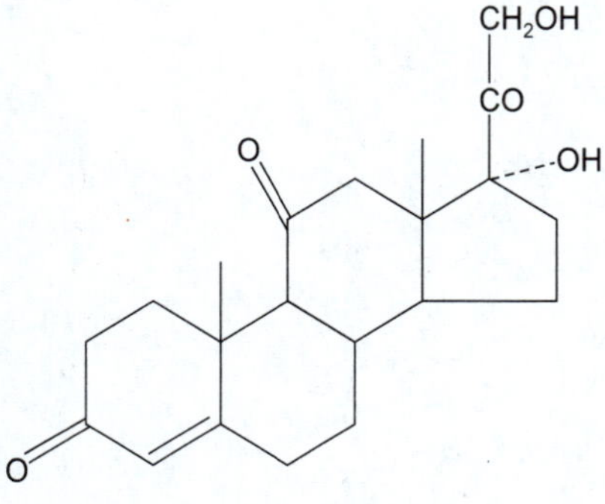

Hydrocortisone

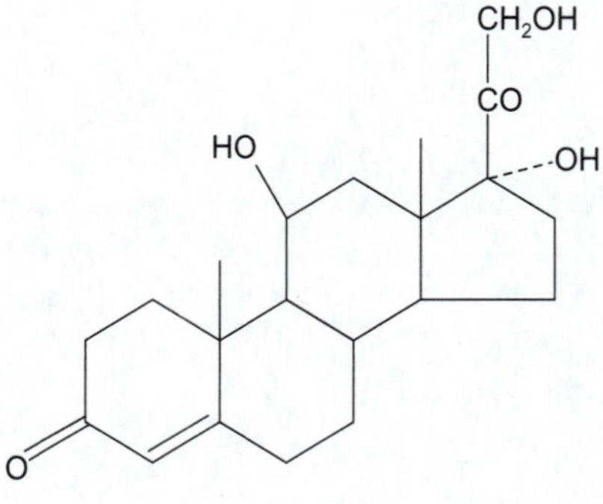

Prednisolone

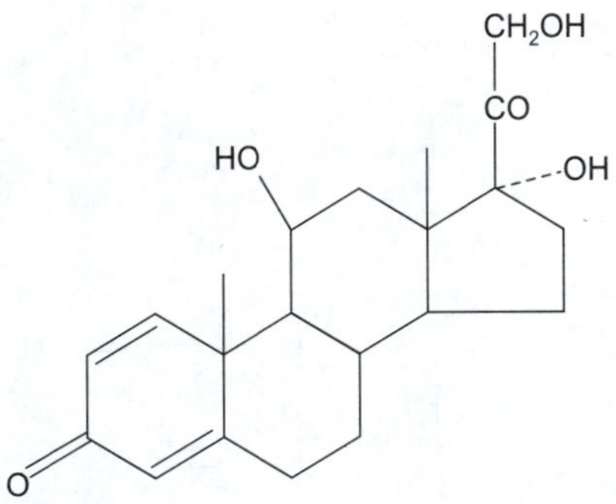

Betamethasone

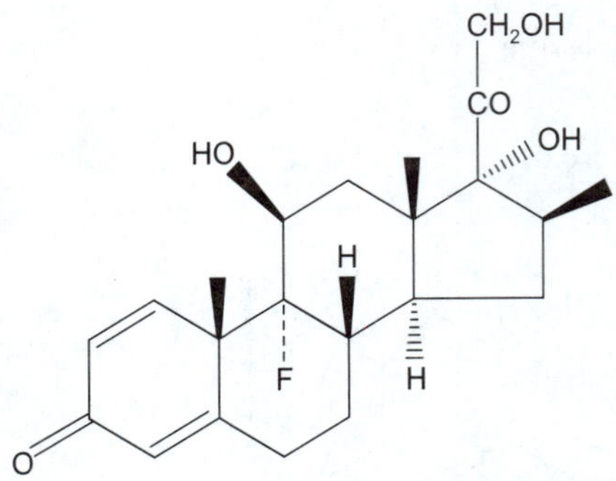

Dexamethasone

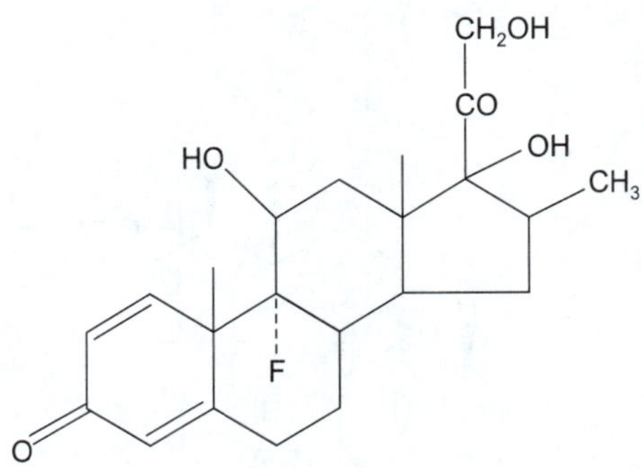

NEWER DRUGS

Macrelin

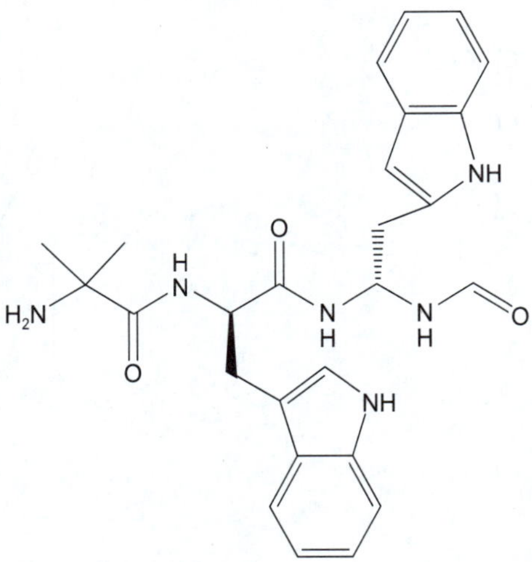

Uses: It is used to diagnose the adult growth hormone deficiency.

Deflazacort

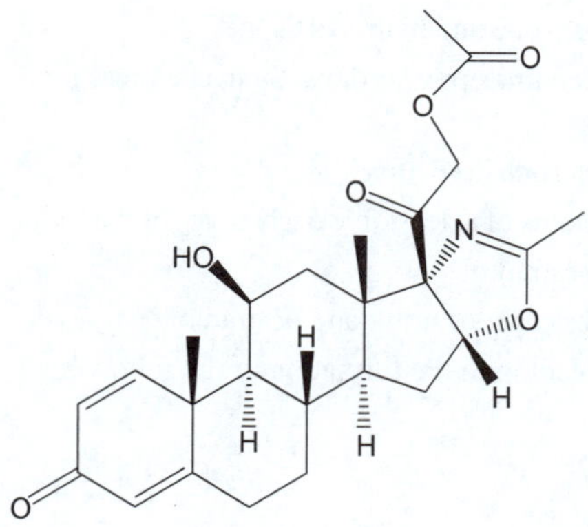

Uses: It is a glucocorticoid used as an anti-inflammatory and immunosuppressant.

Afamelanotide

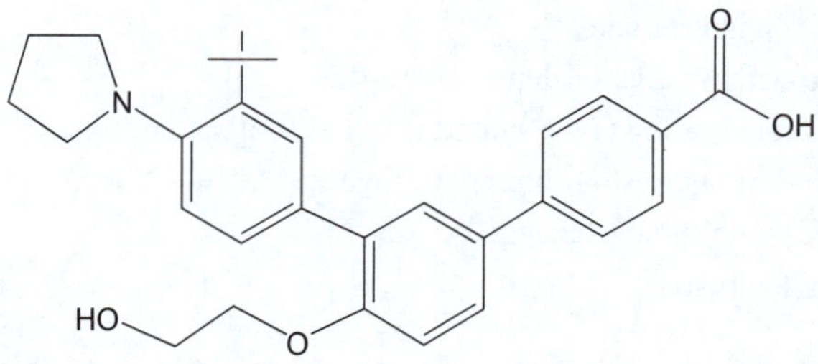

Uses: It is an analogue of α-melanocyte stimulating hormone used to prevent skin damage from the sun in people with erythropoietic protoporphyria.

Clascoterone

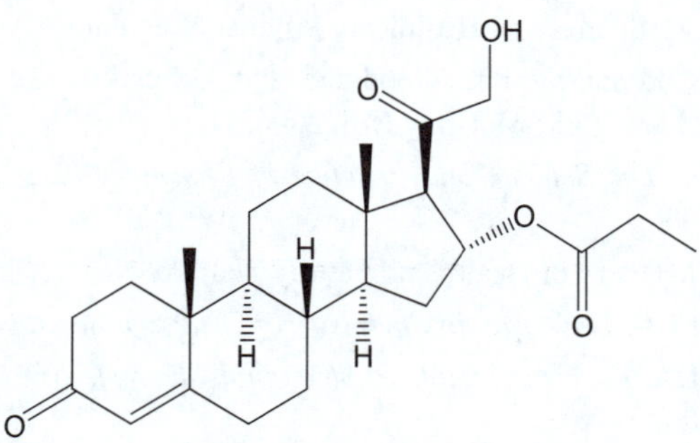

Uses: It is an antiandrogen used to treat acne.

PROBABLE QUESTIONS

1. What are steroids? Provide the nomenclature and stereochemistry of steroids.
2. Classify steroids with suitable examples and mention their therapeutic uses.

3. Write a brief account of the androgens. How will you synthesize testosterone from the following: (a) Cholesterol, (b) dehydroepiandrosterone
4. Describe the synthesis of cortisone and hydrocortisone.
5. Name the steroids used as contraceptives, draw their chemical structure, and write the synthesis of anyone of them.
6. Write a brief note on progesterone derivatives.
7. Give the names and official status of at least five derivatives of the following, which are used in medicine.
   (a) Testosterone, (b) oestradiol
8. Write the inter-relation of oestrone, oestriol, and oestradiol.
9. Outline the synthetic route leading to the formation of the following.
   (a) Oestradiol
   (b) Progesterone
   (c) Testosterone
   (d) Cortisone
   (e) Stilbestrol
10. What are hormones? Classify them with suitable examples and write the synthesis of testosterone.
11. Describe the structure–activity relationship of progesterones.
12. Outline the synthesis of androsterone.
13. Describe the structure–activity relationship of androgens.
14. Outline the synthetic route leading to the synthesis of testosterone or progesterone.
15. Describe the structure–activity relationship of oestrogens.
16. Classify corticosteroids with suitable examples.
17. Outline the synthesis of cortisone.

SUGGESTED READINGS

1. Abraham DJ (ed). *Burger's Medicinal Chemistry and Drug Discovery* (6th edn). New Jersey: John Wiley, 2007.
2. Bhatnagar A, Brodie AMH, et al.(eds.). Fourth International Aromatase Conference. *J Steroid Bio Chem Mol Biol* 61:107–426, 1997.
3. *British Pharmacopoeia*. Medicines and Healthcare Products Regulatory Agency. London, 2008.
4. Bruntan LL, Lazo JS, and Parker KL. Goodman and Gilman's: *The Pharmacological Basis of Therapeutics* (11th edn). New York: McGraw Hill, 2006.
5. Gennaro AR. *Remington: The Science and Practice of Pharmacy* (21st edn). New York: Lippincot Williams and Wilkins, 2006.
6. *Indian Pharmacopoeia*. Ministry of Health and Family Welfare. New Delhi, 1996.
7. Lednicer D and Mitscher LA. *The Organic Chemistry of Drug Synthesis*. New York: John Wiley, 1995.
8. Lemke TL and William DA. *Foye's Principle of Medicinal Chemistry* (6th edn). New York: Lippincott Williams and Wilkins, 2008.
9. Reynolds EF (ed). *Martindale the Extra Pharmacopoeia* (31st edn). London: The Pharmaceutical Press, 1997.
10. Zeelen FJ. *Medicinal Chemistry of Steroids*. Elsevier: Amsterdam, 1990.

CHAPTER 11

Thyroid and Antithyroid Drugs

The thyroid gland present in the human body regulates and maintains the normal growth and maturation by releasing thyroid hormones. The important and the major kind of two thyroid hormones are T_3—tri-iodothyronine (most active form) and T_4—tetraiodothyronine (thyroxine). The other hormone is calcitonin, secreted by the parathyroid gland or parathyroid follicular cells. Thyroxine was first obtained by Kendall as a crystalline powder in 1915. Later, it was synthesized by Harington and Barger in England.

SYNTHESIS AND SECRETION

Thyroid hormones are synthesized by thyroid glands and stored in thyroid follicles. The main source of thyroid is iodine in diet.

Various steps involved in the synthesis of thyroid hormones are depicted as follows.

1. **Iodine uptake:** Thyroid cells uptake plasma iodide by active transport process along with the help of sodium–iodide symporter.
2. **Oxidation of iodide:** The iodide gets oxidized to iodinium ion by the enzyme thyroperoxidase with the usage of hydrogen peroxide. The formed iodinium ion combined with the tyrosine residues of thyroglobulin (TG) leads to the formation of monoiodotyrosine (MIT) and di-iodotyrosine (DIT).
3. **Coupling reaction:** Pairs of MIT and DIT are coupled to generate T_3(MIT + DIT). Coupling of pairs of DIT + DIT leads to the formation of T_4. The entire reaction is catalyzed by the enzyme peroxidase.
4. **Storage and release:** TG containing iodinated tyrosine residues are stored in the follicle and released in to the circulation.

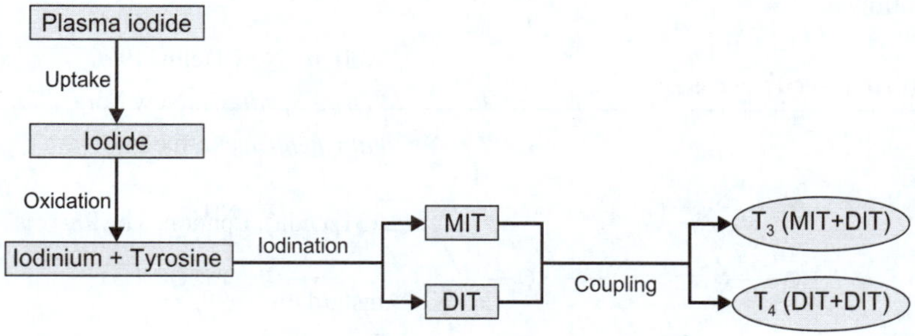

Figure 11.1: Formation of thyroid hormones.

Regulation of secretion

The secretion of thyroid hormone is regulated by TSH (secreted by anterior pituitary) and TRH (secreted from hypothalamus). Normally, 15–30 mcg of T_3 and 70–90 mcg of T_4 secreted in our body daily. Maximum amount of T_4 is converted into $T_{3,}$ in the peripheral tissues.

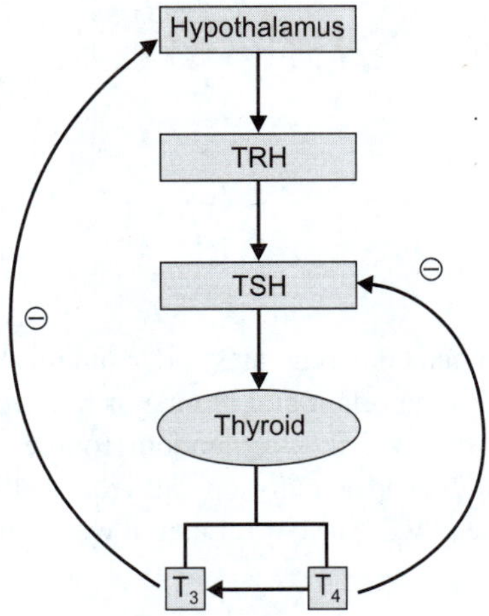

Figure 11.2: Feedback mechanism of thyroid hormone.

Mechanism of action

Thyroid hormones acts on the specific receptors, known as nuclear receptors or steroid receptors.

Thyroid Diseases: There are two types of diseases related to thyroid gland.

1. **Hypothyroidism:** Inadequate secretion of thyroid hormones, known as hypothyroidism. It leads to bradycardia, mental and growth retardation, dwarfism, etc. The therapeutic use of thyroid hormones is for hormone replacement therapy in patients with hypothyroidism or cretinism and for TSH suppression therapy in patients with thyroid cancer.
2. **Hyperthyroidism:** Excess secretion of thyroid hormones and circulation, known as hyperthyroidism. It leads to tachycardia, excess heat production, tremor and cardiac arrythmias. Antithyroid drugs propylthiouracil, methimazole and carbimazole are used to treat this condition.

Thyroid Drugs: Drugs which are used for the treatment of hypothyroidism are called thyroid drugs. They are as follows:

L-Thyroxine or Levothyroxine (T_4)

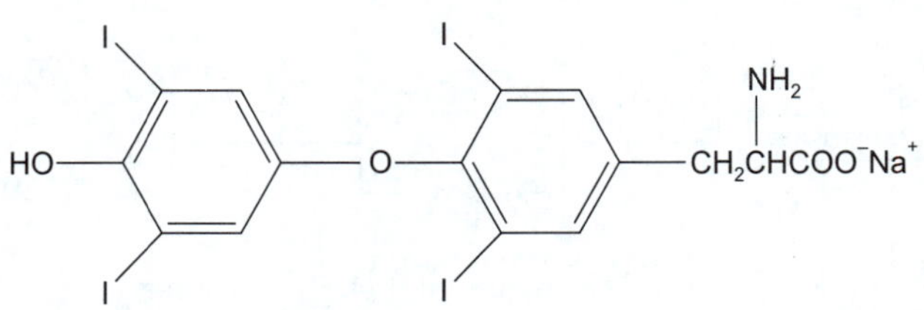

O-[4[Hydroxy-3,5-diiodophenyl]-3,5-diiodo-2-tyrosine]monosodium salt

Properties: It is slightly yellow colour, odourless and tasteless powder. It is hygroscopic in nature, hence stored in dark coloured bottles to prevent spontaneous deiodination. The levo isomer is the active form of the drug.

Uses: It is the drug of choice for the replacement therapy in hypothyroidism. It is also used for the treatment of chronic lymphocytic thyroiditis, non-epidemic goiter, etc. IV administration of T_4 is used to treat myxoedema coma.

Dose: Oral route: 50–100 mg daily, for IV route – 1.5 to 5 ml solution, 100 µg/ml.

L-Thyronine or Liothyronine (T_3)

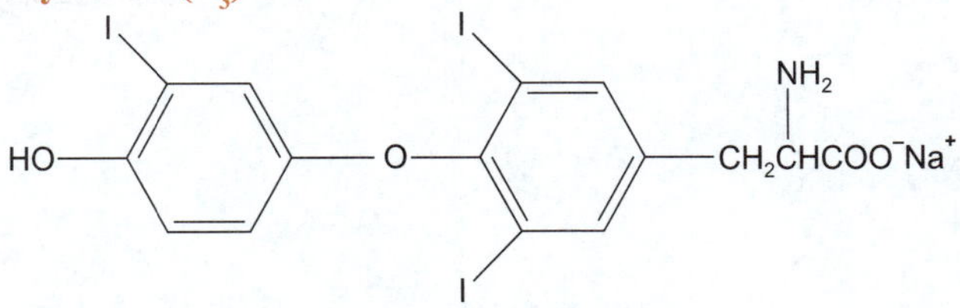

Properties: It is light-tan colour, odourless and tasteless crystalline powder. It is slightly soluble in water.

Uses: It is the drug of choice for the replacement therapy in hypothyroidism. It is also used for the treatment of male infertility, metabolic insufficiency and some kind of metabolic disorders.

Liver is the major site of non-deiodinative degradation of thyroid hormones; T_4 and T_3 are conjugated with glucuronic and sulfuric acids through the phenolic hydroxyl group and excreted into the bile. Some amount of thyroid hormones are liberated by hydrolysis of the conjugates in the intestine and reabsorbed.

ANTITHYROID DRUGS

Introduction

Antithyroid drugs are compounds that act within the thyroid gland to inhibit the biosynthesis of the thyroid hormones. Excessive amount of thyroid hormones in the circulation is associated with a number of diseased states, including Graves disease, toxic adenoma, goitre, and thyroidities among others.

Classification

Antithyroid drugs are classified as follows:

I. Thioureylenes

i. Thiouracil derivatives

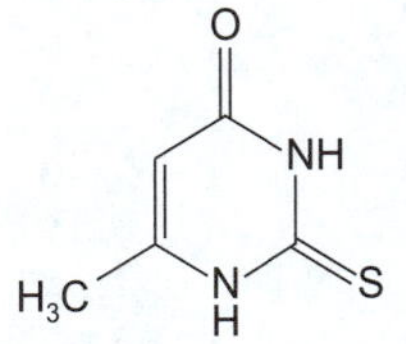

Methylthiouracil

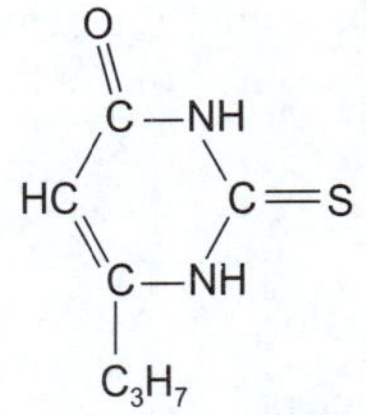

Propylthiouracil

ii. Imidazoles

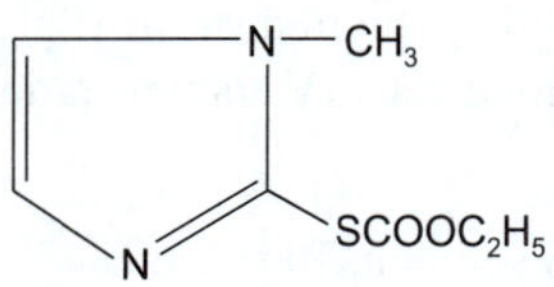

Carbimazole

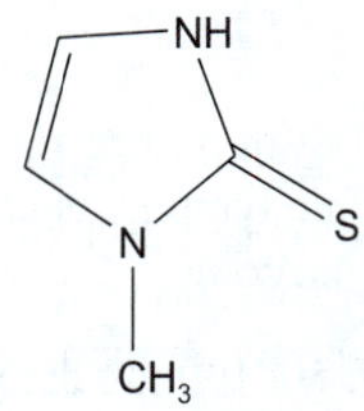

Methimazole

iii. Aniline derivatives

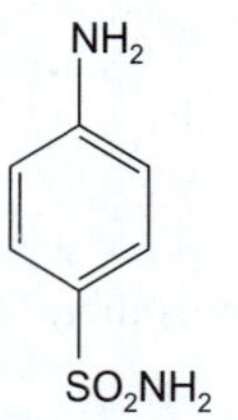

Sulphanilamide

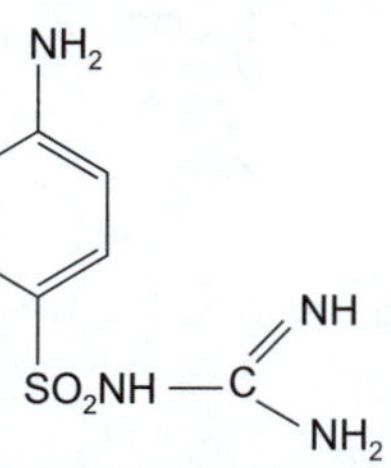

Sulphaguanidine

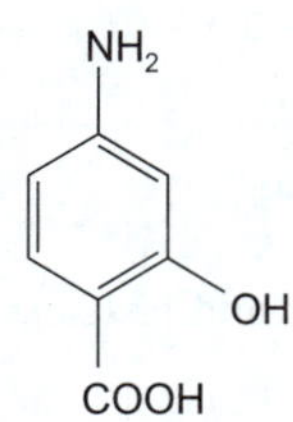

p-Aminosalicylic acid

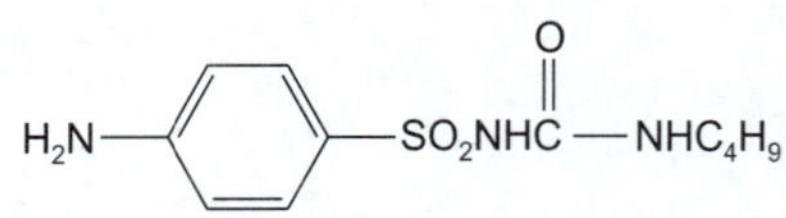

Carbutamide

Mode of action: These agents interfere with some of the process catalyzed by thyroid peroxidase, such as iodide oxidation, organification, and coupling of iodotyrosines.

II. Polyhydric Phenols

i. Resorcinol

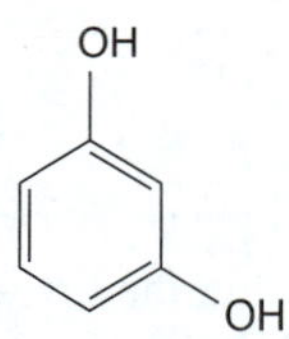

Mode of action: The only clinical agent from this category is resorcinol. It possesses same mechanism of action similar to that of thioamides.

III. Ionic Inhibitors

(a) Potassium perchlorate
(b) Thiocynate

Mode of action: These anions resemble iodide ions and affect the power of thyroid gland to accumulate iodine.

IV. Miscellaneous Agents

(a) Lithium carbonate
(b) Adrenergic blockers

SYNTHESIS AND DRUG PROFILE

I. Thioureylenes

Mode of action: Thiourea and thiouracil derivatives are among the primary drugs to treat thyroid hyperactivity. Methyl and propylthiouracil derivatives are effective drugs in the treatment of thyroid-related problems. They prevent iodine incorporation into the organic form perhaps by antagonizing the iodide oxidation by peroxidase. They are also found to prevent coupling of iodotyrosines to form iodothyronines.

The 2-thiouracil derivatives, that is, 4-keto-2-thio pyrimidines, are undoubtedly tautomeric compounds and can be represented as follows:

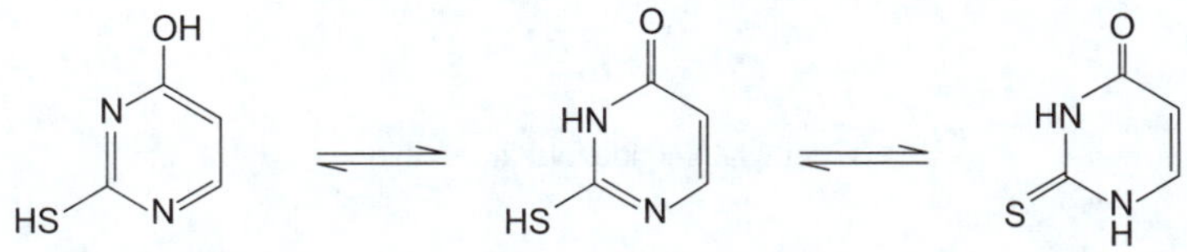

Some 300-related structures have been evaluated for antithyroid activity, but, of these, only the 6-allyl-2-thiouracil and closely related structure possess useful clinical activity. The most serious adverse effect of thiouracil therapy is agranulocytosis.

i. **Propylthiouracil** (Tietil)

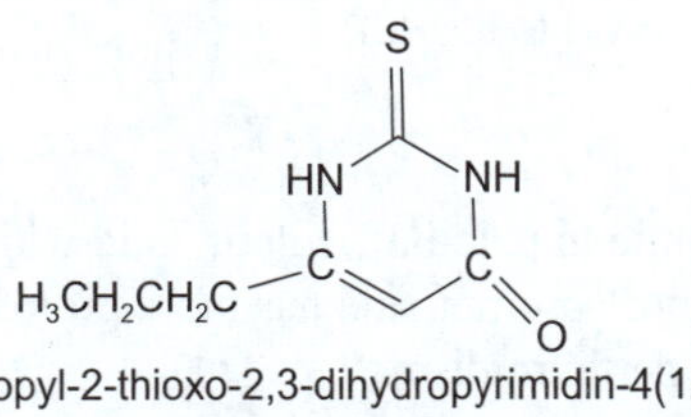

6-Propyl-2-thioxo-2,3-dihydropyrimidin-4(1*H*)-one

Synthesis

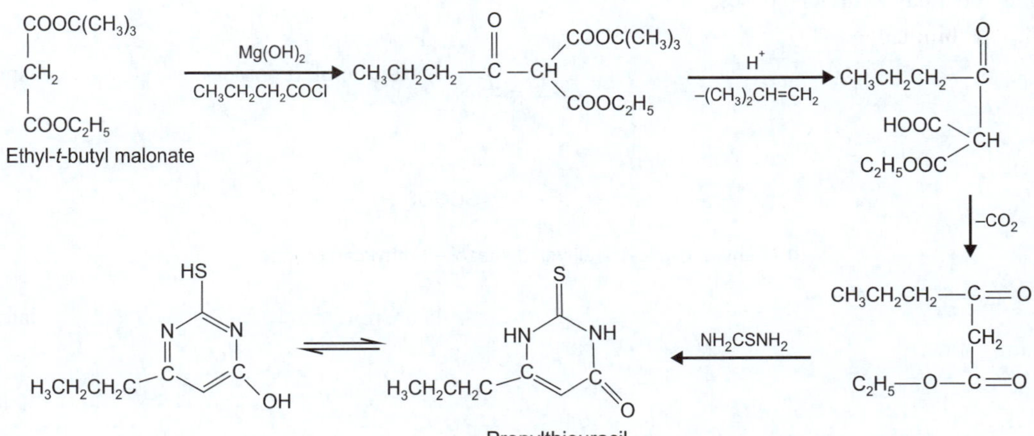

Properties and uses: It is a white powdery crystalline substance with bitter taste, soluble in water, alcohol, chloroform, and ether. Used in the management of hyperthyroidism.

Dose: For hyperthyroidism, the dose for adults initially is 200–300 mg per day in divided doses. When the patient attains normal basal metabolic rate (euthyroidism), the dose is usually reduced to a maintenance dose of 50–75 mg per day in two-to-three divided doses. In children, over 10-years old, initial dose is 150–300 mg per day in four divided doses until the child becomes euthyroid, then, usually, 100 mg daily is given in two divided doses, for maintenance.

ii. Methimazole (Tapazele)

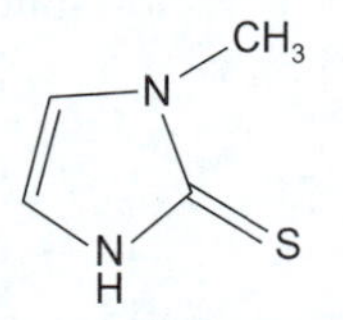

3-Methyl-1H-imidazole-2(3*H*)-thione

Synthesis

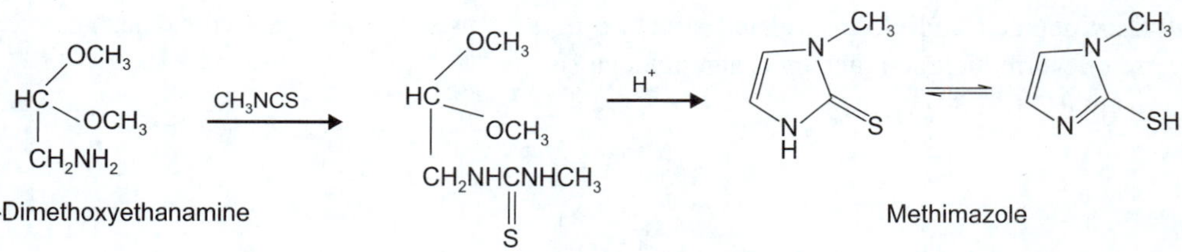

2,2-Dimethoxyethanamine

Methimazole

Properties and uses: It exists as white to pale-buff colour solid with characteristic odour and soluble in water. The drug is more potent, more prompt, and has more prolonged action than propylthiouracil. It is indicated in the treatment of hyperthyroidism.

Dose: Usual initial dose is 5–20 mg every 8 hrs. When condition is stabilized (1–2 months), the dose is reduced to a maintenance dose of 5–15 mg per day. For children, the initial dose is 400 μg/kg body weight per day in divided doses.

iii. Carbimazole

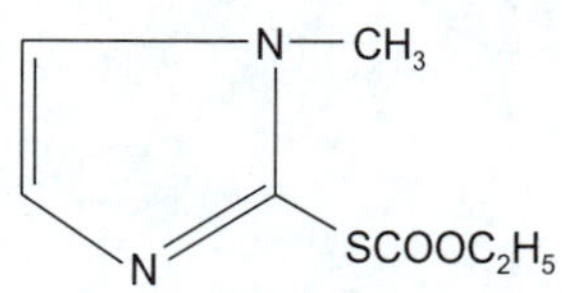

1-Methyl-2-thioxo-1,2-dihydroimidazole-3-ethyl carboxylate

Synthesis

Route I: From: Methimazole

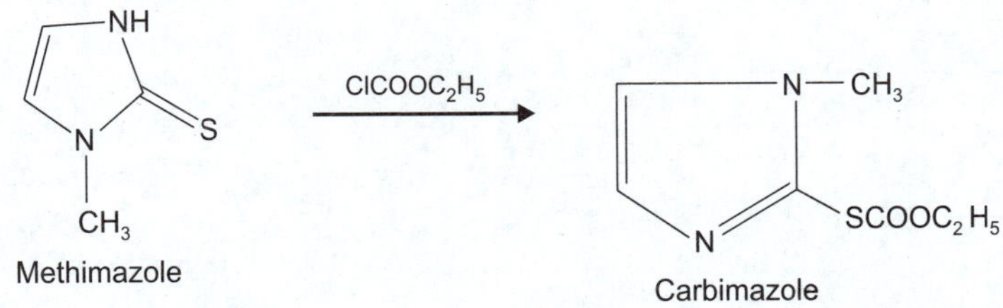

Route II. From: N-Methylamino acetal

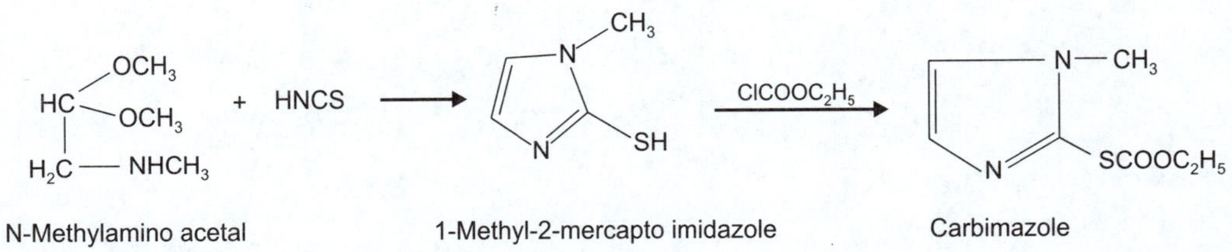

PROBABLE QUESTIONS

1. Define and classify antithyroid agents and write the synthesis and uses of any two of them.
2. Write the synthesis and uses of methylthiouracil and propylthiouracil.

SECTION VI

Chemotherapy

CHAPTER 12

History and Development of Chemotherapy

INTRODUCTION

The term *antibiotic* has its origin in the word *antibiosis* (which means against life), i.e. a process in which one organism may destroy another to preserve itself.

Antibiotics are chemical substances derived from various species of microorganisms (bacteria, fungi, actinomycetes) that suppress the growth of other microorganisms and eventually may destroy them at small concentrations. The probable points of difference amongst the antibiotics may be physical, chemical, pharmacological properties, spectrum of antibacterial activity and mechanism of action. They have made it possible to cure diseases caused by bacteria such as pneumonia, tuberculosis and meningitis and save the lives of millions of people around the world.

As antibiotics are required only in very low concentrations they are also called *chemotherapeutic agents*. Chemotherapy is the treatment of systemic disease or infection with appropriate drugs, which are capable of causing retardation in the multiplication of microorganisms or to suppress their growth without affecting the host system. The word chemotherapy is applicable for the treatment of viral, bacterial, fungal and protozoal infections. However, all chemical substances produced by living cells cannot function as antibiotics. In order to act as antibiotic, the compound must satisfy the following conditions:

1. It should be effective at low concentration against a pathogen.
2. It should be a product of metabolism or structural analogue of the naturally occurring antibiotic.
3. It should not produce significant toxic side effects.
4. The rate of detoxification and elimination from the body must be such that between two successive dosages a proper concentration level is to be maintained.
5. It should be stable so that it can be isolated and formulated suitably.
6. It should be completely eliminated from the system when the administration has been stopped.

HISTORICAL BACKGROUND

There are three phases to explain the history of chemotherapy, such as empirical period, Ehrlich's phase, and the modern phase. In early empirical period of 16th century, Paracelsus used mercury for the treatment of syphilis and during 17th century cinchona bark was used for pyrexia. In 500 to 600 BC, molded curd of soybean was used in Chinese folk medicine for infection and wounds. In early period, during these phases, Hindus used chaulmoogra oil for the treatment of leprosy. In Ehrlich's phase, it was revealed that certain dyes produced toxicity and killed some microorganisms. So neoarsphenamine was developed by Ehrlich for the treatment of syphilis. The word antibiosis was coined after the killing of anthrax bacilli when grown in culture media with other bacteria during the 18th century. The modern phases demonstrated the therapeutic effect of prontosil (a sulphonamide) in pyrogenic infections in 19th century.

In 1929, Sir Alexander Fleming accidentally discovered the antibacterial properties of penicillin by destroying the *staphylococcus* in culture plate; this is broadly cited in modern antibiotic era. Chain and Florey followed up this observation in 1939 and later penicillin was clinically used during1941. In 1942, Waksman proposed the search of *actinomycetes* and discovered streptomycin in 1944. Later, the advance in medicinal chemistry produced synthetic and semisynthetic agents.

SPECTRUM OF ACTIVITY OF CHEMOTHERAPEUTIC AGENTS

The ability of drug with all ranges (gram-positive and gram-negative) of antibiotic action, chloramphenicol, and tetracycline, to antagonize numerous pathogens have resulted mention as broad-spectrum antibiotics. Many of the broad-spectrum antibiotics are active only at high concentration. Some drugs are primarily static and they may exert cidal action at high concentration (e.g. sulphonamides, erythromycin, nitrofurantoin, etc). The bacteriostatic agents are those that interfere with the growth or replication of microorganisms, but does not kill it. The bactericidal drugs are those that kills the microorganisms. Concentration of drugs at the site of infection is an important factor for the therapeutic effect in case of antimicrobials. The classes of antibiotics and their spectrum of activity is detailed in Table 12.1.

Table 12.1: Classes of antibiotics and their spectrum of activity

Class of antibiotics	*Name of the drug*	*Susceptible organism*
Natural penicillins	Penicillin G and V	Gram-positive bacteria—streptococci except viridians. Gram-positive bacilli, i.e. *B. anthracis*, *Corynebacterium diphtheriae*, and all clostridia
Semisynthetic penicillins	Oxacillin	Penicillinase-resistant
	Ampicillin	Broad-spectrum. It is active against all organisms, which are sensitive to penicillin G and many gram-negative organisms, i.e. *Haemophilus influenzae*, *Escherichia coli*, *Proteus*, *Solmonella*, and *Shigella*
	Amoxycillin	Broad-spectrum antibacterial action with penicillinase inhibitor. It is less active against *Shigella* and *H. influenzae*
	Aztreonam	*Pseudomonas* and gram-negative organism
Cephalosporins	Cefazolin	It is active against all organisms and sensitive to penicillin, i.e. streptococci, gonococci, meningococci, *C. diphtheriae*, *H. influenzae*, clostridia, and *Actinomycetes*. Highly active against *Klebsiella* and *E. coli*
	Cephalothin	Similar in spectrum to Cefazolin, but less active against penicillinase producing staphylococci and *H. influenzae*. Parentral administration produces broad-spectrum action
	Cefotaxime	Potent action against aerobic gram-negative and some gram-positive, not active against anaerobes; *Staphylococcus aureus* and *Pseudomonas aeruginosa*

Contd.

Table 12.1: Classes of antibiotics and their spectrum of activity *(Contd.)*

Class of antibiotics	*Name of the drug*	*Susceptible organism*
Glycopeptide antibiotics	Bacitracin	Gram-positive organisms of both cocci and bacilli
	Vancomycin	Gram-positive bacteria. It is useful in case of methicillin-resistant *Staphylococcus aureus*, *Streptococcus viridans*, and *Enterococcus*
	Polymyxin	Gram-negative, including *Pseudomonas* species
Antimycobacterial antibiotics	Isoniazid, ethambutol	*Mycobacterium* species
Inhibitors of protein synthesis	Chloramphenicol	Broad-spectrum
Aminoglycosides	Streptomycin	Broad-spectrum, including *Mycobacterium* species. Primarily active against aerobic gram-negative bacilli
	Neomycin	Broad-spectrum activity
	Gentamycin	Broad-spectrum, including *Pseudomonas* species. Ineffective against *Mycobacterium tuberculosis*, *Streptococcus pyogens*, and *Pneumoniae*
Tetracyclines	Tetracycline, oxytetracycline, doxycycline, minocycline, and chlortetracyclin	All types of pathogens except virus and fungi. Broad-spectrum including *Chlamydia*, spirochetes, and *Rickettsia*. *Mycoplasma* and *Actinomyces* are moderately sensitive
Macrolides	Erythromycin	Gram-positive bacteria, highly active against *Str. pyogens*, *Neisseria gonorrhoeae*, clostridia, *C. diphtheriae*, and *Listera*
	Clarithromycin	Similar to erythromycin, in addition *M. avium* complex. More active against gram-positive cocci, *Moraxella*, *Legionella*, *Mycoplasma pneumoneae*, and *H. pylori*
	Azithromycin	Less effective in gram-positive cocci. Highly active against respiratory pathogens, i.e. *Mycoplasma*, *Chlamydia*, *Moraxella*, *Pneumoniae*, and *Legionella*
Streptogramins	Quinupristin and dalfopristin	Vancomycin-resistant, methicillin-resistant gram-positive bacteria
Oxazolidindione	Linezolid	It is active against methicillin-resistant *Staphylococcus aureus*. Cidal to streptococci, pnemococci, and *Bacteriodes fragilis*
Quinolones and fluoroquinolones	Nalidixic acid, gatifloxacin, peflo-xacin, norfloxacin, ciprofloxacin, etc.	Most susceptible are gram-negative bacilli. At high concentration gram-positive bacteria, highly susceptible bacteria are *E. coli*, *Klebsiella pnemoniae*, *Enterobacter*, *Solmonella typhi*, *Shigella proteus*, *Camphylobacter jejuni*, *Vibrio cholerae*, *Pseudomonas aeruginosa*, *Brucella*, *Listeria*, and *B. anthracis* are little susceptible
Sulphonamides	Cotrimoxazole and other sulpha drugs	Broad-spectrum. Primarily bacteriostatic
Nucleoside and non-neucleoside analogues	Acyclovir, ganciclovir, ribavirin, lamivudine, cidofovir	Herpes virus, cytomegalovirus

Contd.

Table 12.1: Classes of antibiotics and their spectrum of activity *(Contd.)*

Class of antibiotics	*Name of the drug*	*Susceptible organism*
Tricyclic amines	Amantidine, Rimantidine	Influenza virus
8-Hydroxy-quinolones	Quinidochlor	Malarial parasites
Nitrimidazoles	Metronidazole and tinidazole	Broad-spectrum action against protozoa, trichomoniasis, and giardiasis infections
Benzimidazole	Albendazole, mebendazole	*Enterobias*, *Trichuris* infestations
Polyenes	Amphotericin B	Systemic fungal infection, active against wide range of yeasts and fungi, i.e. *Candida albicans*, *Histoplasma capsulatum*, *Blastomyces dermatitidis*, *Cryptococcus neoformans*, *Aspergillus*, *Sporothrix*, and *Torulopsis*
Azole derivatives	Ketaconazole, clotrimaxazole, miconazole	Systemic fungal infection, topical infection. Imidazole and triazole has broad-spectrum antifungal action covering dermatophytes, *Candida*, *Nocardia*, some gram-positive and anerobic bacteria, i.e. *Staphylococcus aureus*, *Bacillus fragilis*, and *Leishmania*
Allylamines	Terbinafine, naftidine	Resistant organisms for azoles
Heterocyclic benzofuran	Griseofulvin	Most dermatophytes of skin fungal infection but not against *Candida*

Bacterial Resistance to Antimicrobial Agents

The bacterial-resistance development depends on three factors. They are as follows:

- The necessary dose or concentration not reached to target.
- The chemotherapeutic agent is not active.
- The target is altered.

The outer membrane of the gram-negative bacteria is a permeability barrier that excludes large polar molecules, including antibiotic, through a protein called porins. Loss of porin channel may prevent the entry of antibiotics and reduces the concentration in target site. If there is an active transport mechanism for the entry of drug into the cell, mutational changes will occur in the transport to produce resistant. For example, passage of gentamycin across the microbial cell membrane by concentration gradient by involving the respiratory electron transport and oxidative phosphorylation. Mutation in this enzyme pathway decreases the concentration to the target.

Inactivation of drugs are seen in case of aminoglycoside and β-lactums. In aminoglycosides, the acquisition of cell membrane-bound inactivating enzymes which phosphorylates/adenylates or acetylates the drug molecule and produces conjugated aminoglycosides. These conjugated aminoglycosides do not bind to target ribosome and so are incapable of enhancing active transport. Nosocomial microbes have rich plasmids producing multidrug resistance and cross-resistance.

In fluoroquinolone, the resistance is occurred by alteration of target. The resistance is noted due to chromosomal mutations producing a DNA gyrase or topoisomerase IV with reduced affinity to the fluoroquinolone or due to reduced permeability of the drug.

Selection of Antimicrobial Agents

The selection is based on thorough knowledge of pharmacological and microbiological factors. Antibiotics are used in three general ways such as empirical therapy, definitive therapy, and prophylactic therapy. When used in empirical, the drug intended should cover all the microorganisms, if the pathogen is exactly not known. In the combination therapy, treatment with a broad-spectrum antibiotic is necessary. After the identification of infecting microorganism, selective drug can be used.

Combination Therapy

It is the combined use of drugs intended to achieve better action; in chemotherapy it is used for the synergistic action (e.g. a sulphonamide used with trimethoprim to produce additive action). Other examples are in the combination of β-lactamase inhibition by clavulanic acid or sulbactum with amoxycillin or ampicillin for β-lacamase producing *H. influenza*, *Neisseria gonorrhoeae*, and other organisms. Combination of a bactericidal with a bacteriostatic drug produces synergistic action. The combination therapy of antimicrobials is also used in the treatment of mixed infection and initial treatment of severe infections.

PROBABLE QUESTIONS

1. Define the term chemotherapy and explain the spectrum of activity of chemotherapeutic agents.
2. Write the classification of antibiotics.
3. Explain in detail about bacterial resistance.

CHAPTER 13

Antibacterial Sulphonamides

INTRODUCTION

The term sulphonamides is employed as a generic name for the derivatives of *para*-amino benzene sulphonamide (sulphanilamide). The sulphonamide drugs were the first effective chemotherapeutic agents to be employed systemically for the prevention and treatment of bacterial infections in humans. The sulphonamides are bacteriostatic antibiotics with a wide spectrum action against most gram-positive bacteria and many gram-negative organisms. Actually it was found to be the metabolic product of prontosil, which is responsible for antibacterial activity, and this has given the initiation to develop sulphonamides as antibacterial agents.

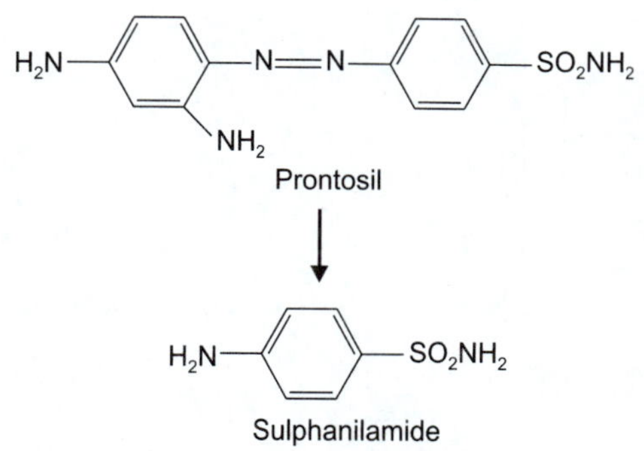

Sulphonamides are total synthetic substances that are produced by relatively simple chemical synthesis. The advent of penicillin and, subsequently of other antibiotics has diminished the usefulness of sulphonamides. Antimicrobial compounds contain sulphonamide (SO_2NH_2) group. This group (SO_2NH_2) is also present in other compounds, such as antidiabetic agents (e.g. tolubutamide), diuretics (e.g. chlorthiazide and its congeners, furosemide, and acetazolamide), and anticonvulsants such as sulthiame. The sulphonamides exist as white powder, mildly acidic in character, and they form water-soluble salts with bases. The pH of sodium salts with some exception, for example, sodium sulphacetamide, is very high when given intramuscular (IM), the marked alkalinity causes damage to the tissues.

Microorganisms that may be susceptible *in vitro* to sulphonamides include *Streptococcus pyogens*, *Streptococcus pneumoniae*, *Haemophilus influenzae*, *H. ducreyi*, *Nocardia*, *Actinomyces*, *Calymmatobacterium granulomatis*, and *Chlamydia trachomatis*. The minimal inhibitory concentration ranges from 0.1 μg/ml for *C. trachomatis* to 4–64 μg/ml for *E. coli*. Sulphonamides are selective drugs used to treat urinary tract infections, bacterial respiratory infections, and gastrointestinal (GI) infections.

Mode of action: Sulphonamides are structure analogues and competitive antagonists of *para*-amino benzoic acid (PABA). They inhibit dihydropteroate synthetase, the bacterial enzyme responsible for the incorporation of PABA into dihydropteric acid, and it is the intermediate precursor of folic acid. Synergistic effect is obtained by a combination of trimethoprim. The compound trimethoprim is a potent and selective inhibitor of microbial dihydrofolate reductase, the enzyme that reduces dihydrofolate to tetrahydrofolate. The simultaneous administration of sulphonamide and trimethoprim blocks the pathway of cell-wall synthesis sequentially.

SAR of Sulphonamides

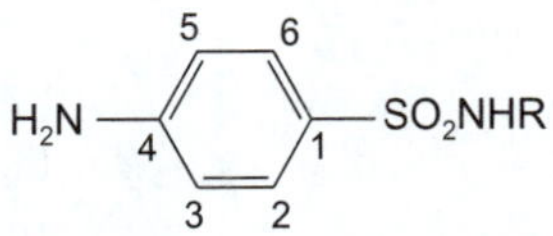

The major features of SAR of sulphonamides include the following:

- Sulphanilamide skeleton is the minimum structural requirement for antibacterial activity.
- The amino- and sulphonyl-groups on the benzene ring are essential and should be in 1 and 4 position.
- The N-4 amino group could be modified to be prodrugs, which are converted to free amino function *in vivo*.

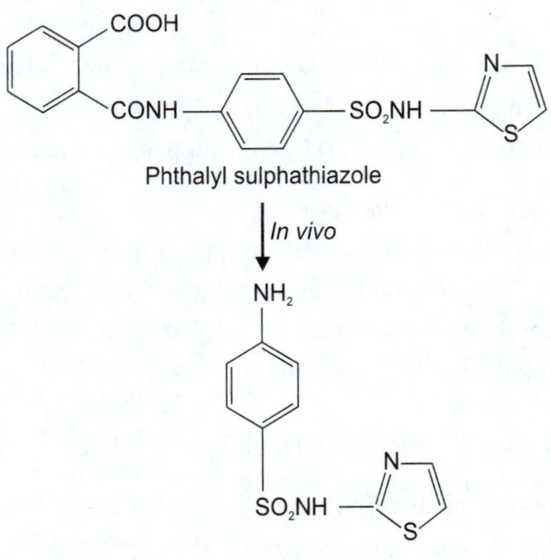

- Sulphur atom should be directly linked to the benzene ring.
- Replacement of benzene ring by other ring systems or the introduction of additional substituents on it decreases or abolishes its activity.
- Exchange of the $-SO_2NH$ group by –CONH reduces the activity.
- On N-1-substituted sulphonamides, activity varies with the nature of the substituent at the amino group. With substituents imparting electron-rich characters to SO_2 group, bacteriostatic activity increases.
- Heterocyclic substituents lead to highly potent derivatives, while sulphonamides, which contain a single benzene ring at N-1 position, are considerably more toxic than heterocyclic ring analogues.

- The free aromatic amino groups should reside *para* to the sulphonamide group. Its replacement at *ortho* or *meta* position results in compounds devoid of antibacterial activity.
- The active form of sulphonamide is the ionized, maximum activity that is observed between the pK_a values 6.6–7.4.
- Substitutions in the benzene ring of sulphonamides produce inactive compounds.
- Substitution of free sulphonic acid ($-SO_3H$) group for sulphonamido function destroys the activity, but replacement by a sulphinic acid group ($-SO_2H$) and acetylation of N-4 position retains back the activity.
- Sulphonamides bind to the basic centres of arginine, histidine, and lysine sites of proteins. The binding groups are alkyl, alkoxy, and halides. The binding affects the activity of sulphonamides; protein binding appears to modulate the availability of the drug and its half-life.
- The lipid solubility influences the pharmacokinetic and antibacterial activity, and so increases the half-life and antibacterial activity *in vitro*.

CLASSIFICATION

Sulphonamides can be classified in various ways:

On the basis of the site of action

- Sulphonamides for general infection: Sulphanilamide, sulphapyridine, sulphadiazine, sulphamethoxacine, sulphamethoxazole.
- Sulphonamides for urinary tract infections: Sulphaisoxazole, sulphathiazole.
- Sulphonamides for intestinal infections: Phthalylsulphathiazole, succinyl sulphathiazole, sulphasalazine.
- Sulphonamides for local infections: Sulphacetamide, mafenamide, silver sulphadiazine.
- Sulphonamides for dermatitis: Dapsone, solapsone.
- Sulphonamides in combination: Trimethoprim with sulphamethoxazole.

On the basis of the pharmacokinetic properties

- Poorly absorbed sulphonamides (locally-acting sulphonamides): Sulphasalazine, phthalylsulphathiazole, sulphaguanidine, salicylazo sulphapyridine, succinyl sulphathiazole.
- Rapidly absorbed and rapidly excreted (systemic sulphanamides): Sulphamethoxazole, sulphaisoxazole, sulphadiazine, sulphadimidine, sulphafurazole, sulphasomidine, sulphamethiazole, sulphacetamide, sulphachlorpyridazine.
- Topically used sulphonamides: Sulphacetamide, mafenide, sulphathiazole, Silver sulphadiazine.

On the basis of the pharamacological activity

- Antibacterial agents: Sulphadiazine, sulfisoxazole.
- Drugs used in dermatitis: Dapsone.

On the basis of the duration of action

- Extra long-acting sulphonamides (half-life greater than 50 hrs): Sulphasalazine, sulphalene.
- Long-acting sulphonamides (half-life greater than 24 hrs): Sulphadoxine, sulphadimethoxine, Sulphamethoxy pyridazine, sulphamethoxydiazine, sulphaphenazole, sulphamethoxine.
- Intermediate-acting sulphonamides (half-life—10–24 hrs): Sulphasomizole, sulphamethoxazole.
- Short-acting sulphonamides (half-life less than 20 hrs): Sulphamethiazole, sulphaisoxazole.
- Injectables (soluble sulpha drugs): Sulphafurazole, sulphadiazine, sulphamethoxine.

On the basis of the chemical structure

- N-1 substituted sulphonamide: Sulphadiazine, sulphacetamide, sulphadimidine.
- N-4 substituted sulphonamides (prodrugs): Prontosil.
- Both N-1 and N-4 substituted sulphonamides: Succinyl sulphathiazole, phthalylsulphathiazole.
- Miscellaneous: Mefenide sodium.

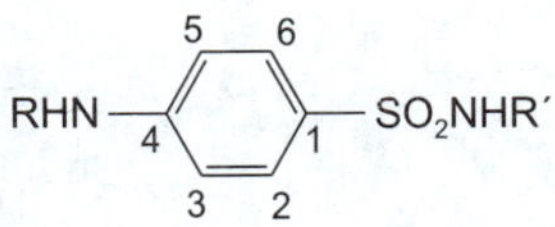

I. N-1 Substituted Sulphonamides

Name	R	R′
Sulphanilamide	–H	–H
Sulphapyridine	–H	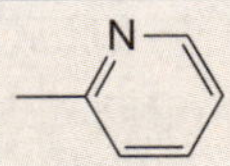
Sulphathiazole	–H	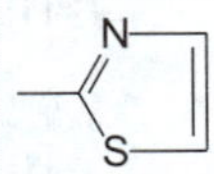
Sulphacetamide	–H	$–COCH_3$
Sulphadiazine	–H	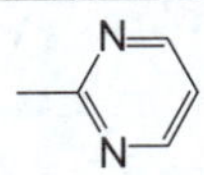
Sulphadimidine	–H	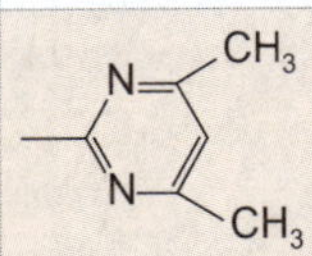

a. Short-acting sulpha drugs

Name	R	R′
Sulphaisoxazol	–H	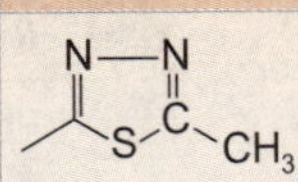
Sulphasomidine	–H	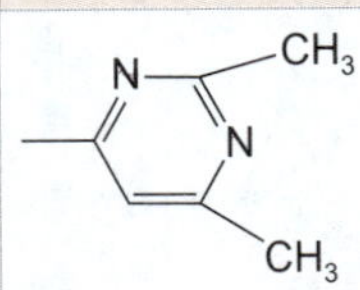
Sulphamethizole	–H	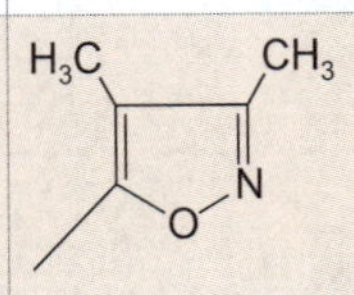

b. Intermediate-acting sulphonamides

Name	R	R′
Sulphasomizole	–H	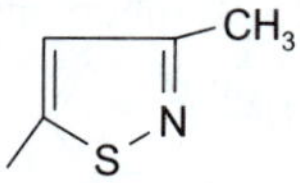
Sulphamethoxazole	–H	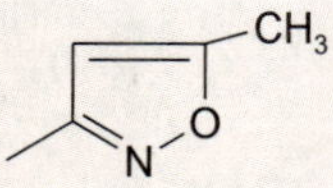

c. Long-acting sulphonamides

Name	R	R′
Sulphamethoxy pyridazine	–H	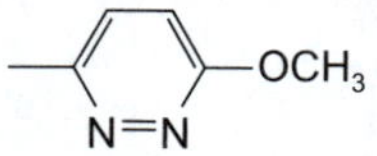
Sulphamethoxy diazine	–H	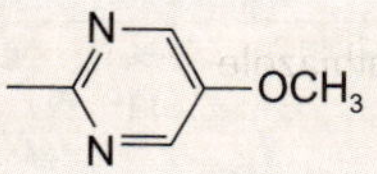
Sulpha dimethoxine	–H	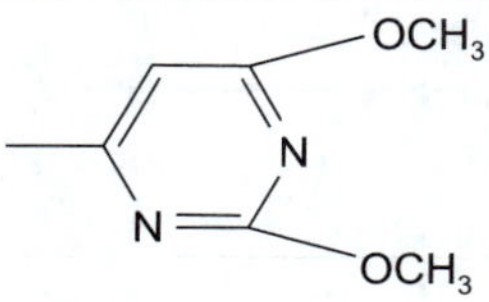
Sulphaphenazole	–H	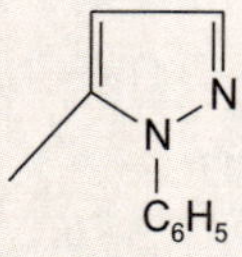

d. Extra long-acting sulphonamides

Name	R	R′
Sulphalene	–H	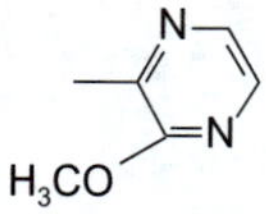
Sulphomethoxine	–H	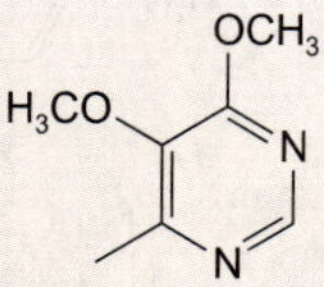

II. N-4 Substituted Sulphonamides

Prontosil

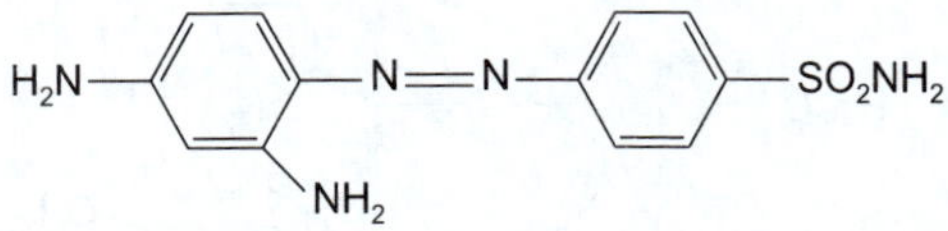

III. Both N-1 and N-4 Substituted Sulphonamides

Name	R	R'
Succinyl sulphathiazole	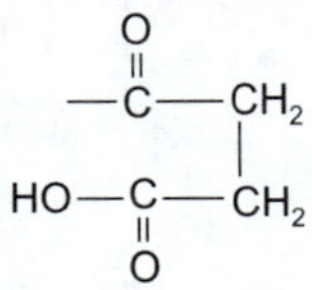	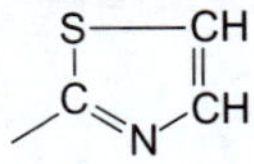
Phthalylsulphathiazole	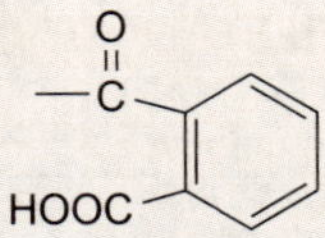	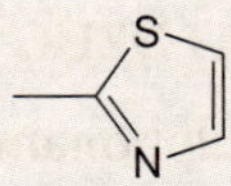

IV. Miscellaneous

a. Topically used sulphonamides

Mafenide

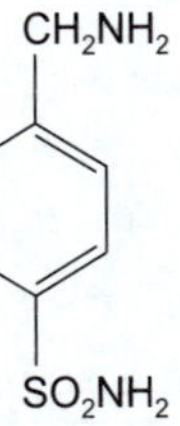

Silver sulphadiazine

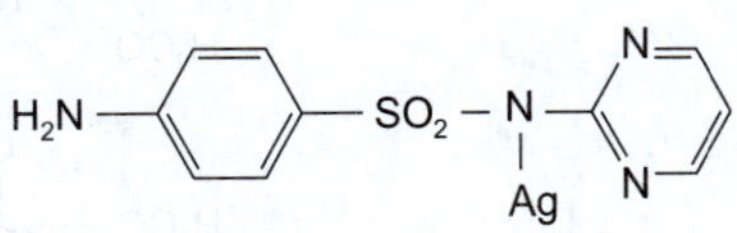

Solapsone

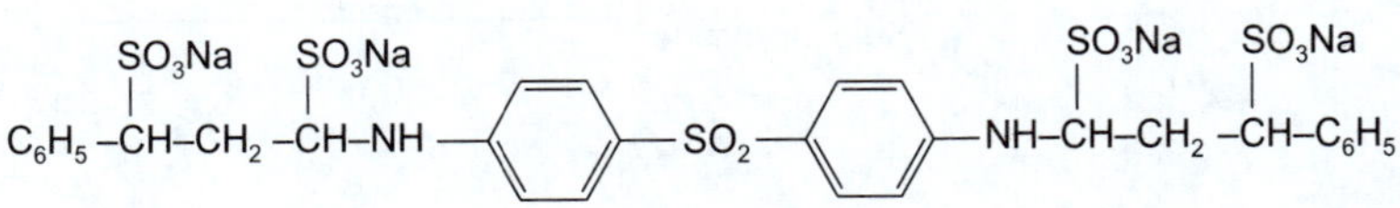

b. Drugs used in combination with sulphonamides

Trimethoprim

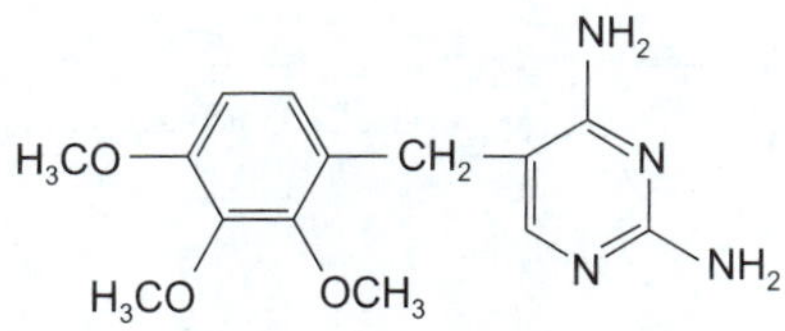

Pyrimethamine

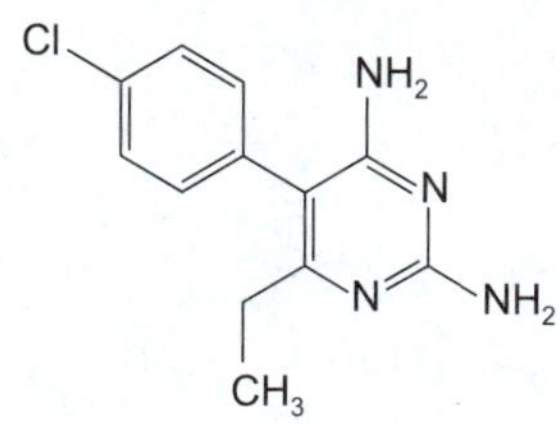

SYNTHESIS AND DRUG PROFILE

I. N-1 Substituted Sulphonamides

i. Sulphanilamide

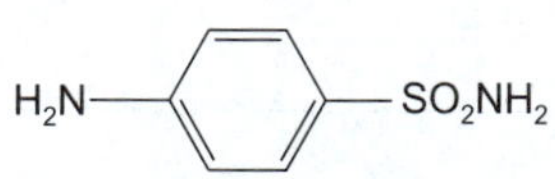

4-Aminobenzene sulphonamide

Synthesis

Route 1. From: Benzene

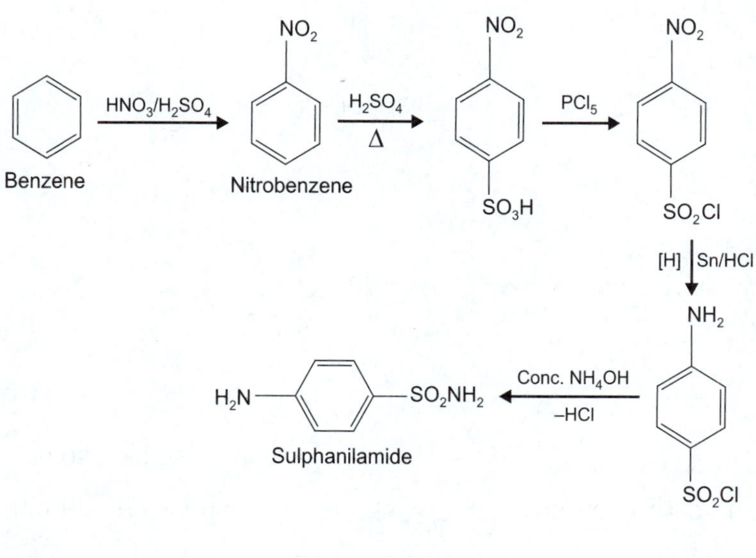

Route 2. From: Nitrobenzene

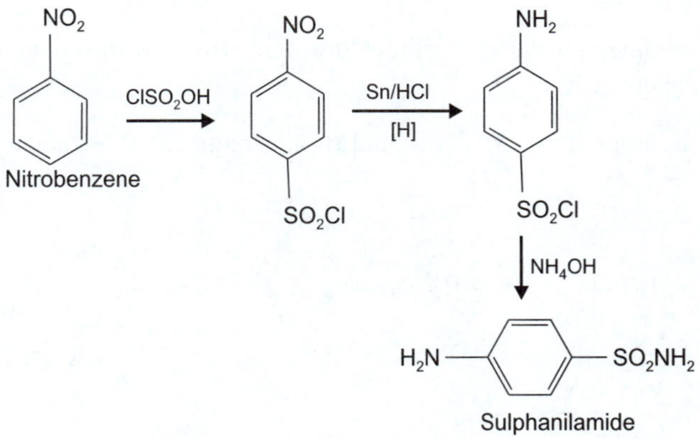

Route 3. From: Aniline

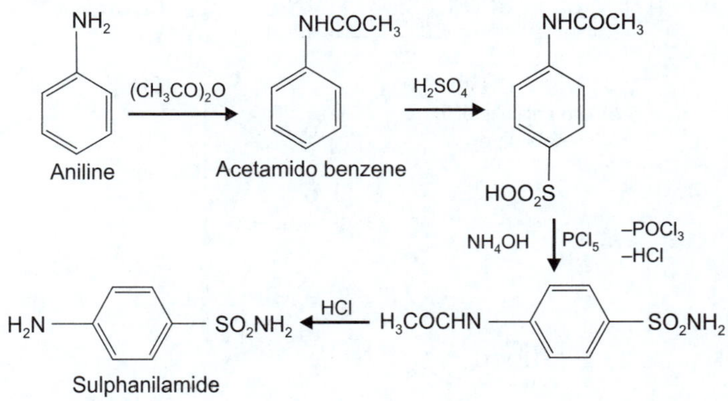

Uses: It is used in veterinary medicine as an antibacterial agent.

ii. Sulphacetamide (Albucid)

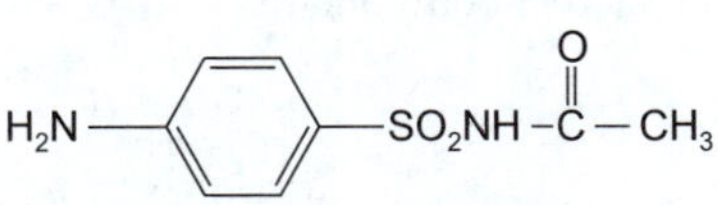

N-Sulphanilyl acetamide

Synthesis

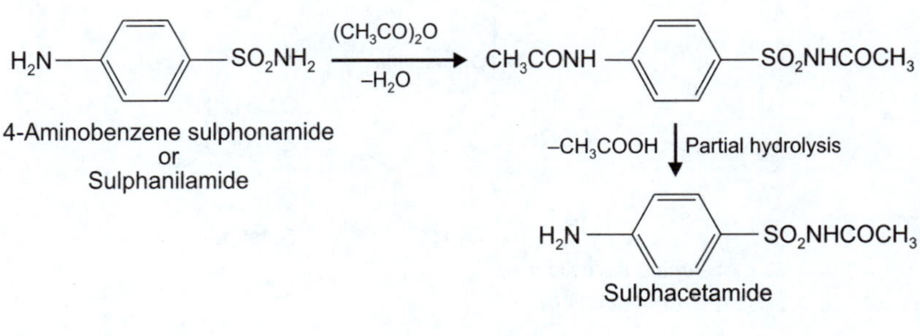

Properties and uses: It exists as white crystalline powder, bitter in taste. Used in the treatment of bacterial infections of urinary tract.

Assay: Dissolve the sample in water and hydrochloric acid. Titrate with sodium nitrite and determine the end point potentiometrically.

Dose: Dose for eyes, as drops 10%, 15%, 20%, and 30%; in ointments 2.5% and 6% of sulphacetamide.

iii. Sulphasalazine

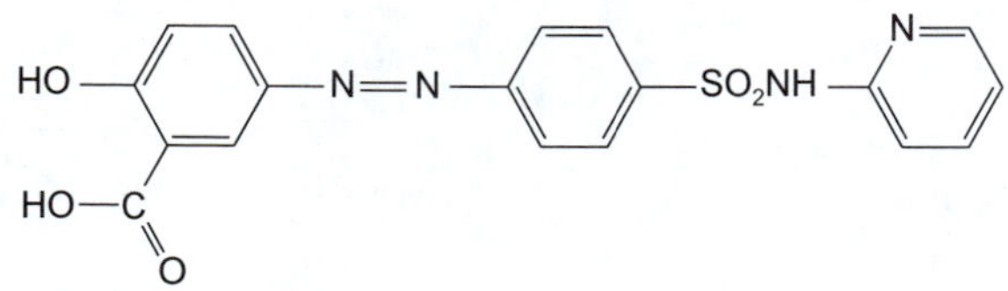

Synthesis

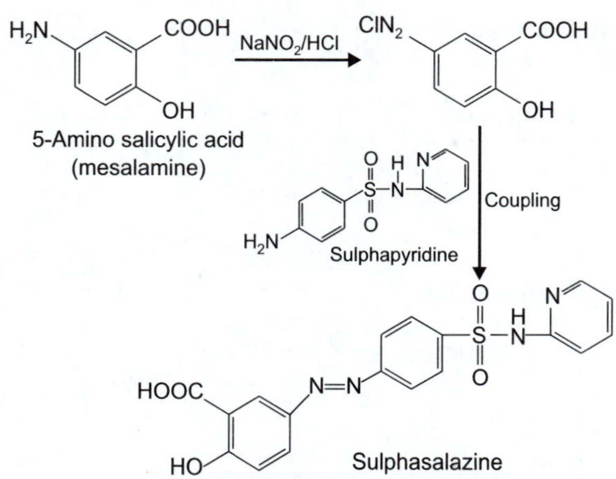

Metabolism: It undergoes reductive metabolism by gut bacteria, converting the drug into sulfapyridine and 5-amino salicylic acid, which are active components.

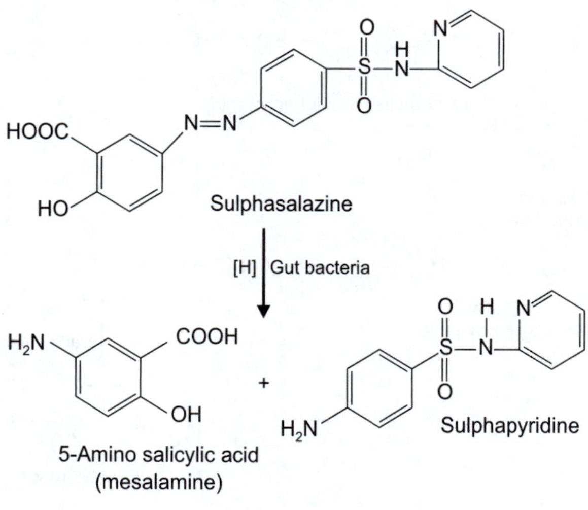

Properties and uses: Sulphasalazine is a bright yellow or brownish-yellow fine powder, very slightly soluble in alcohol, practically insoluble in methylene chloride. It dissolves in dilute solutions of alkali hydroxides. It is used in the treatment of ulcerative colitis.

Assay: Dissolve and dilute the sample in 0.1 M sodium hydroxide and add 0.1 M acetic acid and measure the absorbance at the maxima of 359 nm using ultraviolet spectrophotometer.

Dosage forms: Sulphasalazine tablets BP.

iv. Sulphadiazine

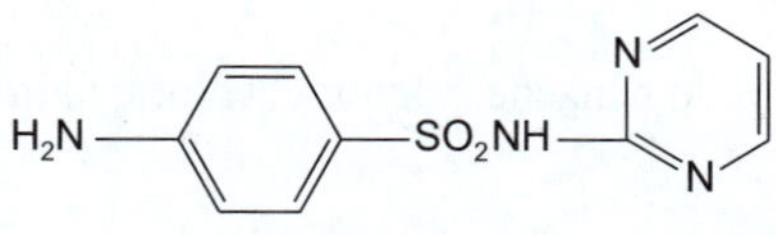

N′-2 Pyrimidinyl sulphanilamide

Synthesis

Step I. Preparation of formyl acetic acid

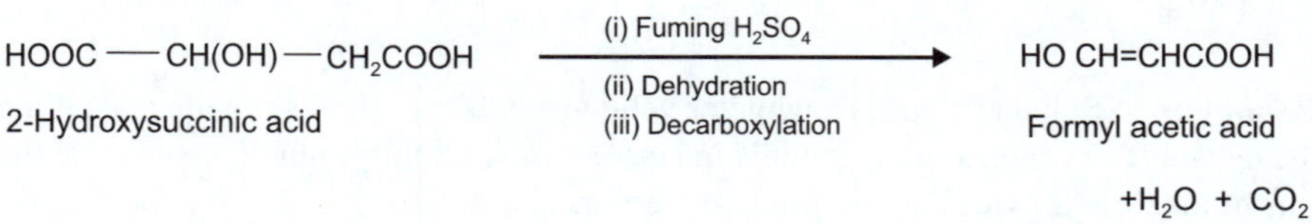

Step II. Synthesis of 2-Aminopyrimidine

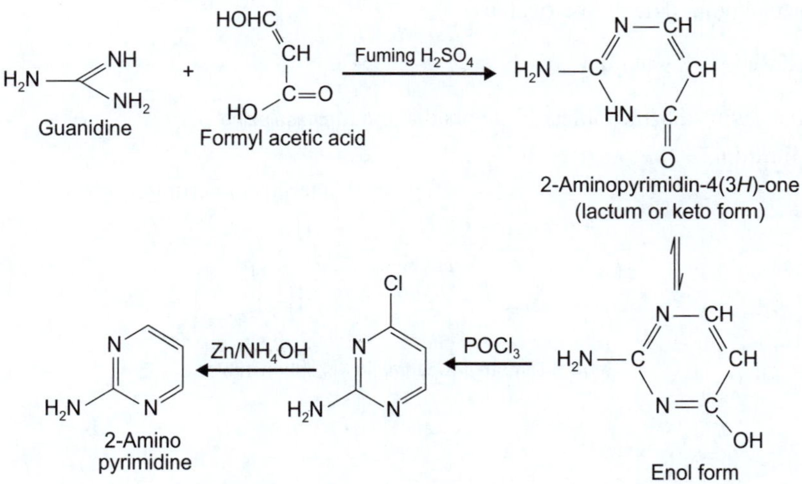

Step III. Synthesis of *p*-acetamido benzene sulphonyl chloride (PABS)

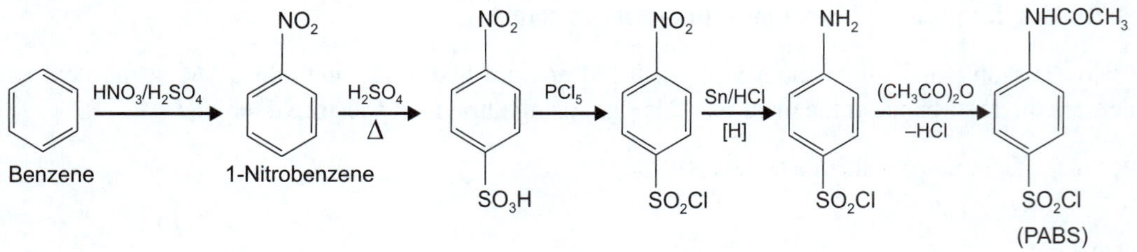

Step IV. Condensation of *p*-acetamido benzene sulphonyl chloride with 2-aminopyrimidine

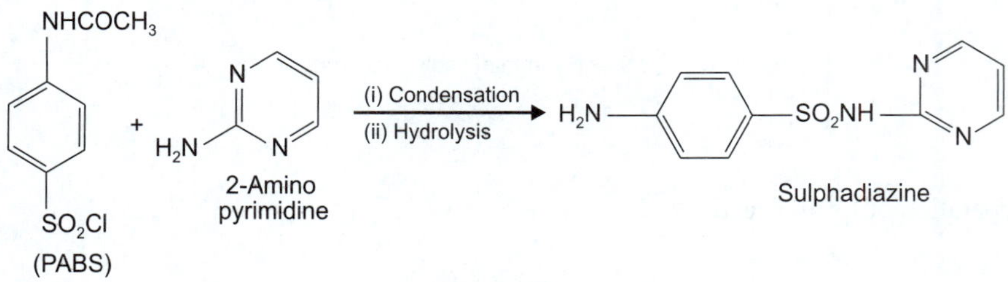

Properties and uses: Sulphadiazine is a white or yellowish-white or pinkish-white crystalline powder or crystals, insoluble in water, slightly soluble in acetone, very slightly soluble in alcohol, and soluble in solutions of alkali hydroxides and in dilute mineral acids. It is used in the treatment of canceroids and rheumatic fever.

Assay: Dissolve the sample in water and hydrochloric acid. Titrate the mixture with sodium nitrite and determine the end point potentiometrically.

Dose: Usual dose is 2–8 g per day.

Dosage forms: Sulphadiazine tablets IP, sulphadiazine injection BP.

v. Sulphadimidine

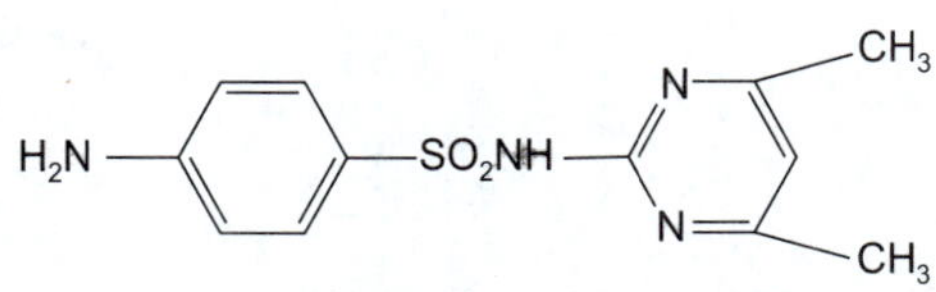

N′(4,6-Dimethyl-2-pyrimidinyl)sulphanilamide

Synthesis

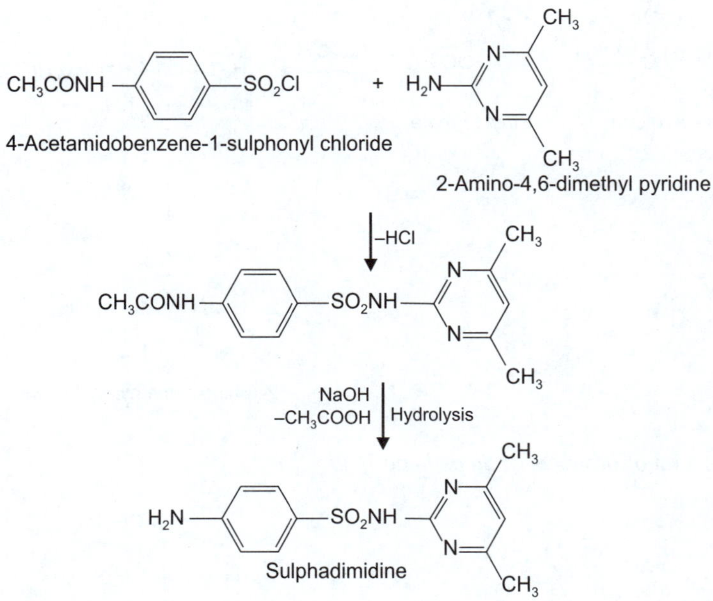

Properties and uses: It exists as white crystalline powder with a bitter taste, insoluble in water, and sparingly soluble in alcohol. It is less effective in meningeal infection because of its poor penetration into the cerebrospinal fluid.

Dose: Dose is 3 g initially and subsequent doses up to 6 g per day in divided doses.

vi. **Sulphamerazine** (Solumedine)

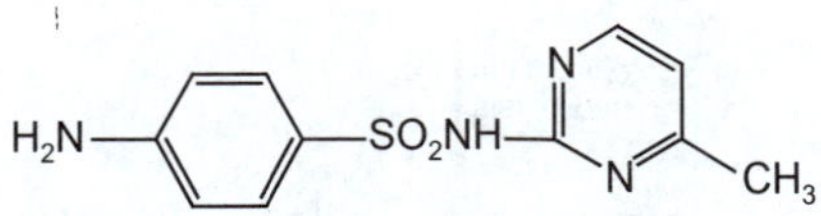

N′-(4-methyl-2-pyrimidinyl)sulphanilamide

Synthesis

Step I. Preparation of PABS

Synthesized as mentioned under *sulphadiazine*.

Step II. Preparation of 2-amino-4-methylpyrimidine

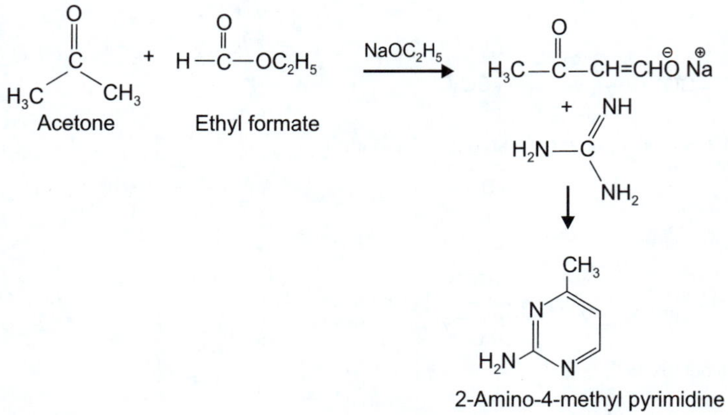

Step III. Condensation of products of *Steps I* and *II*.

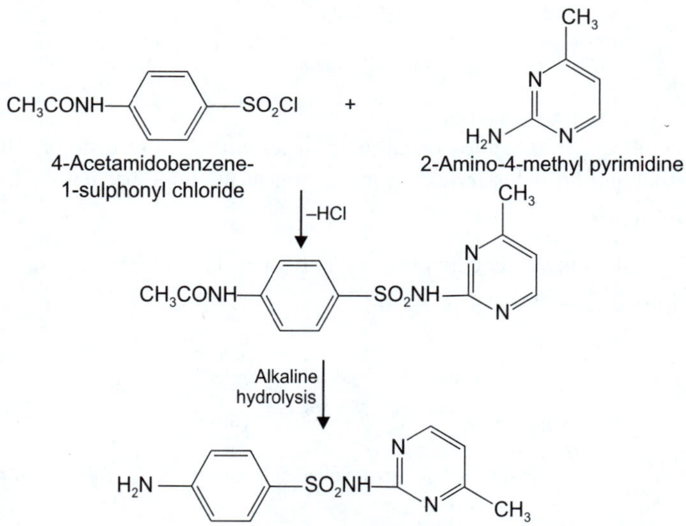

Sulphamerazine

Uses: Used as an antibacterial agent.

Dose: Dose is 4 g initially, and subsequent dose is 1 g every 6 hrs.

vii. Sulphadimethoxine

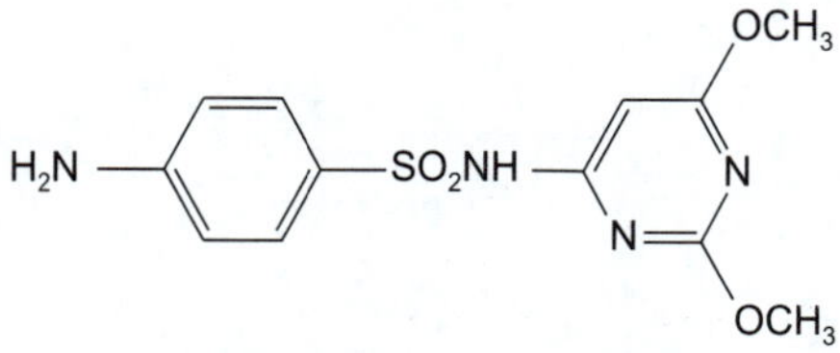

N′-(4,6-Dimethoxy-2-pyrimidinyl)sulphanilamide

Synthesis

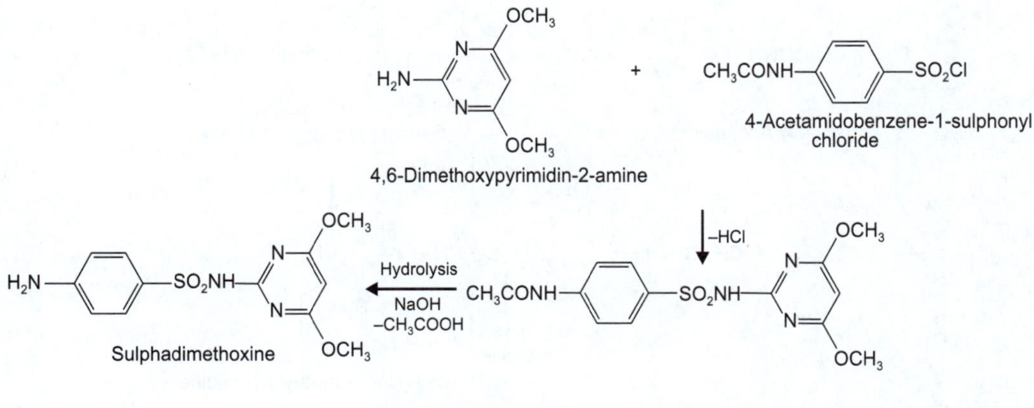

viii. Sulphamethoxy pyridazine

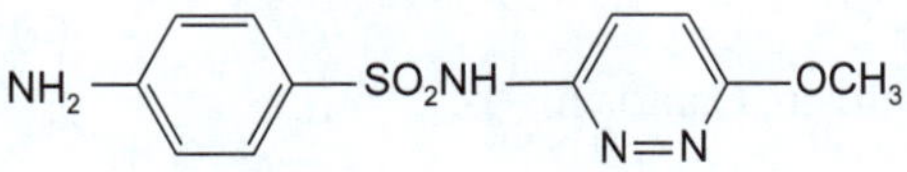

3-(4-Aminobenzene sulphonamido)-6-methoxy pyridazine

Synthesis

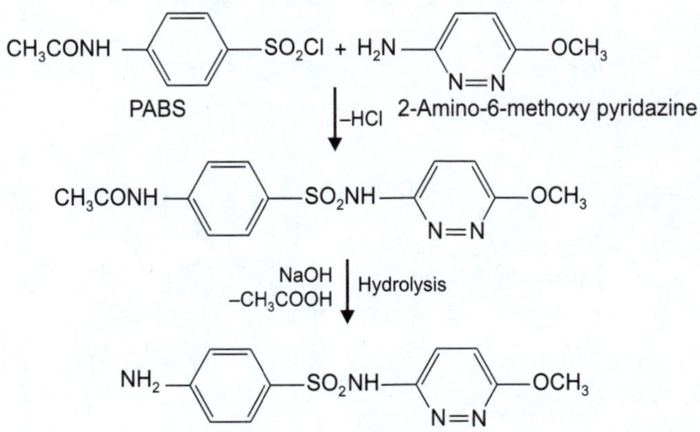

ix. Sulphaphenazole

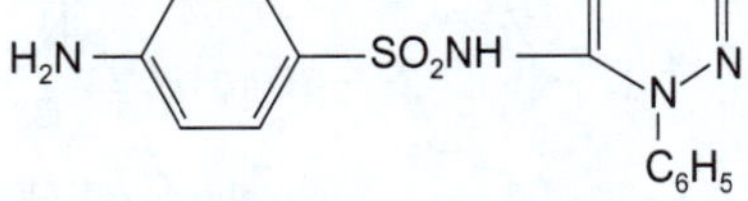

5-(4-Aminobenzene sulphamido)-N-phenyl pyrazole

Synthesis

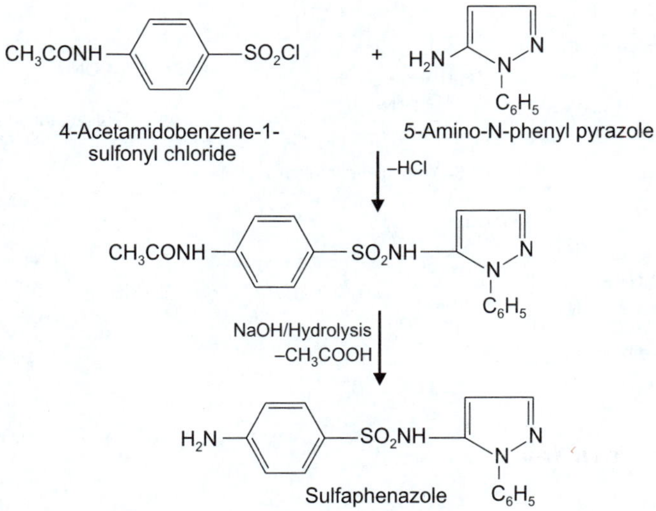

x. Sulphaisoxazole (Lipo Gantrisin, Gantrisin)

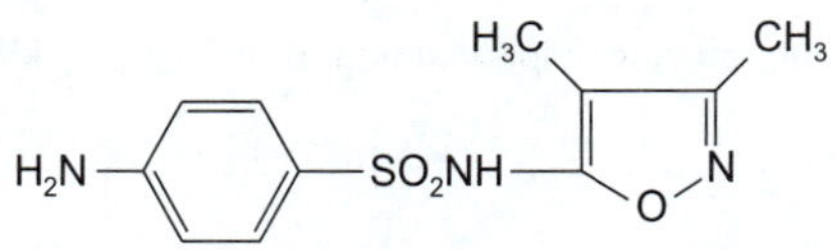

5-(4-Aminobenzene sulphonamido)-3,4-dimethyl isoxazole

Synthesis

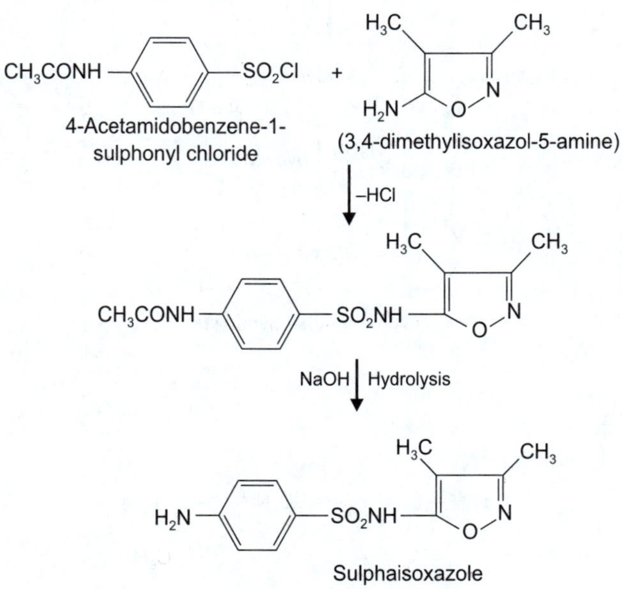

Properties and uses: It exists as white to slightly yellowish crystalline powder and is odourless, soluble in water and in dilute hydrochloric acid. Used in the treatment of urinary tract infections.

Assay: Dissolve the sample in water and hydrochloric acid. Titrate the mixture with sodium nitrite and determine the end point potentiometrically.

Dose: Initial dose is 2–4 g orally for adults and maintenance dose is 4–8 g per day in divided doses.

xi. Sulphamethoxazole (Gantanol)

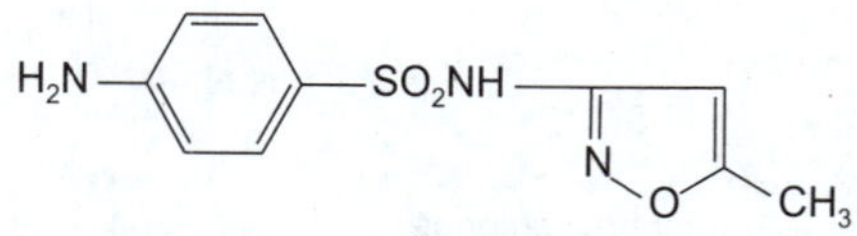

3-(4-Aminobenzene sulphamido)-5-methyl isoxazole

Synthesis

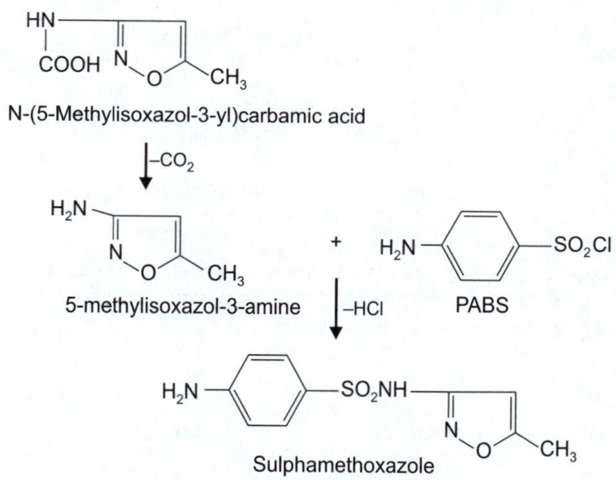

Properties and uses: Sulphamethoxazole is a white or almost white crystalline powder, practically insoluble in water, soluble in acetone, sparingly soluble in ethanol, dissolves in dilute solutions of sodium hydroxide and in dilute acids. Used in the treatment of bacterial infections.

Assay: Dissolve the sample in dilute hydrochloric acid and add potassium bromide. Cool in ice and titrate against 0.1 N sodium nitrite. Determine the end point electrometrically.

Dose: Orally 2 g followed by 1 g every 8 hrs.

Dosage forms: Co-trimoxazole intravenous infusion BP, co-trimoxazole oral suspension BP, paediatric co-trimoxazole oral suspension BP, co-trimoxazole tablets BP, dispersible co-trimoxazole tablets BP, paediatric co-trimoxazole tablets BP.

xii. Sulphaguanidine

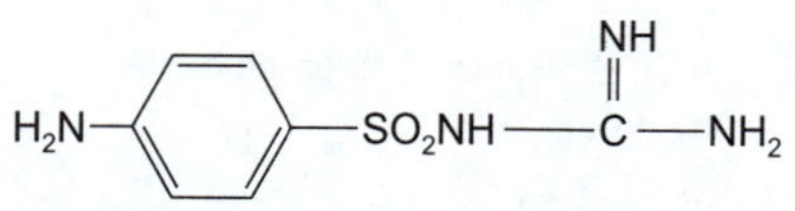

N′-(Diamino methylene)sulphanilamide

Properties and uses: Sulphaguanidine is a white, fine crystalline powder, soluble in dilute mineral acids, very slightly soluble in water and ethanol, slightly soluble in acetone, but insoluble in methylene chloride. Used in the treatment of local intestinal infections, specifically, bacillary dysentery.

Assay: Dissolve the sample in dilute hydrochloric acid and add potassium bromide. Cool in ice and titrate against 0.1N sodium nitrite. Determine the end point electrometrically.

Synthesis

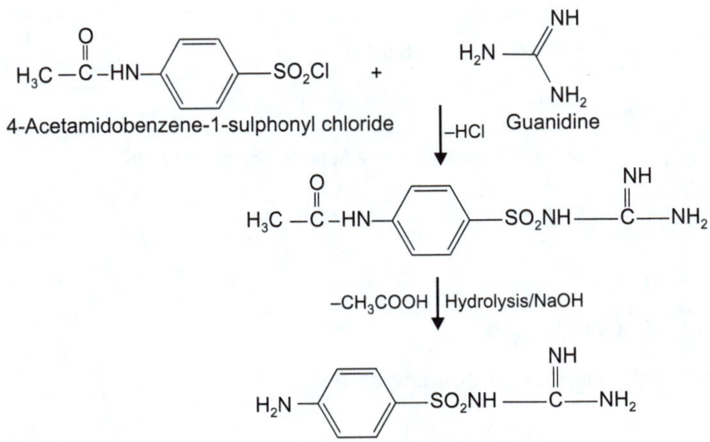

Sulphaguanidine

II. Both N-1 and N-4 Substituted Sulphonamides

i. Succinyl sulphathiazole

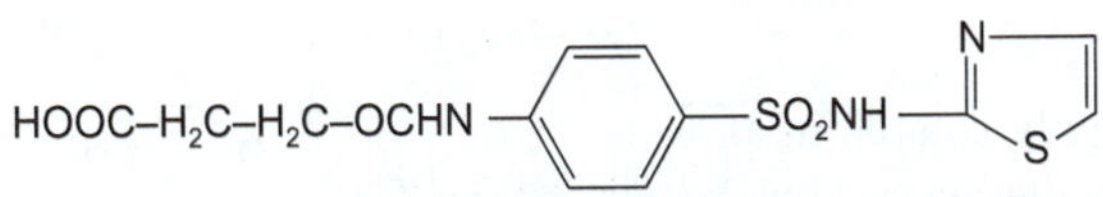

2-[(4-Succinylaminobenzene) sulphonamido] thiazole

Synthesis

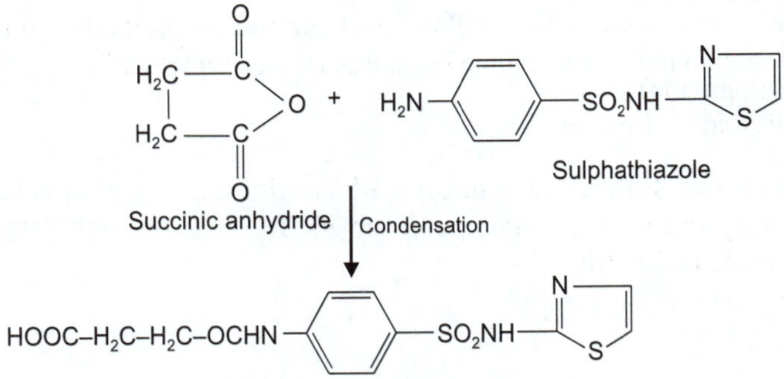

Succinyl sulphathiazole

Uses: Used in bacillary dysentery and cholera.

Dose: Dose is 10–20 g per day in divided doses.

ii. Phthalyl sulphathiazole (Thalazole)

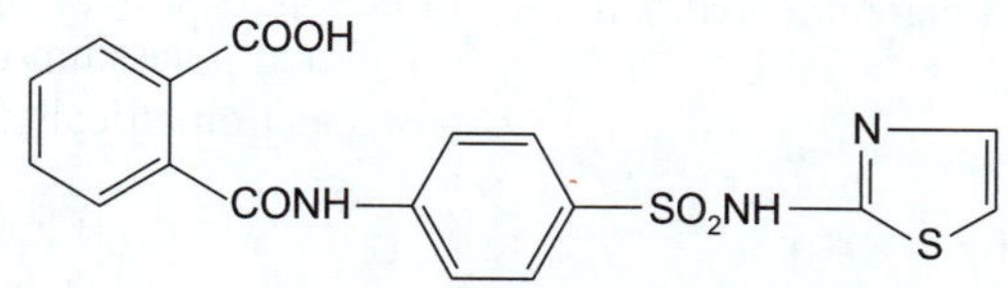

4'-(2-Thiazolyl sulphamoyl) phthalylamino benzene

Synthesis

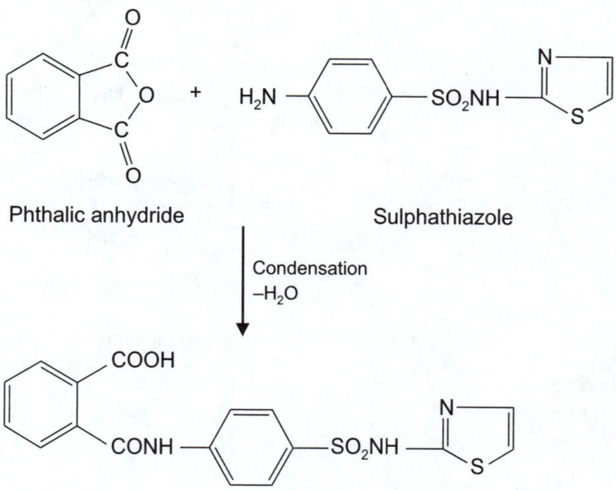

Phthalyl sulphathiazole

Properties and uses: Slightly soluble in alcohol and ether, but insoluble in water. It is used in the treatment of acute bacillary dysentery, bowel irregularities, and ulcerative colitis.

Dose: Dose is 5–10 g per day in divided doses.

III. Miscellaneous

a. Topically used sulphonamides

i. Mafenide (Sulfamylon)

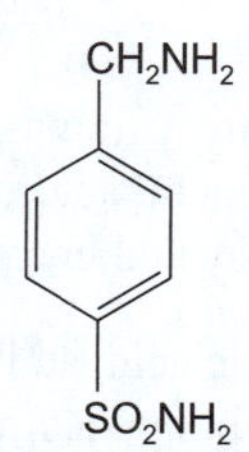

4-(Aminomethyl)benzene sulphonamide

Uses: It is used in the treatment and cure of gas gangrene. It is also effective against *Clostridium welchii* on topical application.

Dose: Dose is 5% solution of mafenide hydrochloride or mafenide propionate for topical use.

Synthesis

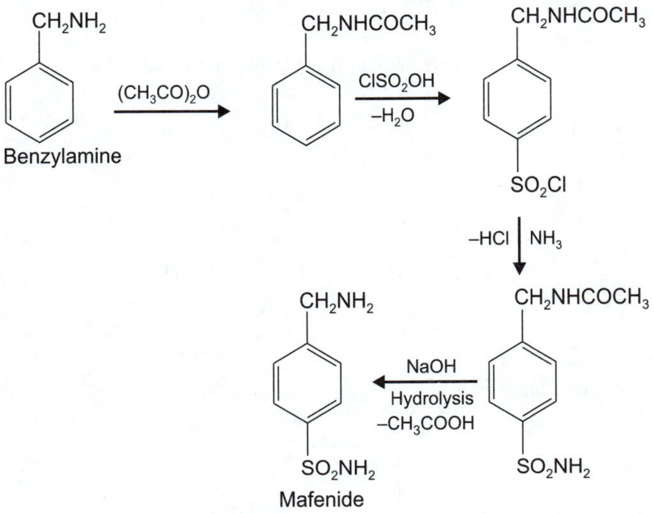

ii. Silver sulphadiazine

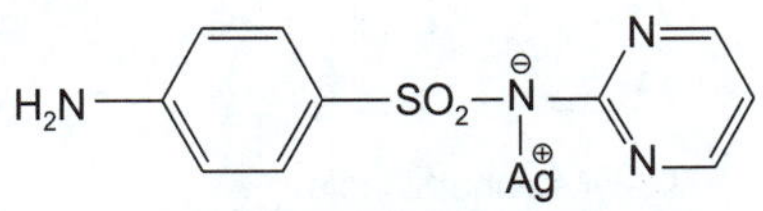

4-Amino-N-(2-pyrimidinyl)mono silver salt of benzene sulphonamide

Uses: It is an effective topical antimicrobial agent, especially, against *Pseudomonas* species; it finds extensive use in burn therapy.

iii. Dapsone (Avcosulfon)

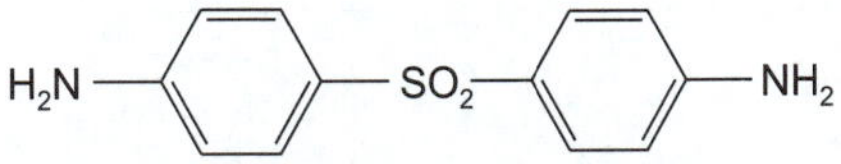

p,p′-Diamino diphenyl sulphone (DDS)

Action and use: Dapsone is a white or slightly yellowish-white crystalline powder, very slightly soluble in water, soluble in acetone and dilute mineral acids, sparingly soluble in alcohol. Used as folic acid synthesis inhibitor in the treatment of leprosy and nocardiosis.

Assay: Dissolve the sample in dilute hydrochloric acid, add potassium bromide, cool in ice, and titrate against 0.1 N sodium nitrite. Determine the end point electrometrically.

Dose: The dose as a leprostatic is 25 mg twice a week initially for 1 month followed by 25 mg per day each month. As suppressant for dermatitis herpetiformis, the dose is 100–200 mg per day.

Dosage forms: Dapsone tablets BP.

Synthesis

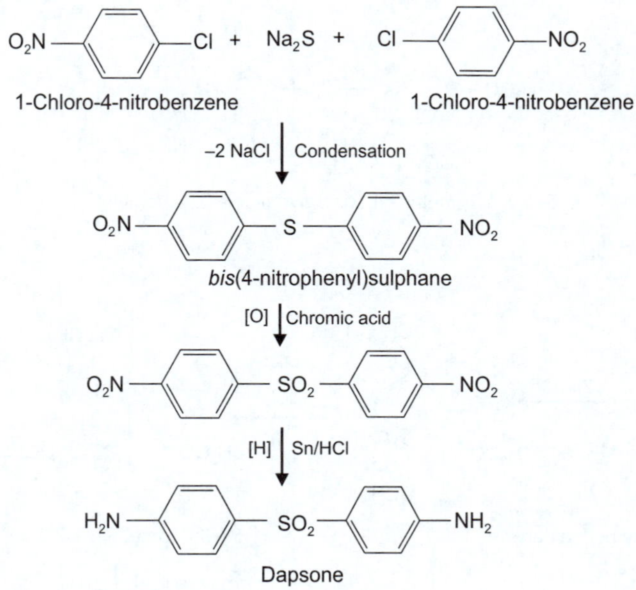

iv. Solapsone

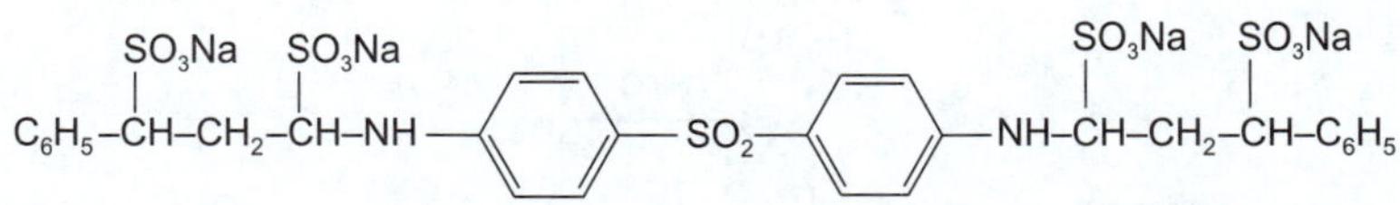

1,1′-[Sulphonyl-*bis*-(4,4-phenyleneimino)]-*bis*-[3-phenyl-1,3-propane disulphonic acid] tetra sodium

Synthesis

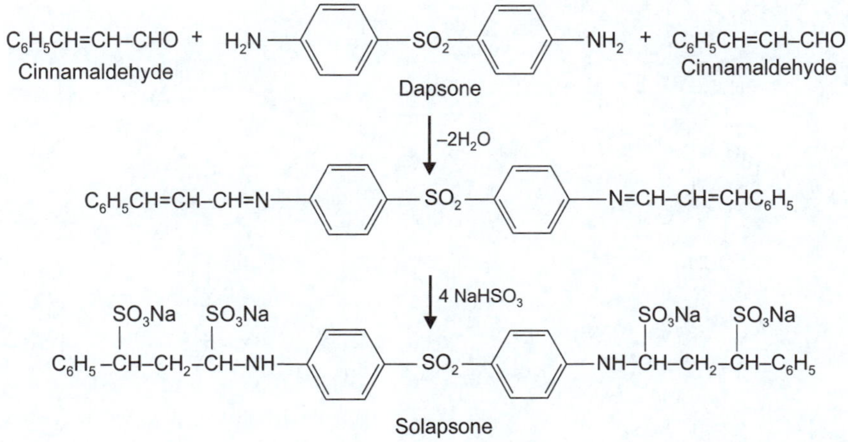

Uses: It is used in the treatment of leprosy.

IV. Drugs Used in Combination with Sulphonamides

i. Trimethoprim

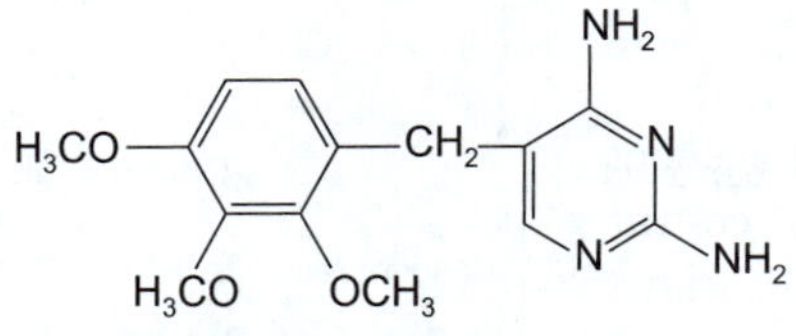

5-(2,3,4-Trimethoxybenzyl)pyrimidine-2,4-diamine

Synthesis

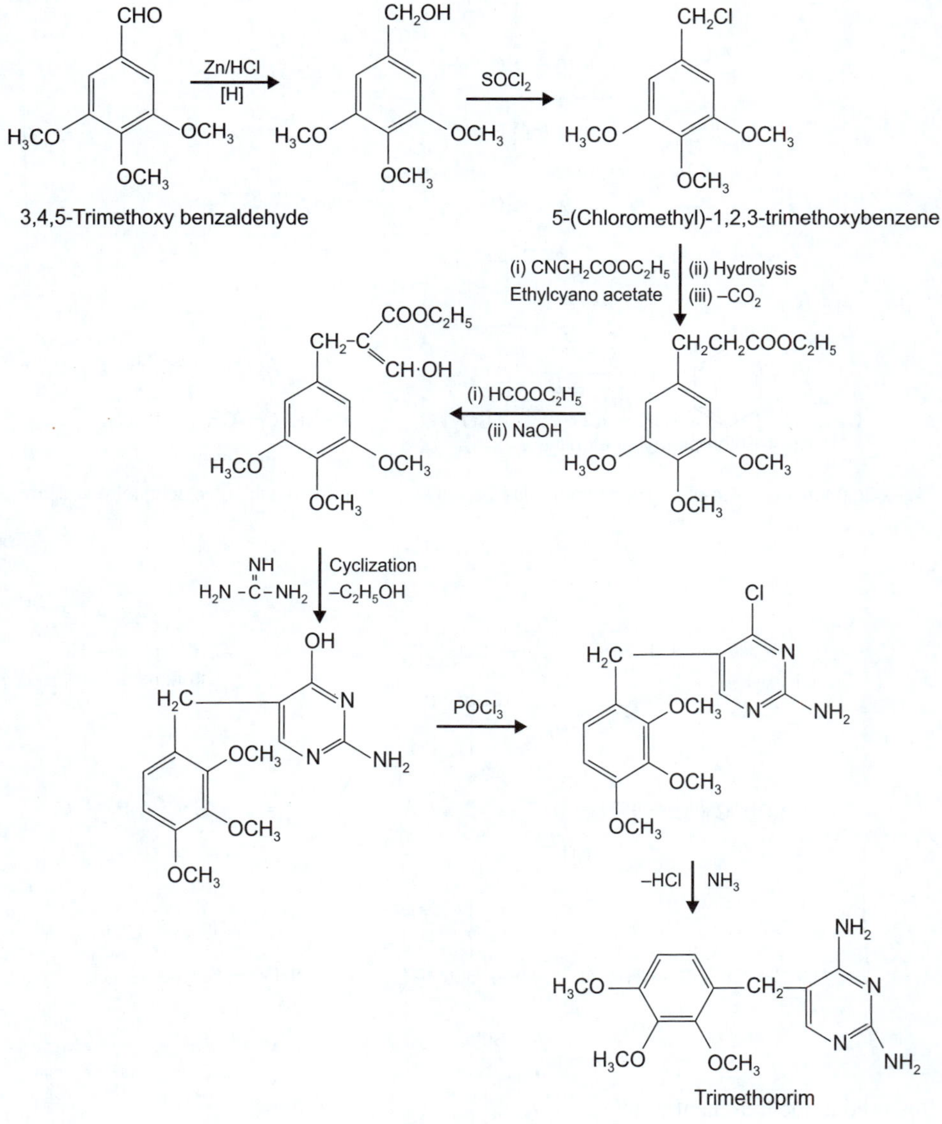

Properties and uses: Trimethoprim is a white or yellowish-white powder, very slightly soluble in water and slightly soluble in ethanol. It is used as dihydrofolate reductase inhibitor, effective against chloroquine and pyrimethamine resistant strains of *Plasmodium falciparum*.

Assay: Dissolve the sample in anhydrous acetic acid and titrate with 0.1 M perchloric acid. Determine the end point potentiometrically.

Dosage forms: Co-trimoxazole intravenous infusion BP, co-trimoxazole oral suspension BP, paediatric co-trimoxazole oral suspension BP, co-trimoxazole tablets BP, dispersible co-trimoxazole tablets BP, paediatric co-trimoxazole tablets BP, trimethoprim oral suspension BP, trimethoprim tablets BP.

ii. Pyrimethamine

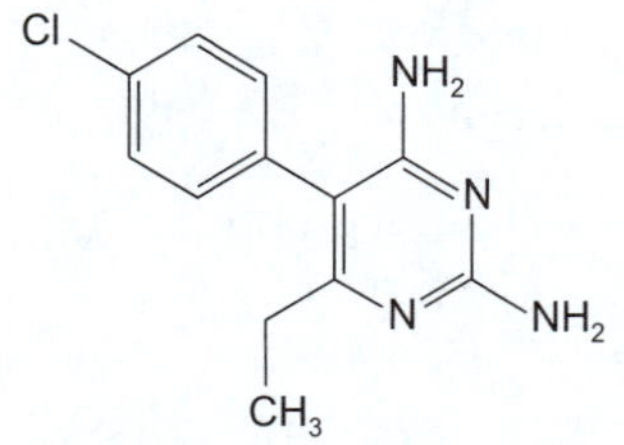

5-(4-Chlorophenyl)-6-ethylpyrimidine-2,4-diamine

Synthesis

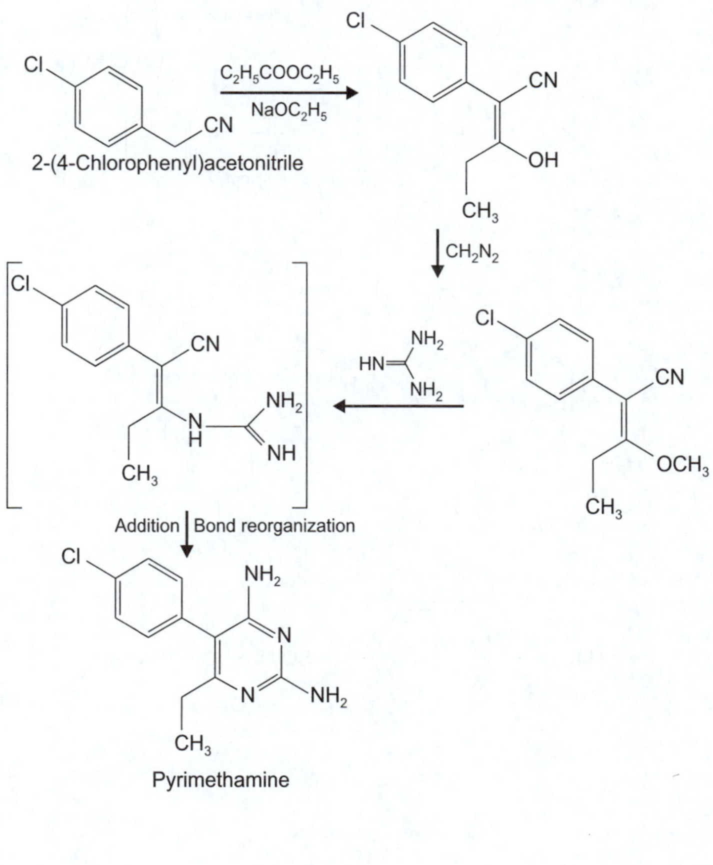

Properties and uses: Pyrimethamine is a white crystalline powder or colourless crystals, practically insoluble in water, and slightly soluble in alcohol. It is used in combination with sulphadoxine for the treatment of malaria.

Assay: Dissolve the sample in anhydrous acetic acid by heating gently. Cool and titrate with 0.1 M perchloric acid. Determine the end point potentiometrically.

Dosage forms: Pyrimethamine tablets IP, pyrimethamine tablets BP.

CLASSIFICATION BASED ON PCI SYLLABUS

Sulphamethizole

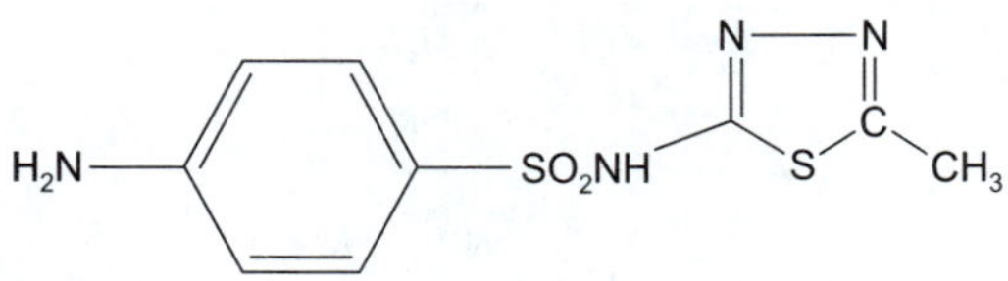

Sulfisoxazole

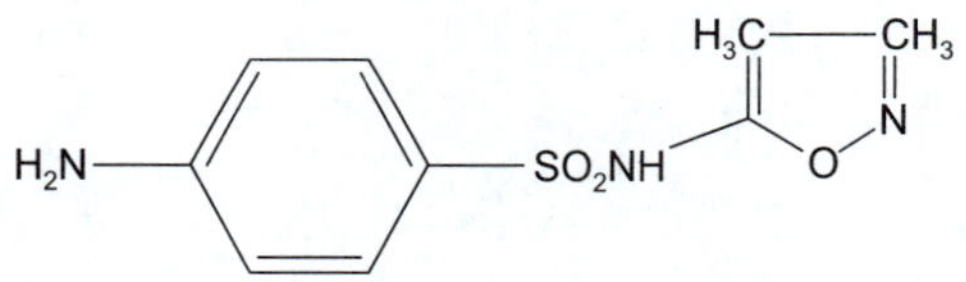

Sulphamethizine

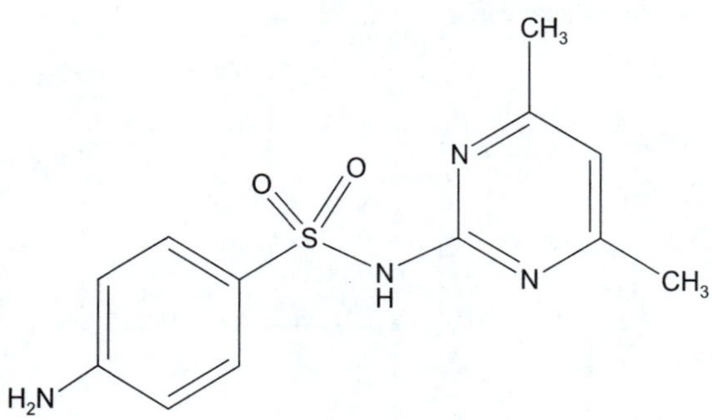

Sulfacetamide

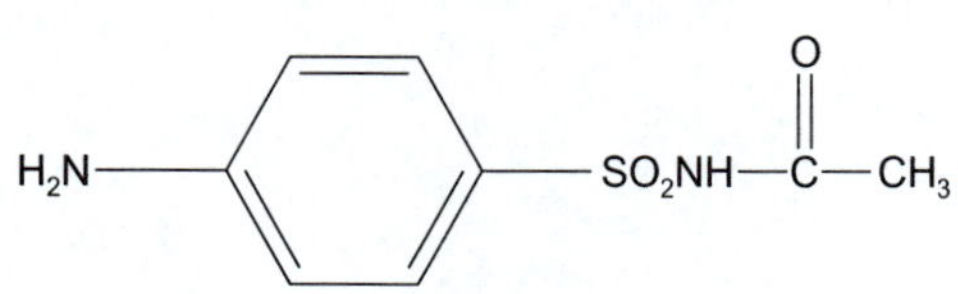

Sulphapyridine

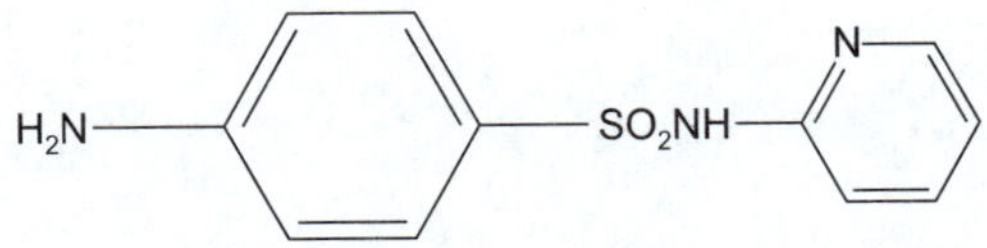

Sulfamethoxazole

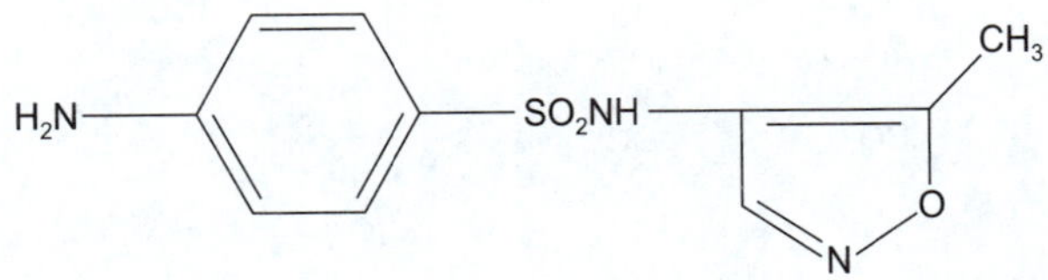

Sulphadiazine

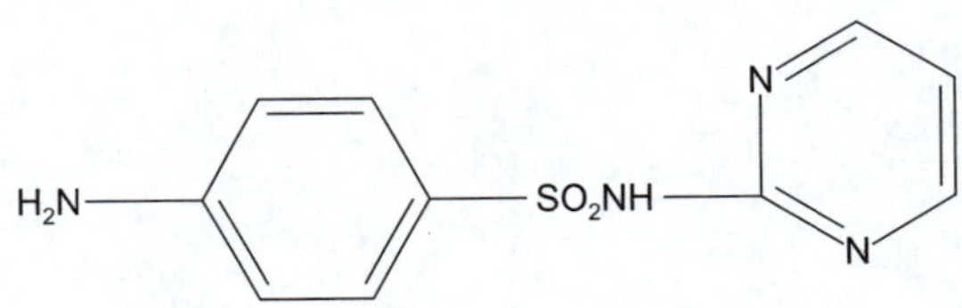

Mafenide acetate

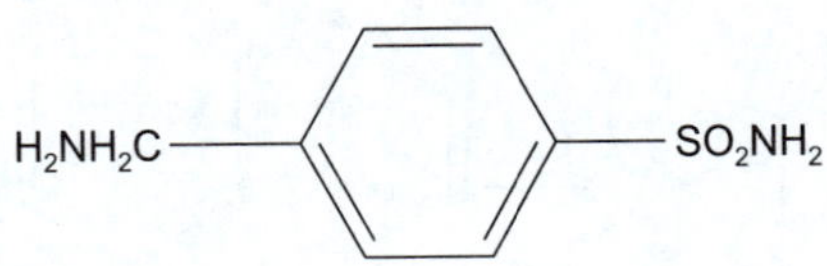

Sulfasalazine

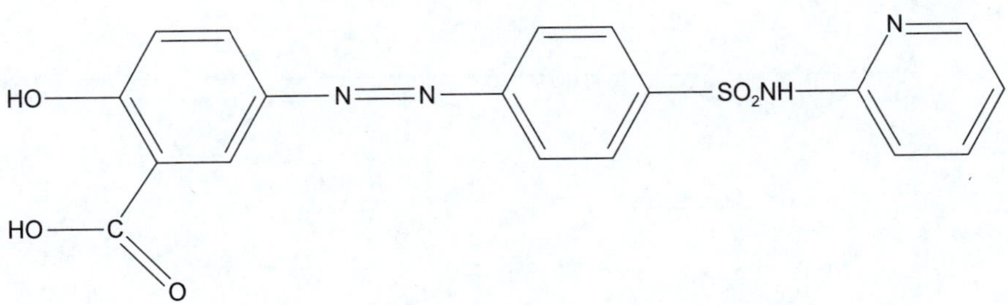

Folate Reductase Inhibitors

Trimethoprim

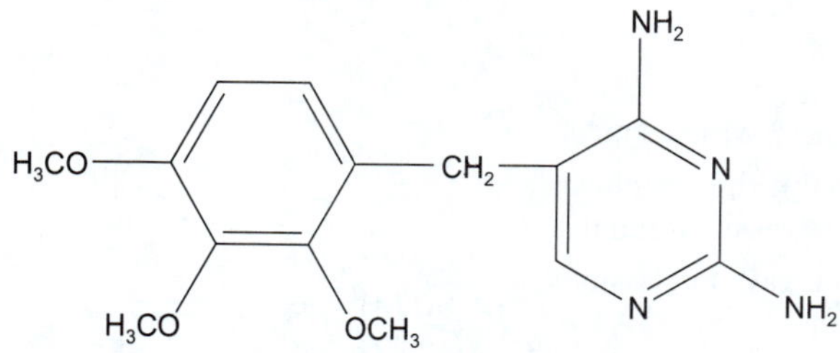

Cotrimoxazole

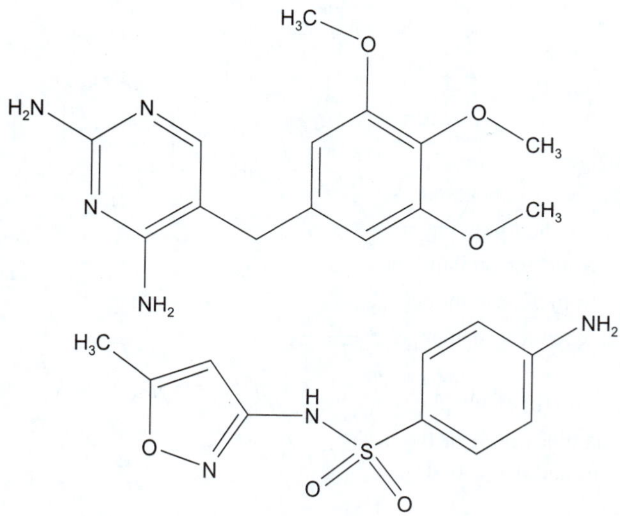

Sulfones

Dapsone

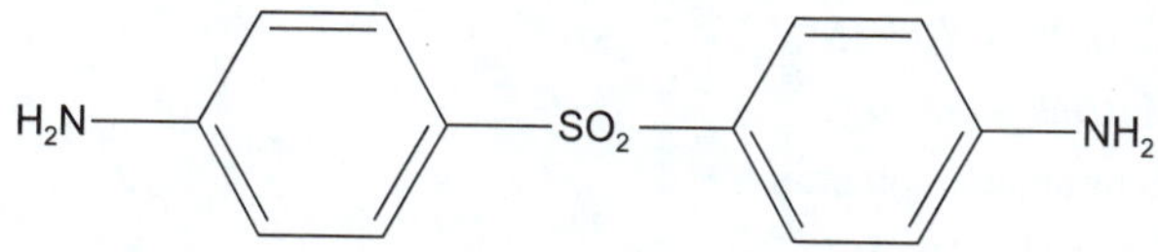

Mafenide acetate

Properties and uses: It is an acetate salt form of mafenide and a synthetic sulphonamide derivative of PABA. It competes with PABA and inhibits dihydropteroate synthase enzyme. By this way it inhibits the binding of PABA to dihydrofolic acid, hence inhibits normal folic acid metabolism. The DNA synthesis is inhibited due to lack of availability of folate metabolites for the synthesis of pyrimidines. It is a bactereostatic agent. It is used to treat infections produced by many kinds of gram-positive and gram-negative organisms such as *Pseudomonas* and some type of anaerobes.

PROBABLE QUESTIONS

1. What are sulphonamides? Write its mode of action and SAR.
2. Explain how an 'azo-dye' breaks down *in vivo* to yield sulphanilamide? N1-Substitution in sulphanilamide is more effective and useful than N4-substitution. Explain.
3. What are the different ways to classify sulphonamides and explain with suitable examples about the chemical classification.
4. Write the synthesis, metabolism, and uses of sulphasalazine and sulphaguanidine.
5. Name the sulphonamides used topically, write the synthesis, and uses of sulphacetamide.
6. How will you synthesize sulphanilamide from the following: (a) Nitrobenzene, (b) benzene, and (c) aniline.
7. Write the structure, synthesis, brand name, assay, dosage forms, and uses of the following:
   (a) Phthalyl sulphathiazole
   (b) Sulphadiazine
   (c) Sulphamethoxazole.
8. Name the poorly absorbed sulphonamides and write the synthesis and uses of any one of them.
9. How will you synthesize the following drugs, employed for urinary tract infections:
   (a) Sulphacetamide from sulphanilamide
   (b) Sulphadimidine from *p*-acetamidobenzene sulphonyl chloride
10. Write the structure, chemical name, synthesis, dose, dosage forms, and uses of the following sulphonamides:
    (a) Sulphaisoxazole and (b) sulphaphenazole.
11. Mention the sulphonamides used in the following and write the synthesis of any one among them. (a) Intestinal infections and (b) second- and third-degree burns.

SUGGESTED READINGS

1. Abraham DJ (ed). *Burger's Medicinal Chemistry and Drug Discovery* (6th edn). New Jersey: John Wiley, 2007.
2. *British Pharmacopoeia*. Medicines and Healthcare Products Regulatory Agency. London, 2008.
3. Bruntan LL, Lazo JS, and Parker KL. *Goodman and Gilman's: The Pharmacological Basis of Therapeutics* (11th edn). New York: McGraw Hill, 2006.
4. Busch H and Lane M. *Chemotherapy*. Chicago: Yearbook Medical, 1967.
5. Goldstein A. 'Antibacterial chemotherapy'. *New England J Med.* 240: 258–61, 1949.
6. Hawking F and Lawrence JS. *The Sulfonamides*. New York: Grune and Stratton, 1961.
7. *Indian Pharmacopoeia*. Ministry of Health and Family Welfare. New Delhi, 1996.
8. Lemke TL and William DA. *Foye's Principle of Medicinal Chemistry* (6th edn.). New York: Lippincott Williams and Wilkins, 2008.
9. Lednicer D and Mitscher LA. *The Organic Chemistry of Drug Synthesis*. New York: Wiley, 1995.
10. Northey EN. 'The sulfonamides and allied compounds'. In *American Chemical Society Monograph Series*, WA Hamor (ed), pp. 46–47. New York: Reinhold Publishing, 1948.

11. Gennaro AR. *Remington: The Science and Practice of Pharmacy* (21st edn). New York: Lippincot Williams and Wilkins, 2006.
12. Reynolds EF. (ed). *Martindale the Extra Pharmacopoeia* (31st edn). London: The Pharmaceutical Press, 1997.
13. Seydel JK. Molecular basis for the action of chemotherapeutic drugs, structure-activity studies of sulfonamides *Proc. III International Pharmacology Congress*. New York: Pergamon, 1966.
14. Schuler FW (ed). *Molecular Modification in Drug Design: Advances in Chemistry.* Series No. 45. Washington, DC: American Chemical Society, 1964.

CHAPTER 14

Quinolone Antibacterials

INTRODUCTION

Quinolones constitute a large class of synthetic antimicrobial agents that are highly effective in the treatment of many types of infectious diseases, particularly those caused by bacteria. Quinolones are potent, broad-spectrum antibacterial agents. The early congeners (non-fluorinated at C-6 position, such as nalidixic acid) were limited to certain gram-negative infections, such as urinary tract infections. However, the modern generation of fluoroquinolones, containing C-6 fluoro substituent and a cyclic basic amine moiety at C-7 position, surpass their predecessors in terms of spectrum of activity and potency. This has allowed for their use against a variety of gram-negative as well as some gram-positive pathogens.

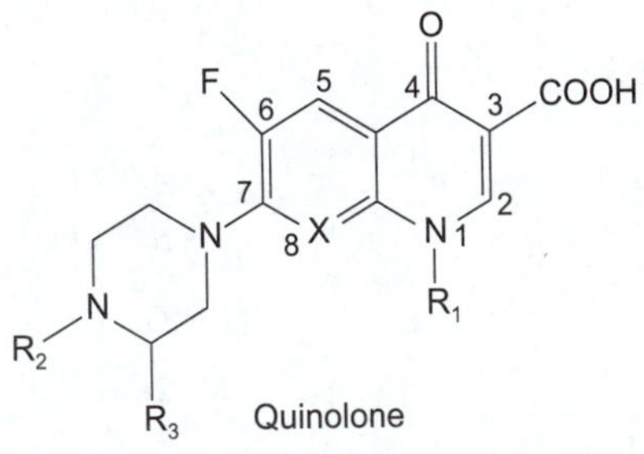

Quinolone

Many analogues have piperazino groups on C-7 because of which they broaden the spectrum, especially to gram-negative organisms, such as *Pseudomonas aeruginosa*, however, they also increase the affinity of the compound for the gamma-aminobutyric acid (GABA) receptor, which contributes to central nervous system (CNS) side effects. Quinolones are easily prepared and administered via parenteral and oral routes, and are well tolerated.

Mode of action: Quinolones inhibit the action of bacterial DNA gyrase enzyme. This enzyme is responsible for supercoiling and compacting bacterial DNA molecules into the bacterial cell during replication. This action is accomplished by modifying the topology of DNA via supercoiling and twisting of these macromolecules to permit DNA replication or transcription.

EFFECTIVE ANTIBACTERIAL QUINOLONE DERIVATIVES

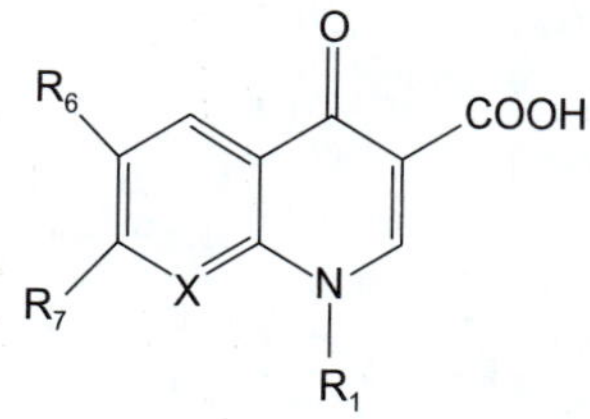

Name	*X*	R_6	R_1	R_7
Nalidixic acid	–N	–H	$-CH_2CH_3$	$-CH_3$
Enoxacin	–N	–F	$-CH_2CH_3$	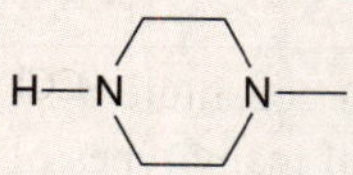
Pipemidic acid	–N	–H	$-CH_2CH_3$	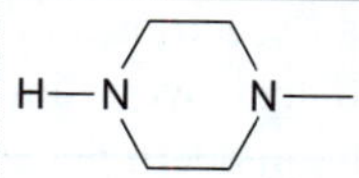
Norfloxacin	–CH	–F	$-CH_2CH_3$	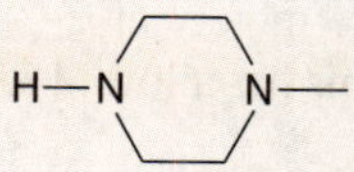
Pefloxacin	–CH	–F	$-CH_2CH_3$	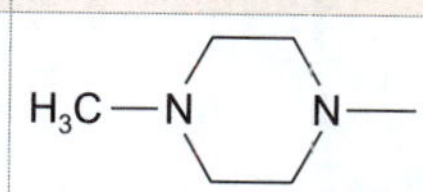
Ciprofloxacin	–CH	–F	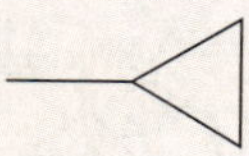	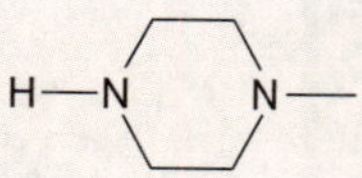
Amifloxacin	–CH	–F	$-NHCH_3$	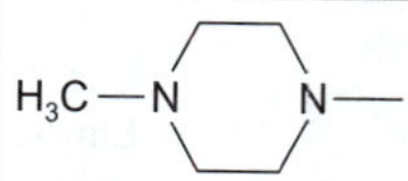
Sparfloxacin	–CF	–F	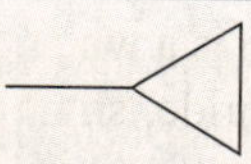	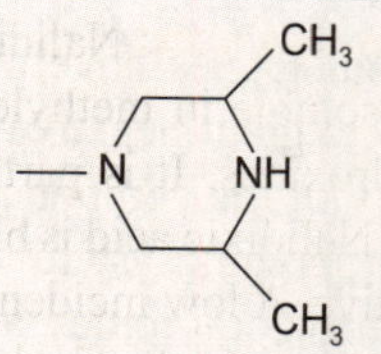
Lomefloxacin	–CF	–F	$-C_2H_5$	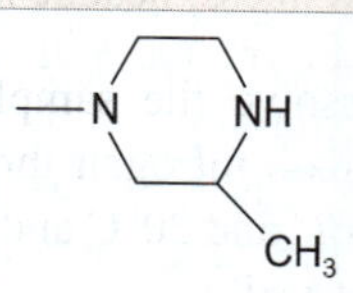
Fleroxacin	–CF	–F	$-CH_2CH_2F$	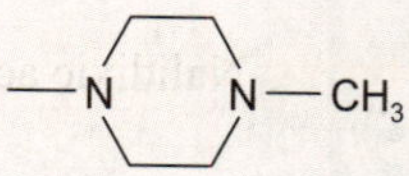

Contd.

Contd.

Name	**X**	R_6	R_1	R_7
Tefloxacin	–CH	–F	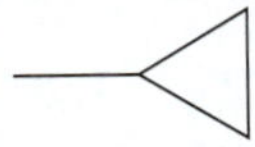	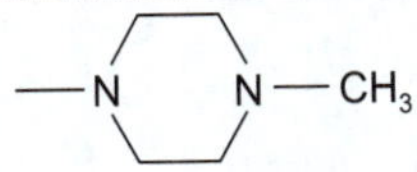
Gatifloxacin	$-COCH_3$	–F	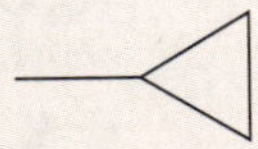	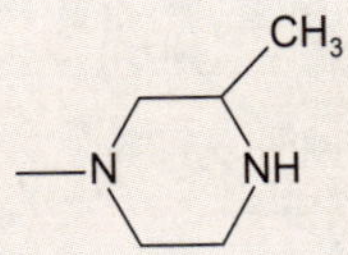
Clinafloxacin	–CCl	–F	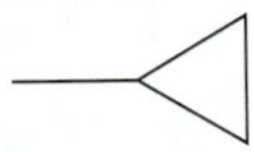	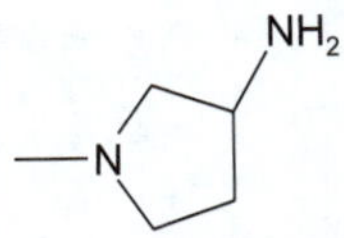
Sitafloxacin	–CCl	–F	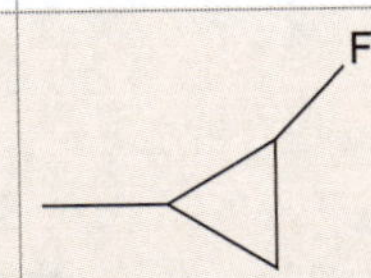	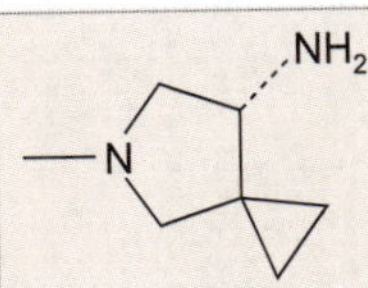

SYNTHESIS AND DRUG PROFILE

i Nalidixic acid

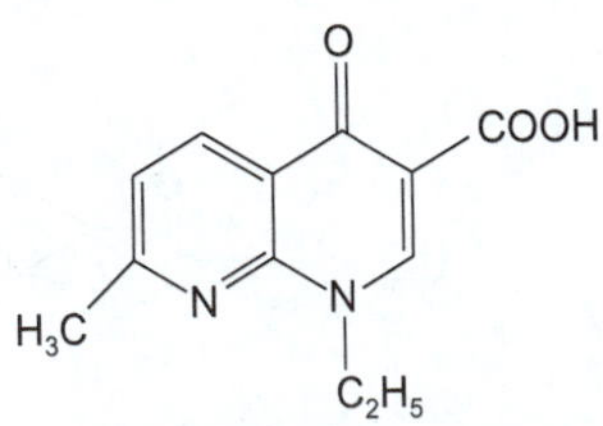

1-Ethyl-1,4-dihydro-7-methyl-4-oxo-1,8-naphthyridine-3-carboxylic acid

Properties and uses: Nalidixic acid is a white or pale yellow crystalline powder, practically insoluble in water, soluble in methylene chloride, slightly soluble in acetone, alcohol, and dilute solutions of alkali hydroxides. It is particularly effective against gram-negative bacteria that cause urinary tract infection. Nalidixic acid is biotransformed into hydroxy methyl derivative at the 7-methyl group, which is also active. A low incidence of adverse effects observed includes gastrointestinal (GI) disturbances, rashes, drowsiness, headache, and visual disturbances.

Assay: Dissolve the sample in methylene chloride and add 2-propanol and carbon dioxide-free water and pass nitrogen through the solution throughout the titration by maintaining a temperature between 15°C and 20°C and titrate against 0.1 M ethanolic sodium hydroxide. Determine the end point potentiometrically.

Dosage forms: Nalidixic acid oral suspension BP, nalidixic acid tablets BP.

Synthesis

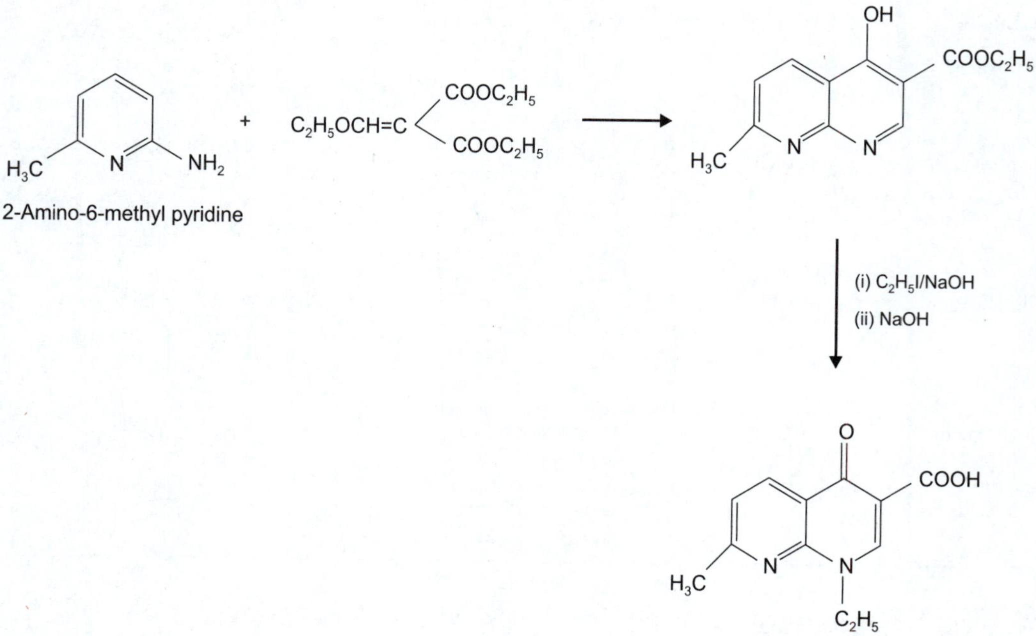

Nalidixic acid

ii. Fluoroquinolones

General Synthesis

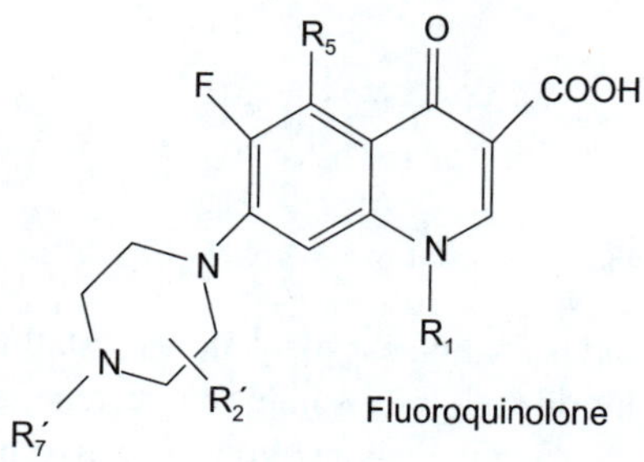

Fluoroquinolone

Synthesis

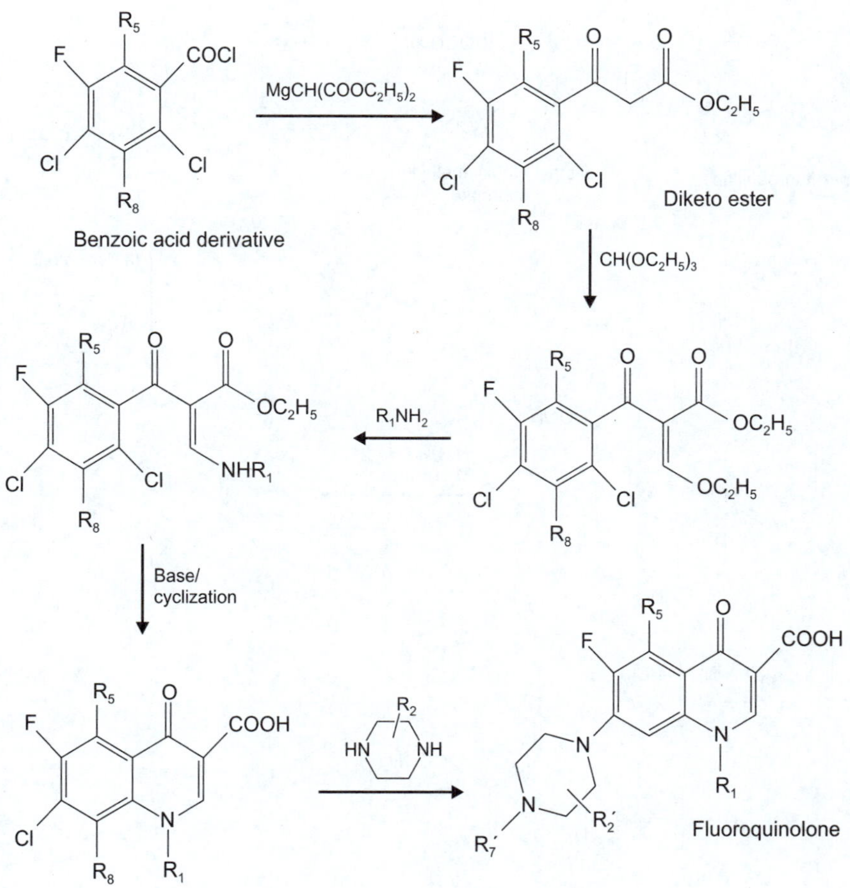
MgCH(COOC2H5)2
Benzoic acid derivative
Diketo ester
CH(OC2H5)3
R1NH2
Base/
cyclization
Fluoroquinolone

iii. Norfloxacin

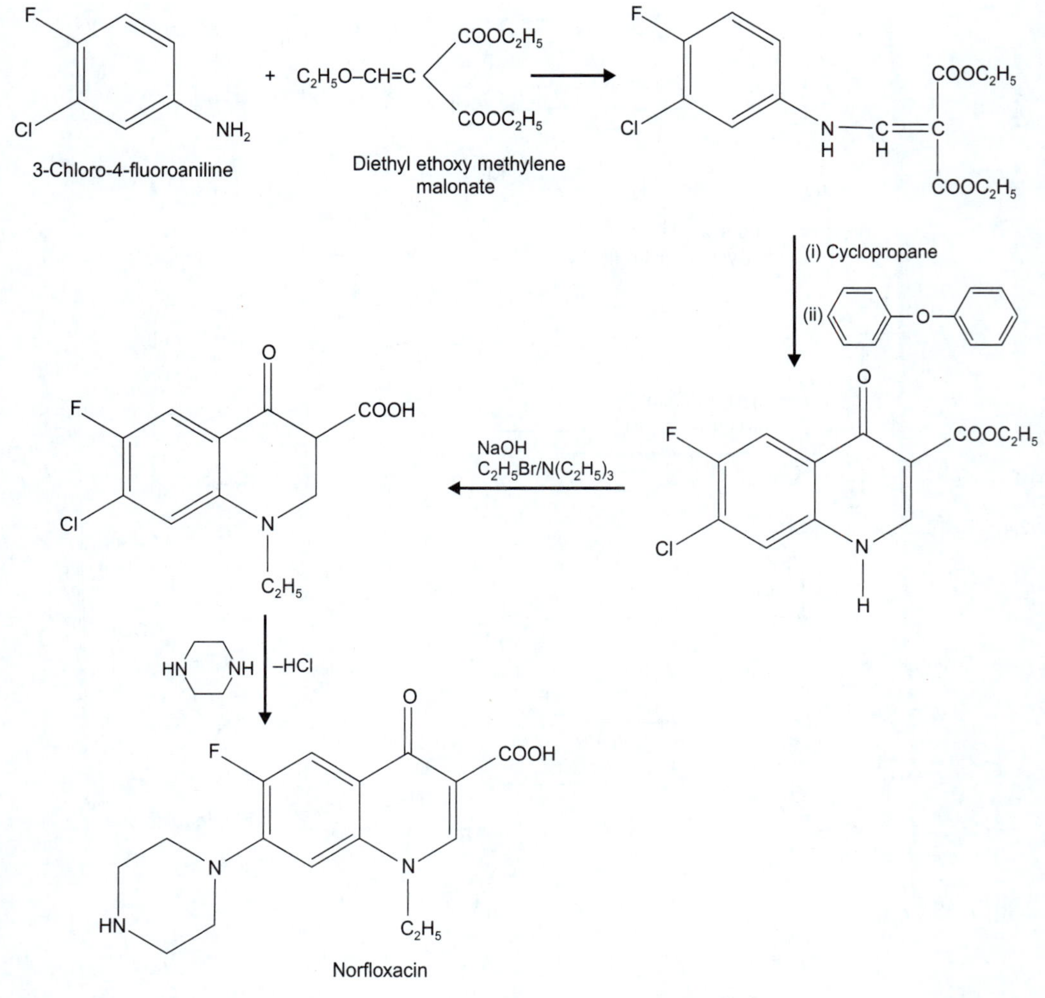

Properties and uses: It is a pale or white, hygroscopic, photosensitive, crystalline powder, which is very slightly soluble in water and slightly soluble in alcohol and acetone. It is used as urinary antiseptic. It is also used to treat typhoid fever and acute gastroenteritis.

Dose: For urinary tract infection 400 mg twice daily for 7–10 days. It should not be given to children or pregnant women.

Assay: Dissolve the sample in anhydrous acetic acid, titrate with 0.1 M perchloric acid, and determine the end point potentiometrically.

iv. Ciprofloxacin

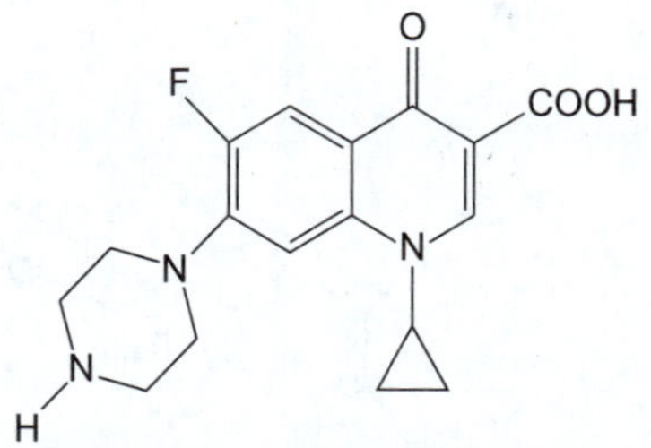

1-Cyclopropyl-6-fluoro-1,4-dihydro-4-oxo-7-piperazine

Synthesis

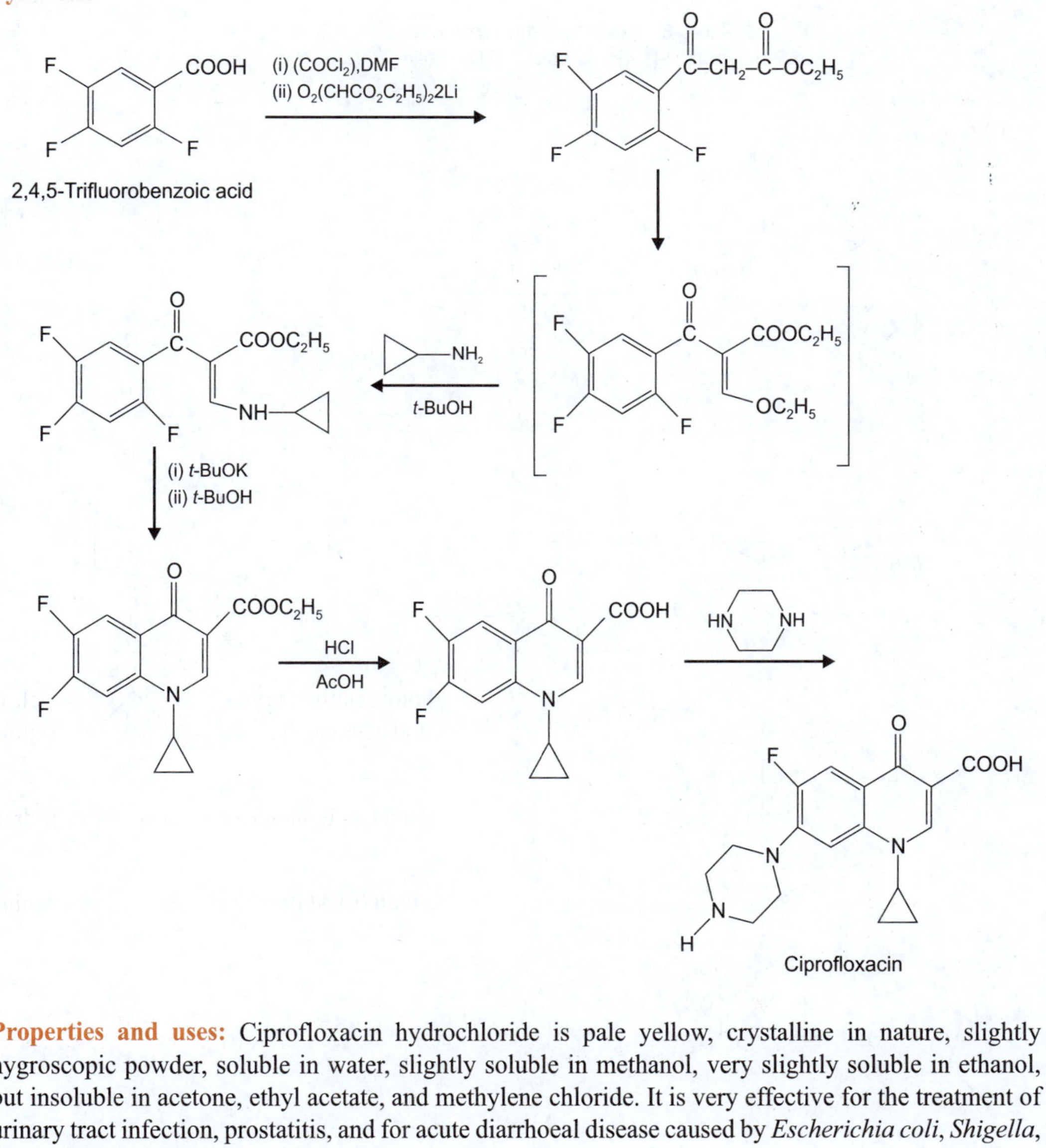

Properties and uses: Ciprofloxacin hydrochloride is pale yellow, crystalline in nature, slightly hygroscopic powder, soluble in water, slightly soluble in methanol, very slightly soluble in ethanol, but insoluble in acetone, ethyl acetate, and methylene chloride. It is very effective for the treatment of urinary tract infection, prostatitis, and for acute diarrhoeal disease caused by *Escherichia coli*, *Shigella*, *Salmonella*, and *Campylobacter*.

Assay: It is assayed by adopting liquid chromatography technique.

Dosage forms: Ciprofloxacin tablets BP.

v. Ofloxacin

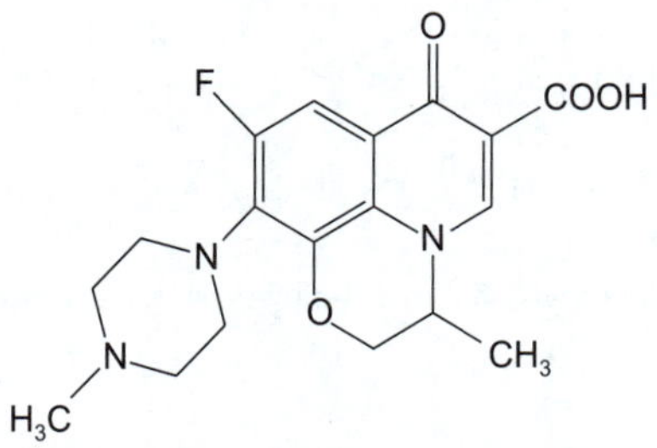

9-Fluoro-3-methyl-10-(4-methylpiperazin-1-yl)-7-oxo-3,7-dihydro-2H-[1,4]oxazino[2,3,4-ij]quinoline-6-carboxylic acid

Synthesis

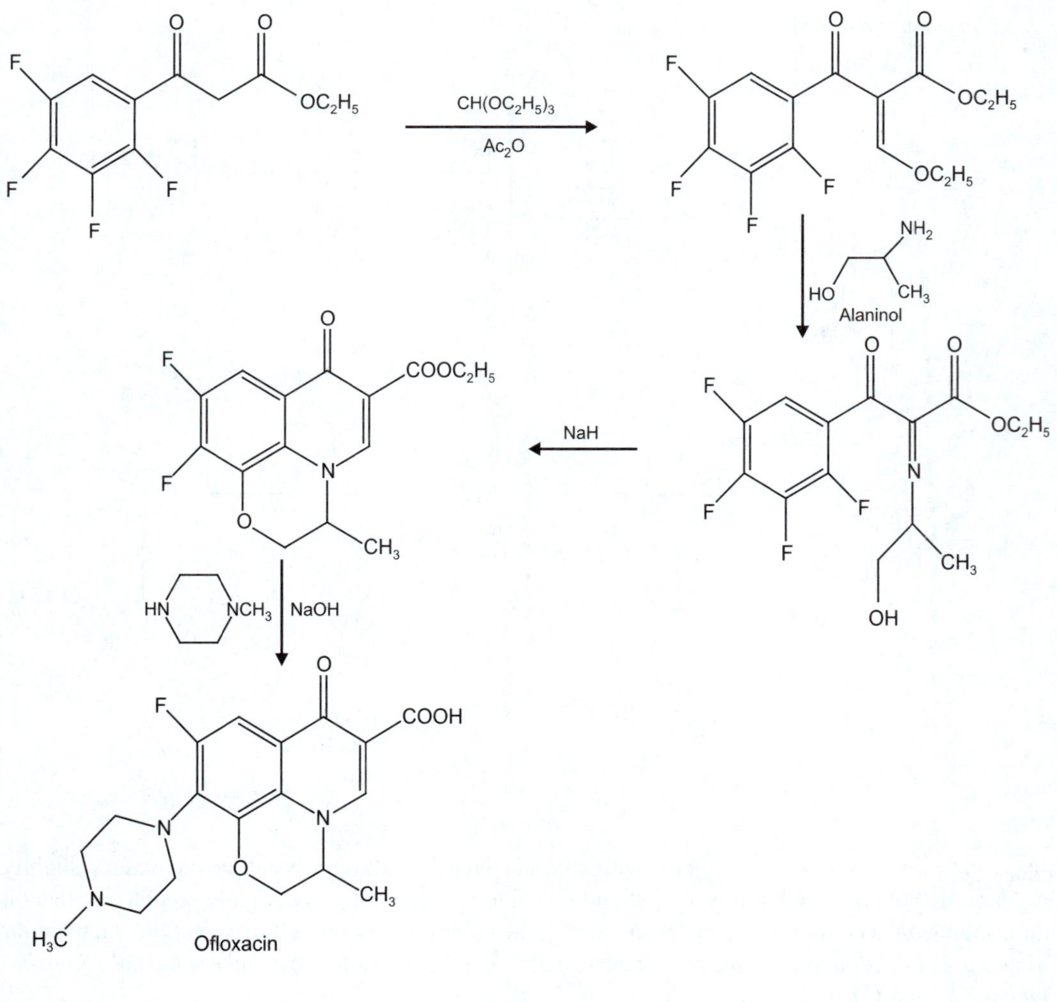

Properties and uses: Ofloxacin is a pale yellow or bright yellow crystalline powder, slightly soluble in water and methanol, and soluble in glacial acetic acid and methylene chloride. It is one of the most promising newer members of the fluoroquionolone family. In this product, N-ethyl moiety has been made rigid by incorporation into a heterocyclic ring. It is useful in the treatment of genitourinary, respiratory, gastrointestinal, skin, soft tissue infections, peridonitis, and gonorrhoea.

Assay: Dissolve the sample in anhydrous acetic acid and titrate against 0.1M per chloric acid. Determine the end point potentiometrically.

vi. Pefloxacin

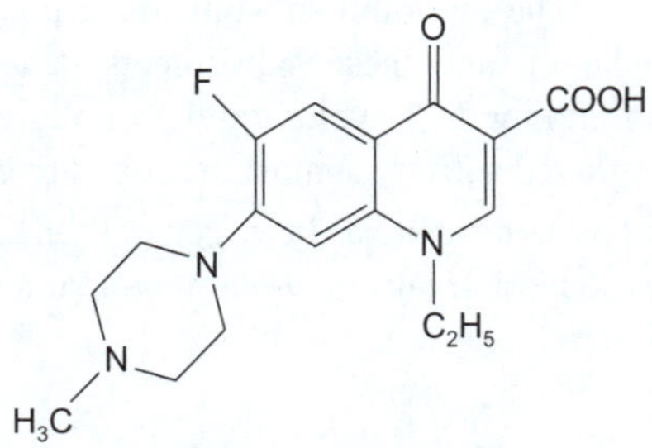

1-Ethyl-6-fluoro-7-(4-methylpiperazin-1-yl)-4-oxo-1,4-dihydroquinoline-3-carboxylic acid

Synthesis

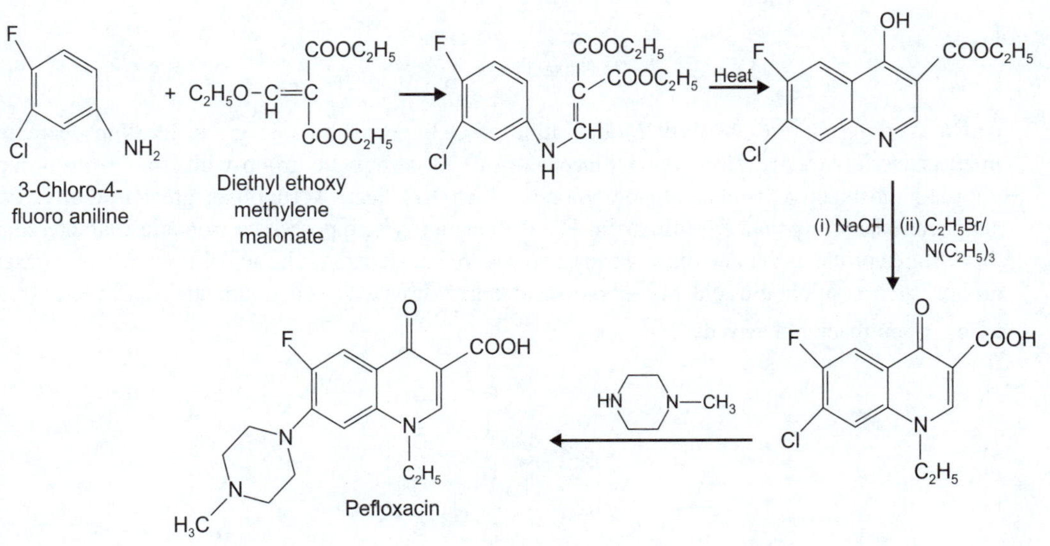

Properties and uses: Pefloxacin mesilate is a white powder, soluble in water, slightly soluble in alcohol, and very slightly soluble in methylene chloride, used as an antibacterial agent.

Assay: Dissolve the sample in anhydrous acetic acid, add acetic anhydride, and titrate against 0.1 M per chloric acid. Determine the end point potentiometrically.

SAR of Quinolones

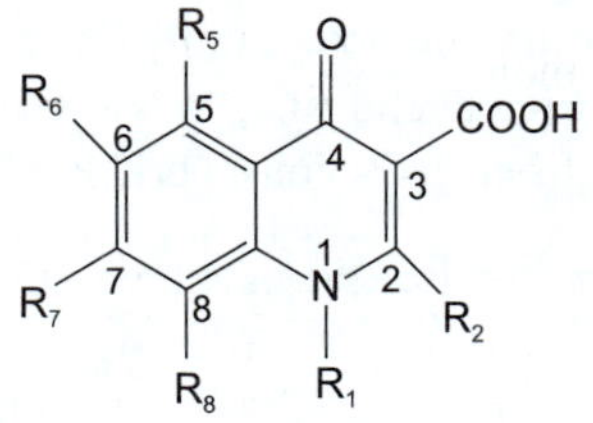

1. **Substituent at N-1 position:** The optimum substituents at position 1 appear to be ethyl, butyl, cyclopropyl, and difluorophenyl, and these substituents have resulted in potent compounds. Addition of a fluorine atom into the N-1 cyclopropyl group or the 1-butyl substituent resulted in compounds with overall improved activity against gram-positive bacteria.
2. The simple replacement of C-2 hydrogen has been generally disadvantageous (e.g. C-2 methyl or hydroxy groups); however, some derivatives containing a suitable C-1, C-2 ring have shown to possess notable activity.

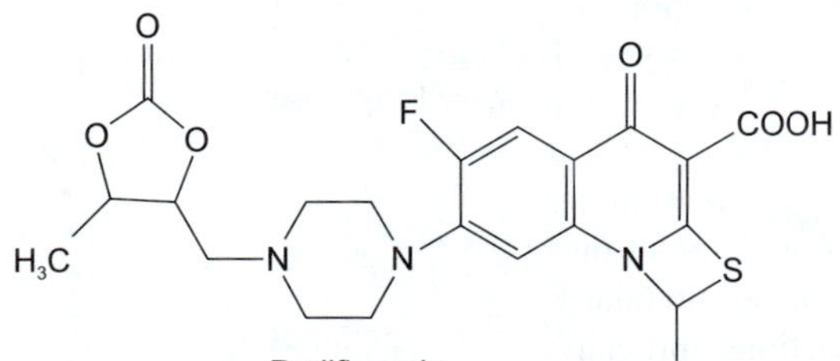

Prulifloxacin

3. **Carboxy functions at position:** Modification of C-3 carboxylic acid group leads to decrease in antibacterial activity. However, replacement of C-3 carboxylic group with isothiazolo group afforded most active isothiazolo quinolone, which has been 4–10 times greater in *in vitro* antibacterial activity than ciprofloxacin. The isothiazolo system possesses aromatic character and the nitrogen proton is very acidic and can be considered as an carboxylic acid mimic, whereas other groups, such as sulphonic acid, phosphonic acid, tetrazole as well as derivatization, as an ester lead to loss of antibacterial activity.

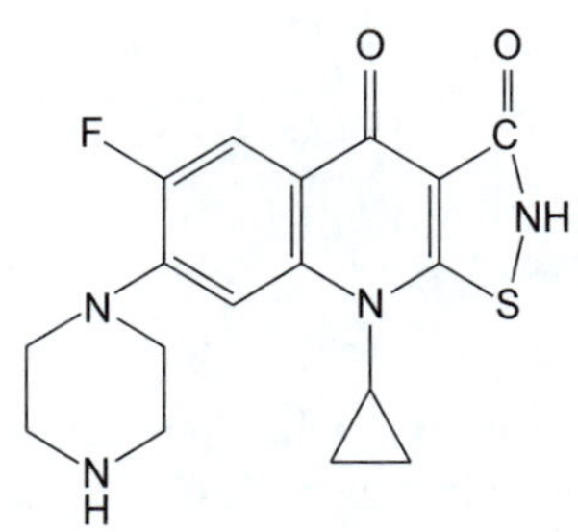

4. The C-4 oxo group of the quinolone nucleus appears to be essential for antibacterial activity. Replacement with 4-thioxo or sulphonyl group leads to loss of activity.
5. The incorporation of a group at the C-5 position has proven beneficial in terms of antibacterial activity. The order of activity is NH_2: CH_3>F, H>OH, or SH, SR.

6. The incorporation of a fluorine atom at the C-6 position of the quinolone is monumental. The order of activity is F > Cl, Br, CH_3 > CN.
7. The introduction of a piperazine moiety at the C-7 position is essential. Other aminopyrrolidines also are compatible for activity.

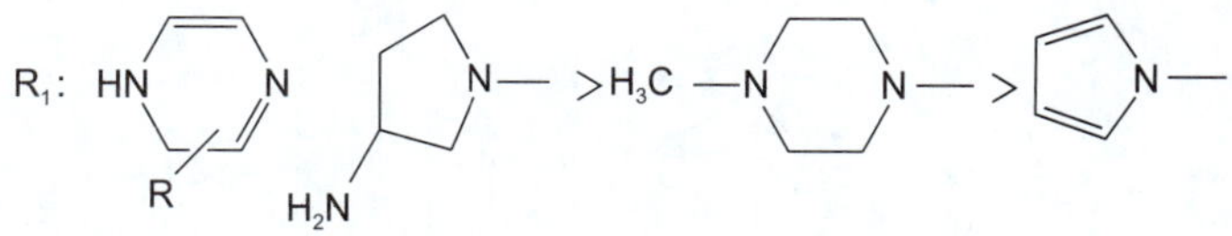

8. In general, a C-8 fluoro substituent offers good potency against gram-negative pathogens, while a C-8 methoxy moiety is active against gram-positive bacteria. The order of activity is F, Cl, OCH_3>H, CF_3>methyl, vinyl, propargyl.
9. A halogen (F or Cl) at the C-8 position improves oral absorption.
10. Linking of N-1 group to the C-8 position with oxazine ring leads to active oflaxacin.

Uses: Fluoroquinolones are used to treat upper and lower respiratory infections, gonorrhoea, bacterial gastroenteritis, skin soft tissue infections, urinary tract infections, bone and joint infections, and against tuberculosis.

Adverse Effects

The most common adverse reactions are nausea, headache, and dizziness. Some CNS problems, such as hallucination, insomnia, and visual disturbances can occur. Some side effects of the quinolones are class effects and cannot be modulated by molecular variation. Most of the fluoroquionolones produce photosensitive reactions and cause convulsions particularly in concurrent administration of NSAID fenopofen. Increasing steric bulk through alkylation ameliorates these effects. Phototoxicity is determined by the nature of the 8-position substituent with halogen causing the greatest photoreaction while hydrogen and methoxy show little light-produced toxicity. These drugs are not recommended for use in prepubertal children or pregnant women.

CLASSIFICATION BASED ON PCI SYLLABUS

Urinary Tract Anti-infective Agents

Quinolones

Nalidixic acid

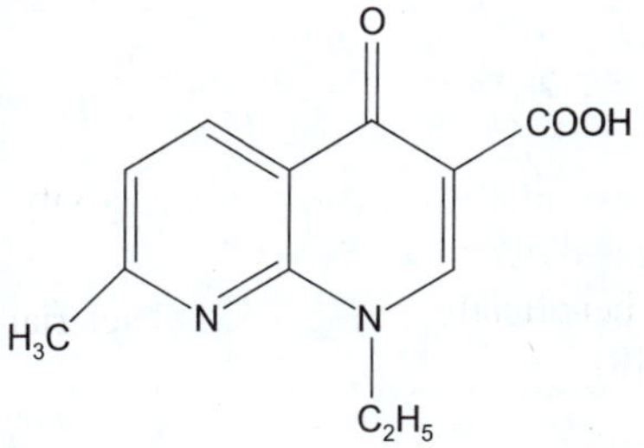

Norfloxacin

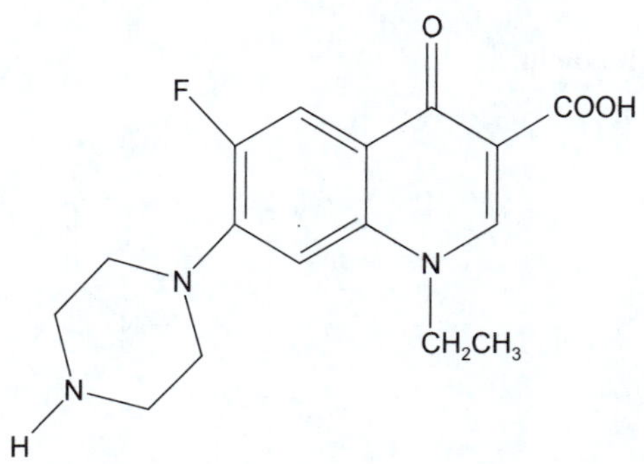

Enoxacin

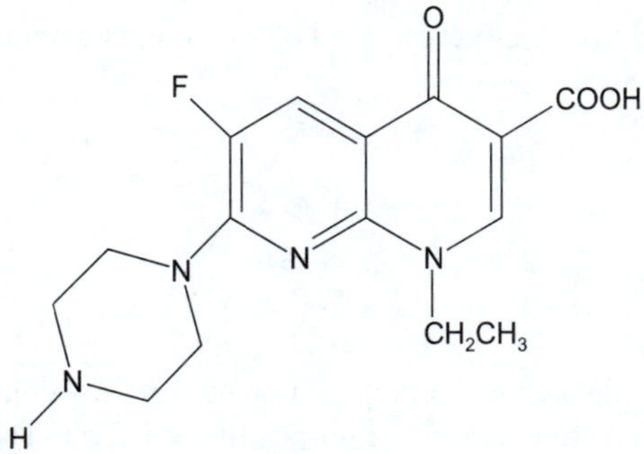

Ciprofloxacin

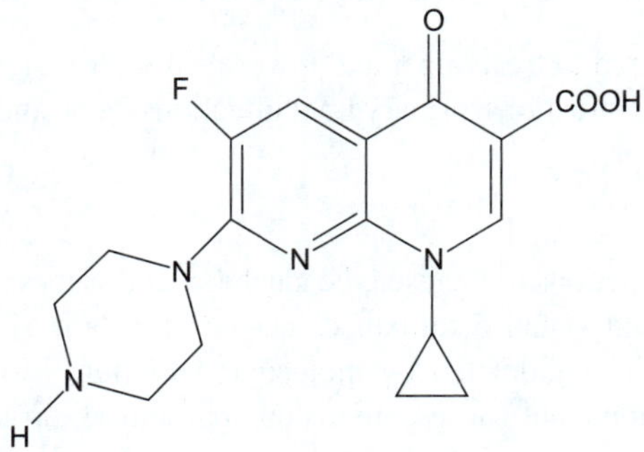

Ofloxacin

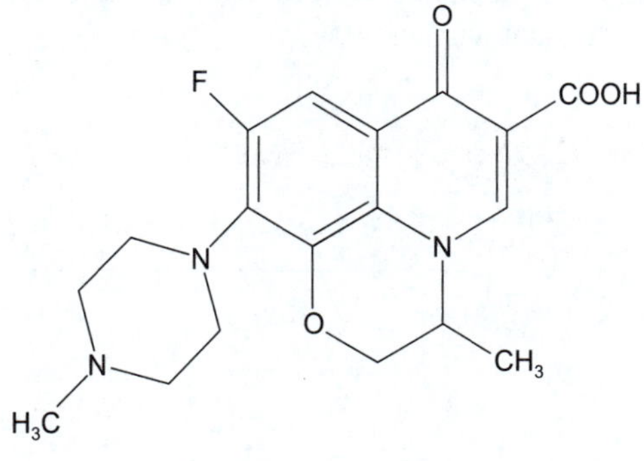

Lomefloxacin

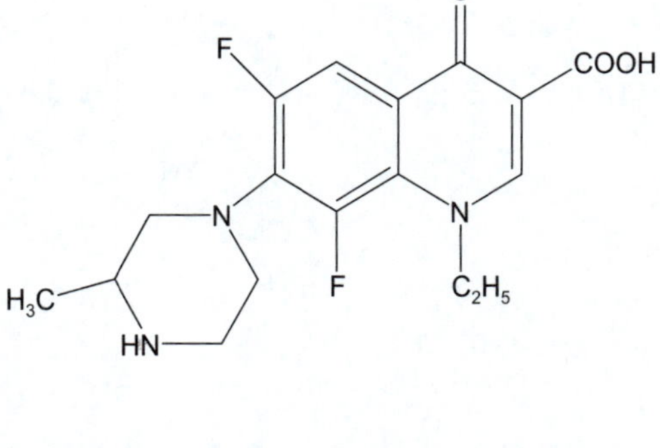

Sparfloxacin

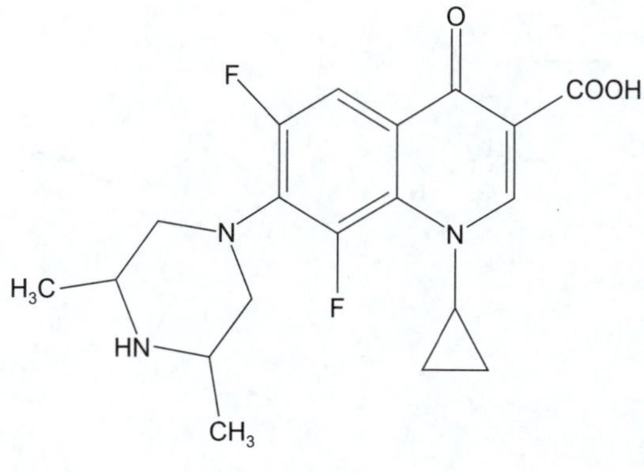

Gatifloxacin

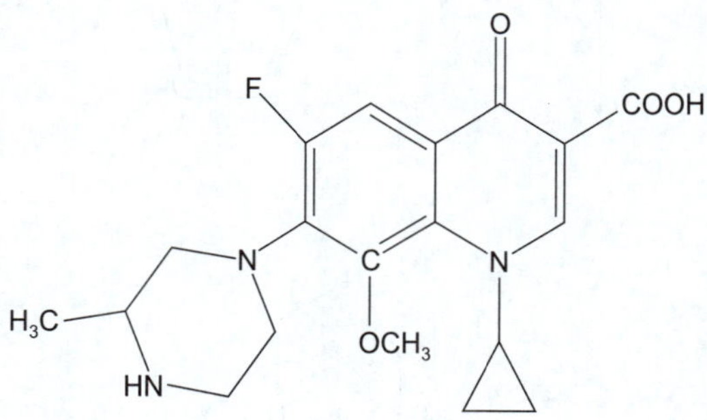

Moxifloxacin

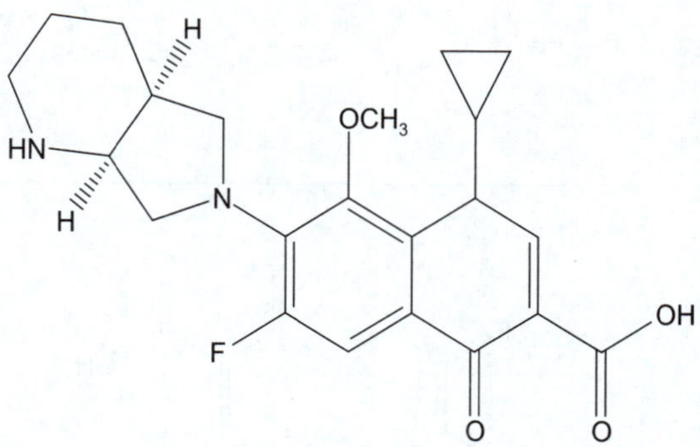

Miscellaneous

Furazolidine

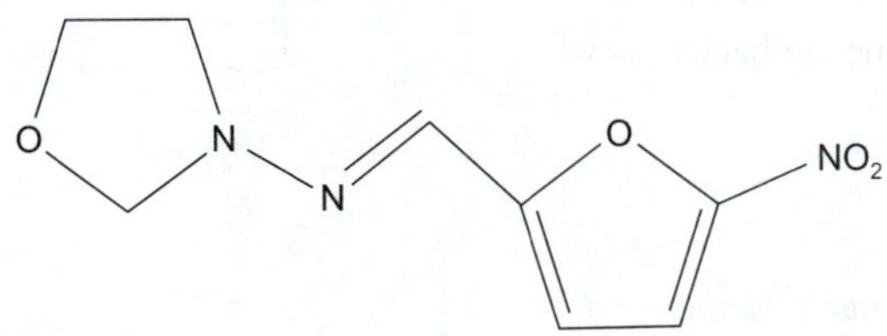

Nitrofurantoin

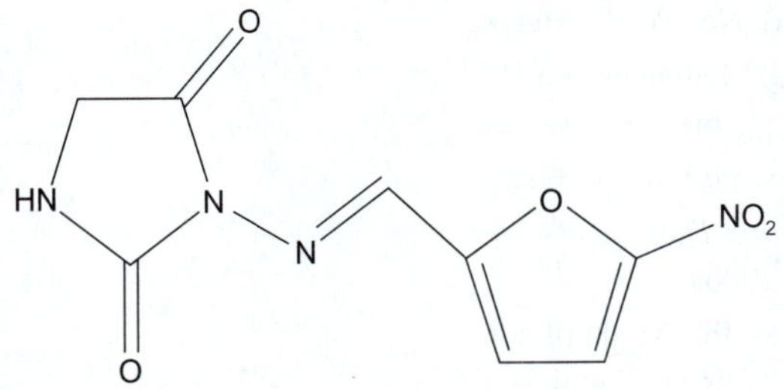

Methanamine

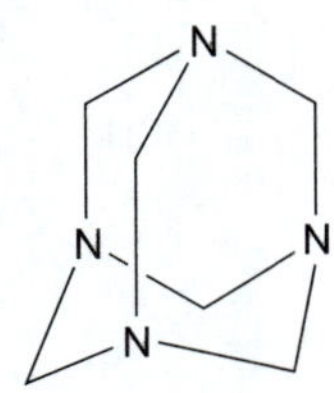

NEWER DRUGS

Delafloxacin

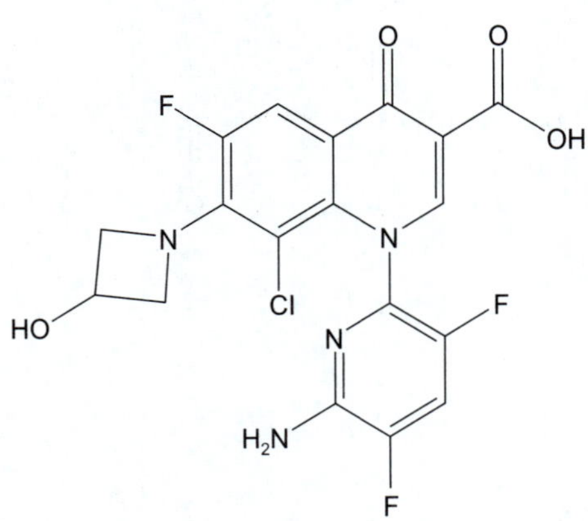

Uses: It is a fluoroquinolone antibiotic used to treat acute bacterial skin infections.

PROBABLE QUESTIONS

1. Draw the structure and number the quinolone nucleus. Mention the position of substituents introduced in quinolone antibacterials. Write the SAR of quinolone antibacterials.
2. Enumerate the quinolone antibacterials with their chemical structures and write the synthesis and uses of ciprofloxacin.

SUGGESTED READINGS

1. Abraham DJ (ed). *Burger's Medicinal Chemistry and Drug Discovery* (6th edn). New Jersey: John Wiley, 2007.
2. Bruntan LL, Lazo JS, and Parker KL. *Goodman and Gilman's: The Pharmacological Basis of Therapeutics* (11th edn). New York: McGraw Hill, 2006.
3. *British Pharmacopoeia*. Medicines and Healthcare Products Regulatory Agency. London, 2008.
4. Chu DTW and Fernandes PB. '*Recent developments in the field of quinolone antibacterial agents*', *in Advances in Drug Research* Vol. 21, Testa B (ed), pp. 39–144. New York: Academic Press, 1991.
5. Gennaro AR. *Remington: The Science and Practice of Pharmacy* (21st edn). New York: Lippincot Williams and Wilkins, 2006.
6. Hooper DC and Wolfson JS. 'Mode of action of the quinolone antimicrobial agents: Review of recent information'. *Rev Infect Dis* 11 (Suppl 5): S902, 1989.
7. *Indian Pharmacopoeia*. Ministry of Health and Family Welfare. New Delhi, 1996.
8. Lednicer D and Mitscher LA. *The Organic Chemistry of Drug Synthesis*. New York: John Wiley, 1995.
9. Lemke TL and William DA. *Foye's Principle of Medicinal Chemistry* (6th edn). New York: Lippincott Williams and Wilkins, 2008.
10. Siporin C, Hefetz CL, and Domagala JM (eds). *The New Generation of Quinolones*. New York: Marcel Dekker, 1990.
11. Suto MJ, Domagala JM, and Miller PF. '*Antibacterial agents, targets and approaches*', *in Annual Reports in Medicinal Chemistry*, Vol. 27, JA Bristol (ed), p. 119. San Diego, CA: Academic Press, 1992.
12. Rosen T. 'The fluoroquinolone antibacterial agents'. Progress in Med Chem 27:235–95, 1990.

CHAPTER 15

Antibiotics

INTRODUCTION

The term antibiotic has its origin in the word antibiosis (i.e. against life). Antibiotics are chemical substances obtained from various species of microorganisms (bacteria, fungi, actinomycetes) that suppress the growth of other microorganisms and eventually may destroy them. The probable points of difference amongst the antibiotics may be physical, chemical, pharmacological properties, antibacterial spectra, and mechanism of action. They have made it possible to cure diseases caused by bacteria, such as pneumonia, tuberculosis, and meningitis, and they save the lives of millions of people around the world.

CLASSIFICATION

Antibiotics are classified on the basis of their mechanism of action and by its chemical nature.

Classification Based on Mechanism of Action

1. **Agents that inhibit the synthesis of bacterial cell walls:** These include the penicillins and cephalosporins that are structurally similar and dissimilar agents, such as cycloserine, vancomycin, bacitracin and the imidazole antifungal agents.
2. **Agents that act directly on the cell membrane of the microorganisms, affecting permeability, and leading to leakage of intracellular compounds:** These include polymyxin, polyene antifungal agents, nystatin, and amphotericin B that bind to cell wall sterols.
3. **Agents that affect the function of 30s and 50s ribosomal subunits to cause reversible inhibition of protein synthesis:** These include tetracyclines, erythromycins, chloramphenicol, and clindamycin.
4. **Agents that bind to the 30s ribosomal subunit and alter protein synthesis:** These include aminoglycosides that leads to cell deaths eventually.
5. **Agents that affect nucleic acid metabolism:** Such as rifampicin, which inhibit DNA-dependent RNA polymerase.

CLASSIFICATION BASED ON CHEMICAL STRUCTURE

1. β-Lactam antibiotics
2. Aminoglycoside antibiotics
3. Tetracycline antibiotics

4. Polypeptide antibiotics
5. Macrolide antibiotics
6. Lincomycins
7. Other antibiotics

1. β-LACTAM ANTIBIOTICS

These consists of two major classes of agents, that is, penicillins and cephalosporins.

Penicillins

Penicillin, the most important of the antibiotics, was first extracted from the mould *Penicillium notatum*. Subsequently, a mutant of a related mould, *P. chrysogenum*, was found to give the highest yield of penicillin and is employed for the commercial production of this antibiotic. Penicillin belongs to a group of antibiotics called β-lactam antibiotics . The basic structure of the penicillins consists of a thiazolidine ring fused with a β-lactam ring, which is essential for antibacterial activity. These two rings constitute the fundamental nucleus of all the penicillins, namely, 6-amino penicillanic acid (6-APA). A variety of semisynthetic penicillins is produced by altering the composition of the side chain attached to 6-APA nucleus. Both the 6-APA nucleus and side chain are essential for the antibacterial activity.

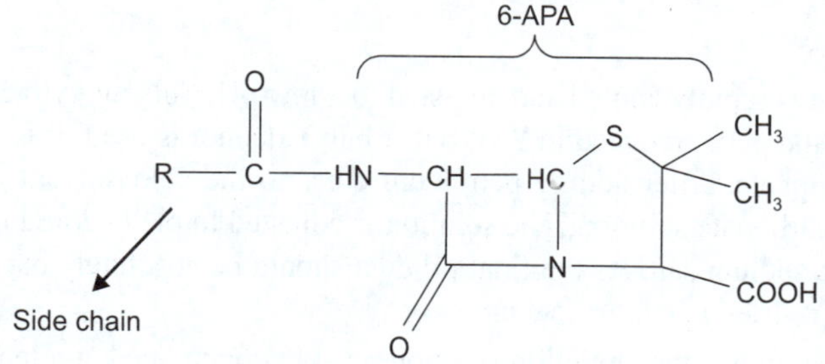

Basic structure of penicillin

Nomenclature: Penicillins are named in the following ways:

a. Chemical abstract

1. The penicillins are described as 4-thia-1-azabicyclo (3.2.0) heptanes.
2. Benzylpenicillin is 6-(2-phenylacetamido)-3, 3-dimethyl-7-oxo-4-thia-1-azabicyclo (3.2.0) heptane-2- carboxylic acid.

b. Penam: In order to simplify the unsubstituted bicylic ring system of penicillin, it is given the name penam. Accordingly, the penicillins are 6-acylamino-2,2-dimethyl penam-3-carboxylates.

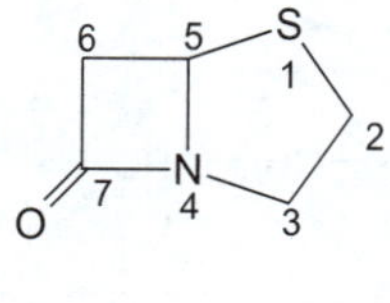

c. Pencillanic acid derivatives

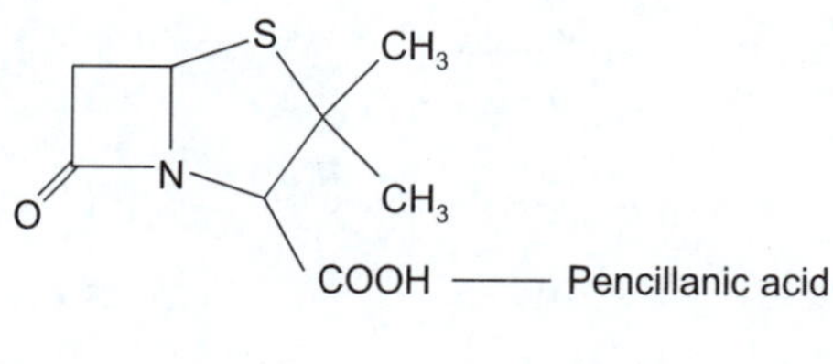

Production of Penicillins

The strains of *Pseudomonas* species are allowed to grow in a nutrient medium obtained from sugary materials (e.g. glucose, sucrose, lactose, maltose, starch) and proteinaceous substance. From this medium, penicillin may be produced by any of the following three methods:

1. **Surface culture method:** An aqueous solution of molasses adjusted to pH 7–8 used as a medium for the microorganism because the molasses under this condition contain sucrose, mineral salts and nitrogenous material almost ideally suited for mould growth. In a few days time, the growth of microorganism begins and after 6 or 7 days, the concentration of penicillin reaches up to 0.3–0.4 mg per cc.
2. **Bran method:** For mould growth, moist bran is a good substrate and the resultant penicillin can be extracted as in liquid production, or the penicillin-containing bran can be used directly. It is difficult to sterilize it, as the bran is a bad conductor of heat.
3. **Submerged culture method:** It is an exclusive method for the commercial production of penicillin. In this process, the inoculums are made into large tanks and the medium usually contains corn steep liquor as an adjuvant and lactose as sugar source. Under the conditions of agitation and aeration, the mould grows throughout the bulk of the liquid as globular pellicles consisting mainly of mycelium. Then temperature is maintained at about 24°C and the medium is agitated by a stream of sterile air.

Isolation of Penicillins

The metabolic solution is rapidly cooled and adjusted to a low pH. Solvent extraction then follows. If amyl alcohol is used, the pH is reduced to 2–3, but if butyl alcohol is used, it is adjusted to 6.4 after adding ammonium sulphate. After adding petroleum ether to the cold solvent extract, it is shaken with dilute sodium bicarbonate solution. The solution is adjusted to pH 6–7 and then rapidly freezed, evaporated to give the sodium salt. As the final product should be absolutely dry as well as pure, the sodium salt penicillin is dried in a high vacuum.

During all these operations, the penicillin solution must be maintained at a temperature just above its freezing point to avoid inactivation. Lastly, since most of the penicillin is administered by injection, the final sample must be non-toxic, sterilized and free from pyrogens for which the concentrated and purified solution of penicillin salt is passed through asbestos pads which absorb microorganisms and pyrogens.

Commercial penicillin consists of a mixture of benzyl, pentenyl and heptyl penicillins. By using certain chemical compounds in the culture medium, it is possible to increase the yield of the desired penicillin. For example, adding 2-phenylethylamine increases the yield of benzyl penicillin.

d. Classification

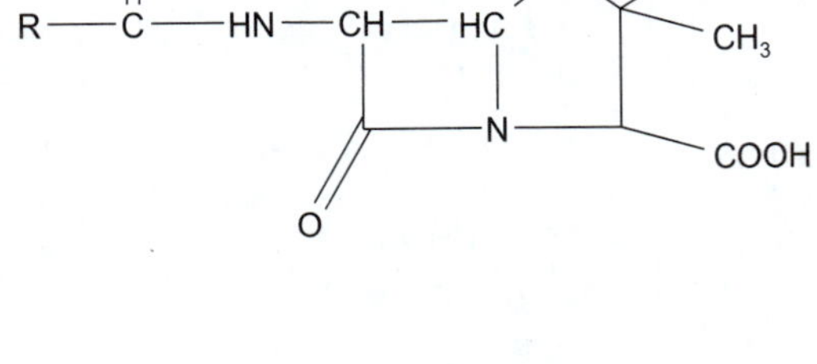

I. Penicillinase-susceptible penicillins

Name	Nature of substituent (R)
Penicillin G (benzyl penicillin)	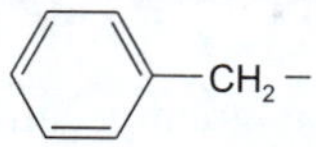
Penicillin V (phenoxy methyl penicillin)	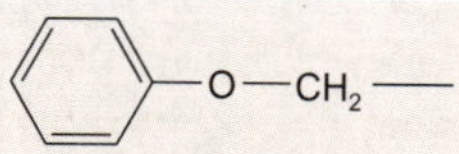
Phenethicillin	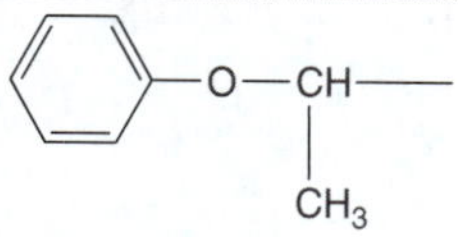

The general impact on antibacterial activity is as follows:

- Excellent gram-positive potency against susceptible staphylococci and streptococci
- Useful against some gram-positive cocci
- Good oral absorption, but relatively acid-labile
- Ineffective against gram-negative bacilli
- Susceptible to deactivation by penicillinase

II. Penicillinase-resistant penicillins

Name	R
(i) Methicillin	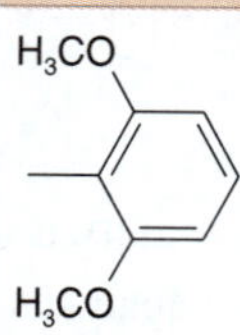
(ii) Oxacillin (R′ = R″ = H)	
(iii) Cloxacillin (R′ = H, R″ = Cl)	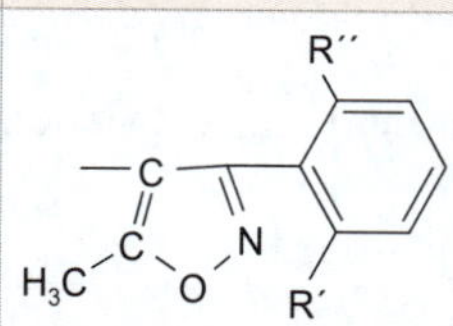
(iv) Dicloxacillin (R′ =, R″ = Cl)	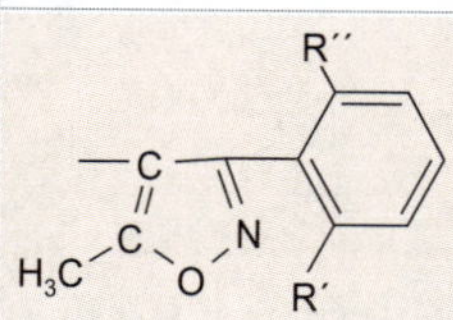
(v) Floxacillin (R′ = F, R″ = Cl)	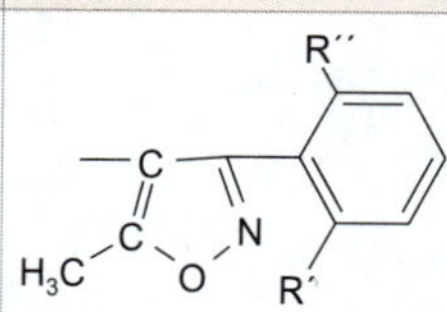
(vi) Nafcillin	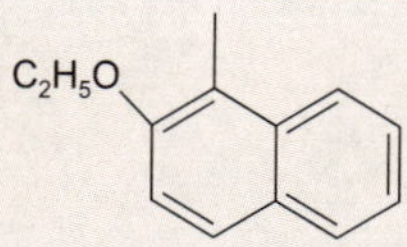

General impact on antibacterial activity is as follows:

- Diminished susceptibility to many penicillinase.
- Active against microrganisms, resistant to early penicillin.
- Oxacillins offer good oral activity.
- Inadequate spectrum against many gram-negative species.

III. Aminopenicillins

Name	*R*
Ampicillin	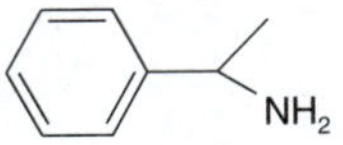
Amoxicillin	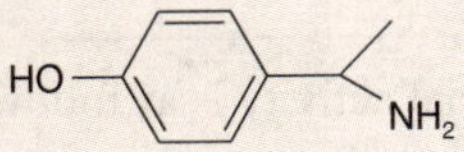
Bacampicillin	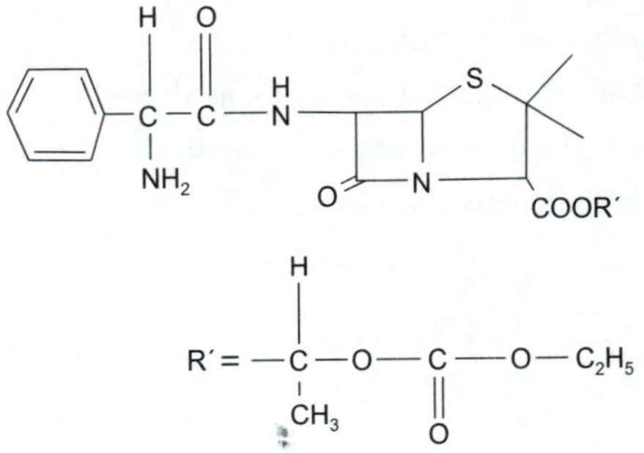

General impact on antibacterial activity is as follows:

- Extended spectrum of activity against some gram-negative bacteria and retention of gram-positive potency
- Ineffective against *Pseudomonas aeruginosa*

IV. Antipseudomonal penicillins (Carboxy penicillins)

Name	*R*
Carbenicillin (R′ = H)	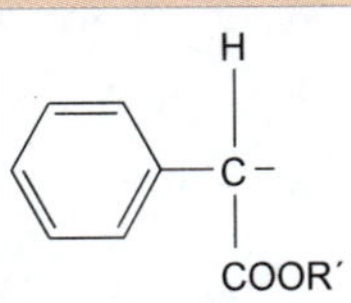
Indanyl carbenicillin (R″ = 5-indanol)	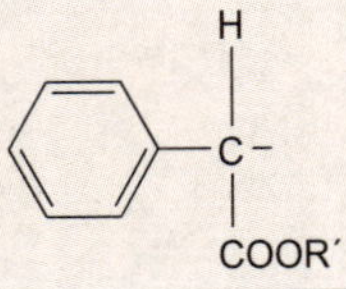
Ticarcillin	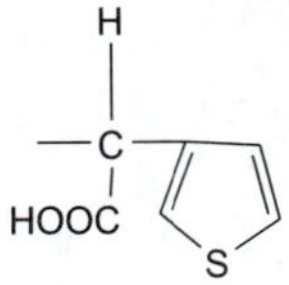

V. Ureidopenicillins

Name	R
Aziocillin	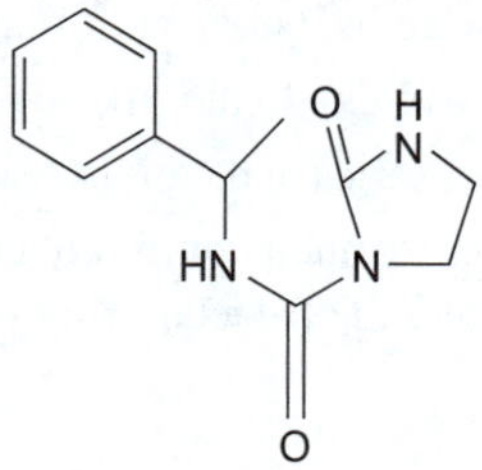
Piperacillin	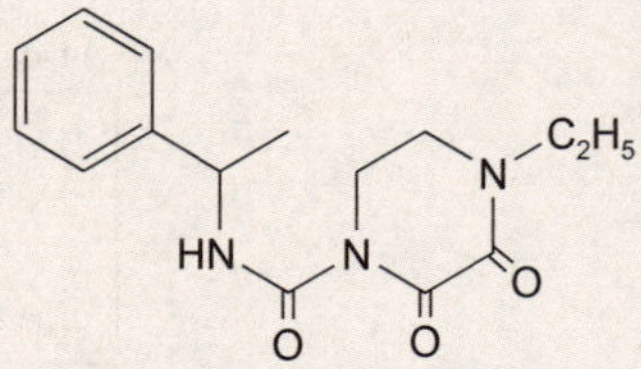

General impact on antibacterial activity is as follows:

- Enhanced spectrum of activity against *P. aeruginosa* and expanded activity against *Klebsiella*.
- Good potency against gram-positive bacteria, but generally not effective against penicillinase producers.
- Good pharmacokinetic profile.
- Good activity against *Escherichia coli*, *Klebsiella*, *Shigella*, *Salmonella*, and many other resistant species.

VI. Miscellaneous penicillins

Name	R
Quincillin	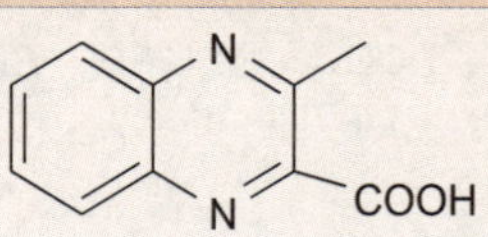
Amidinopencillins (mecillinam)	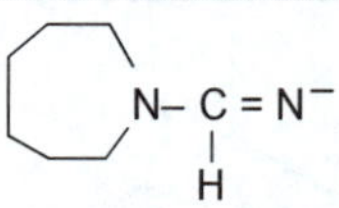
Azidocillin	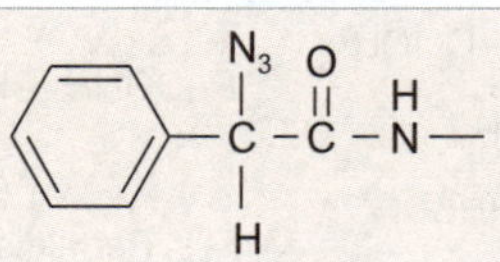
Talampicillin	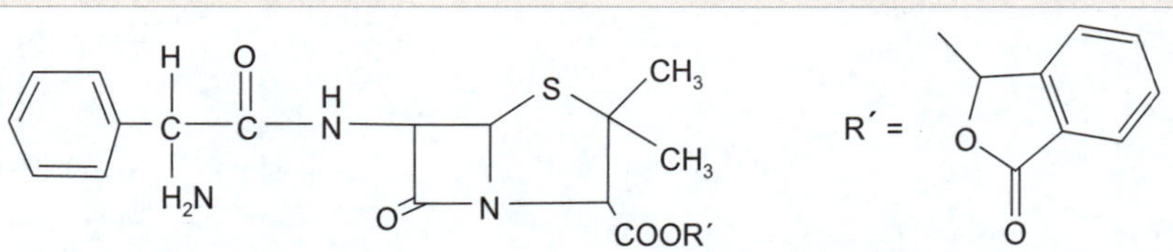

Degradation of Penicillins

The chemical degradation of penicillins is depicted in Figure 15.1.

Inactivation of penicillins by acids, bases, and β-lactamases is as follows:

- The penicillins are very reactive due to the strained amide bond in the fused β-lactum of the nucleus.
- Penicillins undergo a complex series of reactions leading to a variety of inactive degradation products.
- They are extremely susceptible to nucleophilic attack by water or hydroxide ion to form the penicilloic acid. β-Lactamases also cleave the β-lactam ring to give penicilloic acid with a consequent loss of antibacterial activity.

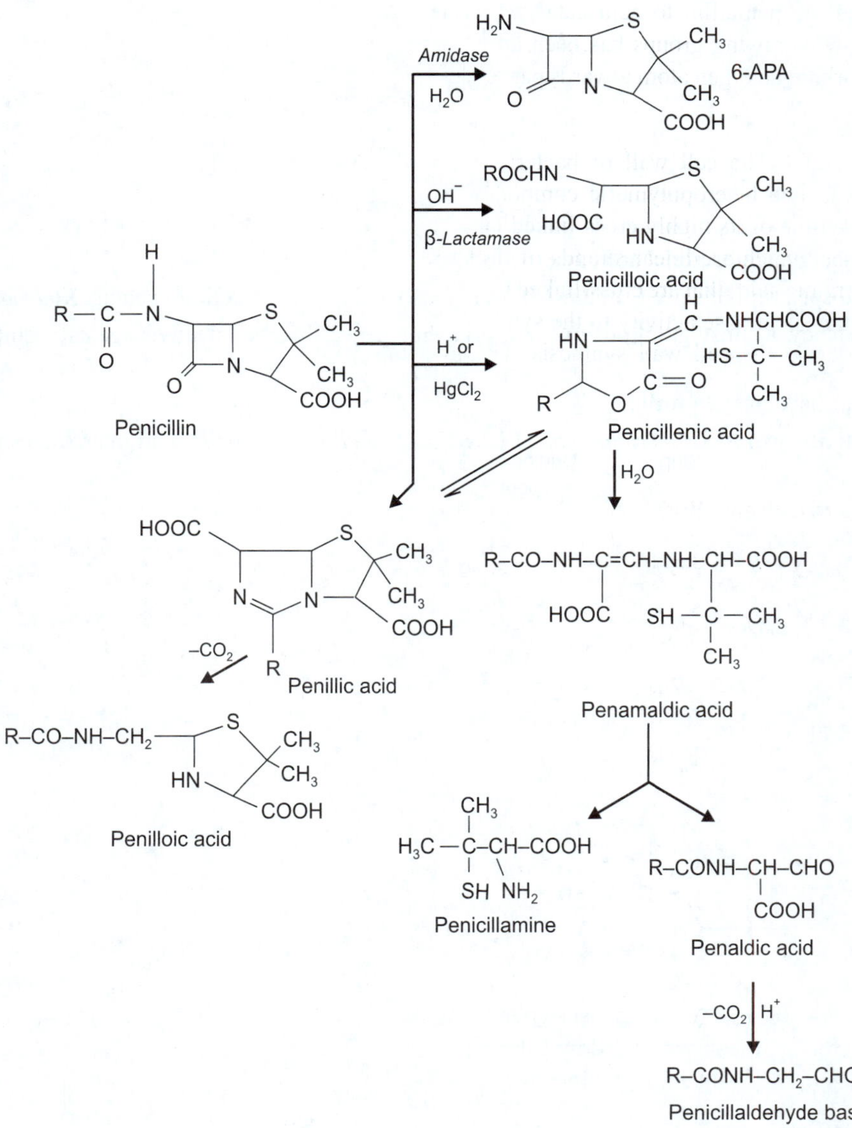

Figure 15.1: Chemical degradation of penicillins.

- In strongly acidic solutions (pH <3), penicillin is protonated at the β-lactam nitrogen, and this is followed by nucleophillic attack of the acyl oxygen atom on the β-lactam carbonyl carbon. The subsequent opening of the β-lactam ring destabilizes the thiazolidine ring, which opens to form penicillenic acid that degrades into two major products penicillamine and penilloic acid. A third product, penicilloaldehyde is also formed.
- Acid-catalyzed degradation in the stomach contributes in a major way to the poor oral absorption of penicillin. Thus, efforts to obtain penicillins with improved pharmacokinetic and microbiologic properties have sought to find acyl functionalities that would minimize sensitivity of the β-lactam ring to acid hydrolysis and at the same time, maintain antibacterial activity.
- Substitution of an electron-withdrawing group for the α-position of the benzyl penicillin has stabilized the penicillin to acid catalyzed hydrolysis. The increased stability imparted by such electron-withdrawing groups has been attributed to a decrease in the reactivity of the side chain amide carbonyl oxygen atom towards participation in β-lactam ring opening to form the penicillenic acid.

Mode of action: The cell wall of bacteria is essential for the normal growth and development. Peptidoglycan is a heteropolymeric component of the cell wall that provides rigid mechanism for stability by virtue of its highly cross-linked lattice-wise structure. The peptidoglycan is composed of glycan chains, which are linear strands of two alternating amino sugars (N-acetyl glucosamine and *N*-acetylmuramic acid) that are cross-linked by peptide chains of an enzyme, transpeptidase. Penicillins inhibit the transpeptidase activity to the synthesis of cell walls. They also block cleavage of terminal D-alanine during the cell wall synthesis. The biosynthesis of peptidoglycan involves three stages (Figure 15.2).

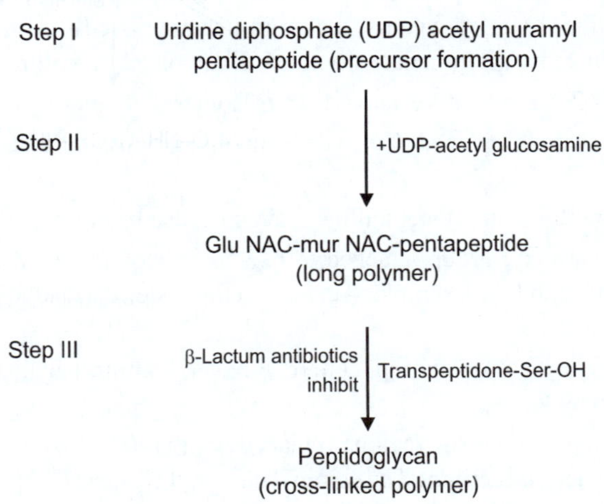

Figure 15.2: Stages involved in the biosynthesis of peptidoglycan.

β-lactam antibiotics inhibit the last step in peptidoglycan synthesis. The transpeptidase enzyme that contains serine is probably acylated by β-lactam antibiotics with the cleavage of –CO-N- bond of the β-lactam ring. This renders the enzyme inoperative and inhibits peptidoglycan synthesis.

SAR of Penicillins

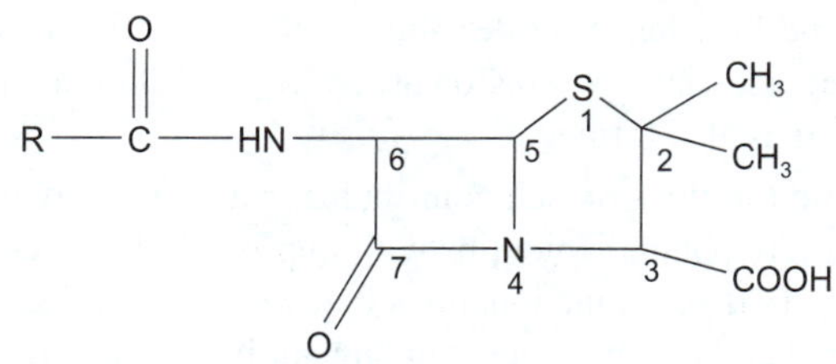

1. **6-Acyl side chain:** Benzyl penicillin has rather serious limitations, that is, narrow spectrum of activity with acids and alkali degradation occurs and is susceptible to all known β-lactamase. The increased latitude in varying the acyl amino side chain through acylation of 6-APA resulted in more significant improvement in the biological properties of penicillins.
   a. Introduction of α-aryloxyalkyl penicillins in the side chain gives increased acid stability and oral absorption. Other substitutents on the α-carbon of the side chain, such as amino (ampicillin), chloro, and guanidine display good resistance to inactivation by acids.
   b. Substitution of the α-carbon atom of the side chain with bulky groups confers β-lactamase resistance. Examples: Methicillin, nafcillin, oxacillin, etc.

      In all these penicillins, an aromatic ring is attached directly to the side chain amide carbonyl, and there is substitution at both positions ortho to the point of attachment. The size of the ring systems plays an important role in determining the ability of the ortho substitutent to confer penicillinase resistance.
   c. Introduction of an ionized or polar group into the α-position of the side chain in the benzyl carbon atom of penicillin-G confers against the gram-negative bacilli. Amino, hydroxyl, carboxyl, and sulphonyl increase gram-negative activity. Example: Ampicillin and carbenicillin.
   d. The D-isomer is 2–8 times more active than L-isomer in ampicillin.
   e. When acyl side chain is replaced with hydroxymethyl groups, increased gram-negative activity is observed.
   f. N-acylated ampicillins (ureidopenicillins) have increased activity against *Pseudomonas*.
2. Many esters of the carboxyl group attached to C-3 have been prepared as prodrugs to increase lipophilicity and acid stability. Example: Acetoxymethyl ester derivatives are used for preparing prodrugs.
3. Introduction of C-6 α-methoxy group confers greater stability against β-lactamase without signifcant loss of potency.
4. The sulphur of the thiazolidine ring can be replaced with O, CH_2, and CH-β-CH_3 with increased broad-spectrum antibacterial activity. The geminal dimethyl group at C-2 position is a characteristic of the penicillin.
5. In general, derivatization of the C-3 carboxylic acid functionality is not tolerated unless the free penicillin carboxylic acid can be generated *in vivo*. Doubly activated penicillin esters, undergo rapid cleavage *in vivo* to generate active penicillin. Example: Pivampicillin and bacampicillin.
6. The N-4 atoms at the ring junction are vital for antibacterial activity; the nitrogen atom contributes to the reactivity of the β-lactam carbonyl centre.

Synthesis and Drug Profile

I. Penicillinase-resistant penicillins

i. Methicillin

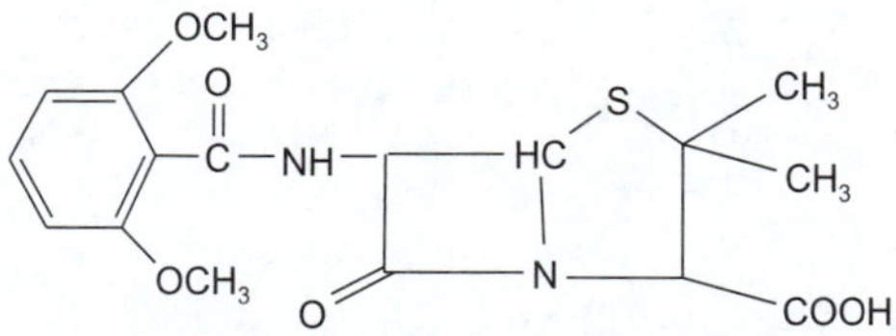

2,6-Dimethoxyphenyl penicillin

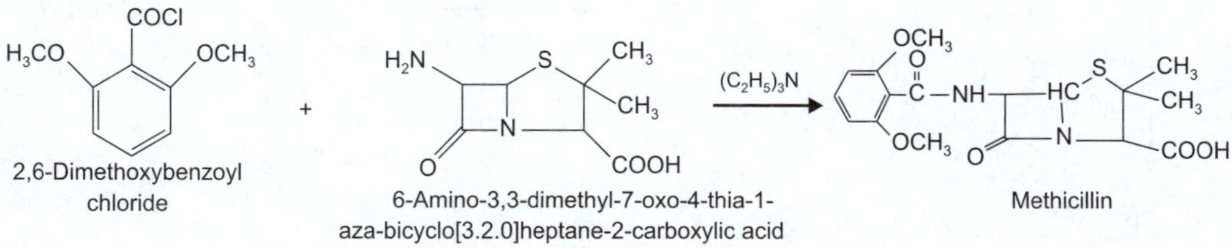

Properties and uses: Methicillin sodium is a white crystalline solid, odourless, soluble in water, slightly soluble in chloroform, but insoluble in ether. It is particularly resistant to inactivation by the penicillinase found in Staphylococci and somewhat more resistant than penicillin G to penicillinase from *Bacillus cereus*. Methicillin sodium has been introduced for use in the treatment of staphylococci infections caused by the strains resistant to other penicillins. It is given by IM or by slow IV infusion every 4–6 hrs.

ii. Oxacillins (Isoxazolyl penicillins)

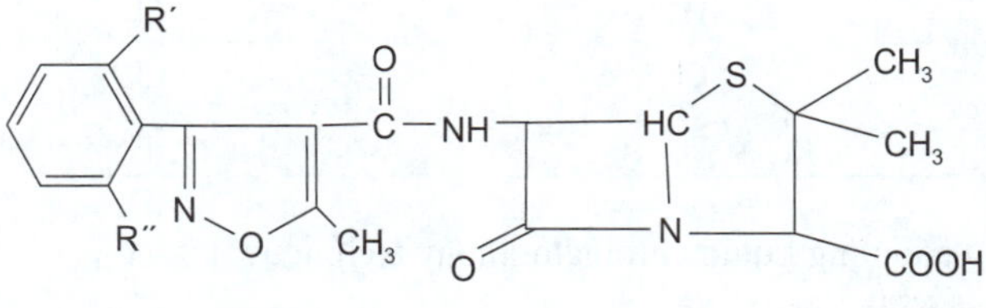

Properties and uses: Oxacillin sodium monohydrate is a white powder, soluble in water and methanol, insoluble in methylene chloride. The use of oxacillin and other isoxazolyl penicillins should be restricted to the treatment of infections caused by staphylococci that are resistant to penicillin G, although their spectrum of activity is similar to that of penicillin G.

Synthesis

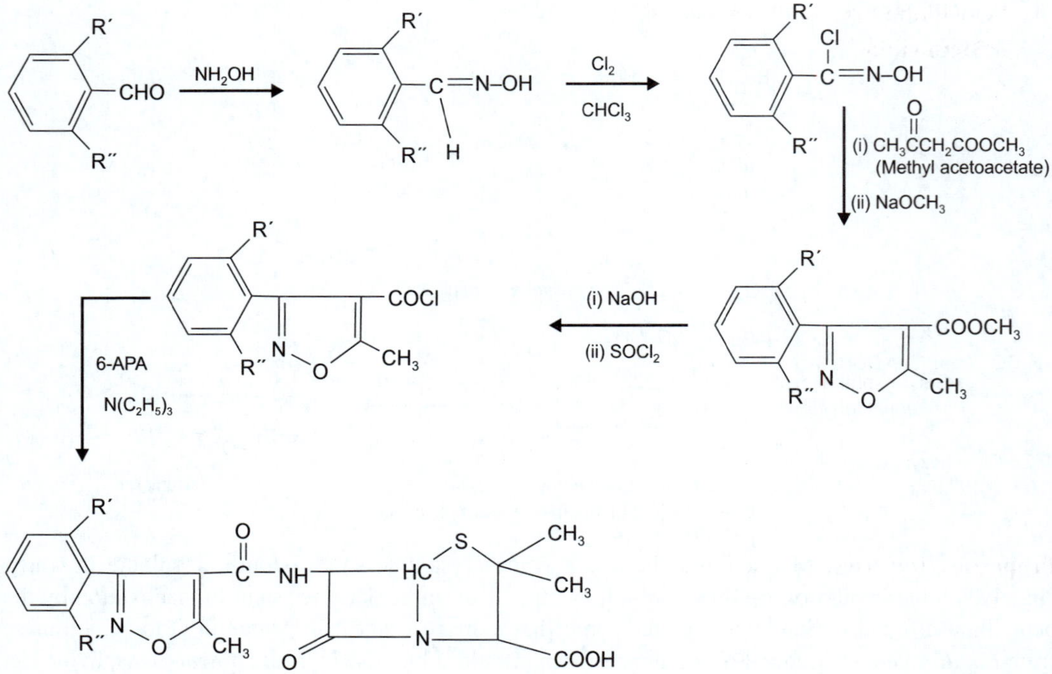

Name	*R′*	*R″*
Oxacillin	–H	–H
Cloxacillin	–H	–Cl
Dicloxacillin	–Cl	–Cl
Floxacillin	–F	–Cl

Assay: It is assayed by adopting liquid chromatography technique.

II. Penicillinase susceptible penicillins

- **Penicillin-V**

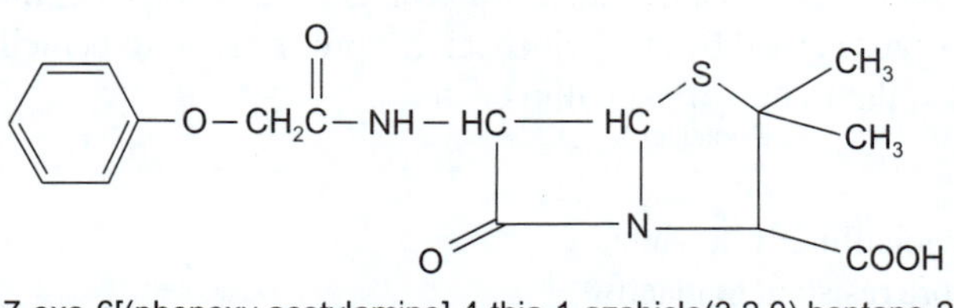

3,3-Dimethyl-7-oxo-6[(phenoxy acetylamino]-4-thia-1-azabiclo(3.2.0) heptane-2-carboxylic acid

Synthesis

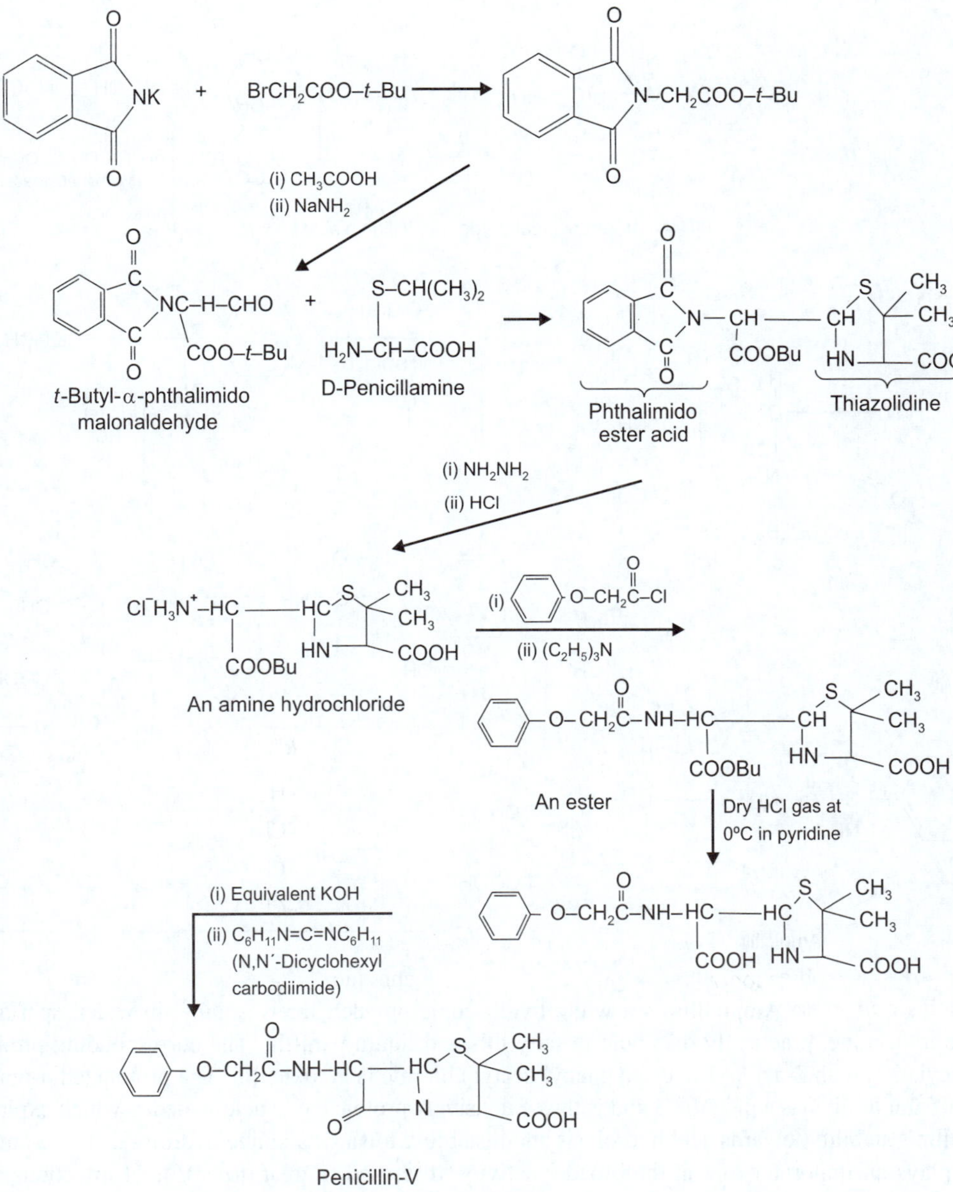

Properties and uses: Penicillin V is a white, odourless, crystalline powder with slightly bitter taste and soluble in water. It is more resistant to inactivation by gastric juice than penicillin G and better absorbed from the gastrointestinal (GI) tract. Equivalent oral doses provide two or five times greater plasma concentration than penicillin G. Penicillin V is given to treat 'trench mouth'. It is useful in the treatment of streptococcal pharyngitis, pneumonia, arthritis, meningitis, and endocarditis caused by *S. pyrogenes*.

Dose: Dose of penicillin V by oral route is 125–500 mg six times daily for 10 days. For prophylaxis of rheumatic fever, the dose is 125–250 mg twice daily.

Assay: It is assayed by adopting liquid chromatography technique.

III. Aminopenicillins

i. Ampicillin (Amcil, Omnipen)

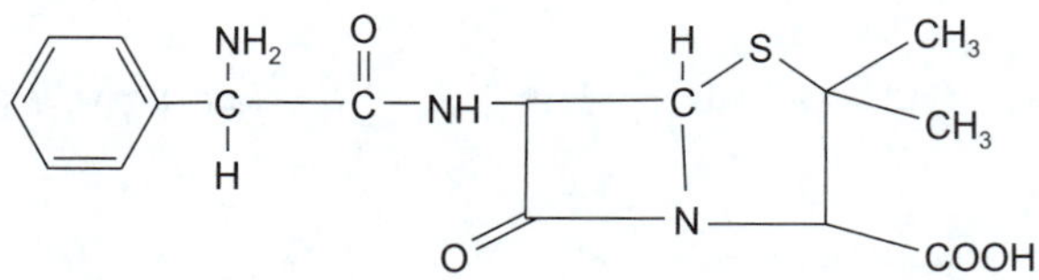

6[D-Aminophenylacetamido] penicillanic acid

Synthesis

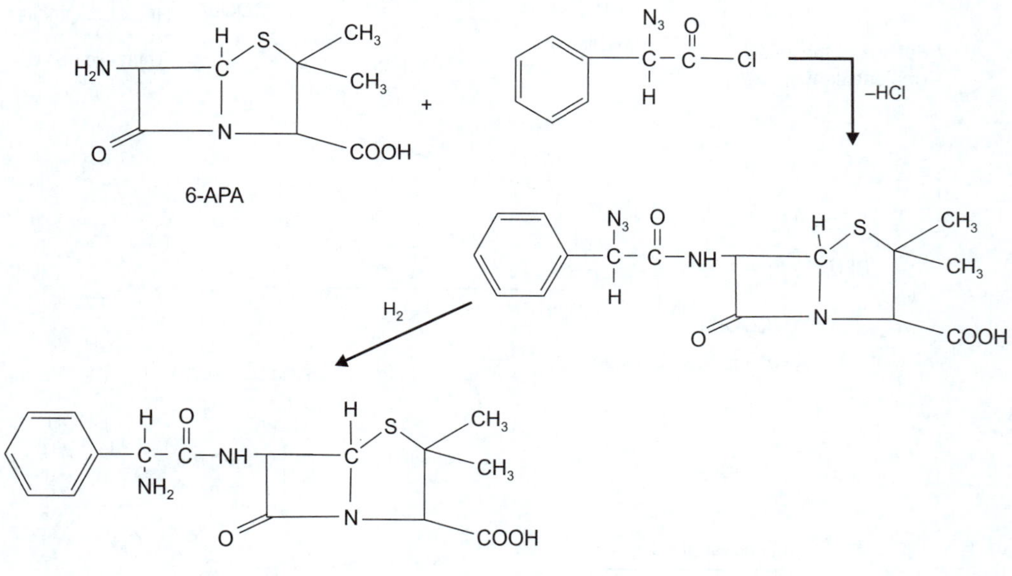

Properties and uses: Ampicillin is a white hygroscopic powder, freely soluble in water, sparingly soluble in acetone, practically insoluble in fatty oils and liquid paraffin. The corresponding product from acylation with 2-azido-4-hydroxyphenyl acetyl chloride is amoxicillin. The protonated α-amino group of ampicillin has a pK_a of 7.3 and is thus extensively protonated in acidic media, which explains ampicillin's stability towards acid hydrolysis and instability towards alkaline hydrolysis. The α-amino group plays an important role in the broader activity. It is used to treat urinary tract infections and respiratory tract infections.

Assay: It is assayed by adopting liquid chromatography technique.

Dose: Available as capsules of 250 or 500 mg, as sodium salt for parenteral use, for oral suspension in strengths of 125–500 mg/5 ml, and in paediatric drops of 100 mg/ml. The consumption dose for adults is 1–4 g per day in divided dose for every 6 hrs, for children the dose is 100–200 mg/kg per day in three portions.

Dosage forms: Ampicillin capsules IP, ampicillin sodium injection IP, ampicillin injection BP.

ii. Pivampicillin

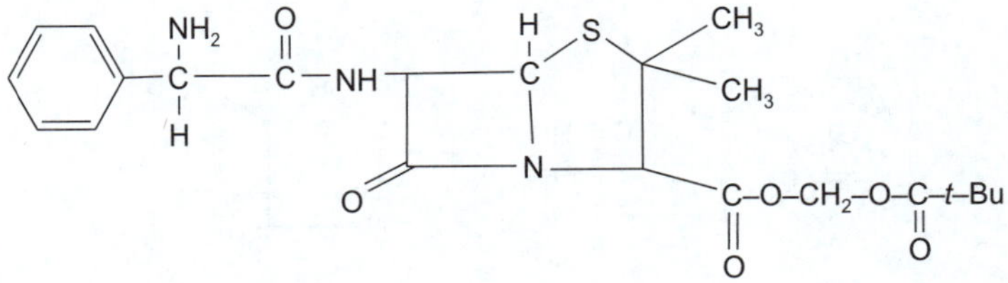

Synthesis

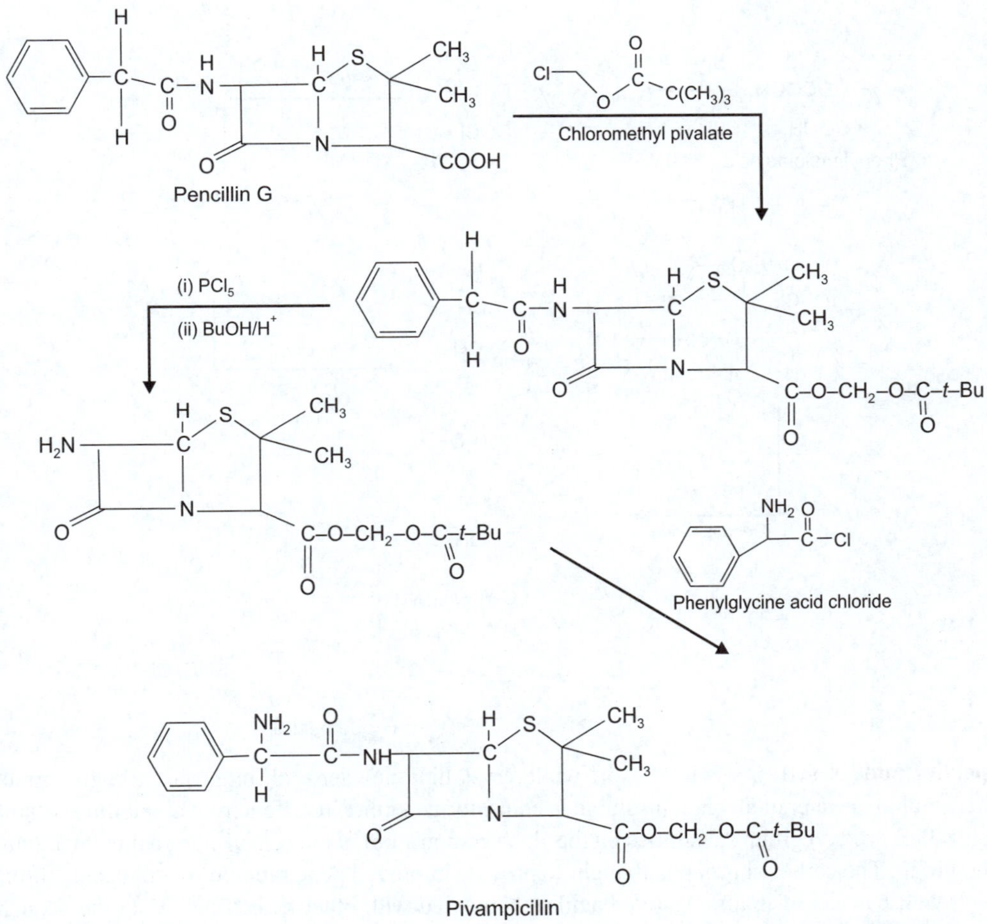

Properties and uses: Pivampicillin is a white crystalline powder, practically insoluble in water, soluble in methanol, ethanol, and dilute acids. It is a produg for ampicillin and in the *in vivo* esters hydrolyzes back to the parent ampicillin. It is used to treat urinary tract infections and respiratory tract infections.

Assay: It is assayed by adopting liquid chromatography technique.

IV. Antipseudomonal penicillins

i. Carbenicillin

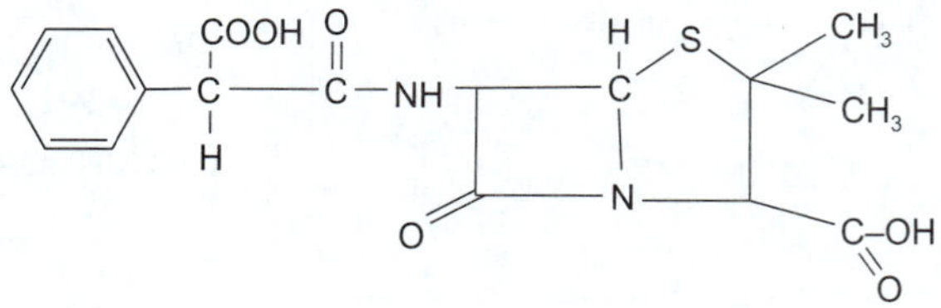

Synthesis

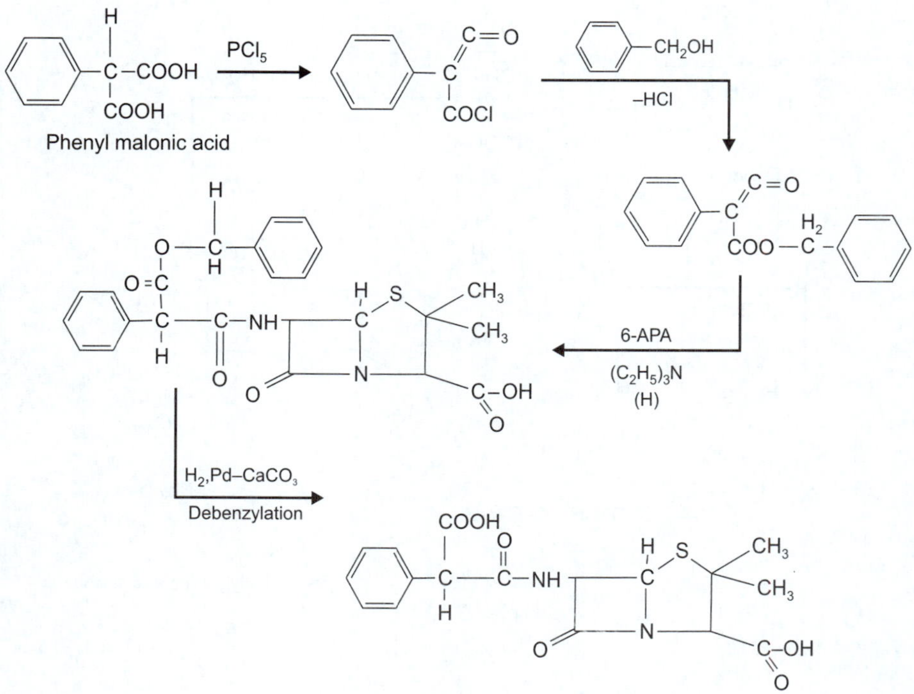

Carbenicillin

Properties and uses: It is a white to off white crystalline powder with bitter taste, hygroscopic in nature, soluble in water or alcohol, insoluble in chloroform or ether. It differs from ampicillin by having an ionizable carboxyl group substituted on the alpha carbon atom of the benzyl side chain rather than an amino group. The carboxyl group is thought to provide improved penetration of the molecule through the cell wall barriers of gram-negative bacillias compared with other penicillins. A similar sequence starting with 3-thiophenylmalonic acid leads to the ticarcillin. It is acid labile being a malonic acid derivative, it decarboxylates readily to penicillin G. It is effective in the treatment of systemic and urinary tract infections. It has low toxicity, except allergic sensitivity, and the drug interferes with platelet function resulting in bleeding.

V. Ureido penicillins

i. Aziocillin (Azlin)

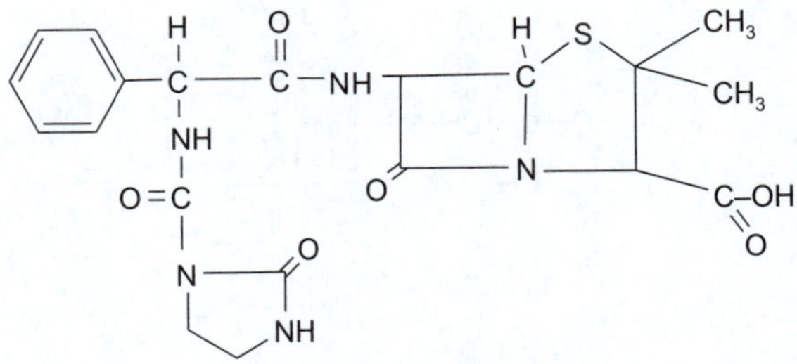

Synthesis

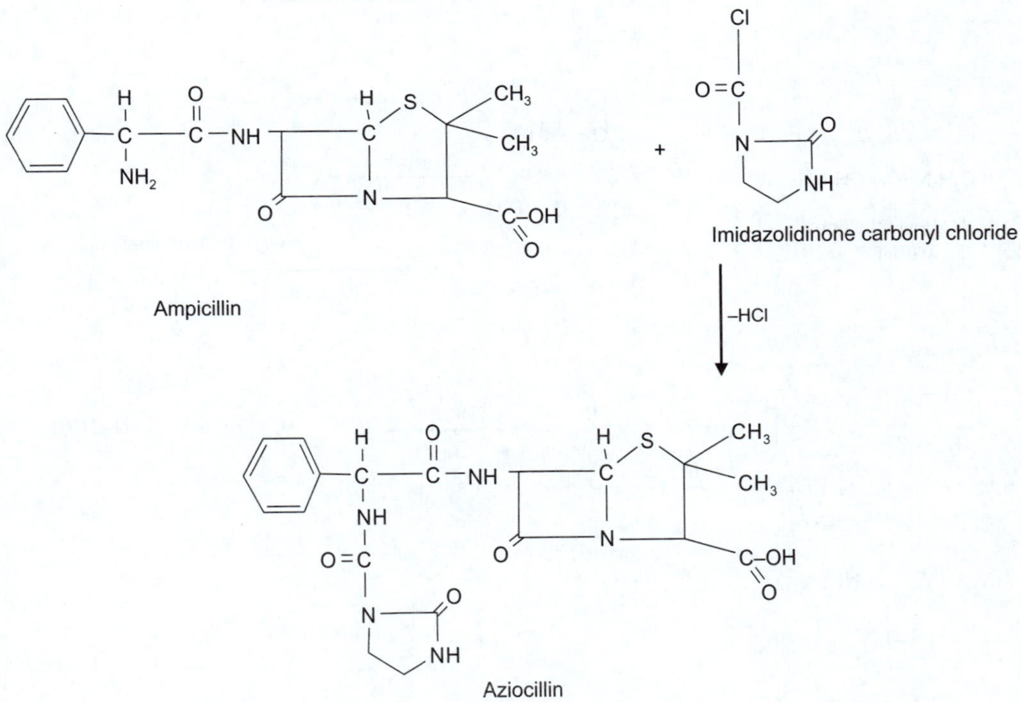

Properties and uses: It is the newest of ureidopenicillins, and is about 10 times more active than carbenicillin against *Pseudomonas* and streptococci.

Dose: The dosage is 8–18 g per day in 4–6 divided doses.

ii. Piperacillin (Pipracil, Pracil)

Synthesis

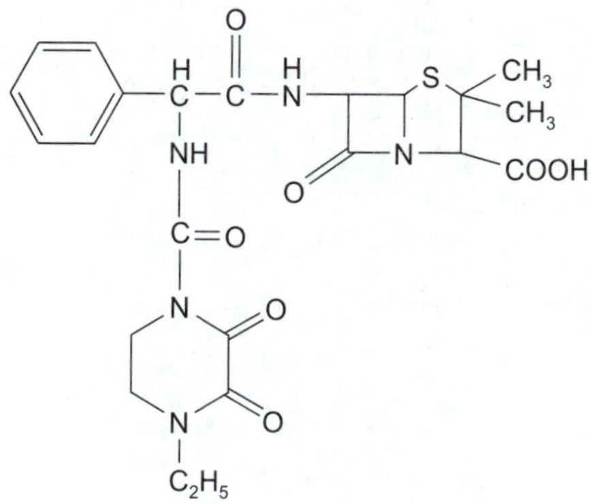

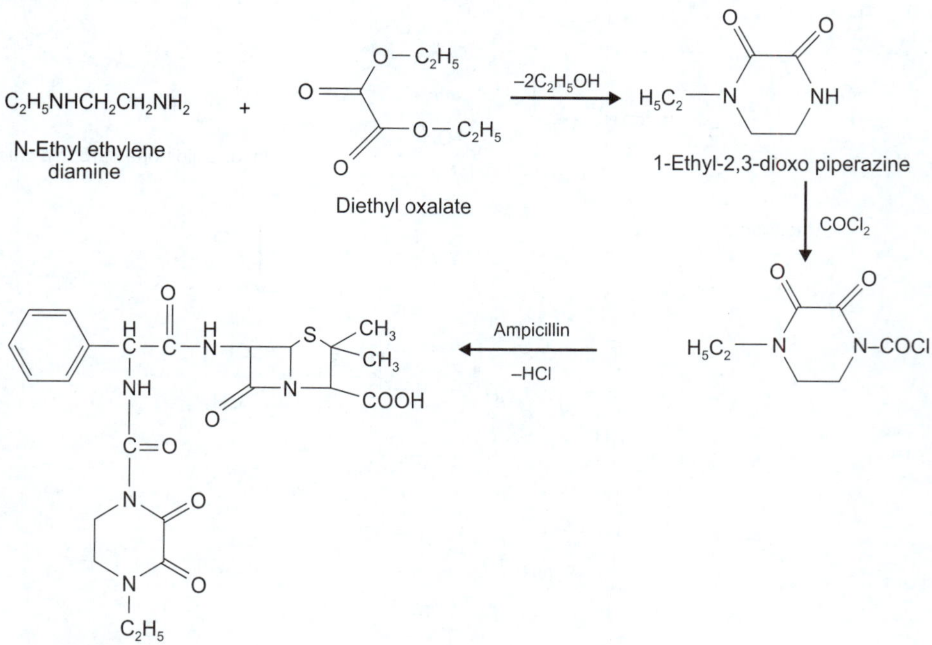

Properties and uses: Piperacillin sodium is a white hygroscopic powder, soluble in water and methanol, practically insoluble in ethyl acetate. It is available as a powder for solubilization and injection. It is best given in combination with an aminoglycoside antibiotic.

Assay: It is assayed by adopting liquid chromatography technique.

Dose: For serious and complicated infections: The adult dose as sodium is 200–300 mg/kg daily in divided doses or 3–4 g per day in divided doses of every 4 or 6 hrs. For life-threatening conditions: Especially those caused by *Pseudomonas* or *Klebsiella* spp, the dose is at least 16 g per day; usual maximum dose is 24 g per day. For children: 1 month–12 years, as sodium 100–300 mg/kg daily in 3–4 divided doses. For neonates: The dose for less than 7 days or lesser than 2 kg, that is, 150 mg/kg daily in 3 divided doses; for more than 7 days and more than 2 kg, that is, 300 mg/kg in 3–4 divided doses, IV route is preferred for infants and children. Single dose more than 500 mg should not be given via IM injection.

Parenteral: For mild or uncomplicated infections: The adult dose as sodium is 100–125 mg/kg daily, the usual dose, if given via IV injection/infusion is 2 g every 6 or 8 hrs or 4 g every 12 hrs, if given via IM injection the dose is 2 g every 8 or 12 hrs. Prophylaxis of infection during surgery, for adults: As sodium, the dose is 2 g just before the procedure or when the umbilical cord is clamped in cesarean section, followed by at least two doses of 2 g at intervals of 4 or 6 hrs within 24 hrs of procedure.

VI. Miscellaneous penicillins

- **Mecillinam** (Amdinocillin)

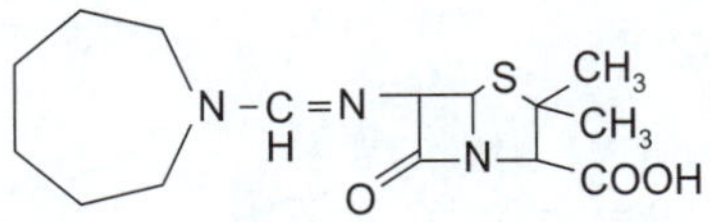

6-β-(Hexahydro-1H-azepin-1-yl)-methylene aminopenicillonic acid

Synthesis

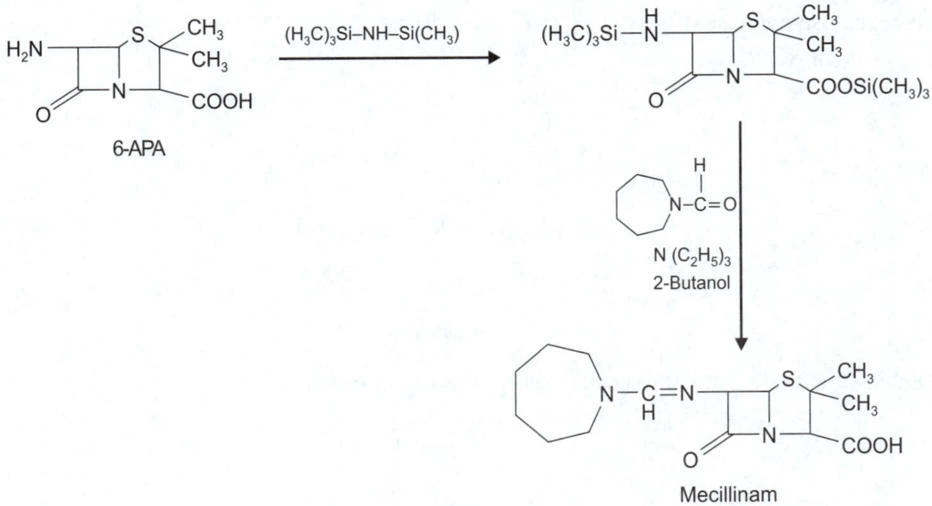

Properties and uses: Mecillinam is particularly active against enterobacteria including some ampicillin-resistant strains and to treat urinary tract infections. It is structurally different from other penicillins, in that, it is not an acyloxy derivative, but rather alkylidene amino-(amidino) derivative of 6-APA, due to this difference, it has significant gram-negative antibacterial activity as compared to gram-positive antibacterial activity.

Cephalosporins

The cephalosporins were isolated from the fungus *Cephalosporium acremonium* in 1945 by Pro Tzu, Newton, and Abraham (1953). The main product being cephalosporin C, the molecular modification of cephalosporin C gave origin to semisynthetic substances. They are β-lactam antibiotics with same fundamental structural requirements as penicillins, the main difference between the two is that cephalosporins contain dihydrometathiazine ring, while penicillin contains a tetrahydrothiazole (thiazolidine) ring. The cephalosporins are much more acid stable than the corresponding penicillins and also have a mechanism of action similar to that of penicillins; they mainly inhibit the cross-linking of the peptidoglycan units in bacterial cell walls by inhibiting transpeptidase enzyme. However, they bind in the target proteins other than penicillins-binding proteins.

Cephalosporins can be divided into three classes:

1. *Cephalosporin N*: It has a penicillin-like structure being a derivative of 6-aminopenicillanic acid.
2. *Cephalosporin P*: An acidic antibiotic, which is steroidal in nature.
3. *Cephalosporin C*: It is a true cephalosporin and it is a derivative of 7 amino-cephalosporanic acid.

Generalized Formula for Cephalosporins

In cephalosporin C

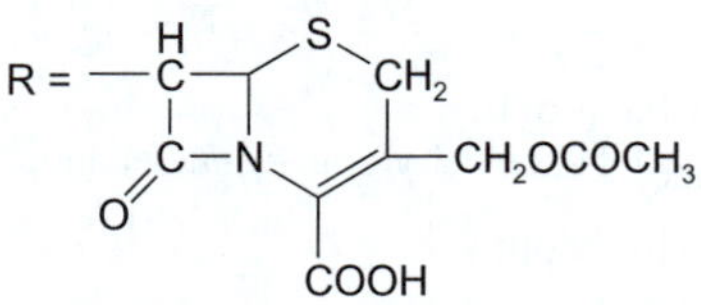

Cephalosporin C contains a side-chain derived from D-α-aminoadipic acid, which is attached to 7-amino-cephalosporanic acid.

In cephalosporin N

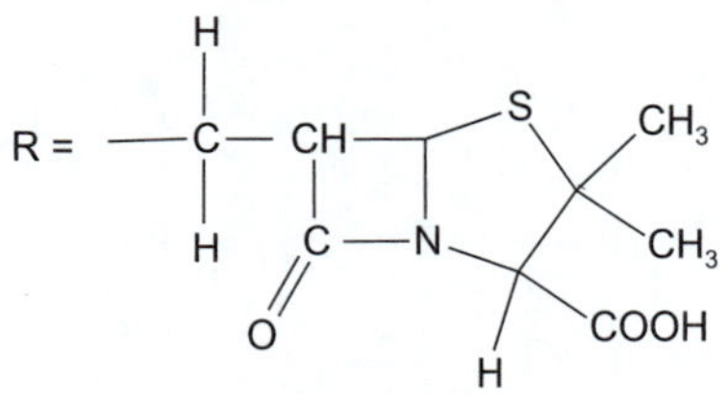

Pencillanic acid

A compound structurally similar to cephalosporin P is called *fusidic acid.*

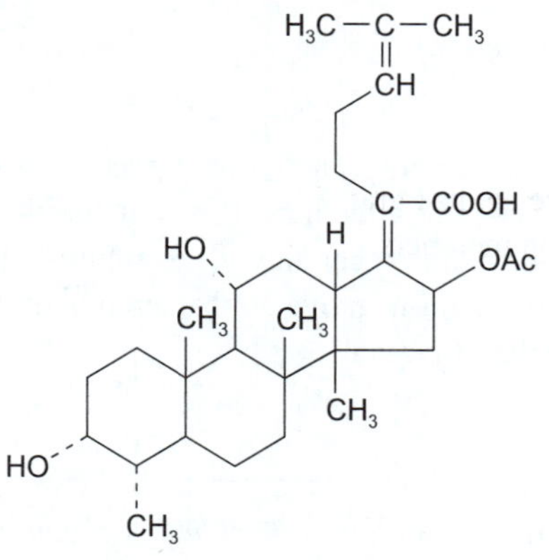

Nomenclatures

Cephalosporins are named in the following ways:

1. **Chemical abstracts:** 5-Thia-1-azobicyclo (4.2.0) octanes. Accordingly, cephalothin is 3-(acetoxy methyl)-8-oxo-7-(2-thienyl) acetamido-5-thia-1-aza-bicyclo[4.2.0]-oct-2-ene-2-carboxylic acid.
2. **Cephem derivatives:** Cephem is the name given to the unsubstituted bicyclic lactam.

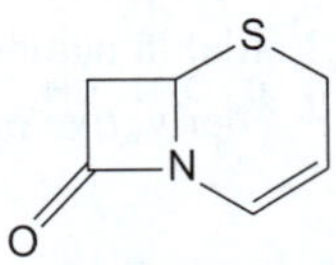

Cephem

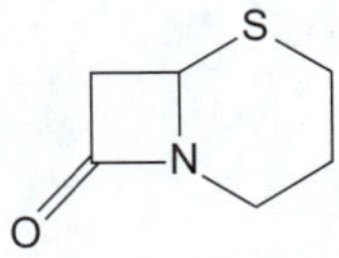

Cephem

Classification

Cephalosporins are classified on the basis of their chemical structure, clinical pharmacology, antibacterial spectrum, or penicillinase resistance.

a. Orally administered: Cephalexin, cephradine, and cefaclor
b. Parentrally administered: Cephalothin, cephapirin, cephacetrile, and cefazedone. These agents are sensitive to β-lactamase.
c. Resistant to β-lactamase and parentrally administered: Cefuroxime, cefamandole, cefoxitin
d. Metabolically unstable: cephalothin and cephairin

Clinically Used Cephalosporins

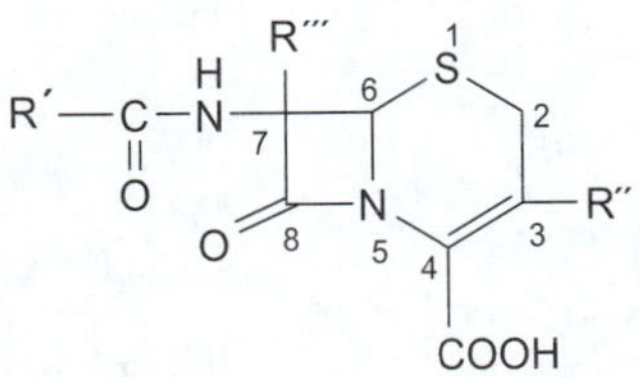

I. **First-generation cephalosporins**

These drugs have the highest activity against gram-positive bacteria and the lowest activity against gram-negative bacteria (Table 15.1).

II. **Second-generation cephalosporins**

These drugs are more active against gram-negative bacteria and less active against gram-positive bacteria than first-generation members (Table 15.2).

III. **Third-generation cephalosporins**

These drugs are less active than first-generation drugs against gram-positive organisms, but have a much-expanded spectrum of activity against gram-negative organisms (Table 15.3).

Table 15.1: First-generation cephalosporins

Name	*R′*	*R″*	*R‴*
Cephaloridine	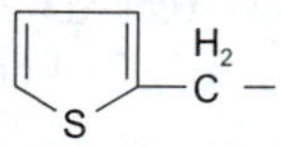	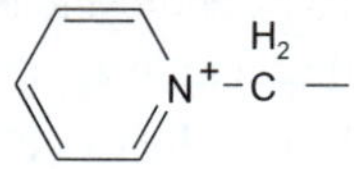	–H
Cephalothin	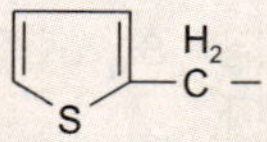	$-H_2C-O-C(=O)-CH_3$	–H
Cephapirin	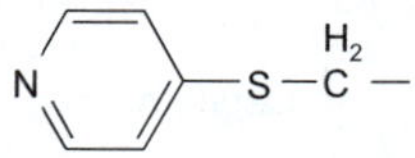	$-H_2C-O-C(=O)-CH_3$	–H
Cephalexin	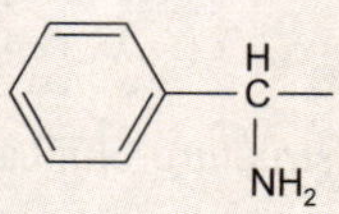	$-CH_3$	–H
Cephaloglycine	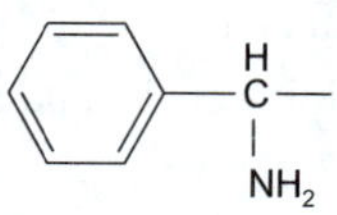	$-H_2C-O-C(=O)-CH_3$	–H
Cefadroxil	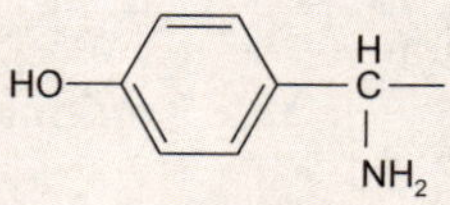	$-CH_3$	–H
Cephradine	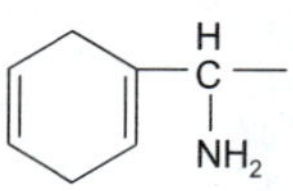	$-CH_3$	–H
Cefazolin	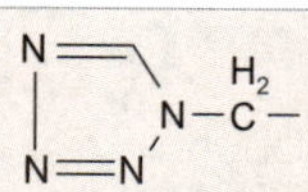	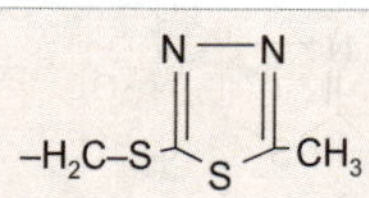	–H

Table 15.2: Second-generation cephalosporins

Name	*R′*	*R″*	*R‴*
Cefamandole	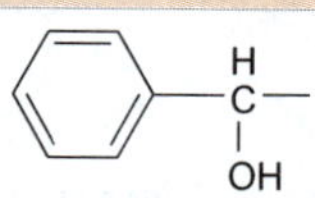	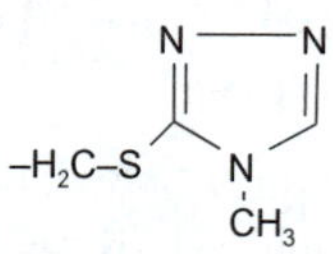	–H
Cefoxitin	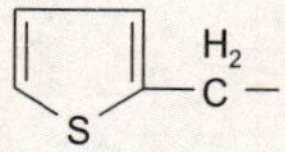	$-H_2C-O-C(=O)-NH_2$	$-OCH_3$

Contd.

Table 15.2: Second-generation cephalosporins *(Contd.)*

Name	*R'*	*R''*	*R'''*
Cefuroxime	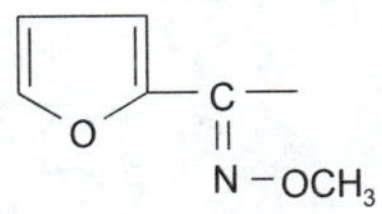	$-H_2C-O-C(=O)-NH_2$	–H
Cefaclor	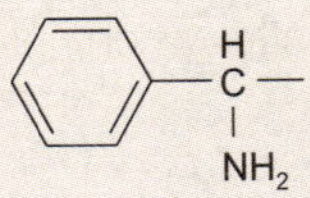	–Cl	–H
Cefonicid	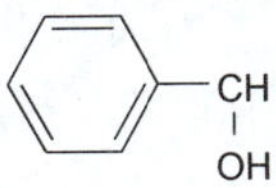	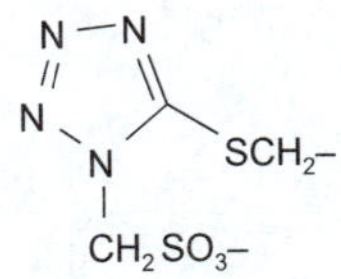	–H

Moxalactam

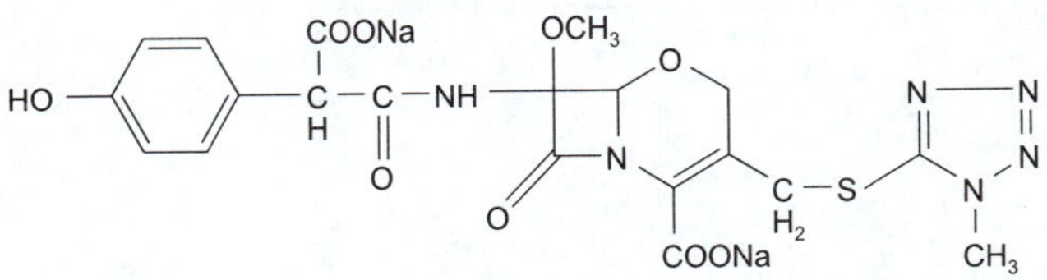

Table 15.3: Third-generation cephalosporins

Name	*R'*	*R''*	*R'''*
Ceftizoxime	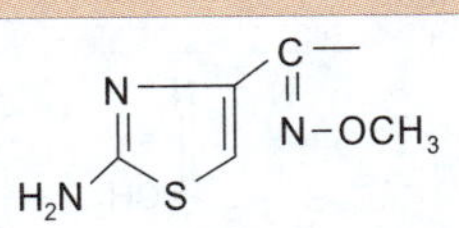	–H	–H
Cefotaxime	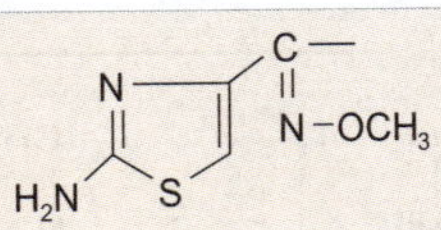	$-H_2C-O-C(=O)-CH_3$	–H
Ceftazidime	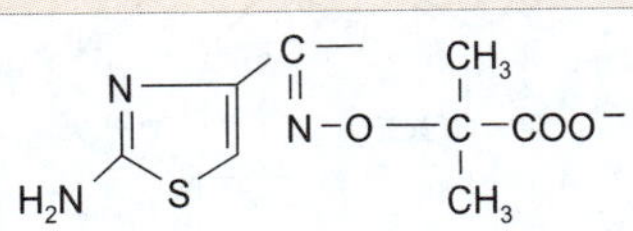	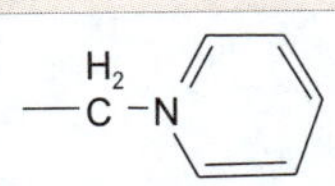	–H
Ceftriaxone	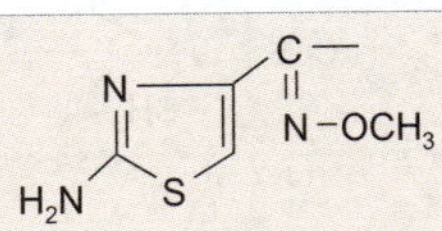	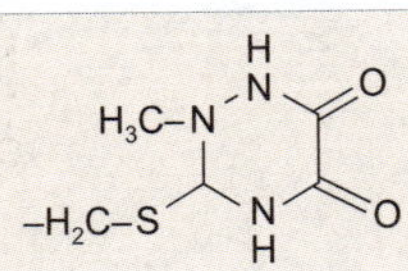	–H
Cefmenoxime	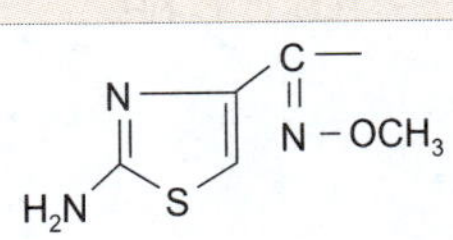	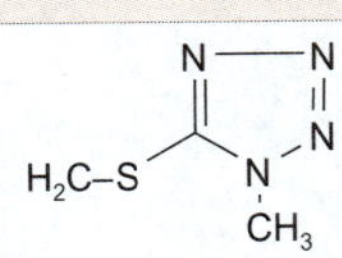	–H

IV. Fourth-generation cephalosporins

Cefepime and cefpirome are new fourth-generation parenteral cephalosporins with a spectrum of activity which makes them suitable for the treatment of infections caused by a wide variety of bacteria (Table 15.4).

Table 15.4: Fourth-generation cephalosporins

Name	*R'*	*R''*	*R'''*
Cefepime	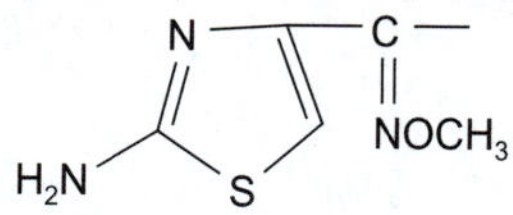	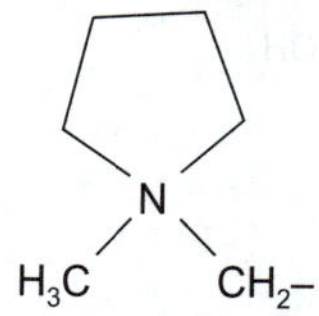	–H
Cefpirome	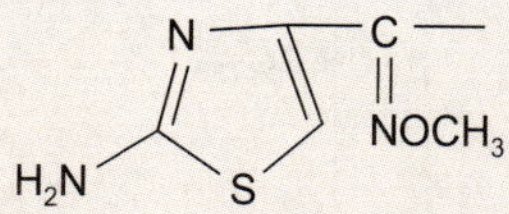	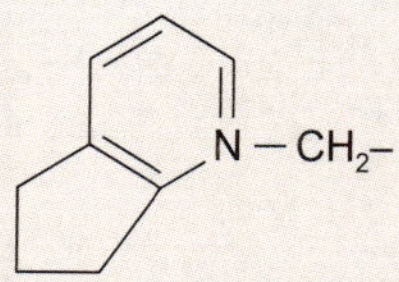	–H

V. Miscellaneous

i. Cefaparole

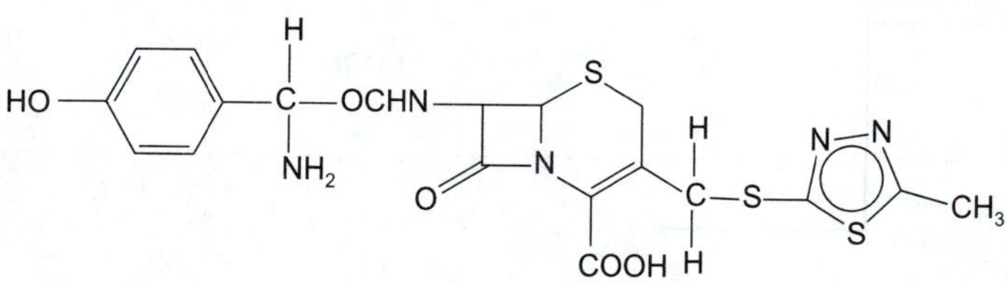

ii. Cefoperazone

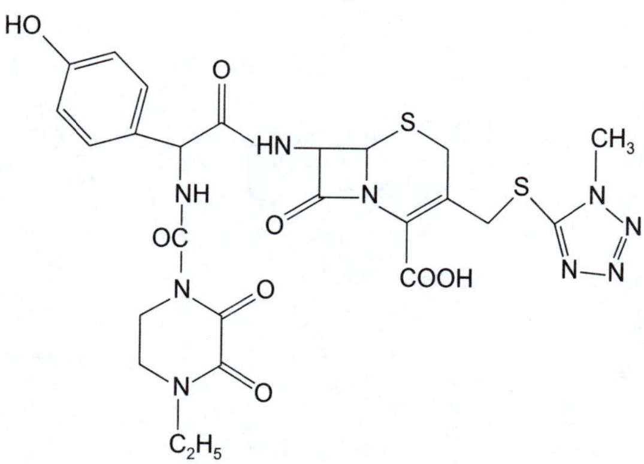

Degradation of Cephalosporins

Cephalosporins experience a variety of hydrolytic degradation reactions.

In strong acid solutions

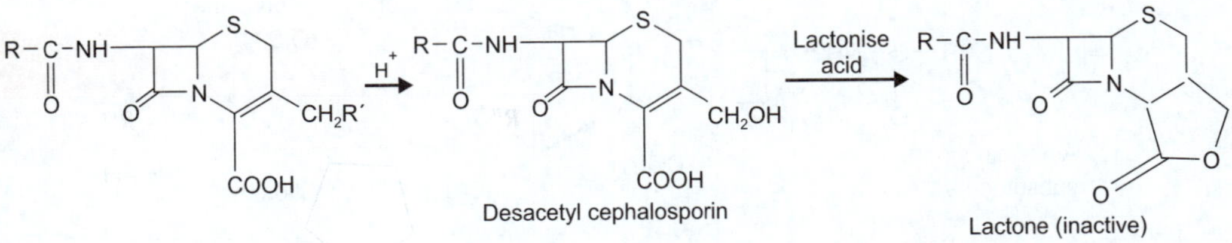

In the presence of β-lactamase

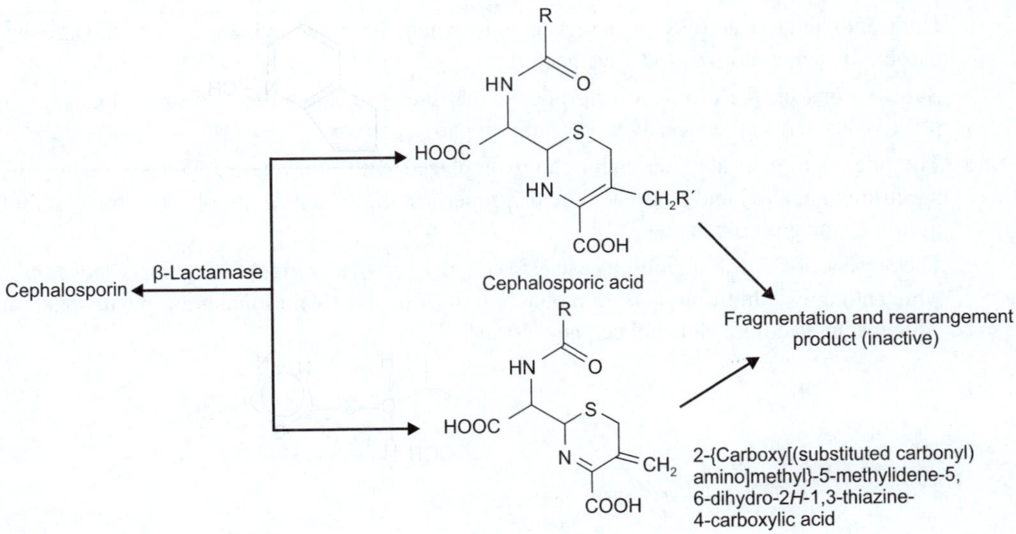

In the presence of acylase

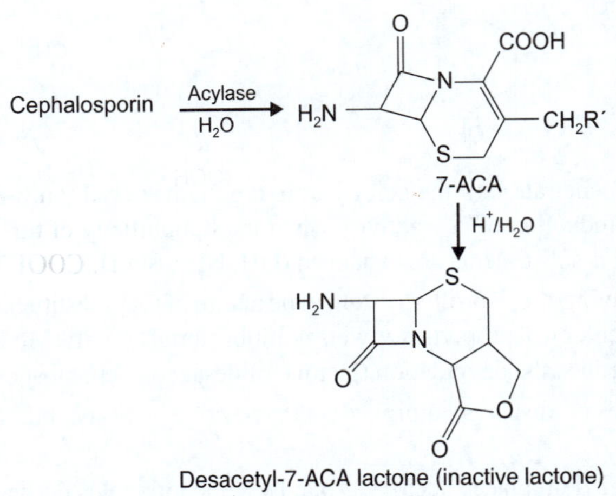

SAR of Cephalosporins

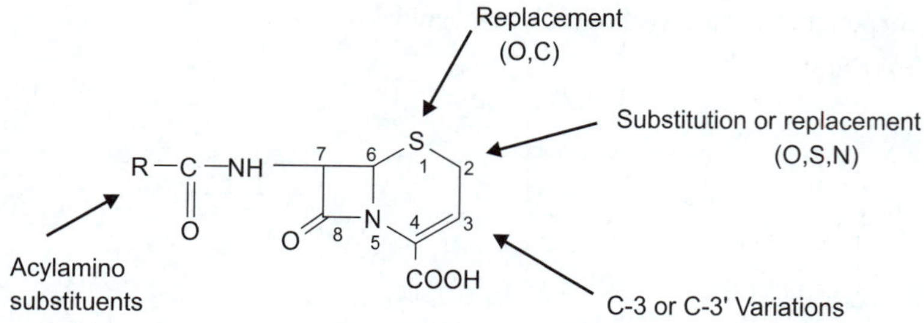

1. **7-Acylamino substitution**
   a. Acylation of amino groups generally increases the potency against gram-positive bacteria, but it is accompanied by a decrease in gram-negative potency.
   b. High antibacterial activity is observed only when the new acyl groups are derived from carboxylic acids for gram-positive bacteria.
   c. Substitutions on the aromatic ring phenyl that increase lipophilicity provide higher gram-positive activity and generally lower gram-negative activity.
   d. The phenyl ring in the side chain can be replaced with other heterocycles with improved spectrum of activity and pharmacokinetic properties; these include thiophene, tetrazole, furan, pyridine, and aminothiazoles.
   e. The presence of catechol grouping can also enhance activity, particularly against *P. aeruginosa*, which not only exhibits antipseudomonas activity, but also retain some gram-positive activity, which is unused for a catechol cephalosporin.

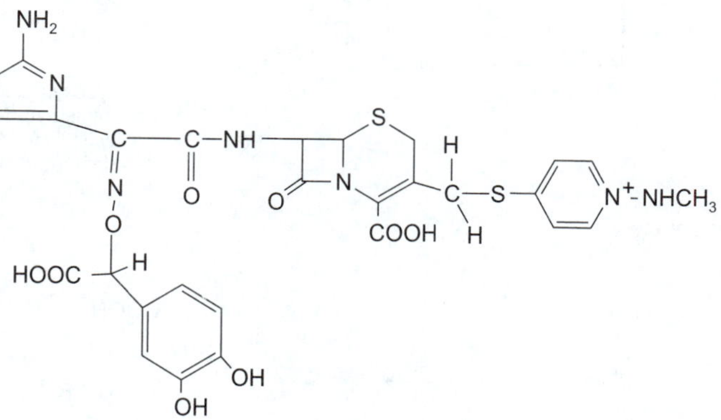

These compounds penetrate into the cell by utilizing the bacterial ion β-dependent ion transport system. There is a reduction of G^{-ve} activity when the lipophilicity of this side chain is increased and effects of polar α-substituents are enhanced (OH, NH_2, SO_3H, COOH).

2. **Modification involving the C-3 substitution:** The nature of C-3 substituents influences pharmacokinetic and pharmacological properties as well as antibacterial activity. Modification at C-3 position has been made to reduce the degradation (lactone of desacetyl cephalosporin) of cephalosporins.
   a. The benzoyl ester displays improved gram-positive activity, but lowered gram-negative activity.
   b. Pyridine, imidaozle-replaced acetoxy group by azide ion yields derivative with relatively low gram-negative activity.

c. Displacement with aromatic thiols of 3-acetoxy group results in an enhancement of activity against gram-negative bacteria with improved pharmacokinetic properties.
d. Replacement of acetoxy group at C-3 position with $-CH_3$, Cl has resulted in orally active compounds.

3. Other modifications

a. Introduction of C-7, a methoxy group, shows higher resistance to hydrolysis by β-lactamases.
b. Oxidation of ring spectrum to sulphoxide or sulphone greatly diminishes or destroys the antibacterial activity.
c. Replacement of sulphur with oxygen leads to oxacepam (latamoxef) with increased antibacterial activity, because of its enhanced acylating power. Similarly, replacement of sulphur with methylene group (loracavet) has greater chemical stability and a longer half-life.
d. The carboxyl group position at C-4 has been converted into ester prodrugs to increase bioavailability of cephalosporins, and these can be given orally as well.
e. Olefinic linkage at C-3 and C-4 positions is essential for antibacterial activity. Isomerization of the double bond to 2nd and 3rd positions leads to great losses in antibacterial activity.

Synthesis and Drug Profile

7-Aminocephalosporinic acid (7ACA)

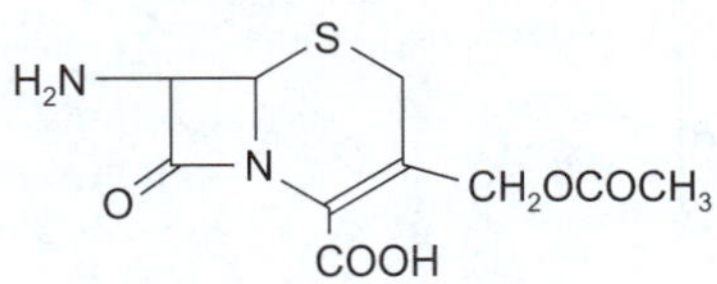

Synthesis

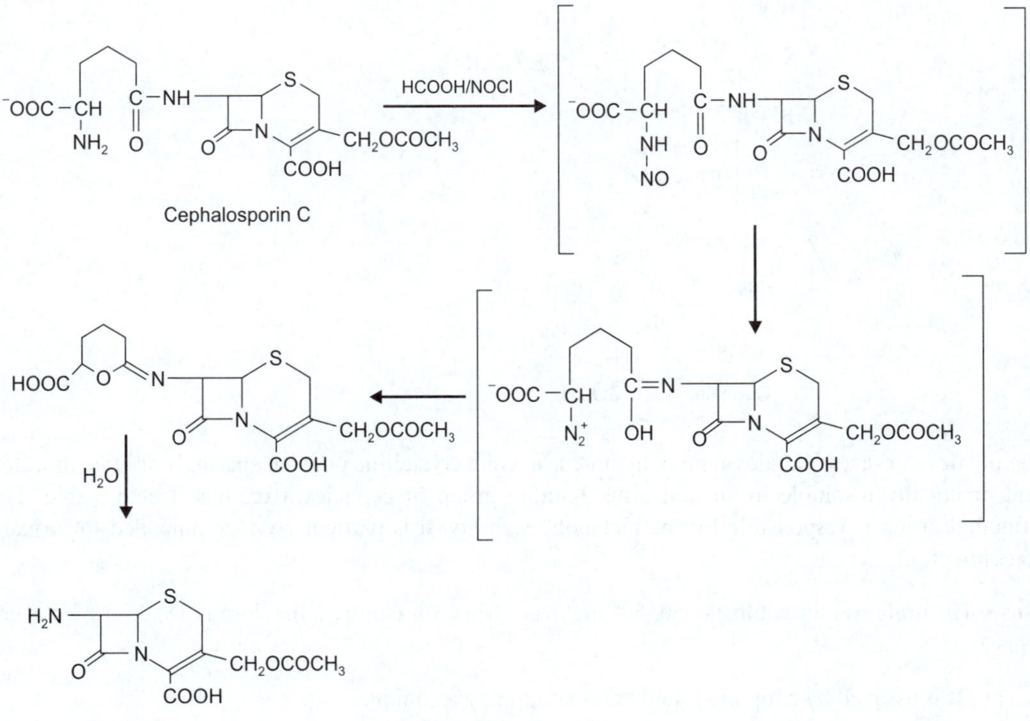

7-ACA

I. First-generation cephalosporins

i. Cephalexin (Keflex, Keforal)

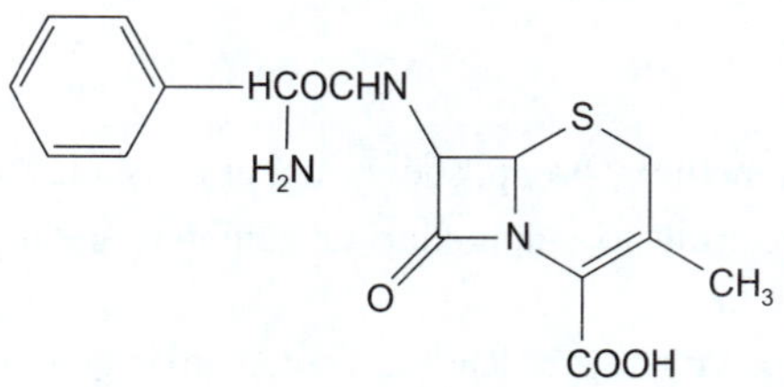

Synthesis

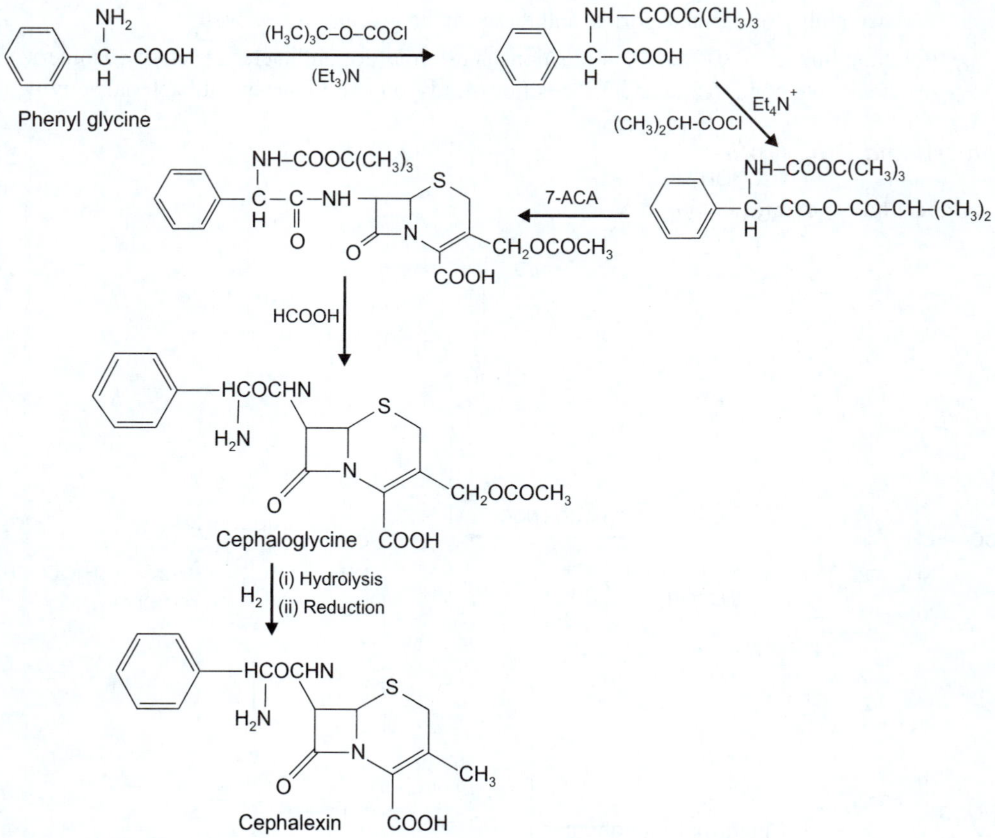

Properties and uses: Cefalexin monohydrate is a white crystalline powder, sparingly soluble in water, and practically insoluble in alcohol. The α-amino group of cephalexin renders it acid stable. The 3-methyl group is responsible for the metabolic stability. It is particularly recommended for urinary tract infection.

Dose: The oral dose for adults is 250–500 mg every 6 hrs, for children, the dose is 18–25 mg/kg every 6 hrs.

Assay: It is assayed by adopting liquid chromatography technique.

Dosage forms: Cefalexin capsules IP, BP, cefalexin oral suspension IP, BP, cefalexin tablets IP, BP.

ii. Cefadroxil (Cefadrox, Droxyl, Codroxil)

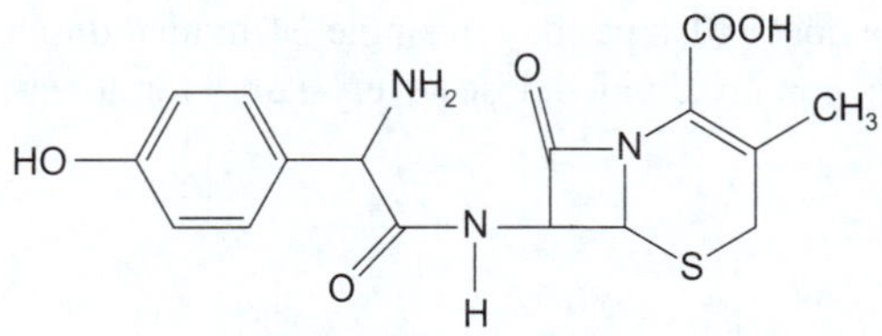

7-(2-Amino-2-(4-hydroxyphenyl)acetamido)-3-methyl-8-oxo-5-thia-1-aza-bicyclo[4.2.0]oct-2-ene-2-carboxylic acid

Synthesis

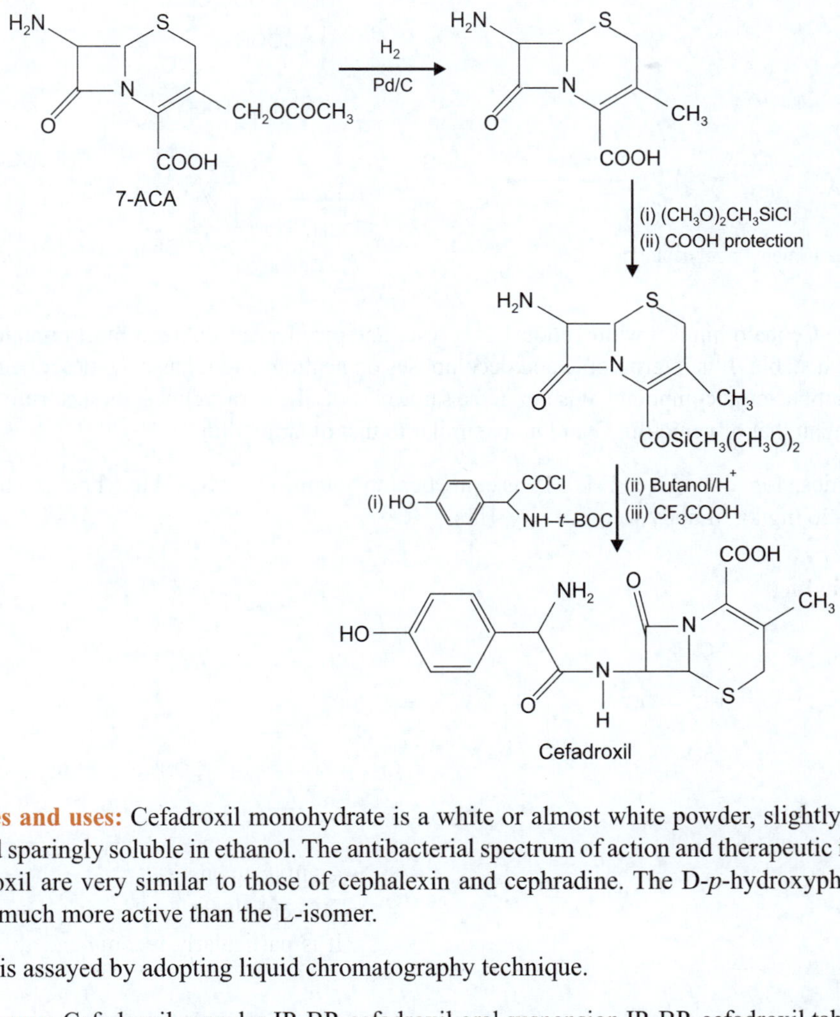

Properties and uses: Cefadroxil monohydrate is a white or almost white powder, slightly soluble in water, and sparingly soluble in ethanol. The antibacterial spectrum of action and therapeutic indications of cefadroxil are very similar to those of cephalexin and cephradine. The D-*p*-hydroxyphenylglycyl isomer is much more active than the L-isomer.

Assay: It is assayed by adopting liquid chromatography technique.

Dosage forms: Cefadroxil capsules IP, BP, cefadroxil oral suspension IP, BP, cefadroxil tablets IP.

Dose: In the case of uncomplicated lower urinary tract infections: For adults, the dose is 1–2 g daily as a single or 2 divided doses. For children more than 6 years, the dose is 500 mg twice a day, whereas for, 1–6 years, 250 mg twice a day; for children less than 1 year, the dose is 25 mg/kg daily in divided doses. In the case of skin and skin structure infections: For adults, the dose is 1 g per day in single or divided doses. For children, the dose is 30 mg/kg per day in equally divided doses every 12 hrs. In the case of pharyngitis and tonsilitis: For adults in the treatment of group A beta-haemolytic streptococcal pharyngitis and tonsilitis, the dose is 1 g per day in single or divided doses for 10 days. In the case of children, 30 mg/kg per day in equally divided doses every 12 hrs for at least 10 days.

iii. Cephalothin (Keflin)

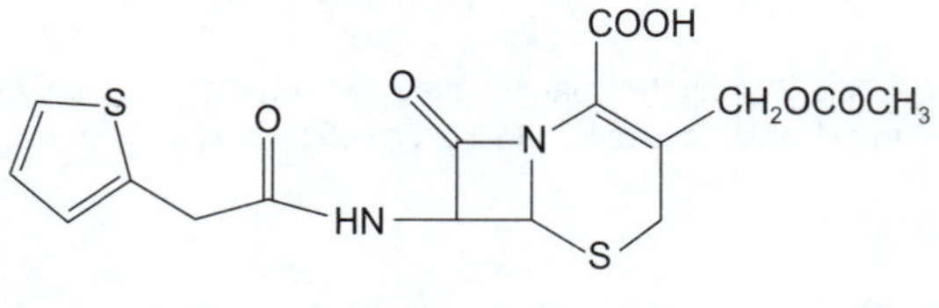

Synthesis

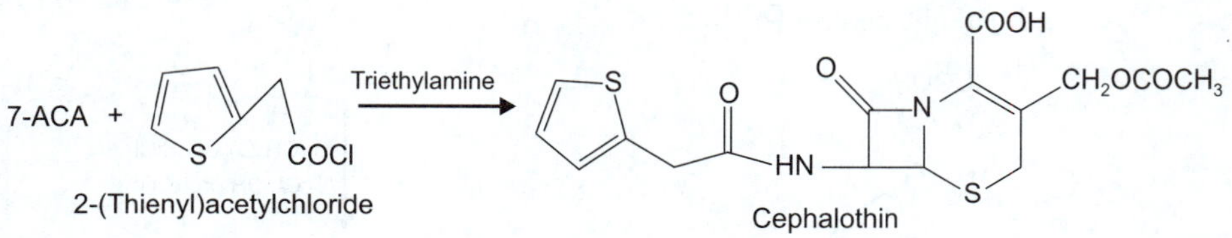

Properties: Cephalothin is a white, odourless, crystalline powder, insoluble in most organic solvents, and it is acid stable. It is hygroscopic and decomposes on heating, and it has been described as broad-spectrum antibacterial compound, it is not in the same class as the tetracyclines. Its spectrum of activity is broader than that of penicillin G and more similar to that of ampicillin.

Dose: The dose for adults given IM or IV is equivalent to 500 mg–1 g every 4 to 6 hrs; for children, the dose is 13–26 mg/kg of body weight every 4 hrs.

iv. Cefsulodin

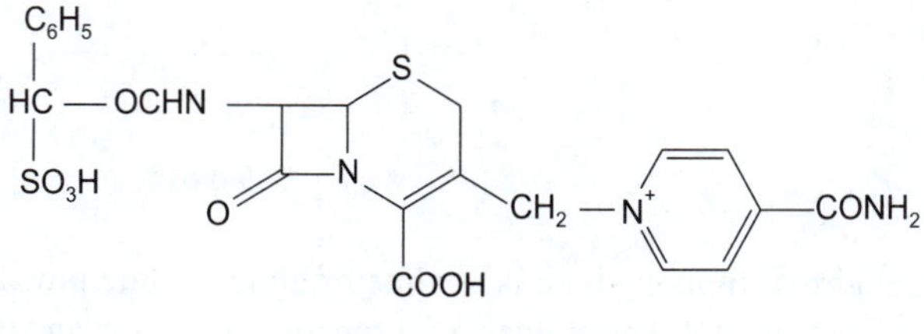

Synthesis

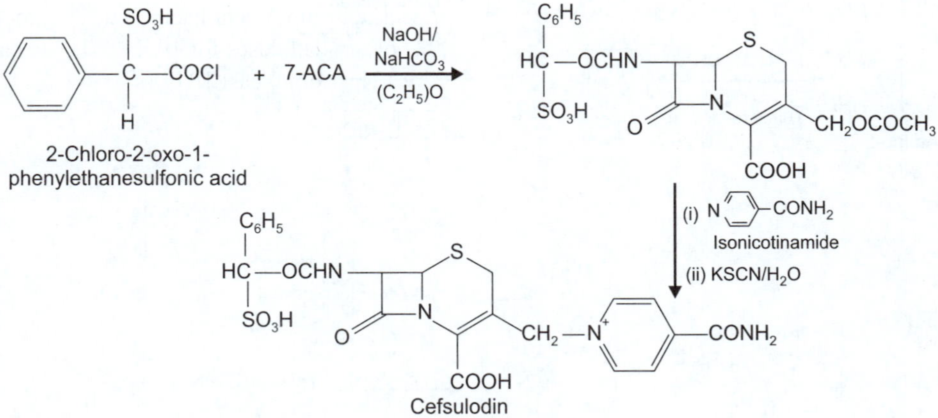

2-Chloro-2-oxo-1-phenylethanesulfonic acid

Properties and uses: It is indicated for use in staphylococcal and pseudomonal infections.

v. Cephradine

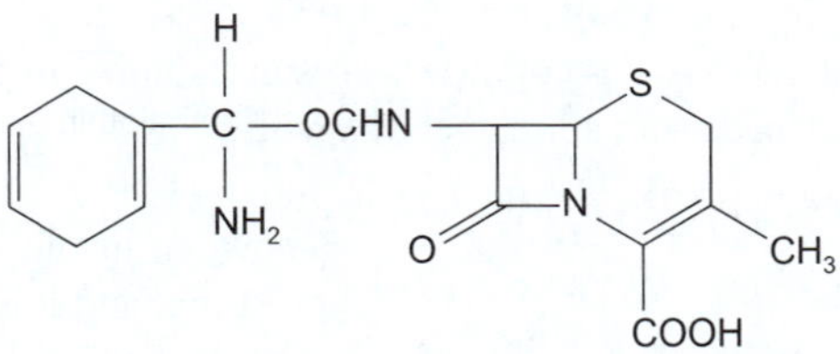

Synthesis

Route-I.

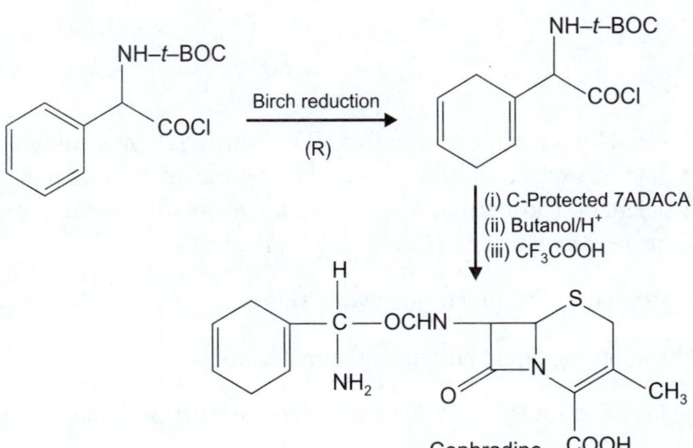

Cephradine

Route-II. From: 2-Amino-2-phenylacetic acid

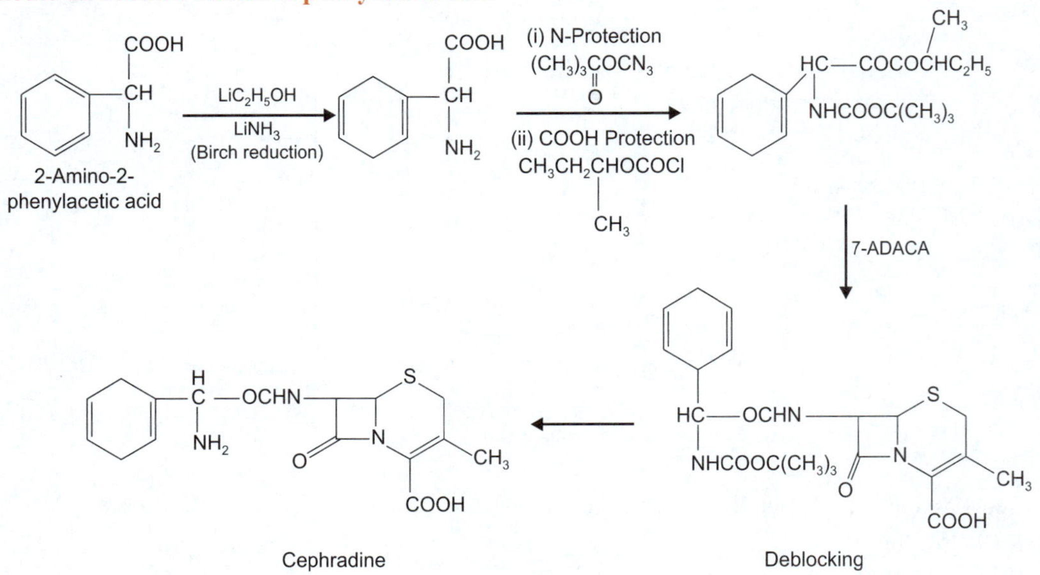

Properties and uses: Cephradine exists as colourless crystals, soluble in propylene glycol, but slightly soluble in acetone or alcohol. Used as an antibacterial agent.

II. Second-generation cephalosporin

i. Cefaclor

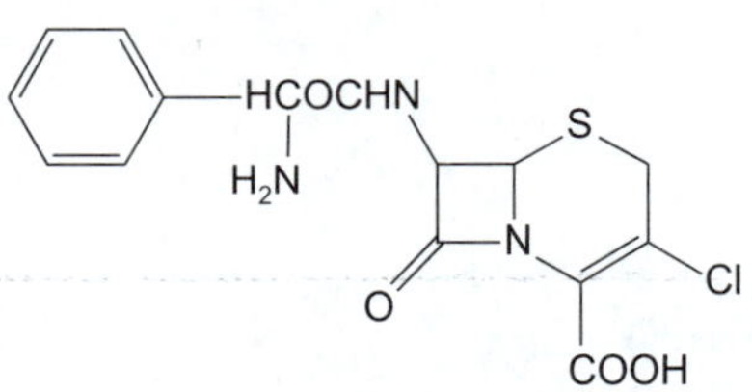

Properties and uses: Cefaclor is a white or slightly yellow powder, slightly soluble in water, practically insoluble in methanol and methylene chloride. It has chloro group at C-3 position, and hence, stable in acid and achieves sufficient oral absorption. Used in the treatment of upper respiratory tract infections caused by *Streptococcus pneumoniae* and *Haemophilus influenzae*.

Dose: The dose orally for adults is 250–500 mg every 8 hrs.

Assay: It is assayed by adopting liquid chromatography technique.

Dosage forms: Cefaclor capsules BP, cefaclor oral suspension BP, prolonged-release cefaclor tablets BP.

Synthesis

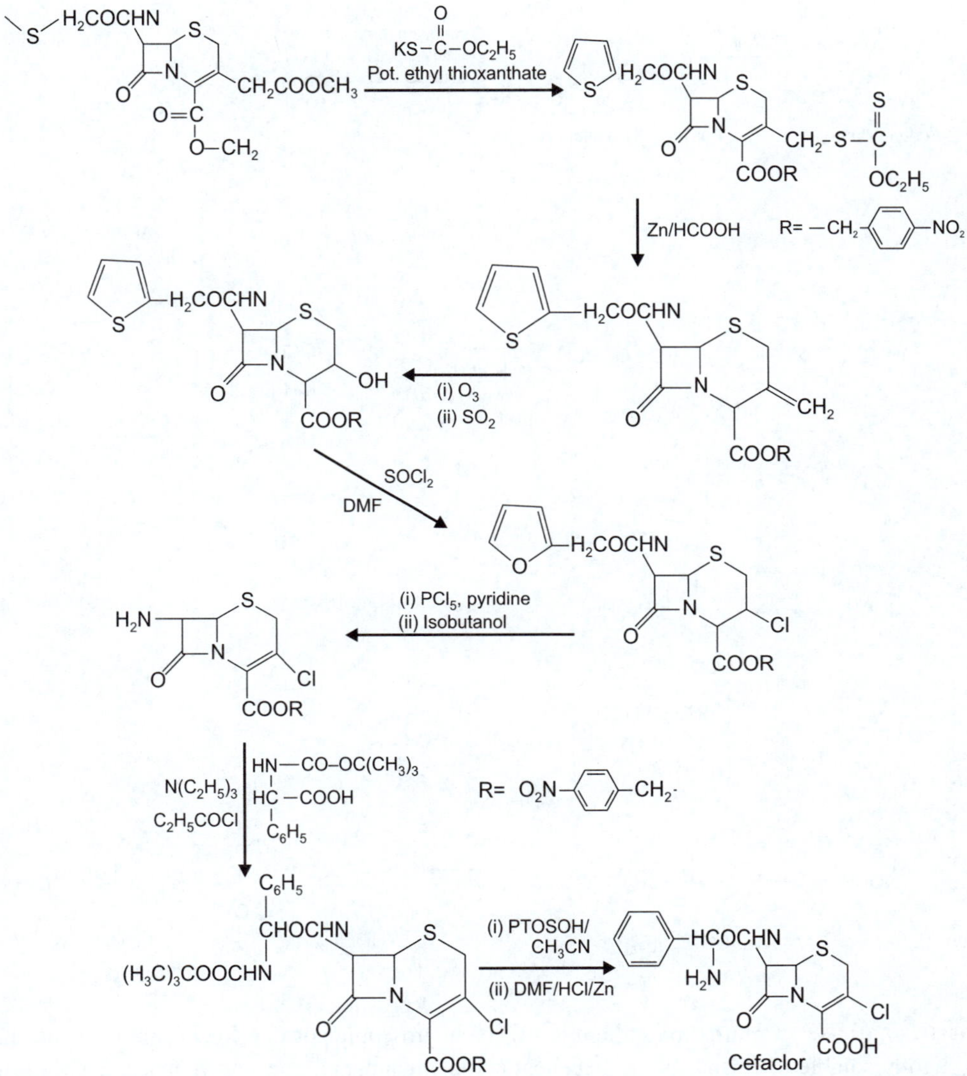

ii. Cefuroxime (Zinacef, Kefurox)

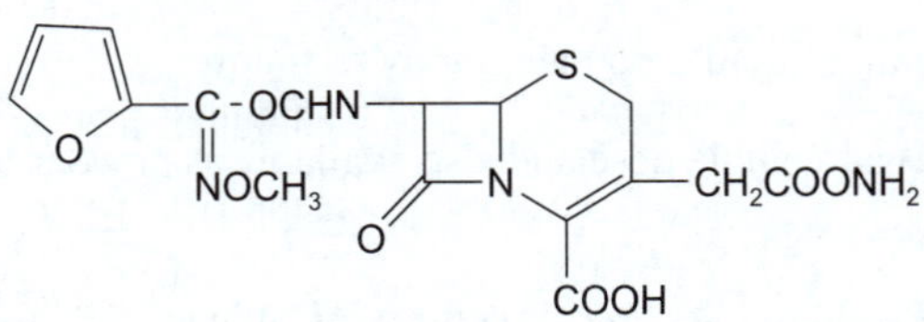

Synthesis

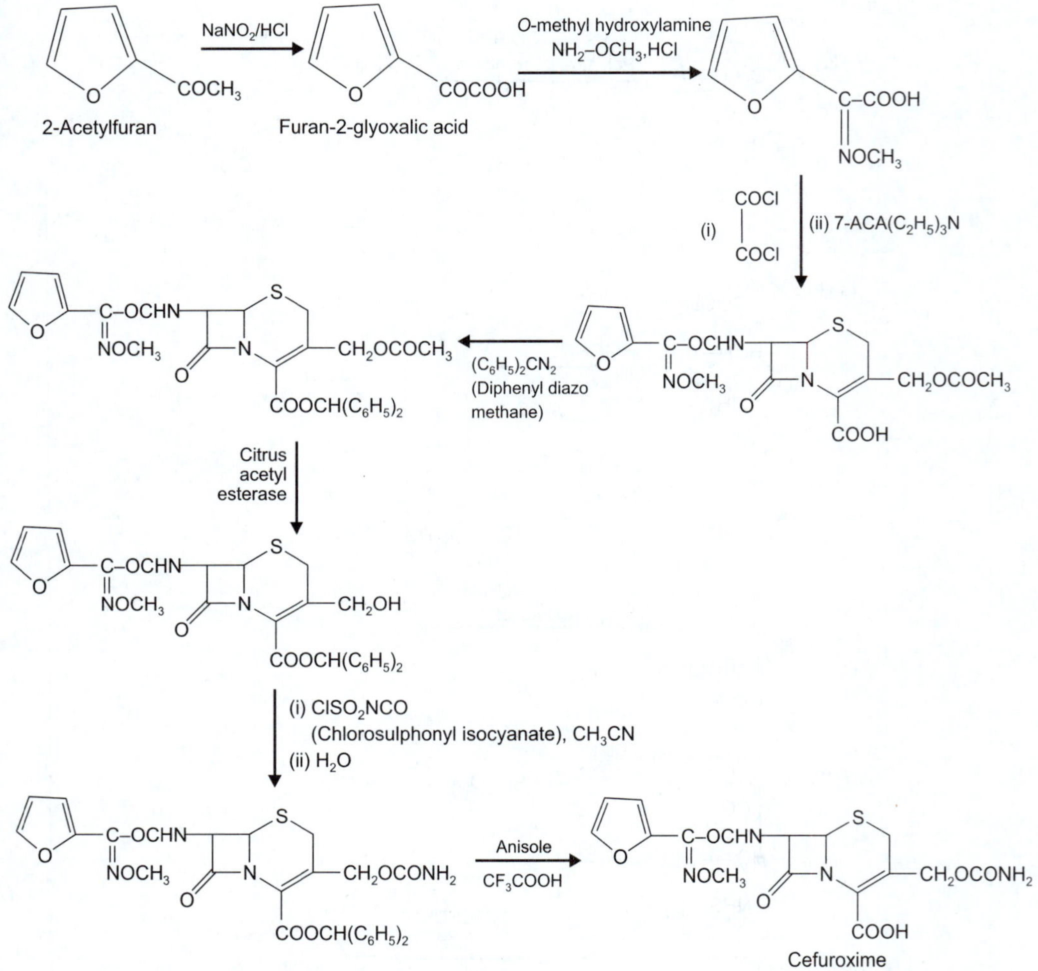

Properties and uses: Cefuroxime sodium is a white hygroscopic powder, freely soluble in water, and very slightly soluble in ethanol. It has excellent activity against all *gonococci*, hence, is used to treat gonorrhoea. It may be used to treat lower respiratory tract infections caused by *H.influenza* and *Para influenzae, Klebsiella* spp. *E. coli, Staphylococcus pneumoniae*, and pyrogens.

Assay: It is assayed by adopting liquid chromatography technique.

Dose: The dose is 1.5 g (IM) as a single dose and also available as powder for injection in strengths of 0.75 and 1.5 g.

Dosage forms: Cefuroxime sodium injection IP, cefuroxime injection BP.

iii. Cefoxitin

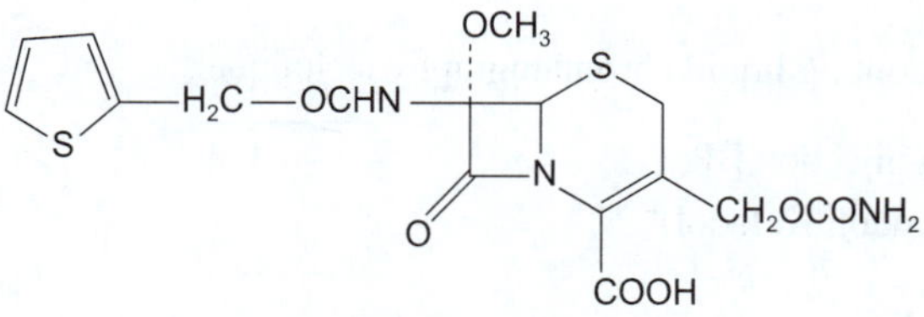

Synthesis

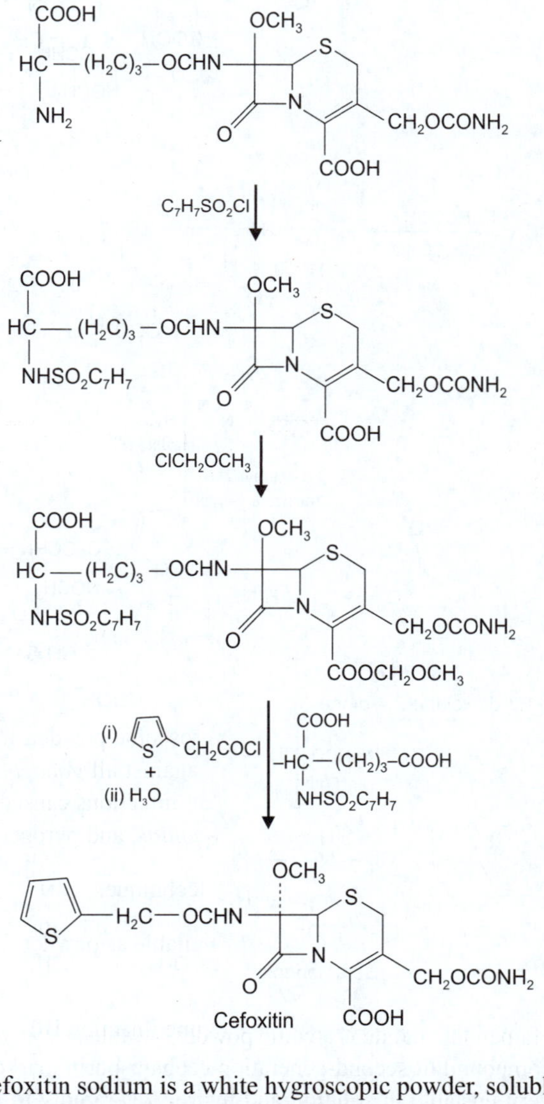

Properties and uses: Cefoxitin sodium is a white hygroscopic powder, soluble in water and sparingly soluble in alcohol. It is not the drug of choice for any infection, but it is an alternative drug for intra-abdominal infections, colorectal surgery, appendectomy, and ruptured viscus because it is active against most enteric anaerobes, including *Bacteroides fragilis*. It is approved for use in the treatment of bone and joint infections caused by *Staphylococcus aureus*, gynaecological and intra-abdominal infections by *Bacteroides* spp.

Assay: It is assayed by adopting liquid chromatography technique.

Dosage forms: Cefoxitin injection BP.

iv. Cefamandole (Mandol, Kefadol)

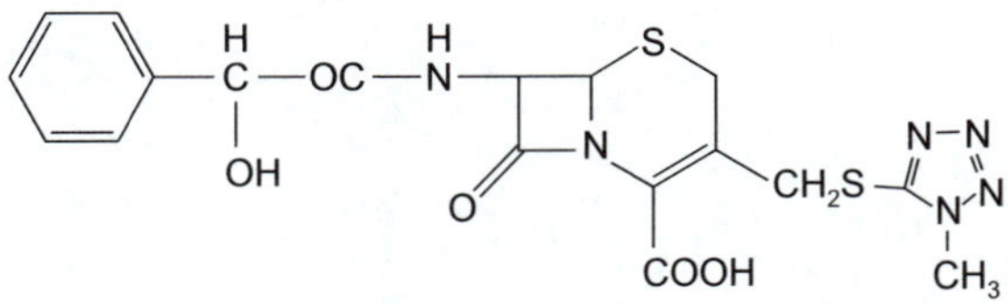

Synthesis

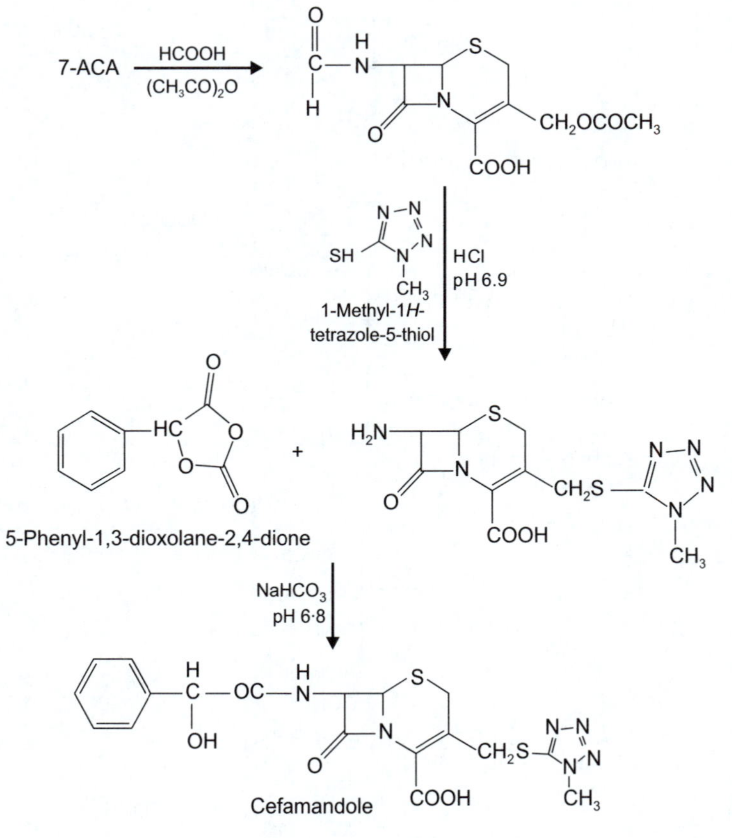

Properties and uses: Cefamandole nafate is a white powder, soluble in water, and sparingly soluble in methanol. It is the first compound of second-generation cephalosporin marketed in the United States. Cefamandole nafate is very unstable in solution and hydrolyzes rapidly to release cefamandole and formate. There is no loss of potency; however, these solutions are stored for 24 hrs at room temperature or up to 96 hrs by refrigeration.

Assay: It is assayed by adopting liquid chromatography technique.

Dose: IV dose is 0.5–2 g every 4 to 6 hrs, also available as injection in strengh of 0.5 and 1 mg/10 ml.

v. Cefonicid

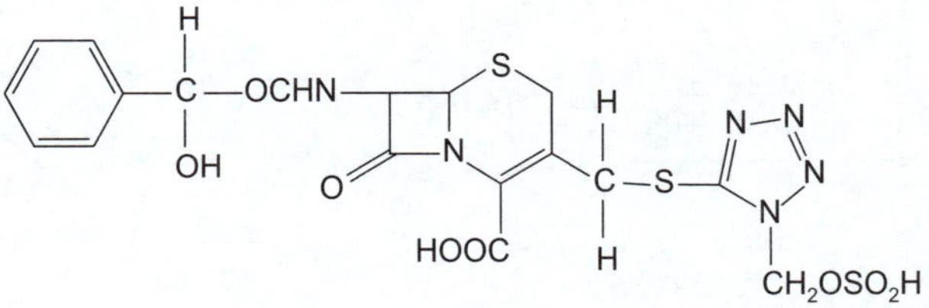

Synthesis

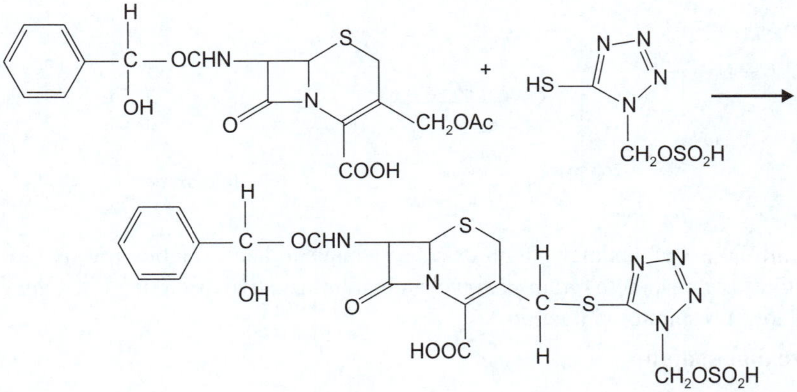

Properties and uses: Monocefonicid is a second-generation cephalosporin that is structurally similar to cefamandole, except that it contains a methane sulphonic acid group attached to the N-1 position of the tetrazole ring. Used in the treatment of bacterial infections.

III. Third-generation cephalosporins

i. Cefotaxime sodium

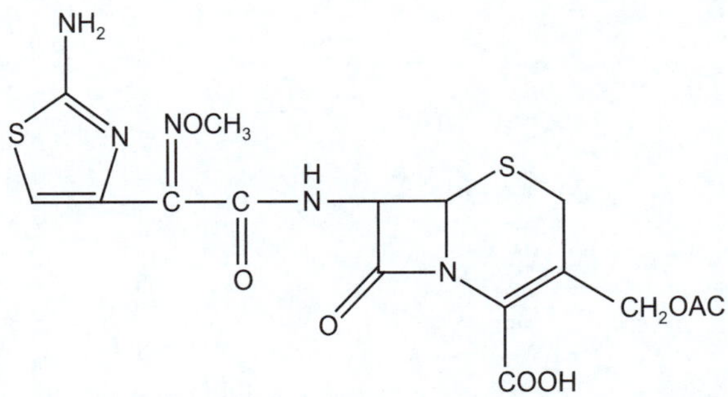

7-(2-(2-aminothiazol-4-yl)-2-(methoxyimino)acetamido)-3-(1-methyl-1*H*-tetrazol-5-ylthio methyl)-8-oxo-5-thia-1-aza-bicyclo[4.2.0]oct-2-ene-2-carboxylic acid

Synthesis

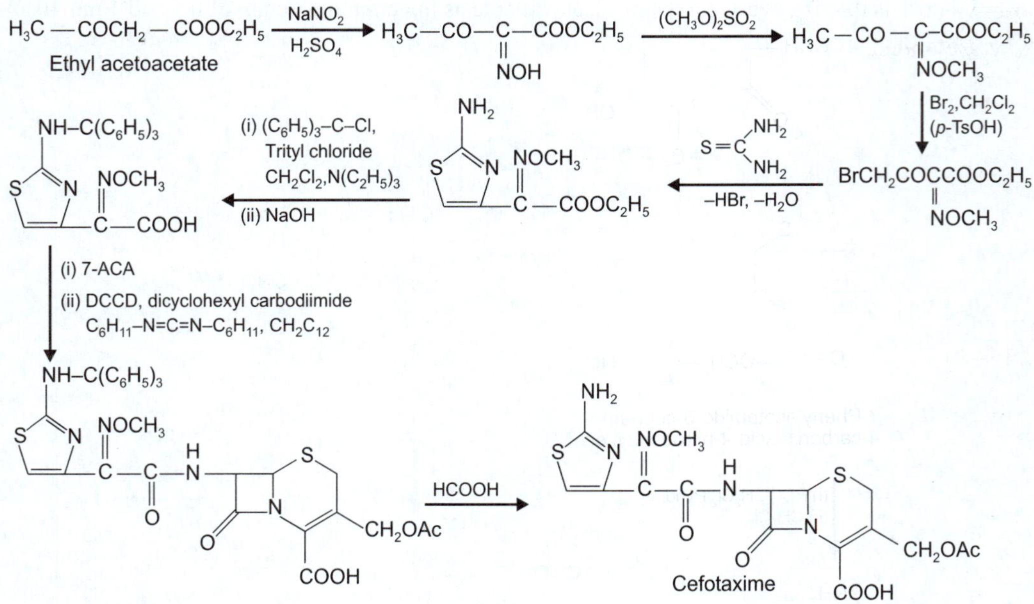

Properties and uses: Cefotaxime sodium exists as white solid and soluble in water, exhibits broad-spectrum activity against both gram-positive and gram-negative bacteria. Used in genitourinary infection and lower respiratory infection.

ii. Ceftizoxime sodium

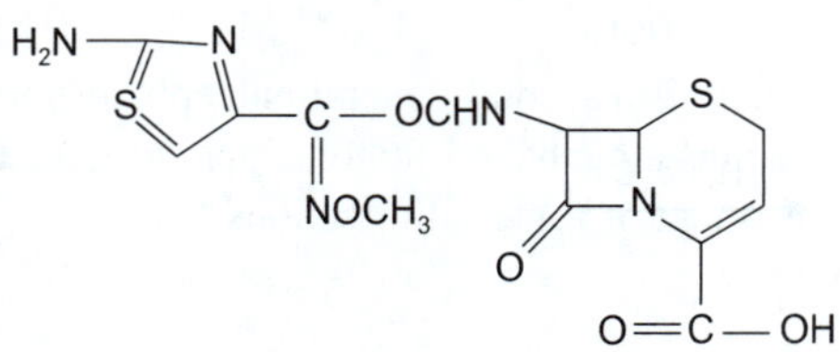

Synthesis

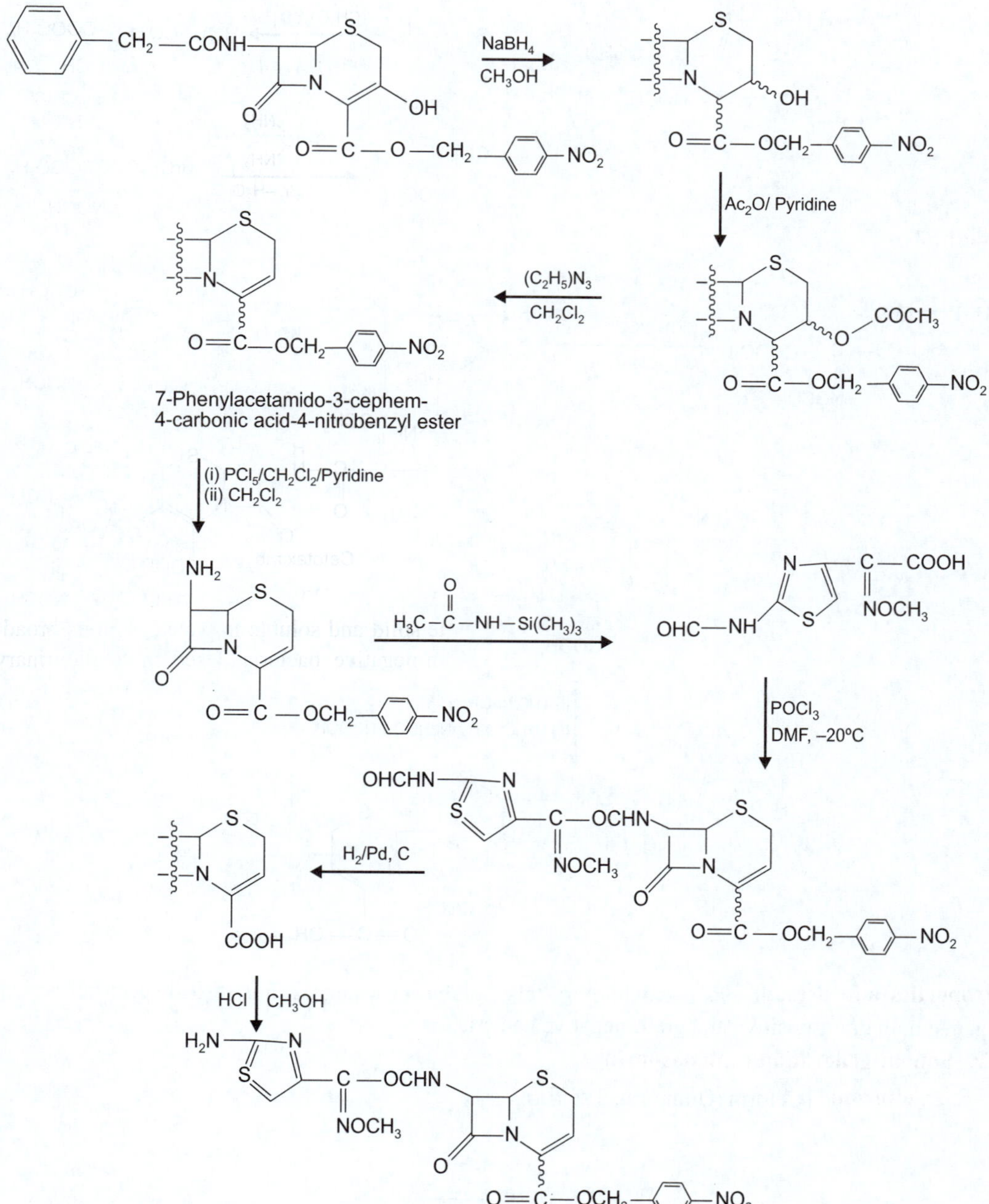

Ceftizoxime

Properties and uses: It is a beta-lactamase-resistant cephalosphorin, used in lower respiratory infection and meningitis.

iii. Ceftriazone

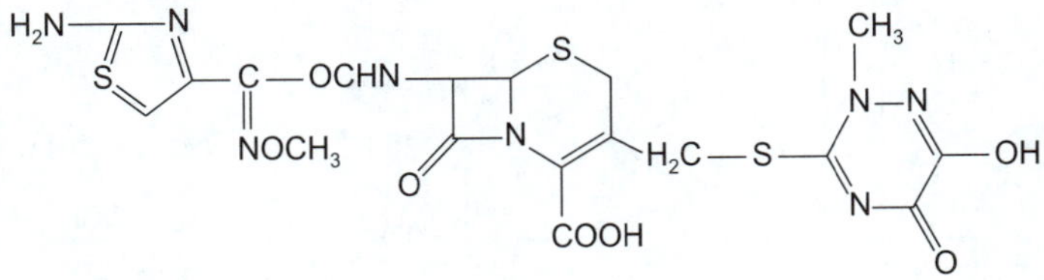

Synthesis

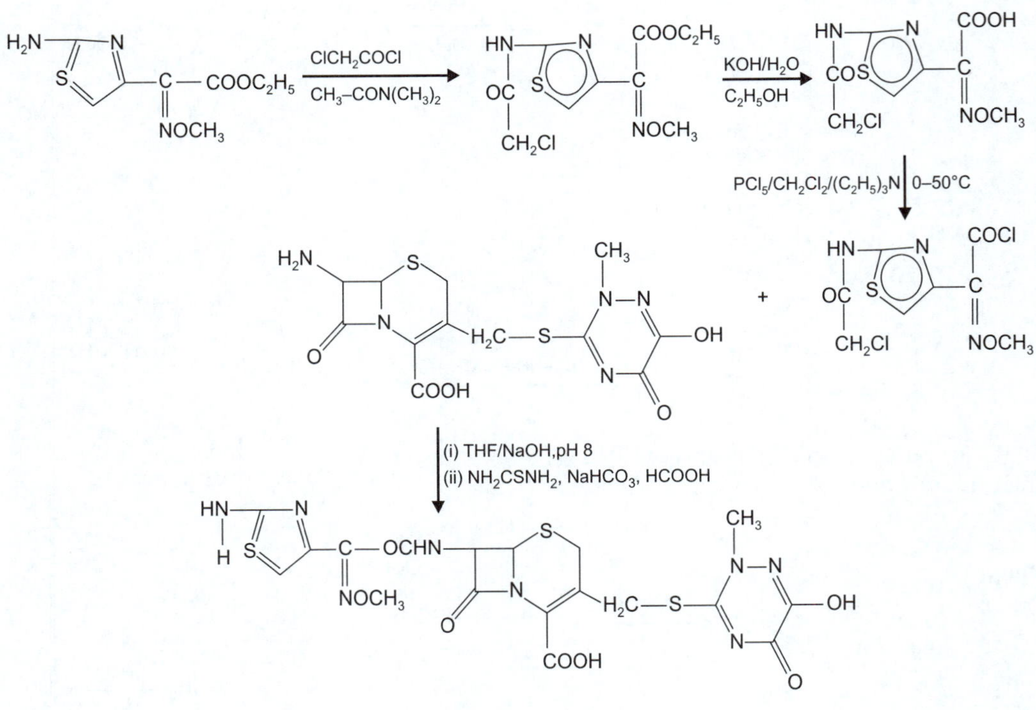

Properties and uses: It exists as white crystals, soluble in water, exhibits broad-spectrum activity against both gram-positive and gram-negative bacteria.

IV. Fourth-generation cephalosporin

i. Cefpirome (Ceform, Ominorm, Taform)

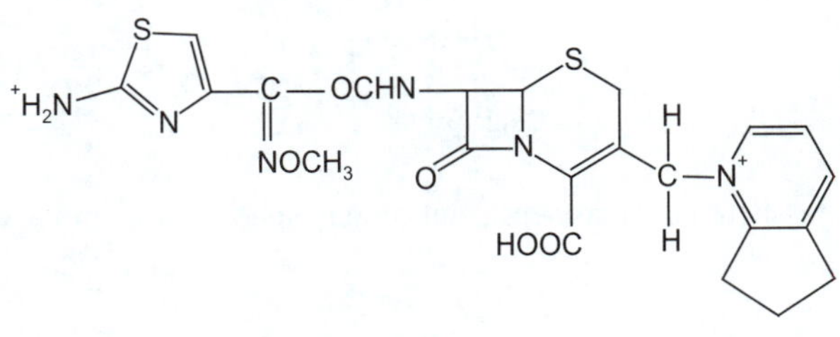

Synthesis

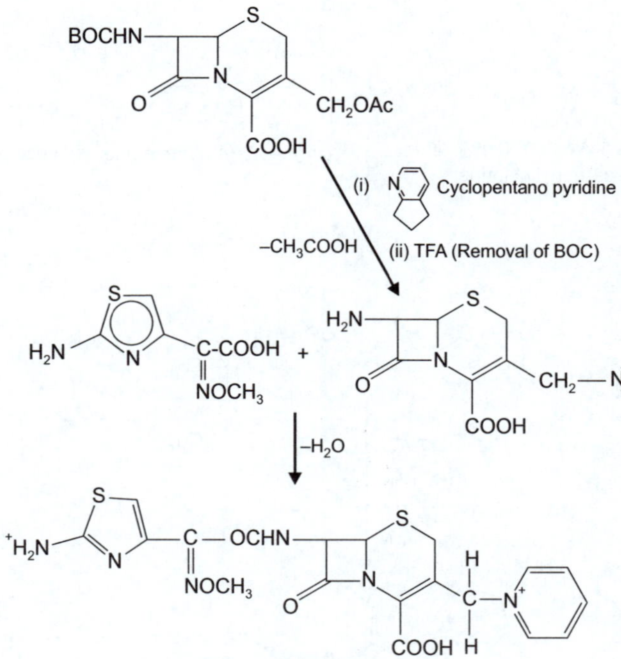

Properties and uses: Cefpirome is used to treat susceptible infections, including urinary and respiratory tract infections, skin infections, septicaemia, and infections in immuno-compromised patients.

Dose: Intravenous dose for adults as sulphate is 1–2 g every 12 hrs over 3–5 min or infuse over 20–30 min.

V. Miscellaneous

i. Cefoperazone

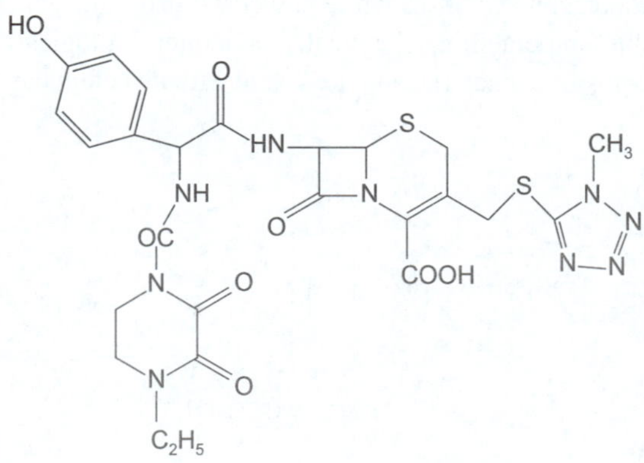

Synthesis

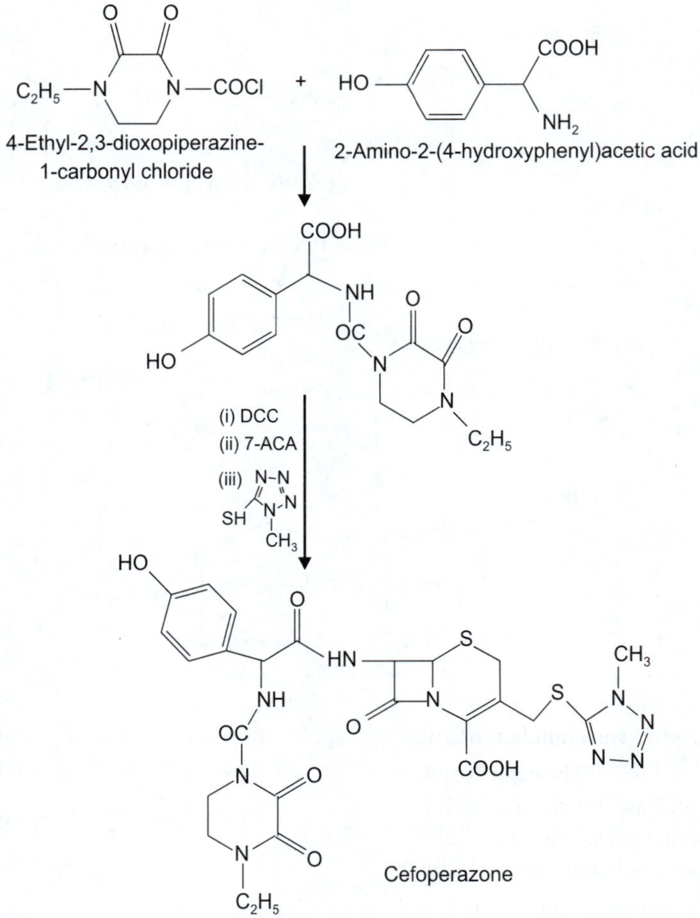

Cefoperazone

Properties and uses: Cefoperazone exists as white powder. It is a third-generation, antipseudomonal cephalosporin that resembles piperacillin, chemically and microbiologically. It is less active than cephalothin against gram-positive bacteria and less active than cefamandole against most of the enterobacteria.

ii. Cefaparole

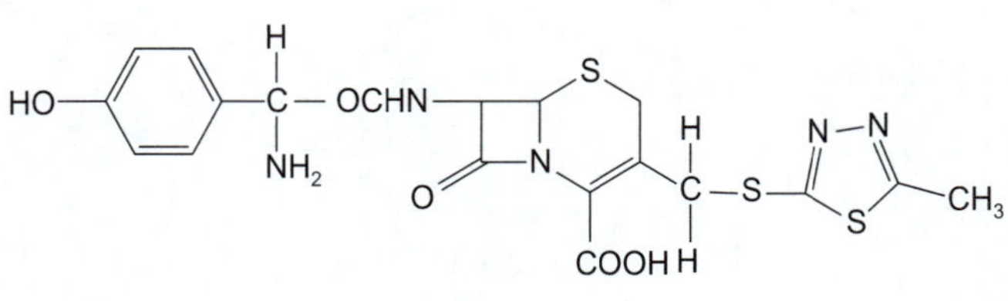

Synthesis

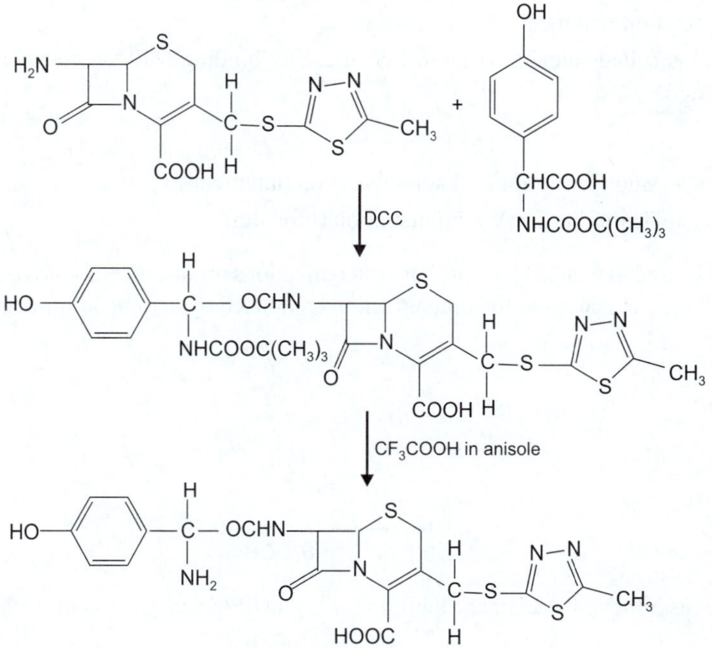

Adverse reactions of the cephalosporins

The cephalosporins produce a number of adverse effects. Examples are the following:

1. **Allergic manifestation:** The cephalosporins should be avoided or used with caution in individuals allergic to penicillins. When cefamandole or cefoperazone is ingested with alcohol, adisulphiram-like effect is seen, because these cephalosporins block the second step in alcohol oxidation, which results in the accumulation of acetaldehyde.
2. **Bleeding:** Bleeding can occur with cefemandole or ceforperazone because of antivitamin K effects. But the administration of the vitamin overcomes this problem.

Lactamase Inhibitors or β-Lactamase Inhibitors

Lactamase inhibitors are structural analogues of β-lactam antibiotics. There are three β-lactamase inhibitors available, they are clavulanic acid, sulbactam and tazobactam.

Clavulanic acid

It is the first β-lactamase inhibitor and discovered in 1970. It was isolated from *Streptomyces clavugerus.*

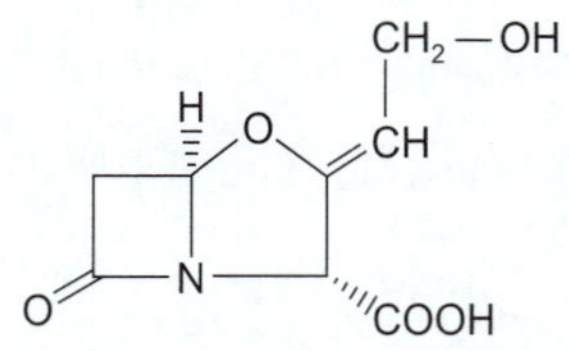

It contains β-lactam ring and effectively binds with β-lactamase enzyme.

Mode of action: It competitively and irreversibly binds with the β-lactamase enzyme and active against various kinds of gram-positive and gram-negative bacteria. It is used along with amoxicillin to treat upper respiratory tract infections.

Clavulanic acid is called suicide inhibitor. Because after binding with the enzyme, clavulanic acid itself gets inactivated.

Dosage forms:

- Clavulanic acid + Amoxycillin for oral administration (augmentin)
- Clavulanic acid + Ticarcillin for IV administration (timentin)

Uses: Augmentin is used to treat UTI, respiratory tract infections produced by *S. aureus*, *E.coli*, *Shigella*, *Salmonella,* etc. Timentin is used to treat the infections produced by aerobic gram-negative bacilli, etc.

Sulbactam

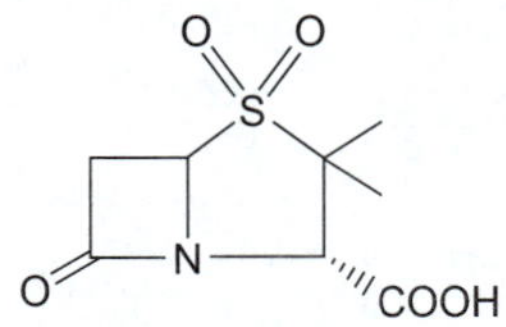

Sulbactam is a semisynthetic β-lactamase inhibitor, it is one of the compound of pencillanic acid.

IUPAC Name: (2S,5R)-3,3-dimethyl-4,4,7-trioxo-4λ^6 -thia-1-aza bicycle(3.2.0)heptane-2-carboxylic acid

Mode of action: It is irreversibly bind with β-lactamase and blocking the enzyme.

Dosage form: It is used along with ampicillin and administered by IM or IV route.

Therapeutic uses: The combination of sulbactam and ampicillin is used to treat intra-abdominal, pelvic infections and soft tissues infections produced by *E.coli/Proteus*, *B. fragilis,* etc.

Tazobactam

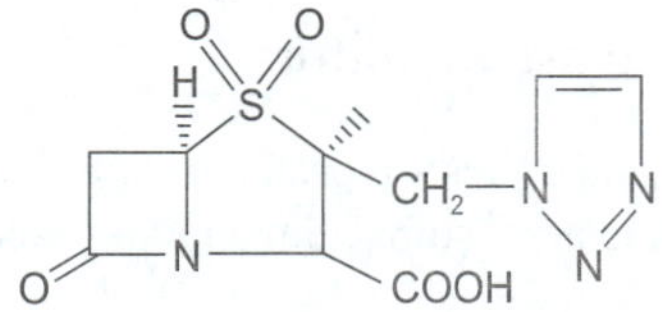

It is a penicillanic acid sulphone derivative and it contains β-lactam ring system. It is more active than salbactam.

Mode of action: Tazobactam irreversibly binds with β-lactamase enzyme and inactivates it.

Therapeutic uses: The combination of tazobactam with piperacillin is used to treat infections produced by *E.coli* and Bacteroides.

Monabactams

Aztreonam

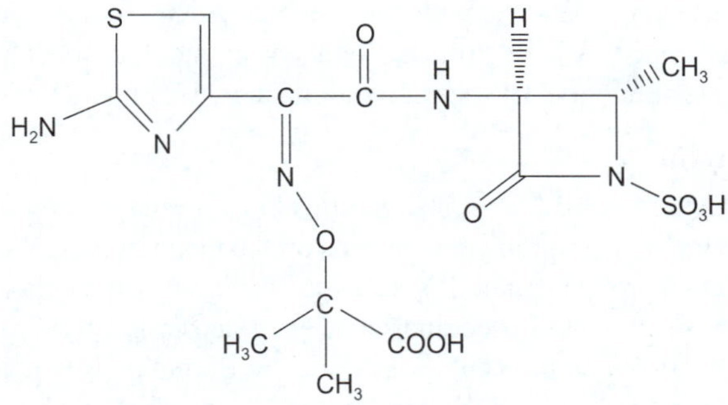

Aztreonam is also β-lactamase inhibitors that constitute a single ring in its basic structure hence known as monobactam.

Mode of action: It also irreversibly binds with β-lactamase and inactivates it. It is the only drug acting against gram-negative bacteria such as *Enterobacteriaceae*, *H. influenza*, but it is inactive against gram-positive bacteria.

Route of administration: It is given by parenteral route of administration.

Advantages: It possesses lack of cross-reactivity with other β-lactam antibiotics.

Newer Drugs

Cefiderocol

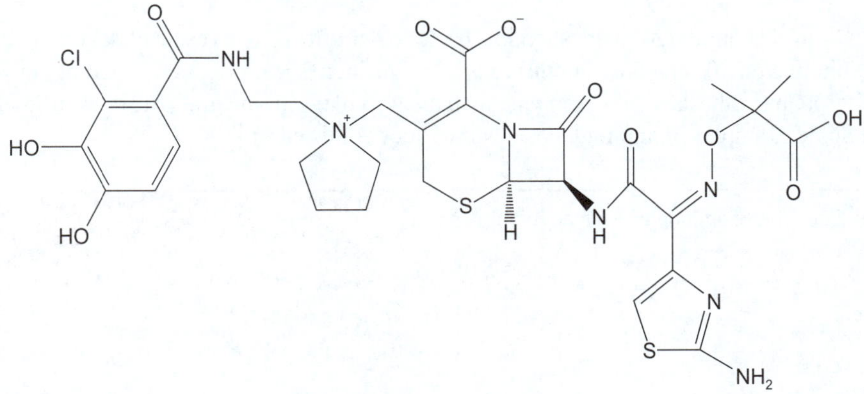

Uses: It is an antibiotic used to treat complicated urinary tract infections when no other drugs are available.

2. AMINOGLYCOSIDE ANTIBIOTICS

The aminoglycoside antibiotics contain one or more amino sugars linked to an aminocytitol ring by glycosidic bonds. These are broad-spectrum antibiotics; ingeneral, they have greater activity against gram-negative than gram-positive bacteria. The development of streptomycin, the first antibiotic of this group, was a well-planned work of Waksman (1944) and his associates, who isolated it from a strain of *Streptomyces griseus*.

The aminoglycoside can produce severe adverse effects, which include nephrotoxity, ototoxicity, and neuro effects. These properties have limited the use of aminoglycoside chemotherapy to serious systemic indications. Some aminoglycosides can be administered for ophthalmic and topical purposes.

Production of streptomycin

Initially, streptomycin was produced by surface cultures but nowadays streptomycin is produced by submerged cultures. The yield of streptomycin depends on the medium used. Again as in penicillin the culture medium must contain protein materials such as soyabean meal and cottonseed meal, in addition to other constituents. The medium used is composed of 1% glucose, 1% peptone, 0.3% meat extract or 1–2% corn steep liquor and 0–5% sodium chloride. The culture solution is kept in large vats, growth of the microorganism begins at 24–28°C and the maximum yield is achieved after 3–5 days.

Isolation of streptomycin

After separating the mycelium and other waste materials, the antibiotic from the filtrate is removed either by adsorption on charcoal or on base-exchange resins. Using dilute aqueous or alcoholic mineral acids, it is eluted from the adsorbent and the acidic eluate is purified by passing it through anion exchange resin. The pure streptomycin is isolated either as sulphate or as the crystalline trihydrochloride with calcium chloride. Aseptic handling must be done during the production and isolation of the drug.

In order to get completely sterile drug, the crystalline compounds (obtained above) are redissolved to give 25% solution, which is free from undesired impurities (heavy metals, colour and other impurities), by passing through a Seitz filter, and then freeze dried. The freeze dried powder is transferred aseptically to small vials as in case of penicillin.

Streptomycin is a colourless, water-soluble, levorotatory base and has not yet been obtained as a crystalline compound. Its aqueous solutions are stable in the pH range 1–10 and streptomycin infact is more stable than penicillin.

Mode of action: The aminoglycosides exhibit bactericidal effects as a result of several phenomena. Ribosomal binding on 30s and 50s subunits as well as the interface produces misreading; this disturbs the normal protein synthesis. Cell membrane damage also plays an integral part in ensuring bacterial cell death. Some examples of aminoglycoside antibiotics are listed in Table 15.5.

Table 15.5: Examples of aminoglycoside antibiotics

Name	Source
Streptomycin	*Streptomyces griseus*
Neomycin	*S. fradiae*
Kanamycin	*S. kanamyeleticus*
Gentamysin	*Micromonospora purpura*
Netilmicin	*Micromonospora* species
Tobramycin (nebramycin)	*S. tenebrarius*
Framycetin (Soframycin)	*S. decaris*
Paromomycin	*S. rimosus* and *S. paramomycinus*
Amikacin	It is 1-L-(–)-4-amino-2-hydroxy butyryl kanamycin

i. Streptomycin and dihydrostreptomycin

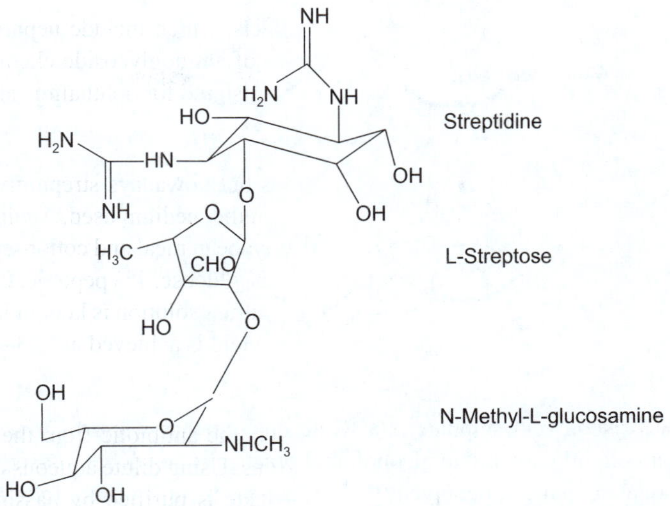

Properties and uses: Streptomycin sulphate is a white hygroscopic powder, very soluble in water, and practically insoluble in ethanol. The organism, *S. griseus*, releases the other substances, such as hydroxy streptomycin, mannisidostreptomycin, and cycloheximide, but do not reach up to the required activity/potency level. The development of resistant strains of bacteria and chronic toxicity constitutes major drawbacks of this category. It is an aminoglycoside antibacterial also used as antitubercular drug.

Assay: It is assayed by microbiological method.

Dosage form: Streptomycin injection BP.

ii. Gentamycins

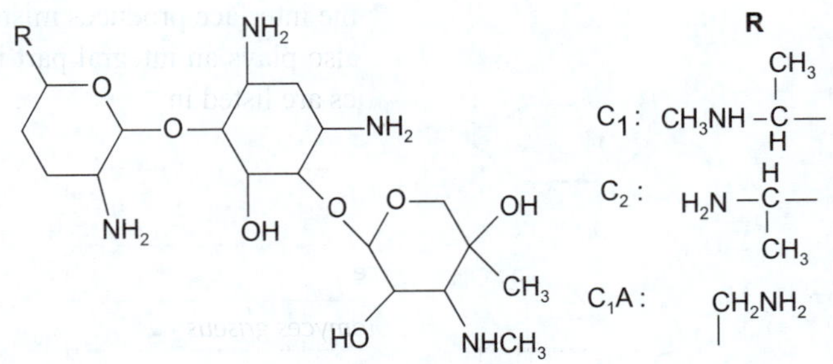

Properties and uses: Gentamycin is a mixture of C_1, C_2, and C_1A compounds, obtained commercially from *Micromonospora purpurea*. Gentamycin sulphate exists as white hygroscopic powder, soluble in water, and practically insoluble in alcohol, although it is a broad-spectrum antibiotic. It is used in the treatment of infections caused by gram-negative bacteria of particular interest and has a high degree of activity against *P. aeruginosa*, where the important causative factor is burned skin. It is used topically in the treatment of infected bed-sores, pyodermata, burns, and in the infection of the external eye.

Assay: It is assayed by microbiological method.

Dosage forms: Gentamicin cream BP, gentamicin eardrops BP, gentamicin and hydrocortisone acetate eardrops BP, gentamicin eyedrops BP, gentamicin injection BP, gentamicin ointment BP.

iii. Neomycin

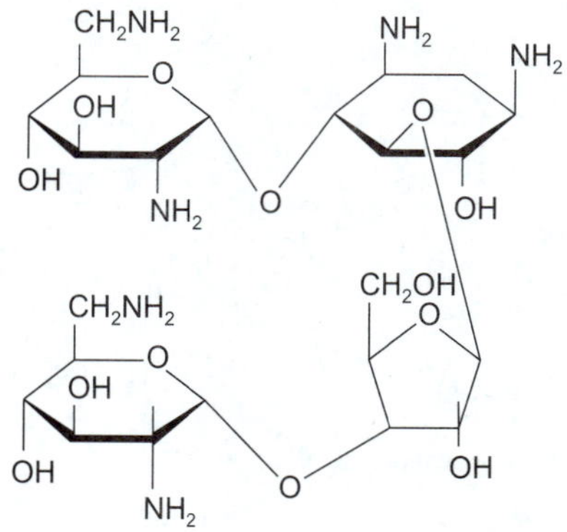

Properties and uses: Neomycin sulphate is a white or yellowish-white hygroscopic powder, very soluble in water, very slightly soluble in alcohol, and practically insoluble in acetone. Neomycin is a mixture of closely related epimers, neomycin B, and C. Neomycin B differs from neomycin C by the nature of the sugar attached terminally to ribose. This sugar called neosamine B differs from neosamine C in its stereochemistry. In neomycin B, the neobiosamine moiety contains β-L-iodopyranosyl, whereas in neomycin C the configuration is inverted and it is 2-D-glucopyranosyl. It is photosensitive and its main use is in the treatment of the ear, eye, and skin infections; these include burns, wounds, ulcer, and infected dermatoses.

Assay: It is assayed by microbiological method.

Dosage forms: Dexamethasone and neomycin ear spray BP, hydrocortisone and neomycin cream BP, hydrocortisone acetate and neomycin eardrops BP, hydrocortisone acetate and neomycin eyedrops BP, neomycin eyedrops BP, hydrocortisone acetate and neomycin eye ointment BP, neomycin eye ointment BP, neomycin oral solution BP, neomycin tablets BP.

iv. Kanamycin

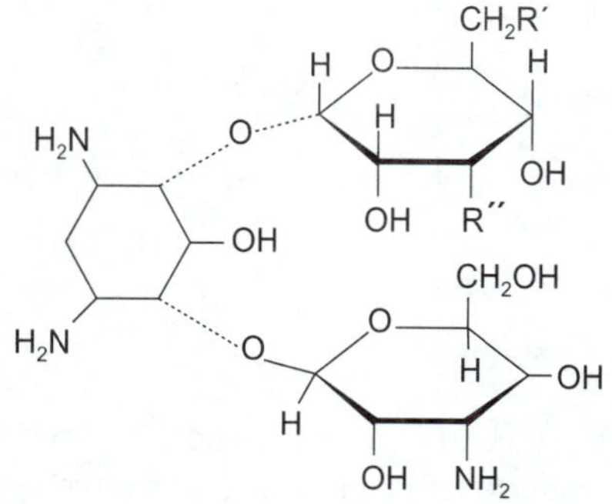

Kanamycin A = R′= NH_2; R″ = OH
Kanamycin B = R′= R″ = NH_2
Kanamycin C = R′=OH; R″ = NH_2

Properties and uses: Kanamycin sulphate is a white crystalline powder, soluble in water, practically insoluble in acetone and in alcohol. The mixture consists of three related structures, that is, kanamycin A, B, and C. The kanamycins do not possess D-ribose molecule that is present in neomycins and paramomycins. The use of kanamycins is restricted to infections of the intestinal tract and to systemic infections.

Assay: It is assayed by microbiological method.

v. Amikacin

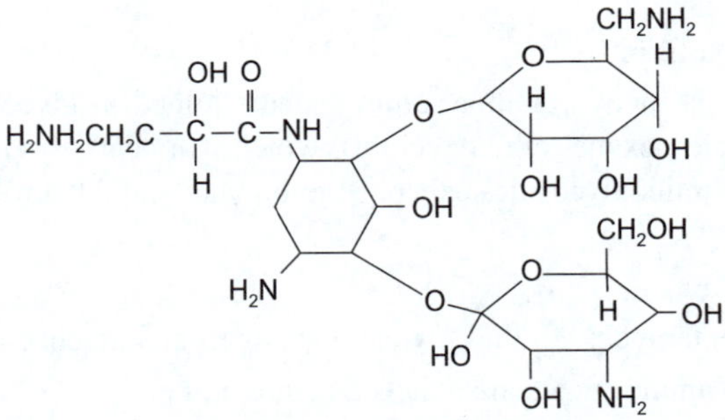

Properties and uses: Amikacin is a semisynthetic drug derived form kanamycin A. It retains 50% of the original activity of kanamycin A. L-Isomer is more active than D-isomer. It resists attack by most bacterial-inactivating enzyme. Therefore, it is very effective and less ototoxic than other aminoglycosides.

Dosage forms: Amikacin sulphate injection IP.

vi. Tobramycin

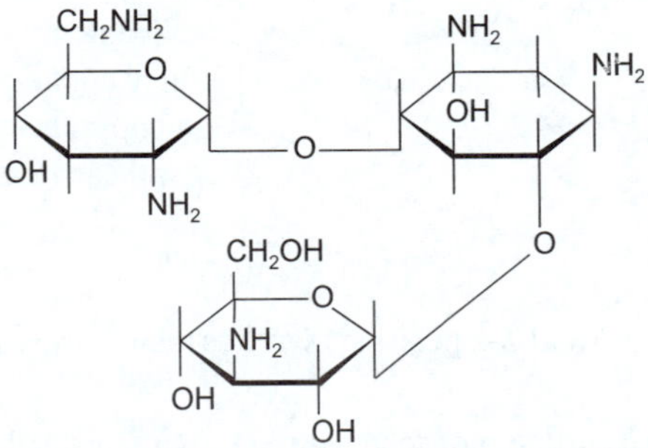

Properties and uses: Its activity is similar to gentamycin. The superior activity of tobramycin against *P. aeruginosa* may make it useful in the treatment of bacterial oesteromyelitis, and pneumonia caused by *Pseudomonas* species.

Dosage form: Tobramycin injection IP.

vii. Netilmicin (1-N-ethylsisomicin)

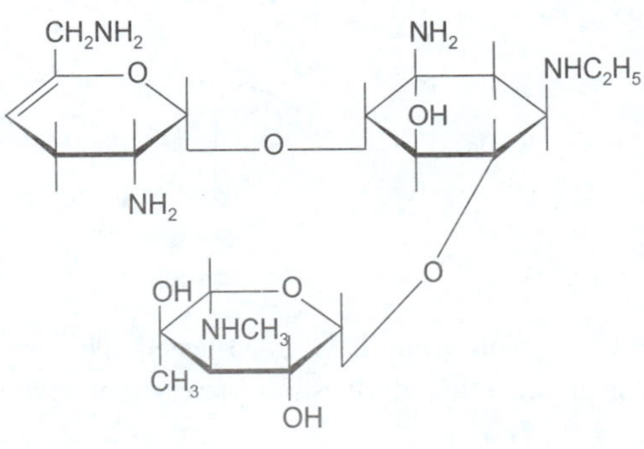

Properties and uses: Netilimycin sulphate is a white or yellowish-white hygroscopic powder, very soluble in water, practically insoluble in acetone and alcohol. It is similar to gentamycin and tobramycin. The majority of the aminoglycoside inactivating enzymes do not metabolize it. It is useful for the treatment of serious infections due to susceptible enterobacteria and other aerobic gram-negative bacilli.

Assay: It is assayed by microbiological method.

SAR of Aminoglycoside Antibiotics

The aminoglycosides consist of two or more amino sugars joined in glycoside linkage to a highly substituted 1,3-diaminocyclo hexane (aminocyclitol), which is a centrally-placed ring. The ring is a 2-deoxy streptamine in all aminoglycosides except streptomycin and dihydrostreptomycin, where it is streptidine.

Thus,

- In kanamycin and gentamycin families, two amino sugars are attached to 2-deoxy streptamine.
- In streptomycin, two amino sugars are attached to strepidine.
- In neomycin family, there are amino sugars attached to 2-deoxy streptamine.

The aminoglycoside antibiotics contain two important structural features. They are amino sugar portion and centrally-placed hexose ring, which is either 2-deoxystreptamine or streptidine.

1. Amino sugar portion

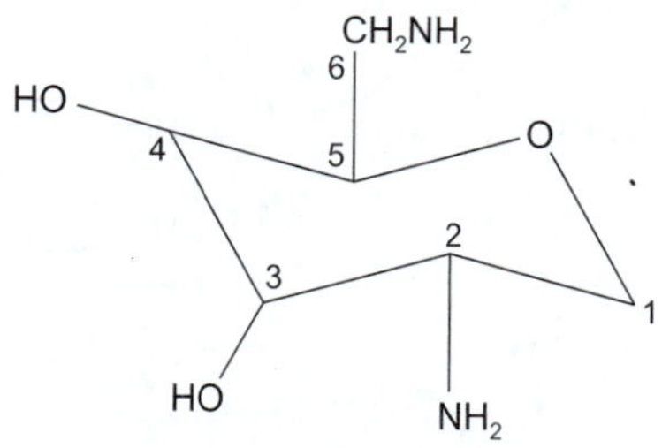

i. The amino function at C-6 and C-2 positions serve as major target sites for bacterial-inactivating enzymes.
ii. Methylation at C-6 position does not decrease the activity; instead, increases enzyme resistance.
iii. Cleavage of 3-hydroxyl or the 4-hydroxyl or both groups does not affect the activity.

2. Centrally-placed hexose ring (aminocyclitol ring)

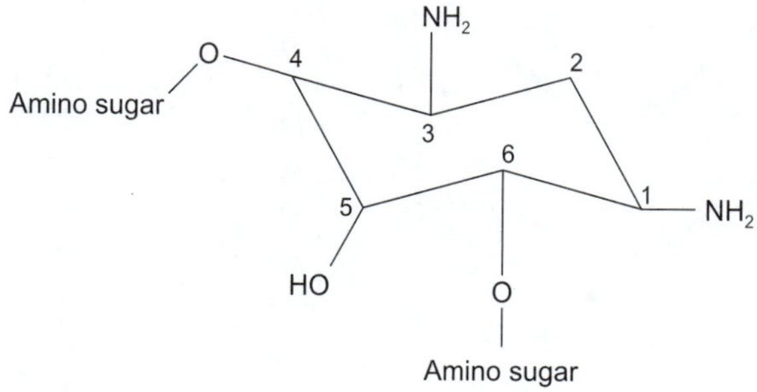

i. Various modifications at C-1 amino group have been tested. The acylation (e.g. amikacyn) and ethylation (e.g.1-N-ethylsisomicin) though does not increase the activity helps to retain the anti-bacterial potency.
ii. In sisomicin series, 2-hydroxylation and 5-deoxygenation result in the increased inhibition of bacterial-inactivating enzyme systems. Thus, very few modifications of the central ring are possible, which do not violate the activity spectrum of aminoglycosides.

Classification Based on PCI Syllabus

Streptomycin

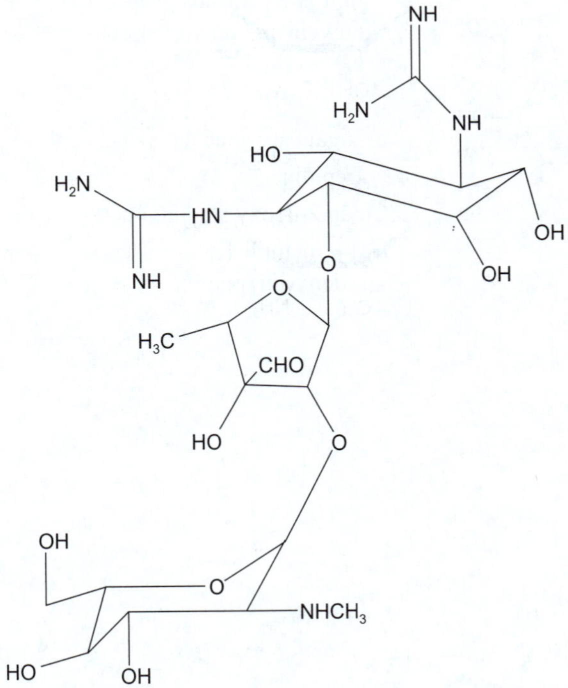

Streptidine

L-Streptose

N-Methyl-L-glucosamine

Neomycin

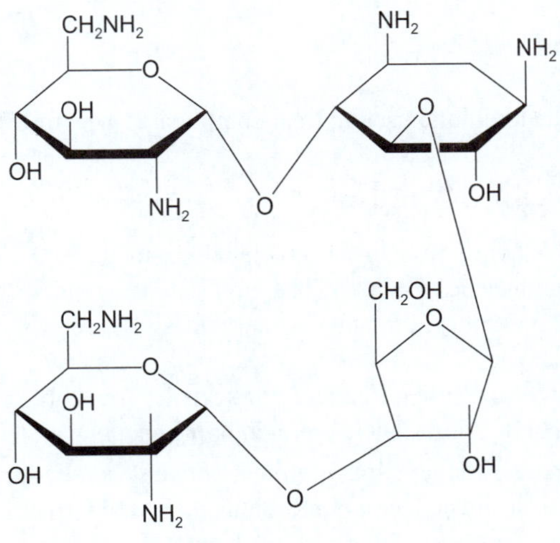

Kanamycin

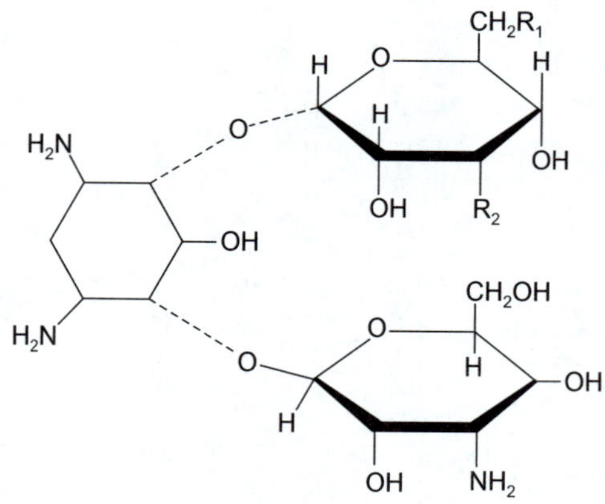

Newer Agents

Plazomicin

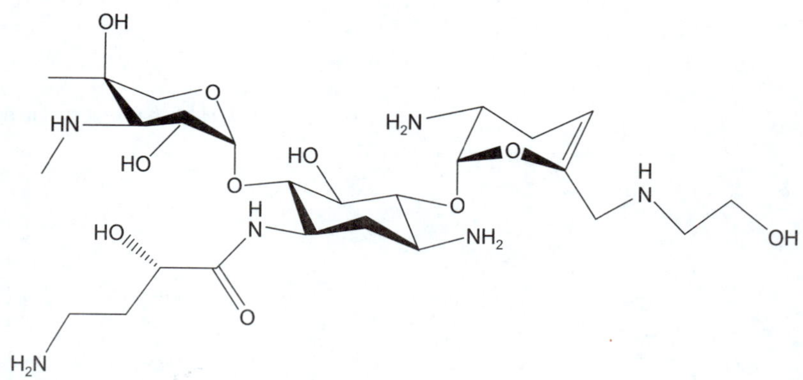

Uses: It is an aminoglycoside antibiotic used to treat complicated type of UTI.

3. TETRACYCLINE ANTIBIOTICS

Tetracyclines have a ring system of four linear annelated six-membered rings and are characterized by a common octahydronaphthacenes skeleton. They are potent, broad-spectrum antibacterial agents effective against gram-positive and gram-negative aerobic and anaerobic bacteria. As a result, the tetracyclines are drugs of choice or well-accepted alternatives for a variety of infectious diseases. Among these, they also play a role in the treatment of sexually transmitted and gonococcal diseases, urinary tract infections, bronchitis, and sinusitis remain prominent.

The majority of the marketed tetracyclines (tetracycline, chlorotetracycline, oxytetracycline, and demeclocycline) are naturally occurring compounds obtained by the fermentation of *Streptomyces* spp. broths. The semisynthetic tetracyclines (methacycline, deoxycycline, minocycline) have the advantage of longer duration of antibacterial action. However, all these tetracyclines exhibit a similar profile in terms of antibacterial potency. In general, their activity encompasses many strains of gram-negative *E.coli*, *Proteus*, *Klebsiella*, *Enterobacter*, *Niesseria*, and *Serratia* spp., as well as gram-negative streptococci and staphylococci. Of particular interest is the potency of tetracylines against *Haemophilus*, *Legionella*, *Chlamydia*, and *Mycoplasma*.

Production of tetracyclines: Chlortetracycline (aureomycin) is produced by a strain of *S. aureofaciens*. It is isolated by the following stages: (i) adsorption on activated charcoal or magnesium silicate; (ii) washing the chromatogram with an acidified organic solvent such as methanol or acetone; (iii) selection of the fraction which appears to be yellow under UV light; (iv) finally recovery of the antibiotic by extraction with butanol, precipitation with dry ether resolution in dilute hydrochloric acid and freezing to remove water. Tetracycline is produced by *S. aureofaciens* as well as other *Streptomyces* organisms; while oxytetracycline (terramycin) is produced by *S. rimosus*.

Classes of Tetracyclines

I. Natural tetracyclines (biosynthetic)
II. Semisynthetic tetracyclines
III. Protetracyclines

I. Natural tetracyclines

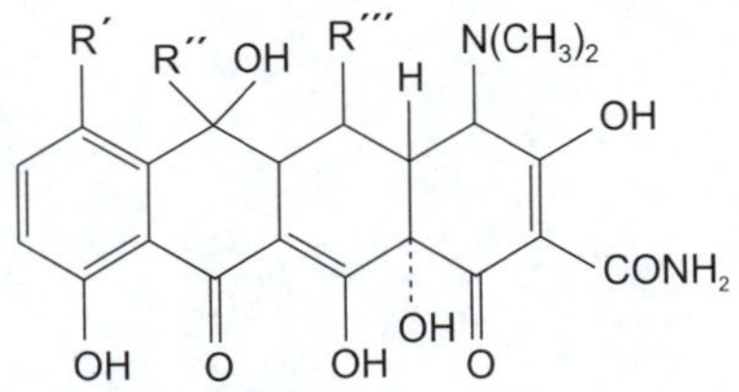

S. No.	Drug	R'	R"	R'''
1.	Tetracycline	–H	$–CH_3$	–H
2.	Chlortetracycline	–Cl	$–CH_3$	–H
3.	Oxytetracycline	–H	$–CH_3$	–OH
4.	Bromotetracycline	–Br	$–CH_3$	–H
5.	Dexamethyltetracycline	–H	–H	–H
6.	Dexamethylchlortetracycline	–Cl	–H	–H

II. Semisynthetic tetracyclines

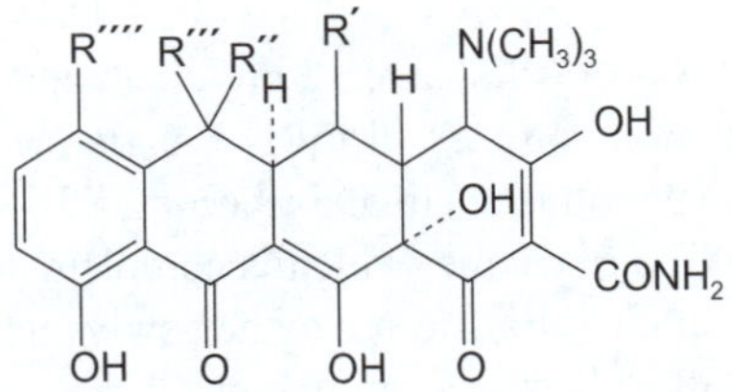

S. No.	Drug	R'	R"	R'''	R''''
1.	Doxycycline	–OH	–H	$–CH_3$	–H
2.	Minocycline	–H	–H	–H	$–N–(CH_3)_2$
3.	Methacycline	–OH	$=CH_2$	–	–H
4.	Meclocycline	–OH	$=CH_2$	–	–Cl
5.	Sancycline	–H	–H	–H	–H

III. Protetracyclines

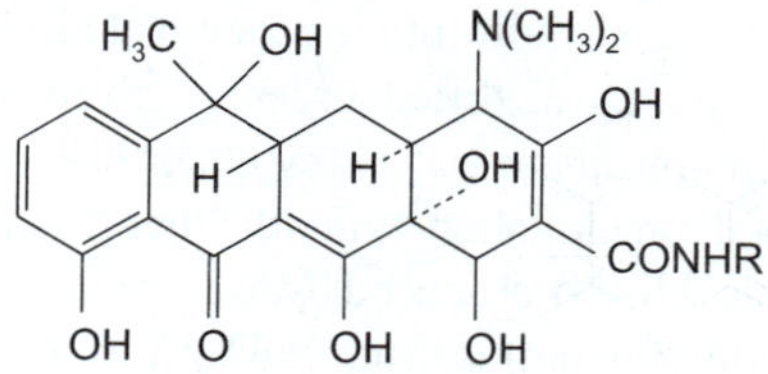

S. No.	Drug	R
1.	Rolitetracycline	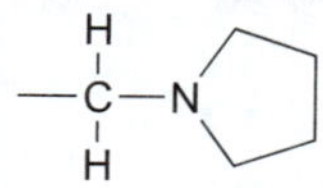
2.	Lymecycline	$-CH_2-NH(CH_2)_4-CH-COOH$ NH_2
3.	Clomocycline	$-CH_2-OH$
4.	Apicycline	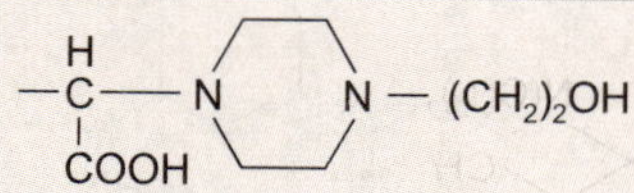
5.	Pipacycline	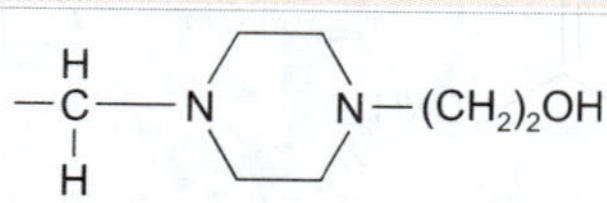
6.	Guamecycline	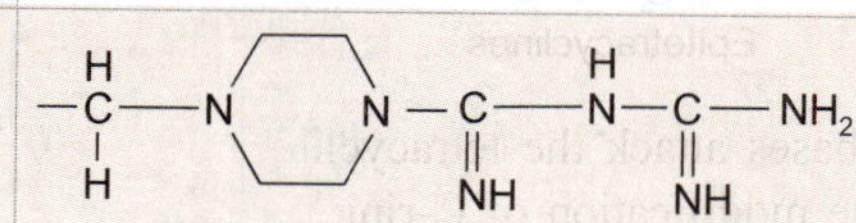
7.	Meglucycline	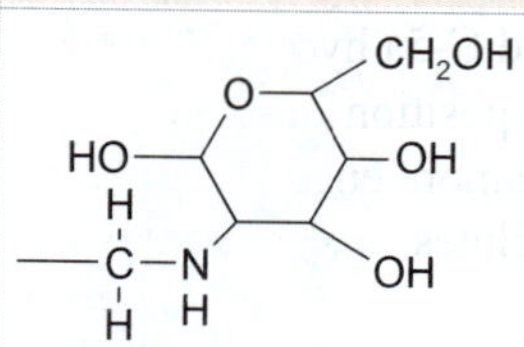

General mode of action of tetracyclines: In bacterial protein synthesis, the messenger RNA attaches itself to 30S ribosomes. The initiation complex of mRNA starts the protein synthesis and polysome formation of the nascent peptide that is attached to 50S ribosomes. Its specific tRNA transports the next amino acid to the acceptor site of the ribosome, which is complementary to the base sequence of the next mRNA codon. The nascent peptide is transferred to the newly attached amino acid by peptide bond formation. Tetracyclines bind to 30S ribosomes and the attachment of aminoacyl-tRNA to mRNA—ribosome complex is interfered.

Physicochemical properties: The tertracyclines are yellow, bitter, odourless, and light-sensitive crystalline compounds. These are amphoteric due to the acidic and the basic substituents, and have low solubility in water (0.5 mg/ml). They form water-soluble salts with strong acids and bases. In each tetracycline, there are present three ionizable groups: Tricarbonyl methane moiety (pK_a3.3), phenol diketone moiety (pK_a7.7), and ammonium cation moiety (pK_a 9.7).

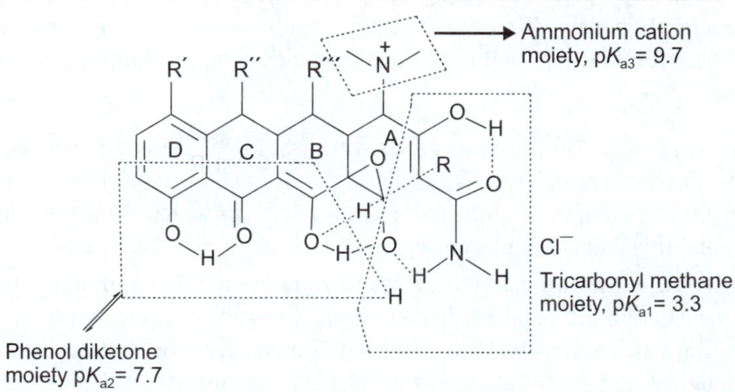

Effect of pH on tetracyclines: An interesting property of tetracyclines is their ability to undergo epimerization at C-4 position in solutions of intermediate pH range. These isomers are called epitetracyclines. Under the influence of the acidic conditions, equilibrium is established in about a day consisting of approximately equal amount of isomers. Epitetracyclines exhibit much less activity than natural isomers.

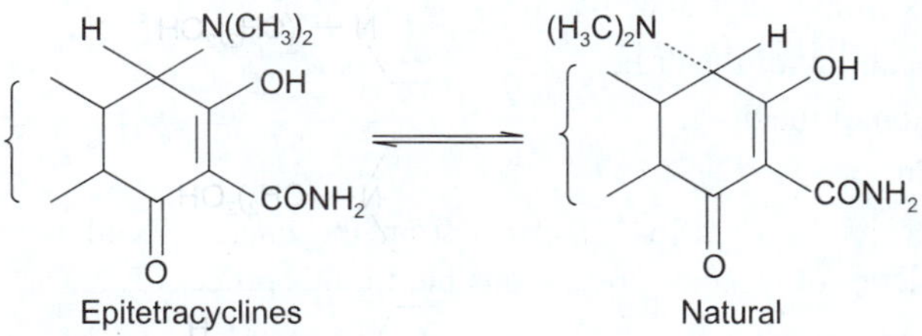

Strong acids and bases attack the tetracyclines having a hydroxyl group on C-6, causing a loss in activity through the modification of C-ring. Strong acids produce dehydration through a reaction involving the C-6 hydroxyl group and C-5a hydrogen. The double bond formed between the positions C-5a and C-6 induces a shift in the position of double bond between C-11a and C-12 to a position between C-11 and C-11a forming the more energetically favoured resonance of the naphthalene group found in the inactive anhydrotetracyclines.

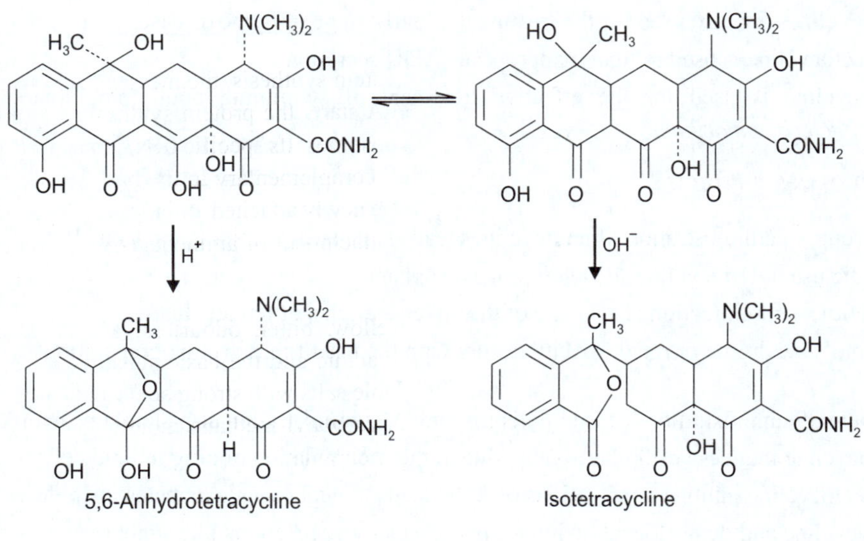

Bases promote a reaction between the C-6 hydroxyl group and the ketone group at the C-11 position, causing the bond between the C-11 and C-11a atoms to cleave and to form the lactone ring found in the isotetracycline.

Effect of metals on tetracyclines: Tetracyclines form stable chelate complexes with many metals, including calcium, magnesium, and iron. The chelates thus formed are insoluble in water accounting for the impairment in absorption of most of the tetracyclines in the presence of milk, calcium, magnesium, and aluminium containing antacids and iron salts.

The affinity of tetracyclines for calcium causes them to be laid down in newly formed bones and teeth as tetracycline calcium orthophosphate complexes. Deposits of these antibiotics in teeth's cause yellow discolouration that darkens because of photochemical reaction. Tetracyclines are distributed into the milk of lactating mothers and also cross the placenta into the foetus. The possible effect of these agents on bones and teeth of the child should be taken into consideration before they are used during pregnancy or in children under 8 years of age.

Resistance to Tetracyclines

Microorganisms develop resistance against tetracyclines by any one of the following methods:

1. Increased drug efflux from bacterial cell.
2. Decreased cell permeability of the drug.
3. Enzymatic inactivation of the drug.
4. Ribosomal protection.

In the all above mechanisms, efflux of drugs from the bacterial cell is an important one and approximately 300 varieties of proteins are responsible for this process.

Common Uses of Tetracyclines

1. Tetracyclines are the drug of choice for the treatment of Rockey Mountain spotted fever.
2. Tetracyclines are used to treat brucellosis.
3. Tetracyclines and metronidazole combination is used to treat amoebiasis.
4. The longer half-life doxycycline is well known or better choice for patients with pre-existing renal failure.
5. Tetracyclines are also used for the treatment of early stage of Lyme disease.
6. Demeclocycline is used to treat inappropriate ADH secretion.
7. Minocycline is used for the effective treatment of swimming pool granuloma caused by *Mycobacterium marinum*.

Common Adverse Effects

1. Oral route of administration of tetracyclines leads to nausea, vomiting and stomatitis.
2. Chronic use of tetracyclines develop fungal esophagitis.
3. Sometime, suprainfection is also one of the adverse effects of tetracyclines.
4. Fanconi's syndrome or renal toxicity occurs with the use of tetracycline preparations with expiry date.
5. IV route of administration leads to phlebitis and IM administration also should be avoided.
6. Minocycline induces vestibular toxicity due to the accumulation of drug in lipid cells of inner ear.
7. Demeclocycline inhibits renal actions of ADH leads to nephrogenic diabetes insipidus.
8. Doxycycline and demeclocycline induce photosensitivity reactions like sunburns.

Synthesis and Drug Profile

I. Natural tetracyclines

i. Chlortetracycline

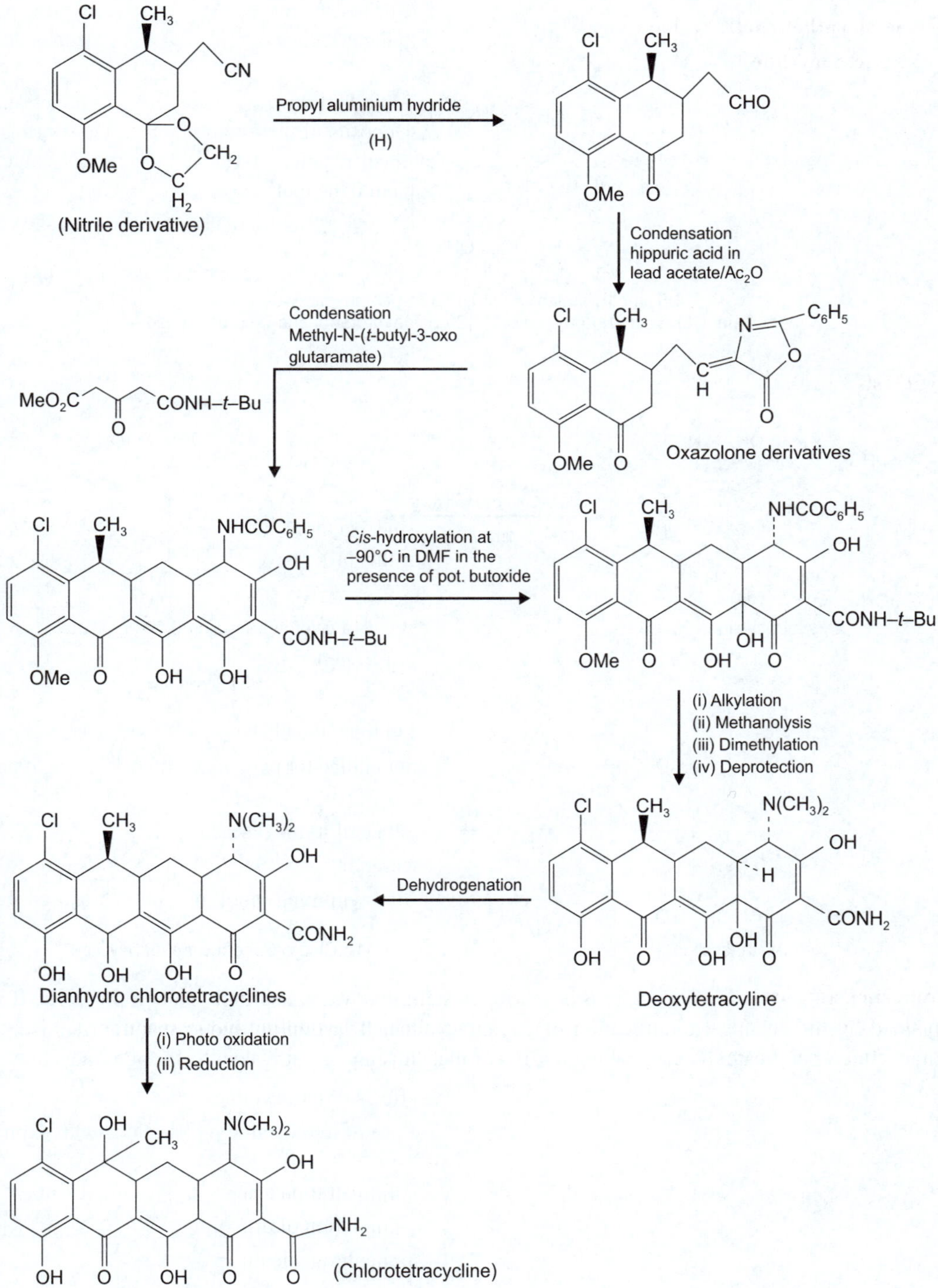

Properties and uses: It is crystalline powder with a bright yellow colour, stable in air but slightly photosensitive and should be protected from light, soluble in water, slightly soluble in alcohol, insoluble in other organic solvents. It is used as an antibacterial agent.

ii. Oxytetracycline: It is produced by *S. rimosus* by fermentation and used as an antibacterial agent.

II. Semisynthetic tetracyclines

i. Methacycline

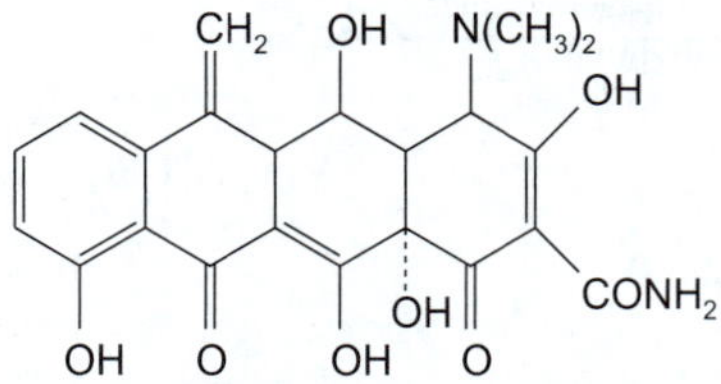

4-(Dimethylamino)-3,5,10,12,12a-pentahydroxy-6-methylene-1,11-dioxo-1,4,4a,5,5a,6,11,12a-octahydrotetracene-2-carboxamide

Synthesis

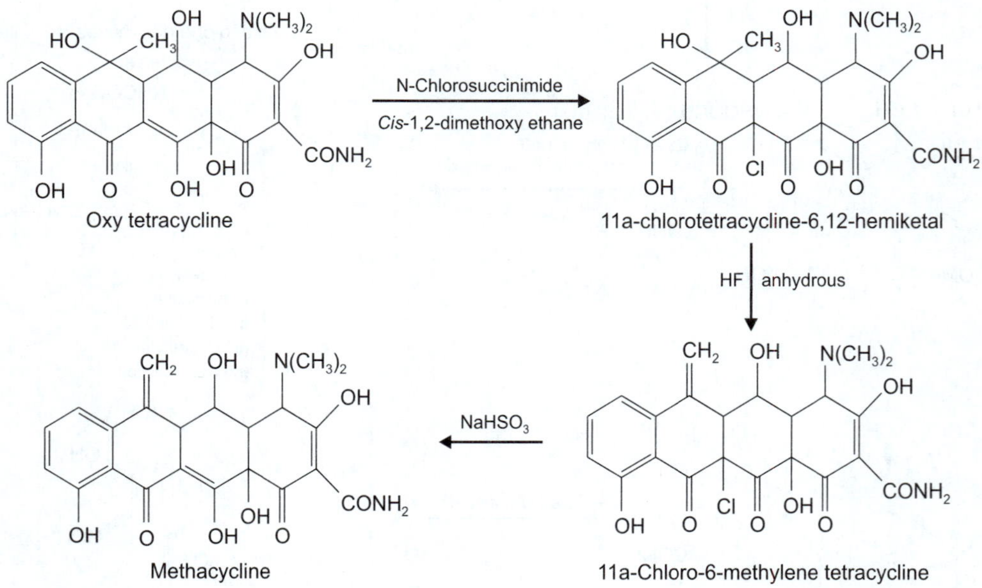

Properties and uses: Methacycline is a yellow crystalline powder, sparingly soluble in water. It is obtained by the chemical modification of oxytetracycline. It has an antibiotic spectrum similar to tetracyclines, but greater potency; about 600 mg of methacycline is equivalent to 1 g of tetracycline.

ii. Doxycycline (Vibramycin)

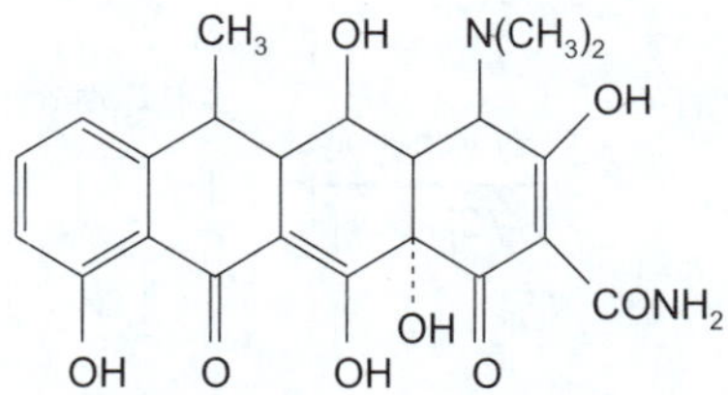

4-(Dimethylamino)-3,5,10,12,12a-pentahydroxy-6-methyl-1,11-dioxo-1,4,4a,5,5a,6,11,12a-octahydrotetracene-2-carboxamide

Synthesis

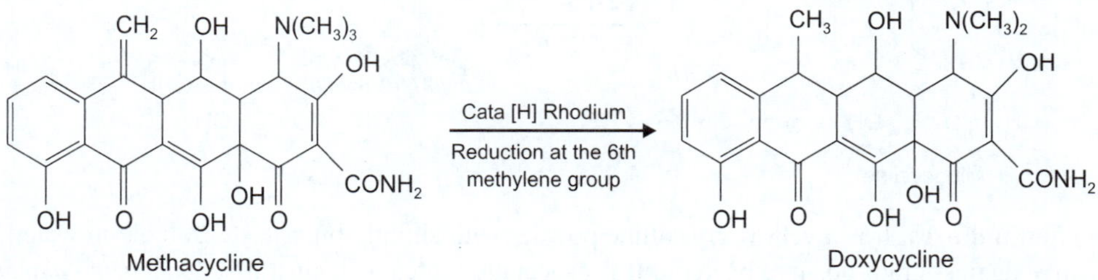

Properties and uses: It was first obtained in small yields by a chemical transformation of oxytetracycline. The 6α-methyl epimer is more than three times as active as its β-epimer.

Dose: In adults, the oral dosage is 100 mg every 12 hrs.

Dosage forms: Doxcycline HCl capsules IP, doxcycline HCl tablets IP.

iii. Minocycline (Cynomycin, Minolox)

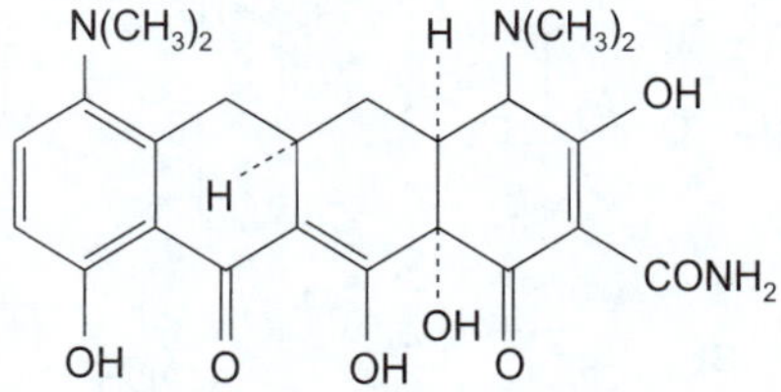

Synthesis

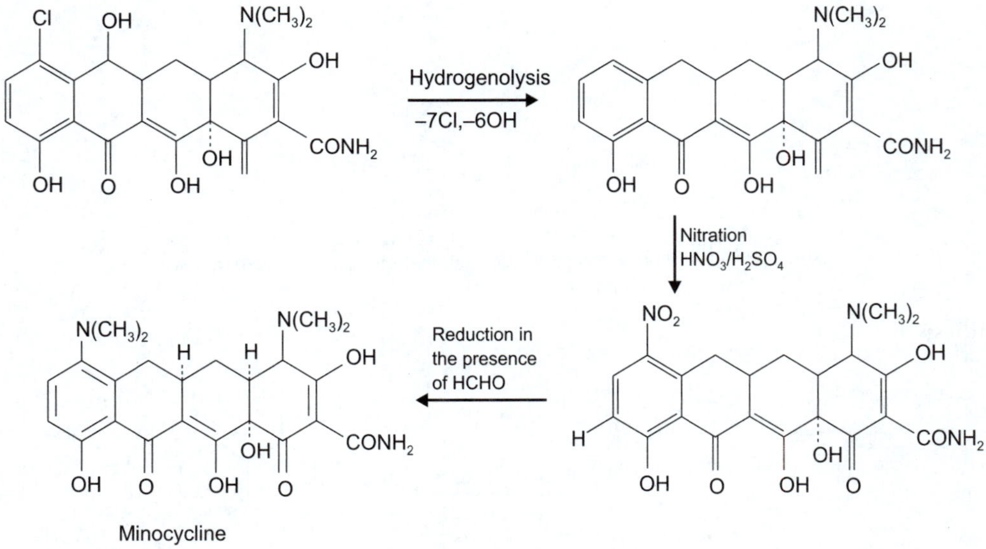

Properties and uses: It is a yellow crystalline powder with slightly bitter taste, soluble in water. It is very active against gram-positive bacteria. It is especially effective against *Mycobacterium marinum*. As a prophylactic against streptococcal infections, it is the drug of choice. It lacks the 6-hydroxyl group, therefore, it is stable to acids and does not dehydrate or rearrange to anhydro or lactone forms.

Dose: The dose orally for adults is 200 mg.

iv. Rolitetracycline

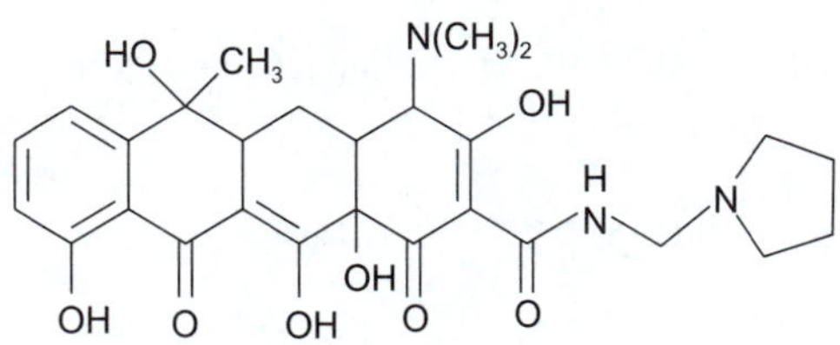

Synthesis

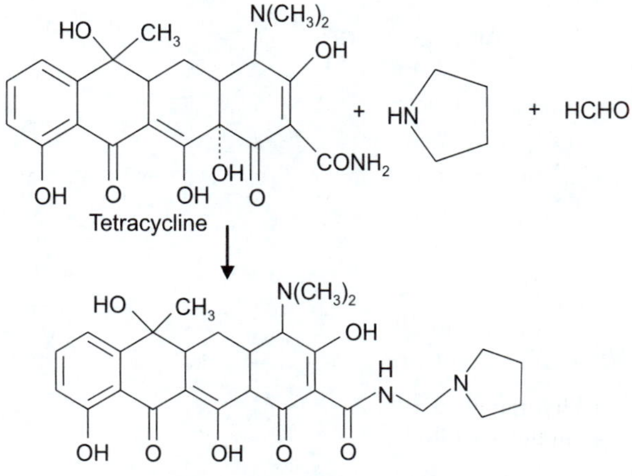

SAR of Tetracyclines

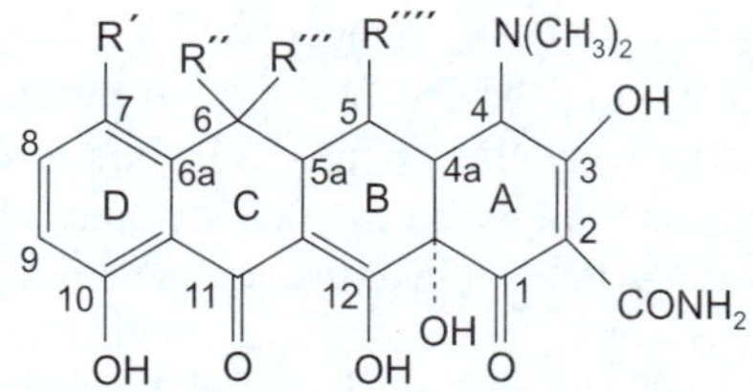

The key structural feature is a linearly fused tetracyclic nucleus and each ring needs to be six membered and purely carbocyclic. A tetracyclic backbone skeleton is essential for activity.

- The D-ring needs to be aromatic and the A-ring must be appropriately substituted at each of its carbon atoms for notable activity.
- The B-ring and the C-ring tolerate certain substitutent changes as long as the keto–enol systems (at C-11, 12, 12a) remain intact and conjugated to the phenolic D-ring.
- The D, C, B-ring phenol, keto-enol system is imperative and the A-ring must also contain a conjugated keto–enol system.
- Specifically, the A-ring contains a tricarbonyl derived keto–enol array at positions C-1, 2, and 3. Other structural requirements for good antibacterial activity include a basic amine function at C-4 position of the A-ring.

Modification of C-1 and C-3 position: The keto-enol system between carbon atom 1 and 3 is highly delocalized and extremely slow to react. The keto-enol tautomerism of ring A is a feature common to all biologically active tetracyclines, blocking this system by forming derivatives at C-1 and C-3 results in loss of antibacterial activity. A–C = O function of C-1 and C-3 is essential for activity.

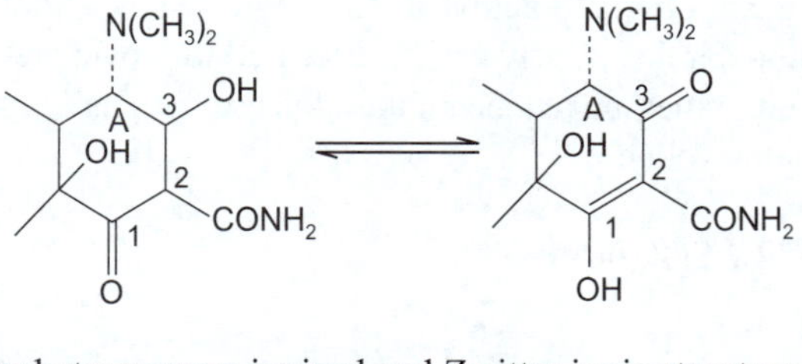

In addition, equilibrium between non-ionized and Zwitter ionic structure of tetracycline is essential for activity.

Modification of C-2 position: The carboxamide moiety is present in all naturally occurring tetracyclines and this group is crucial for antibacterial activity. The amide is best left unsubstituted or monosubstitution is acceptable in the form of activated alkylaminomethyl amide (Mannich bases). An example includes rolitetracycline large alkyl group on the carboxamide that may alter the normal keto–enol equilibrium of the C-1, 2, and 3 conjugated systems and diminishes inherent antibacterial activity. The replacement of carboxamide group or dehydration of carboxamide to the corresponding nitrile results in a loss of activity.

Modification of C-4 position: The naturally occurring tetracyclines contain α-C-4 dimethyl amino substituents that favourably contribute to the keto–enolic character of the A-ring. Replacement of dimethyl amino group with a hydrazone oxime or hydroxyl group leads to a pronounced loss of activity probably due to the increase in heteroatom basicity.

Modification of C-4a position: The α-hydrogen at C-4a position of tetracyclines is necessary for useful antibacterial activity.

Modification of the C-5 and C-5a positions: Many naturally occurring antibacterial tetracyclines have an unsubstituted methylene moiety at the C-5 position. However, oxytetracycline contains C-5 α–hydroxyl group, was found to be a potent compound, and has been modified chemically to some semisynthetic tetracyclines. Alkylation of the C-5 hydroxyl group results in a loss of activity. Ester formation is only acceptable if the free oxytetracycline can be liberated *in vivo*; only small alkyl esters are useful. The configuration of the naturally occurring tetracyclines places the C-5a hydrogen atom in a α-configuration. Epimerization is detrimental to antibacterial activity.

Modification at the C-6 position: The C-6 position is tolerant of a variety of substituents. The majority of tetracyclines has α-methyl group and α, β-hydroxyl group at this position. Demeclocycline is a naturally occurring C-6 demethylated chlortetracycline with an excellent activity. The C-6 methyl group contributes little to the activity of tetracycline. Similarly, the C-6 hydroxyl group also appears to offer little in terms of antibacterial activity and removal of this group affords doxycycline.

C-7 and C-9 substituents: The nature of the aromatic D-ring predisposes the C-7 position to electrophilic substitution. Nitro and halogen groups are introduced in some C-7 tetracyclines, which are among the most potent of all the tetracyclines *in vitro*, but these compounds were potentially toxic and carcinogenic. The C-7 acetoxy, azido, and hydroxyl tetracyclines are inferior in terms of antibacterial activity.

C-10 substituents: The C-10 phenolic moiety is necessary for antibacterial activity.

C-11 substituents: The C-11 carbonyl moiety is part of one of the conjugated keto–enol system required for antibacterial activity.

C-11a substituents: In general, modifications at the C-11a position of tetracycline are not tolerated.

C-12/12a substituents: As with the C-11 position, the C-12 is a part of the keto–enol system that is vital for the drug uptake binding and observed antibacterial activity. The C-12a hydroxyl group is needed for antibacterial activity although this moiety can be esterified to provide tetracyclines with increased lipophilicity. Antibacterial properties are retained if the alkyl ester is small in size and readily undergoes hydrolysis to liberate free tetracycline.

Classification Based on PCI Syllabus

Tetracycline

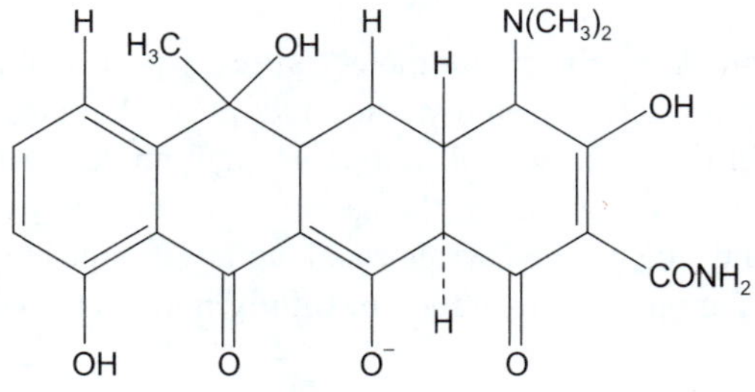

Oxytetracycline

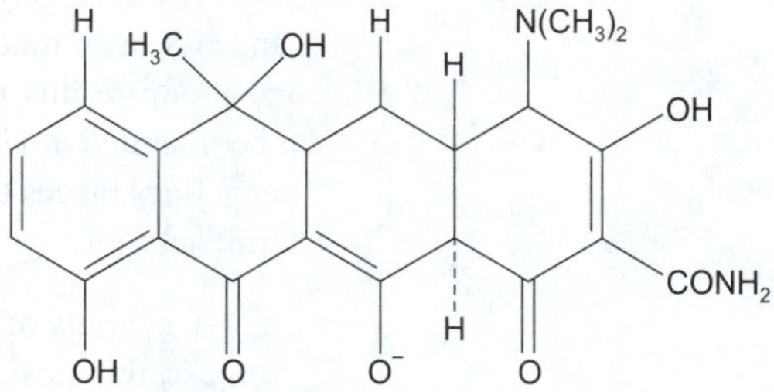

Chlortetracycline

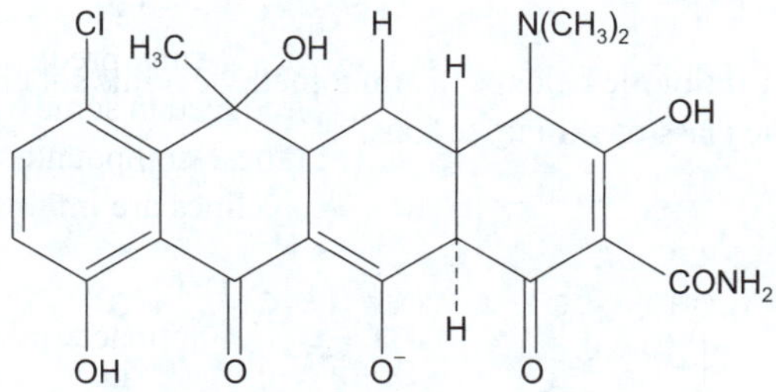

Minocycline

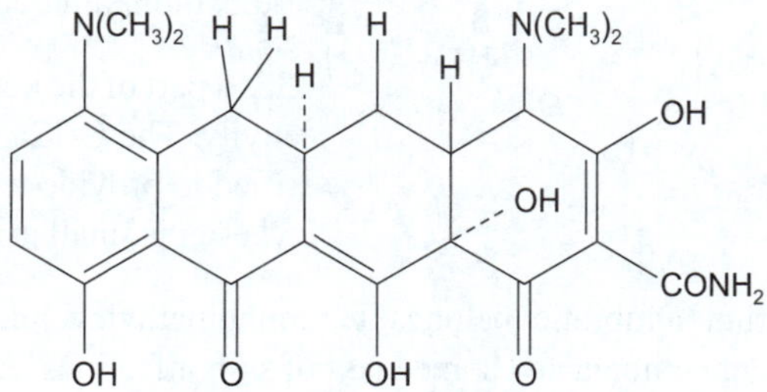

Doxycycline

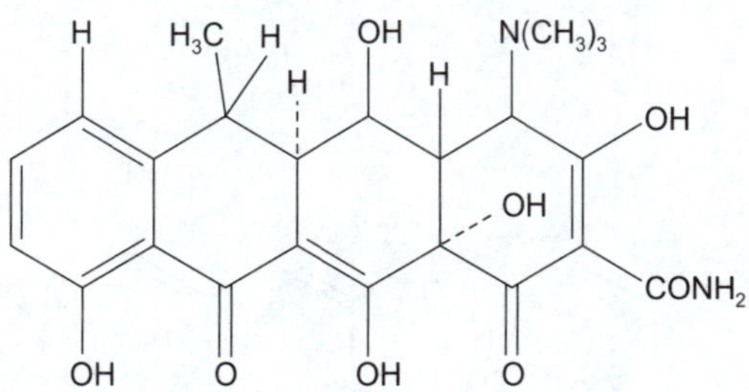

Newer Agents

Omadacycline

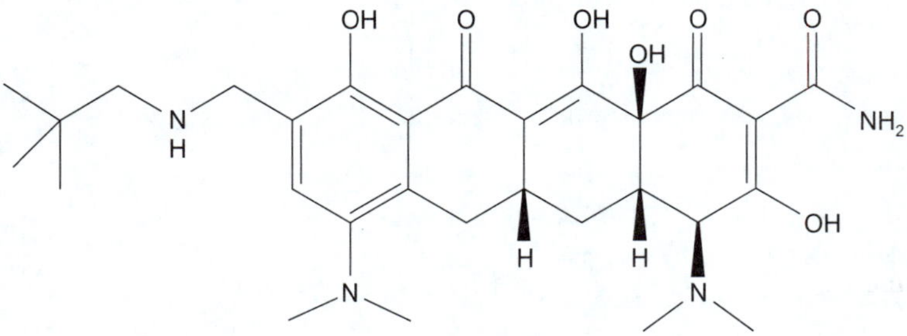

Uses: It is a broad-spectrum antibiotic belongs to aminomethylcycline subclass of antibiotics. It is used to treat pneumonia and some class of skin infections.

Sarecycline

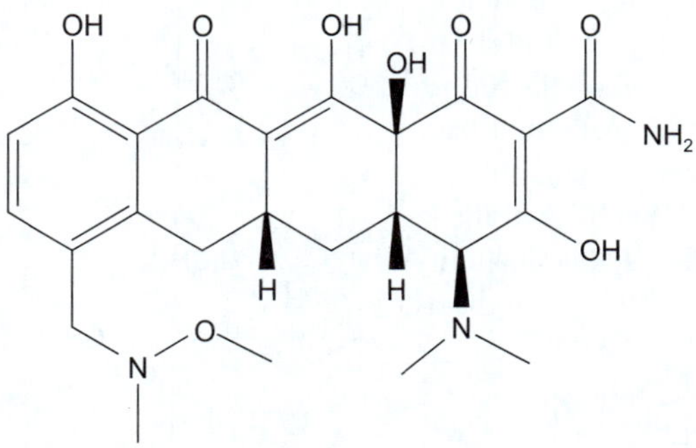

Uses: It is a broad-spectrum antibiotic belongs to aminomethylcycline subclass of tetracycline antibiotics and used to treat pneumonia and some class of skin infections.

Dacomitinib

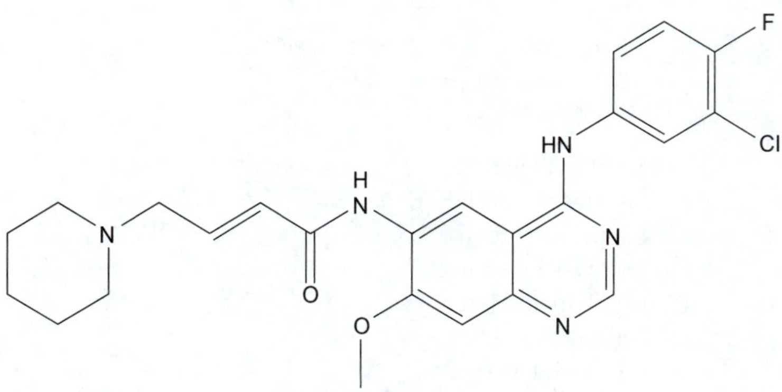

Uses: It is a narrow spectrum tetracyclines-derived antibiotic for the treatment of inflammatory lesions of non-nodular moderate-to-severe acne vulgaris.

4. POLYPEPTIDE ANTIBIOTICS

The compounds have complex polypeptide structure. These are resistant to animal and plant proteases. These contain lipid moieties besides amino acids that are not found in peptides of animal and plant origins. Examples: Bacitracin, polymycin, amphomycin, tyrothricin, and vancomycin.

i. Bacitracin

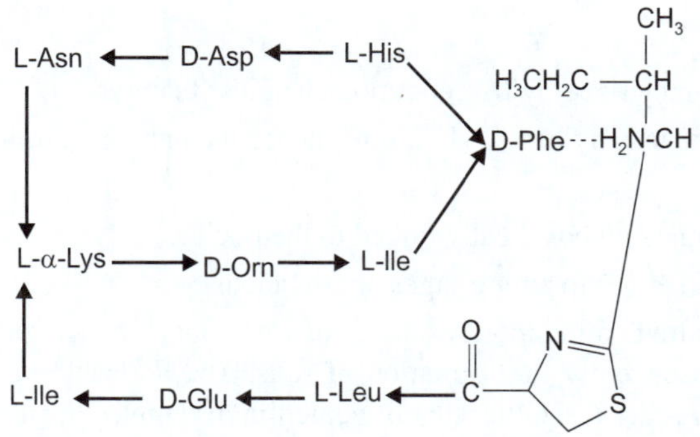

Properties and uses: Bacitracin is a white hygroscopic powder, soluble in water and alcohol. Bacitracin antibiotic is isolated from the fermentation broth of a culture of tracyl-1 strain of *Bacillus subtilis*. It is found to be a complex mixture of at least 10 polypeptides (A, A_1, B, C, D, E, F_1, F_2, F_3, and G), of which bacitracin A fraction is believed to be the most abundant and the most potent. A divalent ion Zn^{2+} enhances its activity. Although bacitracin is occasionally employed for topical application (often in combination with neomycin, polymycin, and tyrothicin) for the treatment of burns, ulcer, and wounds, it can cause serious necrosis of the kidney tubules; if it is given systematically (i.e. IV route) an oral administration is not feasible due to its lack of absorption from the GI tract. A variety of gram-positive cocci and bacilli are sensitive to bacitracin. It should be stored in airtight containers due to its hygroscopic nature.

Assay: It is assayed by microbiological method.

ii. Polymyxin

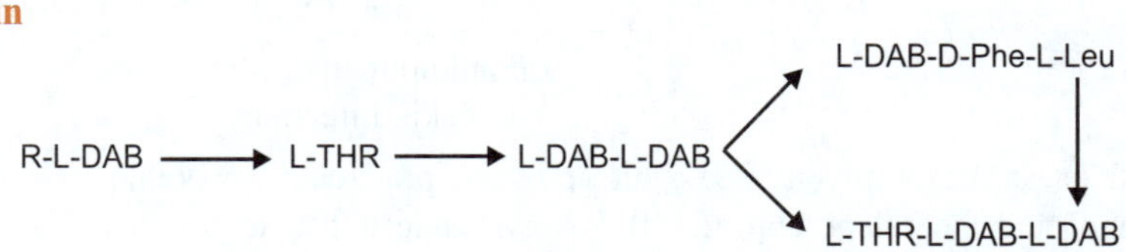

Polymyxin B_1:R = (+)-6-methyloctanoyl
Polymyxin B_2:R = 6-methylpeptanoyl
DAB =α,γ-Diaminobutyric acid

Properties and uses: Polymycin sulphate is a white hygroscopic powder, soluble in water, and slightly soluble in ethanol. The polymyxins are cyclic peptides holding a fatty acid side chain. This is a group of relatively simple basic, cationic, detergent peptides that are produced by *Bacillus polymyxia*. At least, five polymyxins (A, B, C, D, and E) are known, but only polymyxin B and polymyxin E are of clinical utility. Both polymyxin B and polymyxin E (colistin) are mixtures of two components and is used in the treatment of bacterial meningitis, urinary tract infection, burns, wounds, and gastroenteritis. Polymyxin may affect renal tubules and central nervous system (CNS), and because of their nephrotoxicity associated with their systemic use, they are primarily employed to treat topical infections.

Assay: It is assayed by adopting liquid chromatography technique.

5. MACROLIDE ANTIBIOTICS

The macrolide antibacterial agents are extremely useful chemotherapeutic agents for the treatment of a variety of infectious disorders and diseases caused by a host of gram-positive bacteria, both cocci and bacilli; they also exhibit useful effectiveness against gram-negative cocci, specially, *Neisseria* spp. The macrolides are commonly administered for respiratory, skin, tissue, and genitourinary infections caused by these pathogens.

Chemistry: They are characterized by five common chemical features.

1. A macrocyclic lactone usually has 12–17 atoms, hence the name macrolide.
2. A ketone group.
3. One or two amino sugars glycosidically linked to the nucleus.
4. A neutral sugar linked either to amine sugar or to nucleus.
5. The presence of dimethyl amino moiety on the sugar residue, which explains the basicity of these compounds, and consequently the formation of salts. The antibacterial spectrum of activity of the more potent macrolides resembles that of penicillin. Examples: Erythromycin, oleandomycin, clarithromycin, flurithromycin, dirithomycin, azithromycin.

i. Azithromycin

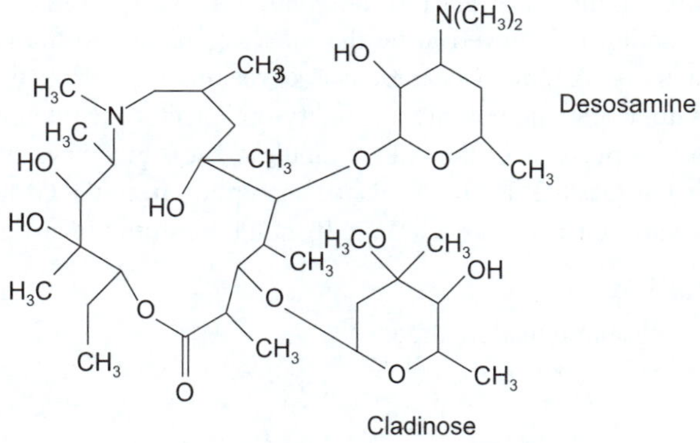

Properties and uses: Azithromycin is a white powder, practically insoluble in water, soluble in anhydrous ethanol and methylene chloride. It is very stable under acidic conditions, is less active against streptococci and staphylococci than erythromycin, and is far more active against respiratory infections due to *H. influenzae* and *Chlamydia trachomatis*.

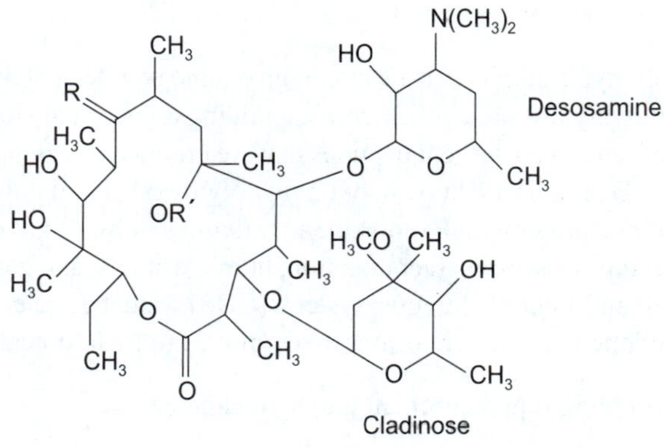

Name	R	R'
Erythromycin	=O	–H
Roxithromycin	$-CH_3OCH_2CH_2OCH_2O=$	–H
Clarithromycin	=O	$-CH_3$

Acid degradation of erythromycin

Erythromycin is unstable in the acid media. The C-6 hydroxyl group reversibly attacks the C-9 ketone giving rise to a hemiketal intermediate. Dehydration prevents regeneration of the parent erythromycin and the C-12 hydroxyl group can subsequently add to produce a spiroketal species. The cladinose group is cleaved from the macrocycle and more harsh conditions lead to the release of desosamine. Useful antibacterial activity lasts till the dehydration of the hemiketal and the spiroketal is weakly active.

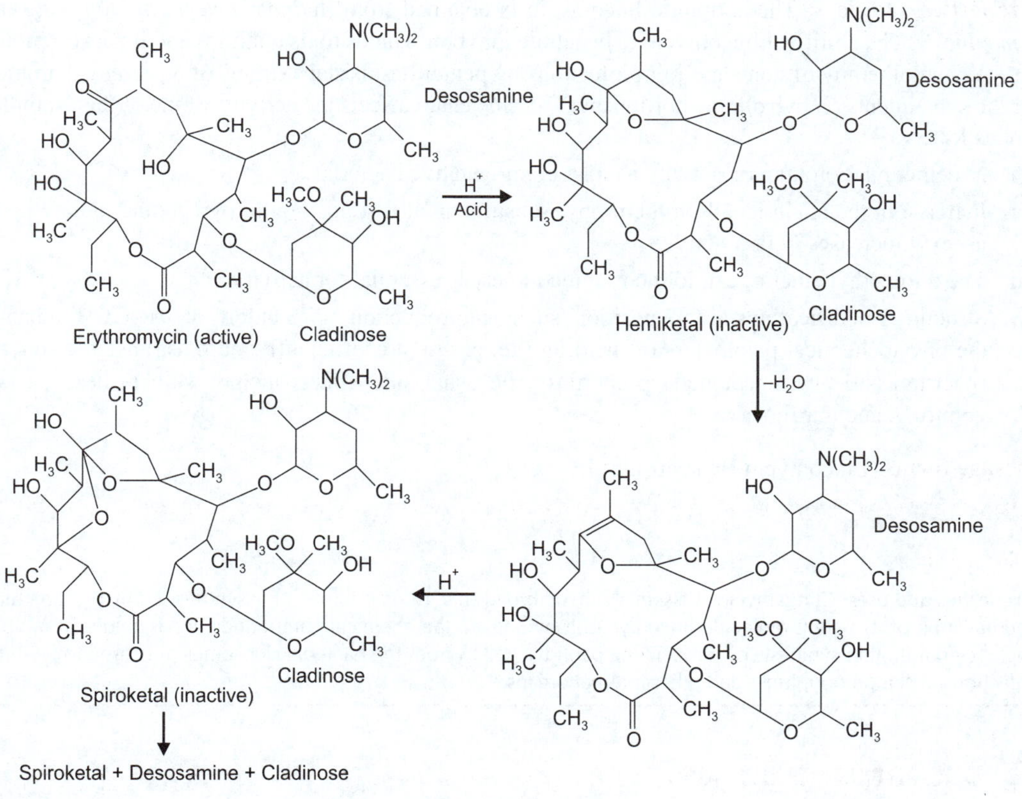

Mode of action: Macrolide antibiotics are bacteriostatic agents that inhibit protein synthesis by binding irreversibly to a site on the 50S subunits of the bacterial ribosome. Thus, inhibiting the translocation steps of protein synthesis at varying stages of peptide chain elongation (hinder the translocation of elongated peptide chain back from 'A' site to 'P' site). The macrolides inhibit ribosomal peptidyl transferase activity. Some macrolides also inhibit the translocation of the ribosome along with the mRNA template.

6. LINCOMYCINS

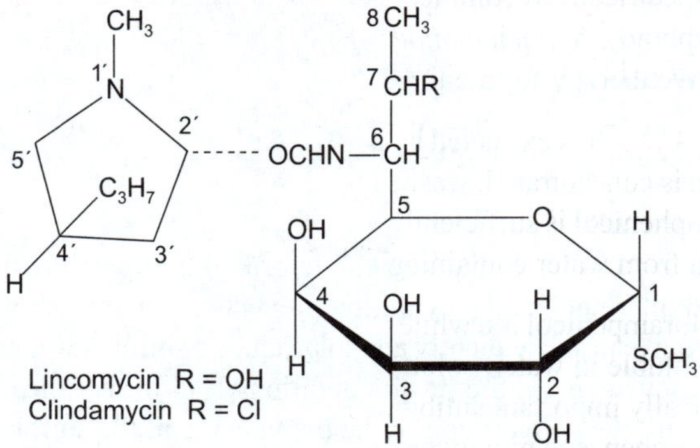

Properties and uses: The antibiotic lincomycin is obtained from *Actinomycetes*, *Streptomyces*, and *Lincolnesis*. The ability of lincomycin to penetrate into bones, adds to its qualities and it gets promoted in the chemotherapy of bone and joint infections by penicillin-resistant strains of *S. aureus*. Variation of the substituents on pyrrolidine portion and C-5 side chain affects the activity. Some of the examples are as follows:

i. N-demethylation imparts activity against gram-negative bacteria.
ii. Increase in the chain length of the propyl substitutent at C-4 position in pyrrolidine moiety up to n-hexyl increases *in vivo* activity.
iii. The thiomethyl ether of α-thiolincosamide moiety is essential for activity.
iv. Structural modifications at C-7 position, such as introduction of 7S chloro or 7 R-OCH_3, change the physiochemical parameters of the drug (i.e. partition coefficient), and thus, alter the activity spectrum and pharmacokinetic properties. The usual side effects include skin rashes, nausea, vomiting, and diarrhoea.

Dosage forms: Lincomycin HCl capsules IP.

Clindamycin

Properties and uses: Clindamycin is a semisynthetic broad-spectrum antibiotic. It is synthesised by the structural modification of its parent molecule lincomycin. It belongs to the chemical compounds lincosamides. It inhibits the bacterial protein synthesis by dissociating peptidyl –tRNA from the bacterial ribosomes. It is used to treat the infections of skin, blood, lungs and other internal organs.

7. OTHER ANTIBIOTICS

Examples of other antibiotics are chloramphenicol, rifampicin and mupirocin.

Chloramphenicol or Chloromycetin

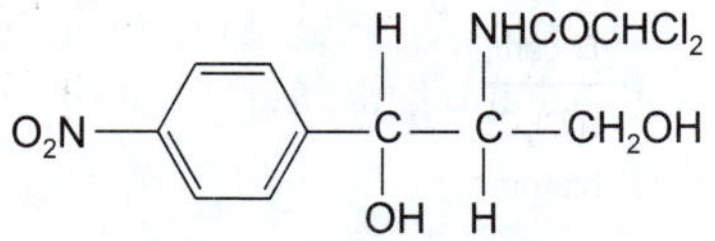

N-(1,3-Dihydroxy-1-(4-nitrophenyl)propan-2-yl)dichloroacetamide

Chloramphenicol has a spectrum of activity resembling that of the tetracyclines except that it exhibits a bit less activity against some gram-positive bacteria. It is isolated from *Salmonella venezuelae* by

Ehrlich et al. in 1947. It contains chlorine and is obtained from an actinomycete, and thus, named as chloromycetin. It is specifically recommended for the treatment of serious infections caused by *H. influnzae*, *S. typhi* (typhoid), *S. pneumoniae, and N. meningitides*. Its ability to penetrate into the CNS presents an alternative therapy for meningitis and exhibits antirickettsial activity.

Isolation of chloramphenicol: It is extracted by adopting counter-current principle using amyl acetate. The amyl acetate solution is concentrated, washed with sulphuric acid, alkali and finally with water and then evaporated. Chloramphenicol is sufficiently stable in hot water to be used at about 93°C. The crude crystals are recrystallized from water containing charcoal.

Properties and uses: Chlorampenicol is a white or greyish-white or yellowish-white crystalline powder or fine crystals, slightly soluble in water, soluble in alcohol and propylene glycol. It was the first, and still is the only therapeutically important antibiotic to be produced in competition with microbiological processes. It contains a nitrobenzene moiety and is a derivative of dichloroacetic acid. Since it has two chiral centres, four isomers are possible. The D-(–) threo is the biologically active form. It is used in the treatment of typhoid fever caused by *S. typhi*. The most serious adverse effect of chloramphenicol is bone marrow depression and fatal blood dyscrasias.

Assay: Dissolve the sample in water, dilute with the same solvent, and measure the absorbance at the maximum of 278 nm using ultraviolet spectrophotometer.

Dose: Usual adult dose is 500 mg every 6 hrs.

Dosage forms: Chloramphenicol capsules IP, BP, chloramphenicol eardrops IP, BP, chloramphenicol eye ointment IP, BP, chloramphenicol eyedrops BP.

Synthesis

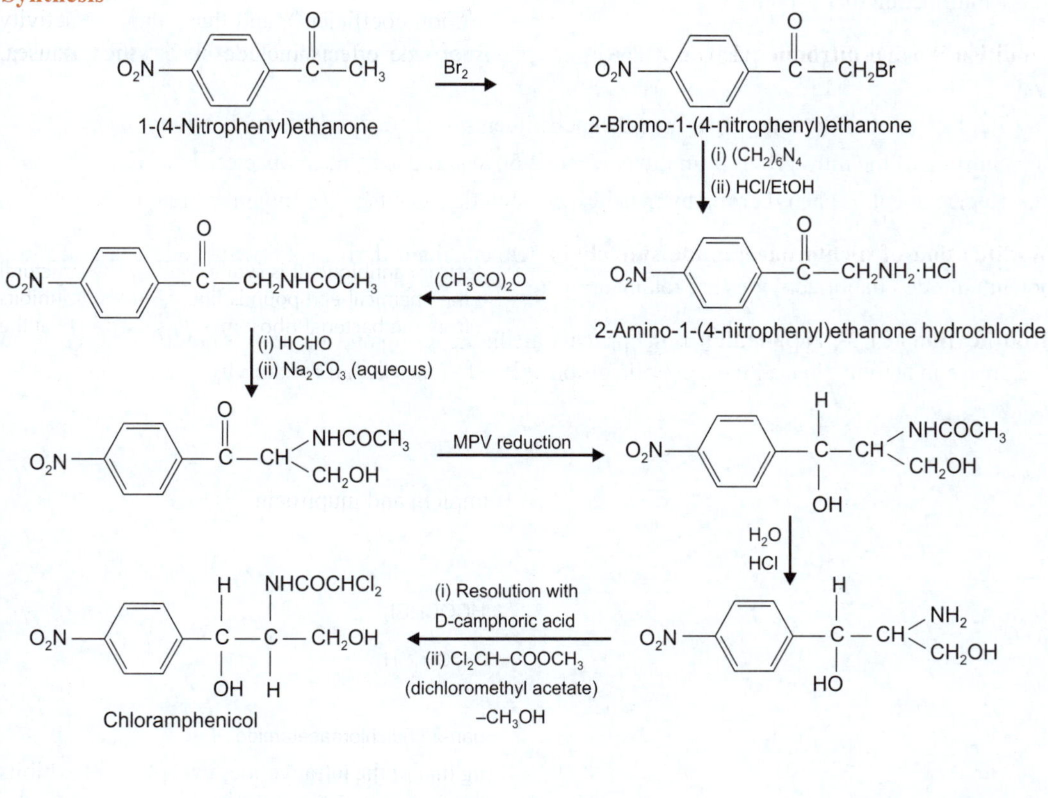

Stereochemistry of chloramphenicol: As chloramphenicol contains two chiral centres, it exists in two possible pairs of enantiomers, namely threo and erythro. Among the four stereoisomers, only the D-threo form is biologically active.

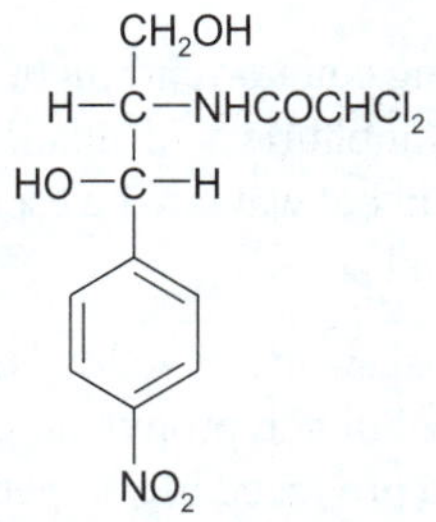

threo-Chloramphenicol

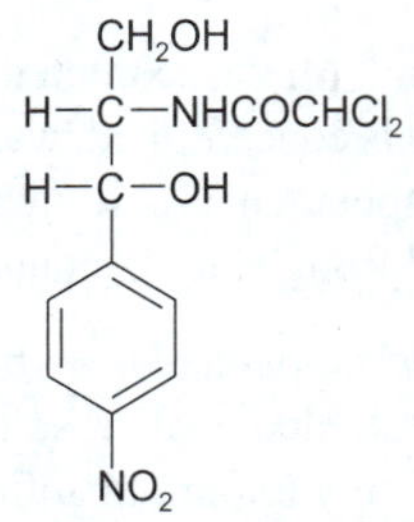

erythro-Chloramphenicol

SAR of Chloramphenicol

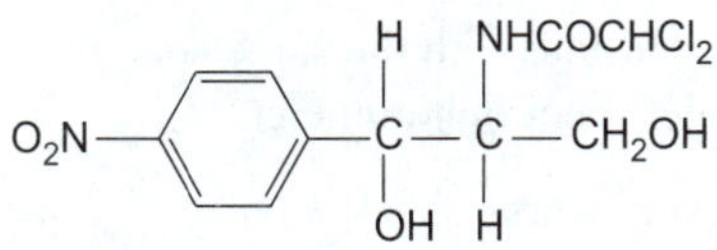

a. Modification of *p*-nitrophenyl group.
b. Modification of dichloroacetamide side chain.
c. Modification of 1,3-prepanediol.

Modification of *p*-nitrophenyl group: The *p*-nitrophenyl group may be modified through the following ways:

a. Replacement of the nitro group by other substituents leads to a reduction in activity.
b. Shifting of the nitro group from the *para* position also reduces the antibacterial activity.
c. Replacement of phenyl group by the alicyclic moieties results in less potent compounds.

Modification of dichloroacetamide side chain: Other dihalo derivatives of the side chain are less potent although major activities are retained.

Modification of 1,3-propanediol: If the primary alcoholic group on C-1 atom is modified, it results in a decrease in activity; hence, the alcoholic group seems to be essential for activity.

✖ Rifampicin

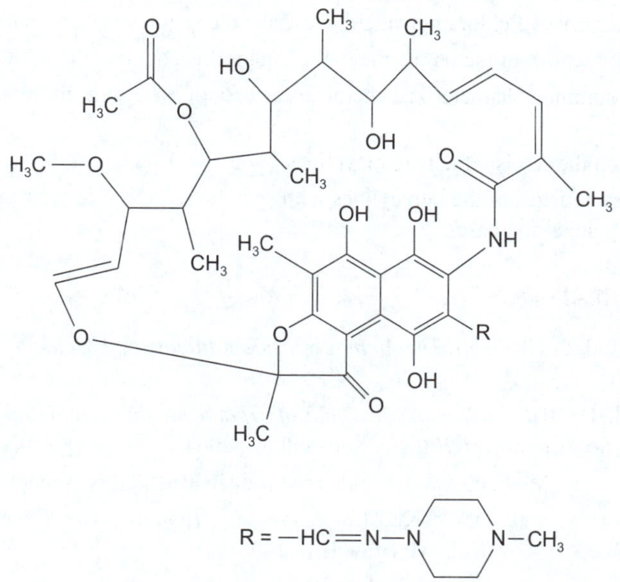

Properties and uses: Rifampicin is a reddish-brown or brownish-red crystalline powder, slightly soluble in water, acetone, and alcohol and soluble in methanol. It is a broad-spectrum bactericidal antibiotic, structurally similar to complex macrocyclic antibiotic obtained from *S. mediterrani*. They belong to a new class of antibiotics called ansamycins. Five types, that is, rifampicin A, B, C, D, and E are present. It penetrates well into cerebrospinal fluid and is, therefore, used in the treatment of tuberculous meningitis.

Assay: Dissolve the sample in methanol and dilute it with the same solvent. Dilute the solution with phosphate buffer solution pH 7.4 and measure the absorbance at the maximum at 475 nm, using phosphate buffer solution pH 7.4 as blank.

PROBABLE QUESTIONS

1. What are penicillins? Classify with suitable examples and write the SAR of penicillins.
2. What are the cardinal requirements of a substance to be called an antibiotic? Draw the structure, chemical name, and other names of the naturally occurring penicillins.
3. Explain the synthesis and the uses of phenoxy methyl penicillin and amoxycillin.
4. Draw the structure, chemical name, and uses of the following:
   (a) Penicillins related to ampicillin, (b) Esters of ampicillin
5. Write short notes on the degradation of penicillins.
6. Write the structure, chemical name, uses, and synthesis of the given category of penicillins: (a) Acid-resistant penicillins, (b) beta-lactamase-resistant penicillins.
7. What are cephalosporins? Explain how they differ from penicillins chemically. Write the SAR of cephalosporins in detail.
8. Write a comprehensive account of cephalosporins with suitable examples.
9. What are aminoglycoside antibiotics? Write the mode of action, structure, and uses of three potent drugs of this category.

10. Name any five aminoglycoside antibiotics and mention their source.
11. What are the reasons for recognizing chloramphenicol as a potent antibiotic? Write in detail about the SAR and stereochemistry of chloramphenicol. Describe the synthesis of chloramphenicol.
12. Explain the salient features of the tetracylines. Write a brief account on the SAR of tetracylines.
13. What are the five common characterized chemical features of macrolide antibiotics? Write its mode of action.
14. Write short notes on the semisynthetic tetracyclines.
15. Elaborate the characteristics of the tetracylines with specific reference to their (a) effect on metals and (b) effect on strong acids and bases.

SUGGESTED READINGS

1. Barnes WG and Hodges GR (eds). *The Aminoglycoside Antibiotics: A Guide to Therapy*. Boca Raton, FL: CRC, 1984.
2. Block JH and Beale JM. *Wilson Gisvold's Text book of Organic Medicinal and Pharmaceutical Chemistry* (11th edn). New York: Lippincott Williams and Wilkins, 2004.
3. *British Pharmacopoeia*. Medicines and Healthcare Products Regulatory Agency. London, 2008.
4. Bruntan LL, Lazo JS, and Parker KL. *Goodman and Gilman's: The Pharmacological Basis of Therapeutics* (11th edn). New York: McGraw Hill, 2006.
5. Bryker AJ, Butzler JP, Neu HC, and Tulken PM (eds). *Macrolides, Chemistry, Pharmacology and Clinical Uses*. Paris: Arnate Blackwell, 1993.
6. Coute JE. *Manual of Antibiotics and Infectious Diseases* (8th edn). Baltimore: Williams & Wilkins, 1995.
7. Ehrlich J, Bartz QR, Smith RM, Joslyn DA, Burkholder PR. 'Chloromycetin: A new antibiotic from a soil actinomycete'. *Science* 106: 417, 1947.
8. Gennaro AR. *Remington: The Science And Practice of Pharmacy* (21st edn). New York: Lippincot Williams and Wilkins, 2006.
9. Havaka JJ and Boothe JH (eds). *The Tetracyclines*. New York: Springer-Verlag, 1985.
10. *Indian Pharmacopoeia*. Ministry of Health and Family Welfare. New Delhi, 1996.
11. Kirsk HA. 'Dirithromycin'. *Drugs of Today* 31: 1–10, 1995.
12. Lednicer D and Mitscher LA. *The Organic Chemistry of Drug Synthesis*. New York: John Wiley, 1995.
13. Lemke TL and William DA. *Foye's Principle of Medicinal Chemistry* (6th edn). New York: Lippincott Williams and Wilkins, 2008.
14. Mandell GL, Douglas RG (Jr), and Bennett JE (eds). *Principles and Practice of Infectious Diseases* Vol. 1 (4th edn). New York: Churchill-Livingstone, 1995.
15. Mitscher L A. *The Chemistry of Tetracycline Antibiotics*. New York: Marcell Dekker, 1978.
16. Neu HC, Young LS, and Zinner SH. *The New Macrolides*. New York: Marcel Dekker, 1995.
17. Omura S (ed). *Macrolide Antibiotics*. Orland, FL: Academic Press, 1984.
18. Progdeu RN and Peters DH. 'Diithromycin: A review'. *Drugs* 48: 599–616, 1994.
19. Schatz A, Bugie E, and Waksman S. 'Streptomycin, a substance exhibiting antibiotic activity against gram-positive and gram-negative bacteria'. *Proc Soc Exptl Biol Med* 55: 66–69, 1944.
20. Wolff M E. *Burger's Medicinal Chemistry and Drug Discovery* (5th edn). New York: John Wiley, 1995.

CHAPTER 16

Antitubercular Agents

INTRODUCTION

Tuberculosis is the most prevalent infectious disease worldwide and a leading killer caused by a single infectious agent, that is, *Mycobacterium tuberculosis*. According to World Health Organization (WHO) report, *M. tuberculosis*, currently infects over 2 billion people worldwide, with 30 million new cases reported every year. This intracellular infection accounts for at least 3 million deaths annually. Common infection sites of the tuberculosis are lungs (primary site), brain, bone, liver, and kidney. The main symptoms are cough, tachycardia, cyanosis, and respiratory failure. Depending upon the site of infection, the disease can be categorized as follows:

- Pulmonary tuberculosis (respiratory tract).
- Genitourinary tuberculosis (genitourinary tract).
- Tuberculous meningitis (nervous system).
- Miliary tuberculosis (a widespread infection).

Drugs used in the treatment of tuberculosis can be divided into two major categories (Figure 16.1):

1. **First-line drugs:** Isoniazid, streptomycin, rifampicin, ethambutol, and pyrazinamide.
2. **Second-line drugs:** Ethionamide, *p*-amino salicylic acid, ofloxacin, ciprofloxacin, cycloserine, amikacin, kanamycin, viomycin, and capreomycin.

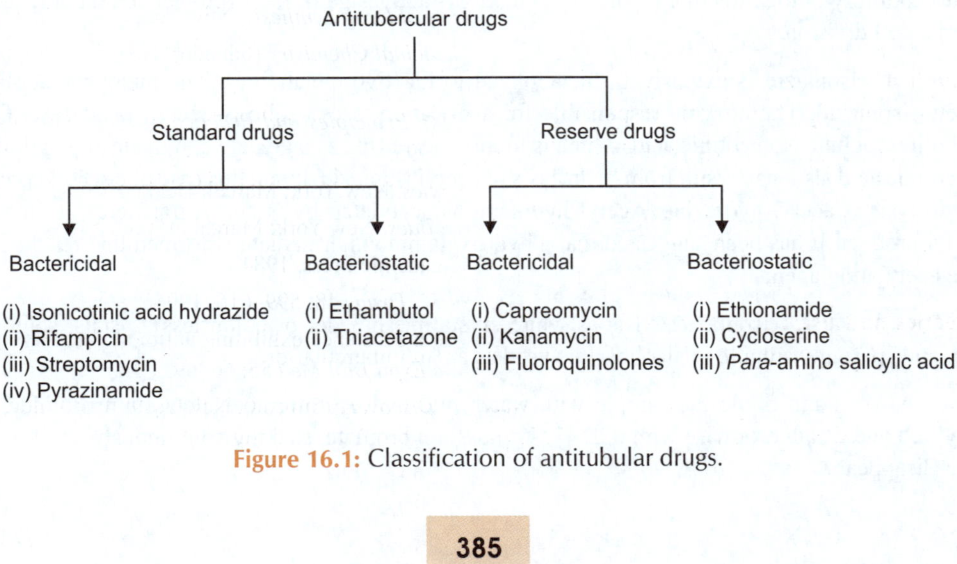

Figure 16.1: Classification of antitubular drugs.

The majority of the patients with tuberculosis are treated with first-line drugs and show excellent results with a 6-month course of treatment. For the first 2 months, isoniazid, rifampicin, and pyrazinamide are given, followed by isoniazid and rifampicin for the remaining 4 months. Second-line drugs are used mainly to treat multidrug resistant *M. tuberculosis* infections.

SYNTHESIS AND DRUG PROFILE

I. Standard Drugs

i. Isoniazid (Continazin, Laniazid, Isonex, Ipcazide, INH, Isokin)

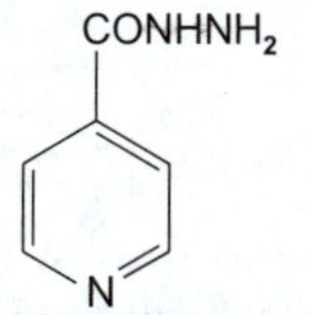

Isonicotinic acid hydrazide (INH)

Synthesis

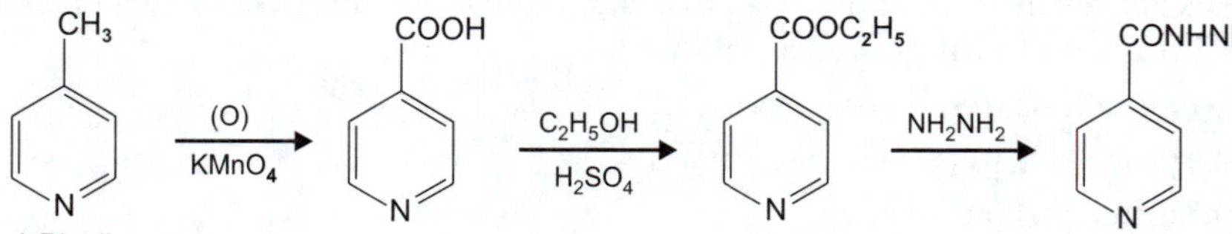

Mode of action: Isoniazid is a prodrug that is activated on the surface of *M. tuberculosis* by katG enzyme to isonicotinic acid. Isonicotinic acid inhibits the bacterial cell wall mycolic acid, thereby making *M. tuberculosis* susceptible to reactive oxygen radicals. Isoniazid may be bacteriostatic or bactericidal in action, depending on the concentration of the drug attained at the site of infection and the susceptibility of the infecting organism. The drug is active against susceptible bacteria only during bacterial cell division.

Metabolism: Isoniazid is extensively metabolized to inactive metabolites. The major metabolite is N-acetyl isoniazid. The enzyme responsible for acetylation is cytosolic N-acetyl transferase. Other metabolites include isonicotinic acid, which is found in the urine as a glycine conjugate and hydrazine. Isonicotinic acid also may result from hydrolysis of acetyl isoniazid, but in this case, the second product of hydrolysis is acetyl hydrazine. Acetyl hydrazine is acetylated by N-acetyl transferase to inactive diacetyl product. It has been suggested that a hydroxylamine intermediate is formed that results in an active acetylating agent.

Properties and uses: Isoniazid exists as white crystalline powder or colourless crystals, soluble in water, and sparingly soluble in alcohol. It is used as an antitubercular drug.

Assay: Dissolve and dilute the sample with water, add hydrochloric acid, potassium bromide, and methyl red and titrate dropwise with 0.0167 M potassium bromate, shaking continuously, until the red colour disappears.

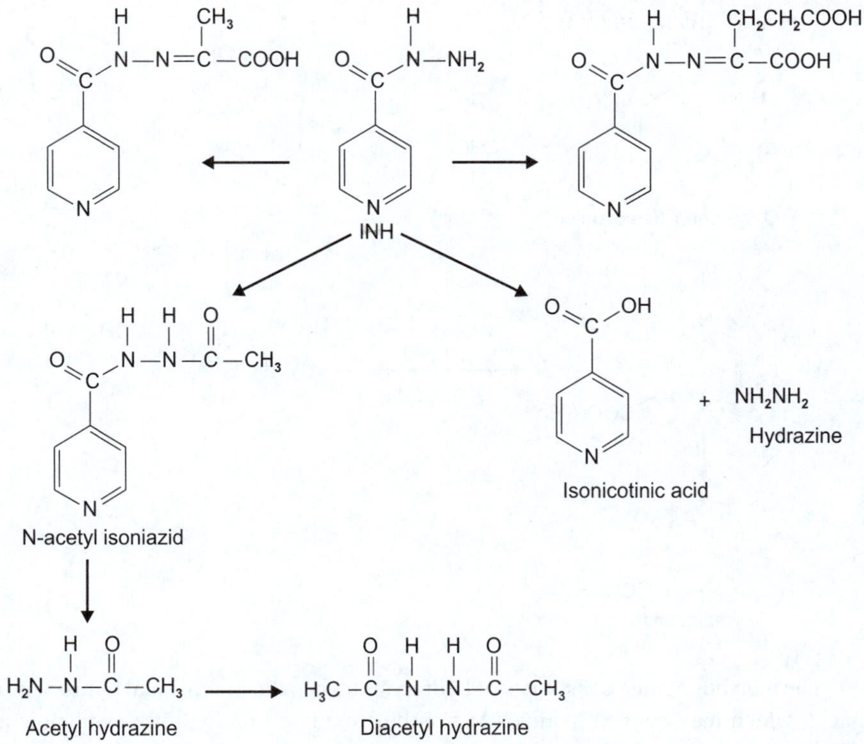

Dose: For the prophylaxis in case of adults is 5 mg/kg, with a maximum of 300 mg. For children: 10–20 mg/kg daily. Combination therapy isoniazid, rifampin and pyrazinamide for 2 months followed by isoniazid (15 mg/kg orally) with rifampin (10 mg/kg up to 600 mg per dose) twice/week for 4 months.

Dose: For the prophylaxis in case of adults 5 mg/kg, with a maximum of 300 mg.

Dosage forms: Isoniazid tablets IP, BP, isoniazid injection BP.

ii. Pyrazinamide

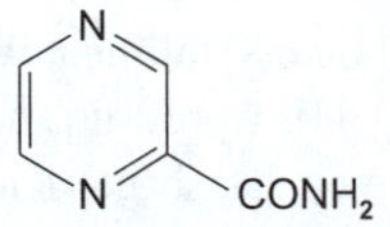

Pyrazine-2-carboxamide

Synthesis

Route I. From: Pyrazine-2,3-dicarboxylic acid

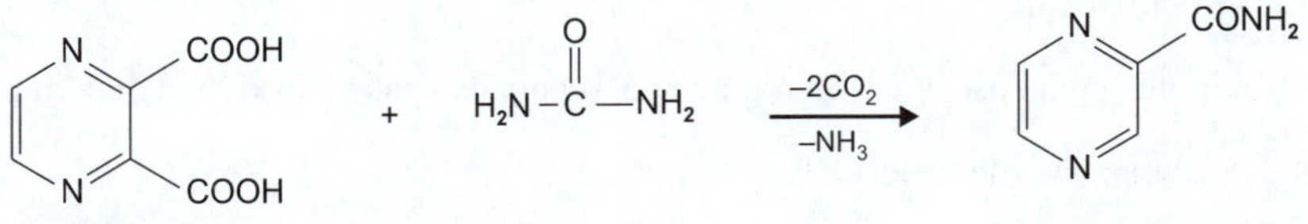

Route II. From: *Ortho*-phenylenediamine

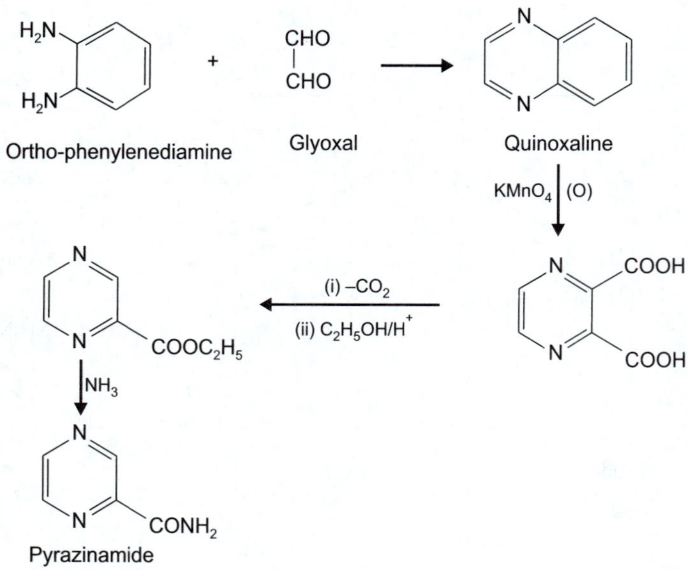

Metabolism: The metabolic route constitutes of hydrolysis by hepatic microsomal pyrazinamidase into pyrazinoic acid, which may be then oxidized by xanthine oxidase to 5-hydroxy pyrazinoic acid. The later compound may appear in the urine either free or as a conjugate with glycine.

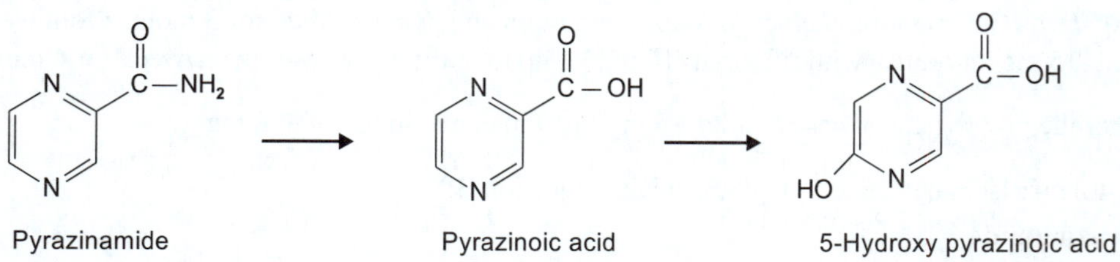

Properties and uses: Pyrazinamide is a white crystalline powder, sparingly soluble in water, slightly soluble in alcohol and in methylene chloride. It is a prodrug and is activated by *M. tuberculosis* amidase enzyme into pyrazine carboxylic acid, which has bactericidal activity. Pyrazinamide has recently been elevated to first-line status in the short-term treatment of tuberculosis regimens because of its tuberculocidal activity and comparatively less short-term toxicity. Pyrazinamide is maximally effective in the low pH environment that exists in macrophages (monocytes). It is used to treat tuberculosis and meningitis. The drug should be used with great caution in patients with hyperuricaemia or gout.

Assay: Dissolve the sample in acetic anhydride and titrate with 0.1 M perchloric acid. Determine the end point potentiometrically.

Dose: Daily administered dose is 20–35 mg/kg in 3–4 equally spaced doses and maximum is 3 g daily.

Dosage forms: Pyrazinamide tablets BP.

iii. Ethambutol HCl (Myambutol)

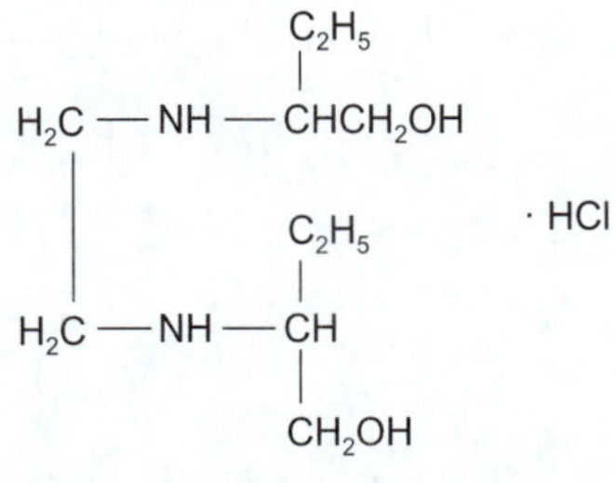

2,2-Ethylene (diamine)-di-(2-butyl-1-ol)

Synthesis

Route I. From: 1,2-Dichloroethane

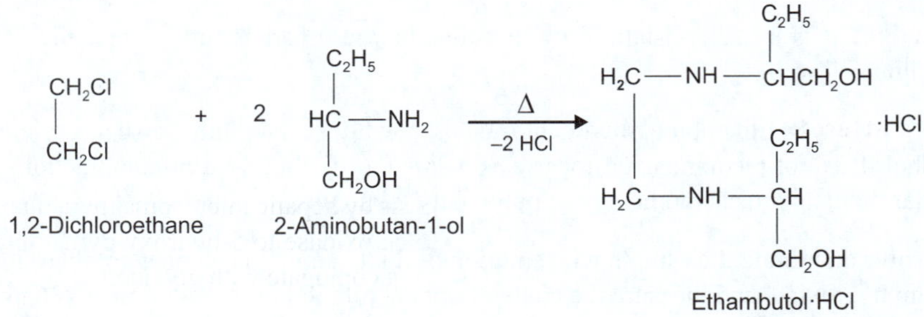

Route II. From: Nitropropane

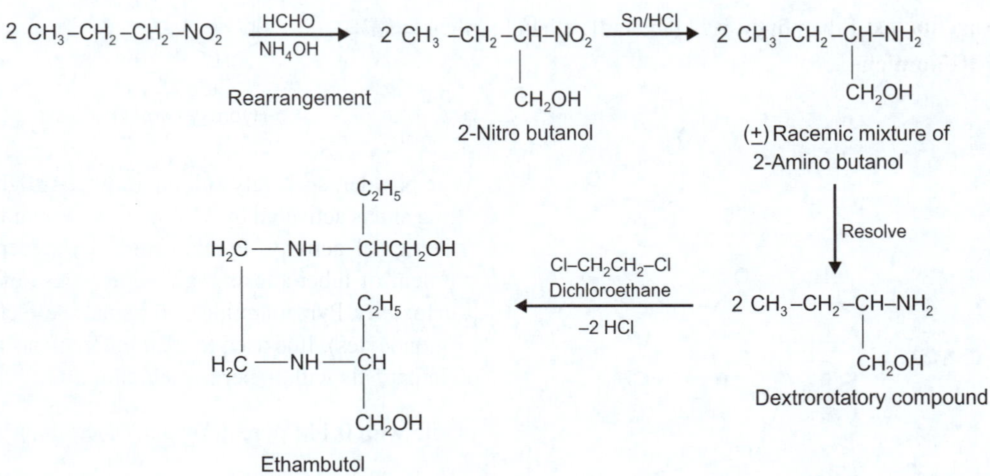

Metabolism: The majority of the administered ethambutol is excreted unchanged and with not more than 15% appearing in the urine as a metabolite, which are devoid of biological activity.

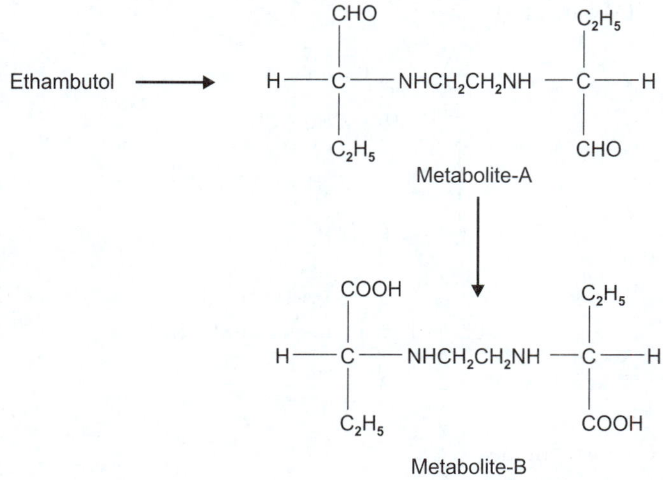

Mode of action: It is a bacteriostatic drug that inhibits the incorporation of mycolic acid into the mycobacterium cell wall.

Properties and uses: Ethambutol hydrochloride is a white crystalline powder, soluble in water and in alcohol. It is not recommended for use as a single drug, but used in combinations with other antitubercular drugs in the chemotherapy of pulmonary tuberculosis.

Assay: Dissolve and dilute the sample with solution of dilute ammonia, copper sulphate solution, and dilute sodium hydroxide, and measure the angle of optical rotation of the solution at 436 nm.

Dose: The administered dose is 15–25 mg/kg once a day; low doses for new cases, and high doses for use in patients who have had previous antitubercular therapy.

Dosage forms: Ethambutol HCl tablets IP, ethambutol tablets BP.

iv. Rifampicin

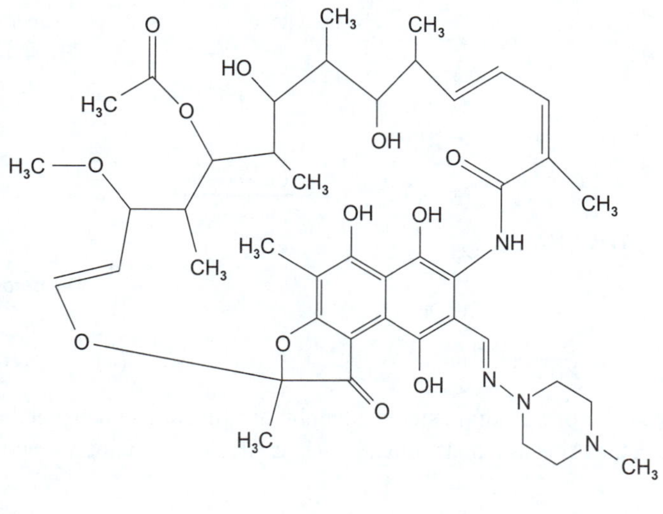

Mode of action: It is an antibiotic obtained from *Streptomyces mediterranei*. Rifampicin inhibits DNA-dependent RNA polymerase of mycobacteria by forming a stable drug–enzyme complex, leading to suppression of initiation of chain formation in RNA synthesis and acts as a bactericidal drug.

Metabolism: The major metabolism of rifampicin and rifapentine is deacetylation, which occurs at the C-25 acetate. The resulting products, desacetyl rifampin, and desacetyl rifapentine are still active antibacterial agents. 3-Formylrifamycin has been reported as a second metabolite following both rifampicin and rifapentine administration.

Properties and uses: Rifampicin is a reddish-brown or brownish-red crystalline powder, slightly soluble in water, acetone, alcohol, and soluble in methanol. Rifampicin is the most active agent in clinical use for the treatment of tuberculosis. It is used only in combination with other antitubercular drugs, and it is ordinarily not recommended for the treatment of other bacterial infections when alternative antibacterial agents are available.

Assay: Dissolve and dilute the sample in methanol. Dilute the solution with phosphate buffer solution pH 7.4 and measure the absorbance at the maxima of 475 nm, using phosphate buffer solution pH 7.4 as blank.

Dosage forms: Rifampicin tablets IP, rifampicin capsules IP, BP, rifampicin oral suspension BP.

v. Rifabutin

It is a semisynthetic rifamycin, structurally similar to rifampicin. It is used against *M. avium*, one of the most common causes of disseminated infections, with patients suffering with Human Immunodeficiency Virus (HIV). *In vitro* activity is attributed to rifabutin's lipophilic nature and its ability to penetrate the cell.

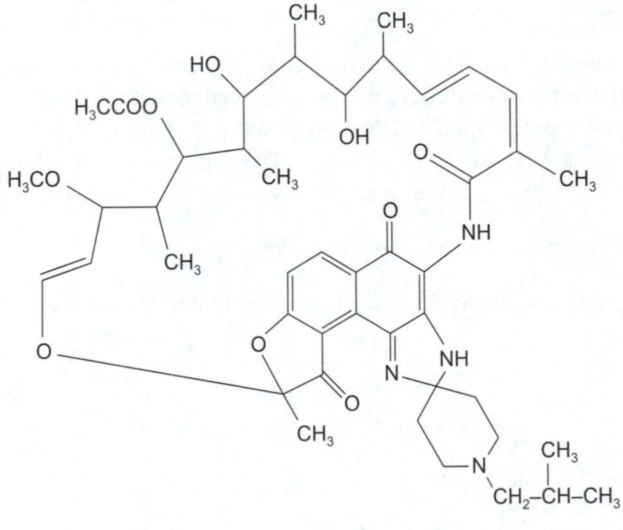

Properties and uses: Rifabutin is a reddish-violet amorphous powder, slightly soluble in water and alcohol, soluble in methanol. It is used as an antitubercular drug.

Assay: It is assayed by adopting liquid chromatography technique.

vi. Streptomycin sulphate

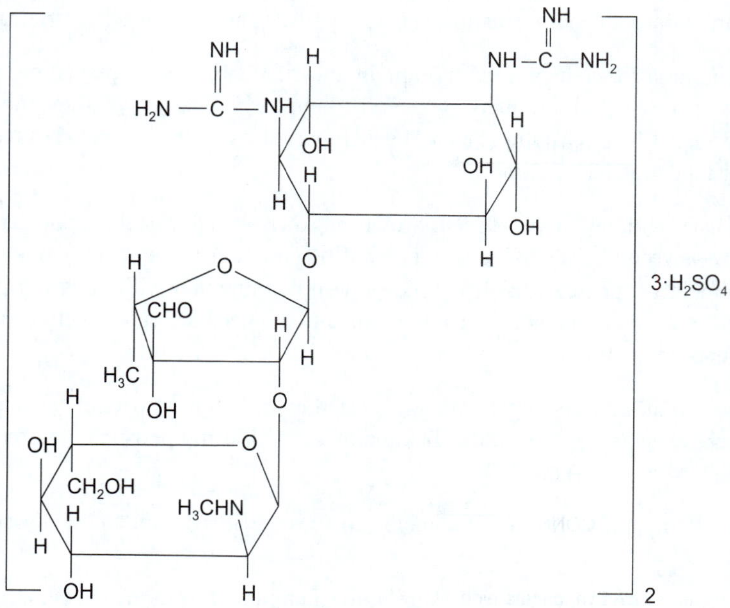

Metabolism: The enzymes responsible for inactivation are adenyltransferase, which catalyzes adenylation of the C-3 hydroxyl group in the N-methyl glucosamine moiety to give the *O*-3-adenylated metabolite and phosphotransferase, which phosphorylates the same C-3 hydroxyl to give *O*-3-phosphorylated metabolite.

Properties and uses: Streptomycin is a white hygroscopic powder, very soluble in water, and practically insoluble in ethanol. It was the first effective drug for the treatment of tuberculosis. It is most often used in combination with other drugs, such as ethambutol and isoniazid, to treat pulmonary infections in patients with organisms that are known to be resistant. There has been an increasing tendency to reserve streptomycin products for the treatment of tuberculosis.

Assay: It is assayed by adopting microbiological assay method.

Dosage forms: Streptomycin sulphate injection IP, streptomycin sulphate tablets IP, streptomycin injection BP.

II. Reserve Drugs

i. Ethionamide (Tridocin)

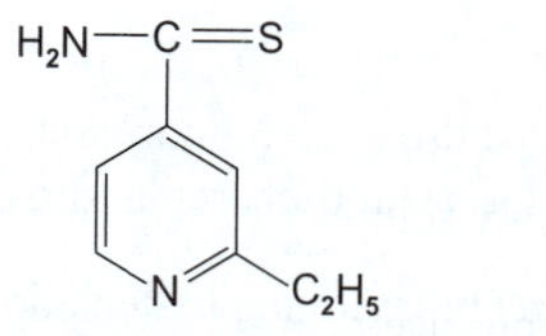

2-Ethylpyridine-4-carbothioamide

Synthesis

Route I. From: 2-Ethyl-4-cyanopyridine

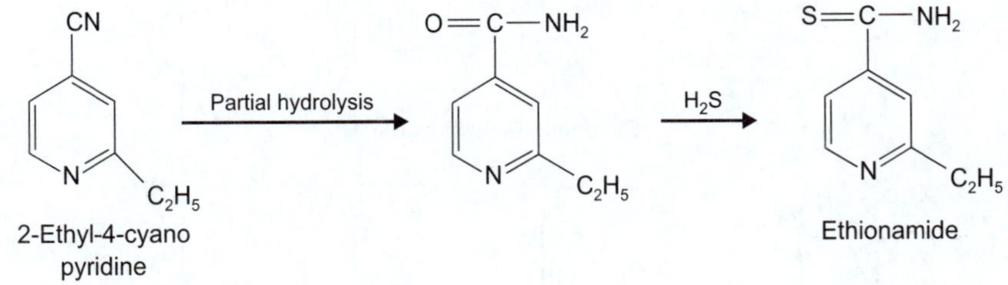

Route II. From: Ethyl propionyl pyruvate

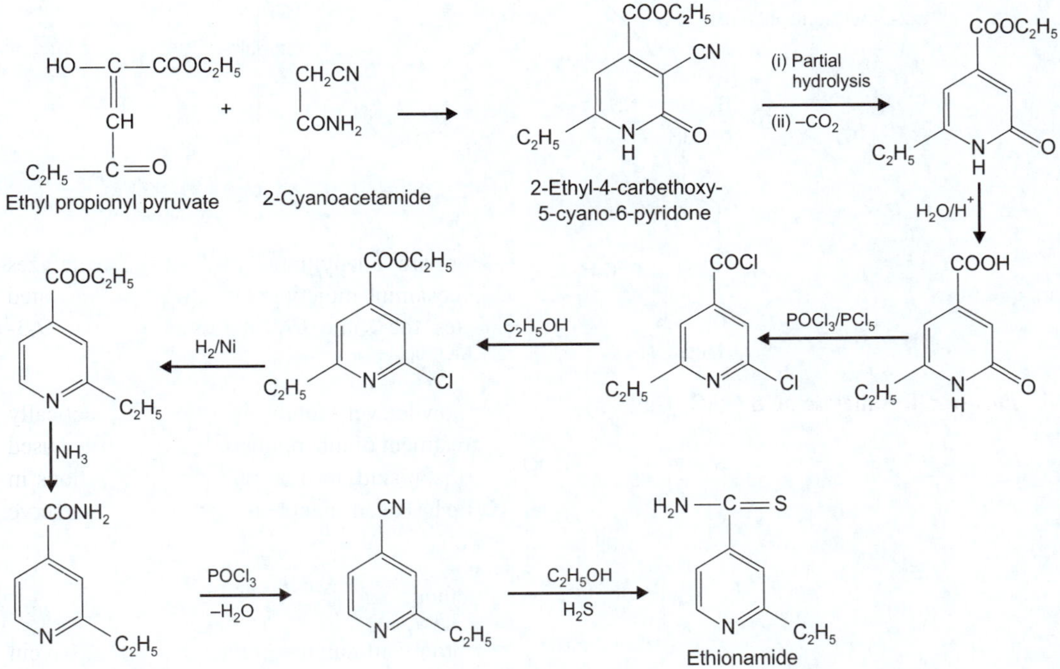

Mode of action: The antimycobacterial action of ethionamide seems to be due to an inhibitory effect on the mycolic acid synthesis.

Metabolism: Less than 1% of the drug is excreted in the free form, and remainder of the drug appear as six metabolites. Among the metabolites, ethionamide sulphoxide, 2-ethyl-isonicotinamide, and the N-methylated-6-oxo-dihydropyridines are the few.

Properties and uses: Ethionamide is a yellow crystalline powder or crystals, practically insoluble in water, soluble in methanol, and sparingly soluble in alcohol. It is used as antitubercular drug.

Assay: Dissolve the sample in anhydrous acetic acid and titrate with 0.1 M perchloric acid. Determine the end point potentiometrically.

Dose: The dose to be administered is 500 mg–1 g per day in three or four divided doses with meals.

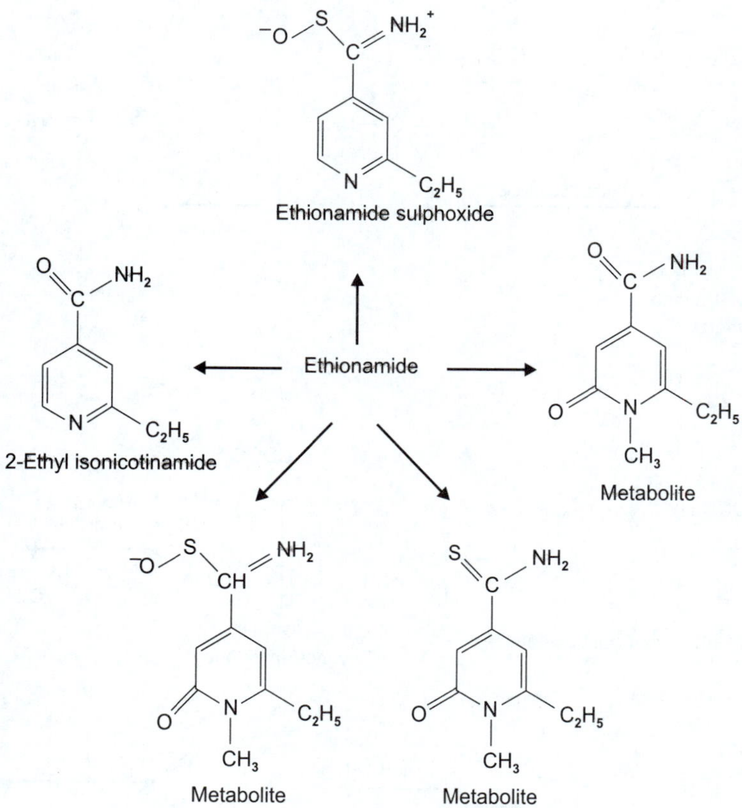

ii. *Para*-aminosalicylic acid (PAS, Tubacin)

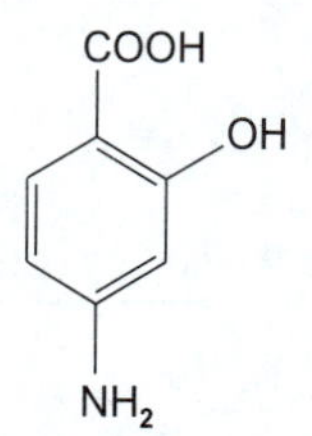

4-Amino-2-hydroxy benzoic acid

Mode of action: *p*-Aminosalicylic acid is an inhibitor of bacterial folate metabolism in a manner similar to the sulphonamide antibacterials.

Properties and uses: *p*-Aminosalicylic acid is bacteriostatic and highly specific for *M. tuberculosis*. Side effects are anorexia, nausea, epigastric pain, diarrhoea, and making poor compliance.

Dose: Dose administered orally is 14–16 g daily after meals in three to four divided doses.

Synthesis

Route I. From: Anthranilic acid

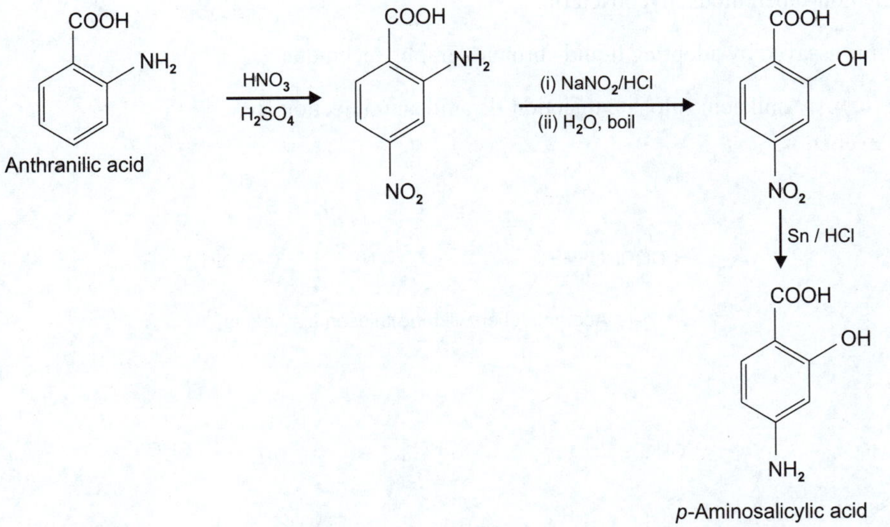

Route II. From: *m*-Nitrophenol

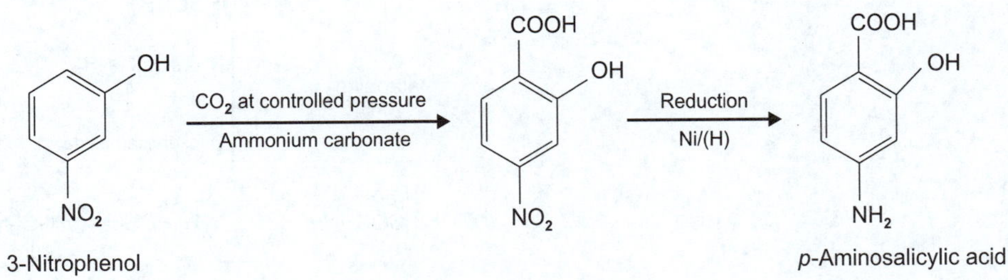

iii. Amikacin

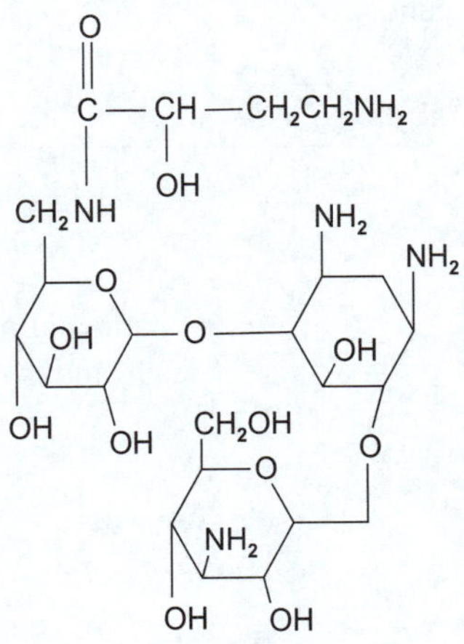

Properties and uses: Amikacin is a white powder, soluble in water, practically insoluble in acetone and in ethanol. It is a semisynthetic aminoglycoside that was first prepared in Japan. It is extremely active against several mycobacterial species, and may become the drug of choice for treatment of diseases caused by non-tuberculous mycobacteria.

Assay: It is assayed by adopting liquid chromatography technique.

Dosage forms: Amikacin sulphate injection IP, amikacin injection BP.

iv. Thiacetazone

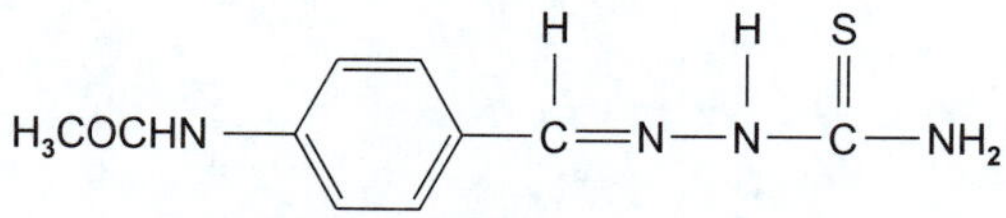

1-(4-Acetamidobenzylidene)thiosemicarbazide

Synthesis

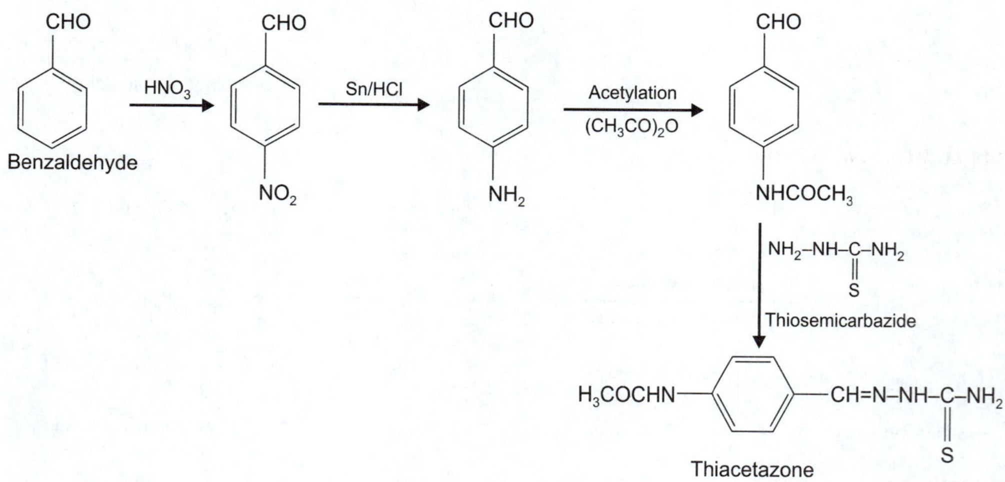

Uses: It is used as an antitubercular agent.

Classification Based on PCI Syllabus

Synthetic Antitubercular Agents

Isoniazid

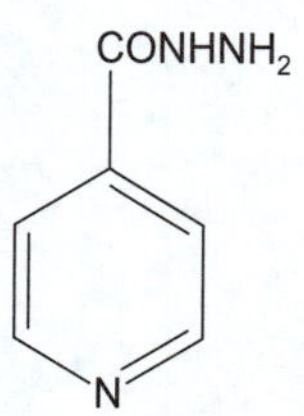

Ethionamide

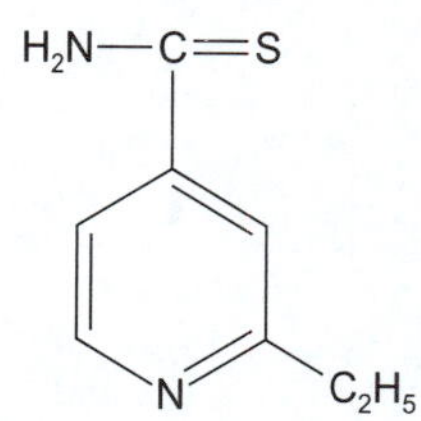

Ethambutol

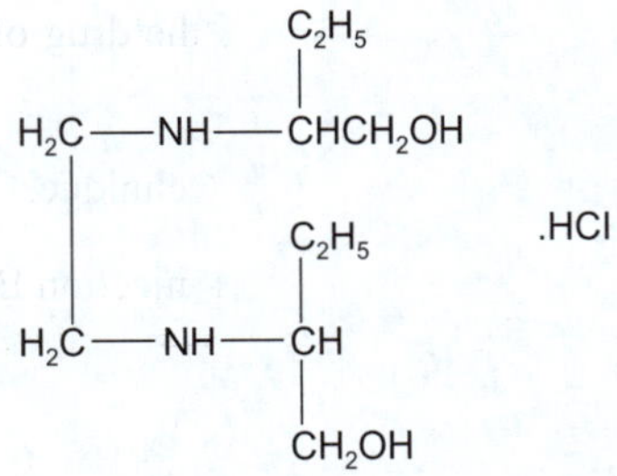

Pyrazinamide

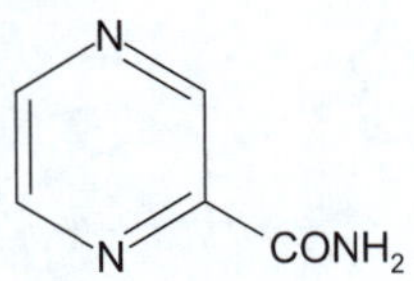

***Para*-Aminosalicylic acid**

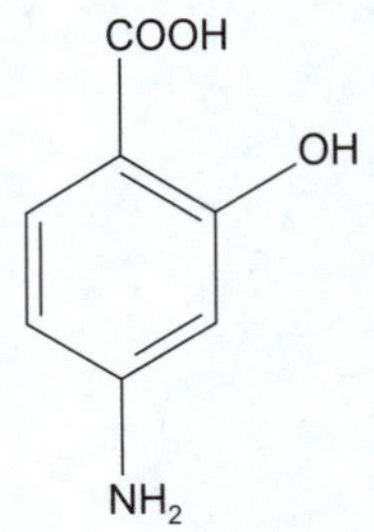

Anti-tubercular Antibiotics

Rifampicin

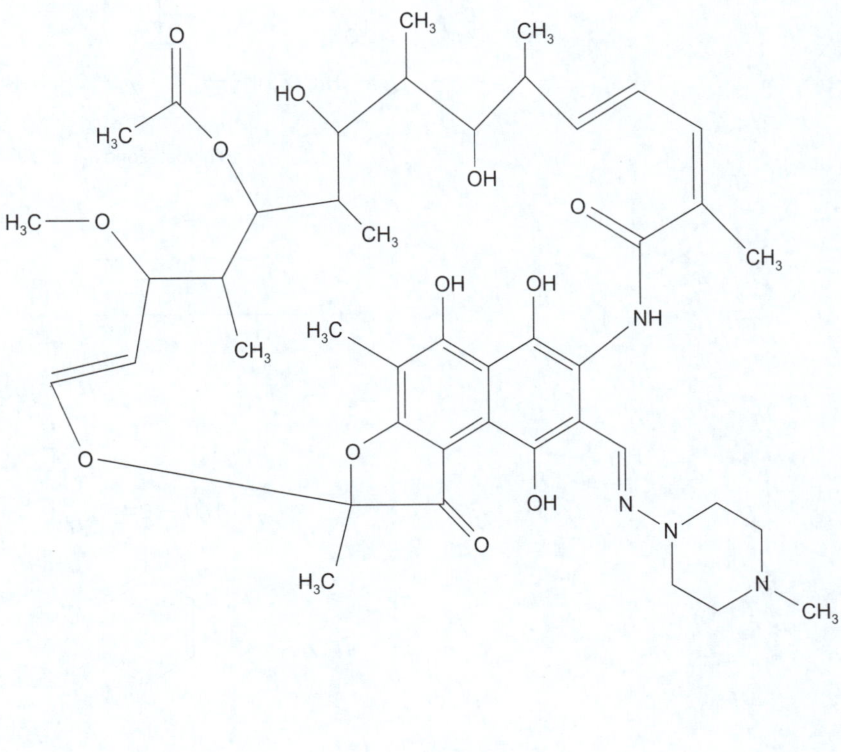

Rifabutin

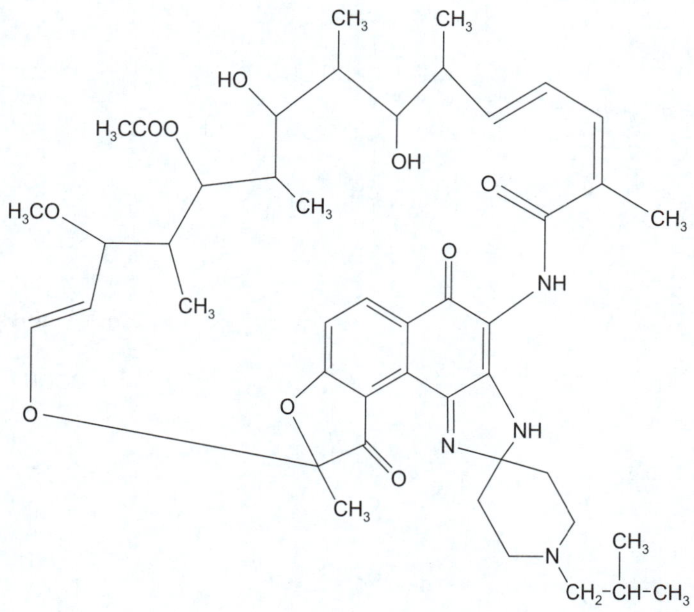

Cycloserine

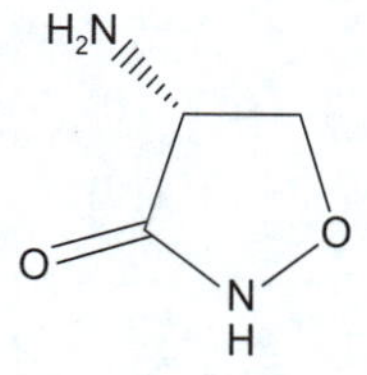

Streptomycin

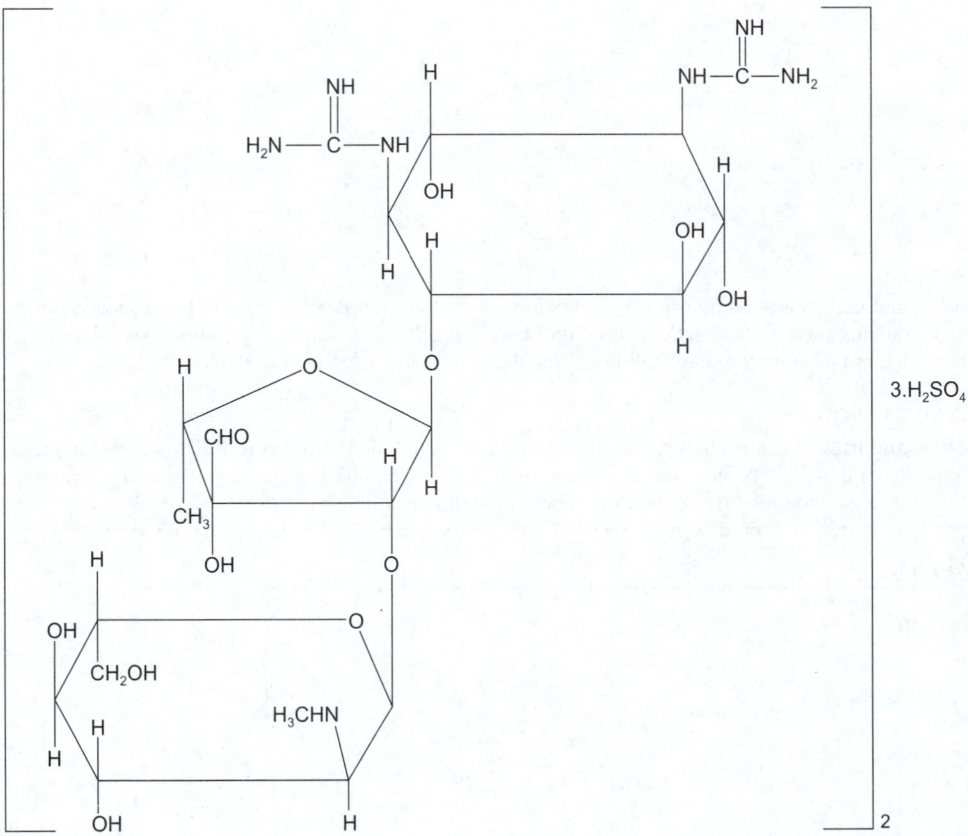

Capreomycin sulphate

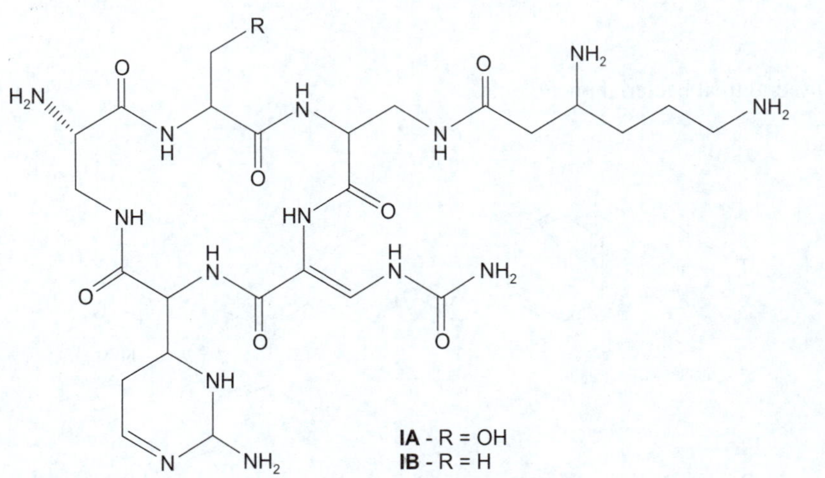

Cycloserine

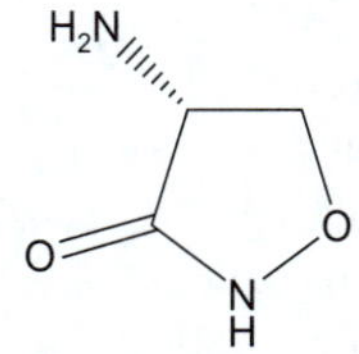

Cycloserine

Properties and uses: It is a 4-amino-1,2-oxazolidinone derivative with R-configuration. It is a second-line anti-TB drug that contains bacteriostatic activity. It inhibits bacterial cell wall synthesis by competitive inhibition of two enzymes such as L-alanine racemase and D-alanine ligase. It is an analogue of D-alanine.

Capreomycin sulphate

Properties and uses: It is a cyclic peptide, broad-spectrum antibiotic produced or isolated from *Streptomyceus capreolus*. It binds with 30s and 50s ribosomal subunits and inhibits protein synthesis and administered by injection. It is a second-line drug for the treatment of multidrug resistant TB.

Newer Drugs

Lefamulin

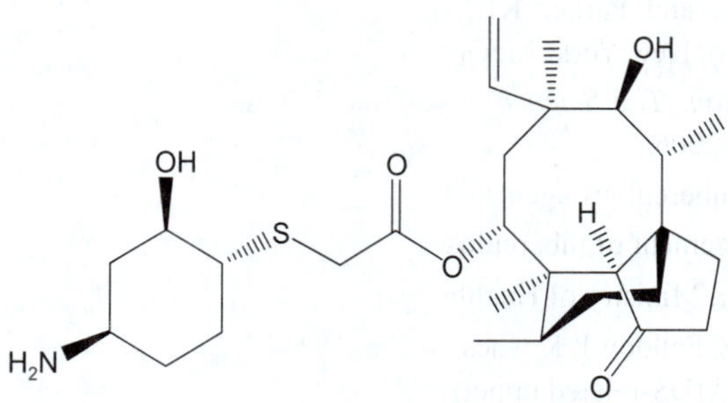

Uses: It is used to treat bacterial pneumonia.

Pretomanid

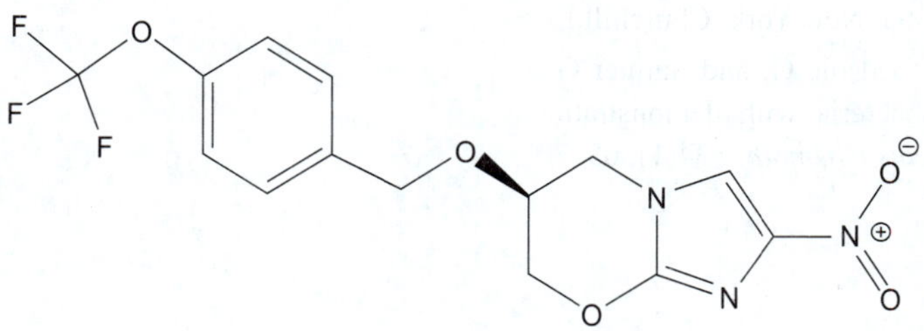

Uses: It is an antibiotic used for the treatment of multidrug-resistant tuberculosis and used together with bedaquiline and linezolid.

PROBABLE QUESTIONS

1. What is tuberculosis? How will you categorize it according to the site of infection? Define antitubercular drugs and classify them with suitable examples.
2. Name the pyridine-containing antitubercular agents. Outline the synthesis, mode of action, metabolism, dose, and dosage forms available for any one of them.
3. Write the structure, chemical name, and uses of at least two most potent drugs from standard drugs and reserve drugs categories.
4. Write a detailed account on pyrazinamide along with its synthesis, mode of action, dosage forms available, and uses.
5. Write the following syntheses:
   (a) Ethambutol, (b) thiacetazone, and (c) PAS.
6. Write a note on antibiotics used in tuberculosis.

SUGGESTED READINGS

1. Abraham DJ (ed). *Burger's Medicinal Chemistry and Drug Discovery* (6th edn). New Jersey: John Wiley, 2007.
2. Banerjee A, Dubnau E, Quemard A, Balasubramanian V, Um KS, Wilson T, Collins D, de Lisle G, Jacobs WR Jr. 'inhA: A gene encoding a target for isoniazid and ethionamide in *Mycobacterium tuberculosis*'. *Science* 263: 227–30, 1994.
3. *British Pharmacopoeia*. Medicines and Healthcare Products Regulatory Agency. London. 2008.
4. Bruntan LL, Lazo JS, and Parker KL. *Goodman and Gilman's: The Pharmacological Basis of Therapeutics* (11th edn). New York: McGraw Hill, 2006.
5. Gennaro AR. *Remington: The Science and Practice of Pharmacy* (21st edn). New York: Lippincot Williams and Wilkins, 2006.
6. Goldberger MJ. 'Antituberculous agents'. *Med Clin North Am* 72: 661, 1988.
7. Holdiners MR. 'Management of tuberculosis meningitis'. *Drugs* 39: 224, 1990.
8. *Indian Pharmacopoeia*. Ministry of Health and Family Welfare. New Delhi, 1996.
9. Lane HC, Laughon BE, Falloon J, Kovacs JA, Davey RT Jr, Polis MA, and Masur H. 'Recent advances in the management of AIDS-related opportunistic infections'. *Ann Intern Med* 120: 945–955, 1994.
10. Lednicer D and Mitscher LA. *The Organic Chemistry of Drug Synthesis*. New York: John Wiley, 1995.
11. Lemke TL and William DA. *Foye's Principle of Medicinal Chemistry* (6th edn). New York: Lippincott Williams and Wilkins, 2008.
12. Mendell GL, Douglas RG Jr, and Bennett JE (eds). *Principles and Practice of Infections Diseases* (3rd edn), pp. 295–303. New York: Churchill Livingstone, 1990.
13. Wallace RJ Jr, Bedsole G, and Sumter G. 'Activities of ciprofloxacin and ofloxacin against rapidly growing mycobacteria with demonstration of acquired resistance following single-drug therapy'. *Antimicrob Agents Chemother* 34(1): 65–70, 1990.

CHAPTER 17

Antifungal Agents

INTRODUCTION

Human–fungi parasitic relationship results in mycotic illnesses. Most fungal infections (mycoses) involve superficial invasion of the skin or mucous membrane of the body orifices. These diseases can usually be controlled by local application of the antifungal agents. Fungi have different shapes and sizes. Some are large while others are minute, parasitic, and saprophytic cells. They differ from the following organisms in some important aspects:

- Algae by lack of photosynthetic ability.
- Protozoa by the lack of motility, possession of chitinuous cell wall, and ease of culture on simple media.
- Bacteria by greater size and having certain intracellular structure such as mitochondria and nuclear membrane.

CLASSIFICATION

On the basis of some differences, fungi may be classified as follows:

a. Phycomyelitis (algae-like)
b. Ascomyelitis (sac-like)
c. Basidiomyelitis (mushrooms)
d. Dueteromyelitis

The potentially effective antifungal compounds are listed in Table 17.1.

Classification Based on the Chemical Structure, Action, and Source

The antifungal agents can be divided into the following classes, based on their chemical structure, mechanism of action, and source:

I. Antibiotics: Amphotericin B, nystatin, griseofulvin
II. Azoles (imidazole, triazole derivatives)
Triazoles: Fluconazole, itraconzole, terconazole
Imidazoles: Clotrimazole, ketoconazole, miconazole, bifonazole, butoconazole, and zinoconazole
III. Fluorinated pyrimidines: Flucytosine
IV. Chitin synthetase inhibitors: Nikomycin Z

V. Peptides/proteins: Cispentacin

VI. Miscellaneous: Ciclopirox, tolnaftate, naftifine, and terbinafine

Classification Based on the Route of Administration

I. Drugs for subcutaneous and systemic mycoses: Amphotericin B, fluconazole, flucytosine, itraconazole, ketoconazole.

II. Drugs for superficial mycoses: Clotrimazole, econazole, griseofluvin, miconazole, nystatin.

Table 17.1: Potentially effective antifungal compounds

Disease	*Compounds*
Dermatophytoses	Azoles (butoconazole, clotrimazole, econazole, itraconazole, miconazole, oxiconazole, sulconazole), griseofulvin, naftifine, terbinafine, tolnaftate
Aspergillosis	Amphotericin B, 5-fluorocytosin, itraconazole
Blastomycosis	Amphotericin B, itraconazole, ketoconazole
Candidiasis	Amphotercin B, 5-fluorocytosine, nystatin azoles (butoconazole, clotrimazole, econazole, fluconazole, itraconazole, ketoconazole, miconazole, terconazole, tioconazole)
Chromomycosis	5-Fluorocytosine, itraconazole, ketocanozole
Coccidiodomycosis	Amphotericin B, fluconazole, itraconazolel, ketoconazole
Cryptococcosis	Amphotericin B, fluconazole
Histoplasmosis	Amphotericin B, itraconazole, ketoconazole
Mucormycosis	Amphotericin B
Paracoccidioidomicosis	Itraconazole, ketoconazole
Pneumocytosis	Trimethoprim, sulphamethoxazole, pentamidine, ecothionate
Pseudallescheriasis	Amphotericin B, miconazole
Sporotrichosis	Amphotericin B, itraconazole, potassium iodide

SYNTHESIS AND DRUG PROFILE

I. Antibiotics

1. Amphotericin B

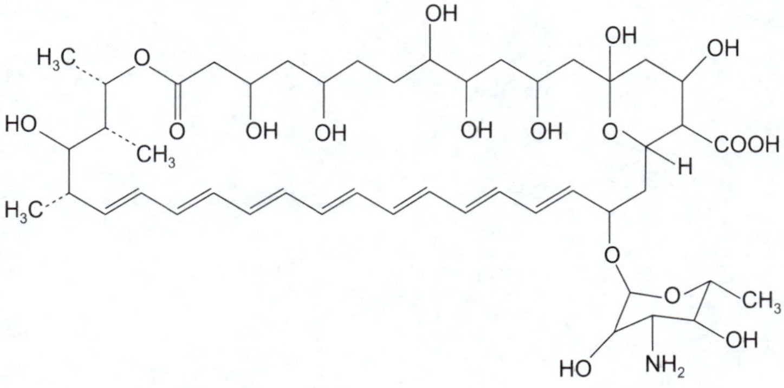

Mode of action: The antifungal activity of this drug depends, at least, in part, on its binding to a sterol moiety. Primarily, ergosterol that is present in the membrane of sensitive fungi, by virtue of their interaction with the sterols of cell membranes and polyenes, appear to form pores or channels. The result is an increase in the permeability of the membrane, allowing leakage of a variety of small molecules, such as intracellular potassium, magnesium, sugars, and metabolites leading to cellular death.

Properties and uses: It is polyene antibiotic obtained from *Streptomyces nodosus*. It is an amphoteric compound that consists of seven-conjugated double bond, an internal ester, a free carbonyl group, and a glycoside side chain with a primary amino group. The carbohydrate moiety is D-mycosamine. The conjugated systems are usually of all *trans* configurations, so that the ring contains a planar lipophilic segment and a less rigid hydrophilic portion. Amphotericin B is an amphoteric, forming soluble salts in both basic and acidic environments, and due to extensive unsaturation, it is unstable, primarily used as antifungal agents.

2. **Griseofulvin** (Fulvicin)

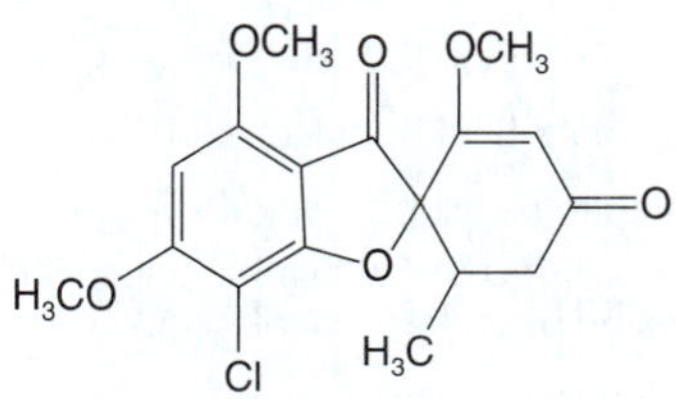

Mode of action: Griseofulvin is a fungi-static drug that causes disruption of the mitotic spindle by interacting with polymerized microtubules.

Properties and uses: Griseofulvin is a white or yellowish-white microfine powder, practically insoluble in water, freely soluble in dimethylformamide and tetrachloroethane, slightly soluble in ethanol and methanol. Used as an antifungal agent.

Synthesis

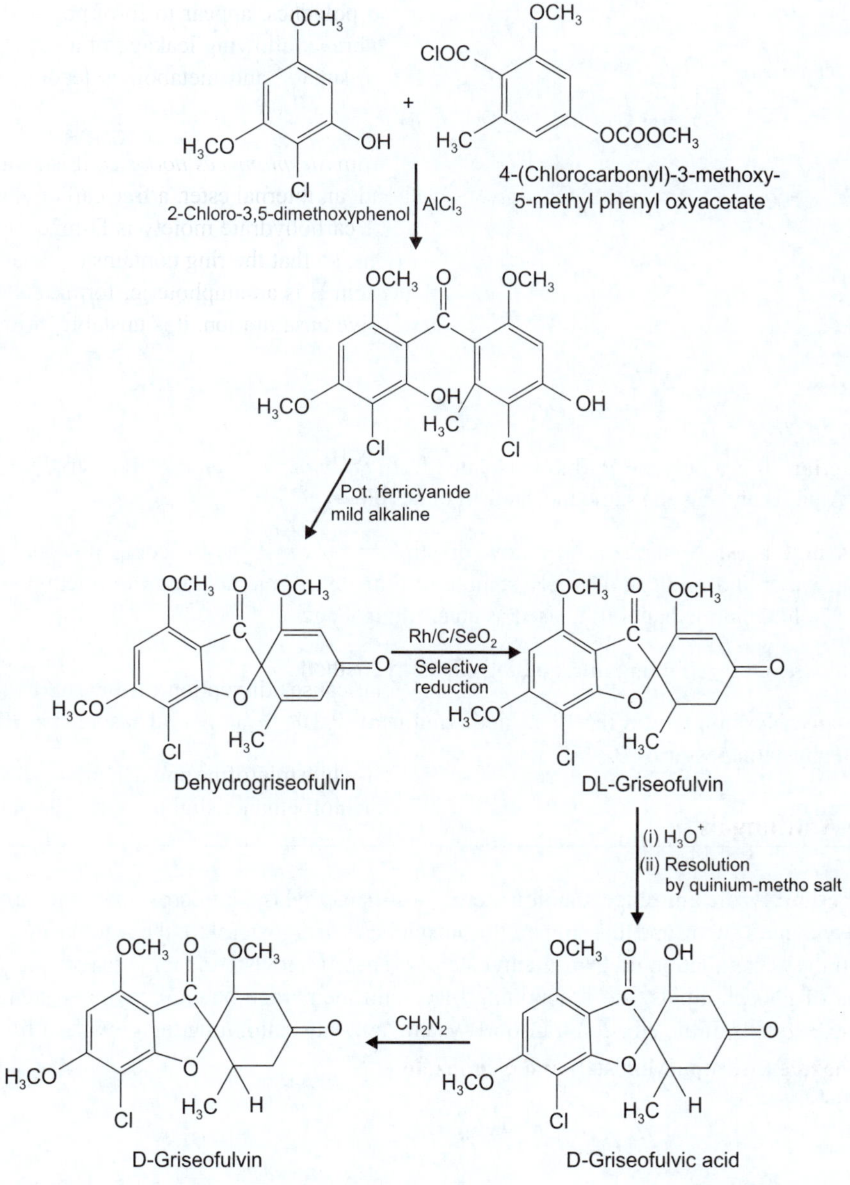

Assay: Dissolve the sample in ethanol and measure the absorbance after dilution with ethanol at the maxima of 291 nm using ultraviolet spectrophotometer.

Dose: As an oral suspension, the administered dose is 125 mg/5 ml; as capsules, 250 or 500 mg as tablets. For adults, in divided doses, the dose is 500 mg/day.

Dosage forms: Griseofulvin tablets IP, BP.

3. Nystatin

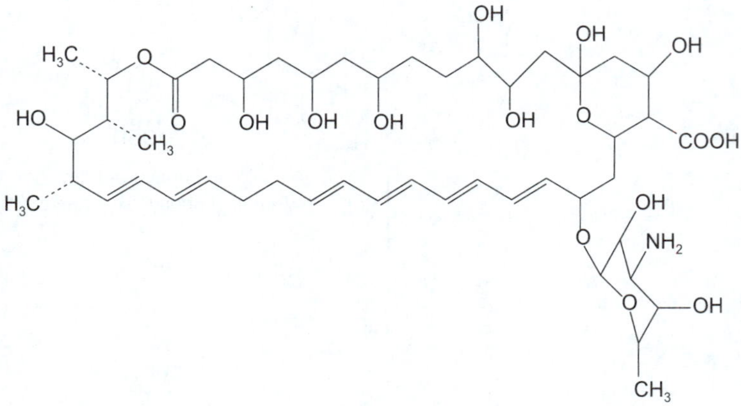

Mode of action: It is a polyene antibiotic isolated from *Streptomyces noursei*. It is structurally similar to amphotericin B and has the same mechanism of action.

Properties and uses: Nystatin is a yellow or slightly brownish hygroscopic powder, practically insoluble in water and in alcohol, freely soluble in dimethylformamide and in dimethyl sulphoxide, and slightly soluble in methanol. It is used as an antifungal agent.

Assay: It is assayed by adopting microbiological assay method.

Dosage forms: Nystatin tablets IP, BP, nystatin ointment IP, BP, nystatin oral suspension BP, nystatin pastilles BP, nystatin pessaries BP.

II. Azole Antifungals

Mode of action: Azole antifungals inhibit sterol 14-α-demethylase, a microsomal cytochrome P450-dependent enzyme system, and thus, impair the biosynthesis of ergosterol for the cytoplasmic membrane and lead to the accumulation of 14-α-methyl sterols. These methylsterols may disrupt the packing of aryl chains of phospholipids, the functioning of certain membrane-bound enzyme systems, such as ATPase and enzymes of the electron transport system, and thus, inhibiting the growth of fungi.

1. Miconazole (Micatin, Monistat) **and Econazole**

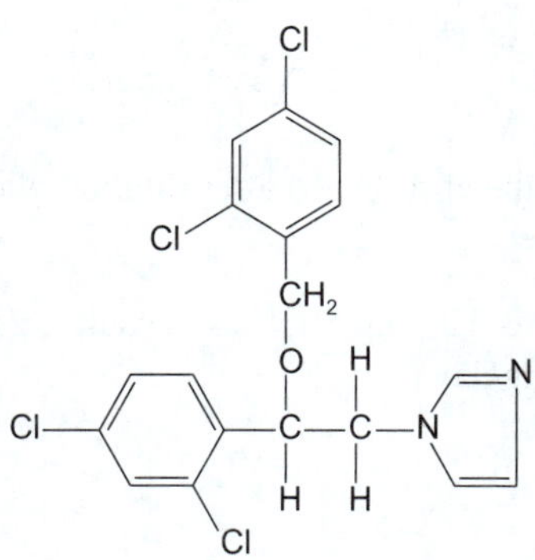

Miconazole

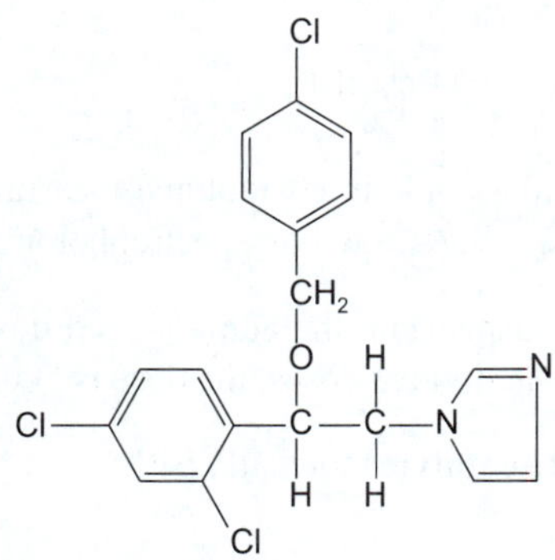

Econazole

Synthesis

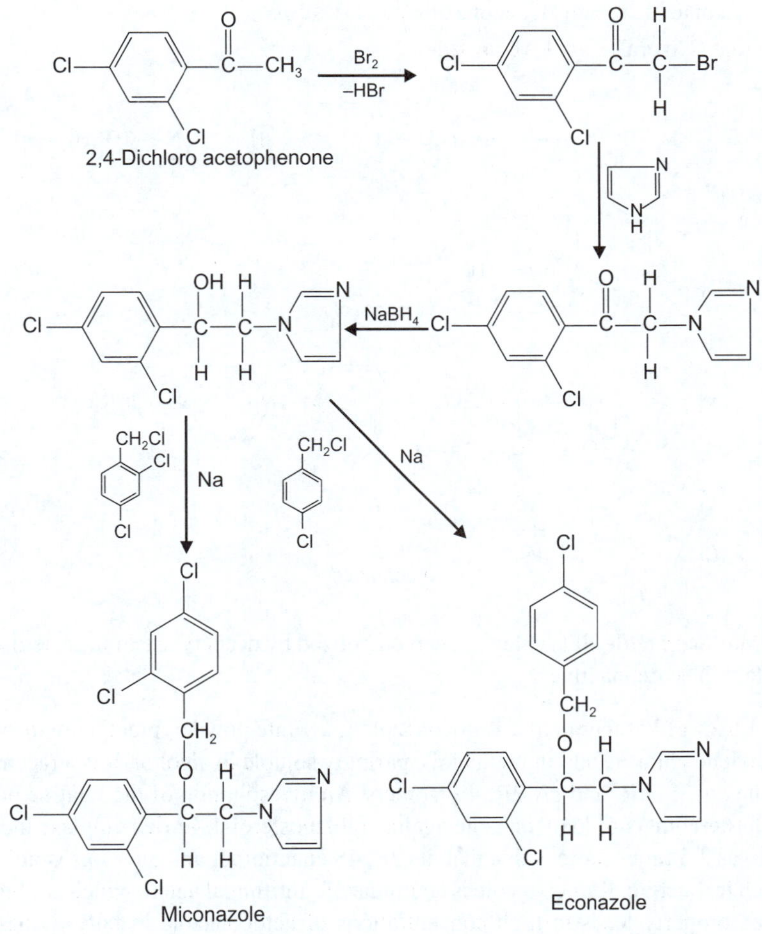

Properties and uses of miconazole: Miconazole is a white or almost white powder, very slightly soluble in water, sparingly soluble in methanol, and slightly soluble in alcohol. It is used as an antifungal agent.

Assay: Dissolve the sample in anhydrous acetic acid, with slight heating, if necessary, and titrate with 0.1 M perchloric acid. Determine the end point potentiometrically.

Dose: It is to be applied in the vagina at bedtime for 7 days, and 200 mg vaginal suppositories for 3 days therapy.

Dosage forms: Miconazole cream IP, BP, miconazole pessaries IP, miconazole tablets IP, miconazole and hydrocortisone cream BP, miconazole and hydrocortisone acetate cream BP, miconazole and hydrocortisone ointment BP.

Properties and uses of econazole: Econazole is white or almost white crystalline powder, very slightly soluble in water, soluble in methanol, sparingly soluble in methylene chloride, and slightly soluble in alcohol. It is used as antifungal agent.

Assay: Dissolve the sample in anhydrous acetic acid and titrate with 0.1 M perchloric acid. Determine the end point potentiometrically.

Dose: It is available as a water insoluble cream (1%) to be applied twice a day.

Dosage forms: Econazole cream BP, econazole pessaries BP.

2. **Ketoconazole** (Nizoral) **and Terconazole**

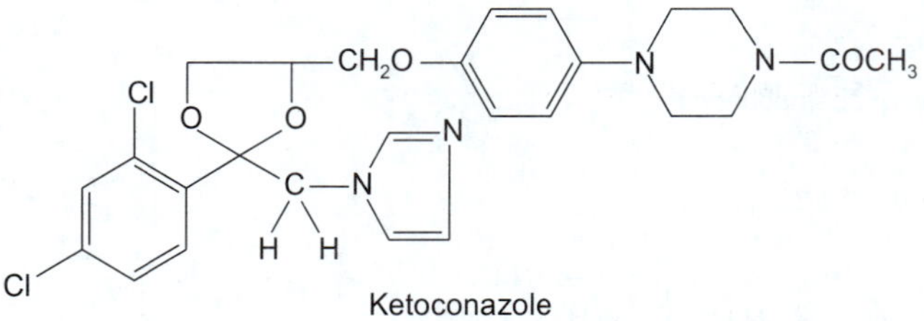

Ketoconazole

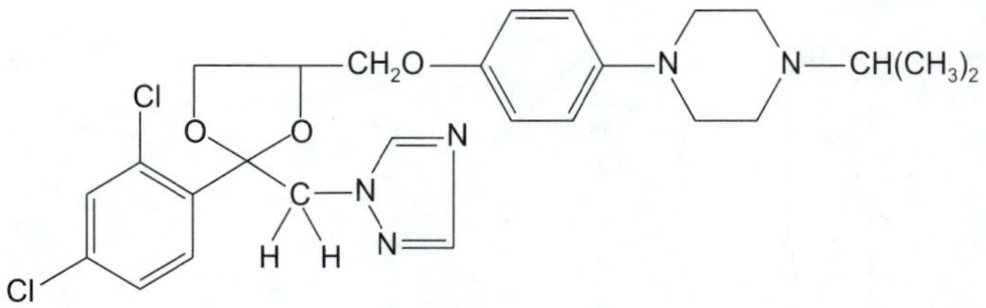

Terconazole

Metabolism of ketoconazole: It is extensively metabolized by deacetylase of the microsomal enzymes and all the metabolites are inactive.

Properties and uses of ketoconazole: Ketoconazole is a white powder, practically insoluble in water, soluble in methylene chloride and in methanol, sparingly soluble in alcohol. It is a racemic compound, consisting of the *cis*-2S, 4R, and *cis*-2R, 4S isomers. An investigation of the relative potencies of the four possible diastereomers of ketoconazole against rat lanosterol-1,4α-demethylase indicated that the 2S, 4R isomer was 2.5 times more active than its 2R, 4S enantiomer and the *trans* isomers, 2S, 4S, and 2R, 4R are much less active. Ketoconazole is an imidazole antifungal agent, which is a highly lipophilic compound. This property leads to high concentrations of ketoconazole in fatty tissues and purulent exudates. Ketoconazole is active against *Candida* spp. and *Cryptococcus neoformans*.

Assay of ketoconazole: Dissolve the sample in a mixture of anhydrous acetic acid and methyl ethyl ketone (1:7) and titrate with 0.1 M perchloric acid. Determine the end point potentiometrically.

Dose: It is administered as 200 mg scored tablets and 2% topical cream.

Synthesis

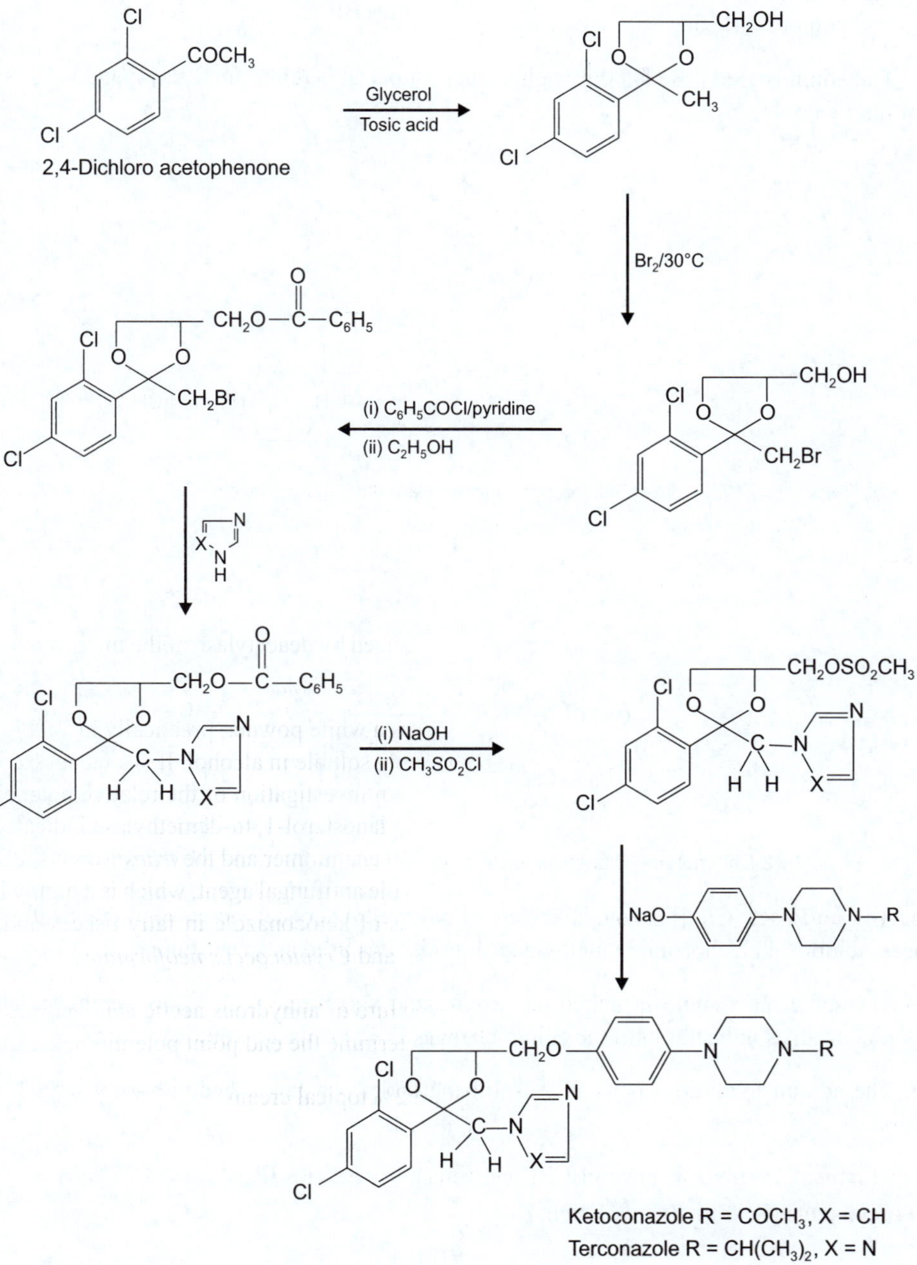

Metabolism of terconazole: It is metabolized by CYP3A4 on oral administration.

Properties and uses of terconazole: Terconazole is a white powder, practically insoluble in water, soluble in methylene chloride and in acetone, sparingly soluble in alcohol. It is a triazole derivative that is used exclusively for the control of vulvovaginal moniliasis caused by *Candida albicans* and other *Candida* spp.

Assay of terconazole: Dissolve the sample in a mixture of anhydrous acetic acid and volumes of methyl ethyl ketone (1:7) and titrate with 0.1 M perchloric acid. Determine the end point potentiometrically at the second point of inflexion.

Dose: The administered dose is 80 g vaginal suppository at bedtime for 3 days; and 0.4% as vaginal cream for 7 days.

3. **Clotrimazole**

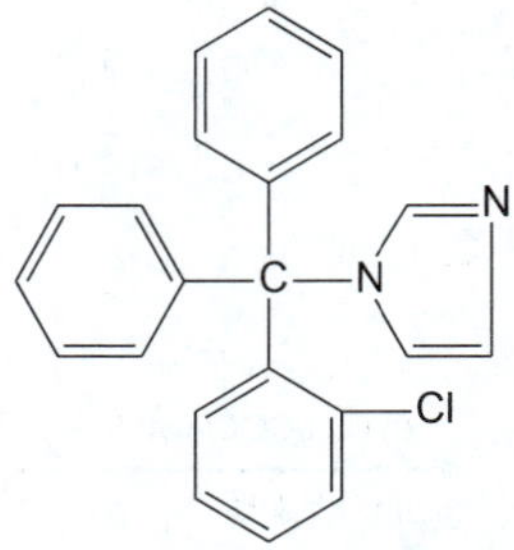

1-((2-Chlorophenyl)diphenylmethyl)-1*H*-imidazole

Synthesis

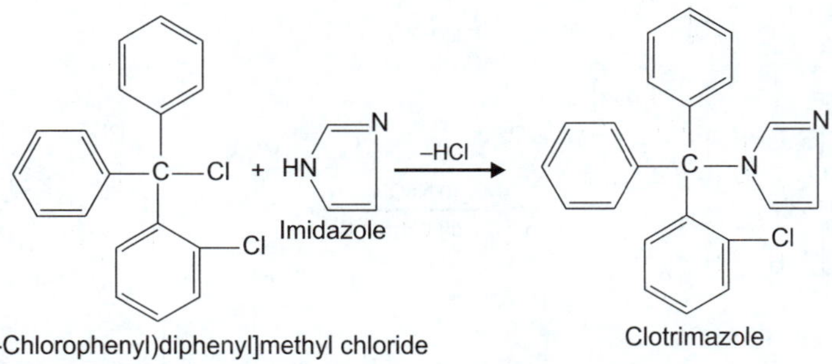

Properties and uses: Clotrimazole is a white or pale yellow crystalline powder, practically insoluble in water, soluble in alcohol and in methylene chloride. It is used as an antifungal agent.

Assay: Dissolve the sample in anhydrous acetic acid and titrate with 0.1 M perchloric acid using naphtholbenzein as indicator until the colour changes from brownish-yellow to green.

Dose: The administered dose is usually as 100 mg tablet per day at bedtime for 7 days for vaginal infection.

Dosage forms: Clotrimazole cream IP, BP, clotrimazole pessaries IP, BP.

4. **Fluconazole** (Syscan, Zocon, Flucos)

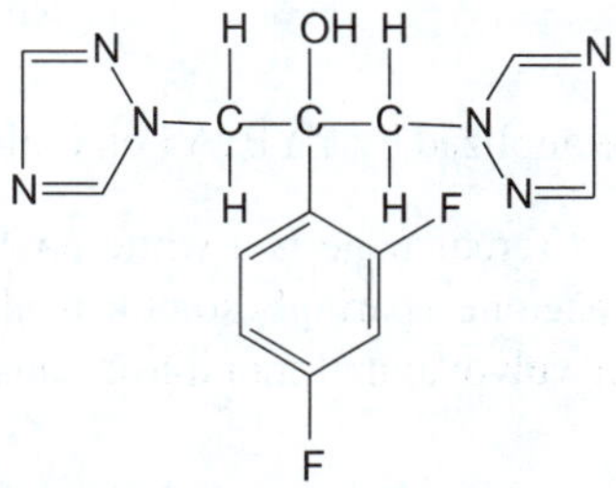

2-(2,4-Difluorophenyl)-1,3-di(1*H*-1,2,4-triazol-1-yl)propan-2-ol

Synthesis

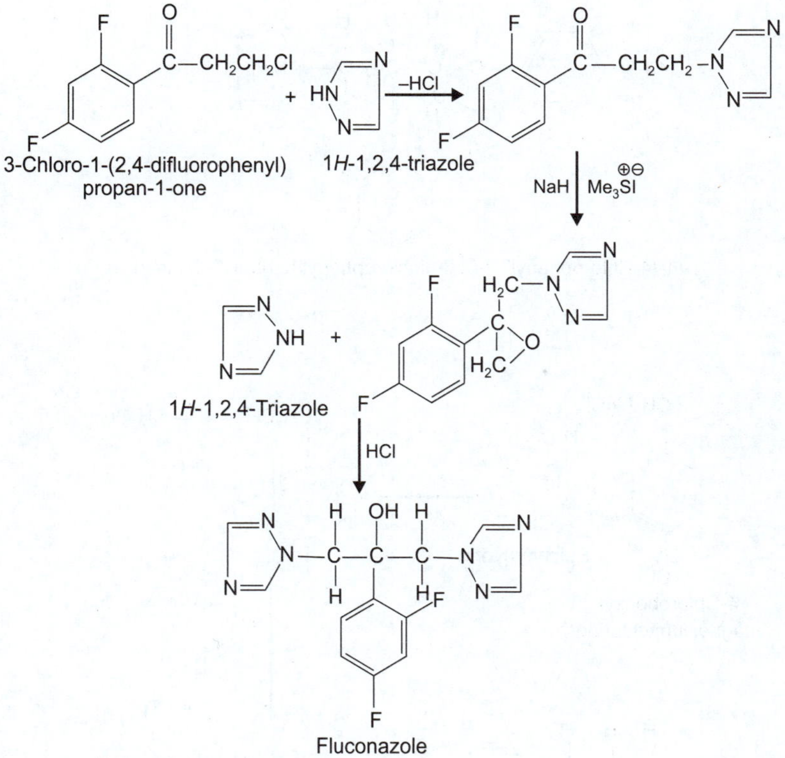

Properties and uses: Fluconazole is a white hygroscopic crystalline powder, slightly soluble in water, and soluble in methanol and in acetone. It is a widely used *bis*-triazole antifungal agent. It is generally considered to be a fungi-static agent, and it is principally active against *Candida* spp. and *Cryptococcus* spp. Fluconazole has useful activity against *Coccidioides immitis*, and is often used to suppress the meningitis produced by the fungus.

Assay: Dissolve the sample in anhydrous acetic acid and titrate with 0.1 M perchloric acid. Determine the end point potentiometrically.

Dose: The administered dose for superficial mucosal candidiasis for adults is 50 mg daily, which is increased to 100 mg daily. Recommended treatment duration is 7–14 days; in the case of oropharyngeal candidiasis, 14 days for atrophic oral candidiasis associated with dentures, 14–30 days for other mucosal candidal infections, including oesophagitis. In the case of children, more than 4 weeks the loading dose is 6 mg/kg followed by 3 mg/kg daily.

The administered dose for dermatophytosis, pityriasis versicolor, and candida infections for adults is 50 mg daily for up to 6 weeks.

The administered dose for cryptococcal infections, including meningitis, systemic candidasis for adults, initially is 400 mg followed by 200–400 mg daily; the maximum dose is 800 mg daily in the case of severe infections. In the case of cryptococcal meningitis, usual treatment duration is at least 6–8 weeks and may also be given via IV infusion. For children more than 4 weeks the dose is 6–12 mg/kg daily; same doses may be given every 72 hrs in neonates up to 2 weeks and every 48 hrs in neonates 2–4 weeks old; the maximum dose is 400 mg daily.

5. Butoconazole

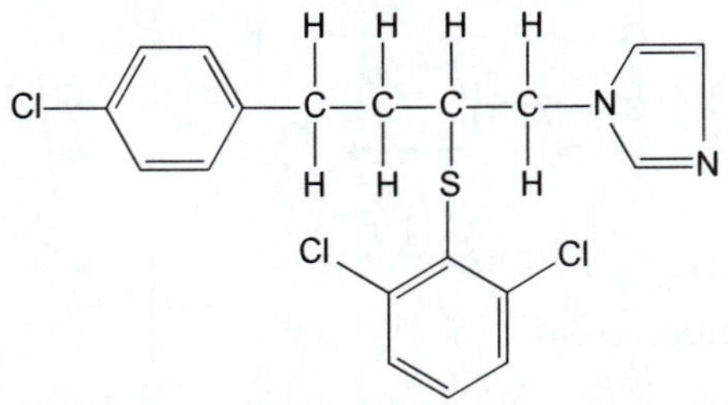

1-(4-(4-Chlorophenyl)-2-(2,6-dichlorophenylthio)butyl)-1*H*-imidazole

Synthesis

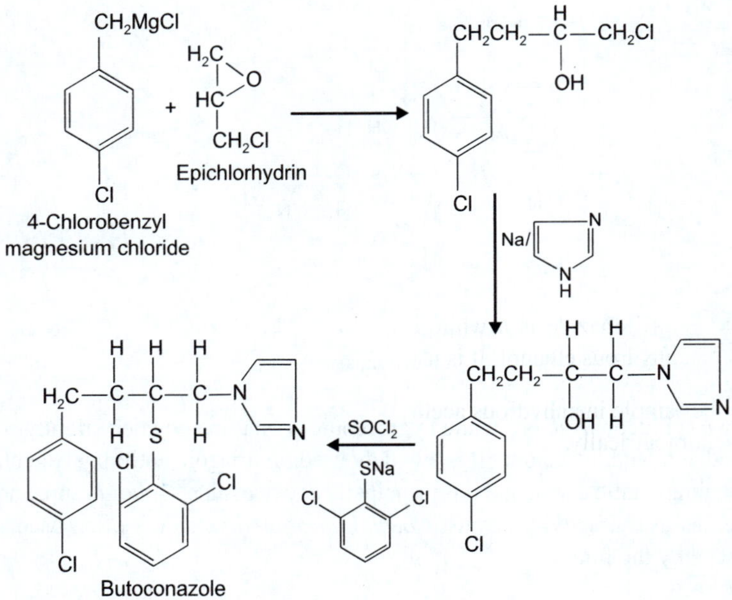

6. Bifonazole

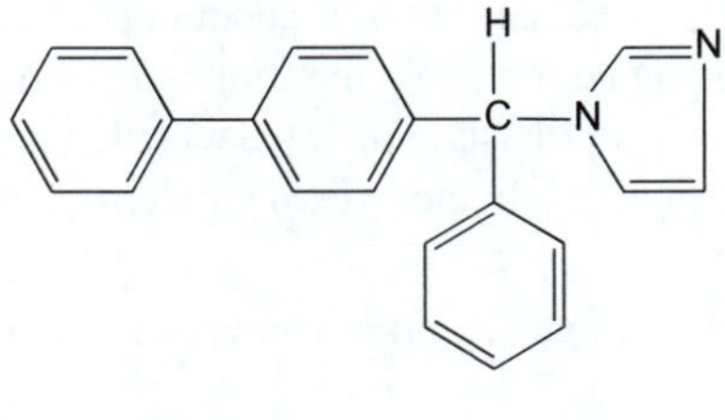

Synthesis

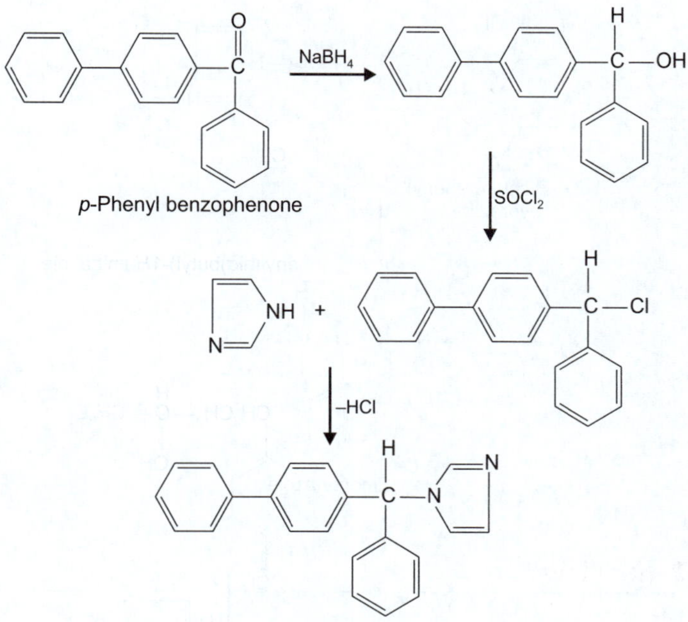

p-Phenyl benzophenone

Bifonazole

Properties and uses: Bifonazole is a white crystalline powder, practically insoluble in water, and sparingly soluble in anhydrous ethanol. It is used as an antifungal agent.

Assay: Dissolve the sample in anhydrous acetic acid and titrate with 0.1 M perchloric acid. Determine the end point potentiometrically.

7. Zinoconazole

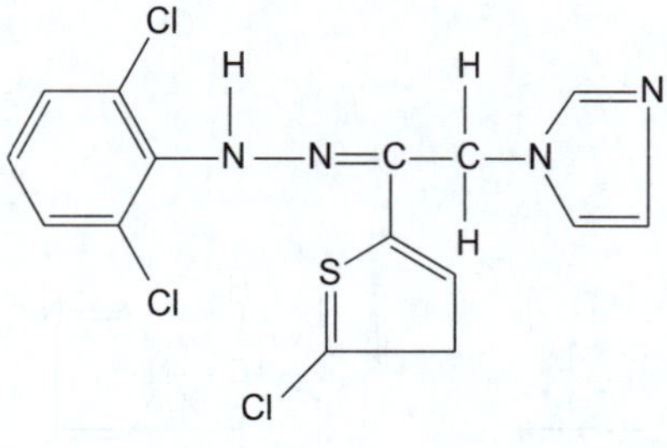

Synthesis

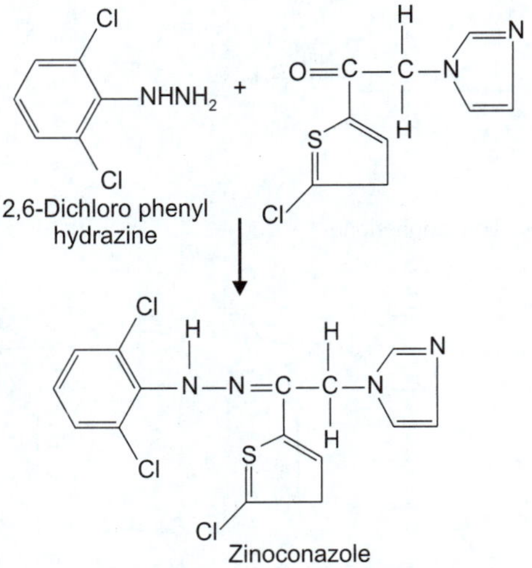

III. Fluorinated Pyrimidines

1. Flucytosine

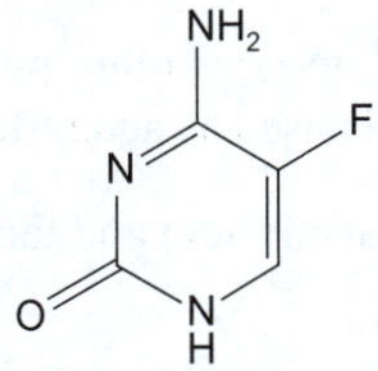

4-Amino-5-fluoropyrimidin-2(1*H*)-one

Synthesis

Route I. From: 5-Fluorouracil

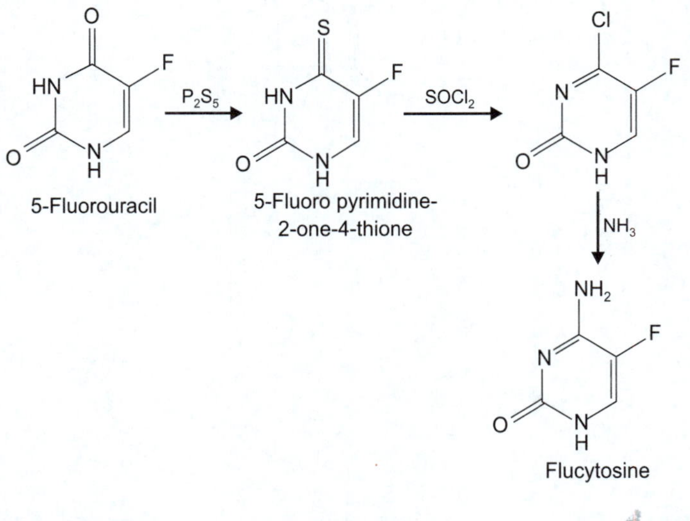

Route II. From: 5-Fluorouracil

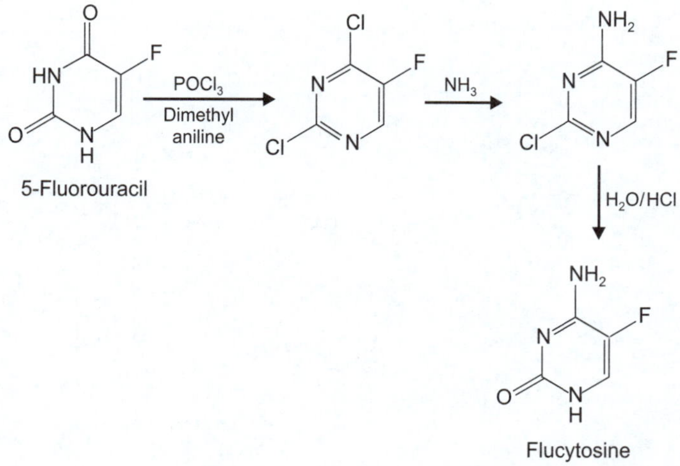

Mode of action: Flucytosine is converted by cytosine deaminase into 5-fluorouracil (5-FU), then, 5-fluoro deoxyuridylic acid is formed. This false nucleotide inhibits thymidylate synthetase, thus, depriving the organism of thymidylic acid, an essential DNA component. It is a potent antimetabolite, which replaces uracil in the pyrimidine pool and thus, disrupts protein synthesis. Mammalian cells do not convert flucytosine to fluorouracil. This fact is crucial for the selective action of this compound. In addition, 5-fluorouracil is metabolized into 5-fluoro uridylic acid by the enzyme uridine monophosphate (UMP) pyrophosphorylase. It is either incorporated into the DNA (via synthesis of 5-fluorouridine triphosphate) or would be metabolized into 5-fluoro deoxyuridylic acid, which is a potent inhibitor of thymidylate synthetase.

Metabolism: It is metabolized to 5-FU by fungal cytidine deaminase. Then 5-FU is converted into 5-fluoro deoxyuridine, which is a thymidylate synthase inhibitor and interferes with both protein and RNA biosynthesis.

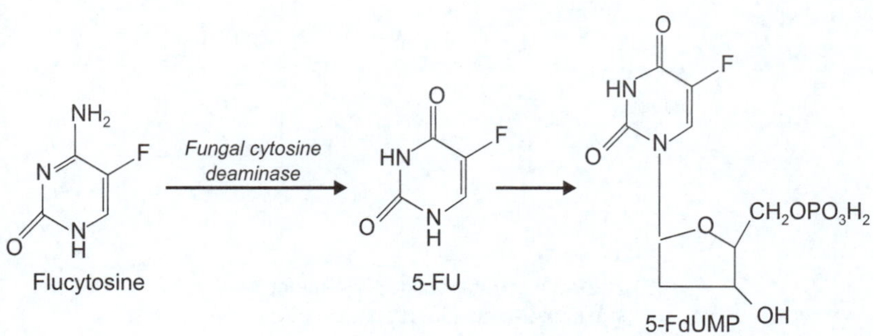

Properties and uses: Flucytosine is a white crystalline powder, sparingly soluble in water, and slightly soluble in ethanol. Flucytosine is the only available antimetabolite drug having antifungal activity.

Assay: Dissolve the sample in anhydrous acetic acid, add acetic anhydride, and titrate with 0.1 M perchloric acid. Determine the end point potentiometrically.

Dosage forms: Flucytosine tablets BP.

IV. Chitin Synthetase Inhibitors

1. Nikomycin

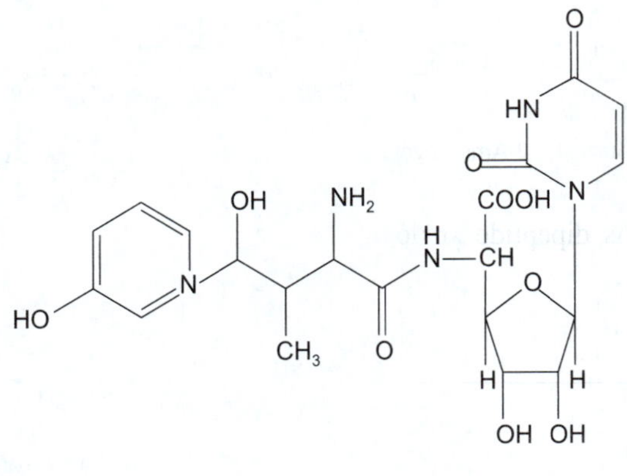

Mode of action: Nikomycin competitively inhibits the chitin synthase, mimicking its substrate uridine diphosphate-*N*-acetyl glucosamine of fungi with *C. albicans* as the primary target organism. The enzyme is an integral membrane protein. Nikomycin Z has shown to act synergistically *in vitro* with fluconazole, ketoconzole, and tioconazole against *C. albicans* at minimum inhibitory concentration (MIC) levels of azoles.

Properties and uses: Nikomycin is a nucleoside peptide antibiotic that is produced by soil strains of *Steptomyces tendae*. It is found to be more potent than most azoles in inhibiting highly chitinous, dimorphic fungal pathogens, such as *Coccidiodes imitis* and *Blastomyces dermatidis*.

V. Peptides/Proteins

Examples: L-Norvalyl FMIP, Cispentacin

i. **L-Norvalyl—FMIP**

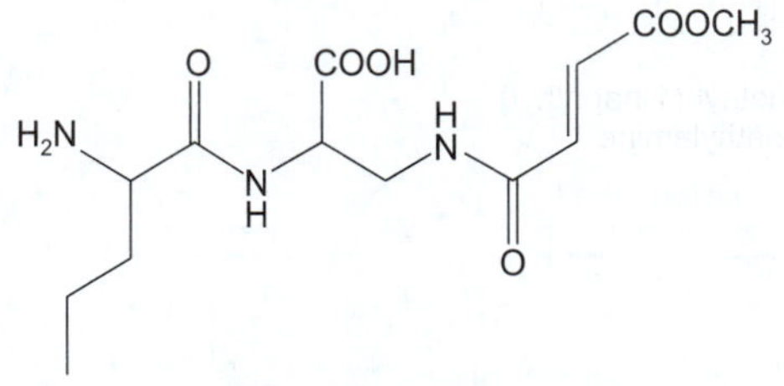

(E)-2-(2-Aminopentanamido)-3-(4-methoxy-4-oxobut-2-enamido) propanoic acid

Mode of action: The inhibitors of glucosamine-6-phosphate synthase delivered through peptide transport systems have been reported as having anticandidal activity.

ii. *cis*-Pentacin

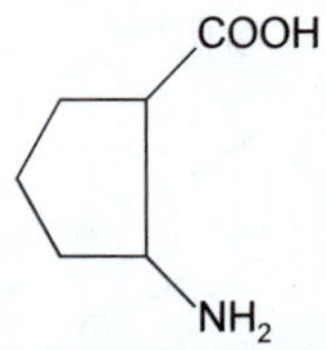

2-Aminocyclopentane carboxylic acid

Properties and uses: It is dipeptide analogue that is shown *in vitro* and *in vivo* activity against *C. albicans*.

VI. Miscellaneous Agents

1. Naftifine (Nabtin)

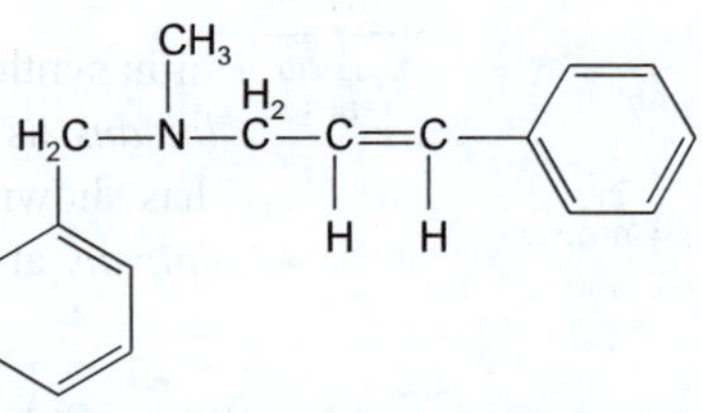

N-Methyl-N-(naphthalen-1-yl-methyl)-3-phenylprop-2-en-1-amine

Synthesis

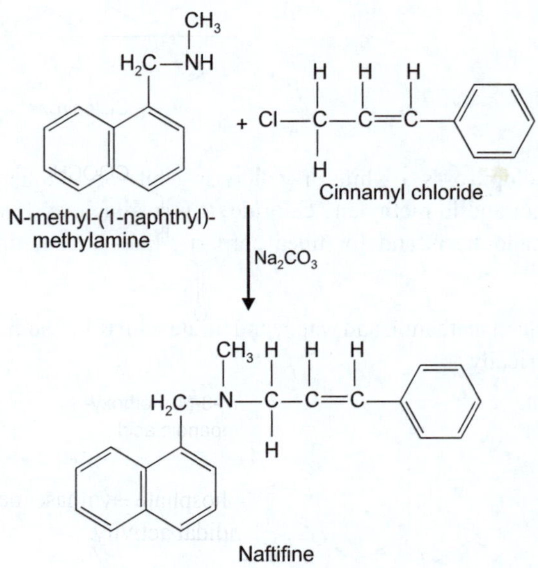

Mode of action: The drug has fungicidal activity against *Tinea cruris* and *Corporis* spp. This inhibits squalene 2,3-epoxidase and thus, inhibits fungal biosynthesis of ergosterol.

Dose: It is administered as 1% cream twice daily.

2. Ciclopirox

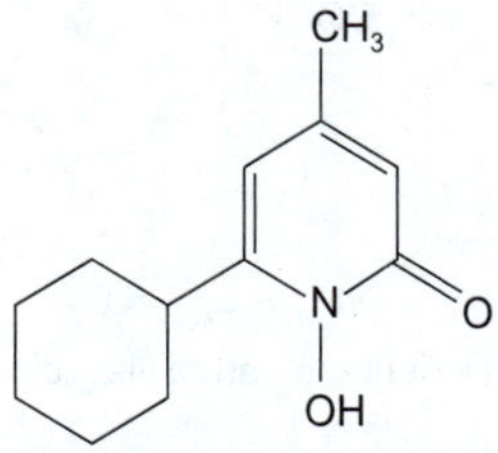

6-Cyclohexyl-1-hydroxy-4-methylpyridin-2(1*H*)-one

Synthesis

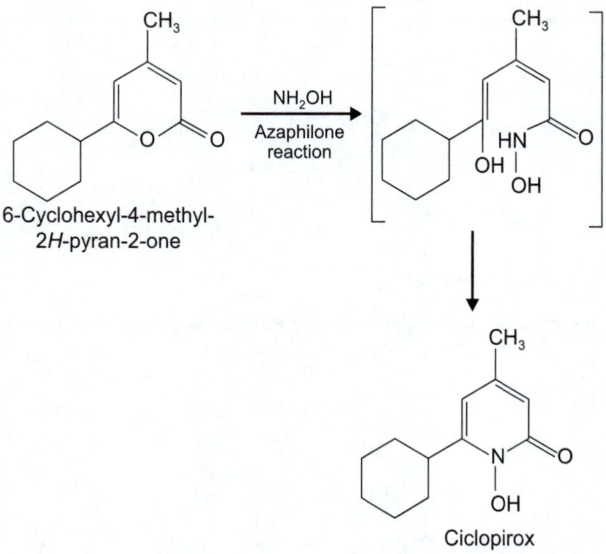

Properties and uses: Ciclopirox is a white or yellowish-white crystalline powder, slightly soluble in water, soluble in ethanol and in methylene chloride. It is available as 1% cream on cotton for the treatment of cutaneous candidiasis and for tinea corporis, tinea cruris, tinea pedis, and pityriasis versicolor.

Assay: Dissolve the sample in methanol, add water, and titrate with 0.1 M sodium hydroxide. Determine the end point potentiometrically.

3. Tolnaftate

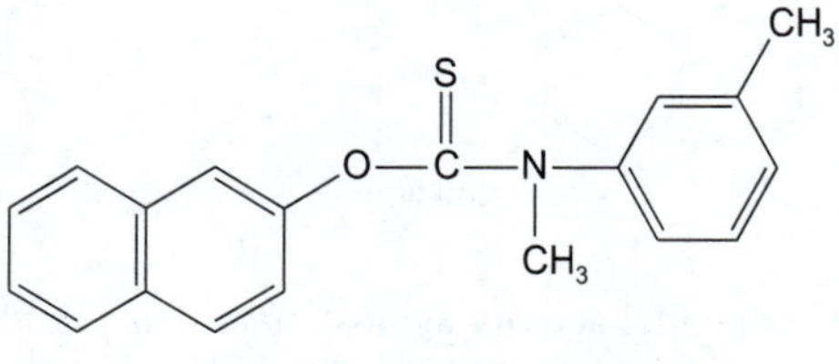

O-(Naphthalen-2-yl)-N-methyl(*m*-tolyl)carbamothioate

Synthesis

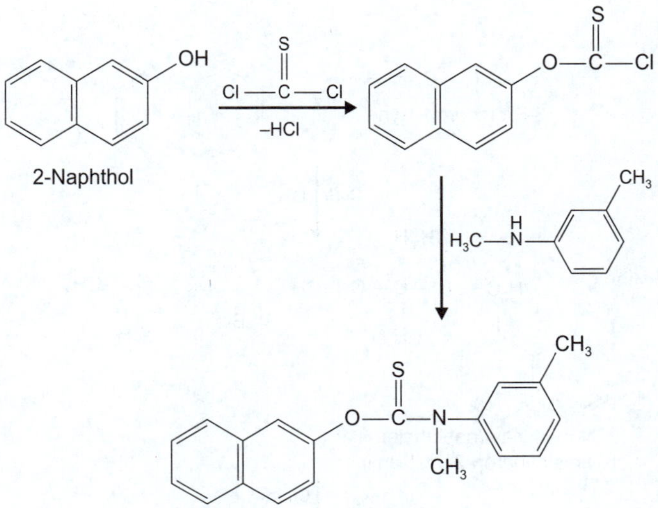

Tolnaftate

Properties and uses: Tolnaftate is a white or yellowish-white powder practically insoluble in water, soluble in acetone and in methylene chloride, and very slightly soluble in alcohol. It is effective for the treatment of most cutaneous mycoses, such as *Trichophytonrubrum* and *Microsporum canis*. Replacement of the aromatic methyl group by hydroxy or methoxy or its removal does not affect potency. Replacement of the complete tolyl group by an α-napthyl or a β-napthyl substituent does not decrease its potency. It is non-toxic.

Dose: The administered dose is 1% as a cream, gel, powder, aerosol powder, and topical solution, applied locally twice a day.

Assay: Dissolve the sample in methanol, measure the absorbance after its dilution with methanol, at the maxima at 257 nm, using ultraviolet spectrophotometer.

4. Terbinafine

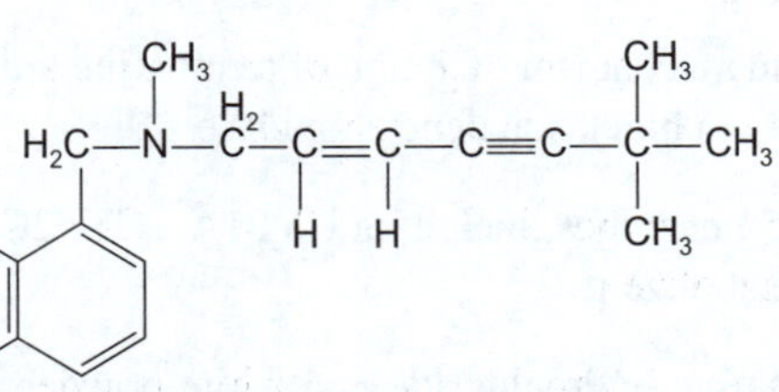

N,6,6-Trimethyl-N-(naphthalen-1-yl methyl)hept-2-en-4-yn-1-amine

Synthesis

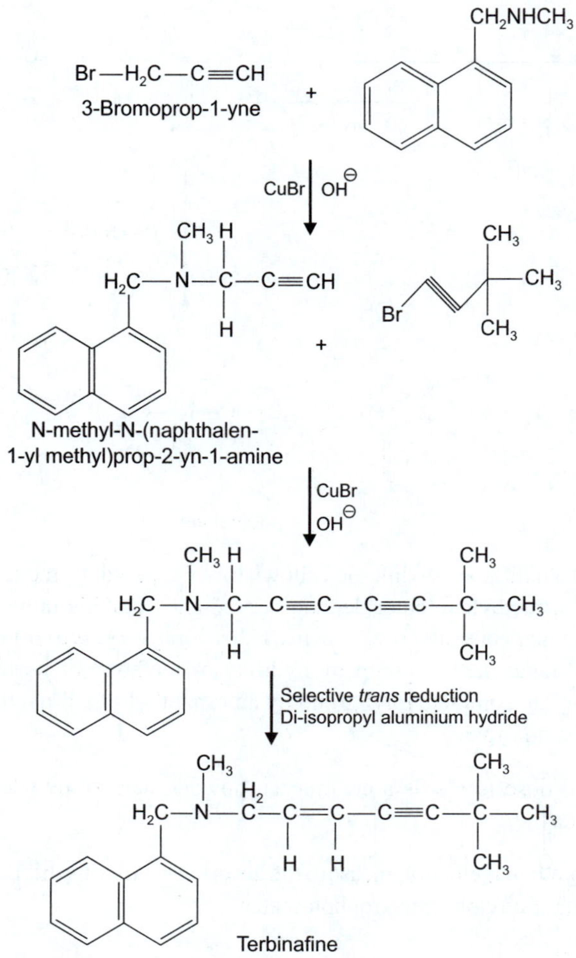

Mode of action: The uses and mechanism of action of terbinafine are the same as those of naftifine. It is active by virtue of its ability to block squalene epoxidase.

Metabolism: Several CYP450 enzymes, including $CYP1A_2$, $CYP2C1_9$, $CYP2C_9$, $CYP2C_8$, $CYP3A_4$, and $CYP2B_6$, extensively metabolize it.

Properties and uses: Terbinafine hydrochloride is a white powder, slightly soluble in water and in acetone, soluble in anhydrous ethanol and in methanol. It is used as an antifungal agent.

Assay: Dissolve the sample in ethanol, add 0.01 M hydrochloric acid, and titrate with 0.1 M sodium hydroxide. Determine the end point potentiometrically.

CLASSIFICATION BASED ON PCI SYLLABUS

Antifungal Antibiotics

Amphotericin-B

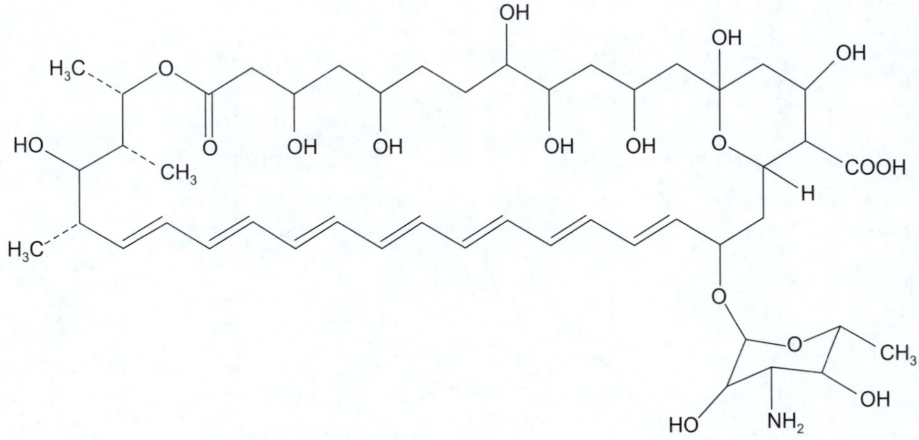

Nystatin

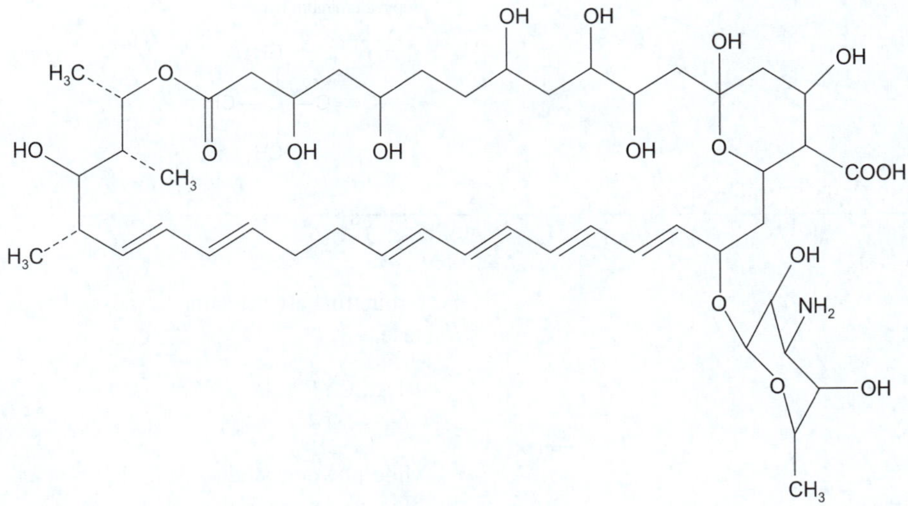

Natamycin

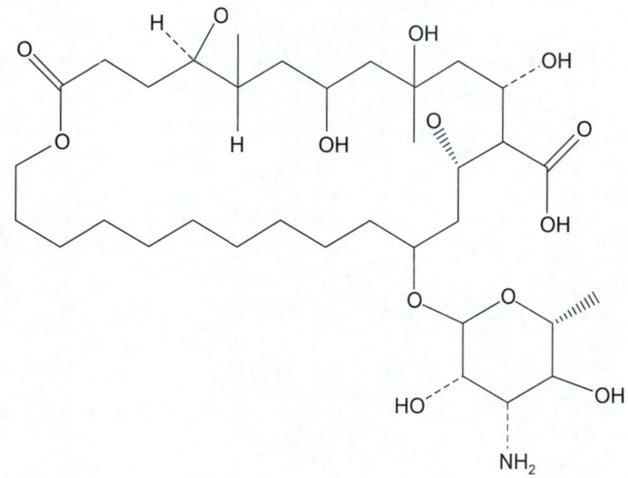

Griseofulvin

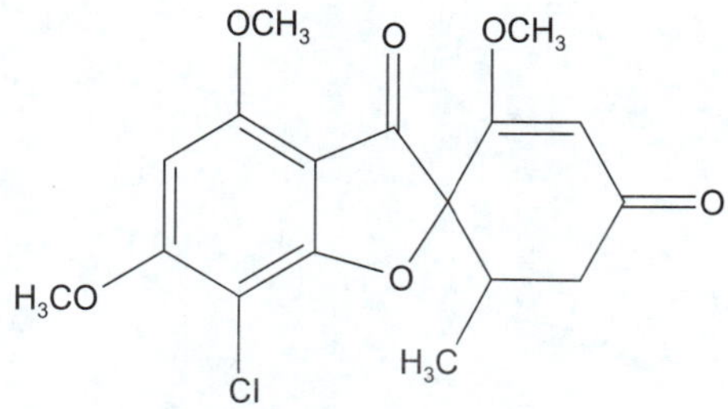

Synthetic Antifungal Agents

Clotrimazole

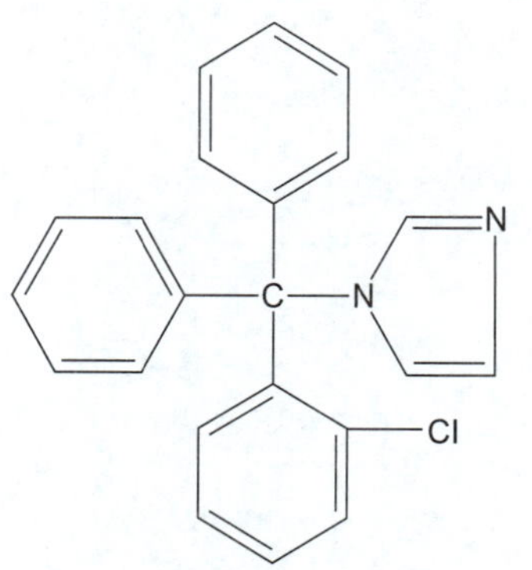

Econazole

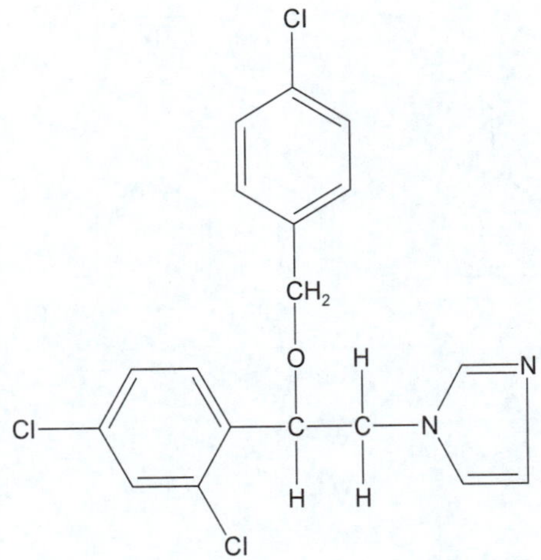

Butoconazole

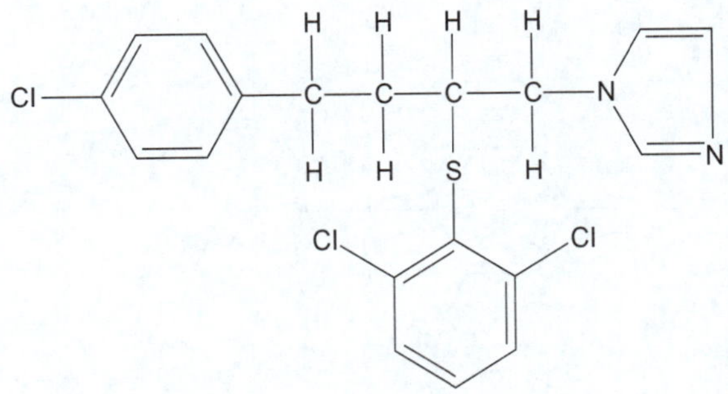

Oxiconazole

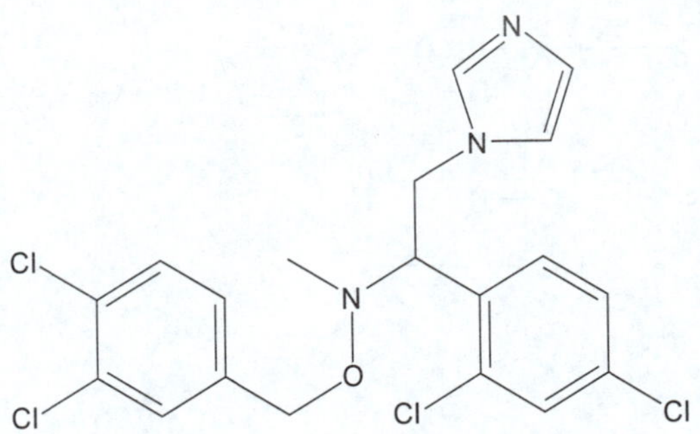

Ticonozole

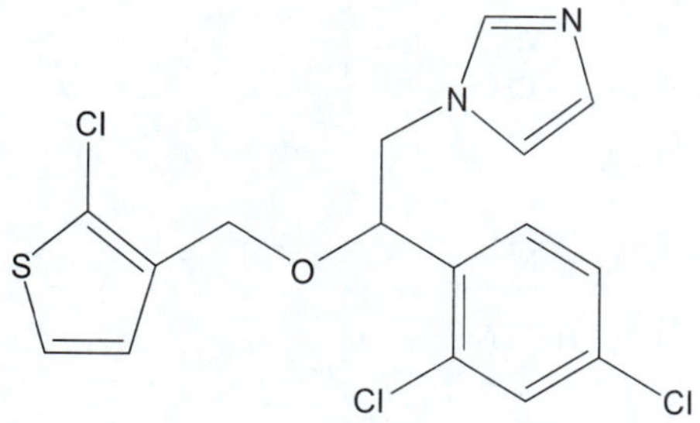

Miconazole

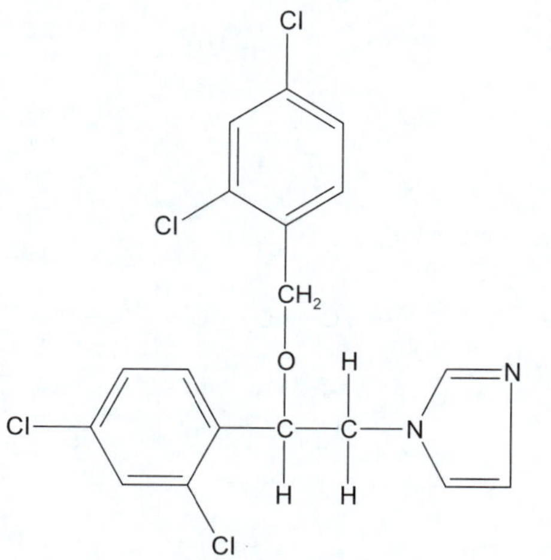

Ketoconazole

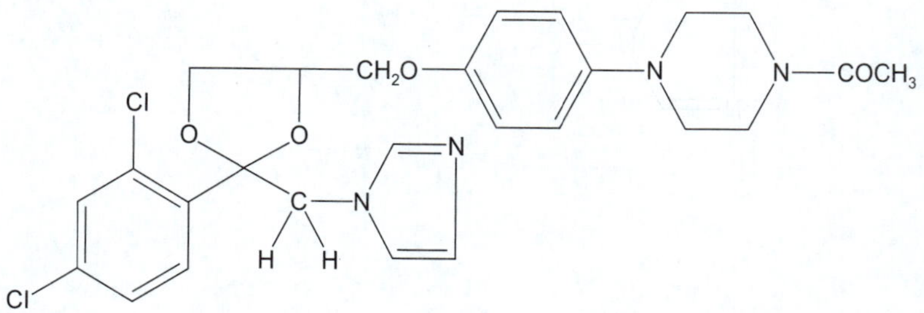

Terconazole

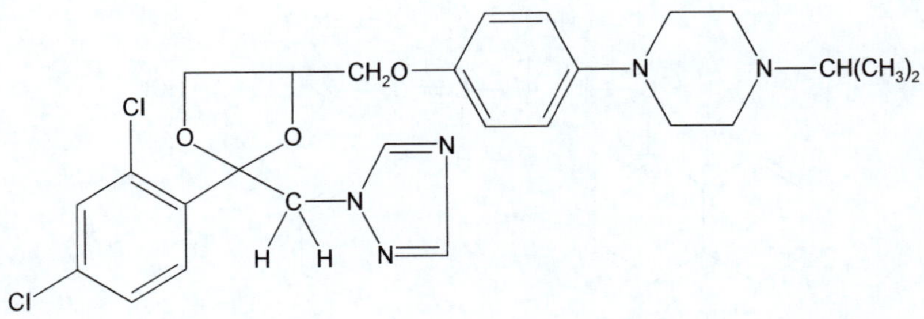

Itraconazole

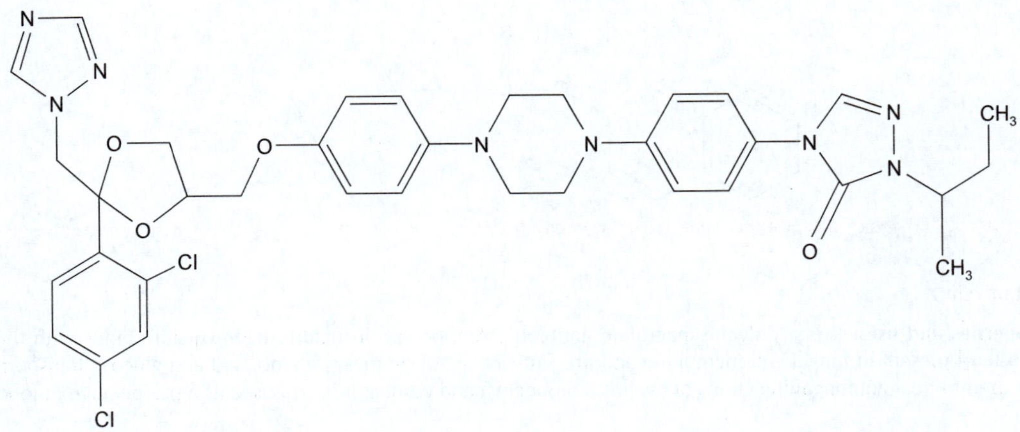

Fluconazole

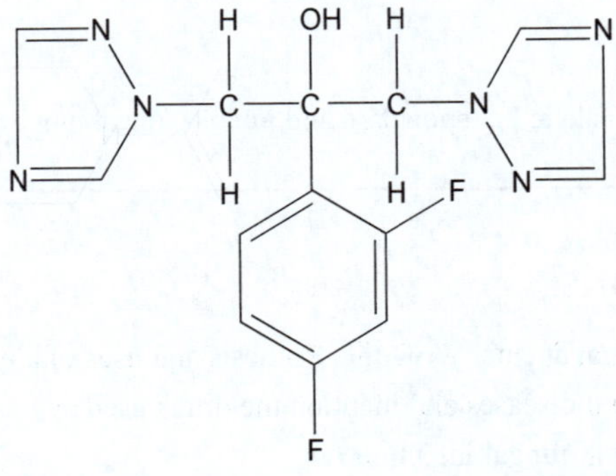

Naftifine hydrochloride

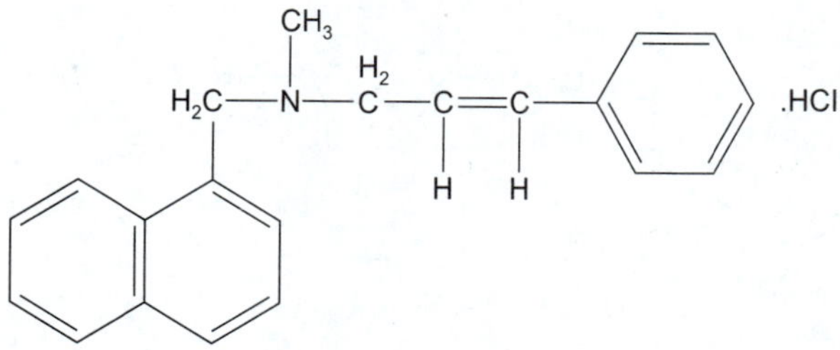

Tolnaftate

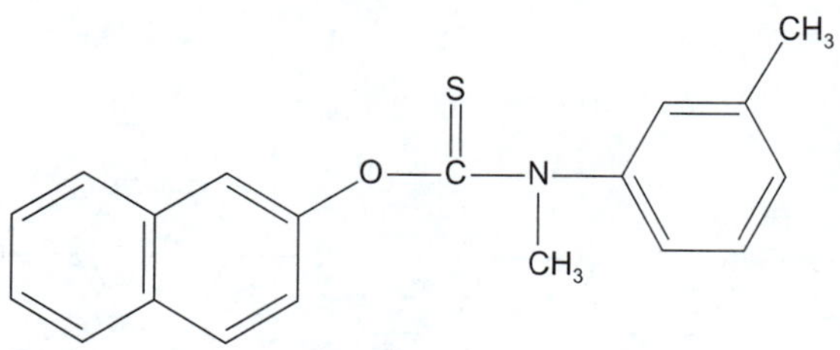

Natamycin

Properties and uses: It is a polyene macrolide antibiotic. Amphoteric in nature. It irreversibly binds with the ergosterol present in fungal cell membrane and prevents the sterol synthesis, amino acid and glucose transport. It is used to treat antifungal infections of eyelids, conjunctiva and cornea. It is also used as a preservative in food industry.

Oxiconazole

Properties and uses: It is used to treat athlete's foot, jock itch, ring worm and tinea versicolor and also used in the form of cream or lotion.

Naftifine

Properties and uses: It inhibits squalene 2,3-epoxidase and inhibits fungal biosynthesis of ergosterol. It is inferior to oxiconazole.

PROBABLE QUESTIONS

1. Define and classify antifungal agents. Write the synthesis and uses of any two of them.
2. Enumerate the various fungal diseases and mention the drugs used against those diseases.
3. Write a note on azoles used in fungal infection.
4. Write the synthesis and uses of tolnaftate, clotrimazole, and griseofulvin.

SUGGESTED READINGS

1. Abraham DJ (ed). *Burger's Medicinal Chemistry and Drug Discovery* (6th edn). New Jersey: John Wiley, 2007.
2. Barrett JF and Klaubert DH. 'Recent advances in antifungal agents'. *Ann Rept Med Chem* 27: 149–58, 1992.

3. *British Pharmacopoeia*. Medicines and Healthcare Products Regulatory Agency. London 2008.
4. Bruntan LL, Lazo JS, and Parker KL. *Goodman and Gilman's: The Pharmacological Basis of Therapeutics* (11th edn). New York: McGraw Hill, 2006.
5. Cohen J. 'Antifungal chemotherapy'. *Lancet* 2: 532, 1982.
6. Debono M and Goordee RS. 'Antibiotics that inhibit fungal cell wall development'. *Annu Rev Microbiol* 48: 471– 497, 1994.
7. Gennaro AR. Remington: *The Science and Practice of Pharmacy* (21st edn). New York: Lippincot Williams and Wilkins, 2006.
8. *Indian Pharmacopoeia*. Ministry of Health and Family Welfare. New Delhi, 1996.
9. Kobayashi GS and Medoff G. 'Antifungal agents—recent developments'. *Ann Rev Microbiol* 31: 291–308, 1977.
10. Lemke TL and William DA. *Foye's Principle of Medicinal Chemistry* (6th edn). New York: Lippincott Williams and Wilkins, 2008.
11. Lednicer D and Mitscher LA. *The Organic Chemistry of Drug Synthesis*. New York: John Wiley, 1995.
12. Lyman CA and Walgh TJ. '*Systemically administered antifungal agents*'. *Drugs* 44(1): 9–35, 1992.
13. McKinley DS and Rapp RP. '*Selecting the right antifungal agent*'. US Pharma 34–36, 1992.
14. Zervos M and Meunier F. 'Flucoazole—a review'. *Int J Antimicrob Agents* 3: 147–70, 1993.

CHAPTER 18

Antiviral Agents

INTRODUCTION

Antiviral agents are substances used in the treatment and prophylaxis of diseases caused by viruses. Viral diseases include influenza, rabies, yellow fever, poliomyelitis, ornithosis, mumps, measles, ebola, human immuno deficiency virus (HIV), herpes, warts, and smallpox. Viruses are not proper living things, but consists of a genome; they are smaller in size with simple chemical composition, sometimes a few enzymes stored in a capsule made up of protein and rarely covered with a lipid layer. The viruses only replicate within the host cell and the viral replication depends primarily on the metabolic processes of the invaded cell. Viruses does not possess cell wall, but they have RNA or DNA enclosed in a shell of protein known as capsid. The capsid is composed of several subunits known as capsomers. In certain cases, capsid may be surrounded by an outer protein or lipoprotein envelope. One group of RNA virus that deserves special mention are reteroviruses. They are responsible for acquired immuno deficiency syndrome (AIDS) and T-leukaemias. Reteroviruses contain reverse transcriptase (RT) enzyme activity that makes a DNA copy of the viral RNA template. Then, the DNA copy is integrated into the host genome, at which it is referred to as provirus and is transcribed into both the genomic RNA and mRNA for translocation into the viral proteins, giving generation to new virus particles. Viral life cycle varies according to the species, but they all share a general pattern that can be sequenced as follows (Figure 18.1):

- **Adsorption:** Attachment of the virus to the host cell.
- **Penetration:** Penetration of virus into the cell.
- **Uncoating:** The genetic material or viral genome (DNA or RNA) passes into the host cell leaving the capsid covering outside the host cell.
- **Transcription :** Production of the viral mRNA from the viral genome.

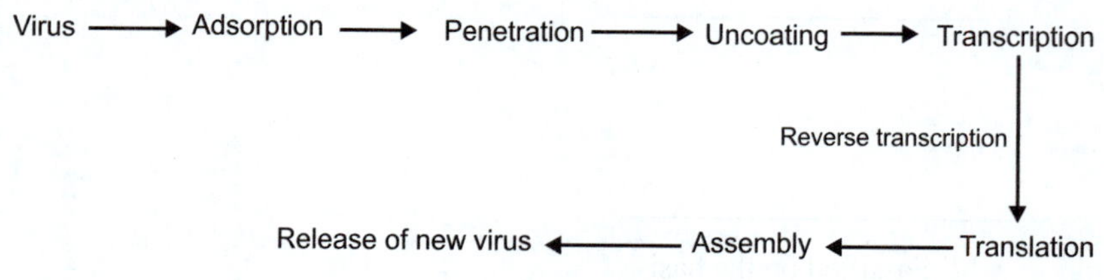

Figure 18.1: Life cycle of virus.

- **Translation:** The viral genome enters the cytoplasm or the nucleoplasma and directs or utilizes the host nucleic acid machinery for the synthesis of the new viral protein and for the production of more viral genome. The viral protein modifies the host cell and allows the viral genome to replicate by using host and viral enzyme. This is often the stage at which the cell is irreversibly modified and eventually killed.
- **Assembly of the viral particle:** New viral coat protein assembles into capsid and viral genomes.
- Release of the mature virus from the cell and the budding process or rupture of the cell and repeat of the process, in a fresh host cell.

Since the host cell machinery is totally utilized for the production of new virions, the normal cell function is affected. Antiviral agents have been developed to act at various stages in the viral replication cycle, such as attachments, replication, and release of the virus.

Some virus types together with diseases that they cause are listed in Table 18.1.

Table 18.1: Examples of viruses with diseases

Virus	*Diseases*
DNA virus	
Pox virus	Smallpox
Herpes virus	Chickenpox, shingles herpes, glandular fever
Adenovirus	Sore throat, conjunctivitis
Papilloma virus	Warts
Parvo virus	Canine distemper
RNA viruses	
Orthomyxovirus	Influenza
Paramn virus	Measles, mumps, rabies
Rhabdo virus	Colds, meningitis
Picor virus	Poliomyelitis
Retrovirus	AIDS, T-cell leukaemia
Arena virus	Meningitis, Lassa fever
Hepadna virus	Serum hepatitis
Reo virus	Diarrhoea
Filo virus	Ebola, Marburg
Bunya virus	Encephalitis, haemorrhagic fever

CLASSIFICATION

Classification According to Its Mechanism of Action

Antiviral drugs may be classified on the basis of its mechanism of action as follows:

I. Nucleoside and nucleotide RT inhibitors

a. Purine nucleosides and nucleotides

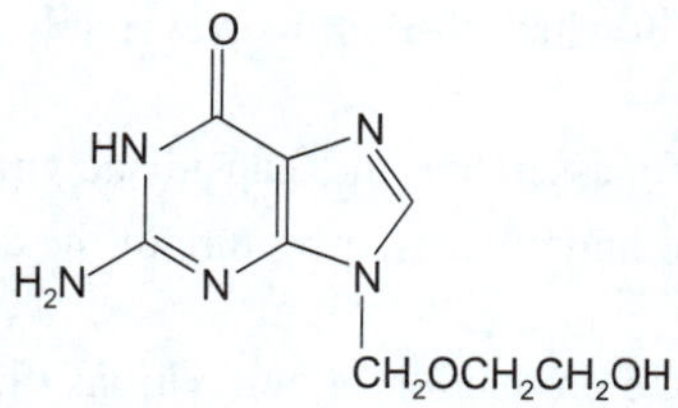

Aciclovir

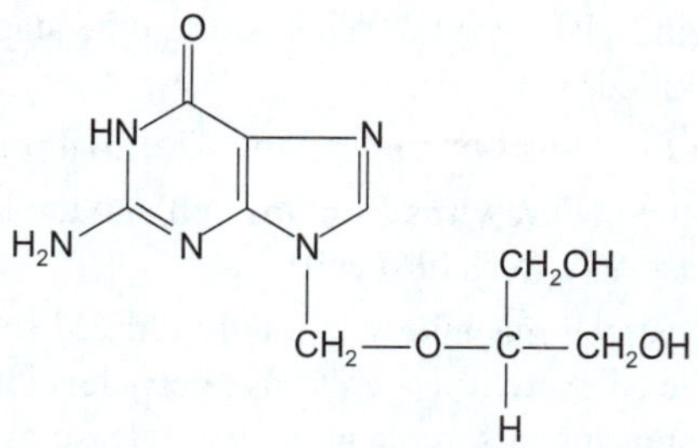

Ganciclovir

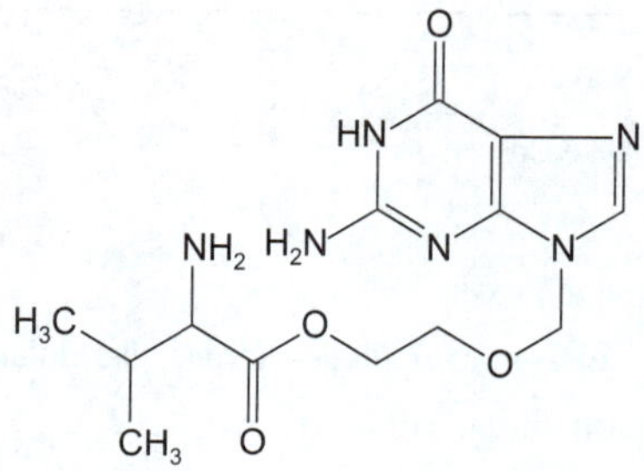

Valaciclovir

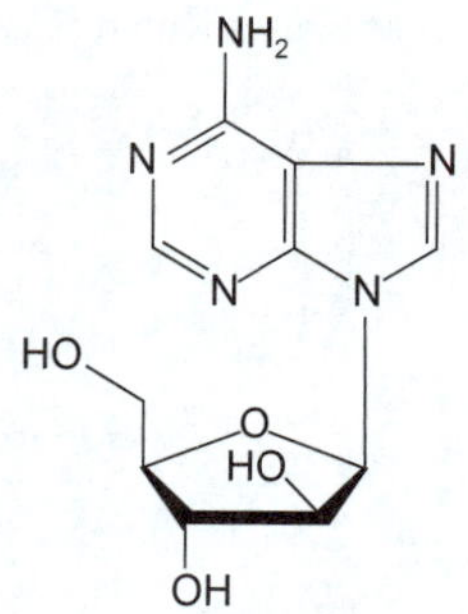

Vidarabine

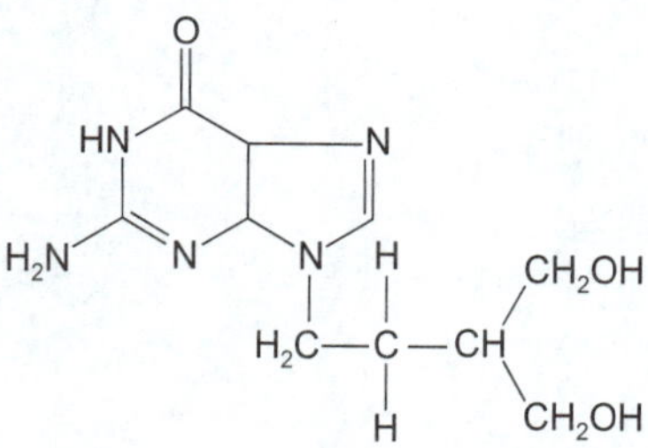

Penciclovir

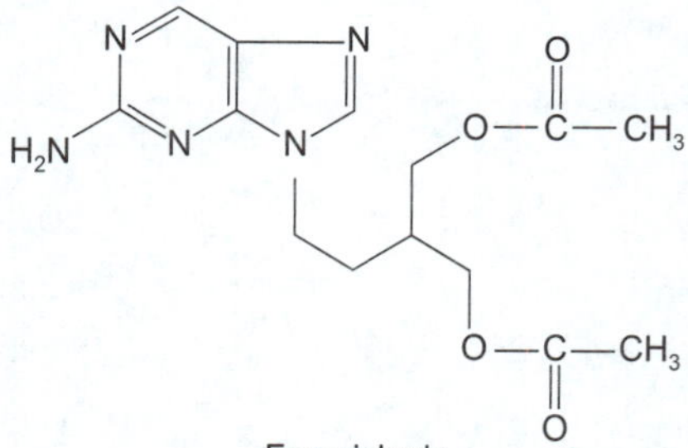

Famciclovir

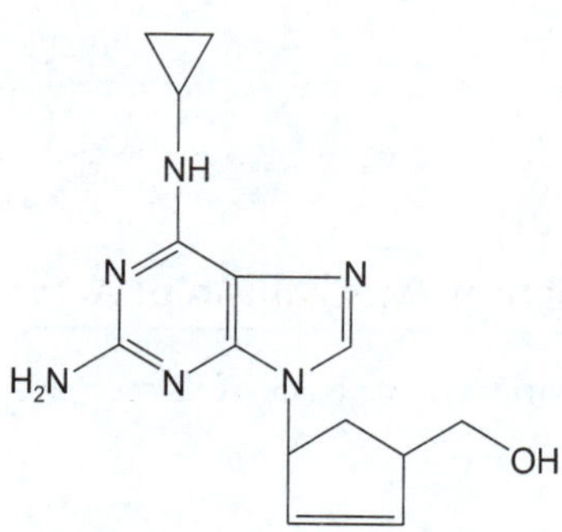

Abacavir

b. Pyrimidine nucleosides and nucleotides

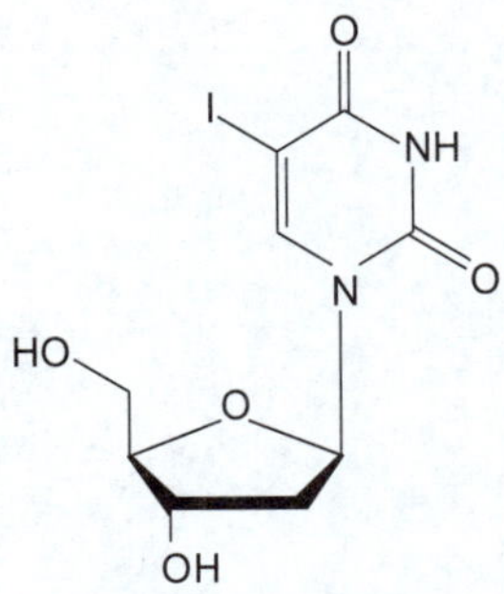

Iodoxuridine

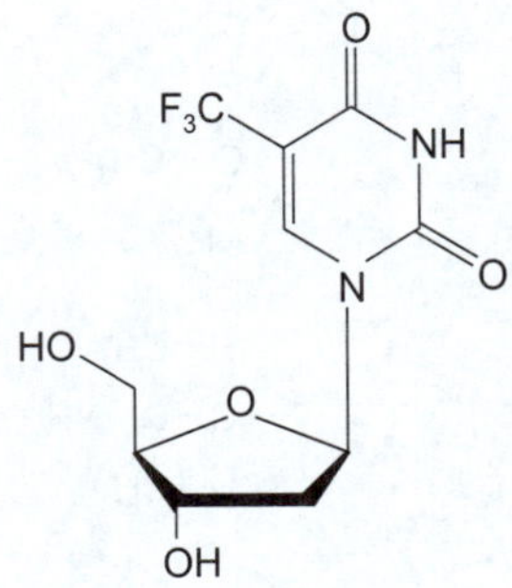

Trifluridine

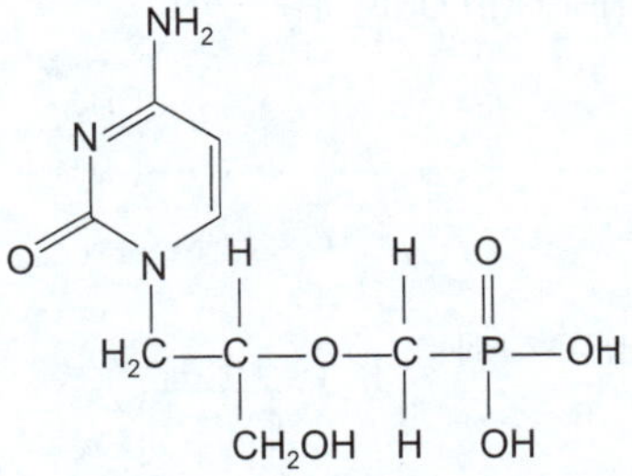

Cidofovir

c. Thiosemicarbazones

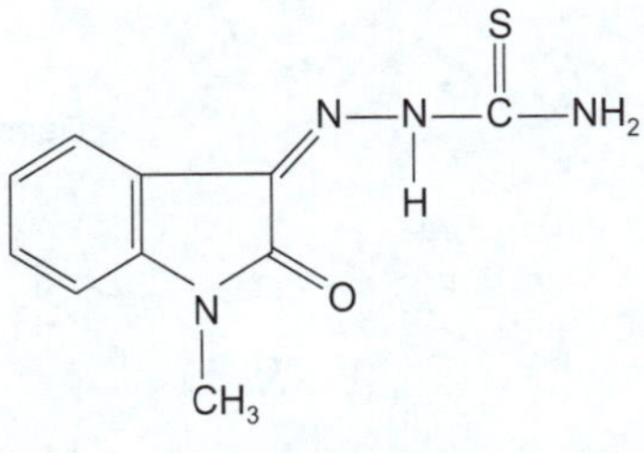

Methisazone

d. Adamantane amines

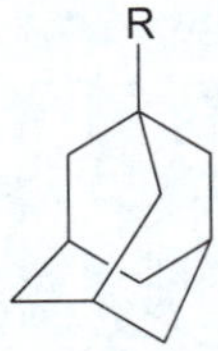

Name	*R*
Amantadine	$-NH_2$
Rimantadine	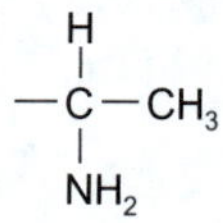
Somantadine	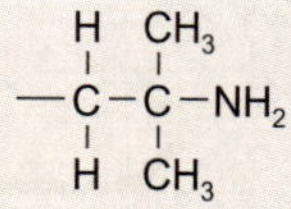
Tromantadine	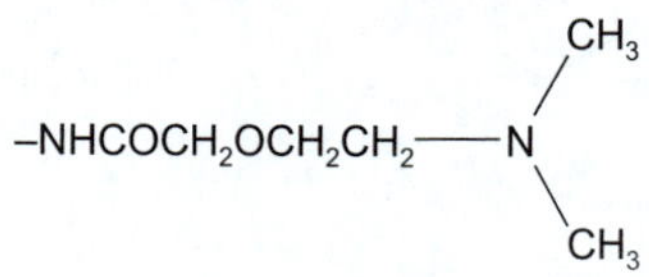

II. Non-nucleoside RT inhibitors

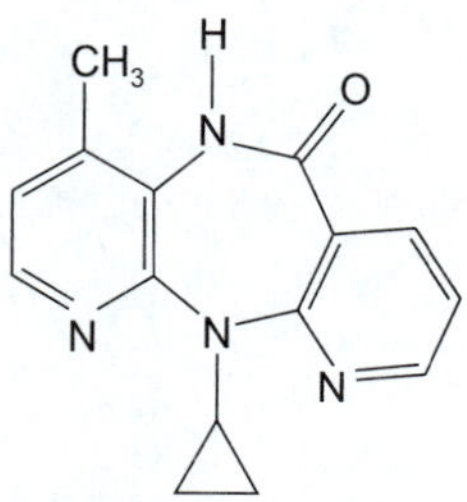

Nevirapine

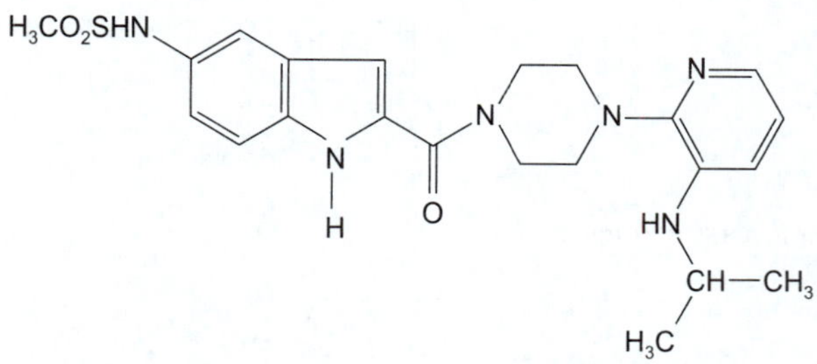

Delavirdine

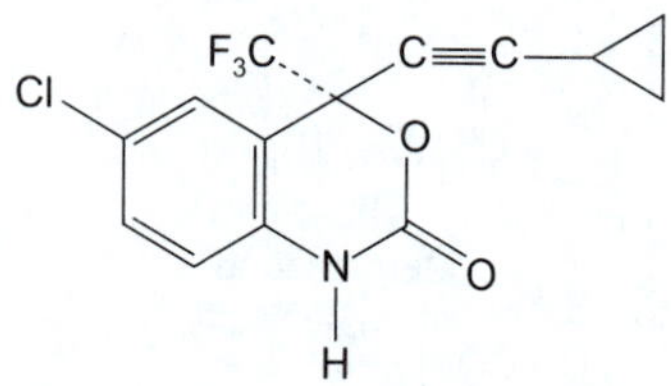

Efavirenz

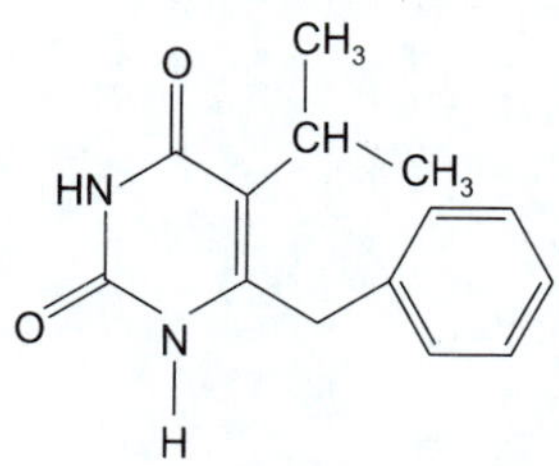

Emivirine

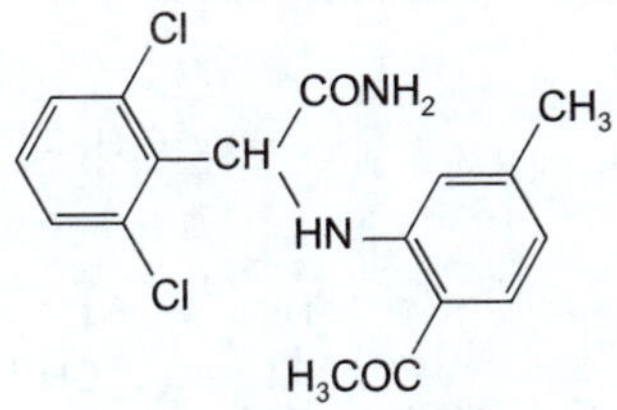

Loviride

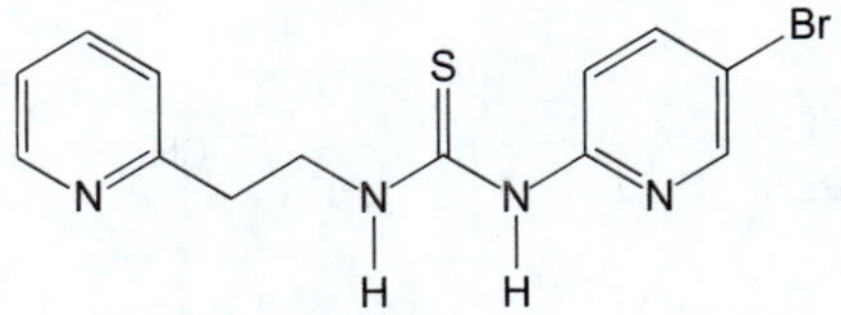

Trovirdine

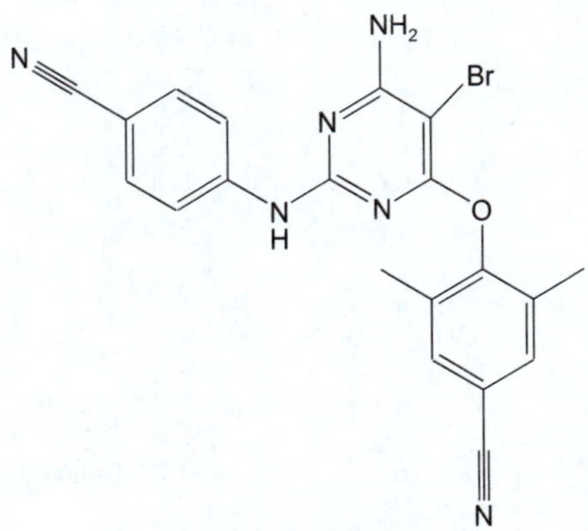

Etravirine

III. Anti-HIV agents—HIV protease inhibitors

Saquinavir

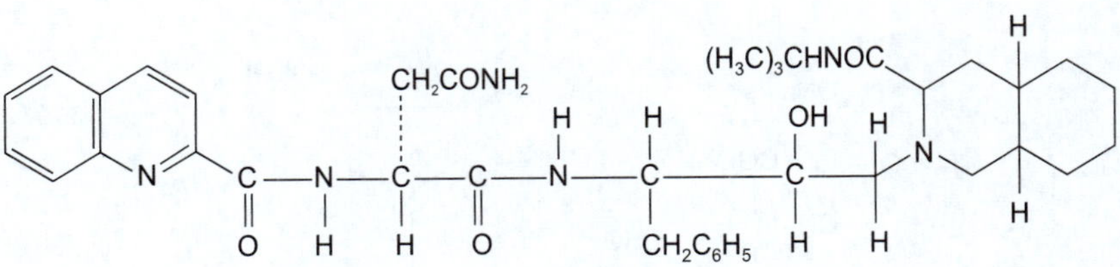

Indinavir

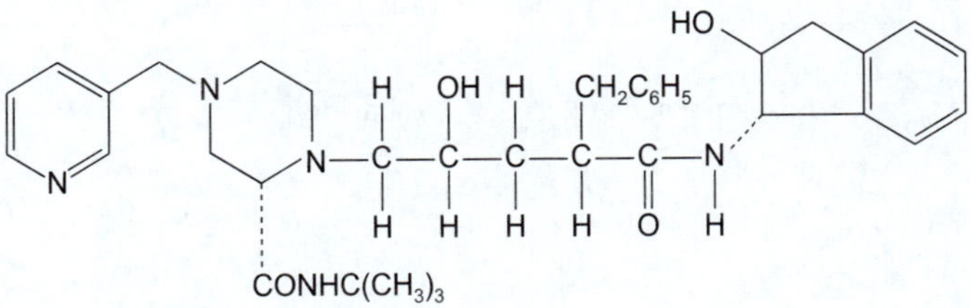

Ritonavir

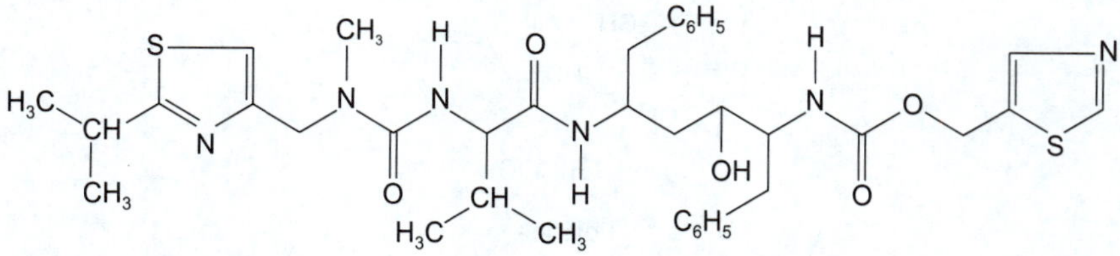

Nelfinavir

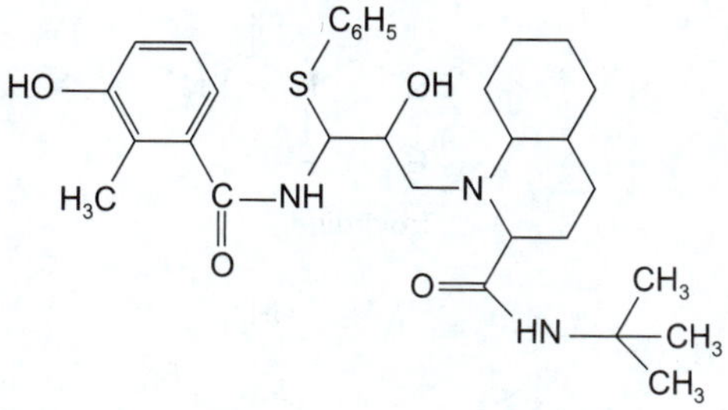

Tipranavir

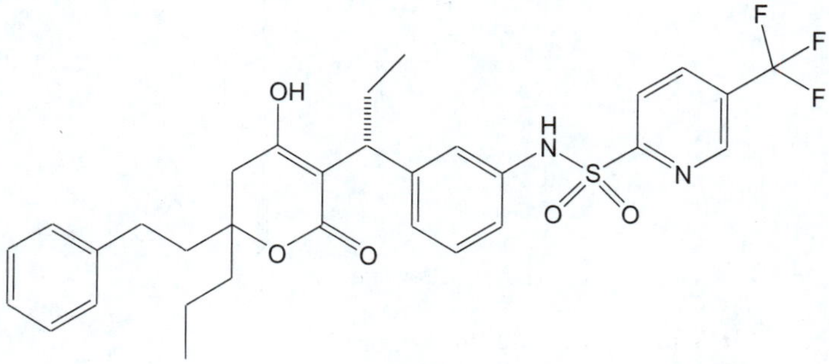

IV. Miscellaneous

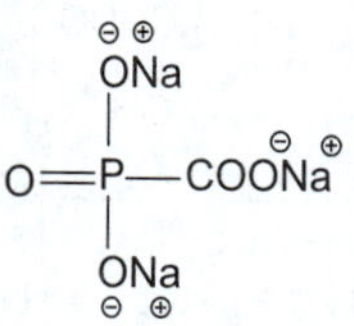

Foscarnet sodium

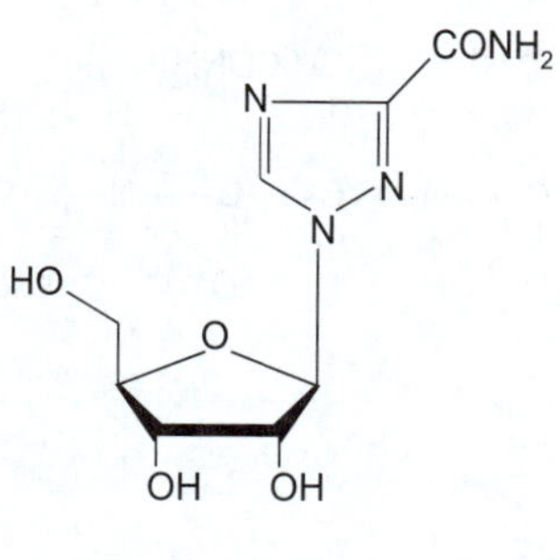

Ribavirin

Classification According to the Enzyme Inhibiton

According to the enzyme inhibition, antiviral agents are classified as follows.

i. DNA polymerase inhibitors: Idoxuridine, trifluridine, vidarabine
ii. RT inhibitors:

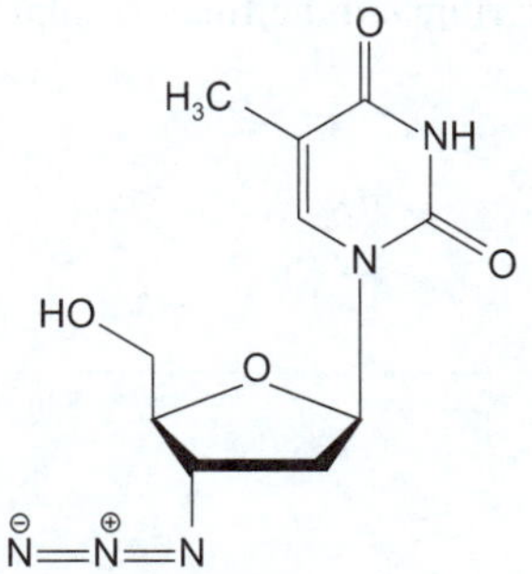

Zidovudine

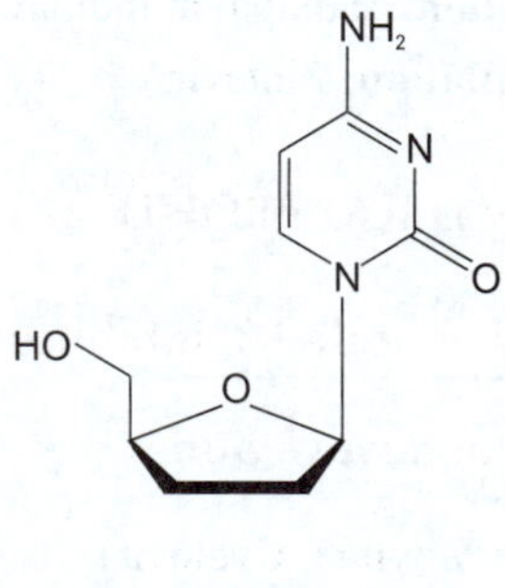

Zalcitabine

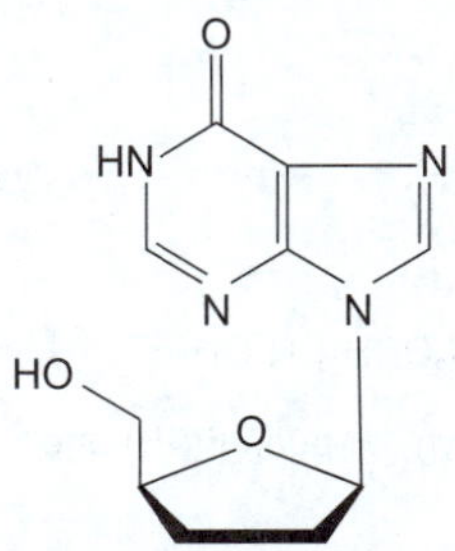

Didanosine

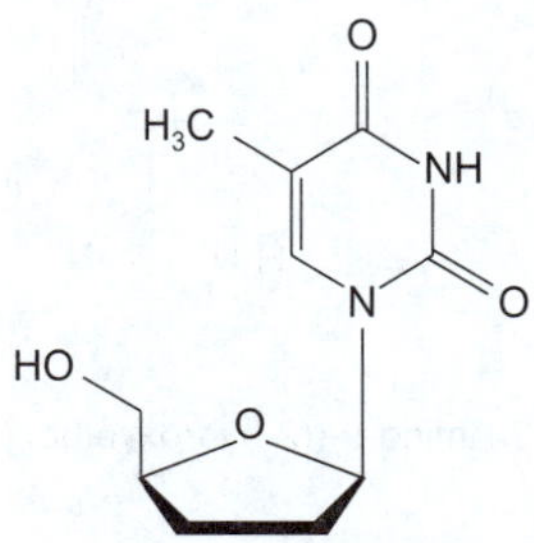

Stavudine

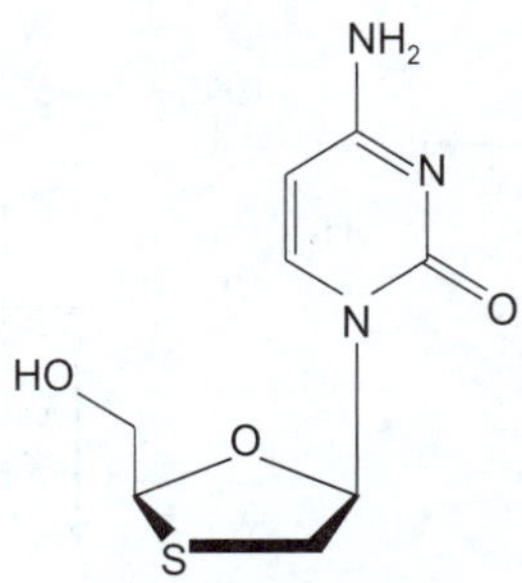

Lamivudine

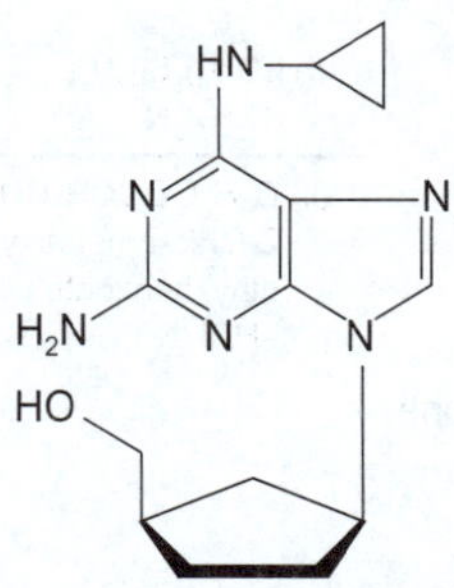

Abacavir

Classification According to the Treatment Protocol

According to the treatment protocol, antiviral agents are classified as follows:

I. Treatment of respiratory virus infection

Adamantane derivatives: Amantadine, rimantadine

II. Treatment of herpes and cytomegalo viruses infection.

a. **Purine nucleotides:** Acyclovir, ganciclovir, vidarabine.
b. **Pyrimidine nucleosides:** Trifluouridine, idoxuridine.
c. **Phosphorus derivatives:** Foscarnet sodium.

III. Treatment of HIV infections

a. **RT inhibition:**
   1. *Purine derivatives:* Didanosine.
   2. *Pyrimidine derivatives:* Zidovudine, stavudine.
   3. *Non-nucleosides:* Nevirapine, delaviridine, efavirenz.

b. **Protease inhibition:** Saquinavir, indinavir, ritonavir, nelfinavir, amprenavir, lopinavir.

c. **Integration inhibition:** Zintevir.

SYNTHESIS AND DRUG PROFILE

I. Nucleoside and Nucleotide RT Inhibitors

a. Purine Nucleosides and Nucleotides

i. Acyclovir (Ocuvir, Zovirax, Cyclovir)

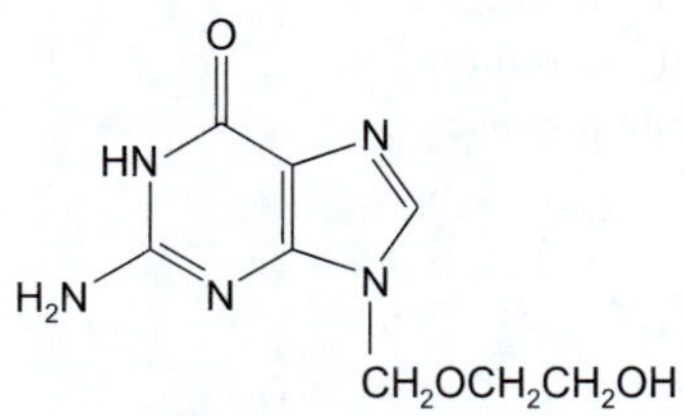

2-Amino-9-((2-hydroxyethoxy)methyl)-1*H*-purin-6(9*H*)-one

Synthesis

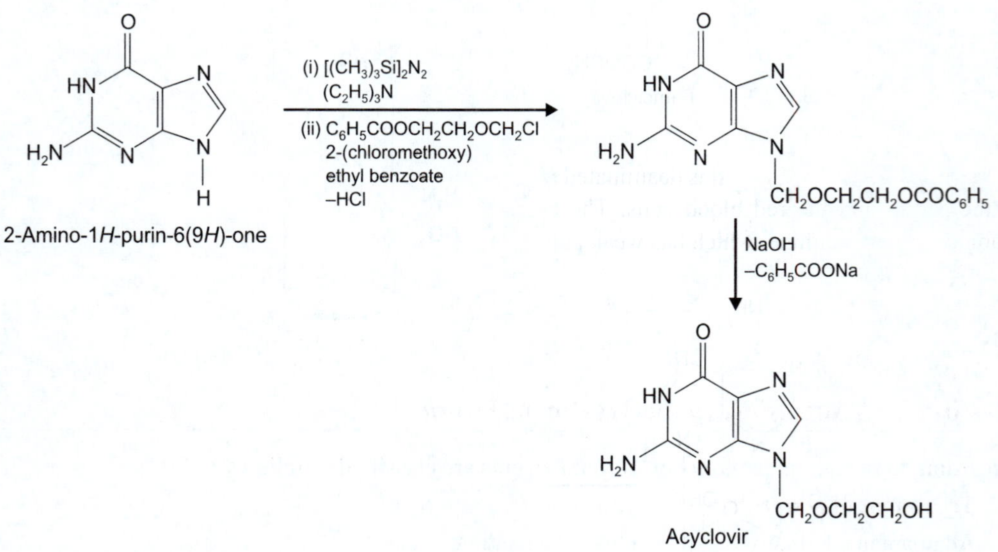

Metabolism: The bioavailability of acyclovir is 15–30% and it is metabolized to 9-carboxymethoxymethyl guanine, which is inactive.

Properties and uses: Acyclovir is a white crystalline powder, slightly soluble in water, soluble in dimethyl sulphoxide and in dilute mineral acids and alkali hydroxides, and very slightly soluble in ethanol. It is a purine nucleoside analogue, used as antiviral agent against herpes viruses.

Assay: Dissolve the sample in anhydrous acetic acid and titrate with 0.1 M perchloric acid. Determine the end point potentiometrically. Perform a blank titration.

Dose: For herpes virus infections the administered dose for immuno-suppressed patients is up to 10 mg/kg body weight every 8 hrs.

Dosage forms: Acyclovir cream BP, acyclovir eye ointment BP, acyclovir intravenous infusion BP, acyclovir oral suspension BP, acyclovir tablets BP, dispersible acyclovir tablets BP.

Metabolism of valacyclovir: The related analogue 6-deoxy acyclovir is a prodrug form of acyclovir that is activated through metabolism by xanthine oxidase.

Metabolism of cidofovir: It is metabolized by phosphorylation and it gives cidofovir diphosphate.

Metabolism of famciclovir: It is a prodrug of penciclovir, which is formed *in vivo* by hydrolysis of acetyl groups and oxidation at the 6th position by the mixed function oxidase. Penciclovir and its metabolite penciclovir triphosphate posseses antiviral activity.

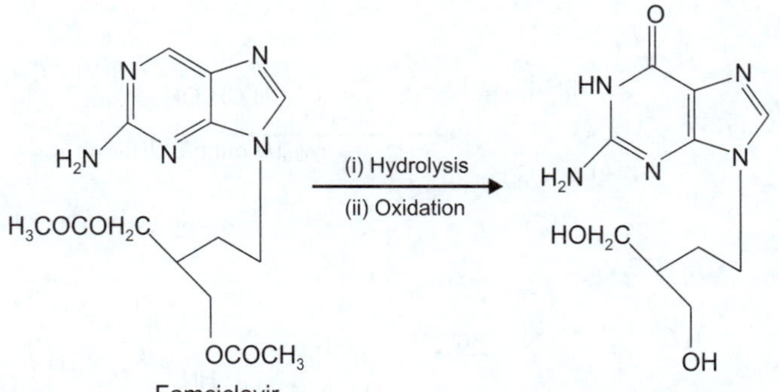

Famciclovir Penciclovir

Metabolism of vidarabine: It is deaminated rapidly by adenosine deaminase enzyme, which is present in the serum and the red blood cells. The enzyme converts vidarabine to its principal metabolite, arabinosyl hypoxanthine, which has weak antiviral activity.

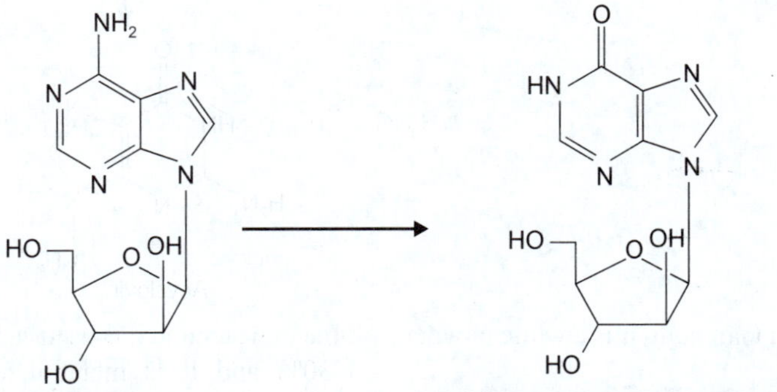

Vidarabine Arabinofuranosyl hypoxanthine

Uses: It is used for the short-term treatment of herpes simplex and chickenpox caused by varicella-zoster virus (VZV).

ii. Ganciclovir (Ganguard)

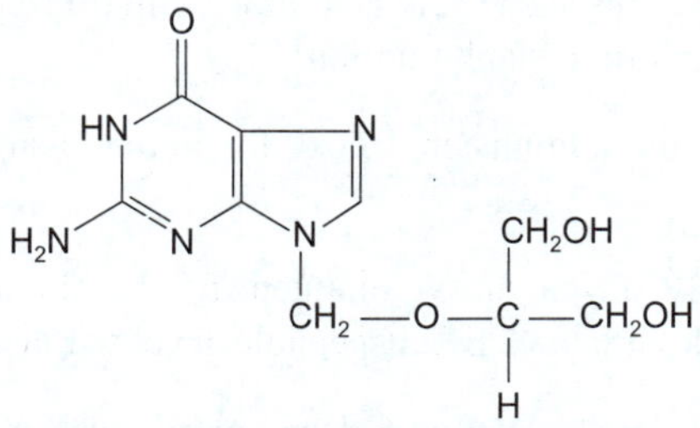

2-Amino-9-((1,3-dihydroxypropan-2-yloxy)methyl)-1*H*-purin-6-one

Synthesis

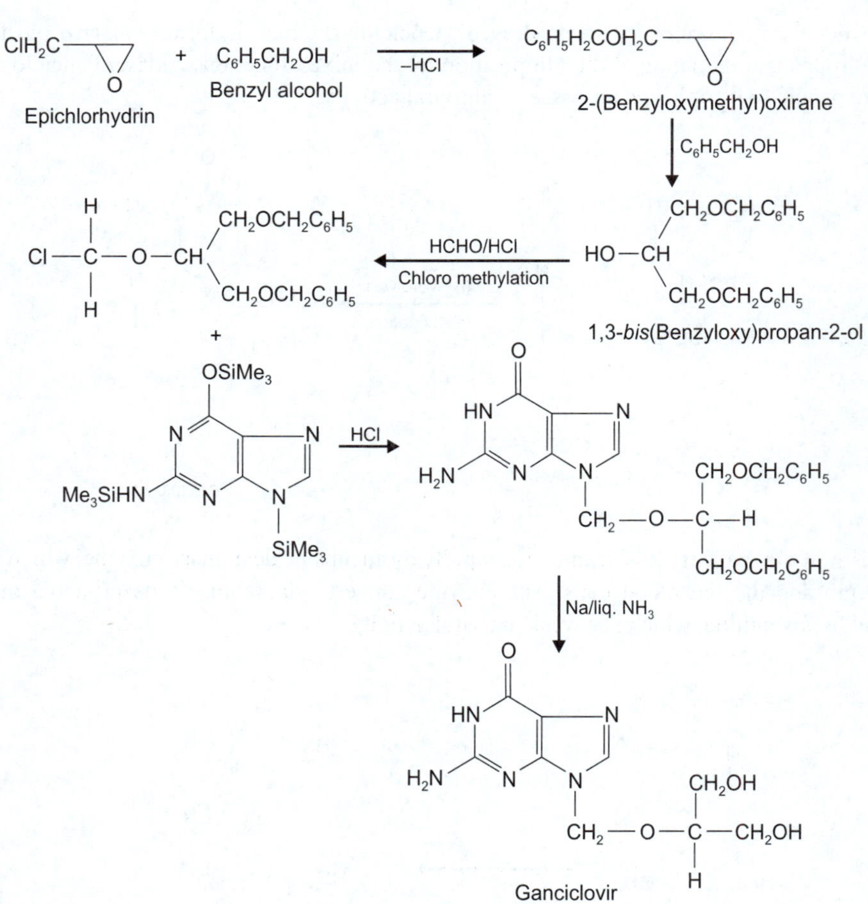

Ganciclovir

Properties and uses: Ganciclovir is a white powder, soluble in water and it is used as an antiviral agent.

Dose: The recommended dose is 5 mg/kg 1 hrs for infusion every 12 hrs for 14 days.

b. Pyrimidine Nucleoside and Nucleotide Inhibitors

i. **Idoxuridine** (Antizona, Dendrid)

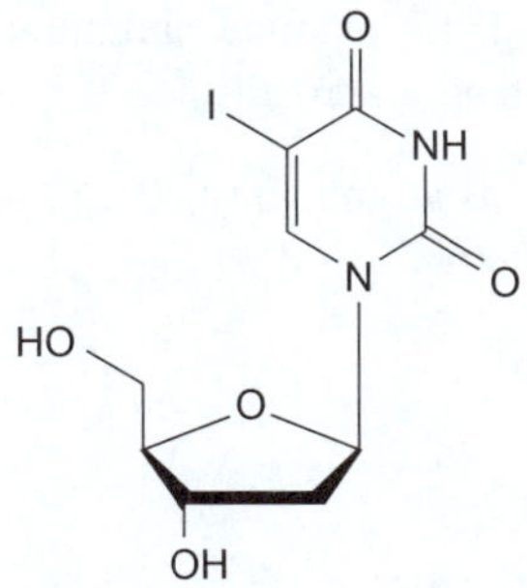

5-Iodo-2-deoxyuridine

Synthesis

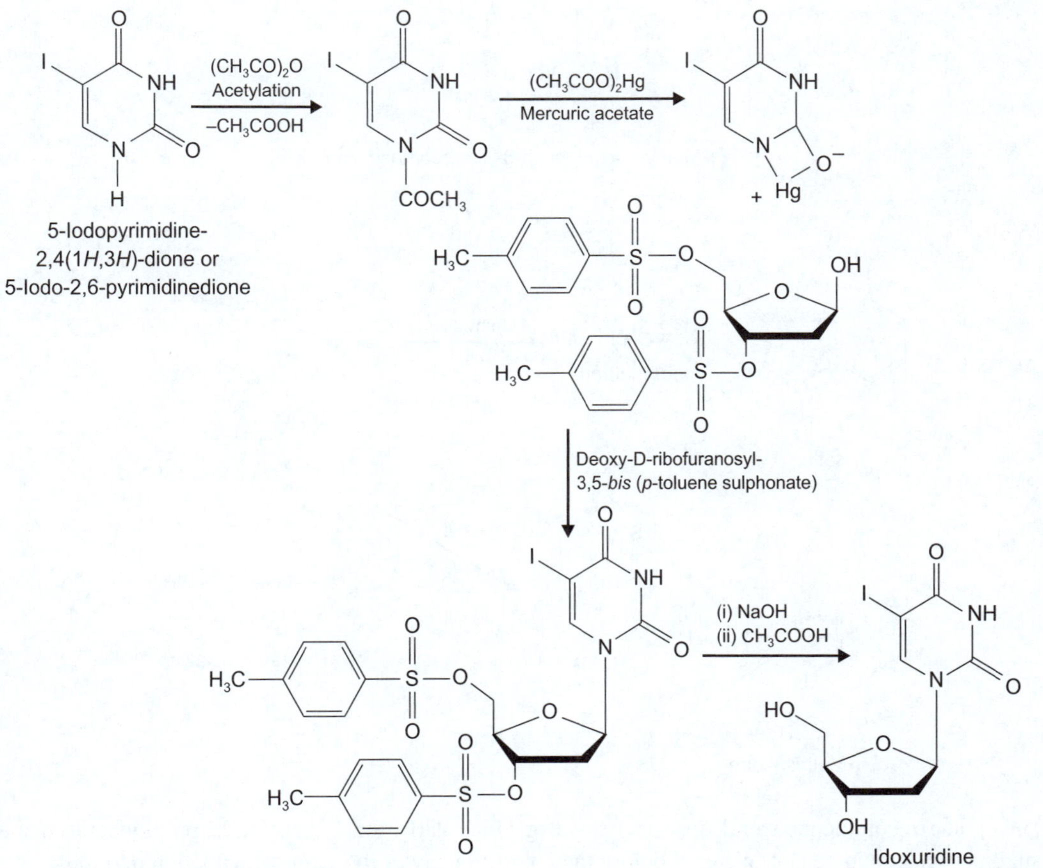

Metabolism: It has a plasma half-life of 30 min and it is rapidly metabolized in the blood to idoxuracil and uracil.

Properties and uses: Idoxuridine is a white crystalline powder, slightly soluble in water and in alcohol. It dissolves in dilute solutions of alkali hydroxides. It is a pyrimidine nucleoside analogue and used as an antiviral agent against herpes virus.

Assay: Dissolve the sample in dimethylformamide and titrate with 0.1 M tetrabutyl ammonium hydroxide. Determine the end point potentiometrically.

Dose: The administered dose topically as a ointment is 0.5%, 4–16 times a day or 0.1 ml of a 0.1% solution every 1 to 2 hrs into the conjunctiva.

Dosage forms: Idoxuridine eyedrops BP.

c. *Thiosemicarbazones*

iv. Methisazone (Marboran)

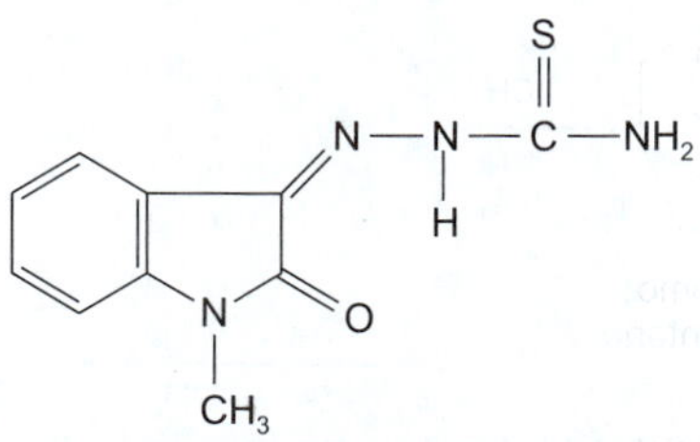

(*Z*)-1-(1-Methyl-2-oxoindolin-3-ylidene)thiosemicarbazide

Synthesis

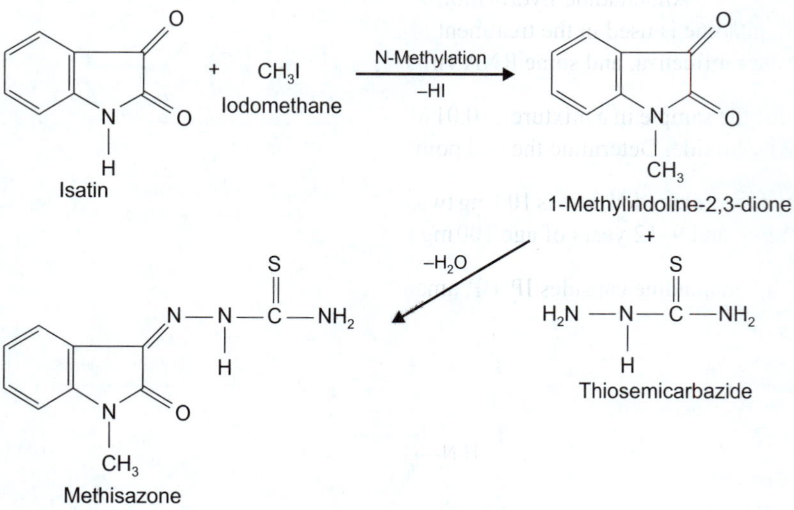

Dose: The recommended oral dose is 1.5–3.0 g twice daily for 4 days. As a prophylactic against smallpox, it should be administered before the 8th or 9th day of the 12-day incubation period.

Uses: Used in the treatment of viral infection.

d. Adamantane Amines

v. **Amantadine** (Symmetrel)

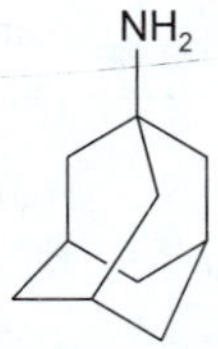

1-Amino adamantane

Synthesis

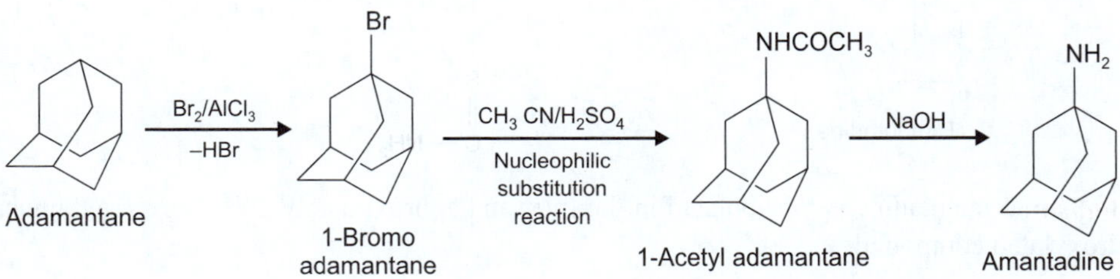

Metabolism: Approximately, 90% of the drug is excreted unchanged by the kidney, primarily through glomerular filtration and tubular secretion, and there are no reports of metabolic products. Acidification of urine increases the rate of amantadine excretion.

Properties and uses: Amantadine hydrochloride is a white crystalline powder, soluble in water and in alcohol. Amantadine is used in the treatment of Parkinson's disease. It is effective against influenza type-A virus, para influenza, and some RNA virus. It is also used as a dopamine receptor agonist.

Assay: Dissolve the sample in a mixture of 0.01 M hydrochloric acid and alcohol (1:10) and titrate with 0.1 M sodium hydroxide. Determine the end point potentiometrically.

Dose: The usual recommended dose is 100 mg twice daily. For children 1–9 years of age the administered dose is 4–9 mg/kg and 9–12 years of age 100 mg twice daily.

Dosage forms: Amantadine capsules IP, BP, amantadine oral solution BP.

vi. **Rimantadine**

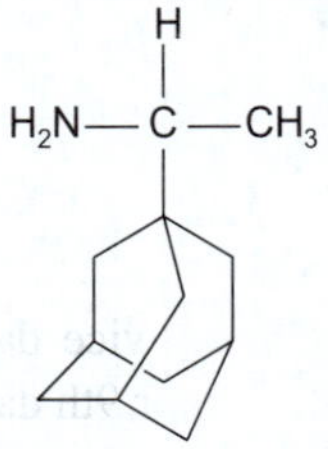

α-Methyl-1-adamatane methylamine

Synthesis

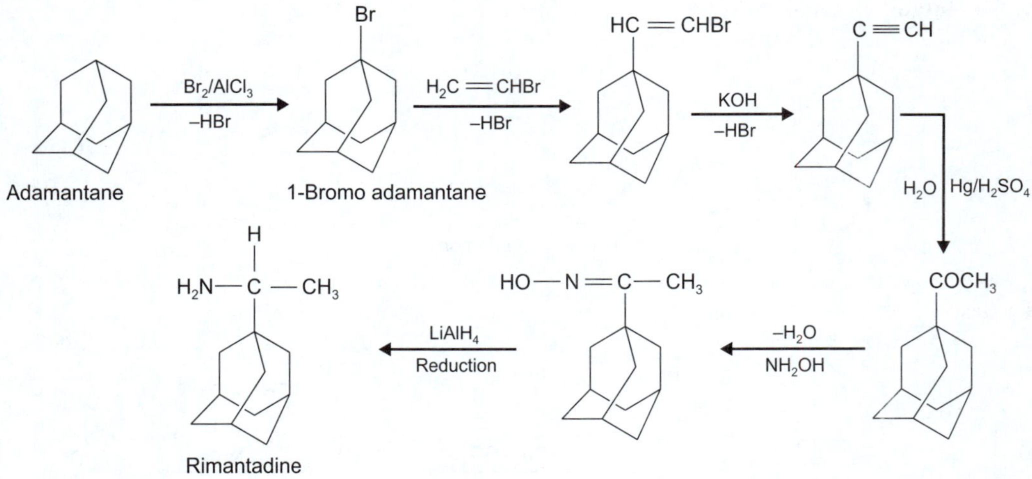

Metabolism: Rimantadine is metabolized in the liver and approximately 20% is excreted unchanged as hydroxylated compound.

Properties and uses: Rimantadine is a white to off-white crystals, soluble in water. It is used for the prevention of infection caused by various strains of influenza virus-A.

Dose: The recommended dose usually is 300 mg.

Miscellaneous

i. **Ribavirin** (Virazole)

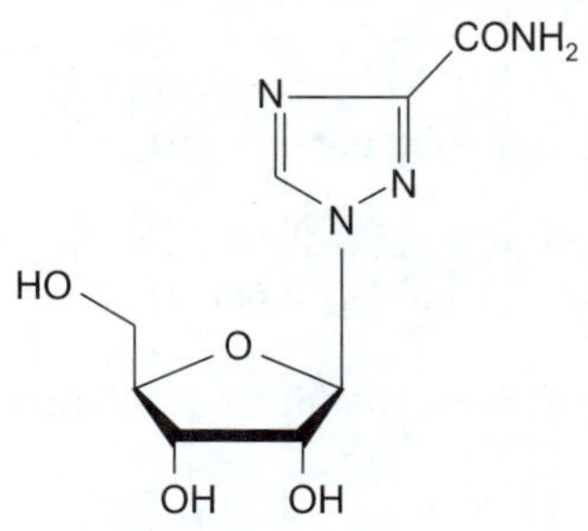

1-(3,4-Dihydroxy-5-(hydroxymethyl)-tetrahydrofuran-2-yl)-1H-1,2,4-triazole-3-carboxamide

Synthesis

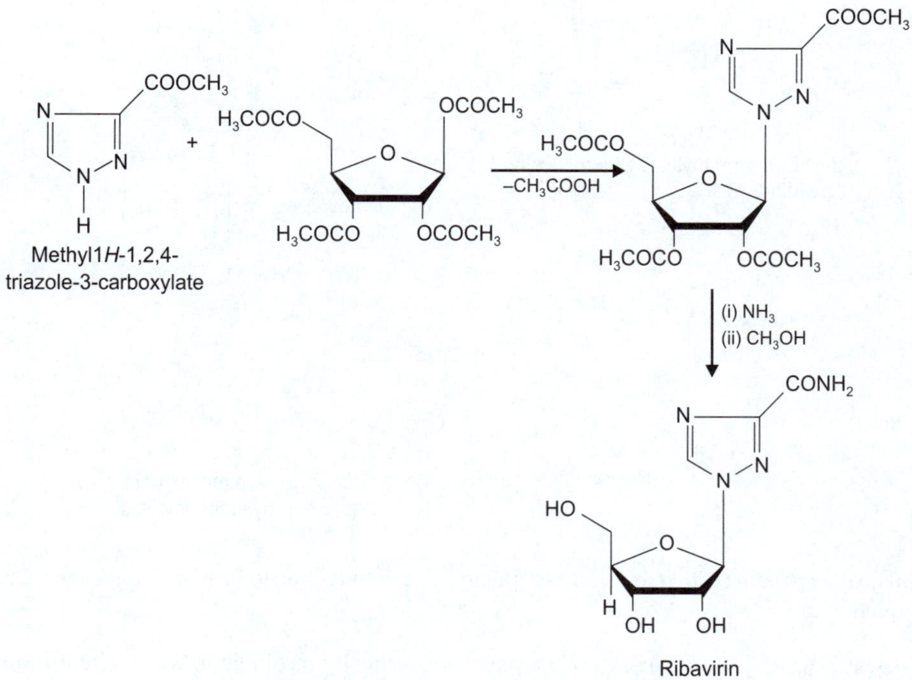

Properties and uses: Ribavirin is a white crystalline powder, soluble in water, slightly soluble in ethanol and in methylene chloride. It is used in the treatment of influenza type-A and -B, hepatitis, genital herpes, and Lassa fever.

Assay: It is assayed by adopting liquid chromatography technique.

Dose: For viral hepatitis, influenza, and herpes virus infections, the recommended dose is up to 1g per day in divided doses.

Dosage forms: Ribavirin nebulizer solution BP.

II. Non-nucleoside RT Inhibitors

i. **Nevirapine** (Neve, Nevipan, Nevimune)

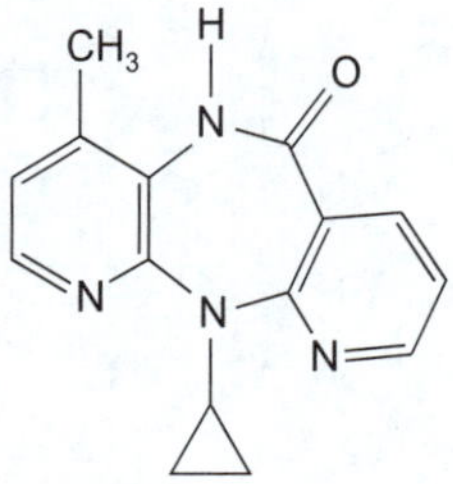

Synthesis

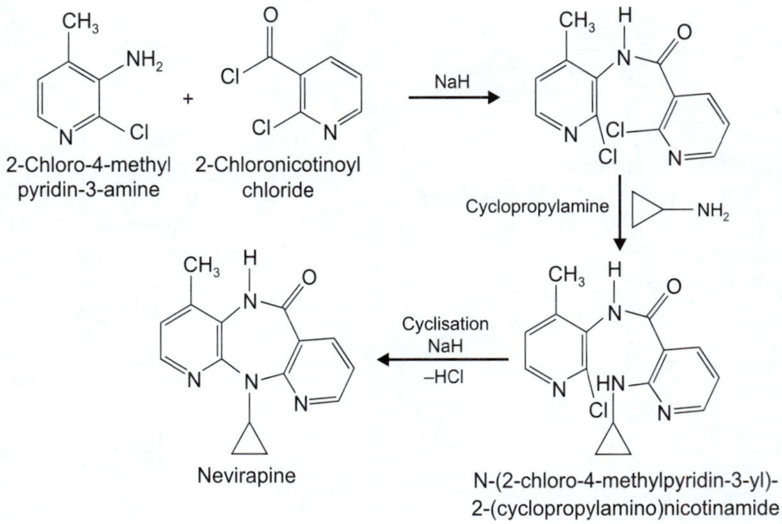

Metabolism: Nevirapine is metabolized as a glucuronide conjugation to form hydroxylated metabolites and excreted in urine.

Properties and uses: Nevirapine is a white powder, practically insoluble in water, slightly soluble in methylene chloride and in methanol. It is a HIV non-nucleoside RT inhibitor, used as an anti-HIV agent. It causes rash fever, nausea, and headache.

Assay: It is assayed by adopting liquid chromatography technique.

Dose: The recommended dose for HIV infection combined with other antiretrovirals in the case of adults is 200 mg once daily for the first 14 days; then, to increase to 200 mg two times/day if rash does not develop. Interrupting the treatment for more than 7 days necessitates reintroduction of the medicine at a lower dose for the first 14 days. For children, 2 months to 8 years the dose is 4 mg/kg once daily for the first 14 days, and increase to 7 mg/kg twice a day, if no rash is present. In the case of patients 8–16 years, the dose is 4 mg/kg once daily for 14 days followed by 4 mg/kg twice/day. Maximum dose that can be administered is 400 mg daily. Interrupting the treatment for more than 7 days necessitates reintroduction at a lower dose for the first 14 days.

ii. Delavirdine

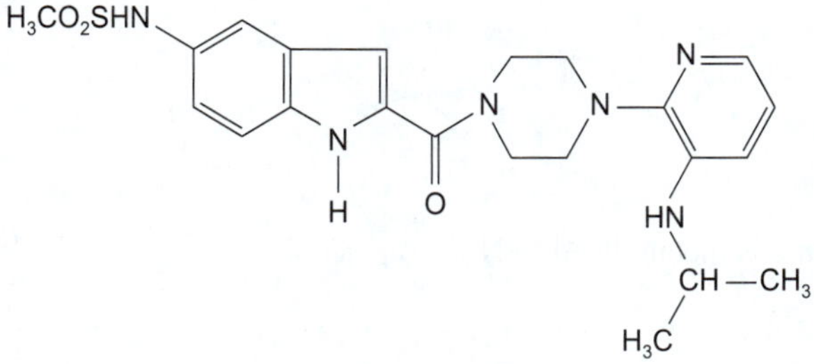

N-(2-(1-(3-(isopropylamino)pyridin-2-yl)piperazine-4-carbonyl)-1*H*-indol-5-ylmethanesulfonamide

Synthesis

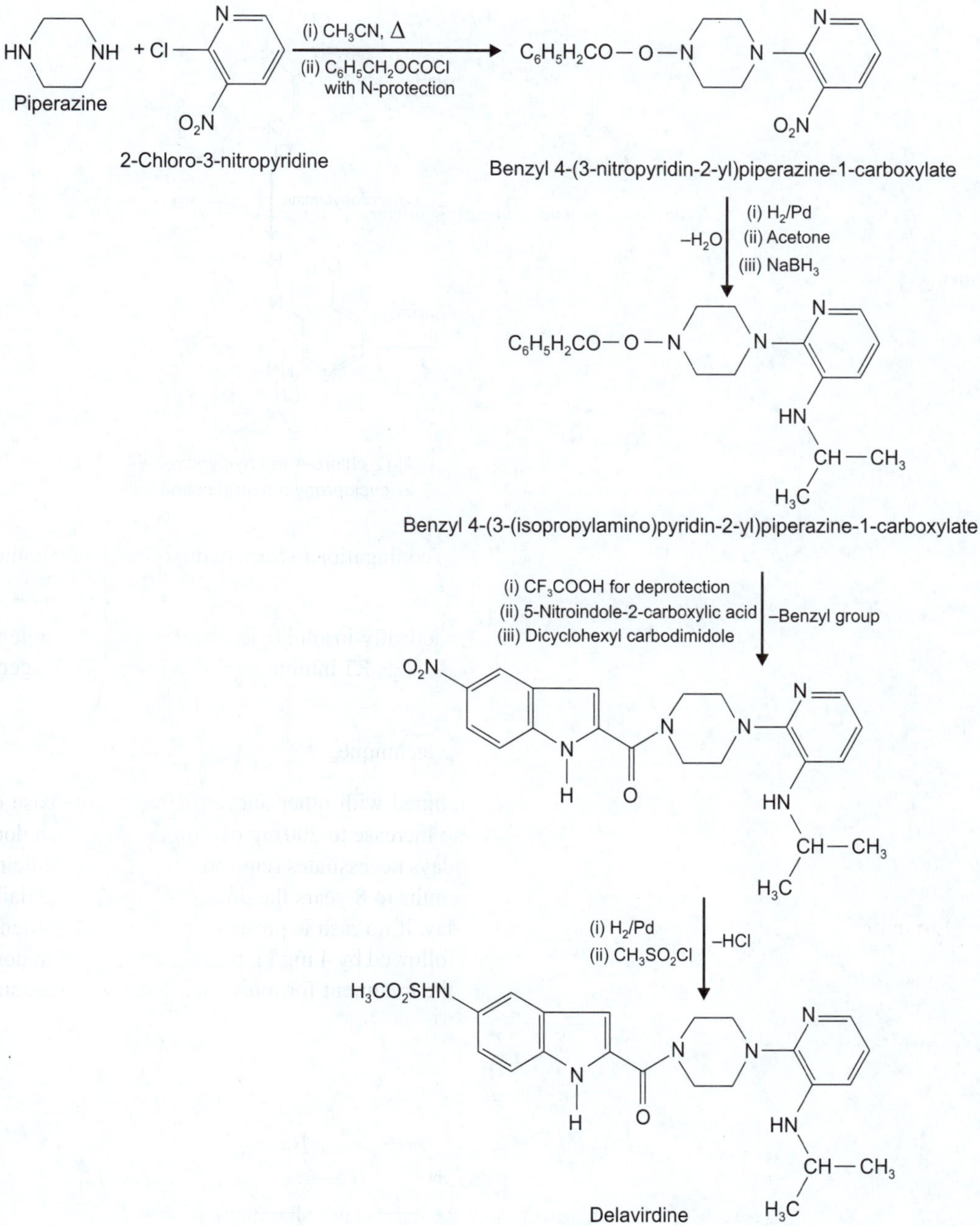

Metabolism: Delavirdine is metabolized to N-desisopropyl metabolite in the liver and the pharmacokinetics is non-linear.

iii. Emivirine

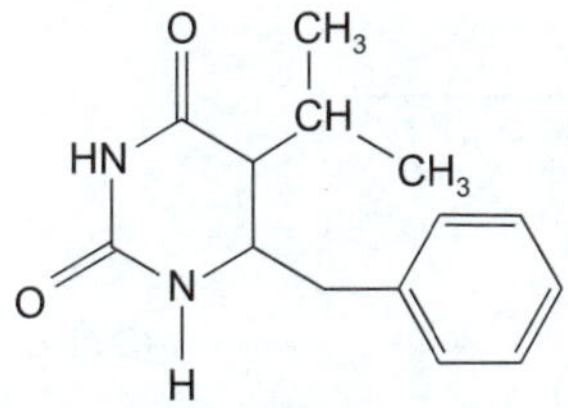

6-Benzyl-5-isopropyl-hexahydropyrimidine-2,4-dione

Synthesis

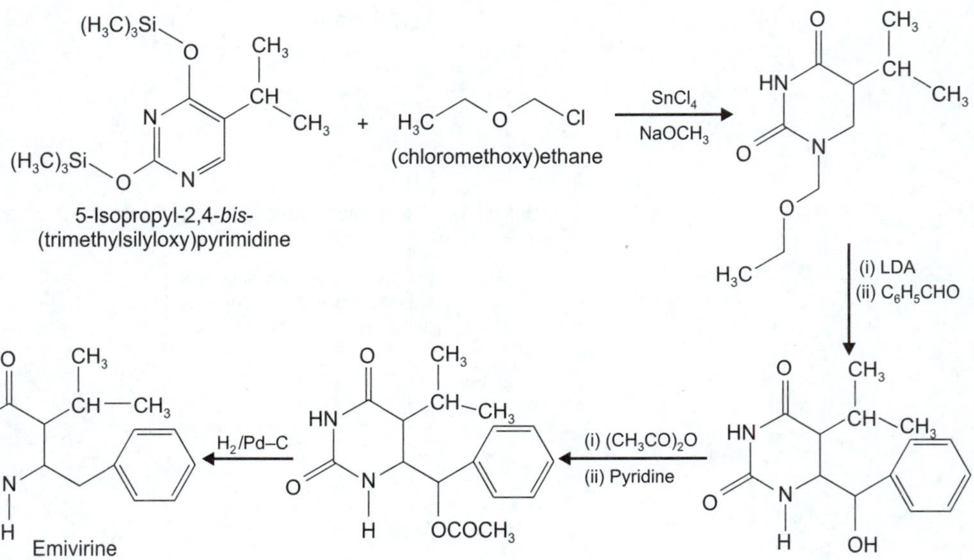

iv. Loviride

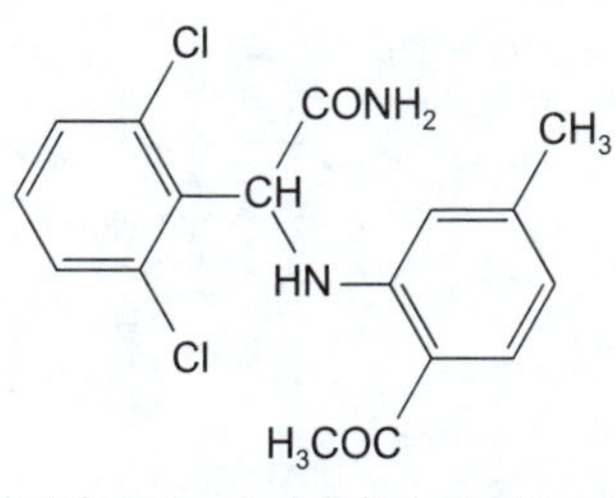

2-(2-Acetyl-5-methylphenylamino)-2-(2,6-dichlorophenyl)acetamide

Synthesis

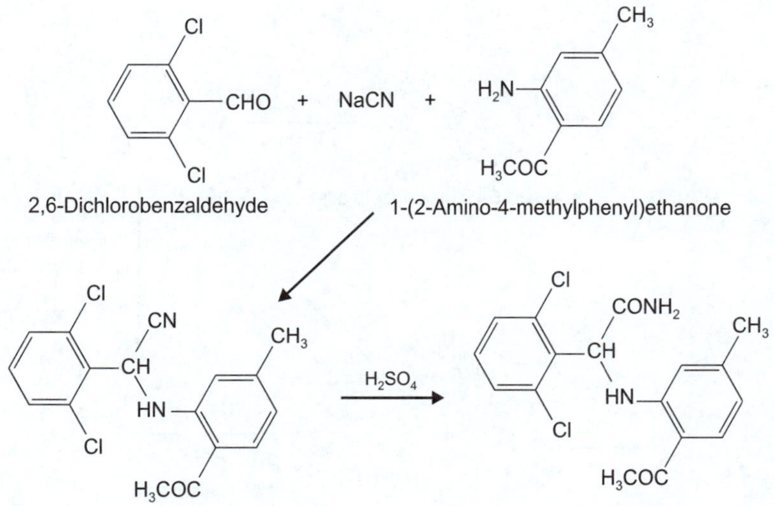

Loviride

v. Trovirdine

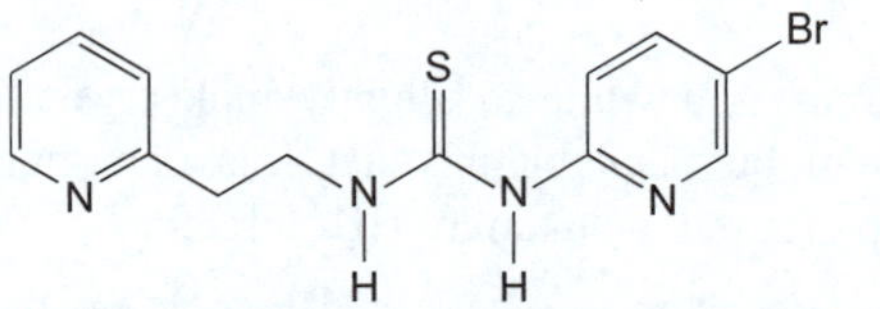

1-(5-Bromopyridin-2-yl)-3-(2-(pyridin-2-yl)ethyl)thiourea

Synthesis

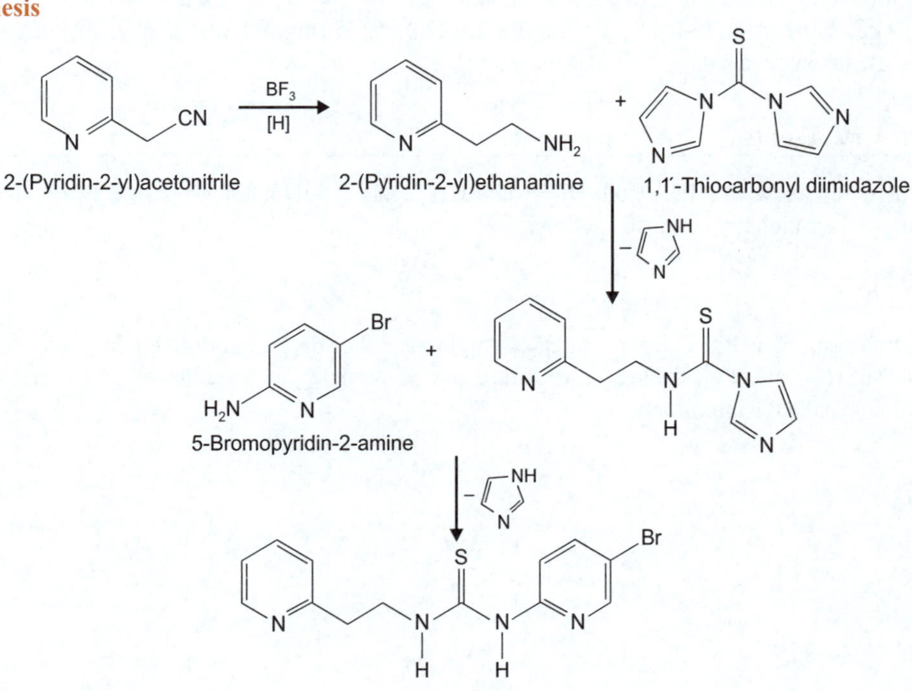

Trovirdine

vi. Efavirenz (Efavir, Efferven, Evirenz)

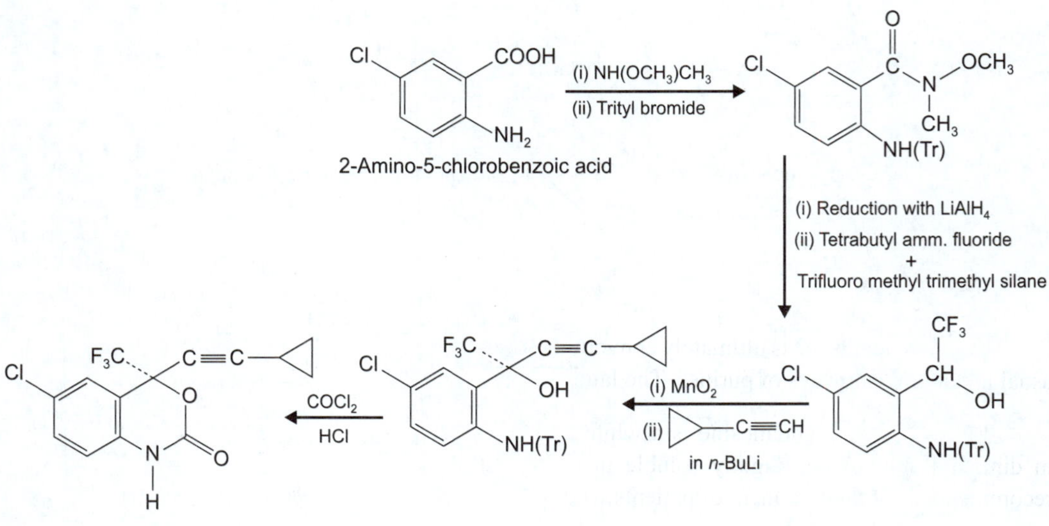

Efavirenz

Properties and uses: Efavirenz is a white to slightly pink crystalline powder, soluble in dilute hydrochloric acid and in ethanol, but insoluble in water. It is a non-nucleoside RT inhibitor used as a part of the combination therapy for the treatment of HIV infection.

Dose: The recommended oral dose for HIV infection combined with other antiretrovirals, in the case of adults is 600 mg, once daily. Dosing at bedtime recommended during first 2–4 weeks of therapy to improve tolerability. In a child above 3 years of age with 10–14 kg of body weight, the dose is 200 mg; for 15–19 kg, 250 mg; for 20–24 kg 300 mg; for 25–32.4 kg, 350 mg; for 32.5–39 kg, 400 mg; ≥40 kg; 600 mg to be taken once a day.

III. Anti-HIV Agents

HIV virus is the cause of AIDS, both HIV-1 and HIV-2 cause AIDS. Anti-HIV agents are classified according to their mode of actions as follows:

RT Inhibitors

Reverse transcription is RNA-dependent DNA polymerase. The drug inhibiting RT interferes with the replication of HIV and stops the synthesis of further viral particle. They are classified into nucleoside and non-nucleoside RT inhibitors.

Didanosine [2′,3′-dideoxyinosine (DDI), Videx]

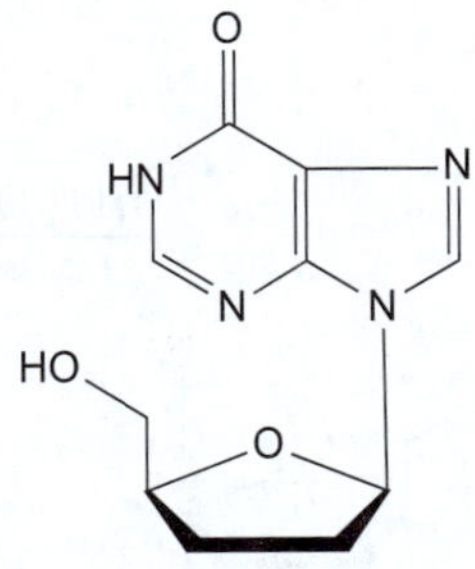

2′,3′-Dideoxyinosine

Metabolism: Didanosine is ultimately converted into hypoxanthine, xanthine, and uric acid through the usual metabolic pathways of purines. The latter is a non-toxic metabolic product.

Properties and uses: Didanosine is a white crystalline powder, sparingly soluble in water, soluble in dimethyl sulphoxide, slightly soluble in methanol and ethanol. It is a nucleoside RT inhibitor recommended for the treatment of patients with advanced HIV infections.

Assay: Dissolve the sample in glacial acetic acid and titrate with 0.1 M perchloric acid. Determine the end point potentiometrically.

Dose: The recommended dose for adults as tablets, which may be chewable and dispersible, for body weight more than 75 kg is 300 mg; for 50–74 kg body weight, 200 mg; for 35–49 kg body weight, 125 mg with antacids.

Synthesis

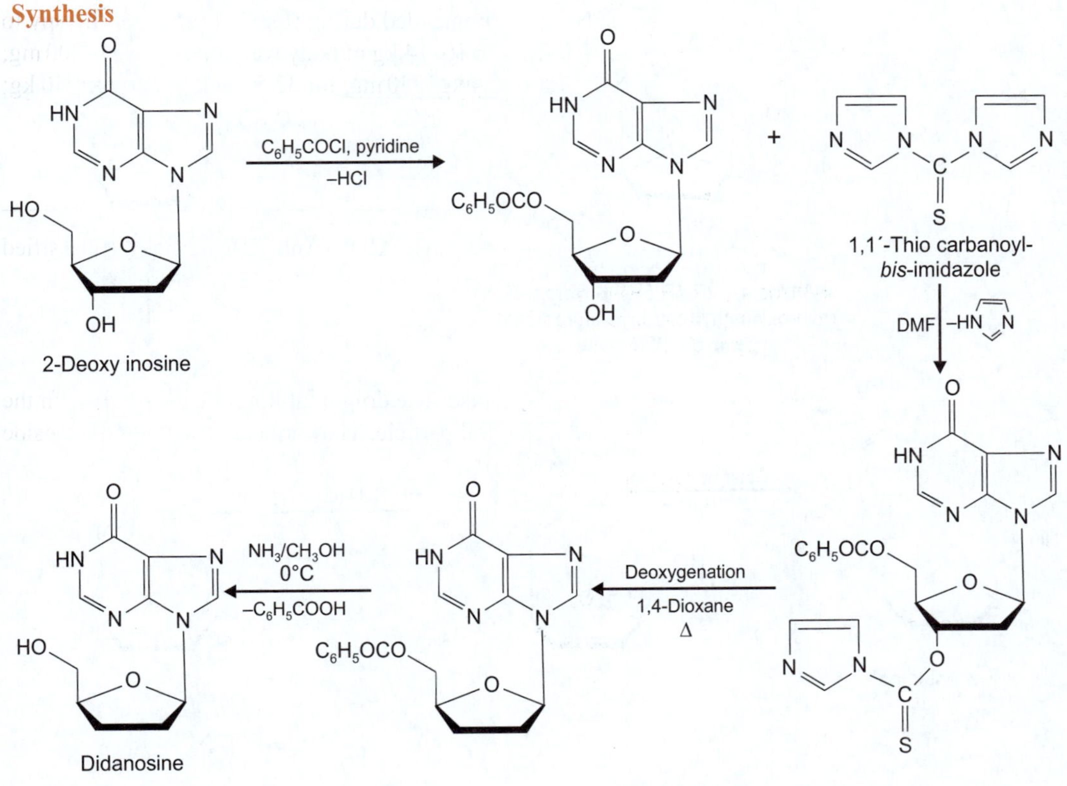

Zalcitabine (DDC, Hivid)

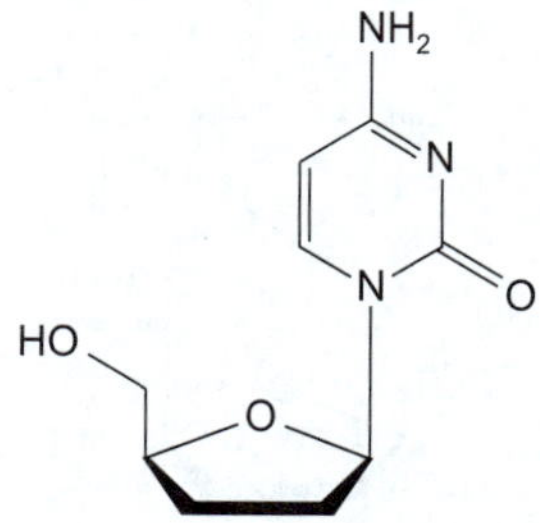

4-Amino-1-((2R,5S)-5-(hydroxymethyl)-tetrahydrofuran-2-yl)pyrimidin-2(1*H*)-one

Properties and uses: Zalcitabine exists as white crystals. It is approved for combination therapy with zidovudine in advanced HIV infection, who has demonstrated significant clinical or immunological deterioration, showing intolerance to zidovudine.

Dose: Zalcitabine is administered with zidovudine at the dose level of 2–25 mg of zalcitabine and 600 mg of zidovudine per day.

Synthesis

Route I.

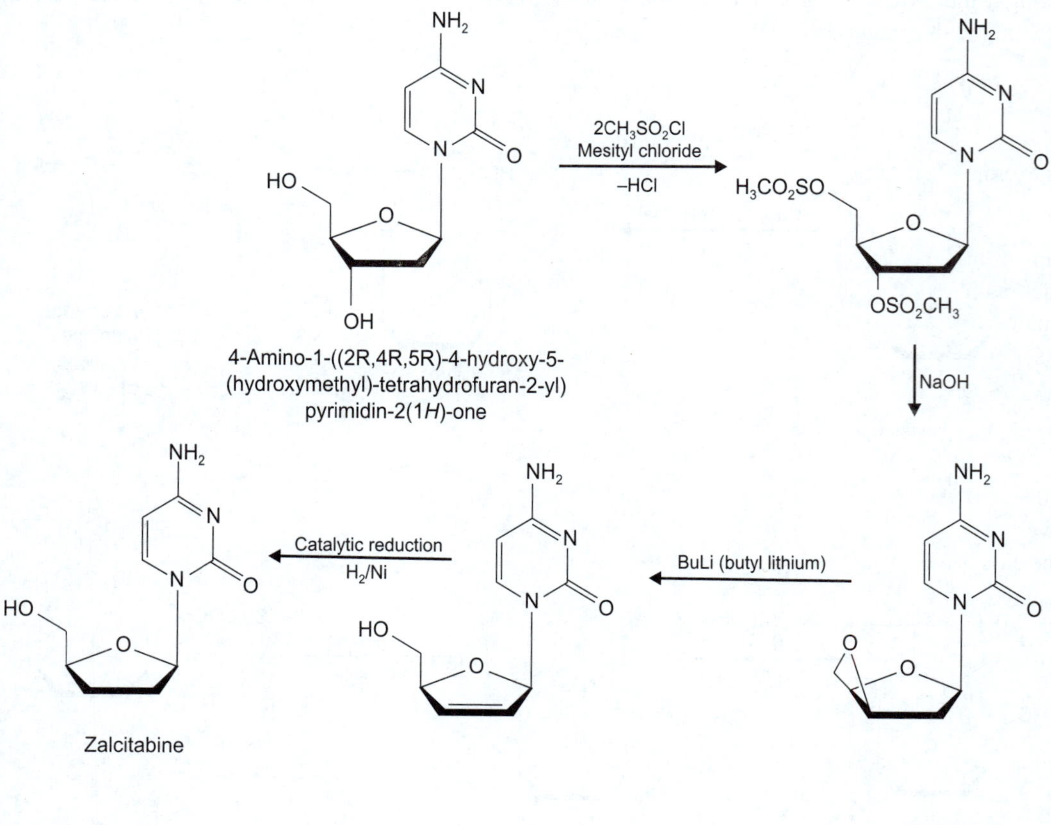

Route II.

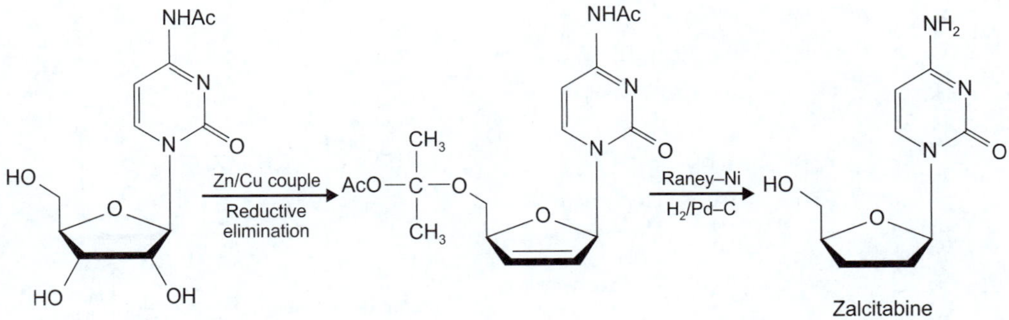

Zalcitabine

Zidovudine (ZDV) [azido-deoxythymidine (AZT), retrovir]

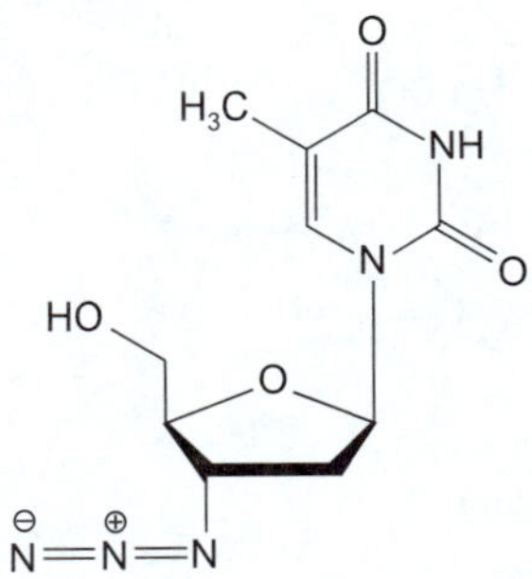

1-((2R,4,5S)-4-azido-5-(hydroxymethyl)-tetrahydrofuran-2-yl)-5-methylpyrimidine-2,4(1*H*,3*H*)-dione

Metabolism: Most of the administered drug is converted to its inactive glucuronide metabolite and it is excreted unchanged through urine.

Properties and uses: ZDV is a white or brownish powder, sparingly soluble in water and soluble in anhydrous ethanol. It is a nucleoside RT inhibitor, having activity against HIV, and hence, it is used for the treatment of AIDS and AIDS-related complex (ARC). It increases the survival and improves the quality of life of patients with complications, such as severe weight loss, fever, and pneumocytosis. As it crosses the blood–brain barrier, it has favourable effect on the neurological symptoms of AIDS.

Assay: It is assayed by adopting liquid chromatography technique.

Dose: The recommended dose for adults in the case of oral asymptomatic HIV-infection initially is 100 mg every 4 hrs, while awake (500 mg a day), after 1 month, the dose may be reduced to 100 mg every 4 hrs. For intravenous infusion, the dose is 1–2 mg/kg infused over 1 hr for every 4 hrs around the clock (6 times a day).

Synthesis

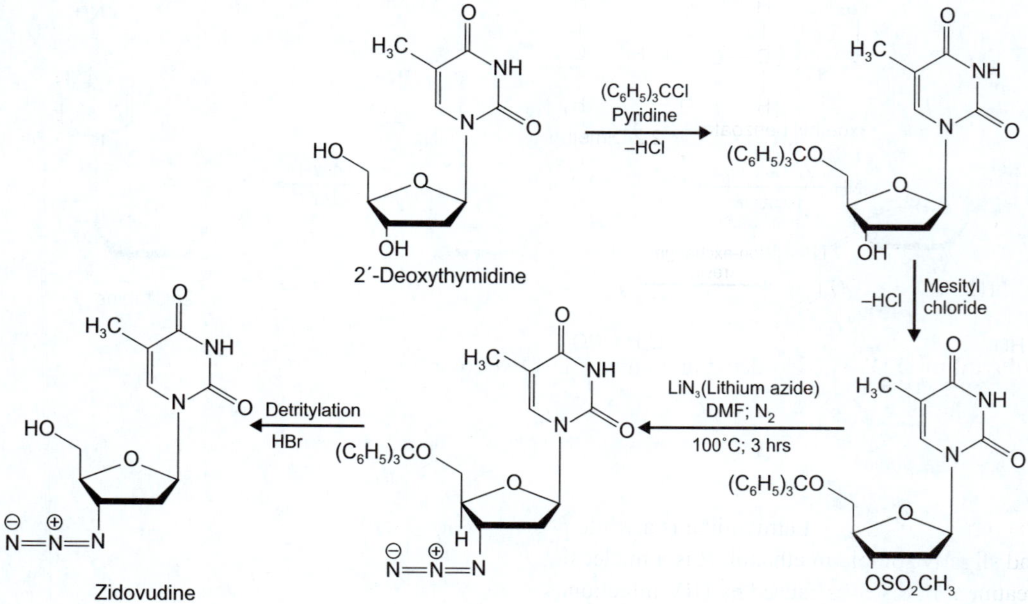

Lamivudine (Lamda, Rolam, Lamvir)

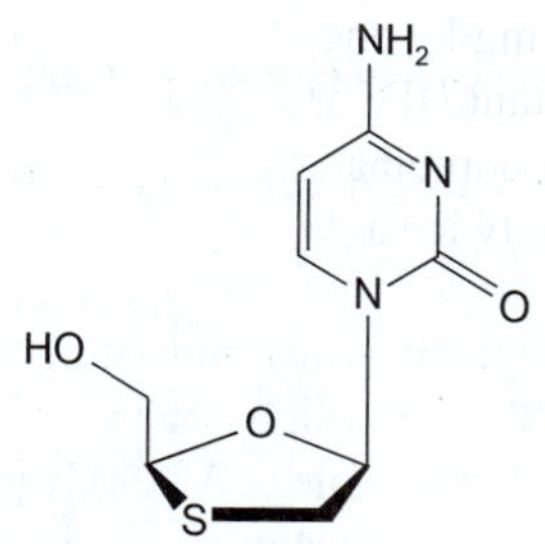

4-Amino-1-((2S,5R)-2-(hydroxymethyl)-1,3-oxathiolan-5-yl)pyrimidin-2(1*H*)-one

Synthesis

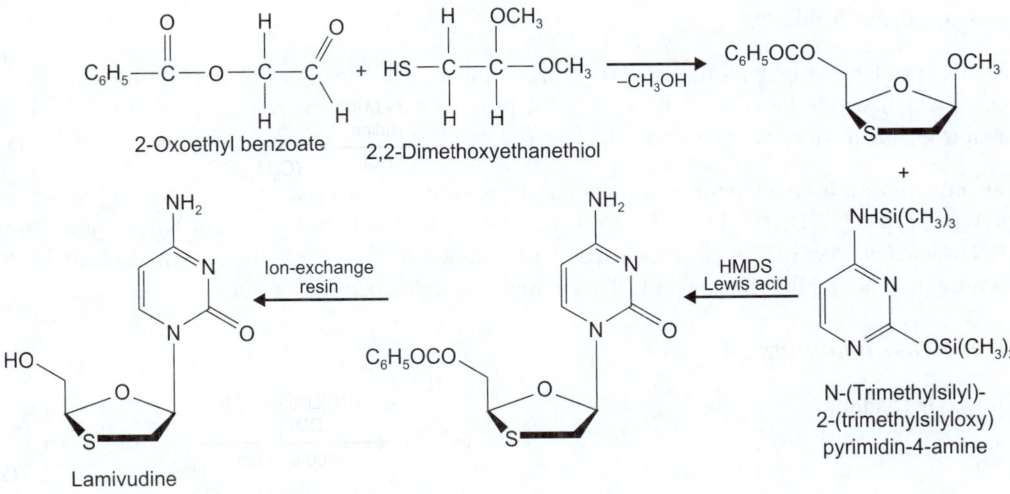

Properties and uses: Lamivudine is a white powder, soluble in water, sparingly soluble in methanol and slightly soluble in ethanol. It is a nucleoside RT inhibitor, used in combination with ZDV for the treatment of diseases caused by HIV infection.

Assay: It is assayed by adopting liquid chromatography technique.

Dose: The recommended dose for chronic hepatitis B in the case of adults is 100 mg once daily. For a child more than 2 years, the dose is 3 mg/kg once daily, maximum is 100 mg per day for HIV infection. The recommended dose for concomitant HIV and hepatits B infection, in the case of adults is 150 mg twice a day or 300 mg once daily, in combination with other antiretrovirals. In the case of a child, 3 months–12 years, the dose is 4 mg/kg twice a day, maximum dose is 300 mg per day.

Etravirine (intelence)

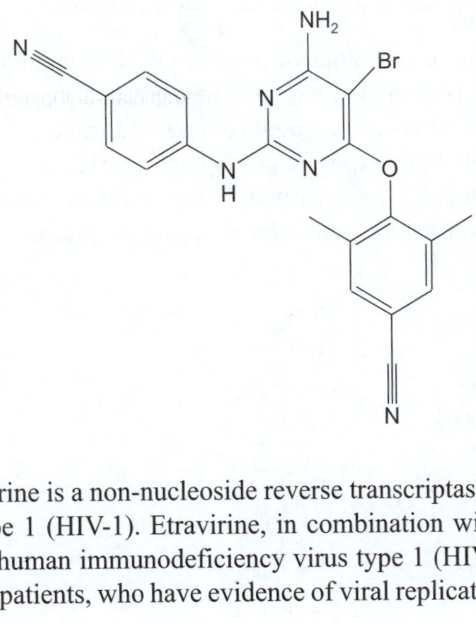

Properties and uses: Etravirine is a non-nucleoside reverse transcriptase inhibitor (NNRTI) of human immunodeficiency virus type 1 (HIV-1). Etravirine, in combination with other antiretroviral agents, is used for the treatment of human immunodeficiency virus type 1 (HIV-1) infection in antiretroviral treatment-experienced adult patients, who have evidence of viral replication and HIV-1 strains resistant to a non-nucleoside reverse transcriptase inhibitor (NNRTI) and other antiretroviral agents. Adverse events associated with the use of etravirine may include rash, diarrhea, nausea, fatigue, abdominal pain, hypertension, and headache.

Dose: It is available as tablet formulated for oral administration. The initial dose is 200 mg (two 100 mg tablets), which should be taken twice daily after meal. It can be dispersed in a glass of water if the patient is unable to swallow the whole tablet.

Mode of action: It is an inhibitor of non-nucleoside reverse transcriptase of human immunodeficiency virus type 1 (HIV-1). The drug binds directly to the enzyme reverse transcriptase and blocks the activities of RNA-dependent and DNA-dependent DNA polymerase by disrupting the enzyme's catalytic site. This drug does not inhibit the human DNA polymerases alpha, beta, and gamma.

HIV Protease Inhibitors

Saquinavir (Saquin)

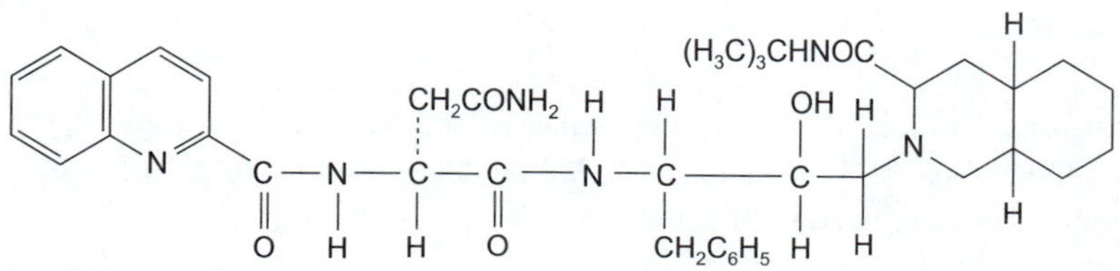

N-((S)-1-(4-(3-(*tert*-butylcarbamoyl)-octahydroisoquinolin-2(1*H*)-yl)-3-hydroxy-1-phenylbutan-2-ylamino)-4-amino-1,4-dioxobutan-2-yl)quinoline-2-carboxamide

Metabolism: Metabolism of saquinavir is catalyzed by CYP3A4 and possibly by CYP3A5. The metabolites mono and dihydroxylated compounds are not active.

Properties and uses: It is a white to off-white fine powder, which is soluble in water. It is a synthetic peptide analogue and inhibitor of HIV-1 and HIV-2 proteases. It is used in combination with RT inhibitors, but it has less cross-resistance with other protease inhibitors.

Dose: The recommended oral dose of saquinavir for HIV infection combined with other antiretrovirals, in the case of adults more than 16 years is 1 g twice a day, when taken with ritonavir 100 mg, it is twice a day. Alternatively, the administered dose of saquinavir could also be 400 mg twice a day with ritonavir 400 mg twice a day. In the case of postexposure prophylaxis, during occupational exposure to HIV, the dose for adults is 1 g of saquinavir twice a day with ritonavir 100 mg twice a day, combined with other antiretrovirals, and should be started as soon as possible and continued for 4 weeks, if tolerated.

Synthesis

Step I. Synthesis of N-*t*-butyl-decahydroisoquinoline-3-carboxamide (A)

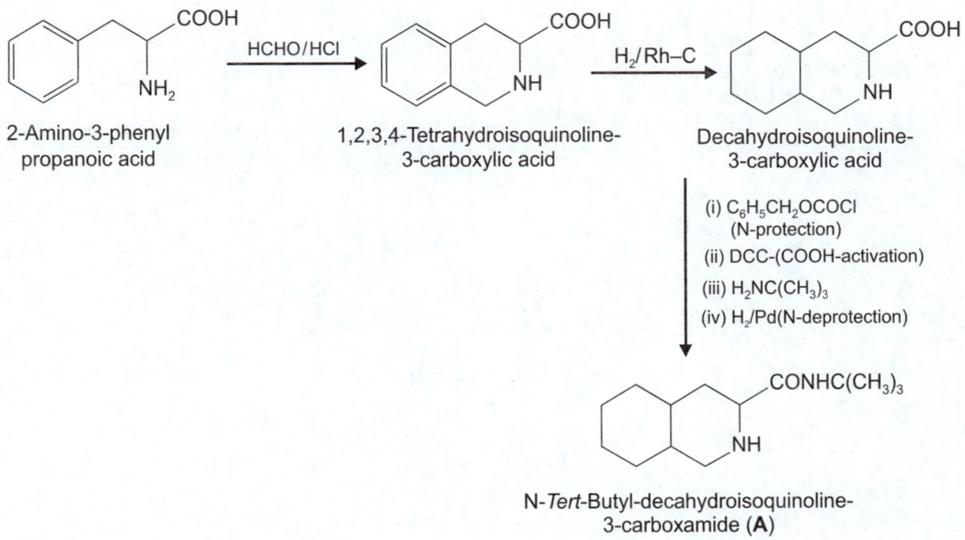

Step II. Synthesis of benzyl 4-chloro-3-hydroxy-1-phenylbutan-2-yl carbamate (B)

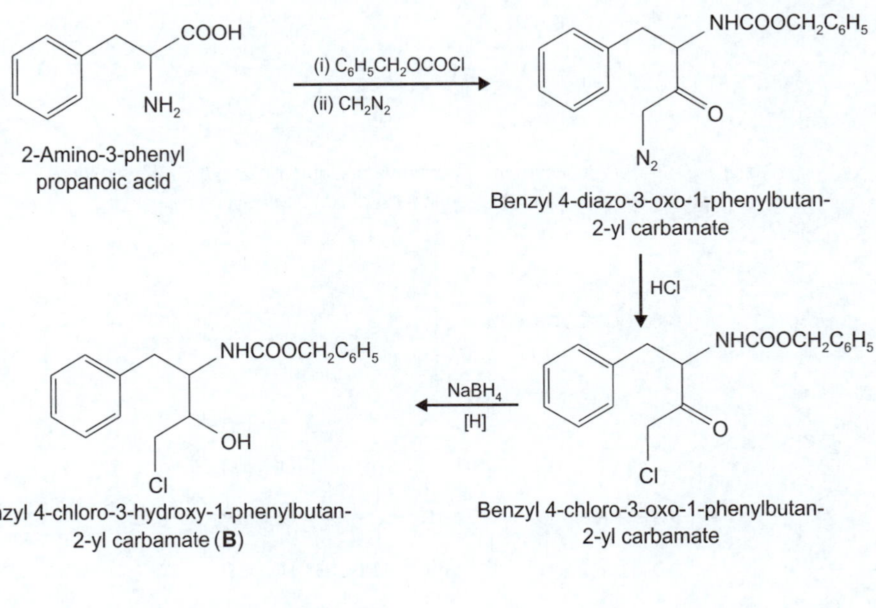

Step III. Condensation of (A) and (B)

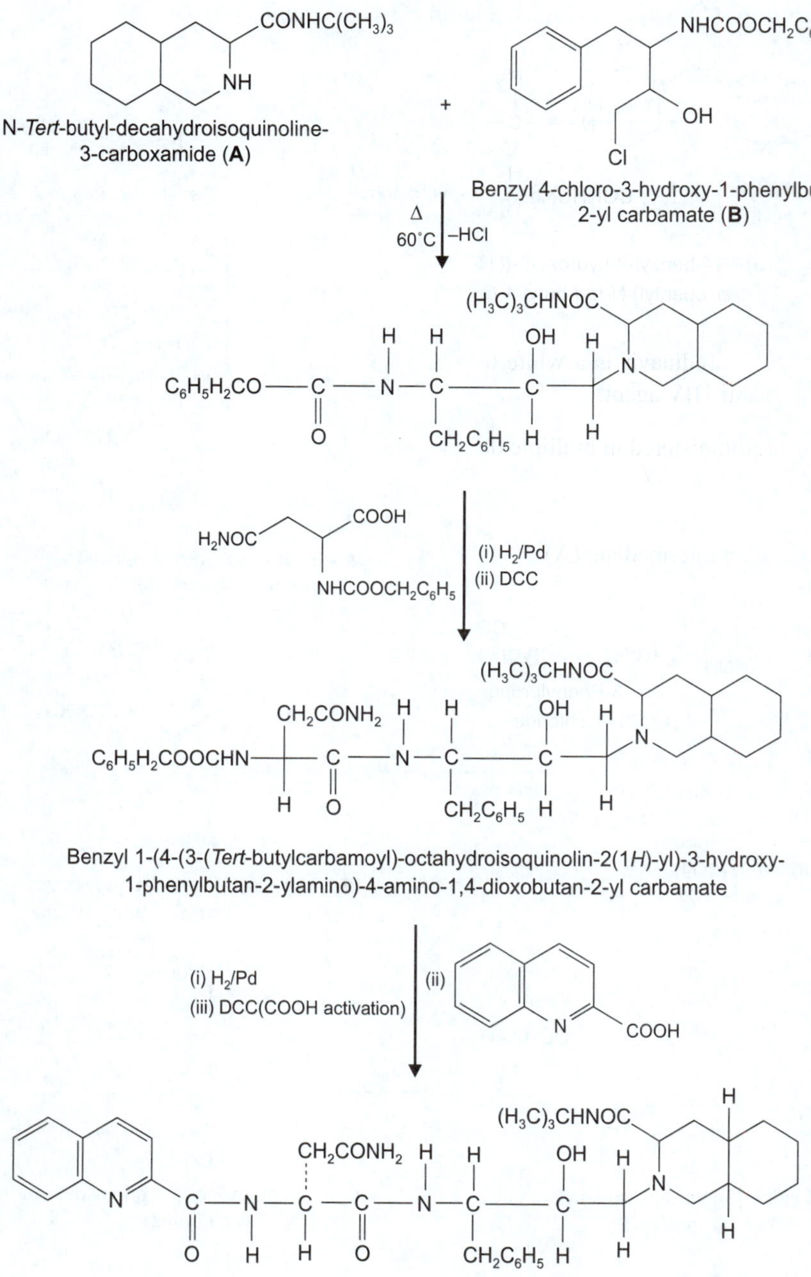

Saquinavir

Indinavir (Crixivan)

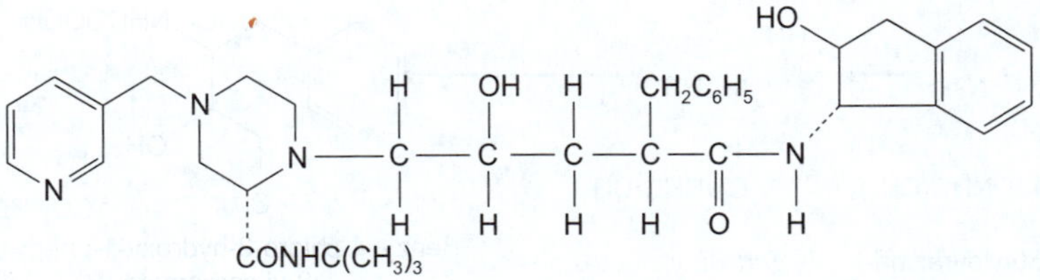

(S)-1-(4-benzyl-2-hydroxy-5-((1S)-2-hydroxy-2,3-dihydro-1*H*-inden-1-ylamino)-5-oxopentyl)-N-*tert*-butyl-4-(pyridin-3-ylmethyl)piperazine-2-carboxamide

Properties and uses: Indinavir is a white to off-white hygroscopic powder, soluble in water or in methanol. Used as anti-HIV agent.

Dose: Indinavir is administered in multiple doses of 100–400 mg every 6 hrs for up to 10 days.

Synthesis

Step I: Synthesis of an intermediate (A)

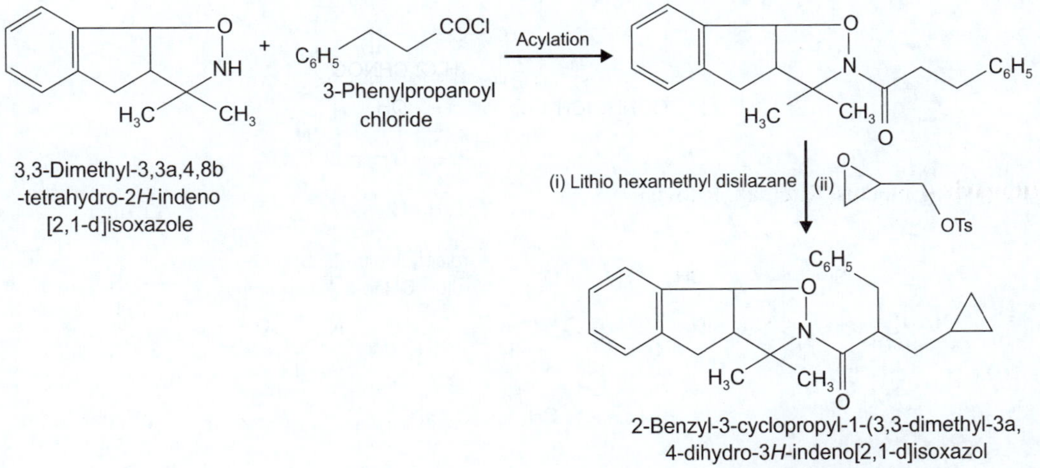

2-Benzyl-3-cyclopropyl-1-(3,3-dimethyl-3a,4-dihydro-3*H*-indeno[2,1-d]isoxazol-2(8b*H*)-yl)propan-1-one

(A)

Step II: Synthesis of indinavir

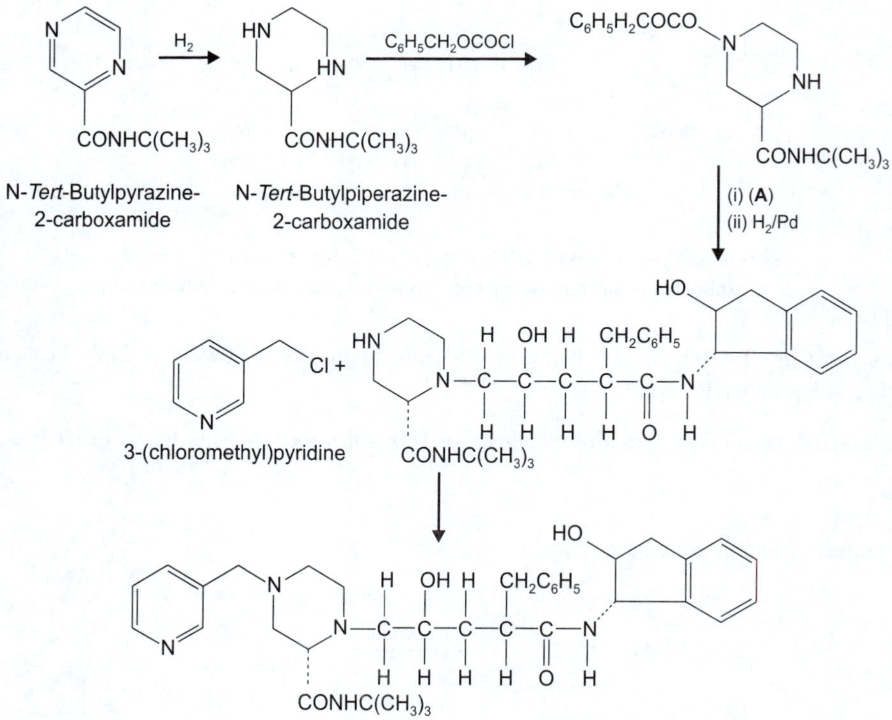

Indinavir

Ritonavir (Empetus, Ritomax, Ritovir)

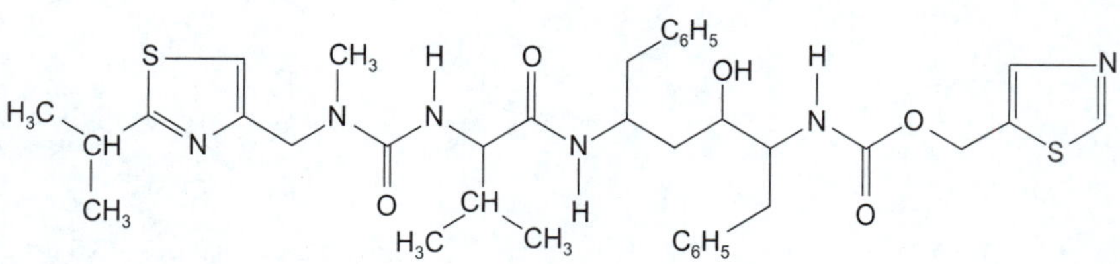

Synthesis

Step I. Synthesis of ritonavir

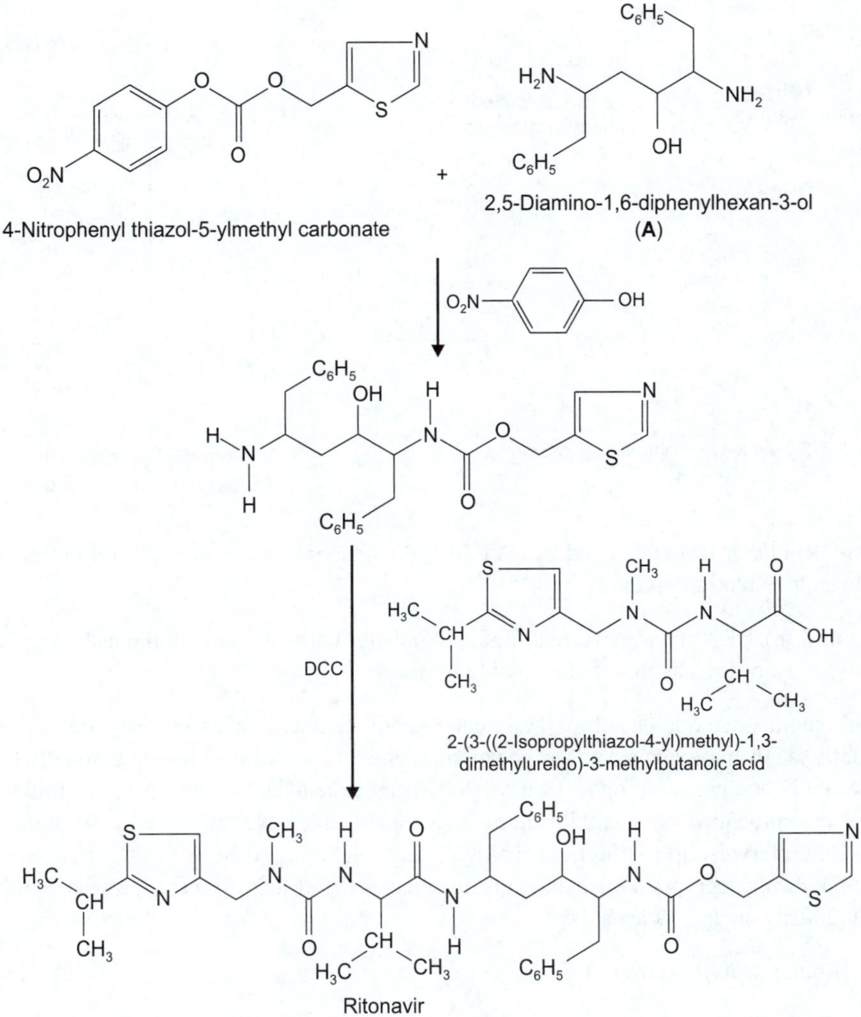

Synthesis of (A)

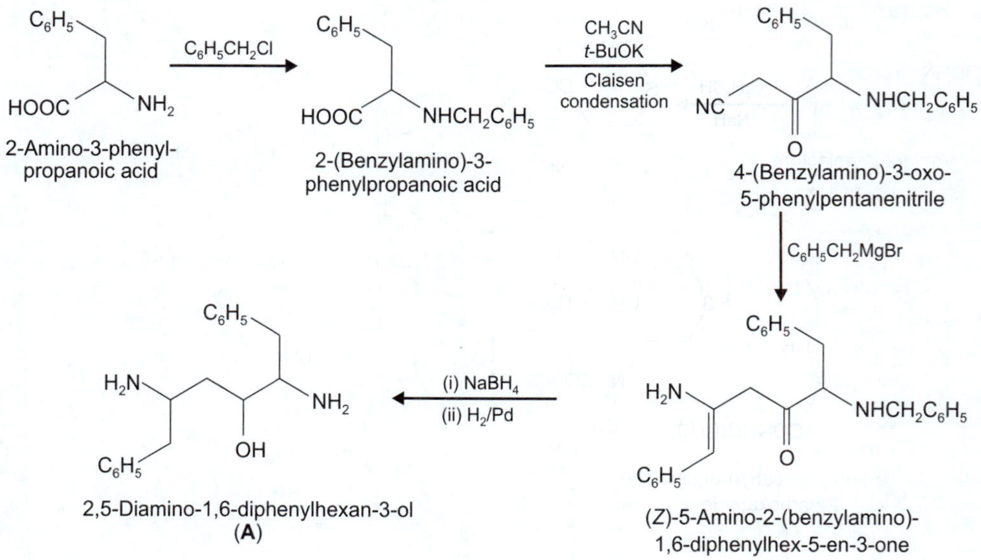

Metabolism: Ritonavir is metabolized by CYP3A4; the metabolites are isolated from urine. They are isopropylthiazole oxidation products.

Properties and uses: Ritonavir is white to light tan powder with a bitter metallic taste. It is soluble in methanol and in isopropyl alcohol, but insoluble in water.

Dose: The recommended oral dose for HIV infection combined with other antiretroviral, in the case of adults, initially is 300 mg twice a day for the day one. The dose may be increased gradually by 100 mg twice a day and over a period of up to 14 days to 600 mg twice a day. In the case of a child more than 2 years, the recommended dose is 250 mg/m^2 twice a day. Increase the dose by 50 mg/m^2 twice a day, at 2–3 day intervals, up to 400 mg/m^2 twice a day. Maximum dose is 600 mg twice a day. As a pharmacokinetic enhancer, in the case of adults, to enhance the efficacy of other protease inhibitors the dose is 100–200 mg once or twice a day.

Nelfinavir (Emnel, Nelvir, Retronel)

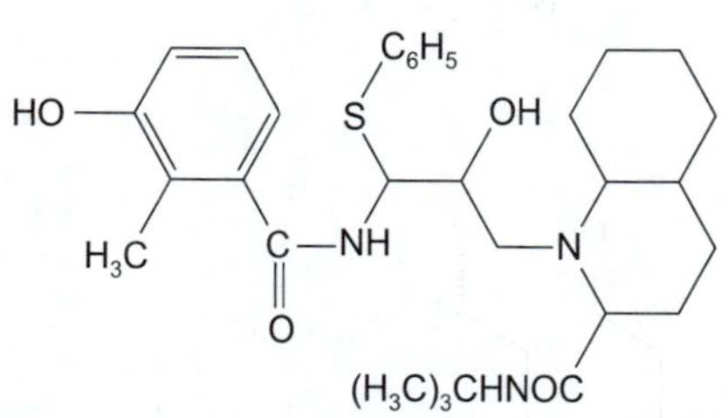

N-*Tert*-Butyl-1-(2-hydroxy-3-(3-hydroxy-2-methylbenzamido)-3-(phenylthio)propyl)-1,2,3,4-tetrahydroquinoline-2-carboxamide

Synthesis

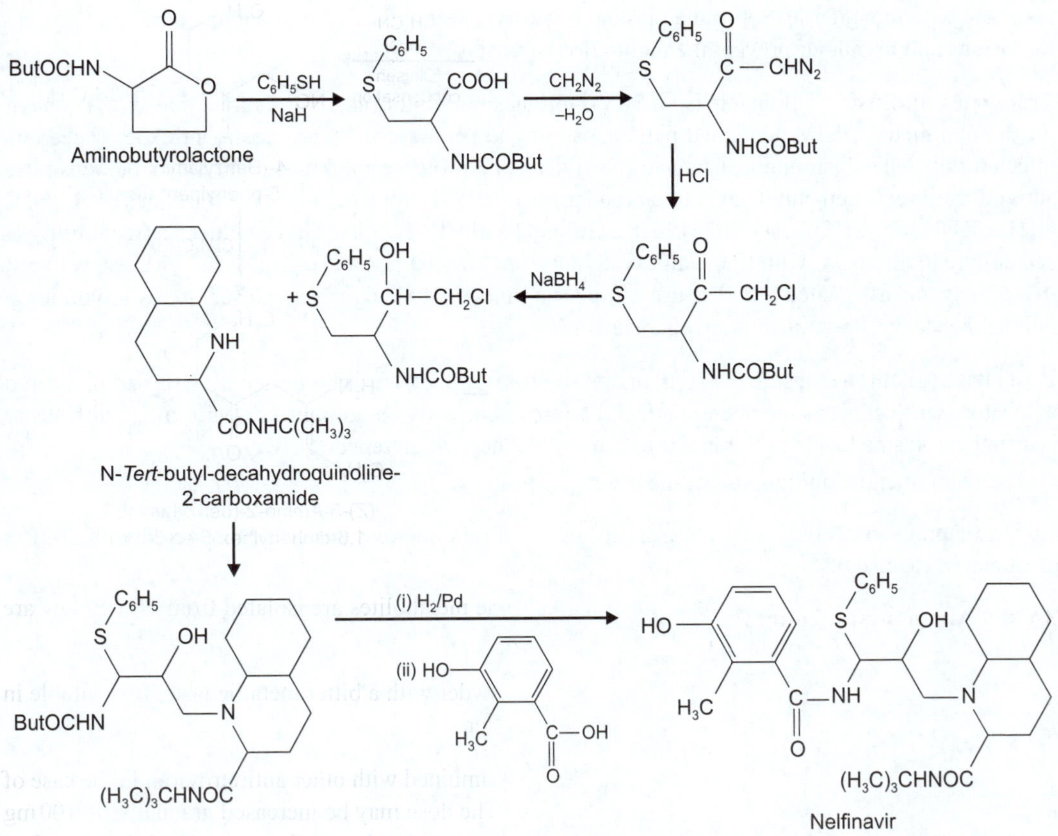

Properties and uses: It is a white to off-white amorphous powder, which is slightly soluble in water, soluble in methanol, ethanol, isopropyl alcohol, or propylene glycol. It is used as an anti-HIV agent.

Dose: The recommended dose for HIV infection combined with other antiretrovirals in the case of adults is 1.25 g twice a day or 0.75 g thrice a day. In the case of a child: For 2–13 years is 45–55 mg/kg twice a day or 25–35 mg/kg thrice a day. Maximum dose for a child is 0.75 g thrice a day.

Tipranavir (Aptivus)

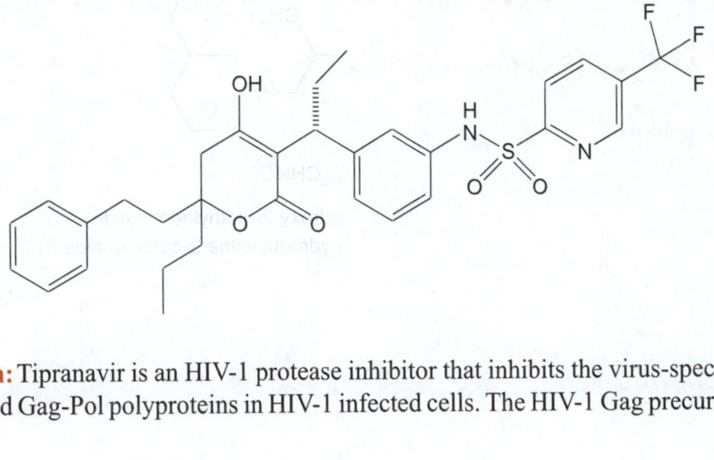

Mode of action: Tipranavir is an HIV-1 protease inhibitor that inhibits the virus-specific processing of the viral Gag and Gag-Pol polyproteins in HIV-1 infected cells. The HIV-1 Gag precursor is synthesized on cytosolic ribosomes and becomes cotranslationally modified by the N-terminal attachment of a myristyl group, which increases its affinity for membranes. Myristylated Gag precursor molecules associate with the inner leaflet of the plasma membrane, where they coalesce into a patch and process for virions and tipranavir prevent the maturation of virions.

Properties and uses: Tipranavir is an HIV-1 protease inhibitor, used in combination with ritonavir for the treatment of HIV-1 infected patients, adult and pediatric, who are treatment-experienced and infected with HIV-1 strains resistant to more than one protease inhibitors. Tipranavir demonstrates antiviral activity in cell culture against a broad panel of HIV-1 group M non-clade B isolates (A, C, D, F, G, H, CRF01 AE, CRF02 AG, CRF12 BF). Group O and HIV-2 isolates have reduced susceptibility in cell culture to tipranavir with EC_{50} values ranging from 0.164–1 μM and 0.233–0.522 μM, respectively. Adverse events associated with the use of this drug may include diarrhea, nausea, pyrexia, vomiting, fatigue, headache, abdominal pain, and anaemia.

Dose: It is available as capsule (250 mg) or oral solution (100 mg/ml). This drug must be co-administered with ritonavir to elicit its therapeutic effect. Failure to correctly co-administer it with ritonavir leads to insufficient plasma levels of tipranavir to achieve the desired therapeutic effect.

The recommended initial dose of the drug is as follows:

Adults: Tipranavir 500 mg (two 250 mg capsules or 5 ml oral solution) co-administered with 200 mg of ritonavir, twice daily.

SAR of Adamantane Amines

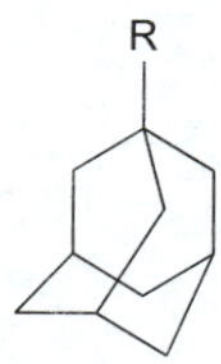

- α-methyl derivative of adamantane produced rimantidine.
- α-methyl-1-adamantane methylamine is flumadine.
- N-Alkyl and N,N-dialkyl derivatives of adamantadine exhibit antiviral activity similar to that of adamantadine HCl. Except glycyl derivatives, N-acyl derivatives show decreased antiviral action and tromantadine possesses efficacy against clinical *Herpes labialis* and *H. genitalis*.
- Replacement of the amino group with OH, SH, CN, or halogen produced inactive compounds.
- Optical isomers and the racemic mixtures of rimantadine are equally active.
- *Influenza A_2* virus, is more susceptible to adamantanespiro-5-pyrrolidine derivative.

CLASSIFICATION BASED ON PCI SYLLABUS

Amantadine hydrochloride

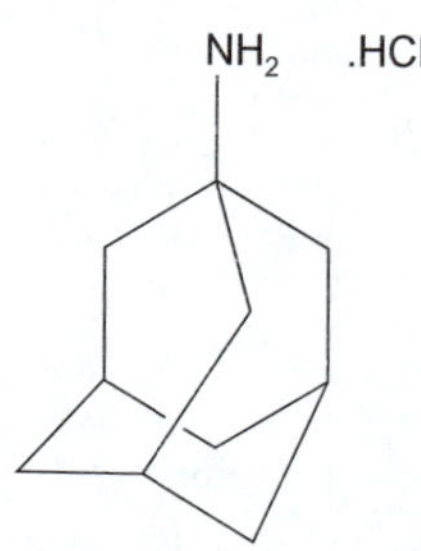

Rimantadine hydrochloride

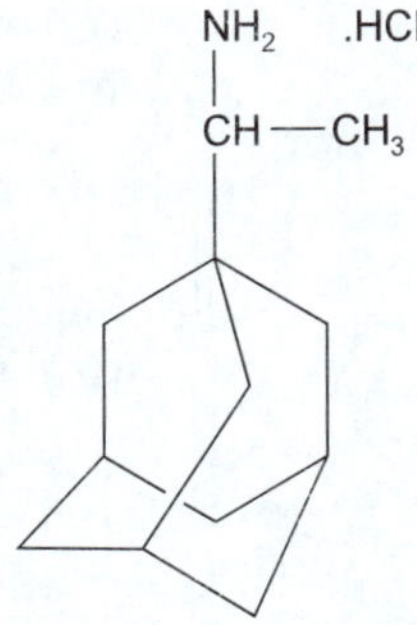

Idoxuridine trifluoride

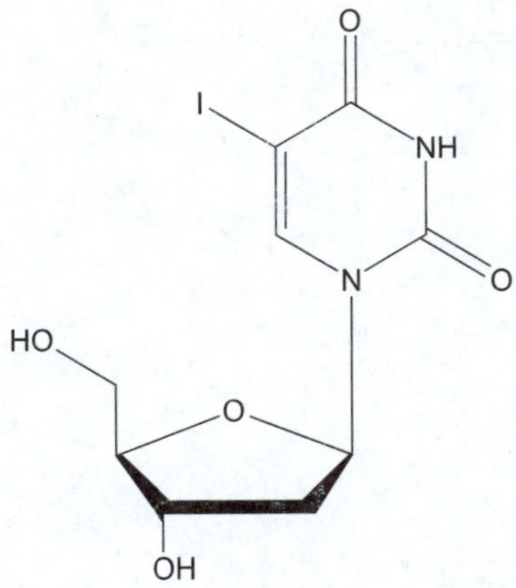

Acyclovir

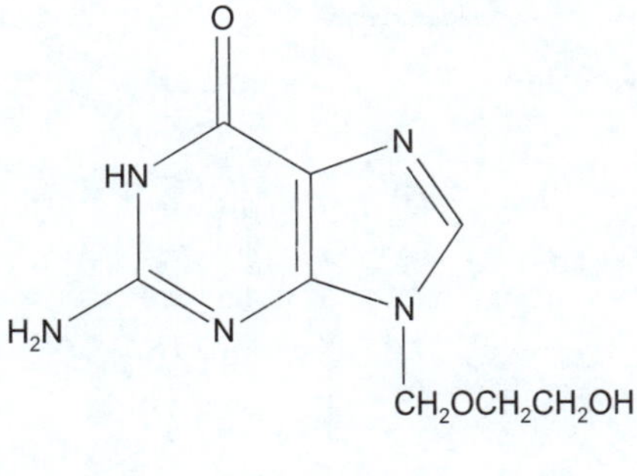

Gancyclovir

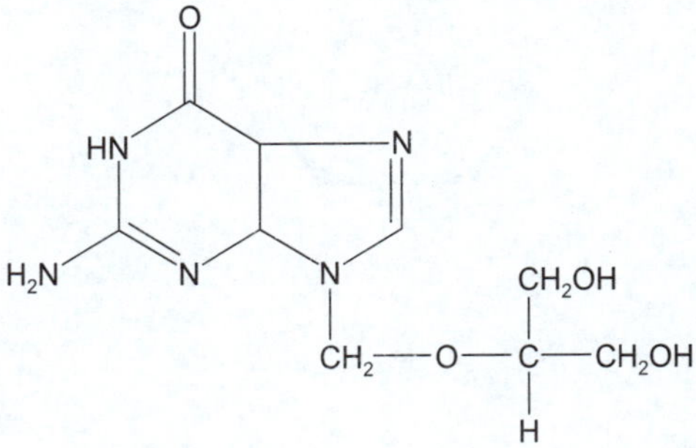

Zidovudine

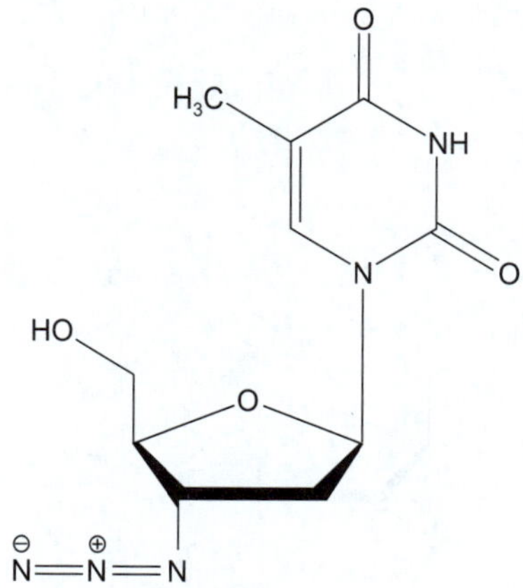

Didanosine

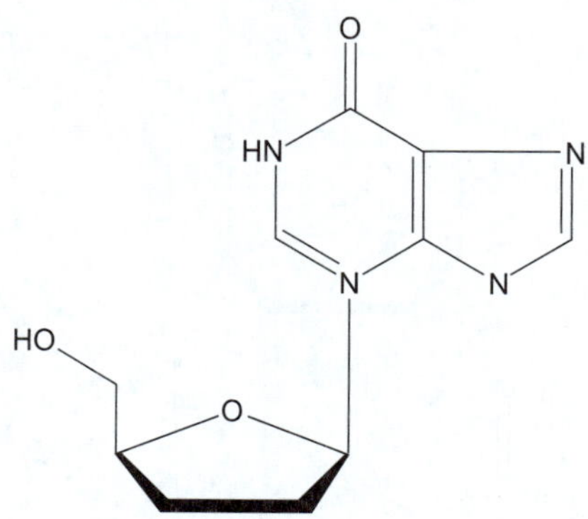

Zalcitabine

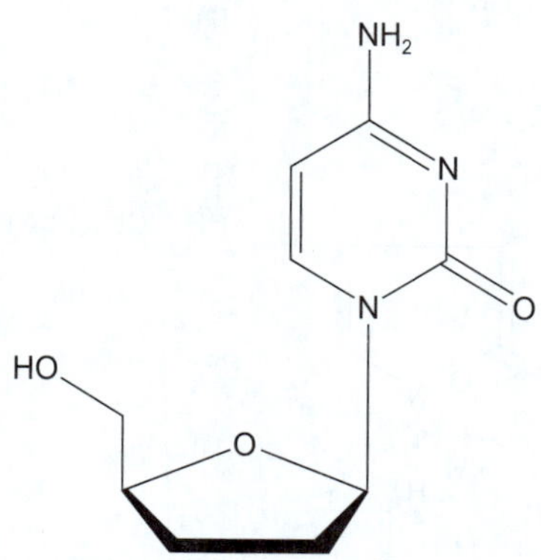

Lamivudine

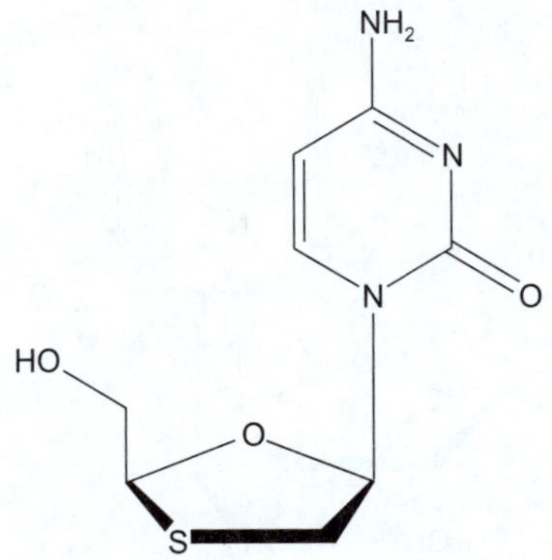

Loviride

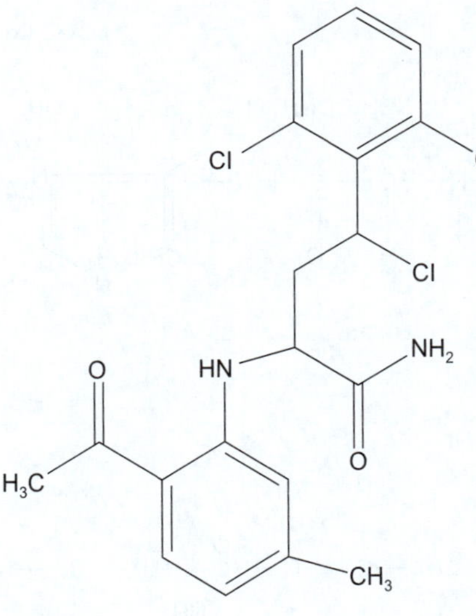

Delavirdin

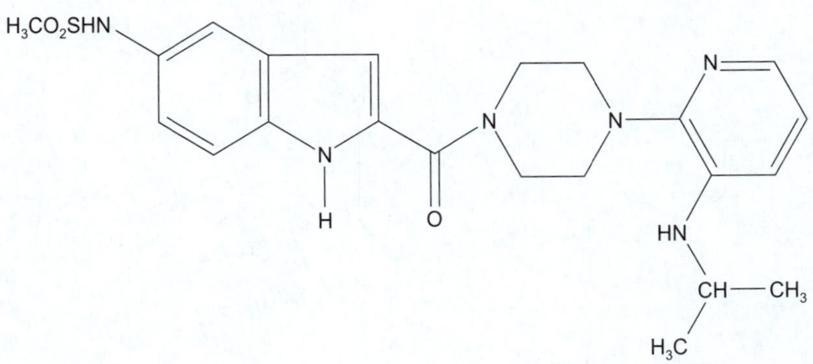

Ribavirin

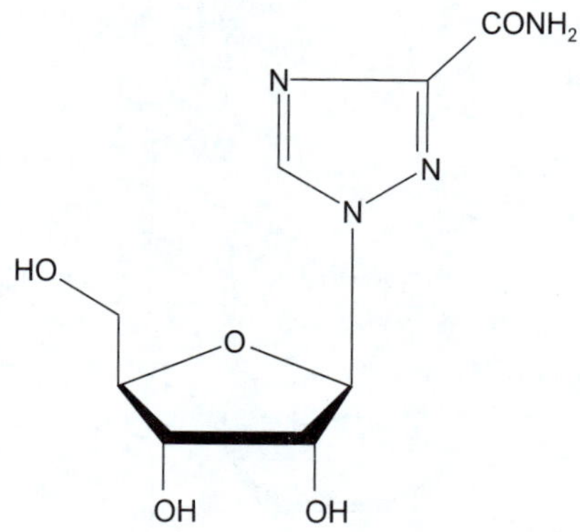

Saquinavir

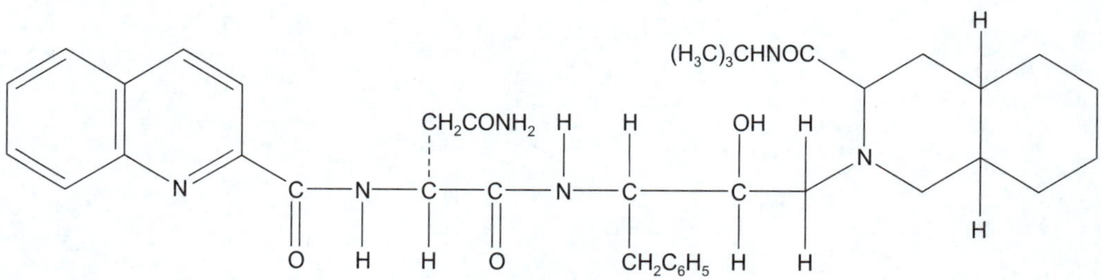

Indinavir

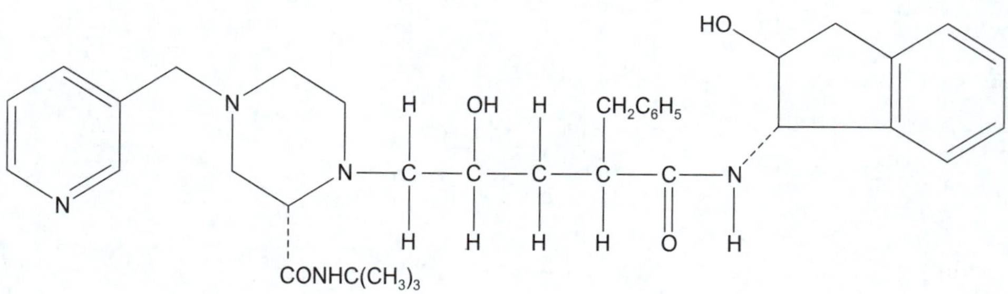

Ritonavir

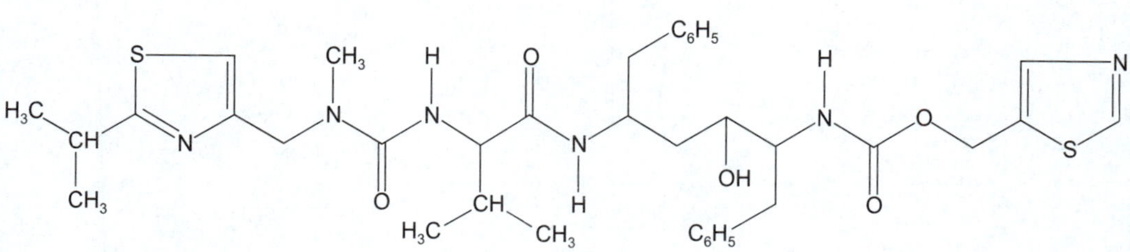

Newer Agents

Letermovir

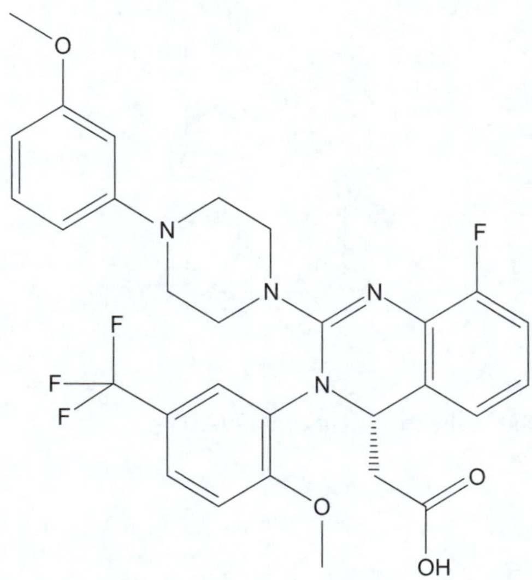

Uses: It is an antiviral drug for the treatment of cytomegalovirus (CMV) infections and may also be useful for other patients with a compromised immune system such as those with organ transplants or HIV infections.

Baloxavirmarboxil

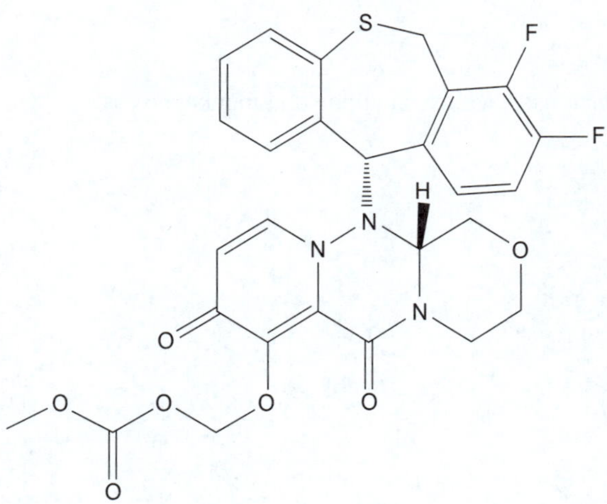

Uses: It is an antiviral drug and used to treat influenza A and influenza B flu.

Doravirine

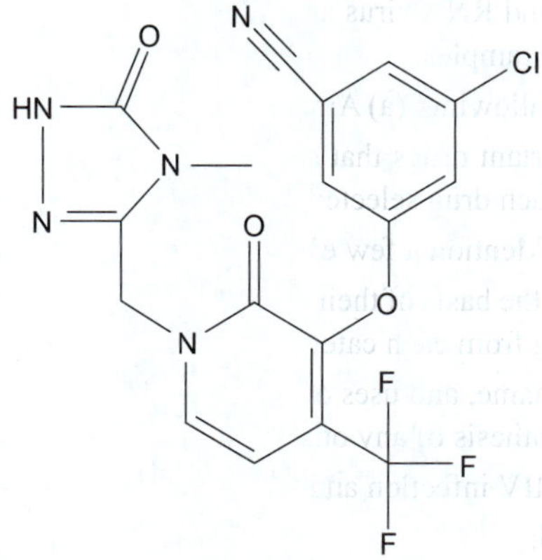

Uses: It is a NNRTIs and used in the treatment of HIV/AIDS.

Tecovirimat

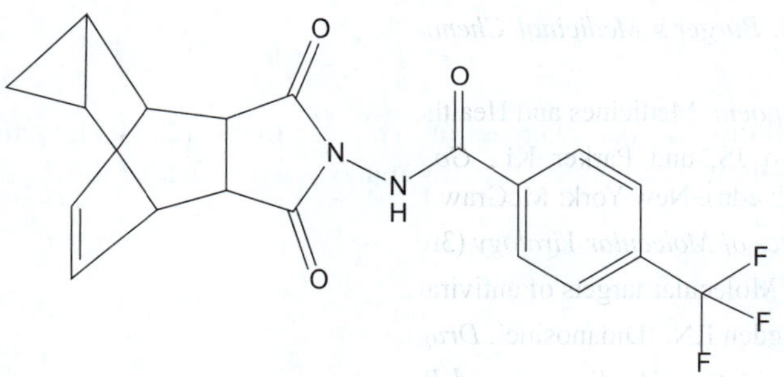

Uses: It is an antiviral agent used against smallpox and monkeypox.

Fostemsavir

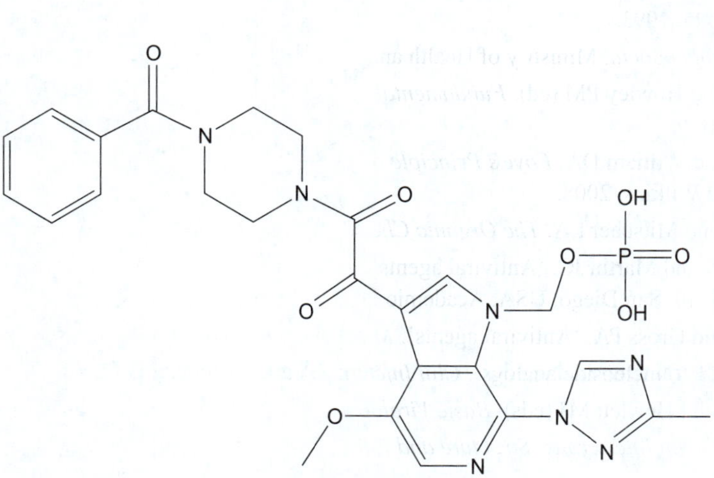

Uses: It is an antiretroviral agent to treat HIV/AIDS co-infection.

PROBABLE QUESTIONS

1. Enumerate a few DNA virus and RNA virus and mention the diseases produced by them. Classify the antiviral agents with suitable examples.
2. How will you synthesize the following: (a) Amantadine HCl, (b) methisazone?
3. Give the names of three important drugs that specifically interfere with viral nucleic acid replication. Discuss the synthesis of one such drug selected.
4. What are protease inhibitors? Mention a few examples and write the synthesis of indinavir.
5. Classify the antiviral drugs on the basis of their mode of action. Draw the structure, chemical name, and uses of at least one potent drug from each category.
6. Write the structure, chemical name, and uses of two important antiviral drugs that affect translation on cell ribosomes. Outline the synthesis of any one of them.
7. Enumerate the drugs used in HIV infection and write the synthesis of any one of them.
8. Discuss the following in detail:
   (a) Important antiviral drugs
   (b) Mode of action of antiviral drugs.

SUGGESTED READINGS

1. Abraham DJ (ed). *Burger's Medicinal Chemistry and Drug Discovery* (6th edn). New Jersey: John Wiley, 2007.
2. *British Pharmacopoeia*. Medicines and Healthcare Products Regulatory Agency. London, 2008.
3. Bruntan LL, Lazo JS, and Parker KL. *Goodman and Gilman's: The Pharmacological Basis of Therapeutics* (11th edn). New York: McGraw Hill, 2006.
4. Cann AJ. *Principles of Molecular Virology* (3rd edn). New York: Academic Press, 2001.
5. Crumpacker CS. 'Molecular targets of antiviral therapy'. *N Engl J Med* 321: 163–72, 1989.
6. Faulds D and Brogden RN. 'Didanosine'. *Drugs* 44(1): 96–116, 1992.
7. Gennaro AR. *Remington: The Science and Practice of Pharmacy* (21st edn). New York: Lippincot Williams and Wilkins, 2006.
8. Havlir DN and Richman DD. 'Antiretroviral therapy'. *Curr Opin Infect Dis* 8: 66–73, 1995.
9. Hirsch MS and D'Aquilla RT. 'Therapy for human immunodeficiency virus infection'. *N Engl J Med* 328: 1686– 695, 1993.
10. *Indian Pharmacopoeia*. Ministr y of Health and Family Welfare. New Delhi, 1996.
11. Knipe DM and Howley PM (ed). *Fundamental Virology* (4th edn). New York: Lippincott Williams and Wilkins, 2001.
12. Lemke TL and William DA. *Foye's Principle of Medicinal Chemistry* (6th edn). New York: Lippincott Williams and Wilkins, 2008.
13. Lednicer D and Mitscher LA. *The Organic Chemistry of Drug Synthesis*. New York: John Wiley, 1995.
14. Mansuri MM and Martin JC. 'Antiviral agents'. In *Annual Reports in Medicinal Chemistry*, Bristol JA (ed), pp. 133–40. San Diego, USA: Academic Press, 1991.
15. Reines EE and Gross PA. 'Antiviral agents'. *Med Clin North Am* 72: 691, 1988.
16. Sommadosi JP. 'Nucleoside analogs'. *Clin Infect Dis* 16: 57–515, 1993.
17. Wagner EK and Hewlett MJ (eds). *Basic Virology*. Malden, MA: Blackwell, 1999.
18. Zoon KC. *Human Interferons: Structure and Function*, pp. 1–12. London: Interferon Academic, 1987.

CHAPTER 19

Antiamoebic Agents

INTRODUCTION

Amoebiasis affects about 10% of the world's population, causing invasive diseases in about 50 million people and death in about 1,00,000 of these annually. This infection is, especially, common in lower socioeconomic groups and institutionalized individuals living under crowded and poor hygienic conditions. Two morphologically identical, but genetically and biochemically distinct, species of *Entamoeba* (*E. histolitica* and *E. dispar*) are the causative organisms. Human beings are the only host for this organisms. Ingested amoebic cysts from contaminated food or water survive and form acid gastric contents and transform them into trophozoites that usually cause colitis which is either acute or chronic (dysentery). In some cases, they target the brain and the liver producing abscesses and systemic diseases.

This parasitic disease is one of the major causes of illness and death in many countries. World Health Organization (WHO) has classified this disease as follows:

1. Asymptomatic
2. Symptomatic
    a. Intestinal amoebiasis
        i. Dysentery
        ii. Non-dysenteric colitis
        iii. Amoeboma
        iv. Amoebic appendicitis
    b. Extraintestinal amoebiasis
        i. Hepatic acute non-supporative
        ii. Liver abscesses
3. Cutaneous involvement of other organs

Lung, brain, and spleen without the obvious liver involvement are some examples under this category. Antiamoebic agents are drugs used to treat amoebiasis. The potential drug should be active within the bowel lumen, in the bowel wall, and particularly in the liver. Worldwide, nearly 480 million people are infected with *E. histolytica*, of whom 10% develope clinical disease. The infection is transmitted exclusively by the faecal–oral route; human beings are the only known hosts.

CLASSIFICATION OF AMOEBICIDES

I. **Luminal amoebicides:** Diloxanide furoate.
   It is active only against intestinal forms of amoeba.

II. **Systemic amoebicides:** Dihydroemetin and chloroquine.
   These agents have been employed primarily to treat severe amoebic dysentery or hepatic abscesses.

III. **Mixed amoebicides:** Metronidazole, tinidazole, and ornidazole.
   These agents are active against both intestinal and systemic forms of amoeba.

SYNTHESIS AND DRUG PROFILE

I. Luminal Amoebicides

i. **Diloxanide Furoate** (Furamide)

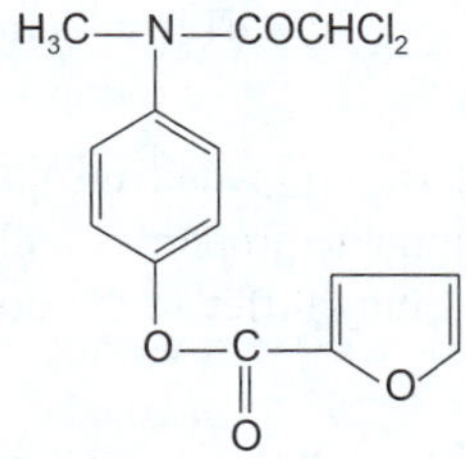

4-(2,2-Dichloro-N-methylacetamido)phenyl furan-2-carboxylate

Synthesis

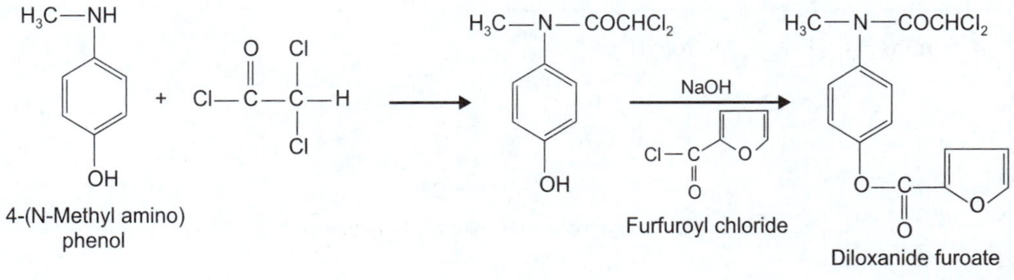

Metabolism: The diloxanide furoate is administered orally and is hydrolyzed in the gut to give diloxanide.

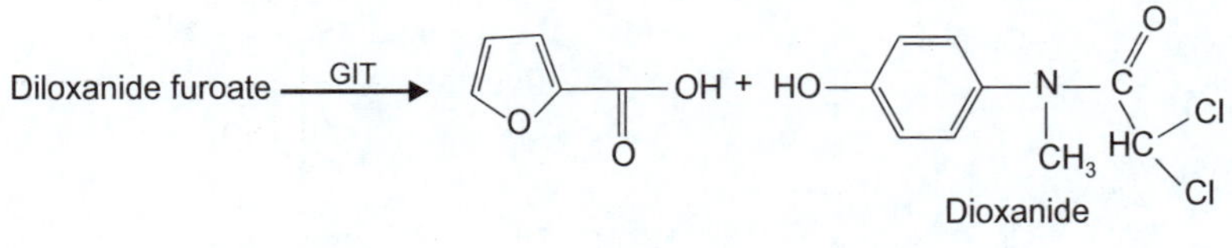

Properties and uses: Diloxanide furoate is a white crystalline powder, very slightly soluble in water, slightly soluble in ethanol and ether. It is dichloro acetamide derivative that is non-toxic, mainly used in the treatment of chronic amoebiasis. It is less effective in the treatment of acute intestinal amoebiasis.

Assay: Dissolve the sample in anhydrous pyridine and titrate against 0.1 M tetrabutylammonium hydroxide. Determine the end point potentiometrically.

Dose: The recommended oral dose is 500 mg three times daily for 10 days (Diloxanide furoate 250 mg + Tinidazole 300 mg) two tablets daily. Diloxanide furoate 250 mg + Metronidazole 250 mg two tablets thrice daily for 10 days.

Dosage forms: Diloxanide tablets BP.

II. Systemic Amoebicides

1. Dihydroemetine

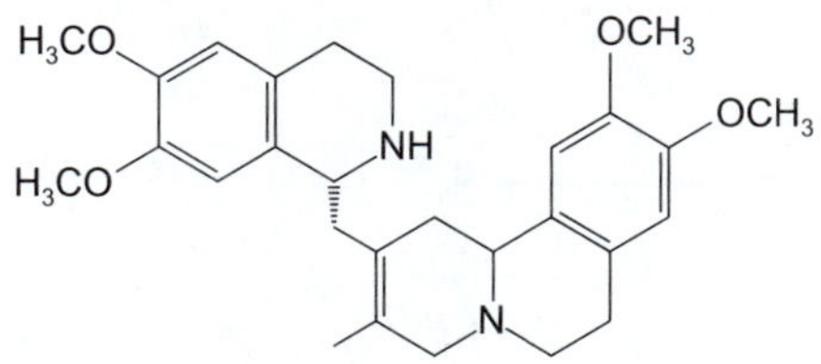

Properties and uses: It is a colorless, odorless powder, insoluble in water but soluble in organic solvents. It is similar to emetine in its antiamoebic properties with fewer side effects. The structure of emetine and dihydroemetine are similar but they differ in the presence of double bond near to ethyl group. It is used as an antiamoebic agent.

2. Chloroquine

Refer 'Antimalarials' Chapter 20 pg no. 480.

III. Mixed Amoebicides

1. Metronidazole (Flagyl, Metrogyl)

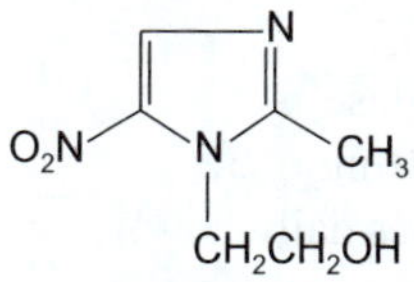

2-(2-Methyl-5-nitro-1*H*-imidazol-1-yl)ethanol

Synthesis

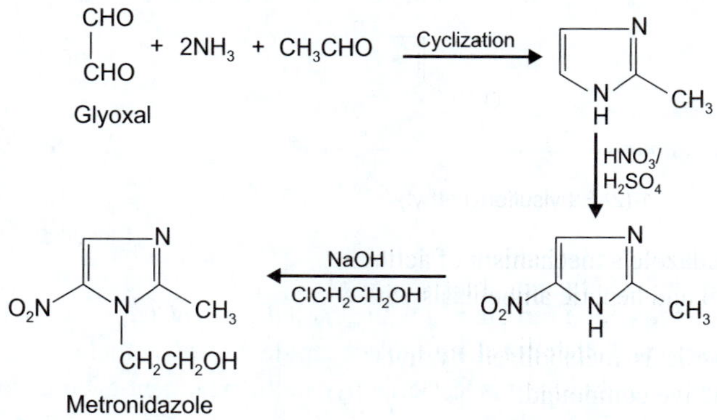

Mode of action: The reactive intermediate formed in the parasital reduction of the 5-nitro group of metronidazole covalently binds to the DNA of the parasite and triggers the lethal effects. Potential reactive intermediates include the nitroxide, nitroso, hydroxylamine, and amine.

Metabolism: In the liver, metabolism of metronidazole leads to two major metabolites, hydroxylation of the 2-methyl group to 2-hydroxymethyl metronidazole and oxidation to metronidazole acetic acid (MAA).

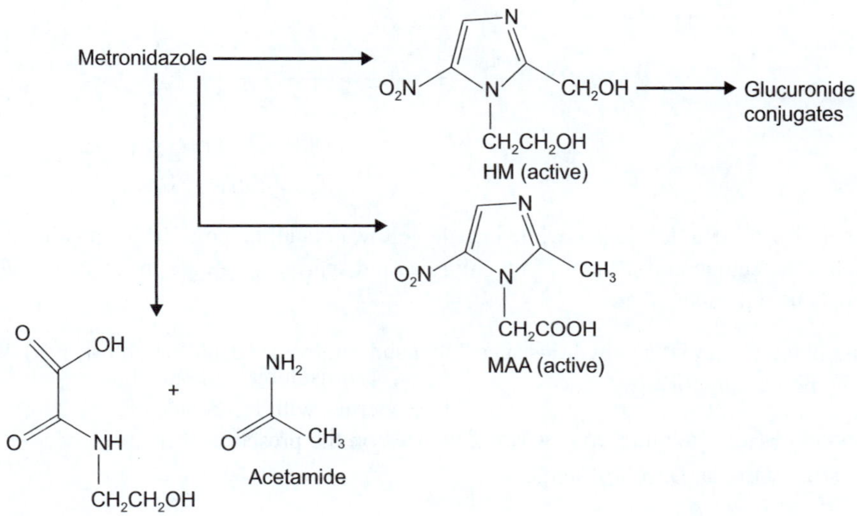

Properties and uses: Metronidazole is a white or yellowish crystalline powder, slightly soluble in water, acetone, alcohol, and methylene chloride. It is used in the treatment of intestinal and hepatic amoebiasis.

Assay: Dissolve the sample in anhydrous acetic acid and titrate with 0.1 M perchloric acid. Determine the end point potentiometrically.

Dose: For amoebiasis, the administered dose is 750 mg orally three times a day for 5–10 days. For trichomoniasis, the prescribed dose is 250 mg orally three times a day for 7 days. For giardiasis, the prescribed dose is 250 mg orally three times daily for 5–7 days.

Dosage forms: Metronidazole gel BP, metronidazole intravenous infusion BP, metronidazole suppositories BP, metronidazole tablets BP.

2. **Tinidazole** (Fasigyn)

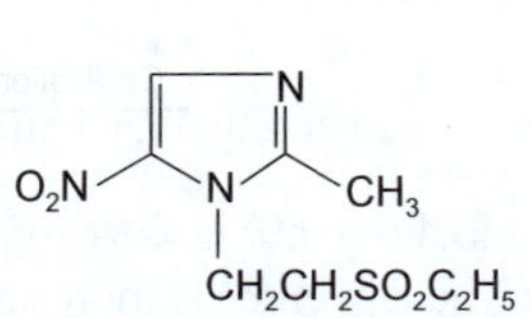

1-(2-(Ethylsulfonyl)ethyl)-2-methyl-5-nitro-1*H*-imidazole

Mode of action: Tinidazole's mechanism of action is similar to that of metronidazole. It is used in the treatment of intestinal and hepatic amoebiasis with a potential greater efficacy than metronidazole.

Metabolism: Tinidazole is metabolized by hydroxylation at the 2-methyl group and catalyzed by CYP3A4 to form inactive compound.

Synthesis

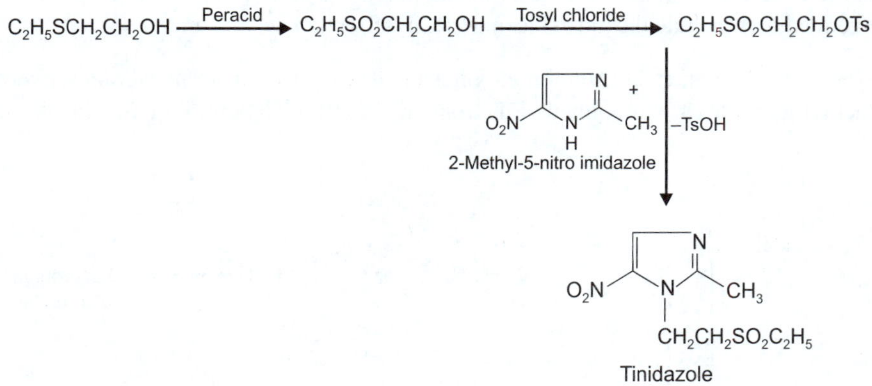

Properties and uses: Tinidazole is a white or pale yellow crystalline powder, practically insoluble in water, soluble in acetone and in methylene chloride, and sparingly soluble in methanol. Used as an antiprotozoal and antibacterial agent.

Assay: Dissolve the sample in anhydrous acetic acid and titrate with 0.1 M perchloric acid. Determine the end point potentiometrically.

Dose: For giardiasis, the administered dose is 2 mg as a single dose.

3. **Ornidazole** (Ornida, Dazolic, Onidaz)

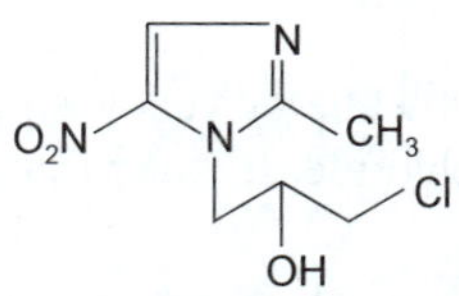

1-Chloro-3-(2-methyl-5-nitro-1*H*-imidazol-1-yl)propan-2-ol

Synthesis

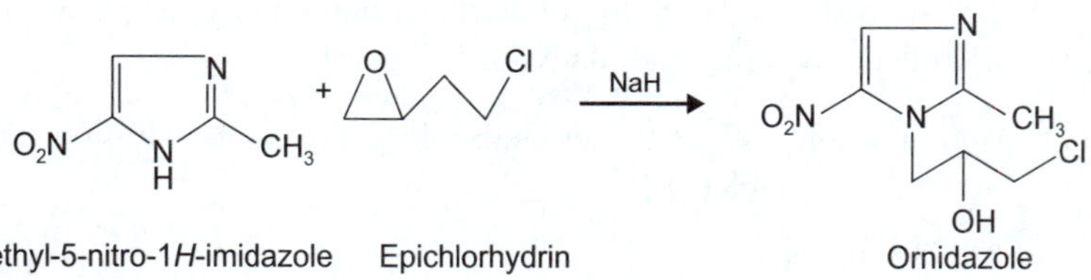

Properties and uses: It has a longer duration of action than metronidazole and used as an antiprotozoal.

Dose: The administered dose for amoebic dysentery in the case of adults is 1.5 g as a single daily dose for 3 days. Alternatively, for patients, whose weight is more than 60 kg, the dose is 1 g two times a day for 3 days. In the case of a child, the administered dose is 40 mg/kg daily. For amoebiasis, the recommended dose for adults is 5 g two times a day for 5–10 days. And in the case of a children, the dose is 25 mg/kg as a single daily dose for 5–10 days.

For giardiasis, in the case of adults, the dose is 1–1.5 g as a single daily dose for 1–2 days. In the case of a child, the dose is 30–40 mg/kg daily. In the case of trichomoniasis, the dose for adults is 1.5 g as a single daily dose or 0.5 g two times a day for 5 days. Treat sexual partners concomitantly. In the case of child, the dose is 25 mg/kg as a single dose. In the case of intravenous administration, during severe amoebic dysentery and amoebic liver abscess the prescribed dose for adults initially is 0.5–1 g infusion followed by 0.5 g every 12 hrs for 3–6 days. For a child, the dose is 20–30 mg/kg body weight daily.

4. Nitazoxanide

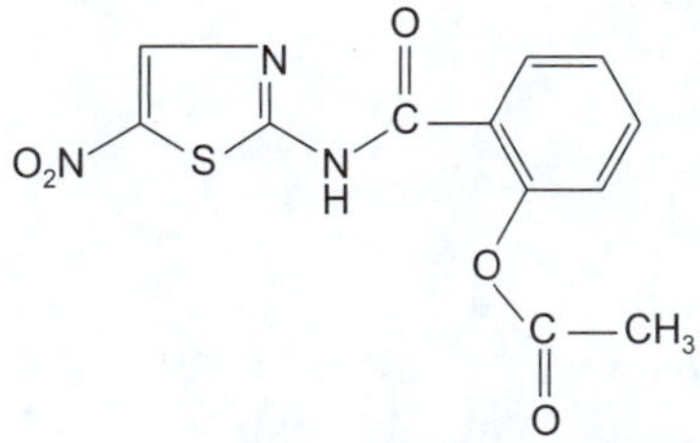

2-((5-Nitrothiazol-2-yl)carbamoyl)phenyl acetate

Synthesis

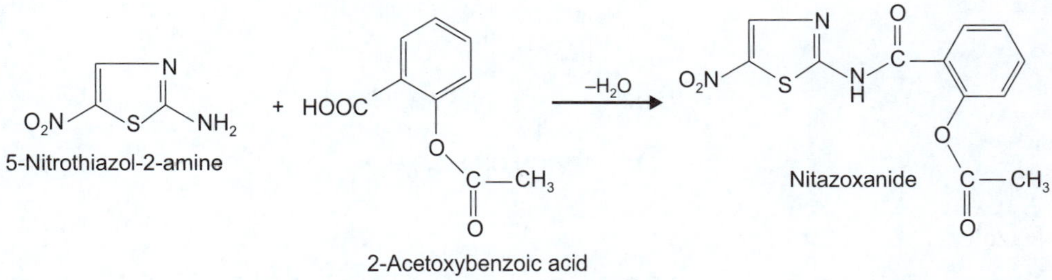

Mode of action: Nitazoxanide is a member of the 5-nitro heterocylces and is a prodrug forming a shortlived redox active intermediate. It appears to be more selective than metronidazole.

Uses: Used as an antiprotozoal agent.

5. Nimorazole (Nitroimidazole)

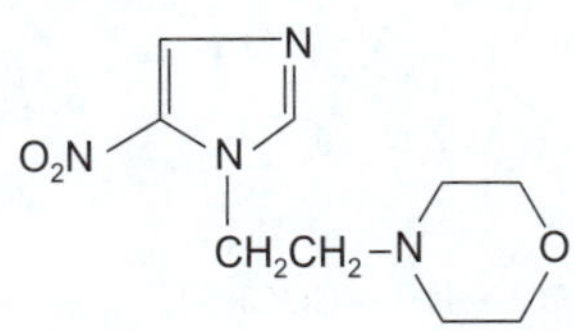

Synthesis

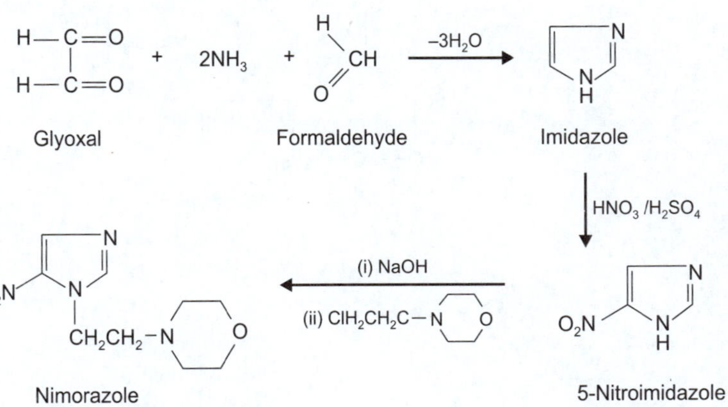

Properties and uses: It possesses antiamoebic activity, and hence, used against intestinal and hepatic amoebiasis.

CLASSIFICATION BASED ON PCI SYLLABUS

Metronidazole

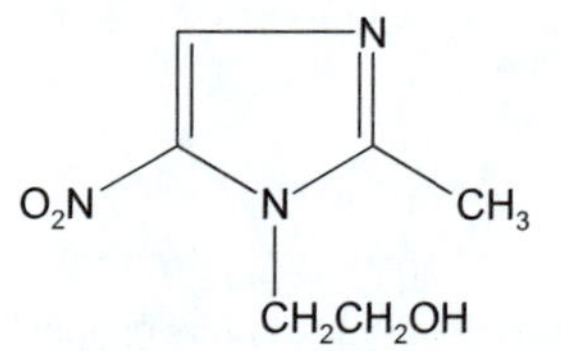

Tinidazole

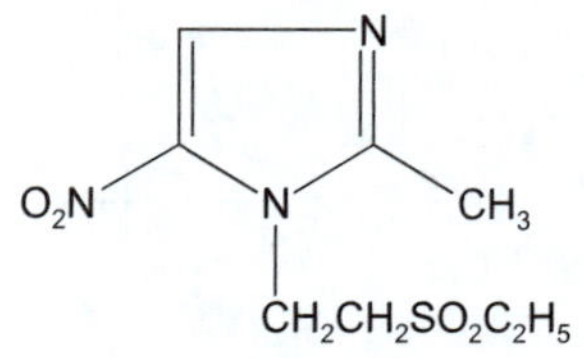

Ornidazole

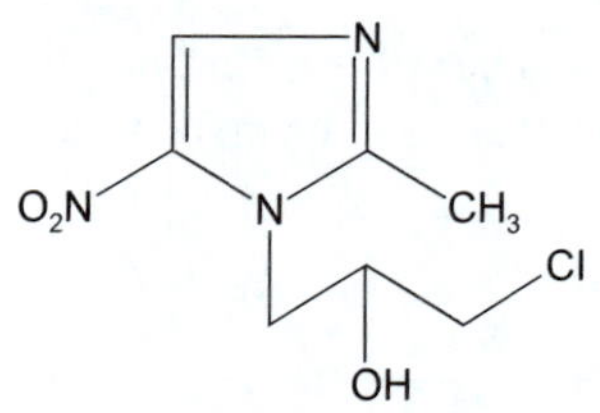

Diloxanide

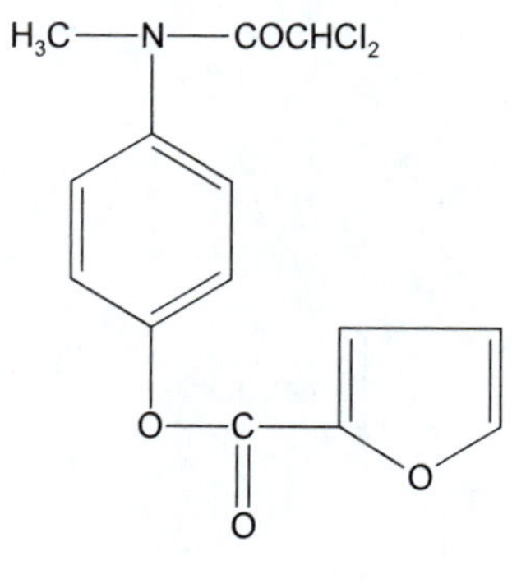

Iodoquinol

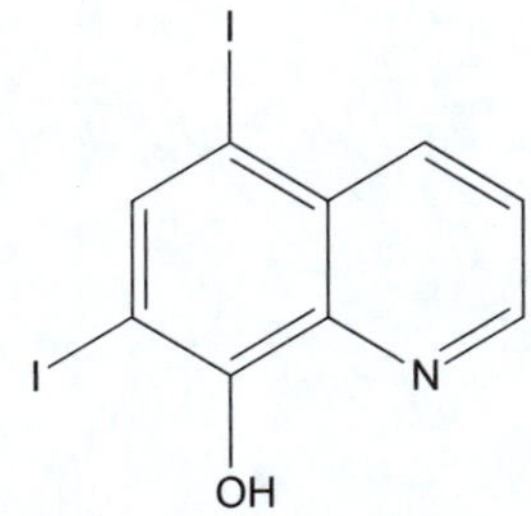

Pentamidine

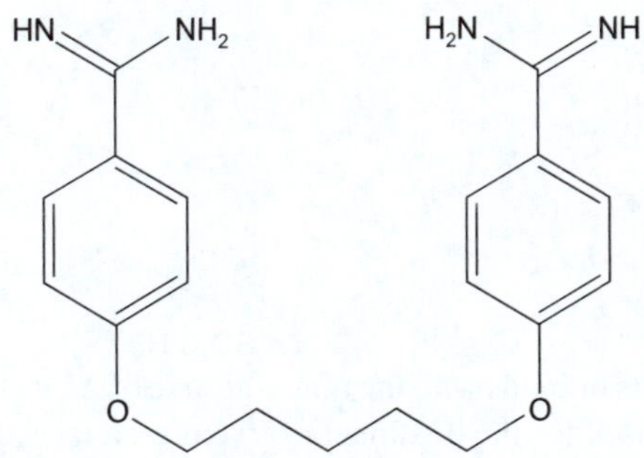

Isethionate

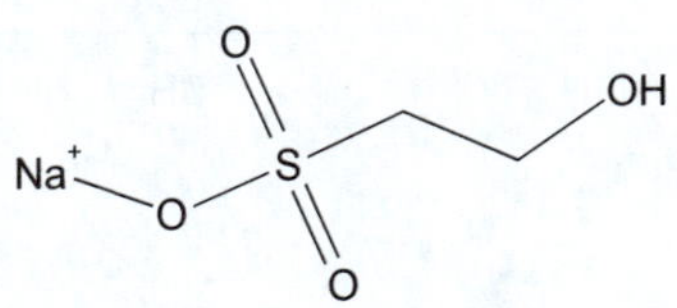

Atovaquone

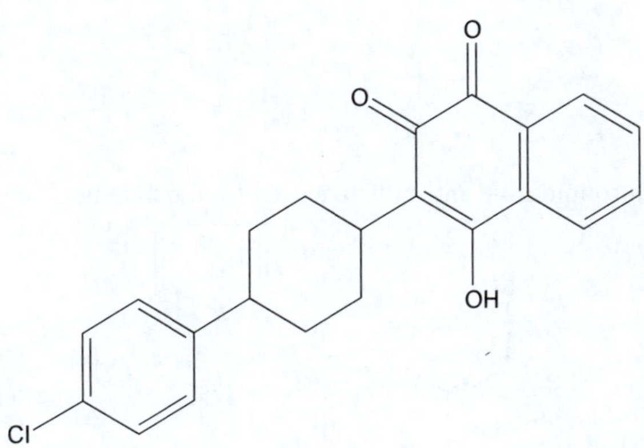

Eflornithine

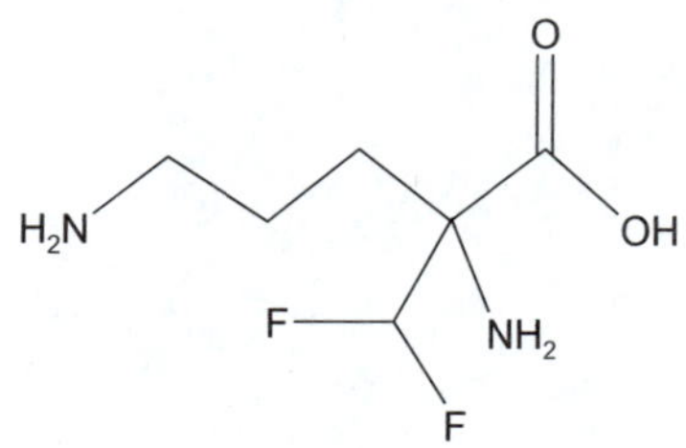

Pentamidine Isothionate

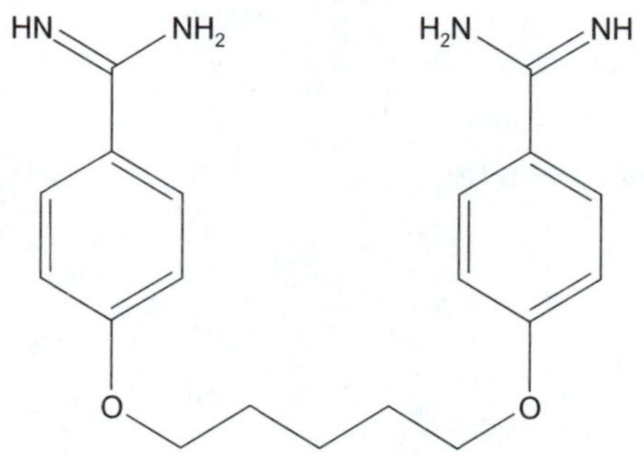

Properties and uses: It interacts or binds with the minor groove of AT-rich DNA and prevents the DNA replication and function. It is used for the treatment of trypanosomiasis, leishmaniasis and few fungal infections. It also used to treat pnemocystis carinii, pneumomia in HIV-infected patients.

Newer Agents

Secnidazole

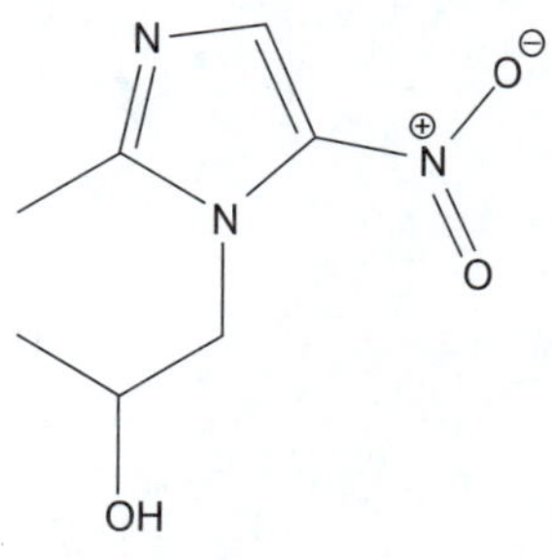

Uses: Secnidazole is a nitroimidazole anti-infective used for the treatment of dientamoebiasis.

Triclabendazole

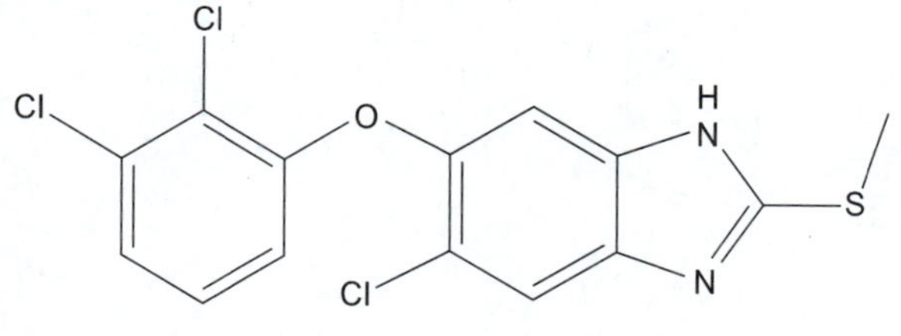

Uses: It is used to treat fascioliasis and paragonimia.

PROBABLE QUESTIONS

1. Classify antiamoebic agents and write the synthesis of any three of them.
2. Write synthesis, metabolism, and uses of diloxanide furoate, metronidazole, and tinidazole.

SUGGESTED READINGS

1. Abraham DJ (ed). *Burger's Medicinal Chemistry and Drug Discovery* (6th edn). New Jersey: John Wiley, 2007.
2. Archer S. 'The chemotherapy of schistosomiasis'. *Ann Rev Pharmacol Toxicol* 25: 485, 1985.
3. Bruntan LL, Lazo JS, and Parker KL. *Goodman and Gilman's: The Pharmacological Basis of Therapeutics* (11th edn). New York: McGraw Hill, 2006.
4. *British Pharmacopoeia*. Medicines and Healthcare Products Regulatory Agency. London, 2008.
5. Freeman CD, Klutman NE, and Lamp KC. 'Metronidazole: A therapeutic review and update'. *Drugs* 54: 679–708, 1997.
6. Gennaro AR. *Remington: The Science and Practice of Pharmacy* (21st edn). New York: Lippincot Williams and Wilkins, 2006.
7. Gutteridge WEE. 'New antiprotozoal agents'. *Int J Parasitol* 17: 121–29, 1987.
8. Harries J. 'Amoebiasis—a review'. *J R Soc Med* 75: 190–97, 1982.
9. *Indian Pharmacopoeia*. Ministry of Health and Family Welfare. New Delhi, 1996.
10. Lednicer D and Mitscher LA. *The Organic Chemistry of Drug Synthesis*. New York: John Wiley, 1995.
11. Lemke TL and William DA. *Foye's Principle of Medicinal Chemistry* (6th edn). New York: Lippincott Williams and Wilkins, 2008.
12. Mandel GL, Bennett JE, and Dolin R (eds). *Principles and Practices of Infectious Diseases*, Vol. I (4th edn). New York: Churchill-Livingstone, 1995.
13. Meshnick SR. 'The chemotherapy of African trypanosomiasis'. In *Parasitic Diseases*, Vol. 2, Mansfield JM (ed), pp.165–99. New York: Marcel Dekker, 1984.
14. Reynolds EF (ed). *Martindale the Extra Pharmacopoeia* (31st edn). London: The Pharmaceutical Press, 1997.
15. Testa B (ed). *Advances in Drug Research*, Vol. 21. New York: Academic Press, 1991.
16. Wilson JD et al. (ed). *Harrison's Principles of Internal Medicine* (12th edn), p. 772. New York: McGraw Hill, 1992.
17. Woolfe G. 'The chemotherapy of amoebiasis'. In *Progress in Drug Research*, Vol. 8, Jucker E (ed), pp. 11–52. Basel, Switzerland: Brikhauser Verlag, 1965.

CHAPTER 20

Antimalarials

INTRODUCTION

Antimalarial agents are drugs used for the treatment or prophylaxis of malaria. Malaria is caused by four species of *Plasmodium*, such as *Plasmodium falciparum*, *P. malariae*, *P. ovale*, and *P. vivax*. Three of which produce the mild forms of malaria by destroying red blood cells in peripheral capillaries and thus, causing anaemia. The bouts of fever correspond to the reproductive cycle of the parasite. However, the most dangerous is the *P. falciparum*. In this case, the infected red blood cells become sticky and form lumps in the capillaries of the deep organs of the body and cause microcirculatory arrest. This disease still affects about 200 millions people and causes at least 2 million deaths per year.

LIFE CYCLE OF *PLASMODIUM*

The different stages of the reproductive cycle (Figure 20.1) of the malarial parasite and the drugs acting at different stages of this cycle are given below.

- Stage I: No drug is effective in this stage.
- Stage II: Primaquine and pyrimethamine can block at this stage.
- Stage III: Primaquine can only prevent because fever occurs at this stage.
- Stage IV: Chloroquine, amodiaquine, santoquine, proguanil.
- Stage V: Primaquine only.

Two important phases of the parasite life cycle are the following:

1. Asexual cycle—occurs in the infected host.
2. Sexual cycle—occurs in the mosquito.

After the insect bite, the parasite forms rapidly. They leave the circulation and localize in the hepatocytes whereby they transform, multiply, and develop into tissue schizonts. The primary asymptomatic tissue stage lasts for 15 days and the tissue schizonts rupture, each releasing thousands of merozites. The released merozites invade more erythrocytes to continue the cycle's synchronous rupture of erythrocytes to continue the cycle. Synchronous rupture of erythrocytes and release of merozytes into the circulation leads to febrile pattern attacks on day 1 and 3; hence, the designation is 'tertian malaria'. Some erythrocyte parasites differentiate into several forms known as gametophytes. After infecting human blood, female mosquito ingests them. Then the exflagellation of male gametocyte is followed by the male gametogenesis and the fertilization of the female gametocytes in the insect's guts. The resulting zygote, which develops as an oocyte in the gut wall, eventually gives rise to infective sporozoite, which invades the salivary glands of the mosquito. The insect then can infect another human by taking a blood meal.

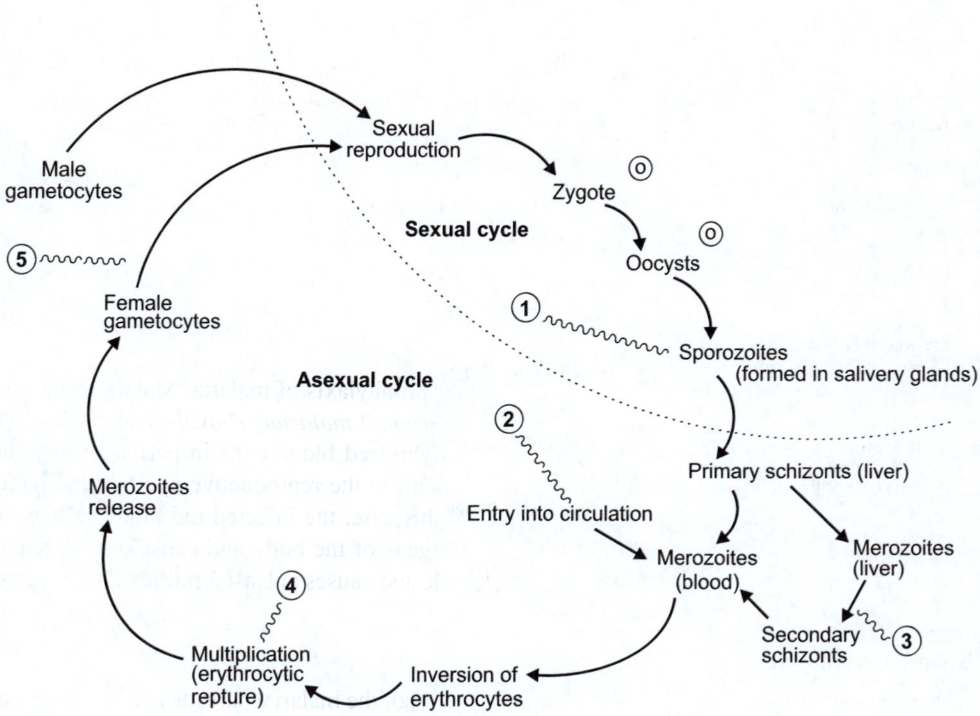

Figure 20.1: Life cycle of *Plasmodium*.

CLASSIFICATION

I. Cinchona alkaloids

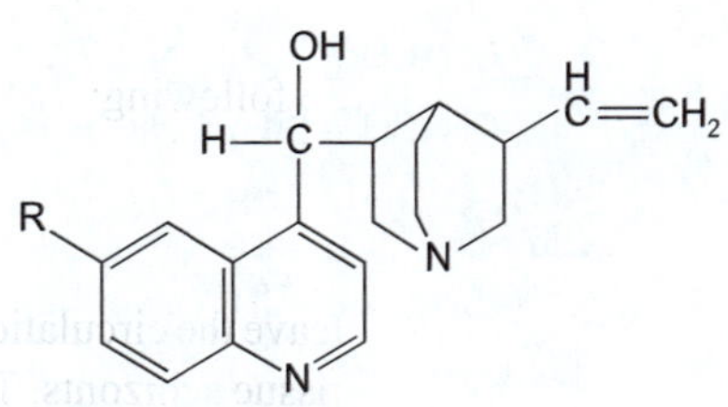

Name	*R*
Quinine	$-OCH_3$, (–)-isomer
Quinidine	$-OCH_3$, (+)-isomer (used as antiarrhythmic)
Cinchonine	–H, (+)-isomer
Cinchonidine	–H, (–)-isomer

II. 7-Chloro-4-amino quinolines

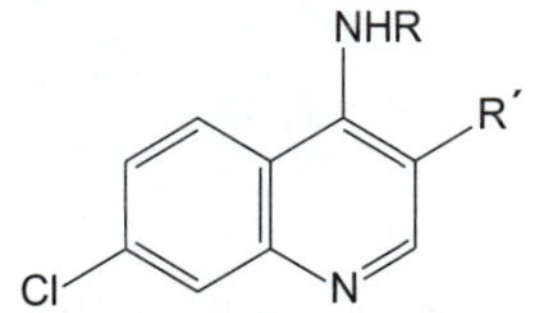

Name	*R*	*R′*
Chloroquine	$-CH(CH_3)(CH_2)_3-N(C_2H_5)_2$	–H
Amodiaquine	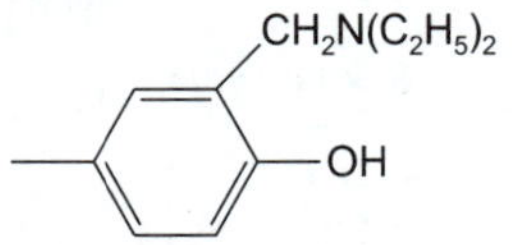	–H
Hydroxychloroquine	$-CH(CH_3)-(CH_2)_3-N(C_2H_5)(CH_2)_2OH$	–H
Sontoquine	$-CH(CH_3)-(CH_2)_3-N(C_2H_5)_2$	$-CH_3$
Amopyroquine	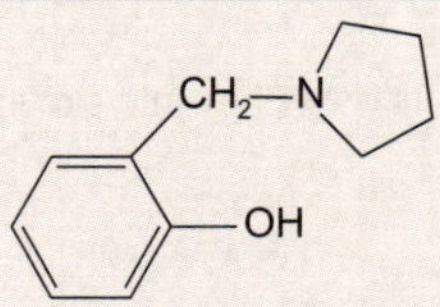	–H

III. 8-Amino quinolines

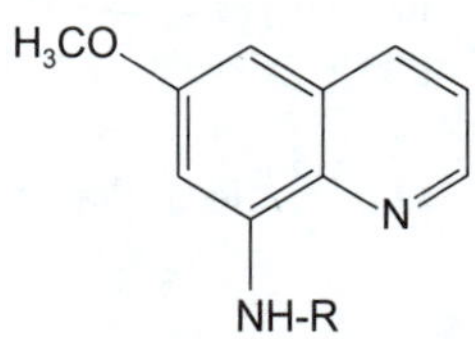

6-Methoxy-8-amino quinoline derivatives

Name	*R*
Primaquine	$-CH(CH_3)-(CH_2)_3-NH_2$
Pamaquine	$-CH(CH_3)-(CH_2)_3-N(C_2H_5)_2$
Pentaquine phosphate	$-(CH_2)_5-NH-CH(CH_3)_2$
Isopentaquine	$-CH(CH_3)-(CH_2)_3-NH-CH(CH_3)_2$
Quinocide HCl	$-(CH_2)_3-CH(CH_3)-N(C_2H_5)_2$

IV. Acridine derivatives (9-amino acridine derivatives)

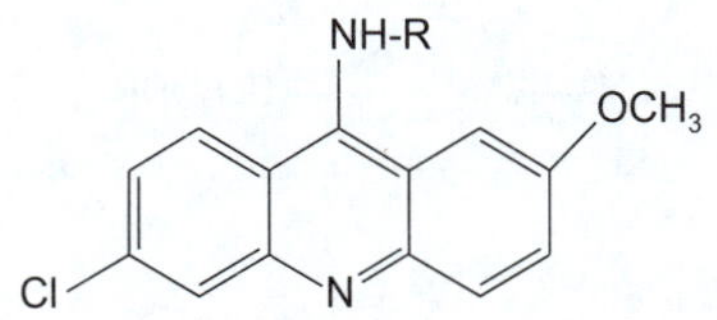

Name	*R*
Quinacrine	$-CH(CH_3)-(CH_2)_3-N(C_2H_5)_2$
Acriquine	$-(CH_2)_4-N(C_2H_5)_2$

V. Antifolates

a. Biguanides

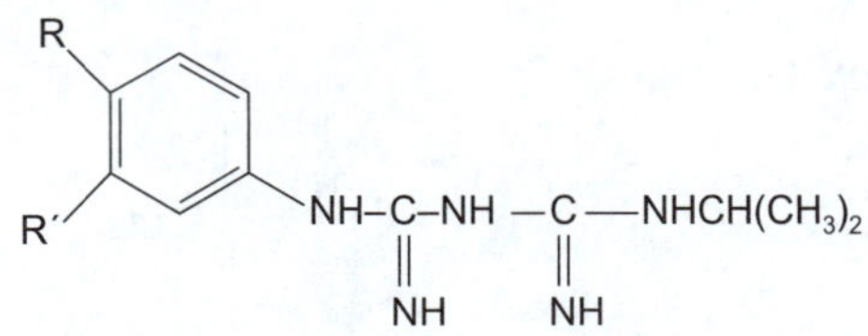

Name	*R*	*R′*
Proguanil	–Cl	–H
Chloro proguanil	–Cl	–Cl
Bromoguanil	–Br	–H
Nitroguanil	$-NO_2$	–H

b. Diamino pyrimidines

Pyrimethamine (Daraprim)

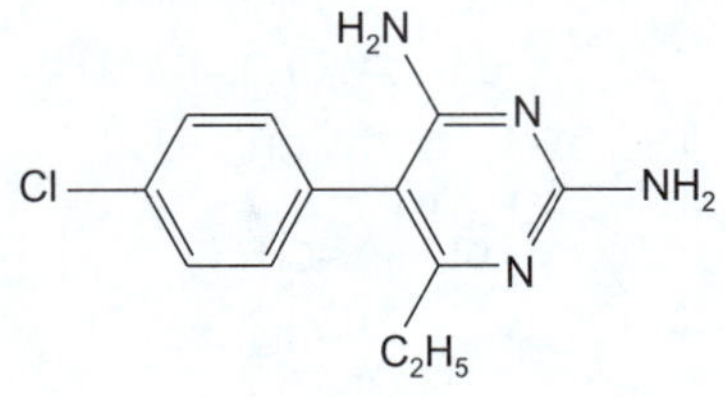

Trimethoprim

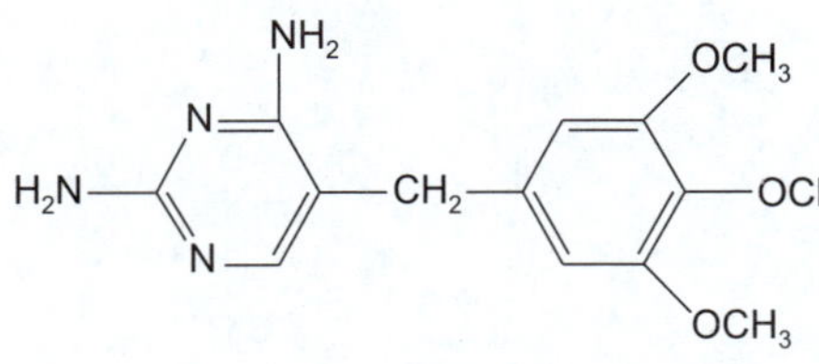

VI. Sulphonamides and sulphones

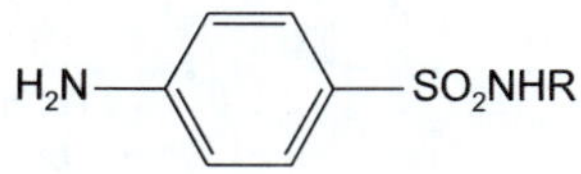

Name	*R*
Sulphadoxine	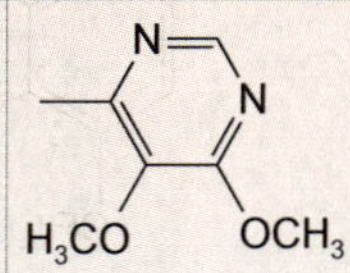
Sulphadiazine	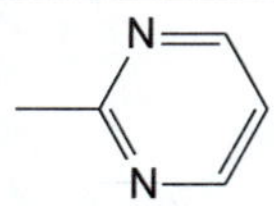
Sulphamethoxazole	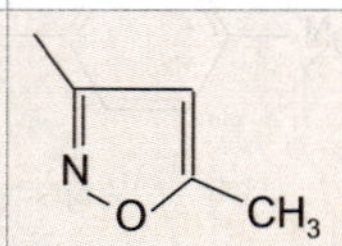
Sulphalene	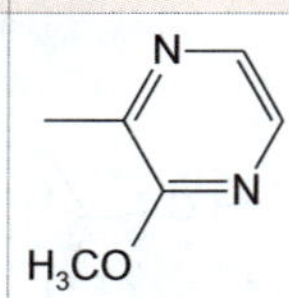

VII. Phenanthrene methanol derivatives

Halofantrine (Hafan)

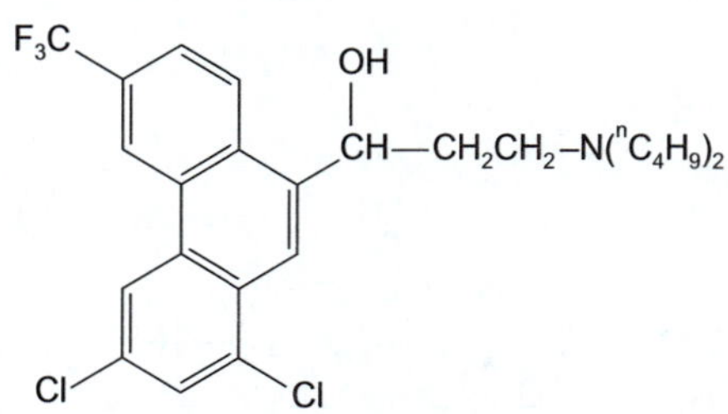

VIII. Miscellaneous drugs

Mefloquine

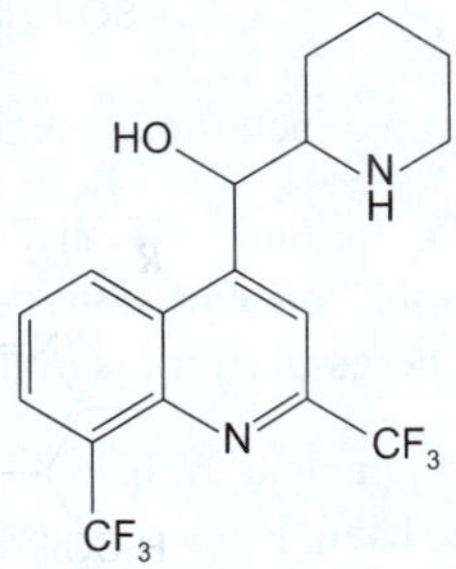

Dapsone

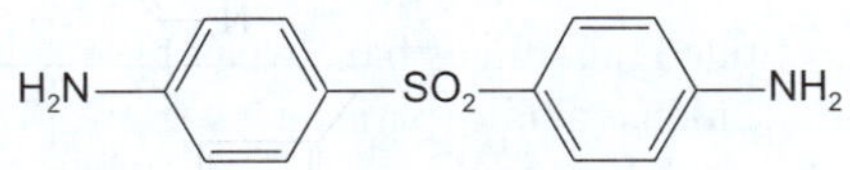

Artemether and artemotil or β-arte-ether

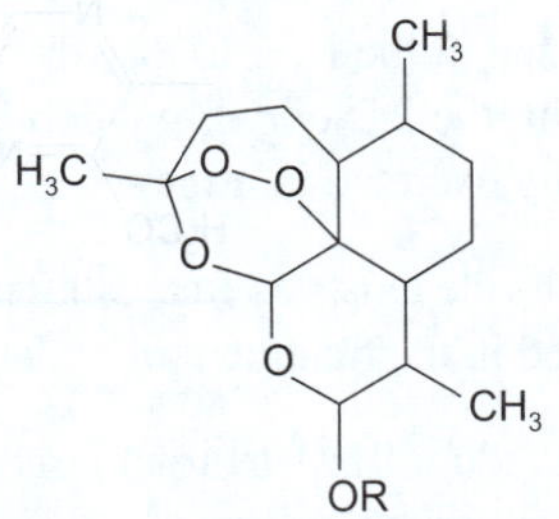

$R = CH_3$; Artemether

$R = C_2H_5$; Arte-ether

Artesunate

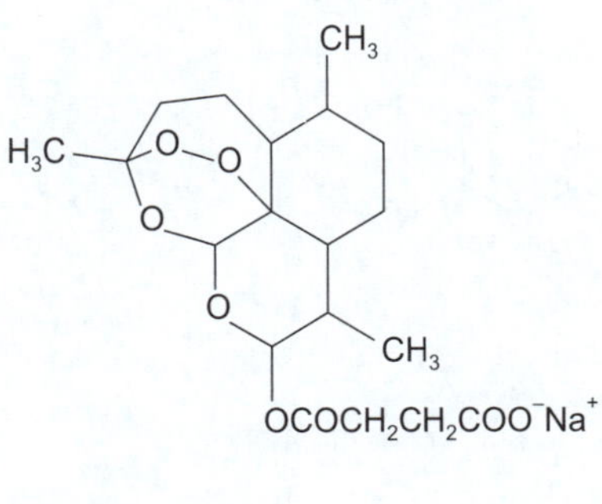

SYNTHESIS AND DRUG PROFILE

I. 4-Substituted Quinolines

Mode of action: Three different mechanism of actions are suggested for these drugs:

DNA interaction: The mechanism of action for quinine is that the drug gets intercalated into the DNA of the parasite. It is based on the fact that the concentration required for the inhibition of nucleic acid synthesis is significantly higher than that necessary for the inhibition of the *Plasmodium* parasite.

Ferriprotoporphyrin IX: The plasmodium parasite utilizes host haemoglobin as a source of amino acid. On digestion of the haemoglobin, the haem is released as ferriprotoporphyrins IX and it produces haemolysis of the erythrocyte parasites. Therefore, ferriprotoporphyrin that is released is converted into non-toxic products and they, in turn, to haemozoites by the polymerase enzyme. The steps involved in the conversion to haemozoites are inhibited by the chloroquine.

Weak base hypothesis: The 4-substituted quinolines have weak base and because of this pK_a they are thought to accumulate in a location, which is acidic (parasite lysozome pH 4.8–5.2). As the extracellular fluid of the parasite is at pH 7.4, the weak base will move towards a more acidic pH of lysosome. Once the acid–base reaction occurs, elevating the pH in the lysozome, that in turn reduces the parasite's ability to digest haemoglobin, thus reducing the availability of amino acids.

Metabolism of quinine: It is metabolized in the liver to 2-hydroxy derivative followed by additional hydroxylation on the quinoline ring with the 2,3-dihydroxy derivative, as the major metabolite. This metabolite has low activity and is rapidly excreted in urine.

Properties and uses: Quinine hydrochloride exists as fine, silky needles, often in clusters, colourless, soluble in water and in alcohol. It is used in the treatment of malaria.

Assay: Dissolve the sample in alcohol, add 0.01 M hydrochloric acid, and titrate with 0.1 M sodium hydroxide. Determine the end point potentiometrically.

Chloroquine (Nivaquin, Aralen, Lariago)

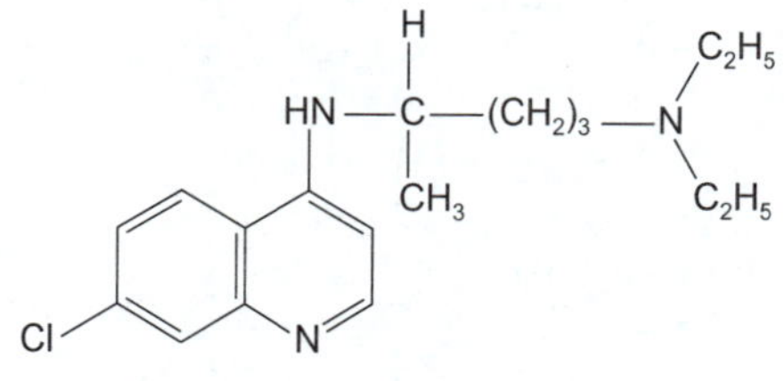

Synthesis

Step I. Synthesis of 4,7-dichloroquinoline

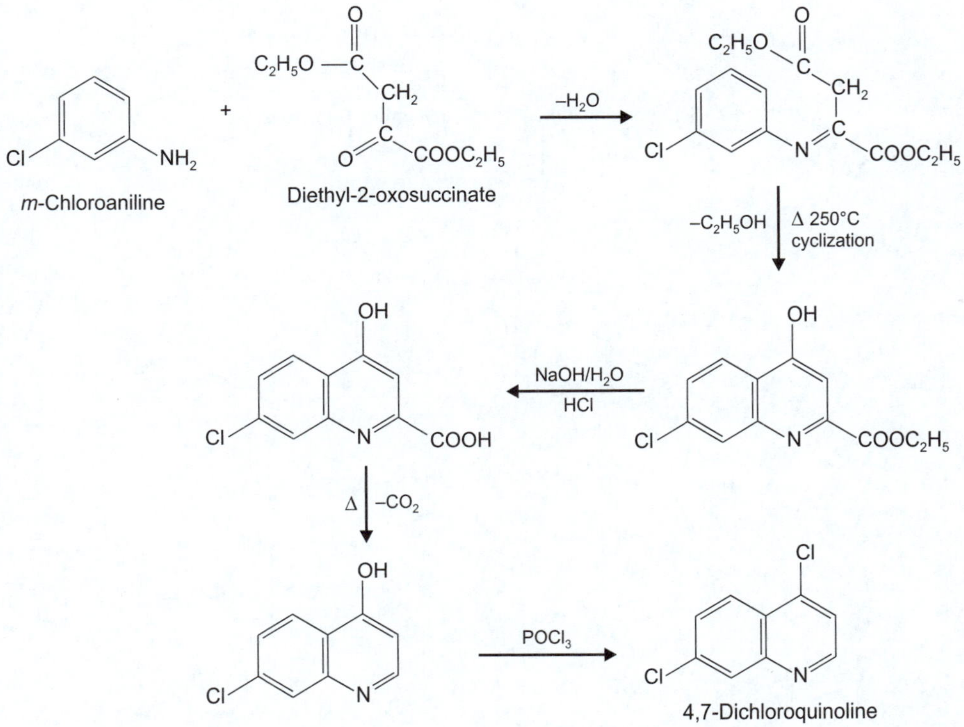

Step II: Preparation of 1-diethylamino-4-amino pentane

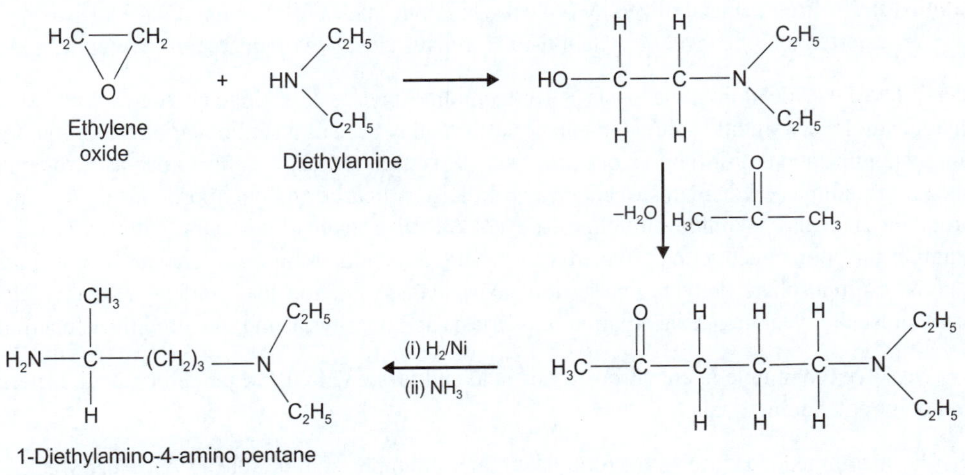

Step III. Condensation of the products of *Steps I* and *II.*

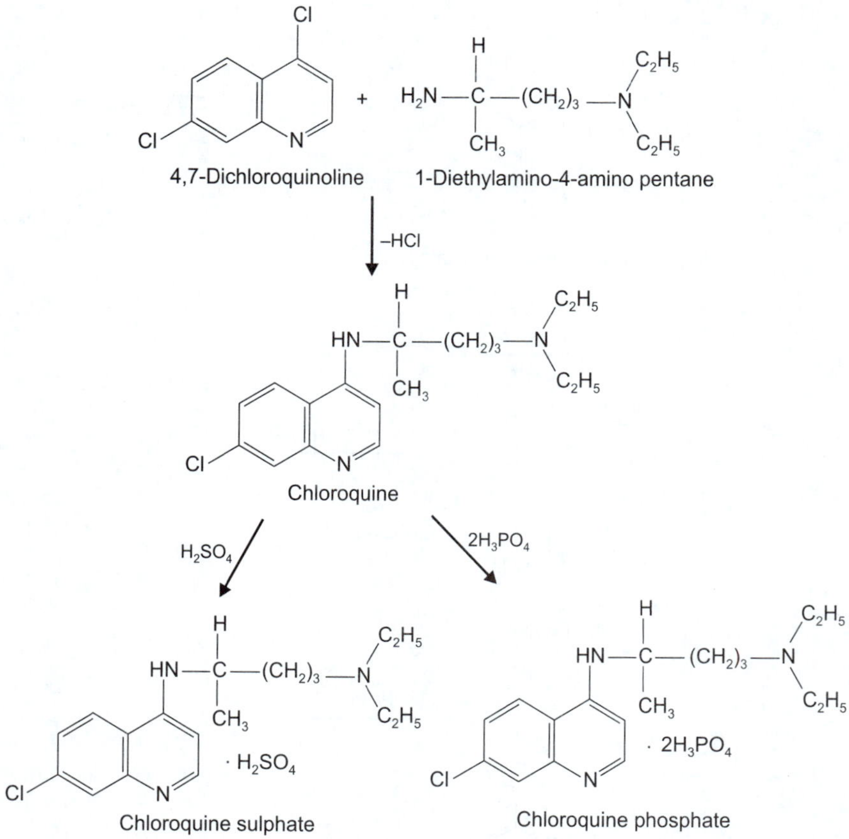

Metabolism: The drug is metabolized by N-dealkylation through CYP2D6 and CYP3A4 isoenzymes. It has been reported that the level of metabolism correlates closely with degree of resistance.

Properties and uses: Chloroquine exists as white or almost white crystalline powder, soluble in water and in methanol, very slightly soluble in ethanol. It is mainly used as an antimalarial. Chloroquine also has antihistaminic and anti-inflammatory properties. It is used to treat hepatic amoebiasis, rheumatoid arthritis, discoid lupus erythematosus, cutanea tards, solar urticaria, and polymorphous light eruptions. Chloroquine and other 4-amino quinolines are not effective against exoerythrocytic parasites. It is an example for poor selective toxicity. Adverse reactions include retinopathy, haemolysis in patients with glucose-6-phosphate dehydrogenase deficiency (same mutation that confers resistance against malaria), muscular weakness, exacerbation of psoriasis and porphyria, and impaired liver function.

Assay: Dissolve the sample in anhydrous acetic acid and titrate with 0.1 M perchloric acid. Determine the end point potentiometrically.

Dose: The recommended dose as a prophylactic and a suppressive is 500 mg once per week. As a therapeutic the dose, initially, is 1 g followed by 500 mg in 6 hrs, and 500 mg on the second and third days.

Dosage forms: Chloroquine sulphate injection IP, BP, chloroquine sulphate tablets IP, BP.

Amodiaquine HCl (Camoquin)

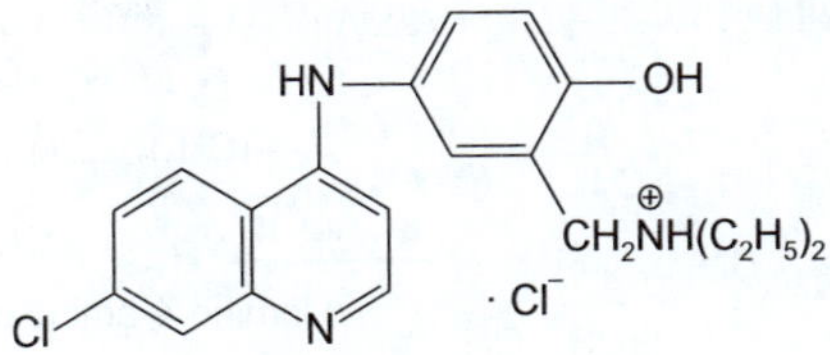

Synthesis

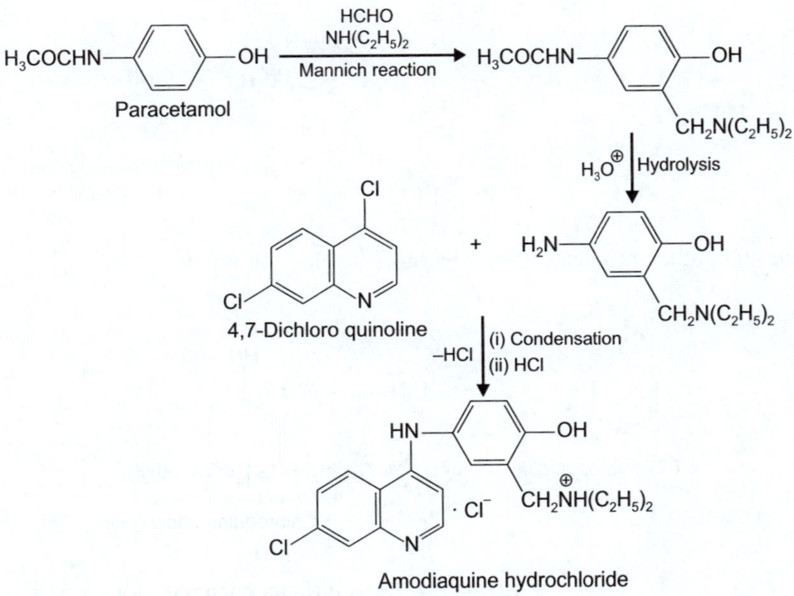

Properties and uses: It exists as yellow crystalline powder with a bitter taste, and is soluble in water. It is very similar to chloroquine and does not have any advantages over the other 4-amino quinoline drugs. It is used for suppressing *P. vivax* and *P. falciparum* infections being 3–4 times more active than quinine.

Dose: The recommended dose initially is 600 mg followed by 300 mg doses 6, 24, and 48 hrs later.

Hydroxychloroquine (Plaquenil)

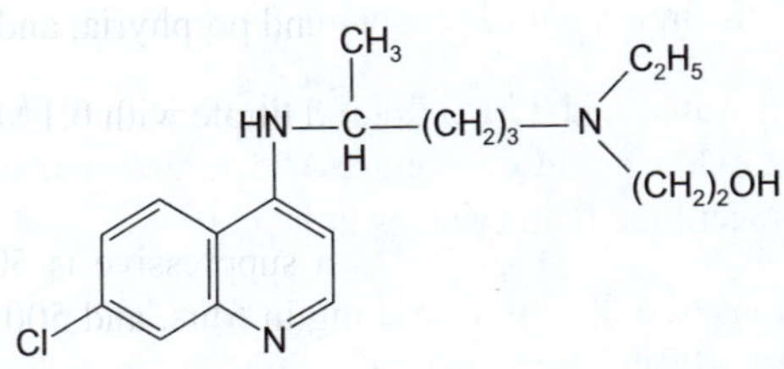

Synthesis

Step I. Preparation of side chain-N-ethyl-N-(2-hydroxyethyl)-4-amino pentylamine

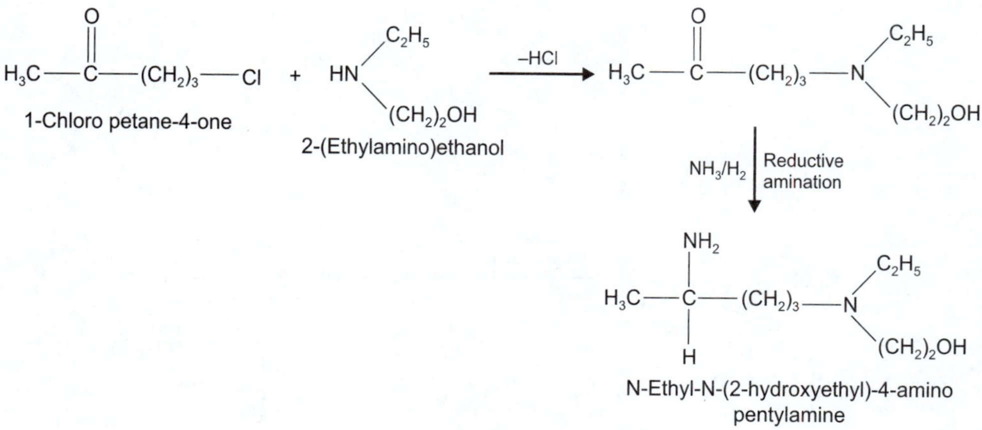

Step II. Condensation of the product of *Step I* with 4,7-dichloro quinoline

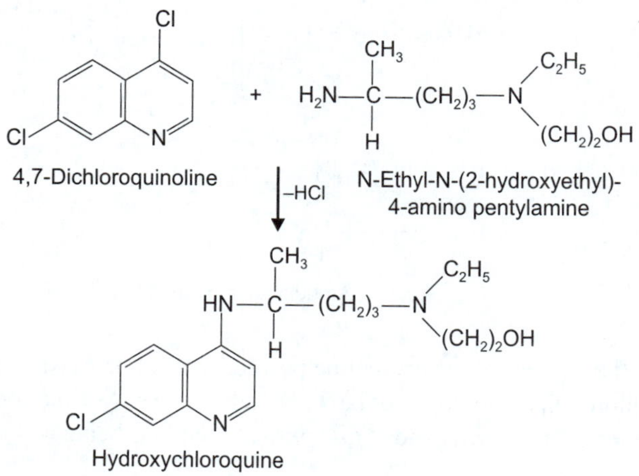

Properties and uses: Hydroxychloroquine is a white or almost white crystalline powder, soluble in water, practically insoluble in ethanol and in ether. It is equivalent to the chloroquine, but it is less toxic and used in the place of chloroquine against normally sensitive strains. It is mainly used as an antimalarial. It is also used for the treatment of rheumatoid arthritis and lupus erythematoses.

Assay: Dissolve the sample in water, add 1 M sodium hydroxide, and extract with dichloromethane. Combine the dichloromethane extracts and evaporate. Add anhydrous acetic acid and titrate against 0.1 M perchloric acid, using oracet blue B solution as indicator.

Dose: In *P. falciparum* infections, the dose is 1.25 g in a single dose or in two divided doses at 6 hrs intervals; in rheumatoid arthritis, 400 mg daily; in lupus erythematosus, 200 to 400 mg one or two times daily.

Dosage forms: Hydroxychloroquine tablets BP.

Structure–Activity Relationship

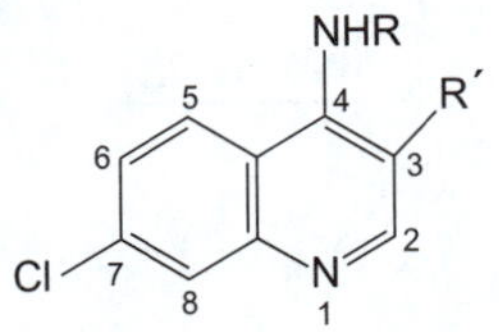

- At C-4 position, the dialkylaminoalkyl side chain has 2–5 carbon atoms between the nitrogen atoms, particularly the 4-diethylaminomethyl butyl amino side chain that is optimal for activity, as in chloroquine and quinacrine.
- The substitution of a hydroxyl group on one of the ethyl groups on the tertiary amine (hydroxy quinoline), reduces toxicity.
- Incorporation of an aromatic ring in the side chain (e.g. amodiaquine) gives a compound with reduced toxicity and activity.
- The tertiary amine in the side chain is important.
- The introduction of an unsaturated bond in the side chain was not detrimental to activity.
- The 7-chloro group in the quinoline nucleus is optimal, the methyl group in position 3 reduces activity, and an additional methyl group in position 8 abolishes activity.
- The D-isomer of chloroquine is less toxic than its L-isomer.

II. 8-Amino Quinolines

Mode of action: While the mechanism of action of the 8-amino quinolines is unknown, it is known that primaquine can generate reactive oxygen species via an autoxidation of the 8-amino quinoline group with the formation of radical anion. As a result, cell destructive oxidants, such as hydrogen peroxide, superoxide, and hydroxyl radical can be formed.

Primaquine (Primaquine phosphate)

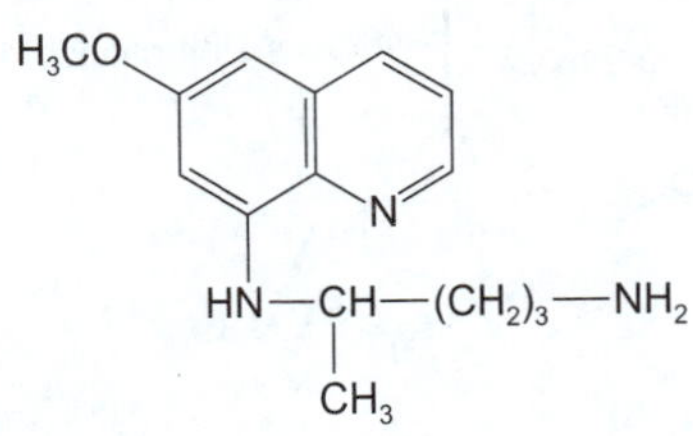

Synthesis

Step I. Preparation of 1-phthalimido-4-bromo pentane

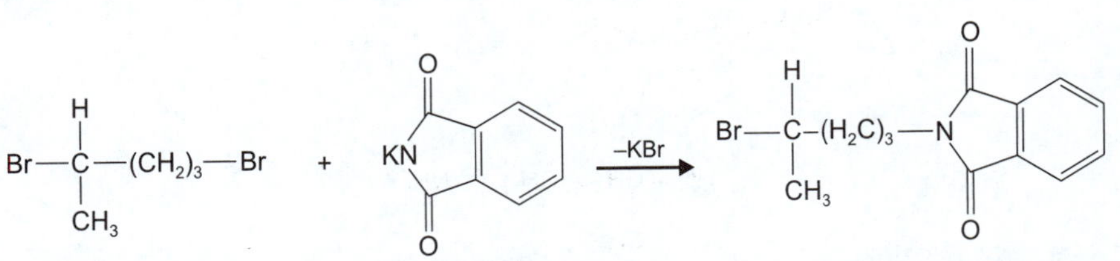

Step II. Synthesis of 8-amino-6-methoxy quinoline

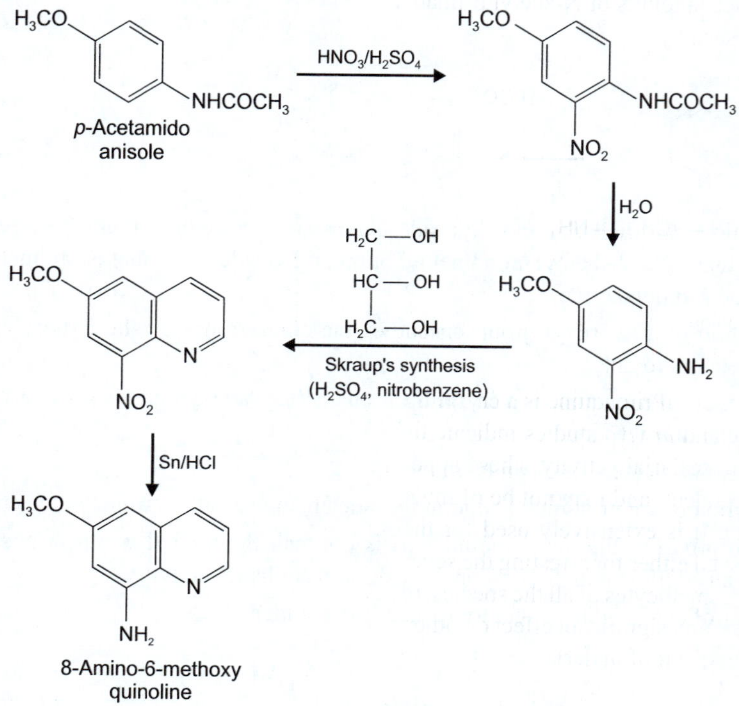

Step III. Condensation of the products of *Steps I* and *II.*

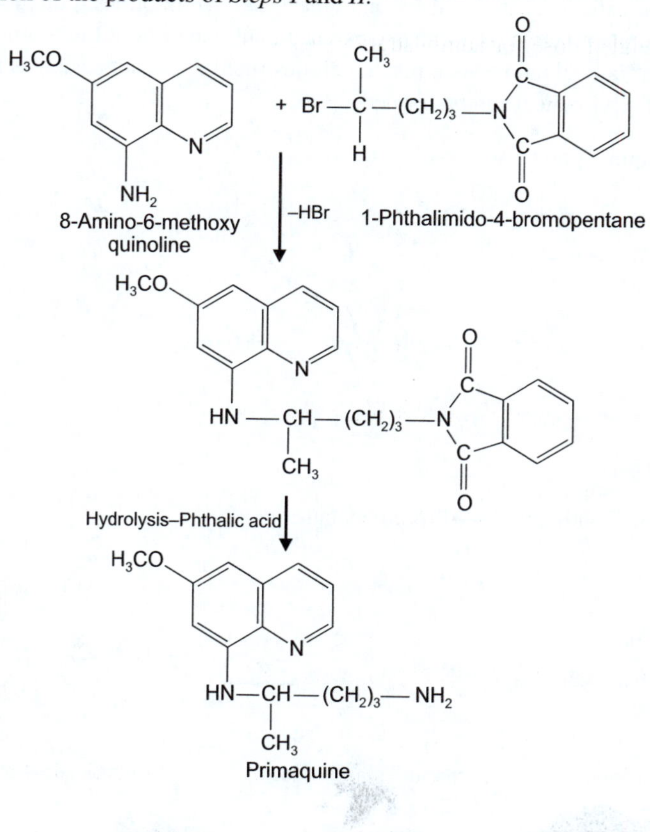

Metabolism: Primaquine is totally metabolized by CYP3A4 with primary metabolites having carboxy primaquine. Trace amounts of N-acetyl primaquine, aromatic hydroxylated products, and conjugation metabolites are seen.

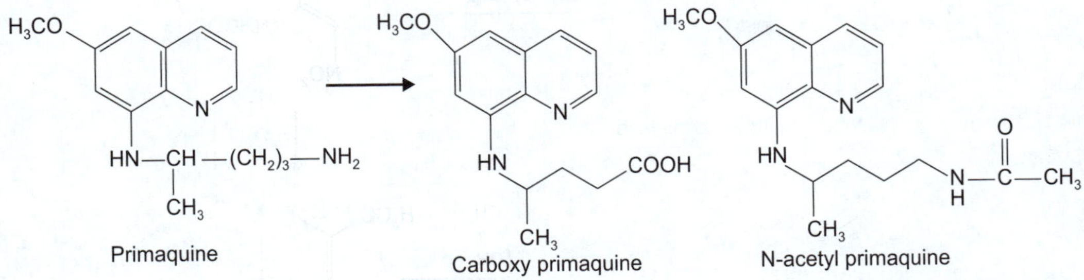

Properties and uses: Primaquine is a crystalline powder, soluble in water, and practically insoluble in alcohol. *In vitro* and *in vivo* studies indicate that the stereochemistry at the asymmetric carbon is not important for antimalarial activity. These appears to be less toxicity with the levorotatory isomer, but this is dose-dependent, and may not be of much importance as the doses used to treat exoerythrocytic *P. vivax* malaria. It is extensively used for the radical cure of relapsing vivax malaria, but it is not normally employed either for arresting the severe attacks of the disease or for the suppressive therapy. It invariably kills gametocytes of all the species, or inhibits their growth and development in the mosquito. It fails to produce any significant effect on other erythrocytic stages, and hence, it must not be employed alone for the treatment of malaria.

Assay: Dissolve the sample in anhydrous acetic acid and heat gently. Allow to cool and titrate with 0.1 M perchloric acid. Determine the end point potentiometrically.

Dose: The recommended dose for administration is 17.5–26.3 mg (10–15 mg of base) once daily for 14 days.

Pamaquine

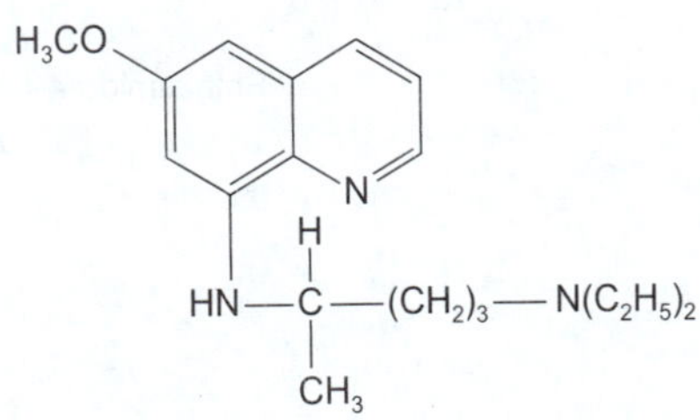

Synthesis

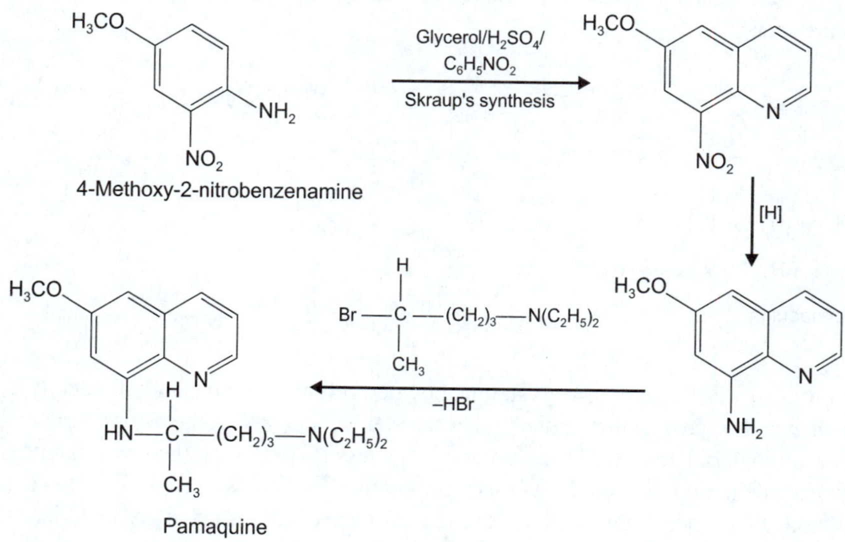

Properties and uses: It was the first 8-amino quinoline marketed, used as an antimalarial agent.

III. Acridine Derivatives

Quinacrine

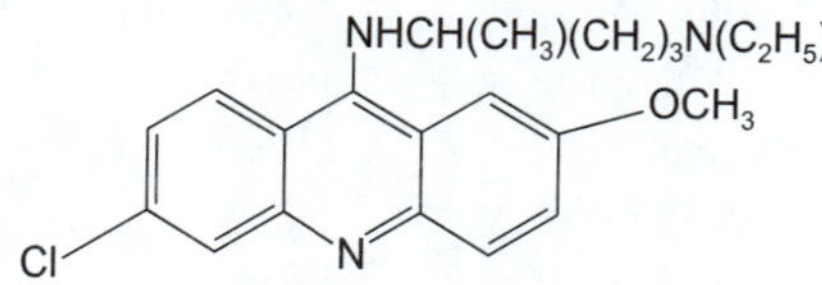

Synthesis

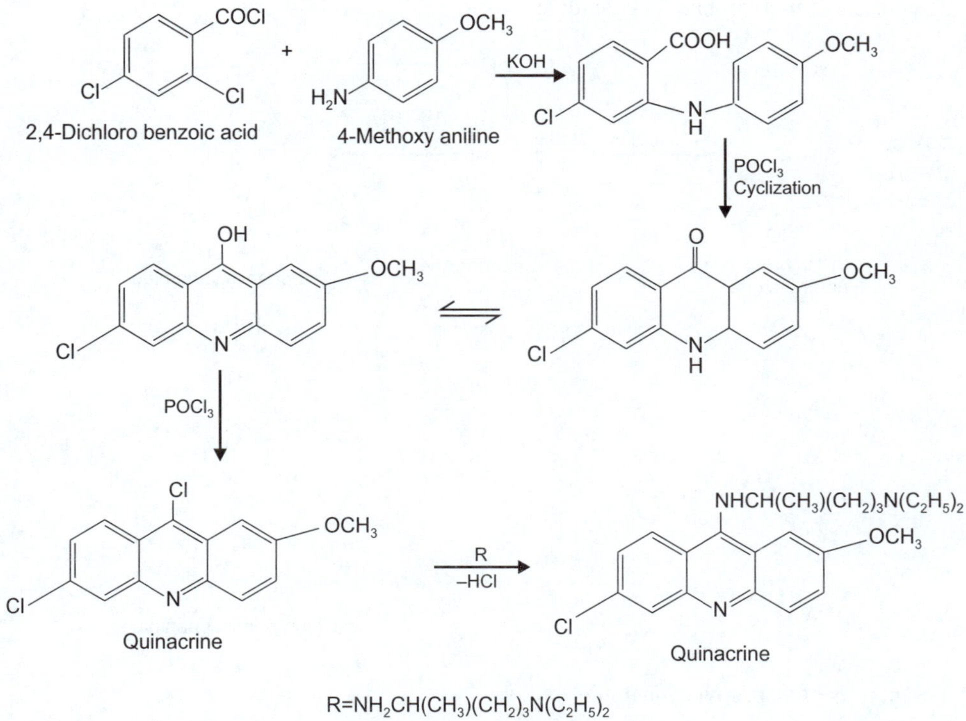

Mode of action: Quinacrine acts at many sites within the cell, including intercalation of DNA strands, succinic dehydrogenase, mitochondrial electron transport, and cholinesterase. It may be tumerogenic and mutagenic and has been used as a sclerosing agent. Because it is an acridine dye, quinacrine can cause yellow discolouration of the skin and urine.

Properties and uses: It acts as a schizontocidal and now it is not used as an antimalarial agent. It is used in the treatment of leishmaniasis and some tapeworm infestations.

IV. a. Biguanides

Mode of action: Biguanides inhibit dihydrofolate reductase enzyme and interfere in the folic acid metabolism. This leads to inhibition of the nuclear division in malarial parasites.

Proguanil HCl (Paludrine)

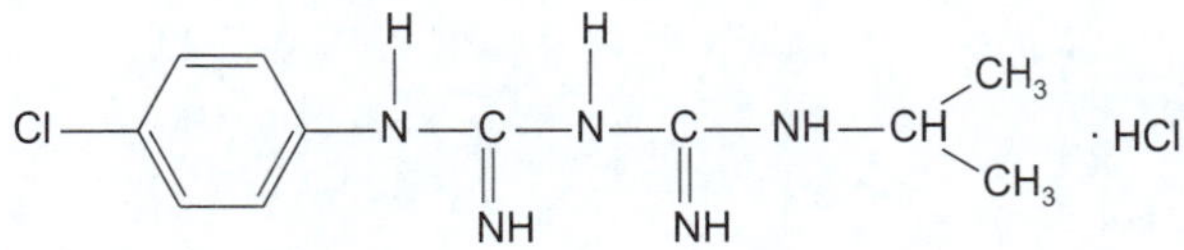

Synthesis

Step I. Synthesis of *p*-chlorophenyl guanidine

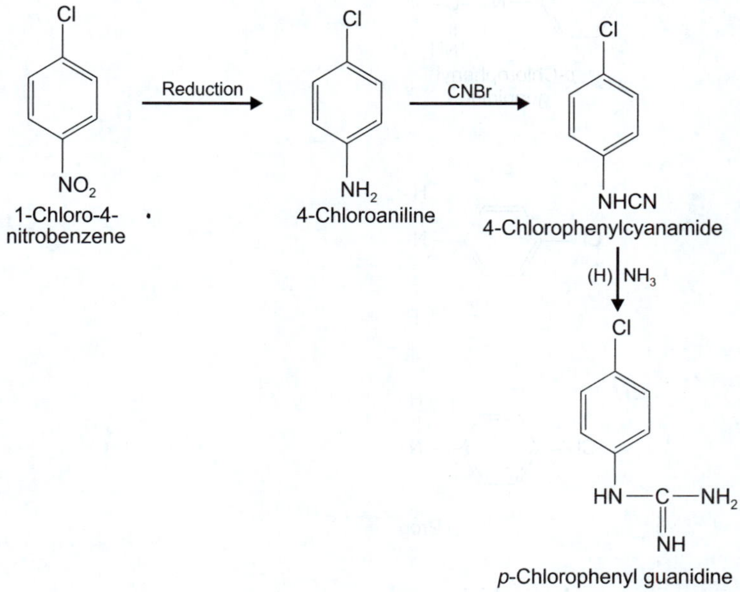

Step II. Synthesis of isopropyl cyanamide

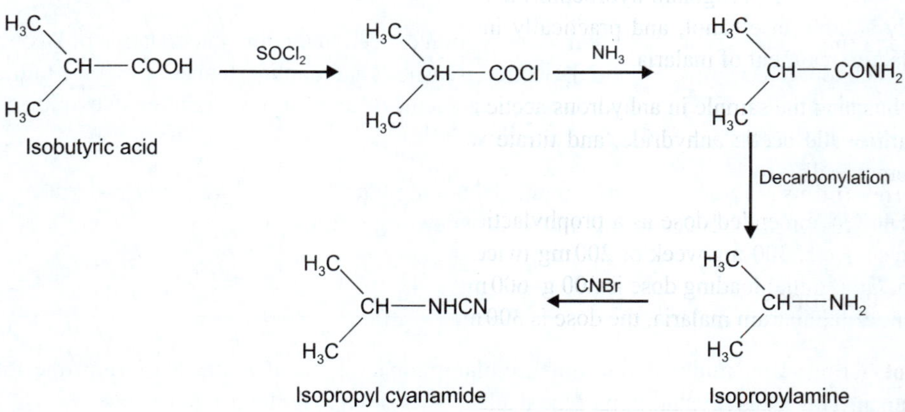

Step III. Condensation of the products of *Steps I* and *II.*

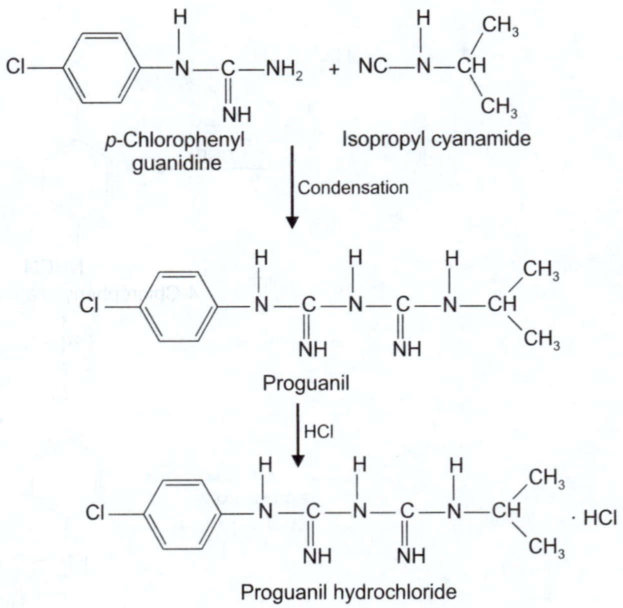

Metabolism: Proguanil is a prodrug, which is metabolized in the liver to diaminotriazine (cycloguanil), that acts as a dihydrofolate reductase inhibitor of *Plasmodium* species and inhibits DNA synthesis.

Properties and uses: Proguanil hydrochloride is a white crystalline powder, slightly soluble in water, sparingly soluble in ethanol, and practically insoluble in methylene chloride. It is used mainly for prophylactic treatment of malaria.

Assay: Suspend the sample in anhydrous acetic acid, shake and heat at 50°C for 5 min. Cool to room temperature, add acetic anhydride, and titrate with 0.1 M perchloric acid. Determine the end point potentiometrically.

Dose: The recommended dose as a prophylactic and a suppressant is 100 to 200 mg per day in non-immune subjects; 300 mg/week or 200 mg twice/week in semi-immune subjects. In the case of acute vivax malaria, initial loading dose is 300 g–600 mg followed by 300 mg per day for 5–10 days. For the treatment of falciparum malaria, the dose is 300 mg two times daily for 5 days.

IV. b. Diaminopyrimidines

Mode of action: It inhibits the reduction of folic acid and dihydrofolic acid to the active tetrahydrofolate coenzyme form.

Pyrimethamine (Daraprim)

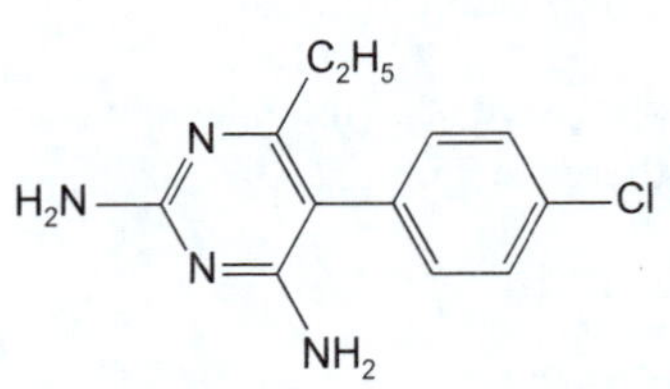

2,4-Diamino-5-(*p*-chlorophenyl)-6-ethyl pyrimidine

Synthesis

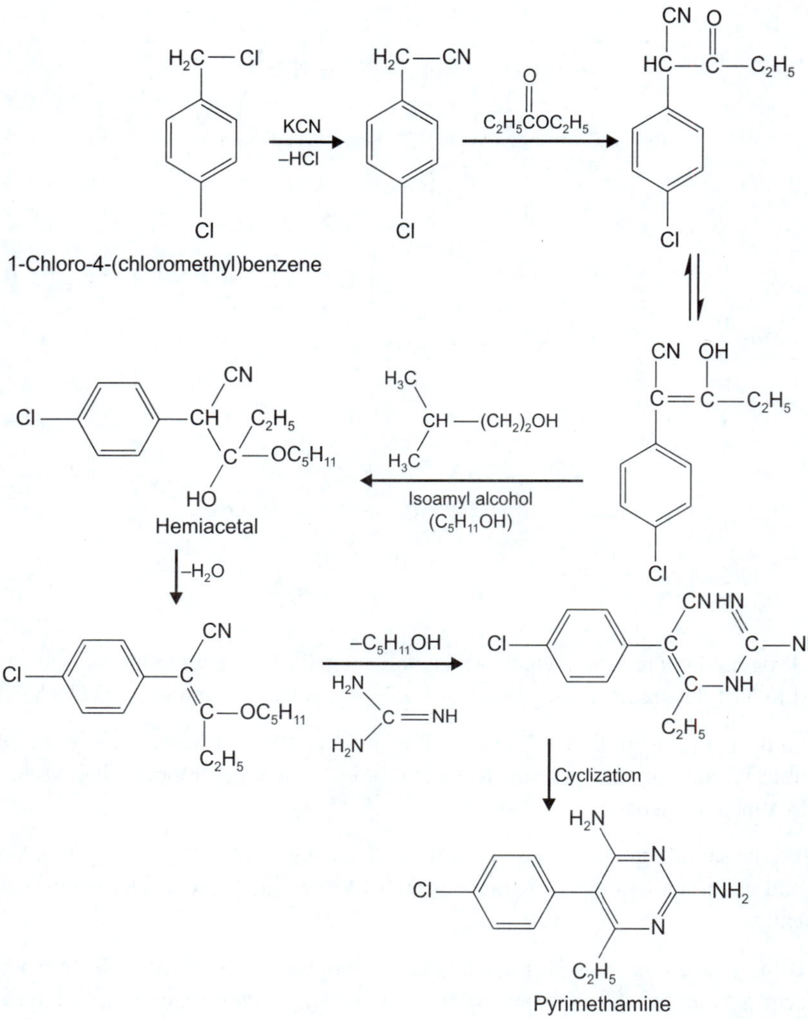

Properties and uses: Pyrimethamine exists as a white crystalline powder or colourless crystals, practically insoluble in water, and slightly soluble in alcohol. Pyrimethamine inhibits the reduction of folic acid and dihydrofolic acid to the active tetrahydrofolate coenzyme form. It finds its extensive use as a suppressive prophylactic for the prevention of severe attacks due to *P. falciparum* and *P. vivax*. It is also used in the treatment of taxoplasmosis and as an immunosuppressive agent.

Assay: Dissolve the sample in anhydrous acetic acid by heating gently. Cool and titrate with 0.1 M perchloric acid. Determine the end point potentiometrically.

Dose: The administered dose as a suppressive is 25 mg once a week, as a therapeutic 50–75 mg once a day for two days when used alone, otherwise 25 mg.

Dosage forms: Pyrimethamine tablets IP, BP.

Trimethoprim (Proloprim)

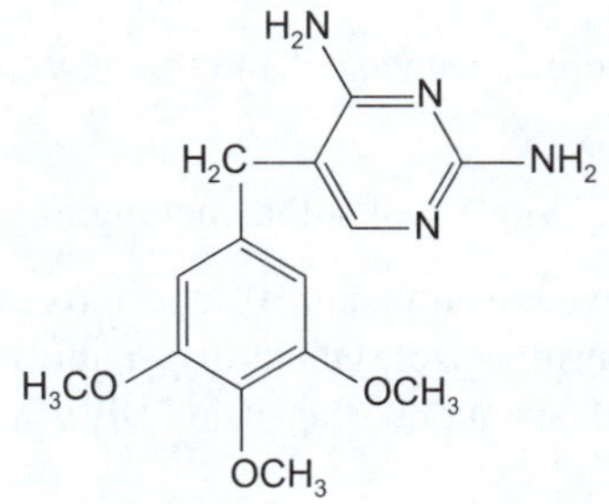

Synthesis

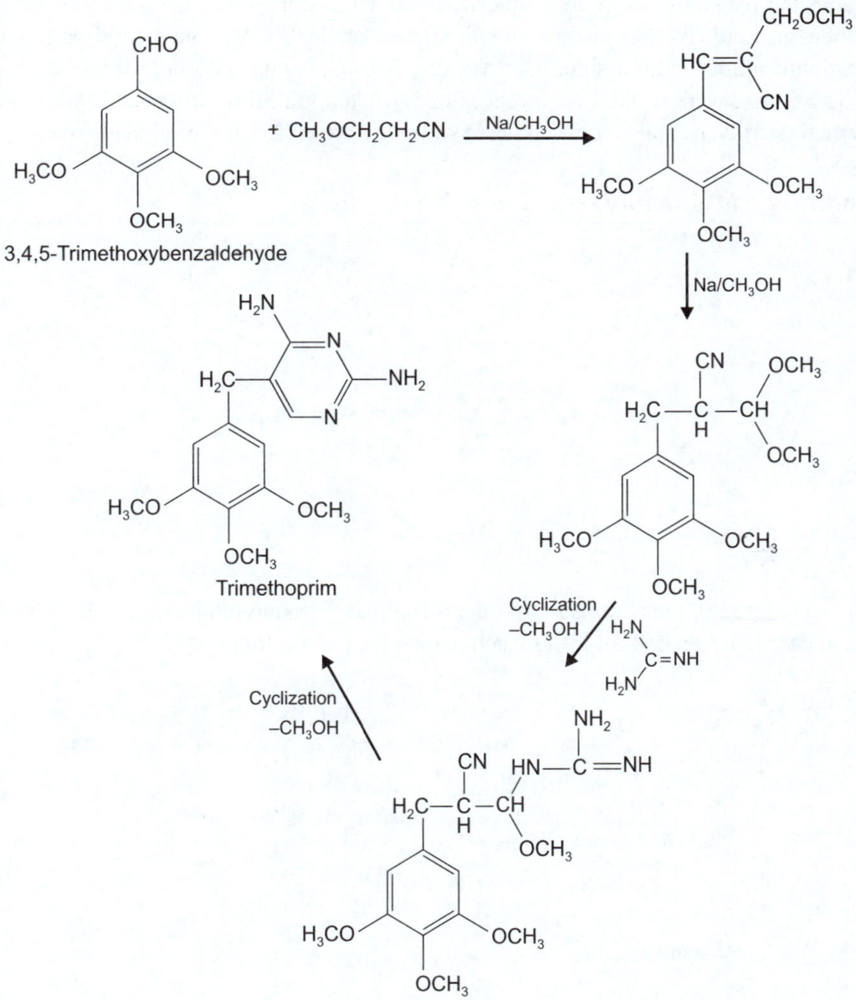

Properties and uses: Trimethoprim exists as a white or yellowish-white powder, very slightly soluble in water, and slightly soluble in ethanol. It is a potent inhibitor of dihydrofolate reductase. It has been employed in conjugation with sulphamethopyrazine in the treatment of chloroquine-resistant malaria.

It has also been used in conjugation with sulphonamides in the treatment of bacterial infections. Trimethoprim is an antibacterial, effective against malarial parasite.

Assay: Dissolve the sample in anhydrous acetic acid and titrate with 0.1 M perchloric acid. Determine the end point potentiometrically.

Dose: The administered dose is 1.5 g with 1 g of sulphametopyrazine per day for 3 days.

Dosage forms: Cotrimoxazole intravenous infusion BP, cotrimoxazole oral suspension BP, paediatric cotrimoxazole oral suspension BP, cotrimoxazole tablets dispersible BP, cotrimoxazole tablets paediatric BP, cotrimoxazole tablets BP, trimethoprim oral suspension BP, trimethoprim tablets BP.

V. Sulphones and Sulphonamides

Mode of action: They only act against the erythrocytic stages of malaria parasite. The sulphadoxine interferes with the parasites ability to synthesize folic acid. Sulphonamides block the incorporation of *p*-aminobenzoic acid (PABA) to form dihydropteroic acid. PABA is the central part of the folate structure. Sulphonamides exhibit significant toxicity because humans do not synthesize the vitamin folic acid. There are severe to fatal occurrences of erythema multiform, Stevens-Johnson syndrome, toxic epidermal necrolysis, and serum sickness syndromes attributed to the sulphadoxine.

VI. Phenanthrene Methanol Derivatives

Halofantrine

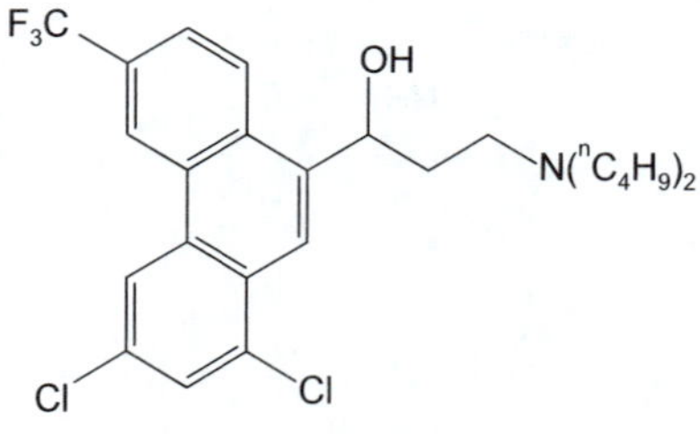

Metabolism: The drug is metabolized by N-dealkylation to desbutyl halofantrine by CYP3A4. The metabolites appear to be several folds more active than the parent drug.

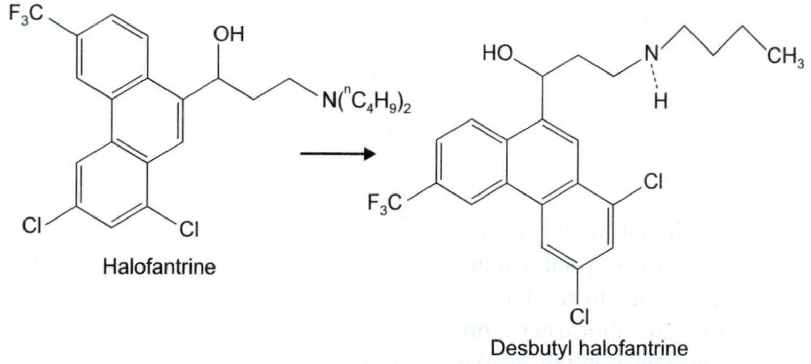

Synthesis

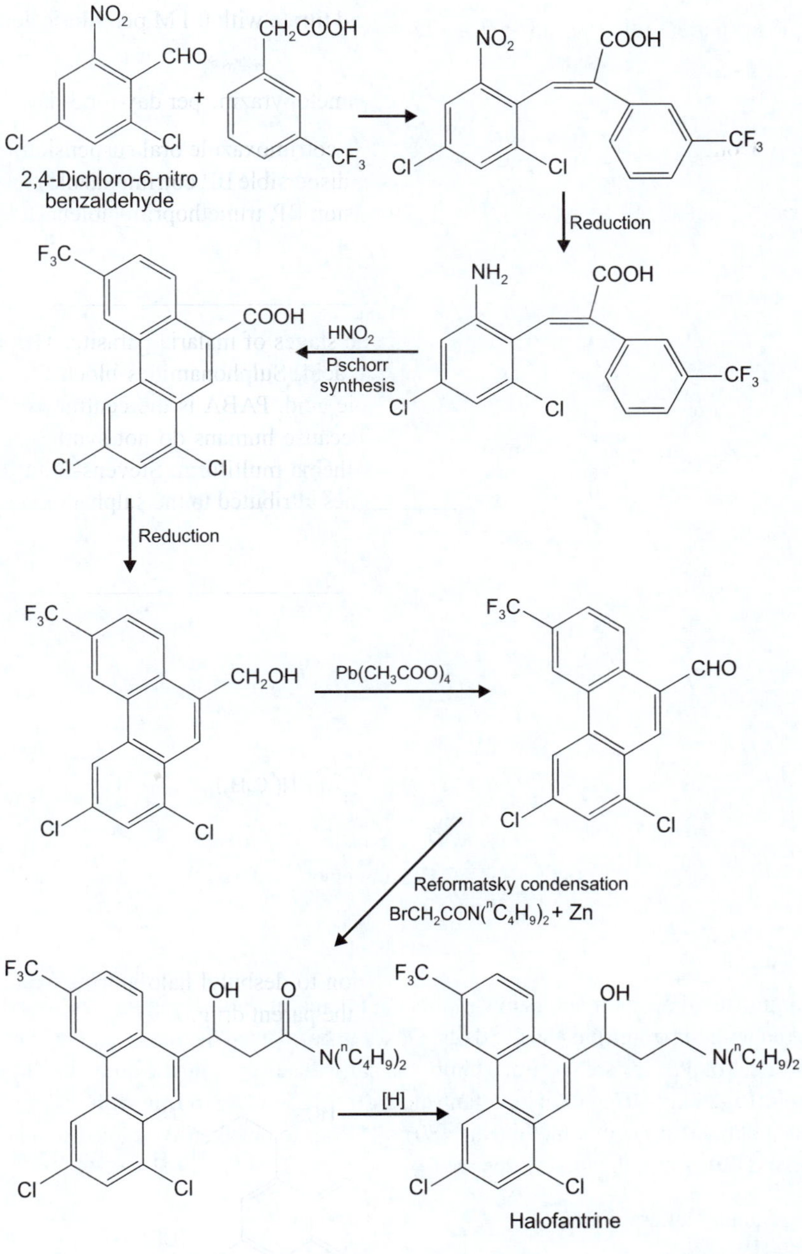

Properties and uses: Halofantrine is a white or almost white powder, practically insoluble in water, soluble in methanol, and sparingly soluble in alcohol. Structurally, halofantrine differs from all other antimalarial drugs and belongs to the latest generation of antimalarials. It is a good example of a drug design that incorporates bioisosteric principles evidenced by the trifluoromethyl moiety. It is schizonticidal and has no effect on the sporozoite, gametocyte, or hepatic stages. It is effective in the treatment and prophylaxis of chloroquine and multidrug-resistant *P. falciparum*.

Assay: It is as assayed by adopting liquid chromatography technique.

VII. Miscellaneous Drugs

Artemether (Larither, Paluther) **and β-arte-ether**

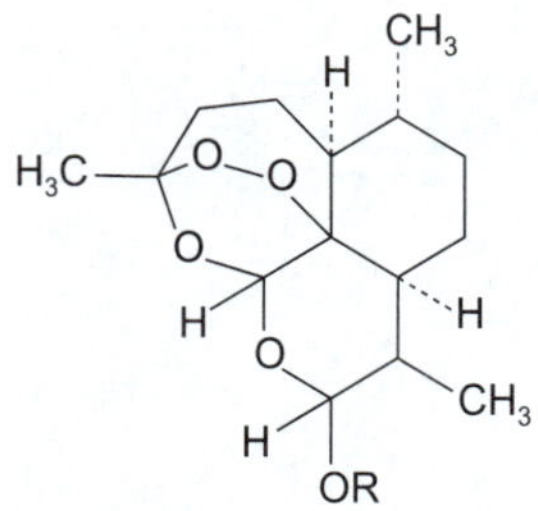

Synthesis

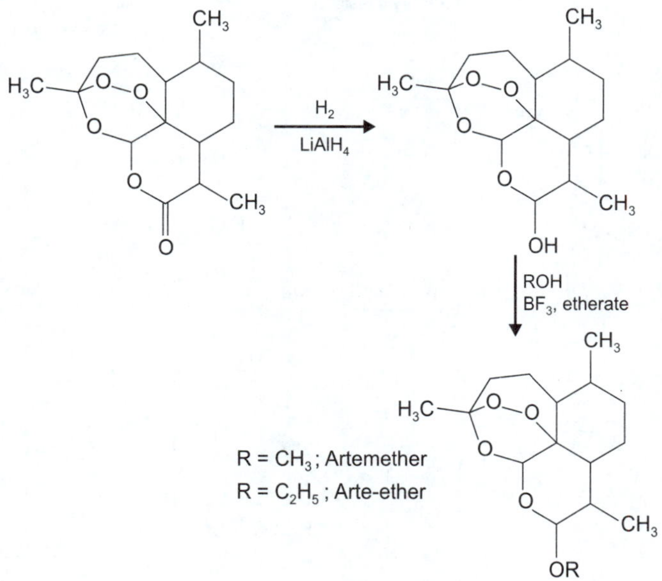

Dose: The administered dose for acute uncomplicated falciparum malaria in the case of adults is 80 mg daily to be taken with lumefantrine 480 mg daily. Doses to be taken at diagnosis and repeated after 8, 24, 36, 48, and 60 hrs. Total doses are six. For a child, the daily dose based on the body weight is as follows: 5–14 kg: 20 mg; 15–24 kg: 40 mg with lumefantrine 240 mg; 25–34 kg: 60 mg with lumefantrine 360 mg and more than 34 kg: 80 mg with lumefantrine 480 mg. Doses to be taken at diagnosis and repeated after 8, 24, 36, 48, and 60 hrs and the total doses are 6.

Artesunate (Asunate, Ultera, Falcigo)

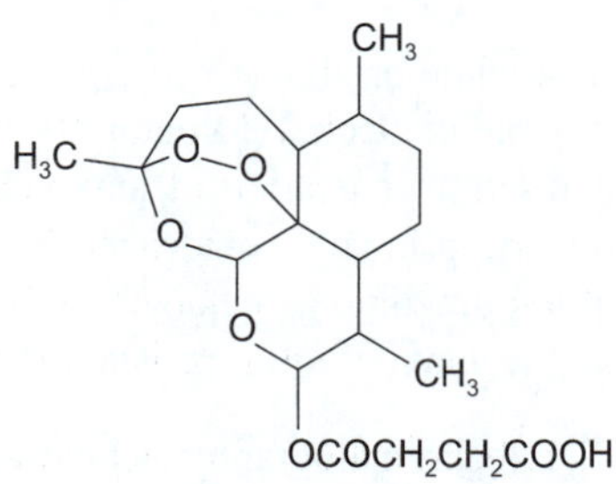

Synthesis

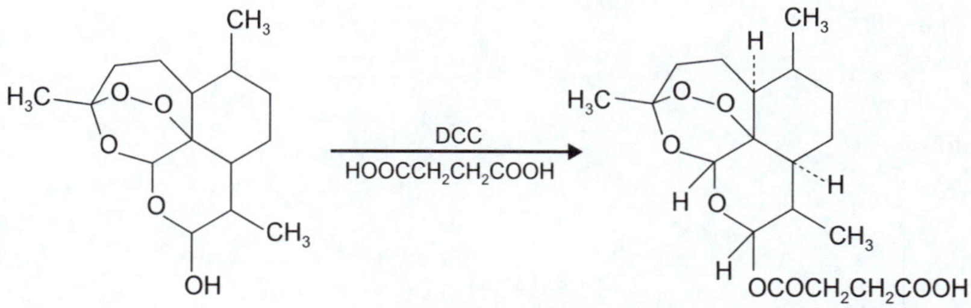

Artesunate

Dose: The dose in the case of falciparum malaria for adults is 2.4 mg/kg via IM or IV administration to be repeated after 12 hrs and 24 hrs later; then, once daily thereafter. For a child, the dose is 2.4 mg/kg via IM or IV administration and to be repeated after 12 hrs and 24 hrs later; then, once daily thereafter.

Mefloquine

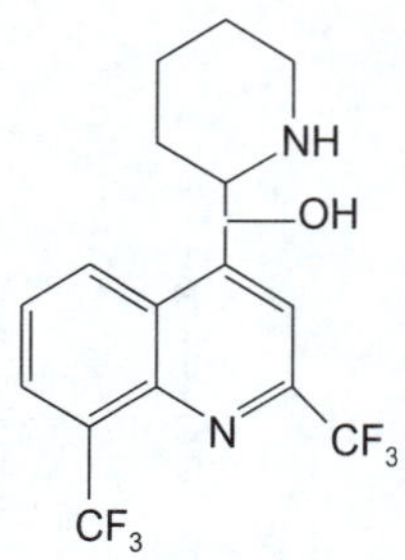

Metabolism of mefloquine: It is metabolized through CYP3A4 oxidation to its major inactive metabolite called carboxy mefloquine and rest of the amount is excreted unchanged in urine.

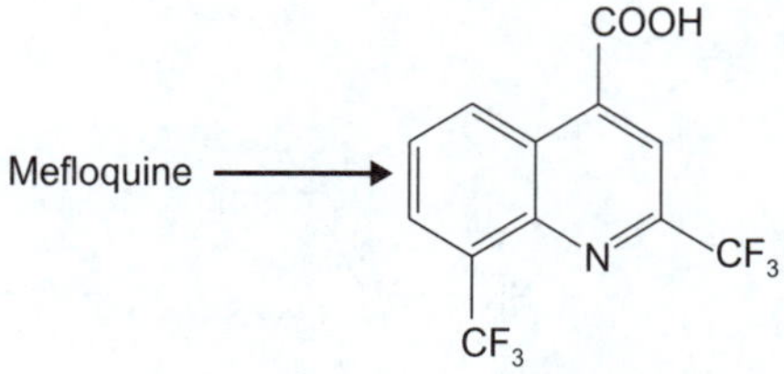

Metabolite

Properties and uses: Mefloquine hydrochloride is a white or slightly yellow crystalline powder, very slightly soluble in water, soluble in methanol and in alcohol. It is used as an antimalarial agent.

Assay: Dissolve the sample in anhydrous formic acid, add acetic anhydride and titrate with 0.1 M perchloric acid. Determine the end point potentiometrically.

CLASSIFICATION BASED ON PCI SYLLABUS

Quinolines

Quinine sulphate

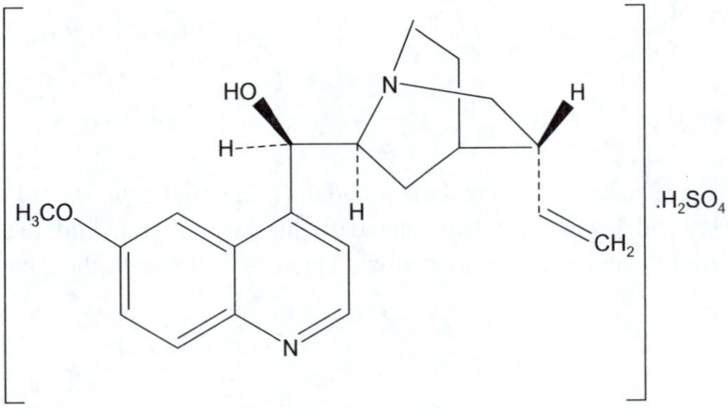

Chloroquine

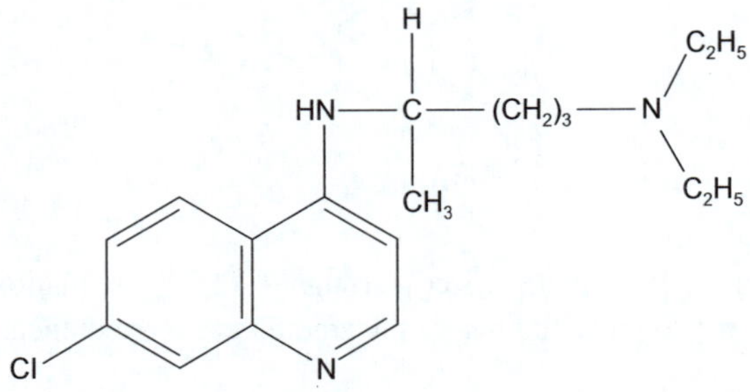

Amodiaquine

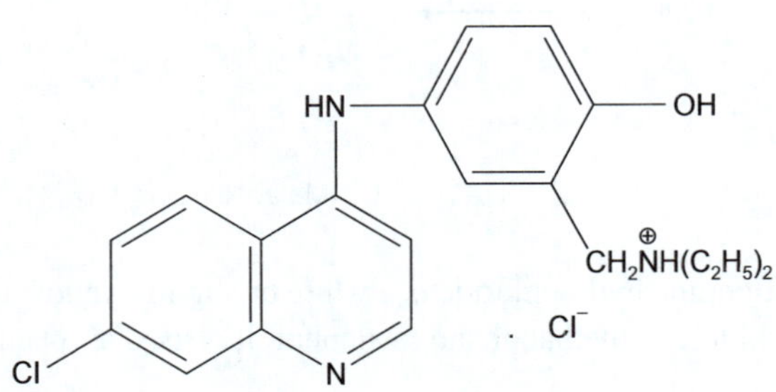

Primaquine phosphate

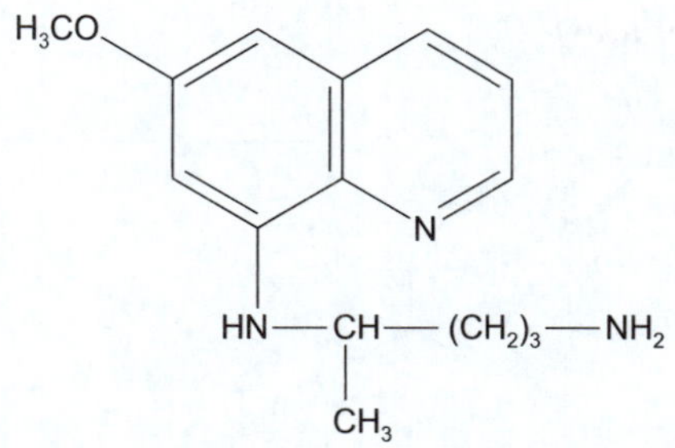

Pamaquine

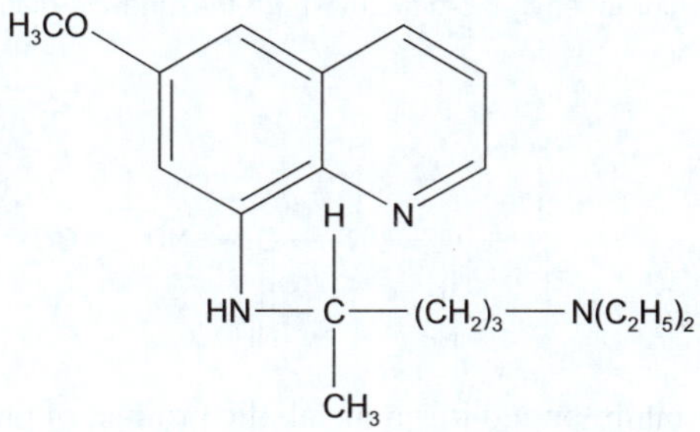

Quinacrine hydrochloride

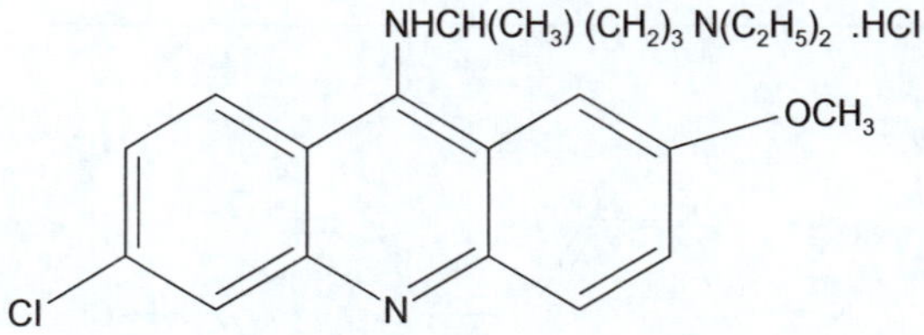

Mefloquine

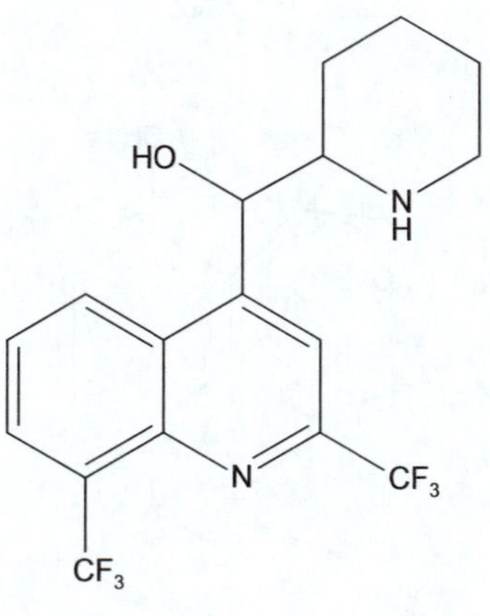

Biguanides and Dihydrotriazines

Cycloguanil Pamoate (Biguanides)

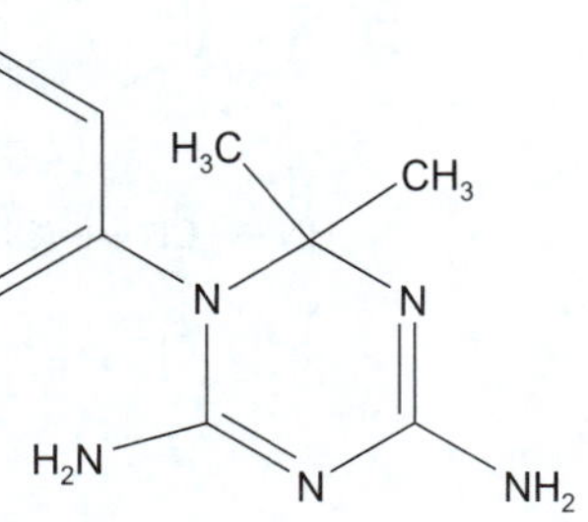

1-(4-chlorophenyl)-6,6-dimethyl-1,3,5-triazane-2,4-diamine

Proguanil

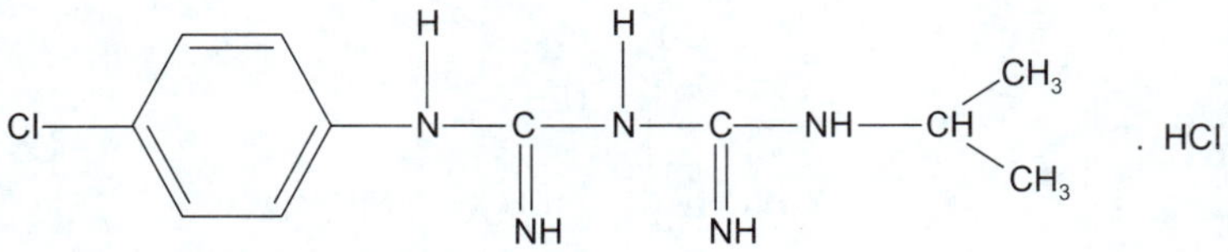

It is a dihydrofolate reductase inhibitor and it is a metabolic product of proguanil.

Uses: The current use of this drug is stopped recently because the development of resistance.

Miscellaneous

Pyrimethamine

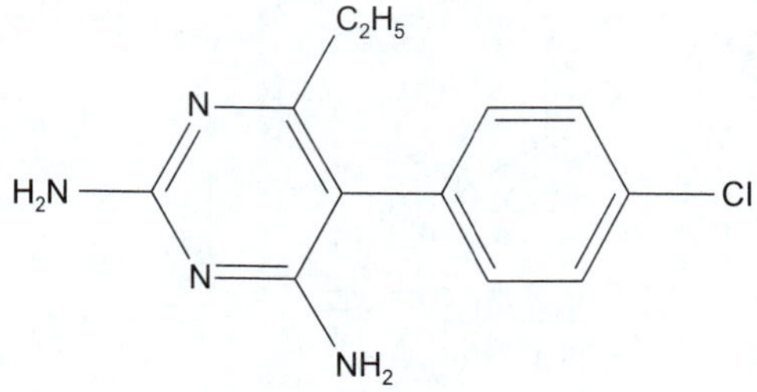

Artesunate

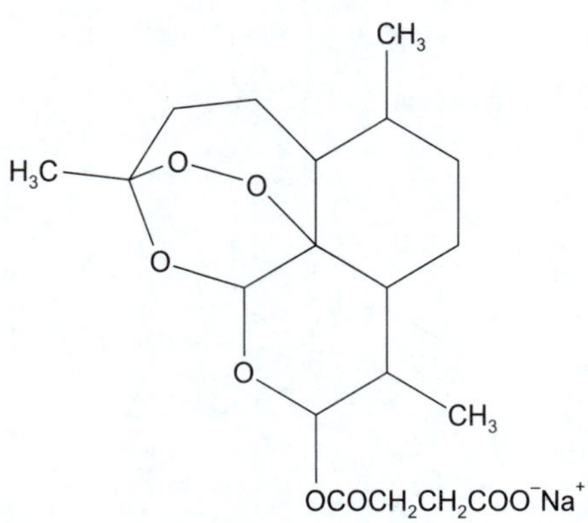

Artemether

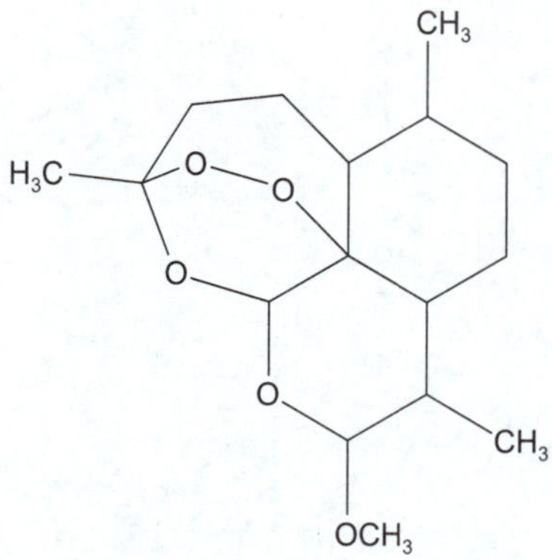

Atovaquone

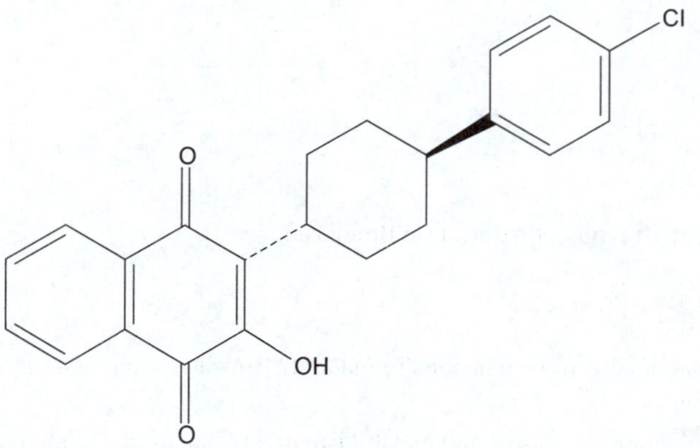

Atovaquone

It is a naphthoquinone derivative that contains 4-(4-chlorophenyl) cyclohexyl group at the 2nd position and hydroxyl group at the 3rd position. It is a synthetic antimalarial agent. It locks the mitochondrial electron transport at the respiratory chain of protozoa, hence inhibits pyrimidine and DNA synthesis leading to death of the protozoa. It is rapidly-acting against blood schizonticide.

Properties and uses: It is used along with proguanil (malarone) for prophylaxis and treatment of chloroquine-resistant malaria. It is also used for the treatment of infections produced by *P. carinii* and *T. gondii*.

Newer Agents

Afenoquine

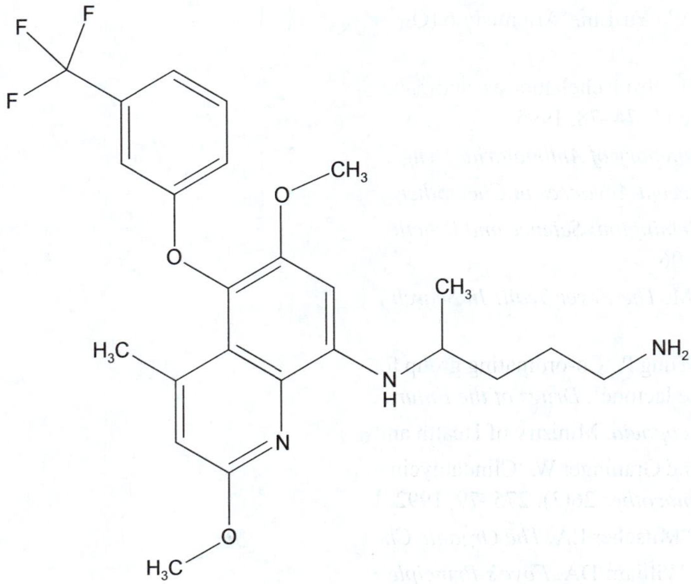

Uses: It is used to treat all types of malaria (antimalarial agent).

PROBABLE QUESTIONS

1. What are the causal organisms responsible for malaria? How do the antimalarials affect the life cycle of mosquito? Explain.
2. Write the mode of action, synthesis, and metabolism of any one of the 4-amino quinoline derivatives.
3. Discuss the synthesis of one important antimalarial drug belonging to the class: (a) Diaminopyrimidines and (b) sulphones.
4. Write the SAR of 4-amino quinolines.
5. Classify the synthetic antimalarials based on their basic chemical nucleus. Provide examples of at least one of the two compounds from each class.
6. Mention the name of drugs obtained upon modification of the side chain at C-4 position on the 4-amino-7-chloroquinoline nucleus.
7. Outline the synthesis of proguanil hydrochloride from *p*-chlorophenyl guanidine and isopropyl cyanamide. Write their structure, synthesis, and the dosage forms available.
8. Name the three important antimalarials derived from 8-amino-6-methoxy quinoline nucleus, their structure, chemical name, uses, and the synthesis of any one drug.
9. Elaborate the synthesis of mepacrine hydrochloride, the uses, and the dosage forms available.
10. Proguanil hydrochloride is the wonder drug for malaria that gets metabolized to its active form cycloguanil *in vivo*. Explain its biotransformation.

SUGGESTED READINGS

1. Abraham DJ (ed). *Medicinal Chemistry and Drug Discovery* (6th edn). New Jersey: John Wiley, 2007.
2. *British Pharmacopoeia*. Medicines and Healthcare Products Regulatory Agency. London, 2008.

3. Bruce-Chwatt LJ (ed). *Chemotherapy of Malaria*, Rev (2nd edn). Geneva: WHO, 1986.
4. Bruntan LL, Lazo JS, and Parker KL. *Goodman and Gilman's: The Pharmacological of Therapeutics* (11th edn). New York: McGraw Hill, 2006.
5. Butler AR and Wu Yu-Lin. 'Artemisinin (Qinghaosu). A new type of antimalarial drug'. *Chem Soc Rev* 85–90, 1992.
6. Cabantchuik ZI. 'Iron chelators as antimalarials: The biochemical basis of selective cytotoxicity'. *Parasitol Today* 11: 74–78, 1995.
7. Cooper WC. *Summary of Antimalarial Drugs*, Report No. 64. U.S. Public Health Service, 1949.
8. Findlay GM. *Recent Advances in Chemotherapy* (2nd edn), Vol. 2. Philadelphia: Blakiston, 1951.
9. Gennaro AR. *Remington: Science and Practice of Pharmacy* (21st edn). New York: Lippincot Williams and Wilkins, 2006.
10. Honingsbaum M. *The Fever Trail: In Search for the Cure for Malaria*. New York: Farrar, Straus, and Girous, 2001.
11. Hsuch KO and Tung P. 'Co-ordinating group for research on the structure of Quing Hau Sau: A new type of sesquiterpene lactone'. *Drugs of the Future* 22(3): 142, 1977.
12. *Indian Pharmacopoeia*. Ministry of Health and Family Welfare. New Delhi, 1996.
13. Kremsner PG and Graninger W. 'Clindamycin in the treatment of experimental and human malaria'. *Rev Contemp Pharmacother* 26(3): 275–79, 1992.
14. Lednicer D and Mitscher LA. *The Organic Chemistry of Drug Synthesis*. New York: John Wiley, 1995.
15. Lemke TL and William DA. *Foye's Principle of Medicinal Chemistry* (6th ed). New York: Lippincott Williams and Wilkins, 2008.
16. Pratt WB. *Fundamentals of Chemotherapy*. London: Oxford University Press, 1973.
17. Panisko DM and Keystone JS. 'Treatment of malaria'. *Drugs* 39: 160, 1990.
18. Rozman RS and Canfield CJ. 'New experimental antimalarial drugs'. *Adv Pharmacol Chemother* 16: 1, 1979.
19. Reynolds EF (ed). *Martindale the Extra Pharmacopoeia* (31st edn). London: Pharmaceutical Press, 1997.
20. Stec EA. *The Chemotherapy of Protozoan Diseases*, Vols I–IV. Washington DC: Walter Reed Army Institute of Research, 1971.
21. Saxena AK and Saxena M. 'Advances in chemotherapy of malaria'. *Prog Drug Res* 30: 221, 1986.
22. Slater AFG and Cerani A. *Nature* 355: 167–69, 1992.
23. Thompson PE and Werbal LM. *Antimalarial Agents Chemistry and Pharmacology*. New York: Academic Press, 1972.

CHAPTER 21

Anthelmintics

INTRODUCTION

Anthelmintics are drugs used to treat parasitic infections due to worms. Worms that are pathogenic to human beings, namely, metazoa are conventionally classified into round worms (nematodes) and two types of flatworms, that is, flukes (trematodes) and tapeworms (cestodes). Anthelmintics act locally either to expel the worms from the gastrointestinal tract or systemically to eradicate the species and the developing forms of helmintics that invade the organs and tissues. This class of agents has added significance due to their wide prevalence in third-world countries and it is estimated over 2 billion people are affected. No cheaper medicines are available for this disease, even now, although the primitive Chinese and Egyptians have started treating this disease 3500 years ago.

CLASSIFICATION

The anthelmintic agents comprise of drugs of chemically diverse structures and their mechanism of action differs from one agent to another.

I. Benzimidazoles

These are versatile anthelmintic agents particularly effective against gastrointestinal nematodes. These are highly effective against *ascaris*, *enterobius*, *trichuris*, and hookworm infections as single or mixed infections.

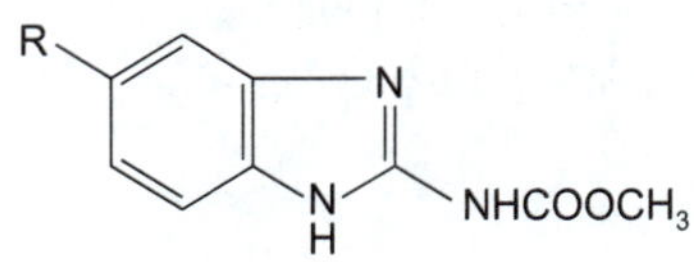

S. No.	*Drug*	*R*
1.	Albendazole	$—S—CH_2CH_2CH_3$
2.	Mebendazole	$—COC_6H_5$
3.	Flubendazole	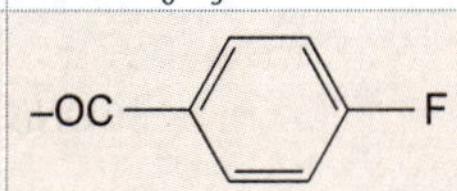

Contd.

S. No.	Drug	R
4.	Cyclobendazole	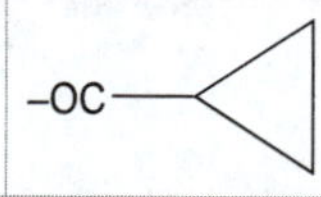
5.	Dribendazole	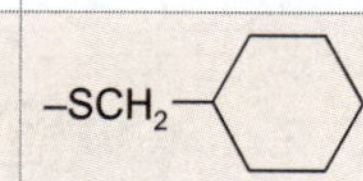
6.	Fenbendazole	S–C_6H_5
7.	Oxibendazole	$OCH_2CH_2CH_3$
8.	Parbendazole	$CH_2CH_2CH_2CH_3$

II. Quinolines and isoquinolines

Oxamniquine

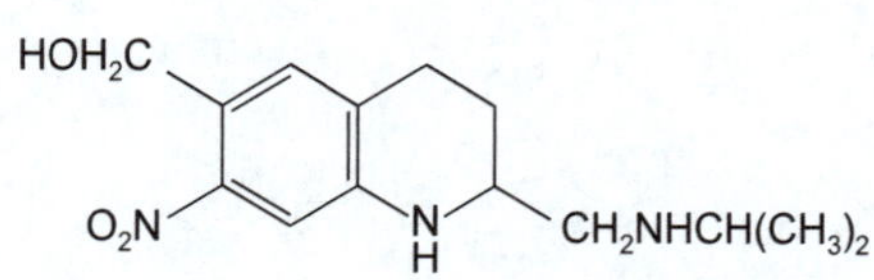

Praziquantel

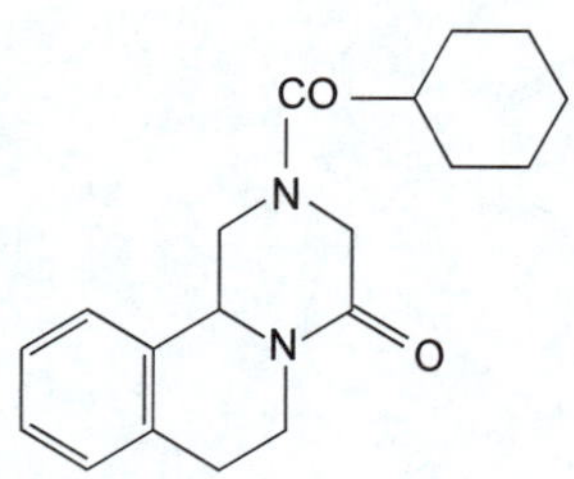

III. Piperazine derivatives

Piperazine citrate

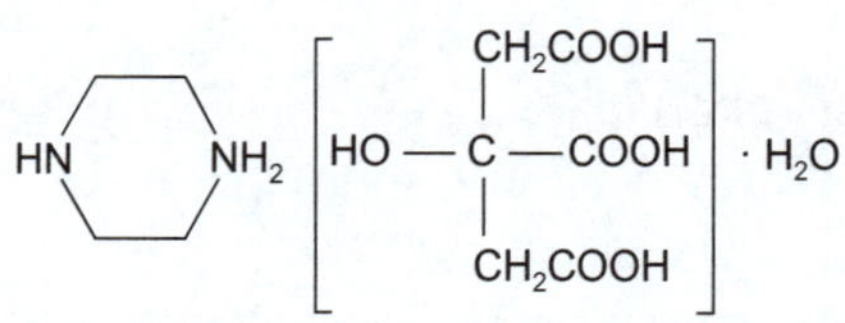

Diethyl carbamazine citrate

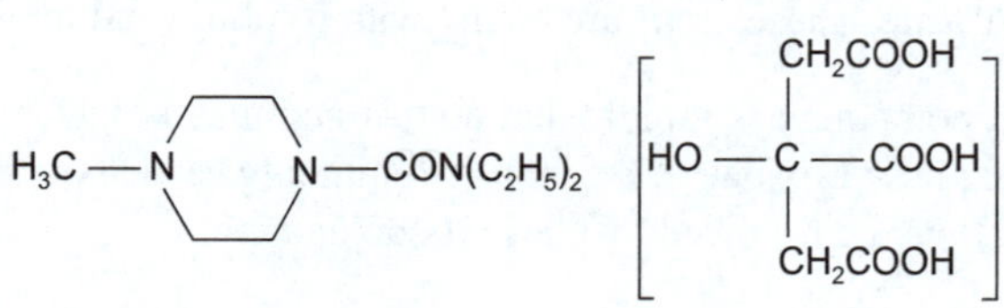

IV. Vinyl pyrimidines

Pyrantel pamoate

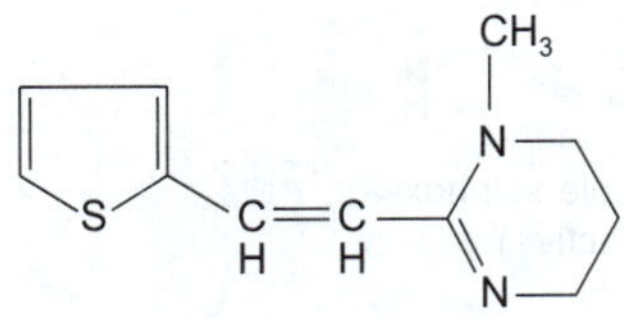

Oxantel

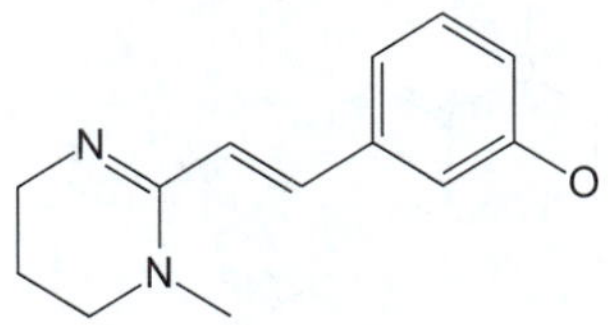

V. Amides

Niclosamide

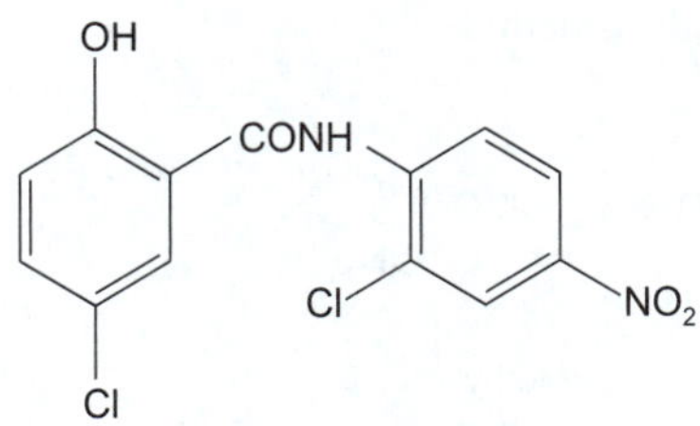

VI. Natural products: Avermectins
VII. Organo phosphorus: Metrifonate
VIII. Imidazothiazoles: Levamisole
IX. Nitro derivatives: Niridazole

SYNTHESIS AND DRUG PROFILE

I. Benzimidazoles

Mode of action: These drugs act by blocking the glucose transportation in the parasites and lead to the depletion of glycogen storage of the intracellular microtubules in the cells of the worms, thereby arresting the nematodes and cell division in the metaphase. The major site of action is microtubular protein β tubilin of the parasite. These drugs are bound with β-tubilin and inhibit the polymerization.

Metabolism: The parent compound is rapidly and almost completely metabolized by oxidative and hydrolytic processes. The phase I oxidative reaction is commonly carried out by the cytochrome P450 catalyzed reaction, which may be followed by phase II conjugation.

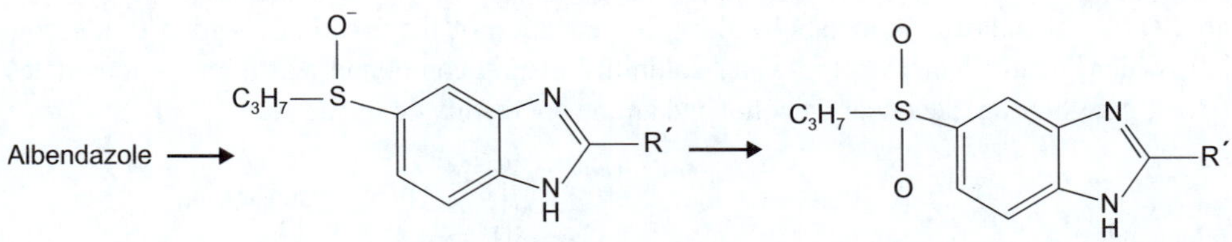

Albendazole sulphoxide
(active)

Mebendazole (Vermox)

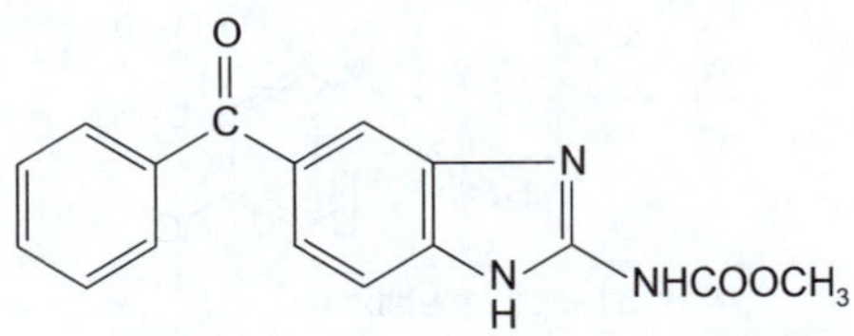

Methyl-5-benzoly-2-benzimidazole carbamate

Synthesis

Step I. Synthesis of an intermediate-S-methyl thiourea arboxylate

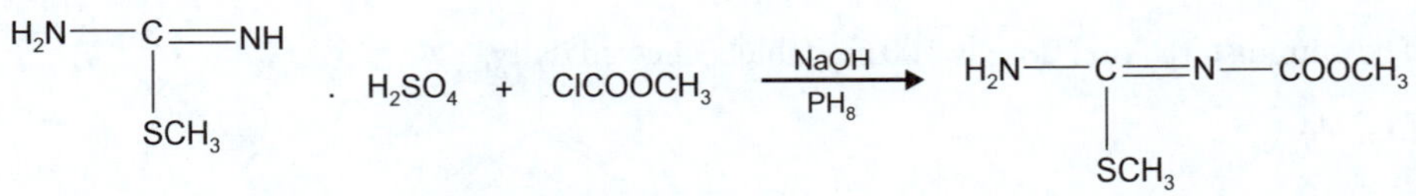

S-methyl thio-urea sulphate | Methyl chloro formate | Methyl-*S*-methyl thiourea carboxylate

Step II. Synthesis of mebendazole

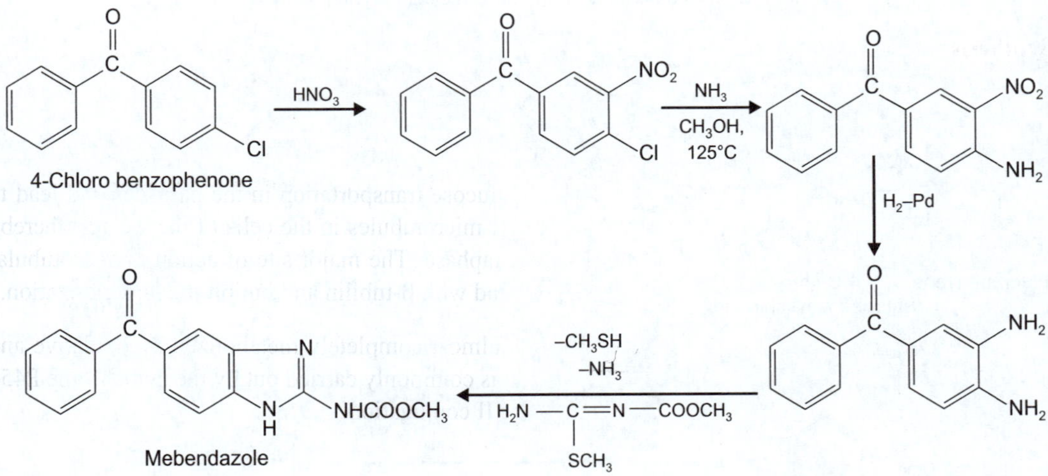

Metabolism: Mebendazole is metabolized by the reduction of the 5-carbonyl group to a secondary alcohol, which greatly increases the water solubility of this compound and thereby potentiates the excretion through urine. Secondary alcohol and amine are readily conjugated.

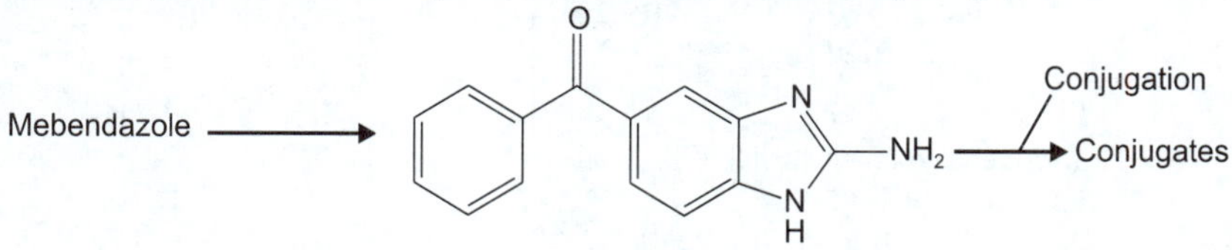

Amino metabolite

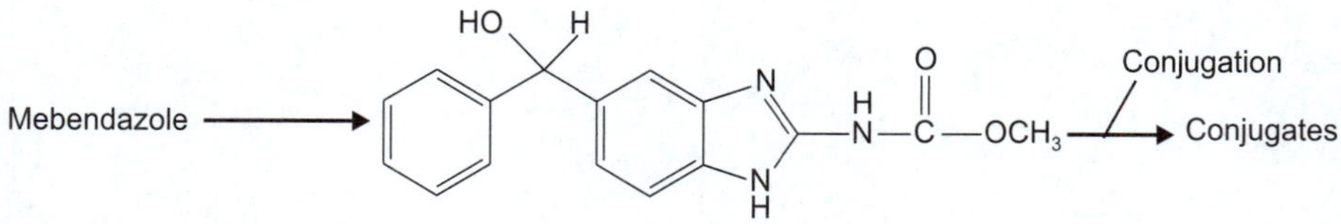

Hydroxy metabolite

Properties and uses: Mebendazole is a white powder, practically insoluble in water, in alcohol, and in methylene chloride. It is used as an anthelmintic agent.

Assay: Dissolve the sample in anhydrous formic acid, add the mixture of anhydrous acetic acid and methyl ethyl ketone (1:7), and titrate against 0.1 M perchloric acid. Determine the end point potentiometrically.

Dose: The administered oral dose is 100 mg tablets chewed daily.

Flubendazole

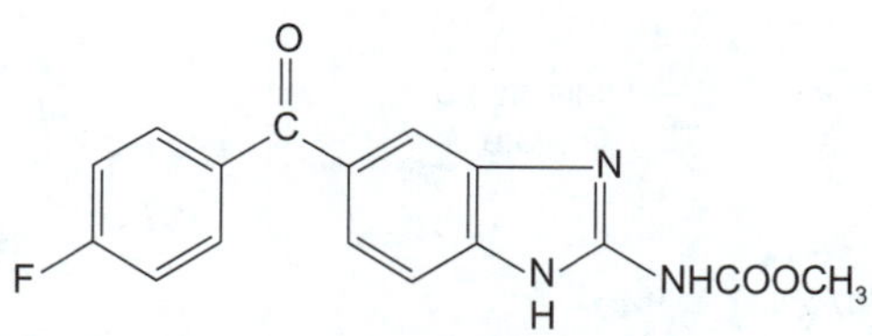

Methyl 5-(4-fluorobenzoyl)-1*H*-benzimidazol-2-yl-carbamate

Synthesis

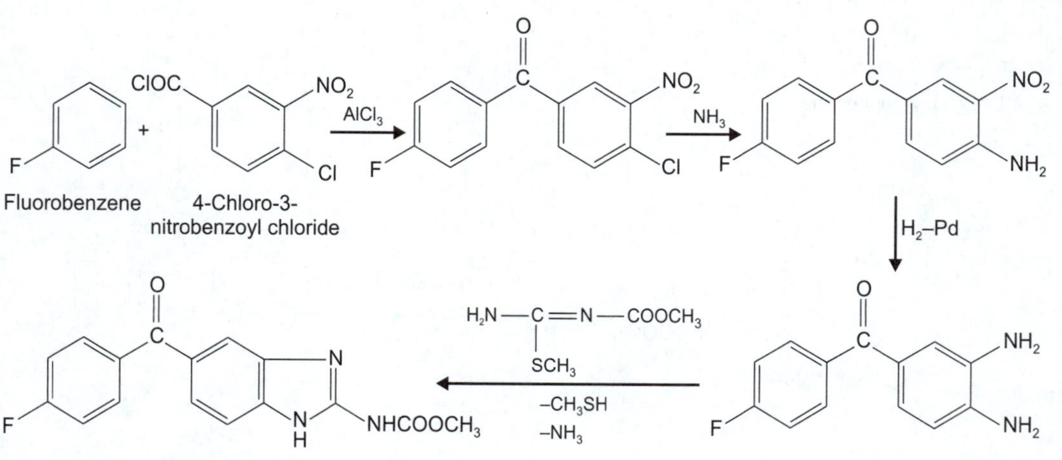

Properties and uses: Flubendazole is a white powder, practically insoluble in water, in alcohol, and in methylene chloride. It is used as an anthelmintic agent.

Assay: Dissolve the sample in anhydrous formic acid, add the mixture of anhydrous acetic acid and methyl ethyl ketone (1:7), and titrate against 0.1 M perchloric acid. Determine the end point potentiometrically.

Albendazole (Valbazen, Bentex, Zental)

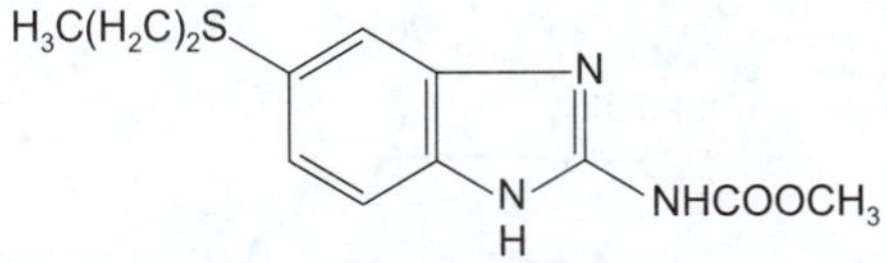

Methyl 5-(propylthio)-1*H*-benzoimidazol-2-yl-carbamate

Synthesis

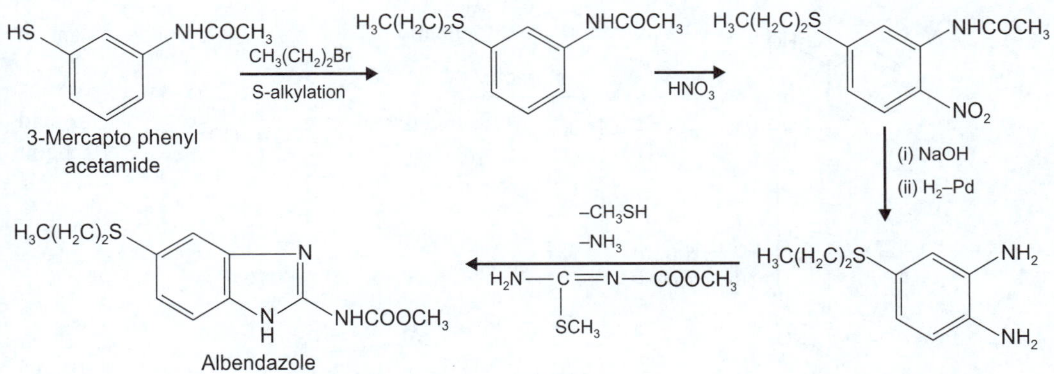

Properties and uses: Albendazole is a white or faintly yellowish powder, practically insoluble in water and alcohol, soluble in anhydrous formic acid, very slightly soluble in methylene chloride. It is used as an anthelmintic agent.

Assay: Dissolve the sample in anhydrous formic acid, add anhydrous acetic acid, and titrate against 0.1 M perchloric acid. Determine the end point potentiometrically.

Dose: The dose for controlling cysticercus cellulose is 5 mg/kg thrice daily for 30 days.

Thiabendazole (Mintezol)

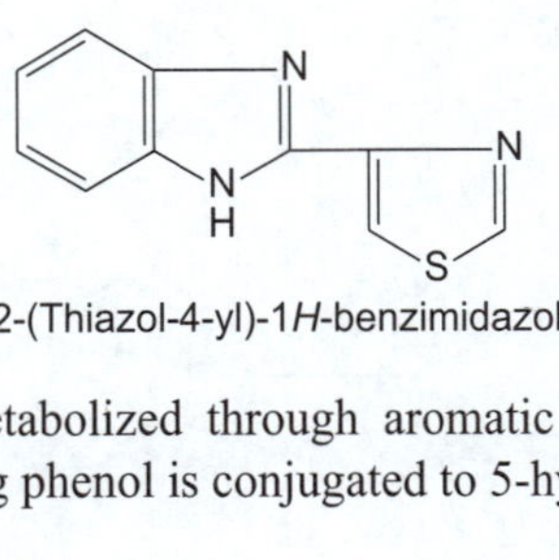

2-(Thiazol-4-yl)-1*H*-benzimidazole

Metabolism: Thiabendazole is metabolized through aromatic hydroxylation at the fifth position catalyzed by CYP1A2. The resulting phenol is conjugated to 5-hydroxythiabendazole glucuronide.

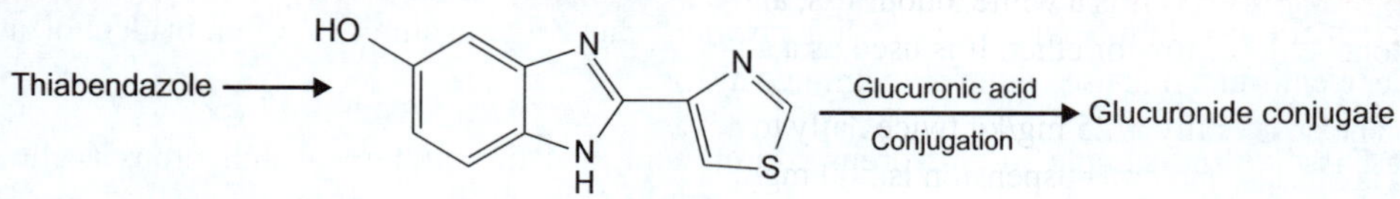

Synthesis

Route I. From: *o*-Nitroaniline or 2-Nitrobenzenamine

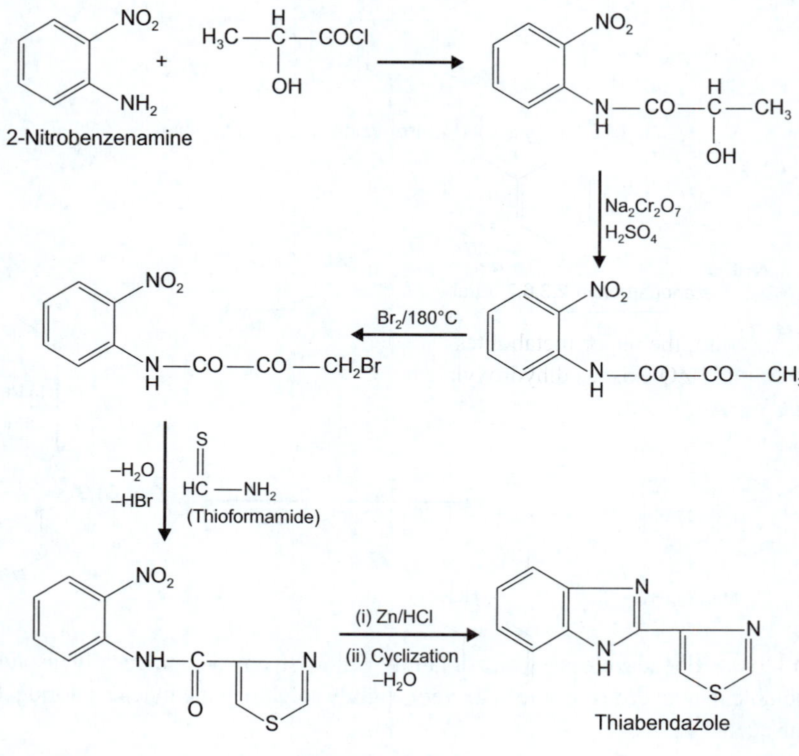

Route II. From: Thiazolonitrile

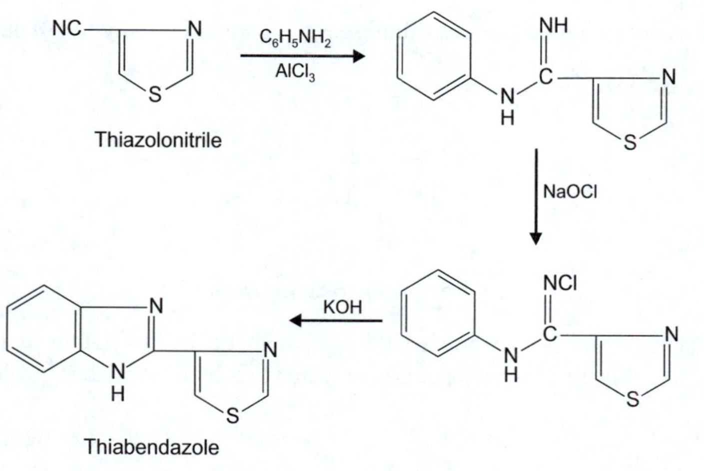

Properties and uses: It is a white, odourless, and tasteless powder, insoluble in water, slightly soluble in acetone, chloroform, or ether. It is used as a anthelmintic.

Dose: The dose orally is 25 mg/kg twice daily to a maximum of 3 g after meals. The dose for chewable tablets is 500 mg and oral suspension is 500 mg/5 ml.

II. Quinolines and isoquinolines

Praziquantel (PZQ, Biltricide)

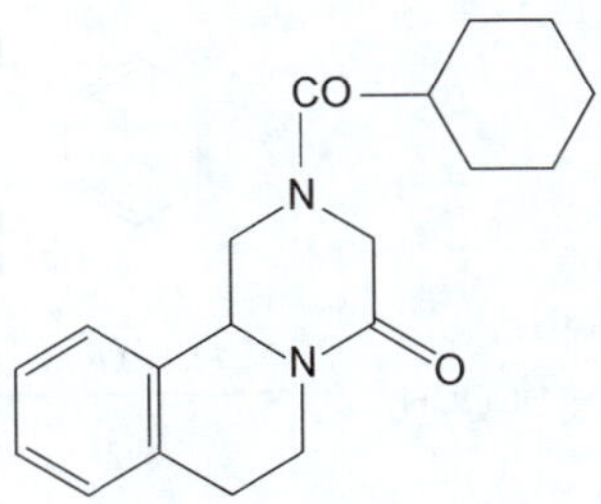

2-(Cyclohexanecarbonyl)-2,3,6,7-tetrahydro-1*H*-pyrazino[2,1-*a*]isoquinolin-4(11b*H*)-one

Metabolism: In serum, the major metabolites are 4-hydroxycyclohexyl carboxylate, but in the urine, 50–60% of the initial PZQ exist as dihydroxylated products. Hydroxylation reactions are catalyzed by CYP2B6 and CYP3A4.

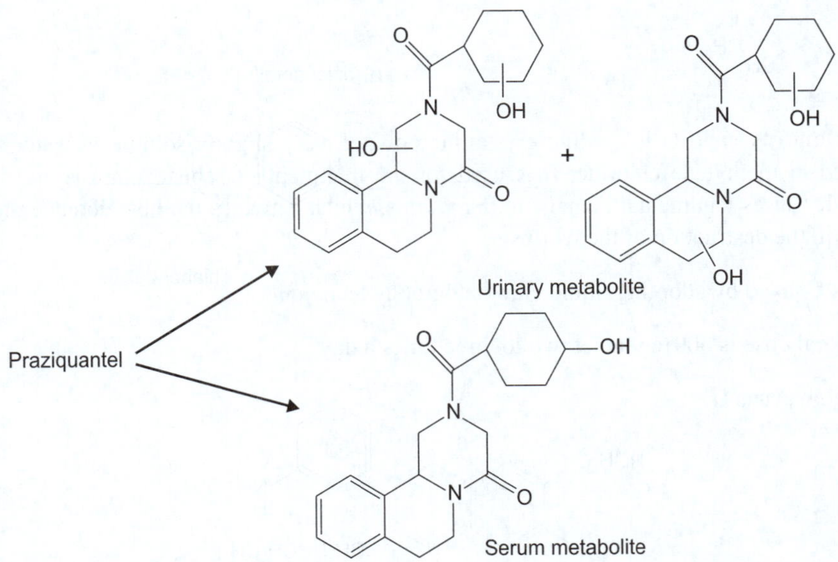

Synthesis

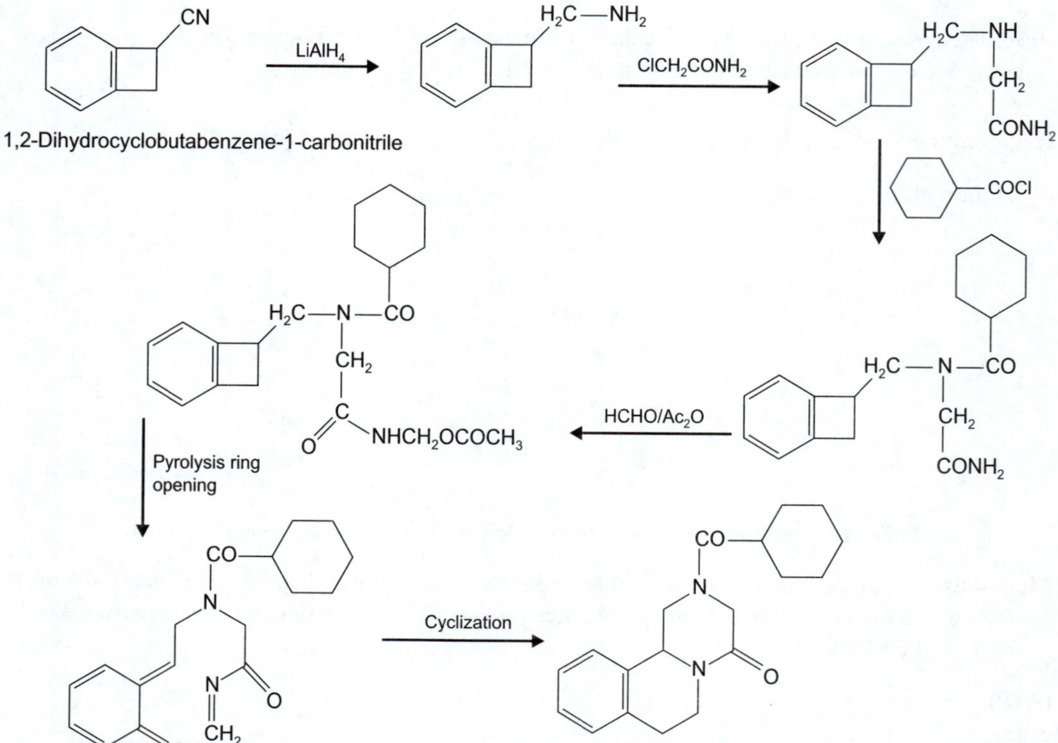

Praziquantel

Properties and uses: PZQ is a white crystalline powder, very slightly soluble in water, soluble in alcohol, and in methylene chloride. It is used for the treatment of schistosomiasis and liver fluke infections. It causes legumental damage to the worms, which activates the host defence mechanisms and results in the destruction of the worms.

Assay: It is assayed by adopting liquid chromatography technique.

Dose: The oral dose is 600 mg tablet two to three times a day.

Oxamniquine (Vansil)

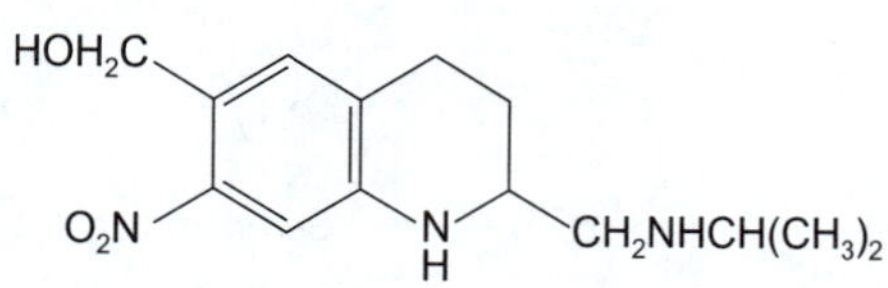

(2-((Isopropylamino)methyl)-7-nitro-1,2,3,4-tetrahydroquinolin-6-yl)methanol

Synthesis

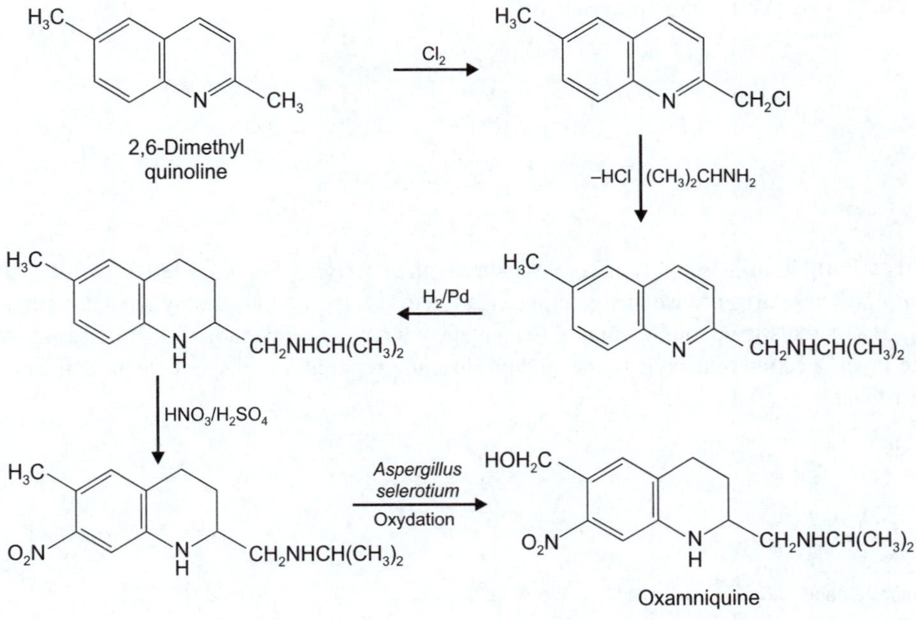

Mode of action: *Schistosoma mansoni* is highly susceptible to oxamniquine. Adenosine-5′-triphosphate (ATP)-dependent enzymatic activation of the drug in susceptible schistosomes forms unstable phosphate esters, which disassociate to yield a chemically reactive carbocation, this intermediate alkylates the DNA.

Metabolism: It is metabolized by oxidative reaction and it gives inactive metabolites of acid and alcohol derivatives.

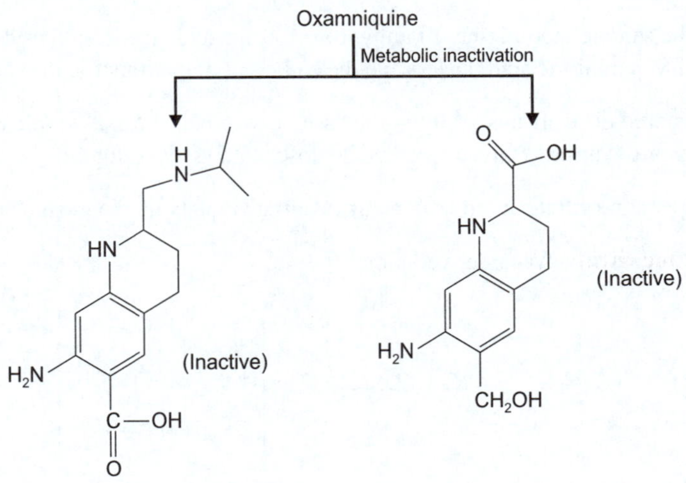

Dose: The dose for oral route after meals depends upon geographical areas. In the western hemisphere, the dose is 15 mg/kg as a single dose, in Africa 15–60 mg/kg over 1–3 days.

III. Piperazine derivatives

Piperazine citrate (Vermizine, Antepar)

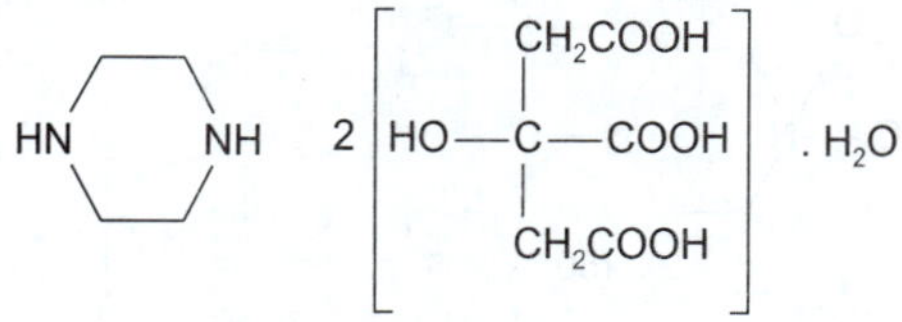

Mode of action: The drug is highly effective against both *Ascaris lumbricoides* and *Enterobius (oxyuris) vermicularis*. These drugs cause the hyperpolarization of the ascaris muscles by gamma-aminobutyric acid (GABA) agonistic action, opening Cl-channels, which cause relaxation, depress responsiveness to the contractile action of acetylcholine, and produce the suppression of spontaneous spike potentials with peristalsis.

Synthesis

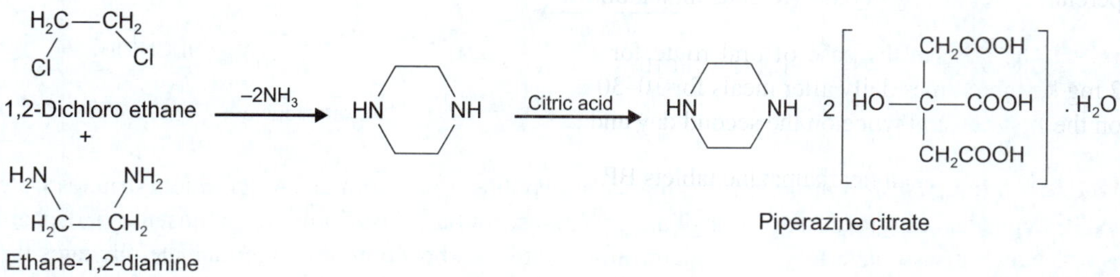

Properties and uses: Piperazine citrate is a white granular powder, soluble in water, and practically insoluble in alcohol, used as an anthelmintic. It can cause gastrointestinal and allergic reactions. It is contraindicated in epileptic patients.

Assay: Dissolve the sample in a mixture of anhydrous formic acid, acetic anhydride (2:3), and titrate quickly against 0.1 M perchloric acid. Determine the end point potentiometrically.

Dose: The administered dose always orally in the case of ascaris is 3.5 g as single dose daily for two consecutive days. For oxyuriasis (thread worms) the dose is 2.5 g given for 7 days.

Dosage forms: Piperazine citrate syrup IP, piperazine citrate tablets IP, piperazine citrate elixir BP.

Diethyl carbamazine citrate (Vanaide, Vellcome)

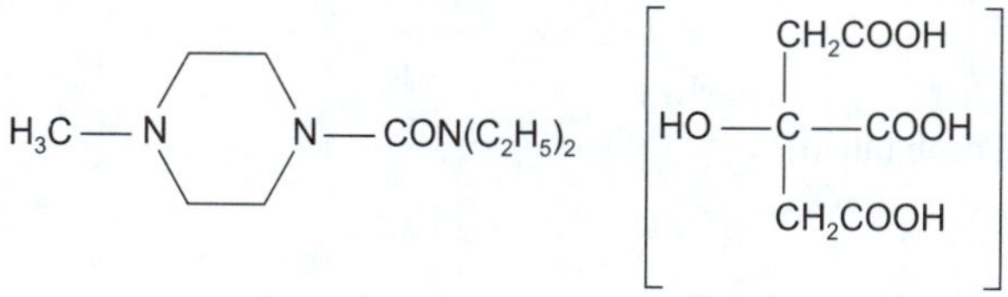

Mode of action: It selectively acts on the microflora, causes attraction, and therefore, is readily phagocytosed by the tissue fixed monocytes. It also has an effect on the muscular activity of the microflora and causes hyperpolarization to destroy the worms.

Metabolism: The metabolism of diethyl carbamazepine leads to the compounds of methyl piperazine and piperazine. Nearly, all of the metabolites appear in the urine.

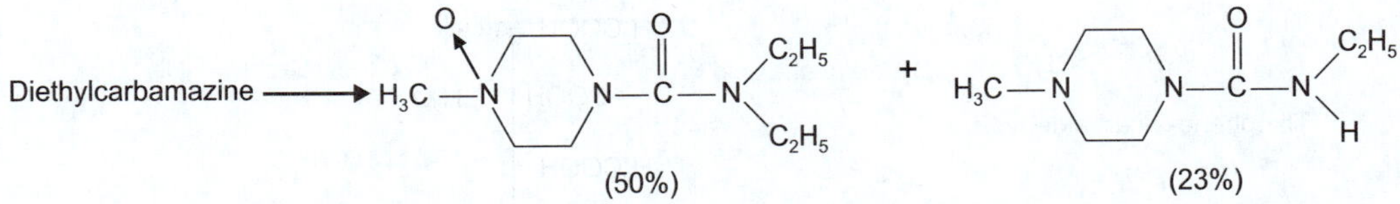

Properties and uses: Diethylcarbamazine citrate is a white crystalline slightly hygroscopic powder, very soluble in water, soluble in alcohol, and practically insoluble in acetone. It is the drug of choice for treating filariasis infections. In adequate dosage, it clears the blood rapidly of the microfilariae and appears to be curative. Antihistamines or corticosteroids may be needed to control the allergic reaction caused by the disintegration of microfilariae. It is active against microfilariea of *Loa loa*, but may cause encephalopathy.

Assay: Dissolve the sample in anhydrous acetic acid, add acetic anhydride, and titrate with 0.1 M perchloric acid using crystal violet as indicator, until a greenish-blue colour is obtained.

Dose: The dose in the case of oral route for *Brugia malayi*, *Loa loa*, and *Wuchereria bancrofti* is 2 mg/kg three times daily after meals for 10–30 days. For *Caecal volvulus*, the dose is 0.5 mg/kg once on the first day and twice on the second day and the adverse effects limit the use of this drug.

Dosage forms: Diethylcarbamazine tablets BP.

Synthesis

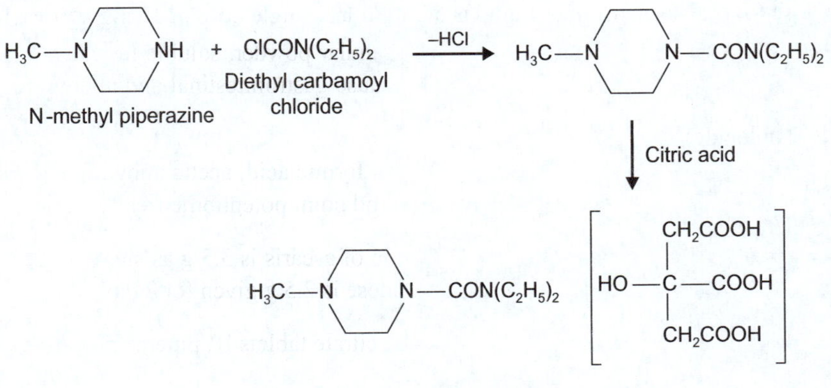

Diethylcarbamazine citrate

IV. Vinyl pyrimidines

Pyrantel (Antiminth, Combantrin)

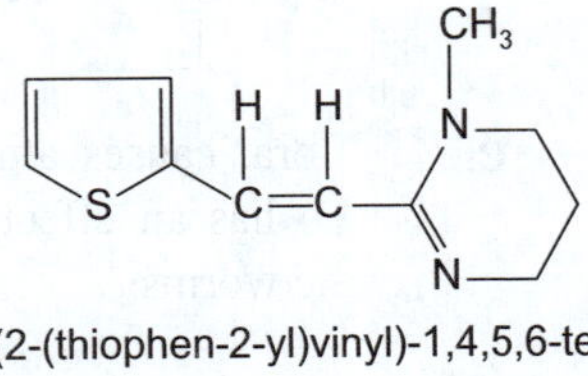

1-Methyl-2-(2-(thiophen-2-yl)vinyl)-1,4,5,6-tetrahydropyrimidine

Synthesis

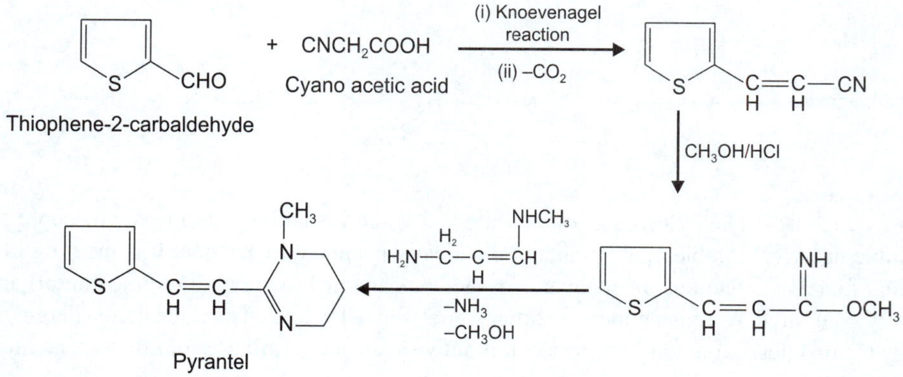

Mode of action: Pyrantel is a depolarizing neuromuscular blocking agent. It induces marked persistent activation of the nicotinic receptors, which result in spastic paralysis of the worm. It is an alternative to mebendazole in the treatment of ascariasis and enterobiasis.

Properties and uses: It is a pale yellow or yellow powder, practically insoluble in water and in methanol, soluble in dimethyl sulphoxide. It is also as investigational drug for the treatment of hookworms, moniliformis, and trichostrongylus infections.

Assay: To the sample add acetic anhydride and glacial acetic acid, heat and stir. Allow to cool and titrate with 0.1 M perchloric acid. Determine the end point potentiometrically.

Doses: The dose for oral suspension or liquid is 50 mg/ml. A single dose of 11 mg/kg for ascarasis and enterobiasis.

V. Amides

Niclosamide (Niclocide)

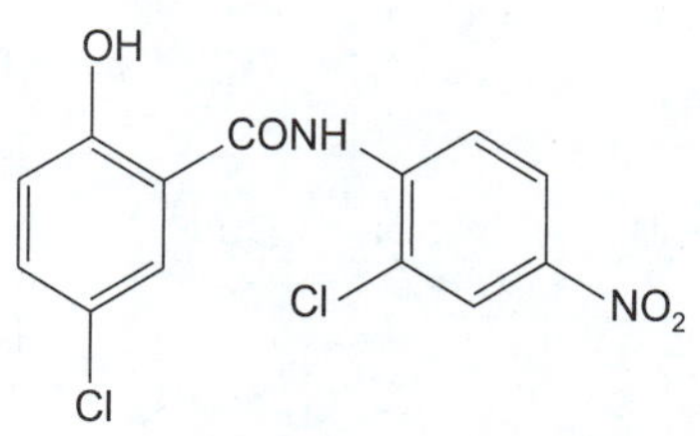

Synthesis

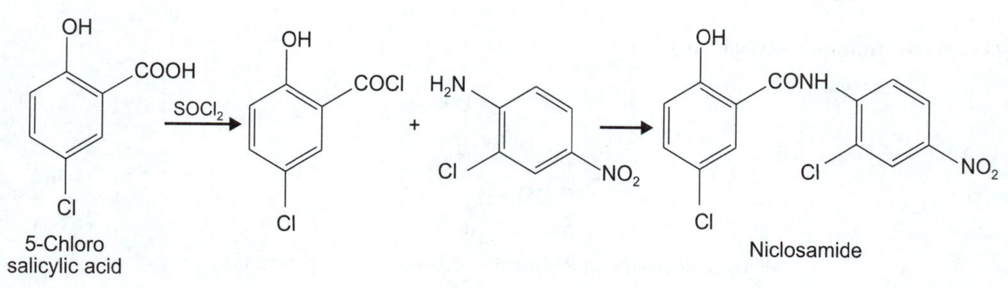

Mode of action: Niclosamide is also a potent mollusicide, which is effective against *Biomphaloria glabrata*, the principle action of the drug may be to inhibit anaerobic phosphorylation of adenosine diphosphate (ADP) by the mitochondria of the parasite, an energy producing process.

Properties and uses: Niclosamide exists as yellowish fine crystals, practically insoluble in water, sparingly soluble in acetone, and slightly soluble in ethanol. It is used as an anthelmintic.

Assay: Dissolve the sample in a mixture of equal volumes of acetone and methanol and titrate with 0.1 M tetrabutylammonium hydroxide. Determine the end point potentiometrically.

Dose: The dose orally to be taken after meals is 2 g chewable tablets.

Dosage forms: Niclosamide tablets BP.

VI. Natural products

Avermectins (Mectizan)

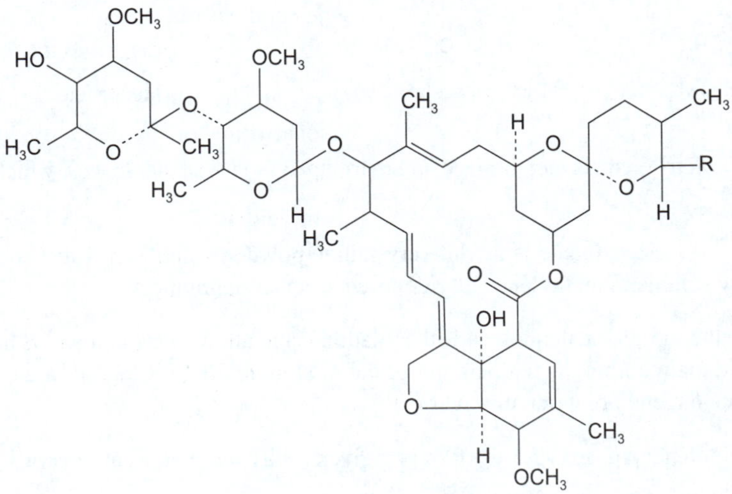

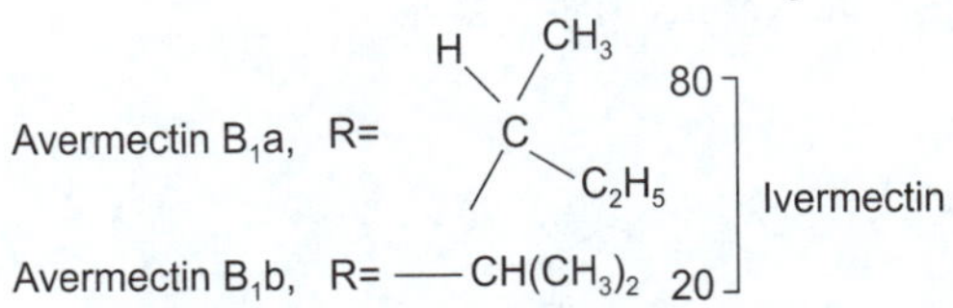

Mode of action: Avermectins specifically open the chloride channels in the invertebrate system distinct from the GABA-gated and glutamate-gated chloride channels.

Metabolism: It is metabolized and it gives 3-*O*-demethyl-22,23-dihydroavermectin $B_{1\alpha}$ monosaccharide.

Properties and uses: Avermectins are macrocyclic lactones with broad antinematocidal activity. This class of compound was isolated from a fermentation broth of a soil actinomycetics (*Streptomycin avermitils*). The drug avermectin is now effectively being used to treat and control *Onchocera volvulus*, the filarial infection responsible for liver blindness. Ivermectin is a mixture of B_1a and B_1b (80:20) and is prepared by catalytic reduction of ivermectin B1 (Abamectin).

VII. Organophosphorus compounds

Metrifonate (Bilacil)

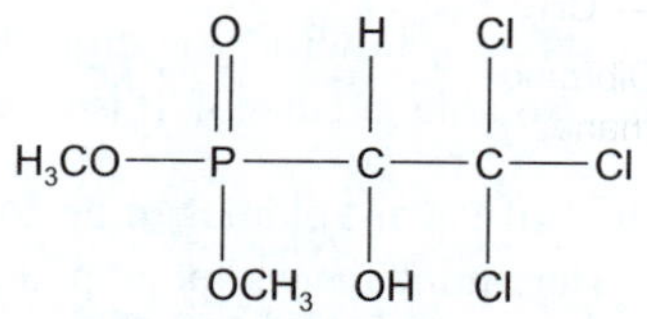

Dimethyl-2,2,2-trichloro-1-hydroxyethylphosphonate

Synthesis

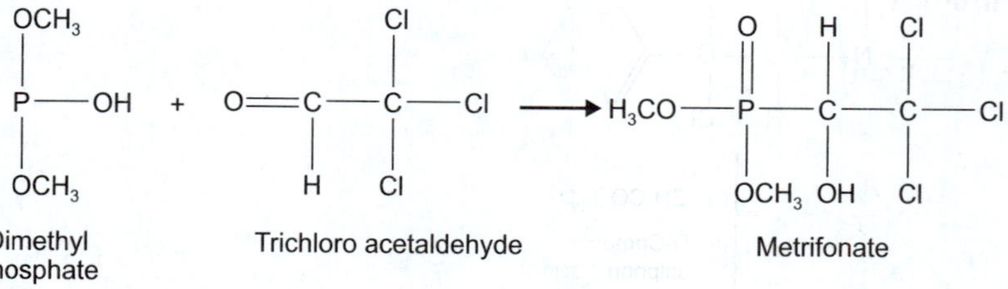

Mode of action: Metrifonate is metabolized and rearranged *in vivo* to dichlorvos, which inhibits acetyl cholinesterase.

Properties and uses: Metrifonate is a white crystalline powder, soluble in water, in acetone, and in alcohol, and very soluble in methylene chloride, used as an anthelmintic.

Assay: Dissolve the sample in alcohol, add ethanolamine, and allow to stand for 1 hrs at 20–22°C. Add chilled nitric acid maintaining the temperature of the mixture at 20–22°C and titrate with 0.1 M silver nitrate. Determine the end point potentiometrically.

Doses: The recommended dose is 7.5 to 10 mg/kg given orally three times at intervals of 2 weeks.

VIII. Midazothiazoles (Bizole, Vermisol)

Levamisole

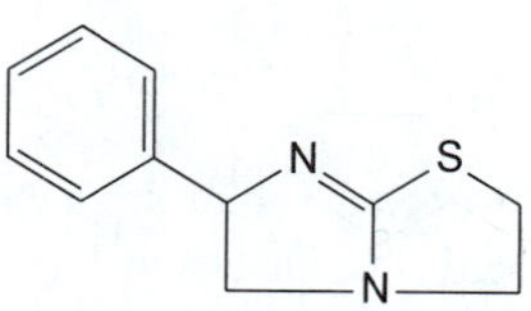

6-Phenyl-2,3,5,6-tetrahydroimidazo[2,1-*b*]thiazole

Synthesis

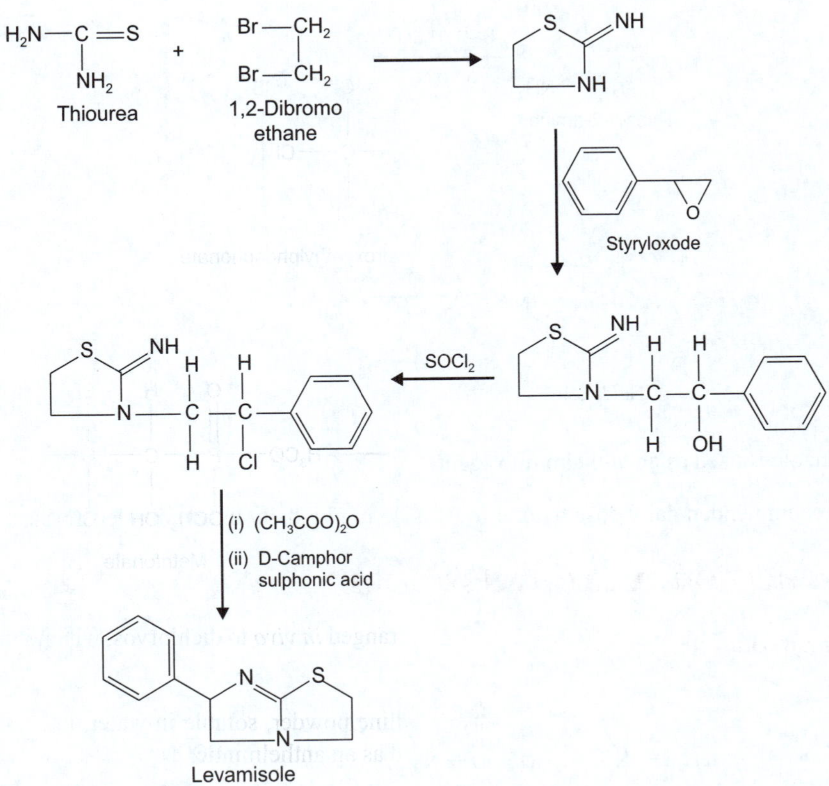

Mode of action: It stimulates the ganglion in the worms, causes tonic paralysis, which results in the expulsion of live worms. These also interfere with the carbohydrate metabolism by inhibiting fumarate reductase.

Dose: The administered dose is 15 mg as a single dose, repeated after 1 month to prevent recurrence.

IX. Nitro derivatives

Niridazole (Ambilhar)

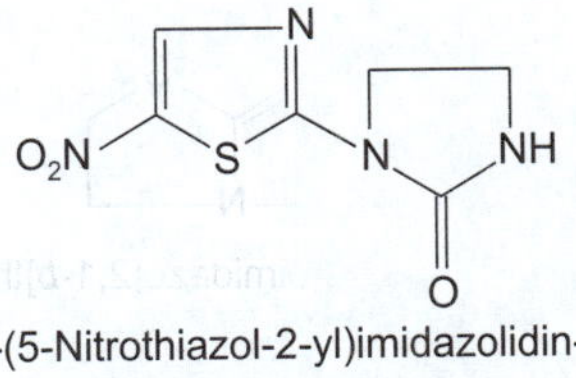

1-(5-Nitrothiazol-2-yl)imidazolidin-2-one

Synthesis

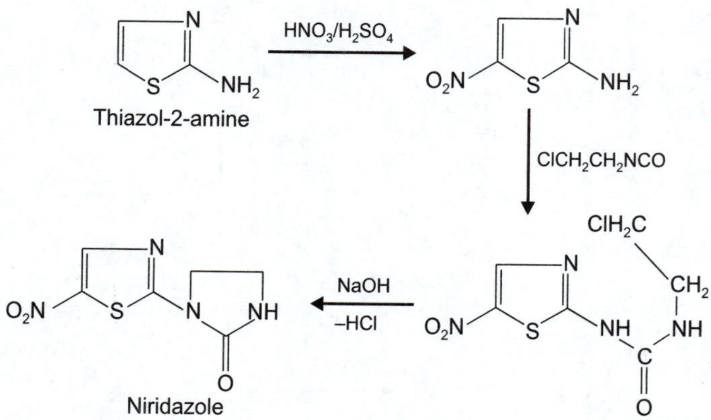

Uses: Niridazole is used as an anthelmintic agent.

Dose: The recommended daily dose by oral route is 25 mg/kg daily in two divided doses.

CLASSIFICATION BASED ON PCI SYLLABUS

Diethylcarbamazine citrate

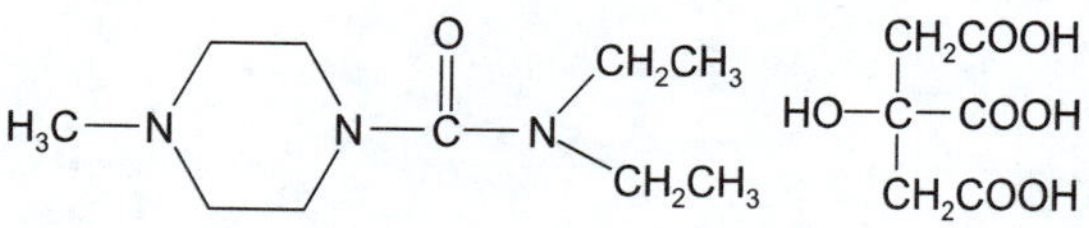

Thiabendazole

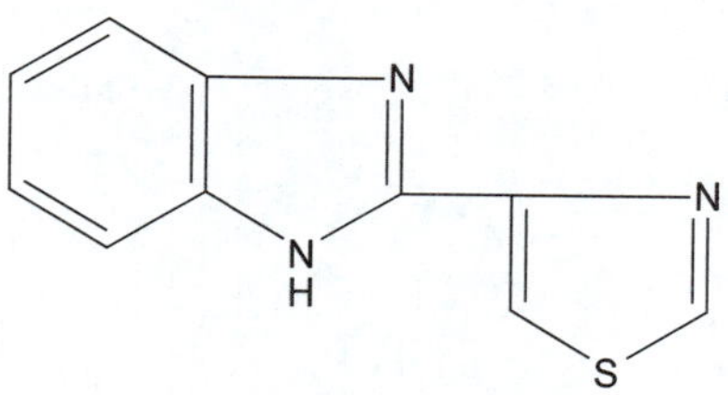

Mebendazole

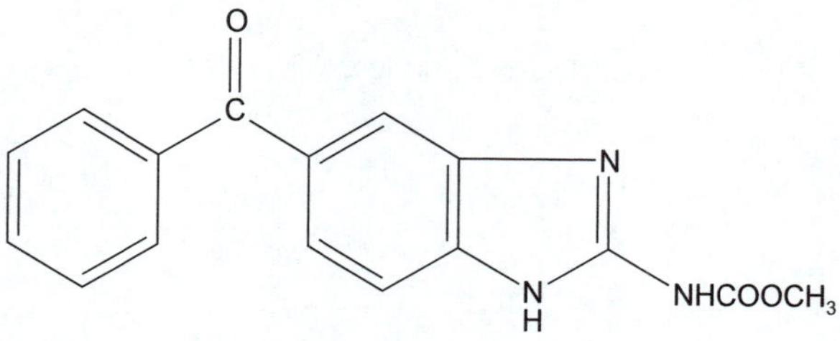

Albendazole

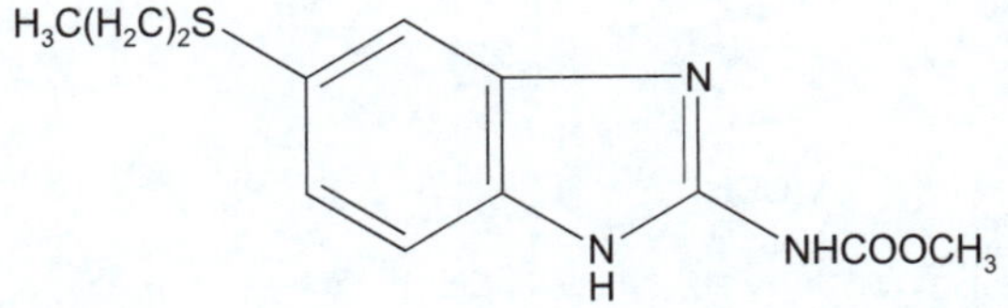

Niclosamide

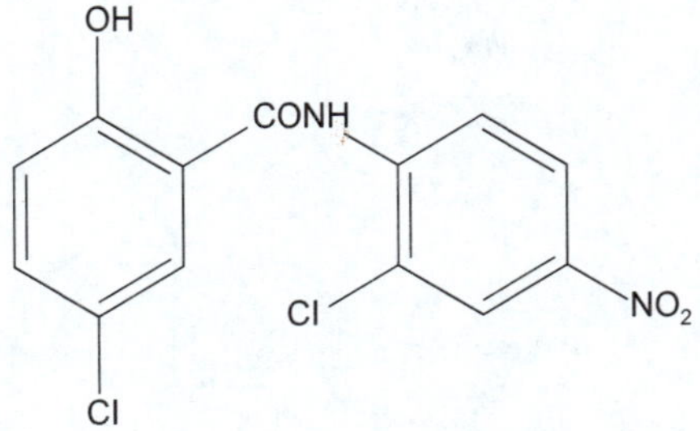

Oxamniquine

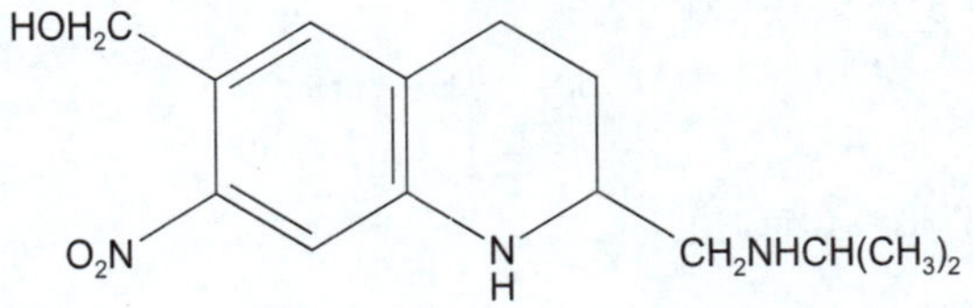

Praziquantal

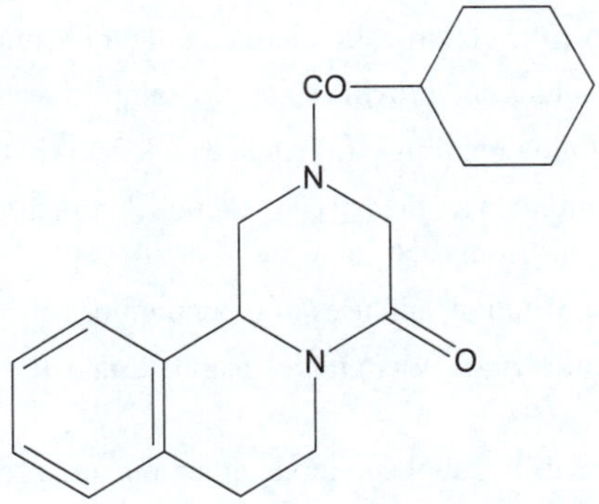

Ivermectin

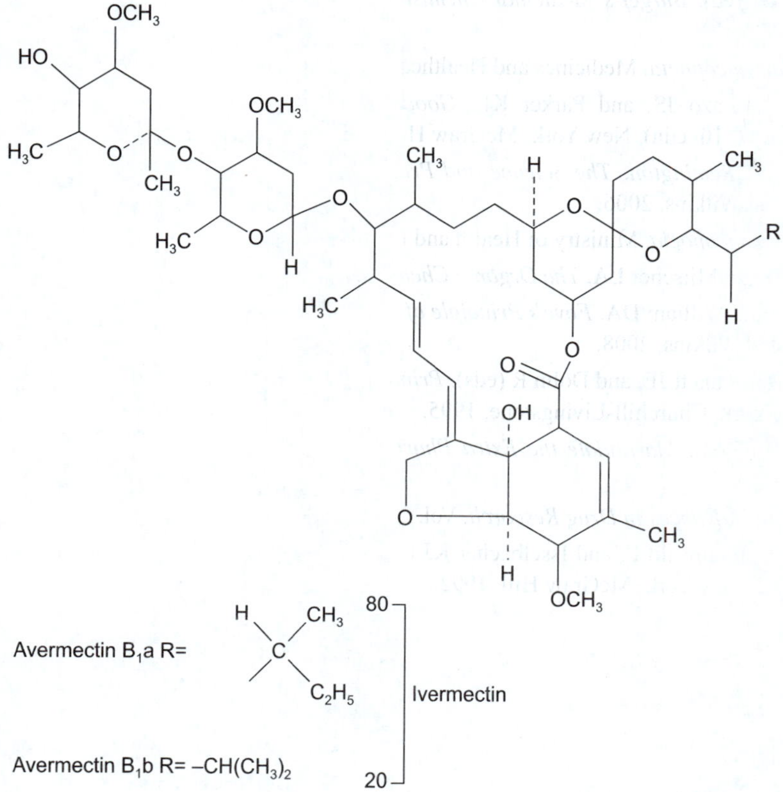

PROBABLE QUESTIONS

1. Define anthelmintics and write the classification based on their chemical structure.
2. Write in detail about anthelmintics and provide suitable examples wherever necessary.
3. Outline the synthesis of the following drugs: (a) Albendazole and (b) thiabendazole.
4. How will you classify anthelmintics on the basis of chemical structures? Write the structure, chemical name, and uses of two examples from each category.
5. Describe the synthesis, mode of action, and uses of oxaminquine.
6. Write a short note on the following: (a) Pyrantel pamoate and (b) organophosphorus anthelmintic compounds.
7. What is avermectin? Describe its metabolism, mode of action, and uses.
8. Enumerate the various benzimidazoles derived from anthelmintics with their chemical structure, and write the synthesis, metabolism, and uses of mebendazole.
9. Mention an anthelmintic drug possessing quinoline nucleus, describe its synthesis, metabolism and uses.
10. Write a note on piperazine-derived anthelmintics.

SUGGESTED READINGS

1. Abraham DJ (ed). *Burger's Medicinal Chemistry and Drug Discovery* (6th edn). New Jersey: John Wiley, 2007.
2. *British Pharmacopoeia*. Medicines and Healthcare Products Regulatory Agency. London, 2008.
3. Bruntan LL, Lazo JS, and Parker KL. *Goodman and Gilman's: The Pharmacological Basis of Therapeutics* (11th edn). New York: McGraw Hill, 2006.
4. Gennaro AR. *Remington: The Science and Practice of Pharmacy* (21st edn). New York: Lippincot Williams and Wilkins, 2006.
5. *Indian Pharmacopoeia*. Ministry of Health and Family Welfare. New Delhi, 1996.
6. Lednicer D and Mitscher LA. *The Organic Chemistry of Drug Synthesis*. New York: John Wiley 1995.
7. Lemke TL and William DA. *Foye's Principle of Medicinal Chemistry* (6th edn). New York: Lippincott Williams and Wilkins, 2008.
8. Mandel GL, Bennett JE, and Dolin R (eds). *Principles and Practices of Infectious Diseases*, Vol. I (4th edn). New York: Churchill-Livingstone, 1995.
9. Reynolds EF (ed). *Martindale the Extra Pharmacopoeia*. (31st edn). London: The Pharmaceutical Press, 1997.
10. Testa B (ed). *Advances in Drug Research*, Vol. 21. New York: Academic Press, 1991.
11. Wilson JD, Braunwald E, and Isselbacher KJ (eds). *Harrison's Principles of Internal Medicine* (12th edn), p. 772. New York: McGraw Hill, 1992.

CHAPTER 22

Antineoplastic Agents

INTRODUCTION

Antineoplastic agents are drugs used for the treatment of cancer, malignancy, tumour, carcinoma, sarcoma, leukaemia, or neoplasm (Greek *neo* = new, *plasm* = formation). Neoplasm refers to a group of diseases caused by several agents, namely, chemical compounds and radiant energy. Cancer is characterized by an abnormal and uncontrolled, division of cells, which produces tumours and invades adjacent normal tissues. Often, cancer cells separate themselves from the primary tumour, and are carried by the lymphatic system to reach distant sites of the organs, where they divide and form secondary tumours (metastasis).

Cell Cycle Kinetics

Two key aspects of cellular life are the following:

1. DNA synthesis and mitosis to produce new cells.
2. Cell differentiation that produces specialized cells.

Limitations of Therapy

- Cancer cells very rapidly develop resistance to antineoplastic drugs.
- Differences between normal and neoplastic human cells are merely quantitative.
- Biochemical and morphological differences between normal and neoplastic cells are slight; therefore, antineoplastic agents are devoid of selective toxicity to tumour cells.
- Antineoplastic agents kill cells by first-order kinetics, that is, they kill a constant fraction of cells. However, some of the cancer cells elude killing and one of these cells may restablize the tumour. It is extremely difficult to kill all the malignant cells.
- Most antineoplastic drugs are highly toxic to the patients.

Adverse Effects

The prominent adverse effects of antineoplastic drugs are exerted on rapidly proliferating normal tissues, in addition, to their chronic and cumulative toxicities.

- **Bone marrow toxicity:** Bleomycin and L-asparaginase.

- **Hair follicle toxicity:** Methotrexate, vincristine, cyclophosphamide, and doxorubicin.
- **Hepatotoxicity:** Azathiopurine, mercaptopurine, and L-asparaginase.
- **Skin rashes:** Vinca alkaloids, nitrosourea, anthracyclins, and mitomycin C.
- **Pulmonary toxicity:** Bleomycin, methotrexate, and busulfan.
- **Cardiac toxicity:** Doxorubicin, daunorubicin, and anthracyclins.
- **Other toxicities:** Intestinal epithelium, central nervous system (CNS) toxicity, nephrotoxicity, immunosuppression, fever, anaphylaxis, cataracts, haemolytic anaemia, pancreatitis, pituitary insufficiency, adrenal insufficiency, coagulation problems, suppression of growth, and carcinogenicity.

CLASSIFICATION

Antineoplastic agents are classified as follows:

I. Alkylating agents
II. Antimetabolites
III. Antibiotics
IV. Plant products
V. Enzymes
VI. Hormones
VII. Immunotherapy
VIII. Monoclonal antibodies
IX. Radio-therapeutic agents
X. Cyto-protective agents
XI. Miscellaneous
XII. Newer Drugs

I. Alkylating Agents

a. Nitrogen mustards

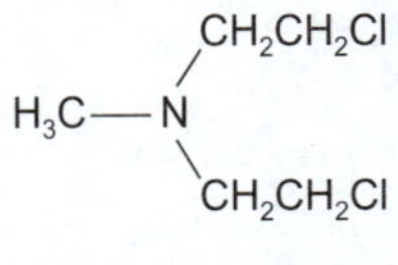

Mechlorethamine

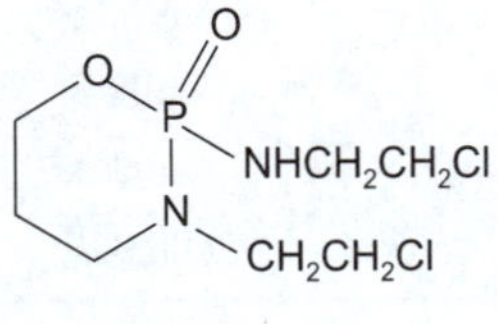

Ifosamide

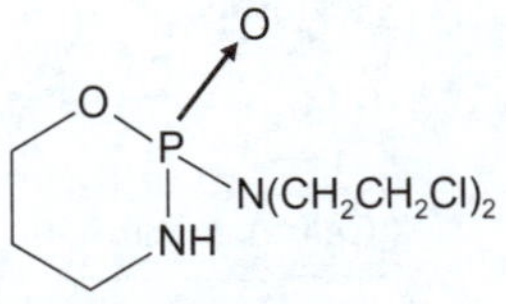

Cyclophosphamide

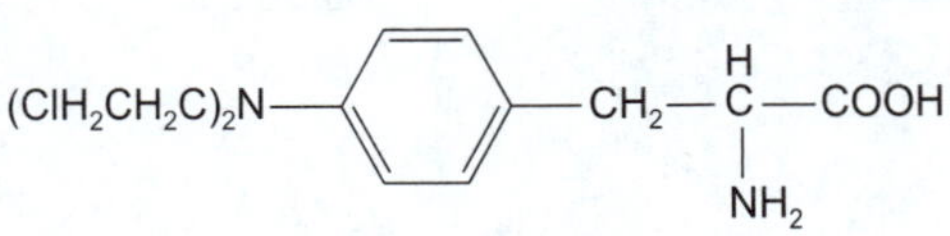

Melphalan

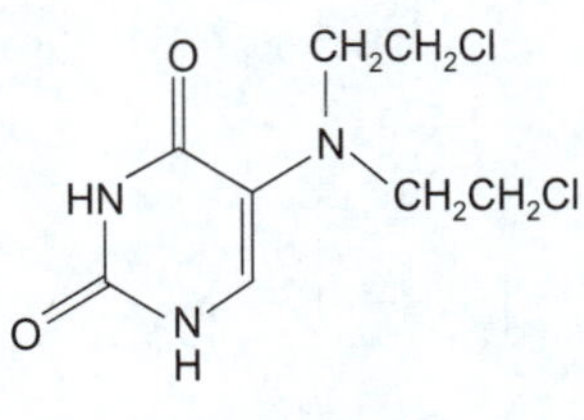

Uracil mustard

Chlorambucil

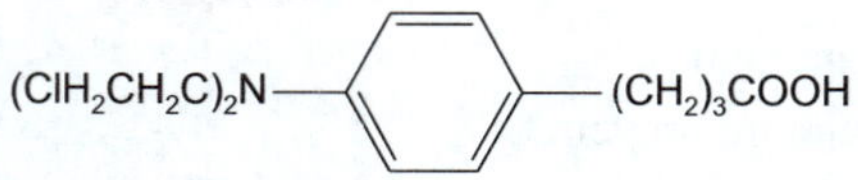

Estramustine

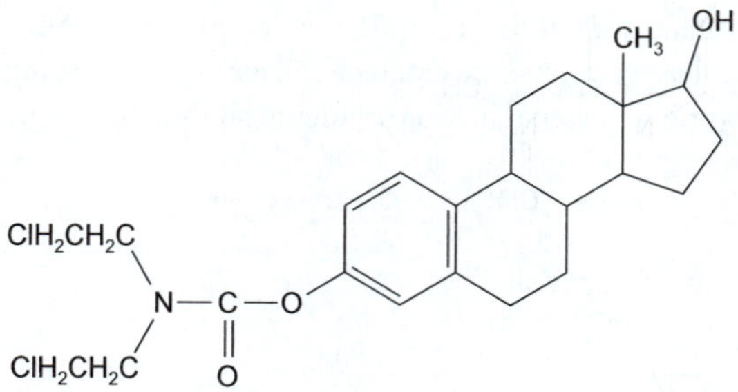

b. Alkyl sulphonate

Busulfan

$CH_3SO_2O(CH_2)_4OSO_2CH_3$

c. Nitrosoureas

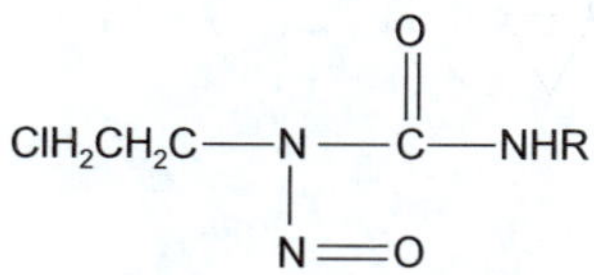

Name	***R***
Carmustine	$-CH_2CH_2Cl$
Lomustine	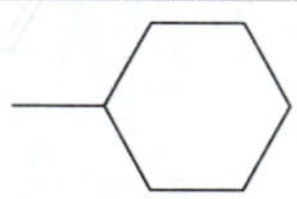
Semustine	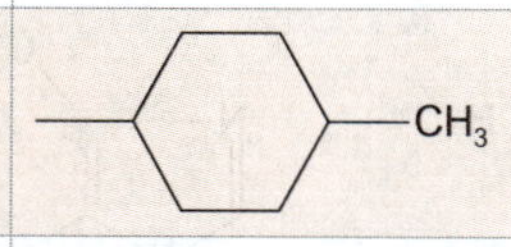
Chlorozotocin	Glucose

d. Aziridines

Thiotepa

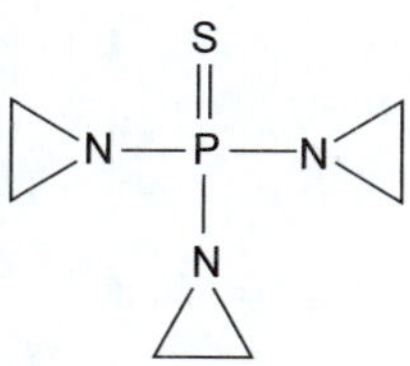

Benzotepa

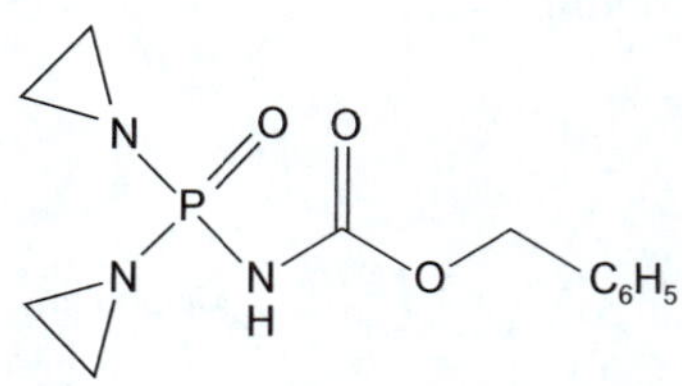

Altretamine

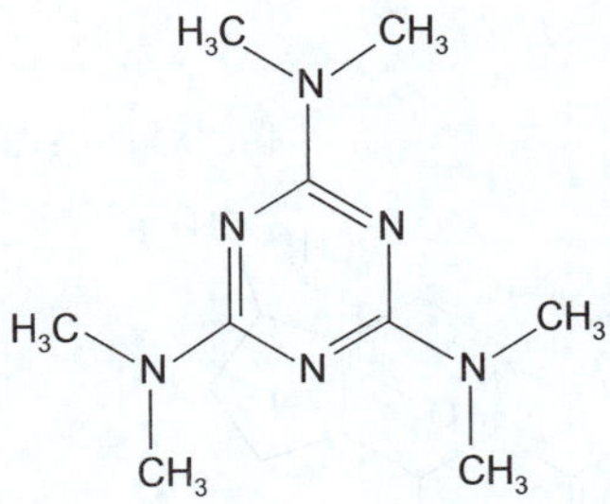

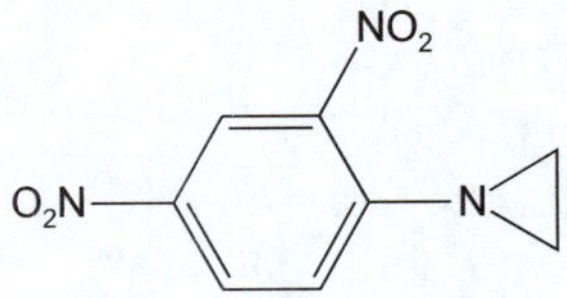

1-(2,4-dinitrophenyl) aziridine

Triethylene melamine

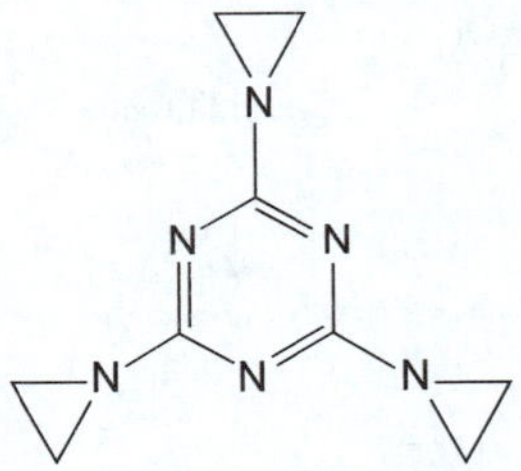

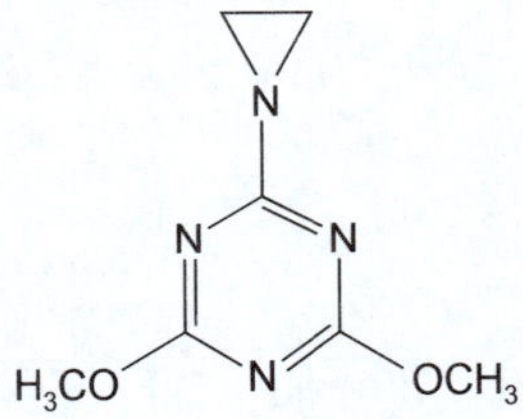

4-(1-aziridinyl)-2,6-dimethoxy triazine

e. Methylhydrazines

Procarbazine

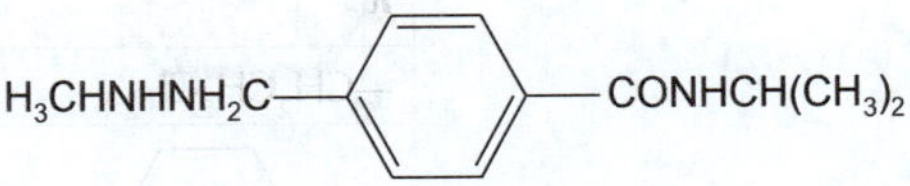

Dacarbazine

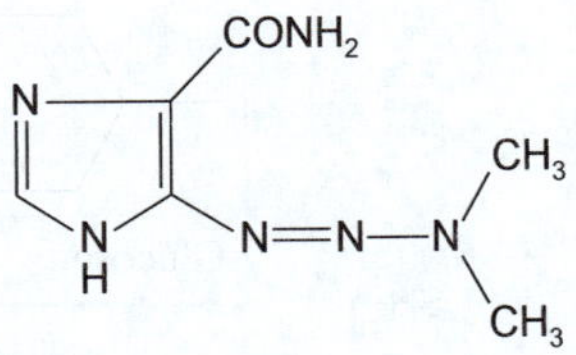

II. Antimetabolites

a. Pyrimidine analogues

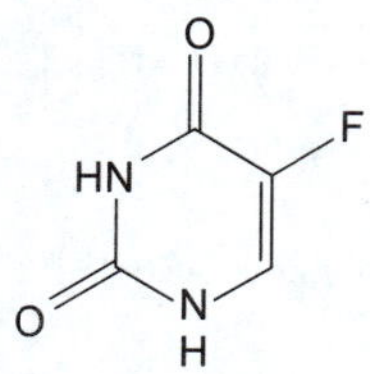

5-Fluorouracil (5-FU)

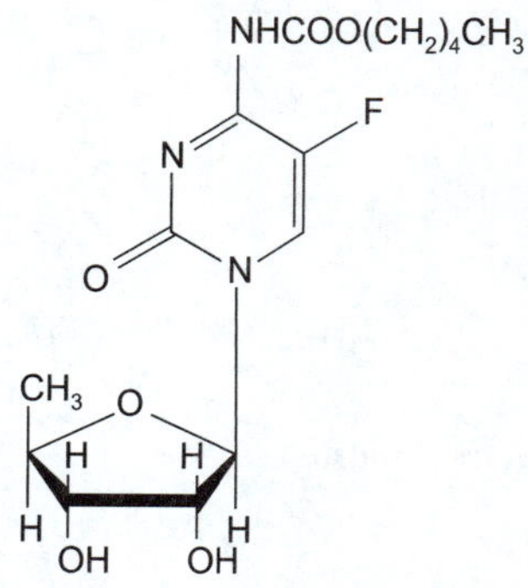

Capectitabine

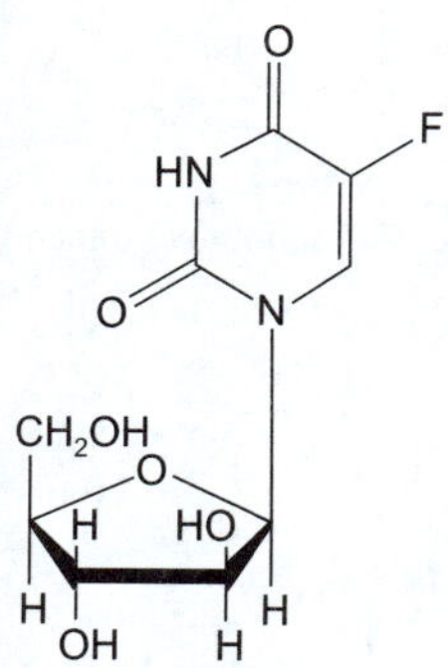

Floxuridine

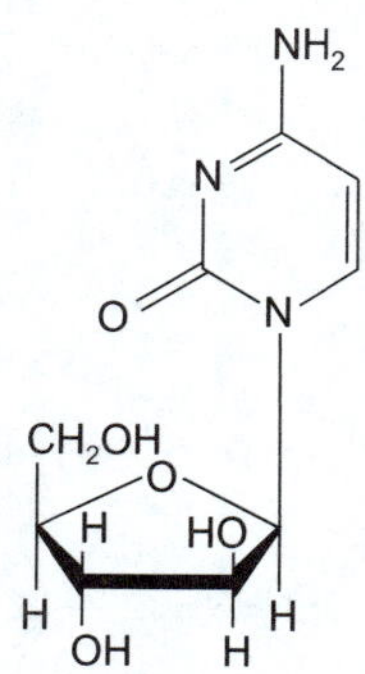

Cytarabine

b. Purine analogues

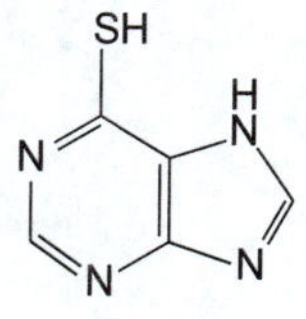

6-Mercaptopurine

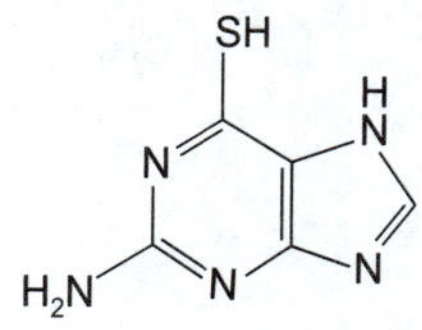

6-Thioguanine

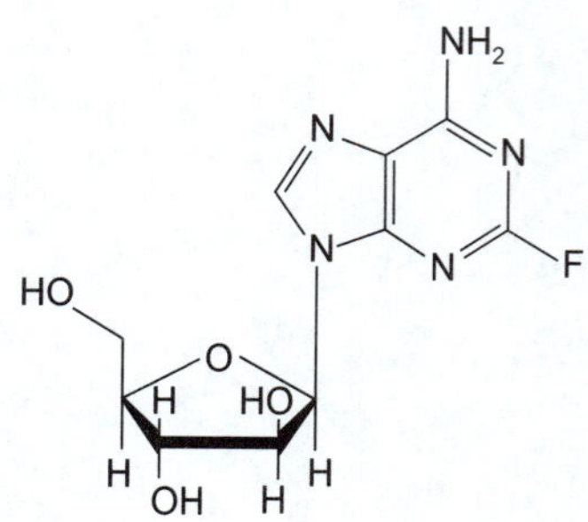

Fludarabine

c. Folic acid analogues

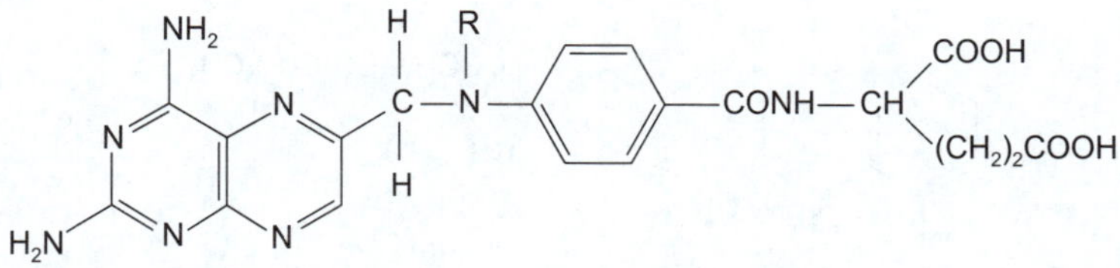

R = H (Aminopterin)
R = CH_3 (Methotrexate)

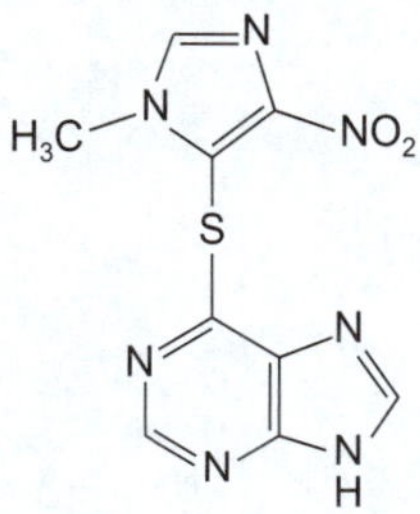

Azathiopurine

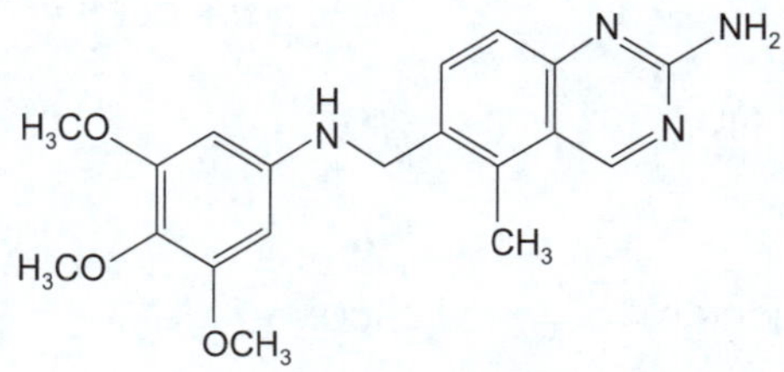

Trimetrexate

III. Antibiotics

a. Anthracyclines

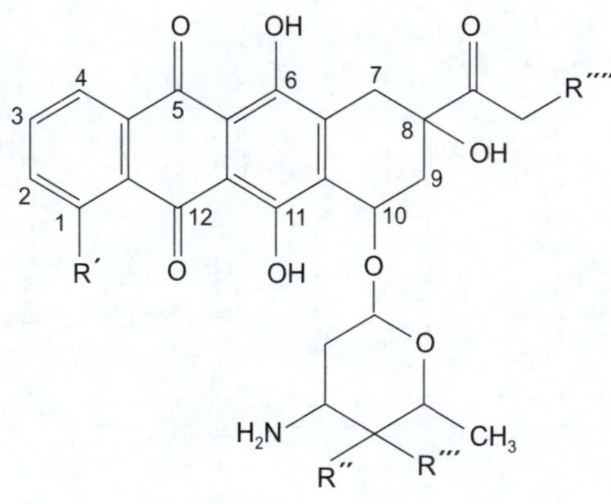

Name	*R'*	*R''*	*R'''*	*R''''*
Daunorubicin	$-OCH_3$	–H	–OH	–H
Doxorubicin	$-OCH_3$	–H	–OH	–OH
Carminomycin	–OH	–H	–OH	–OH
Idarubicin	–H	–H	–OH	–H
Epirubicin	$-OCH_3$	–OH	–H	–OH

Valrubicin

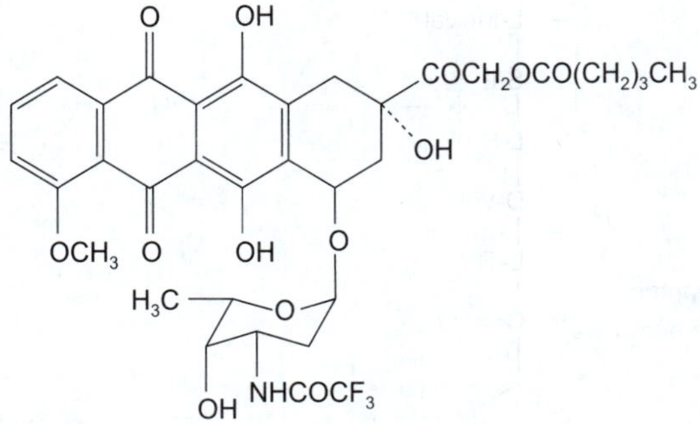

b. Bleomycins

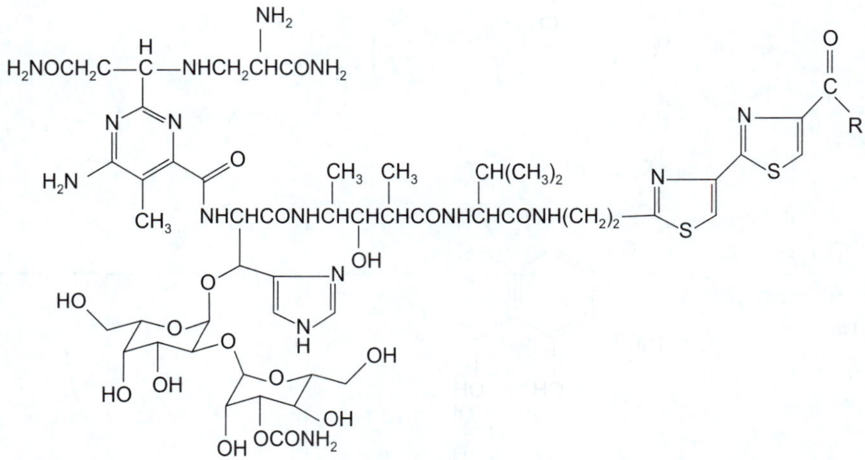

Name	*R*
Bleomycinic acid	–OH
Bleomycin A_2^-	$-NH(CH_2)_3\overset{\oplus}{S}(CH_3)_2$
Bleomycin B_2^-	$-NH(CH_2)_4NH-C(=NH)-NH_2$

c. Mitomycins

Mitomycin C

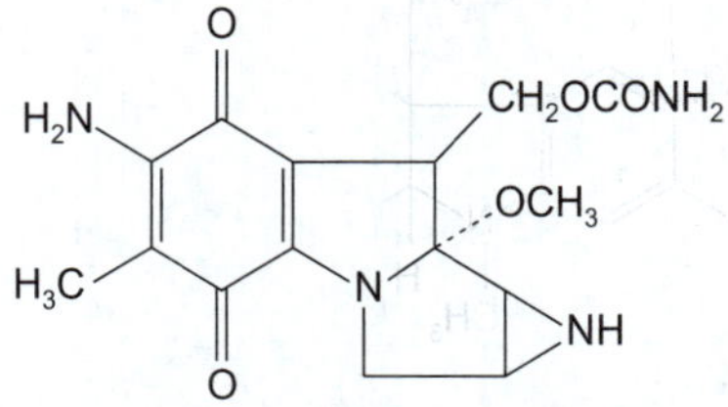

Dactinomycin C or actinomycin D

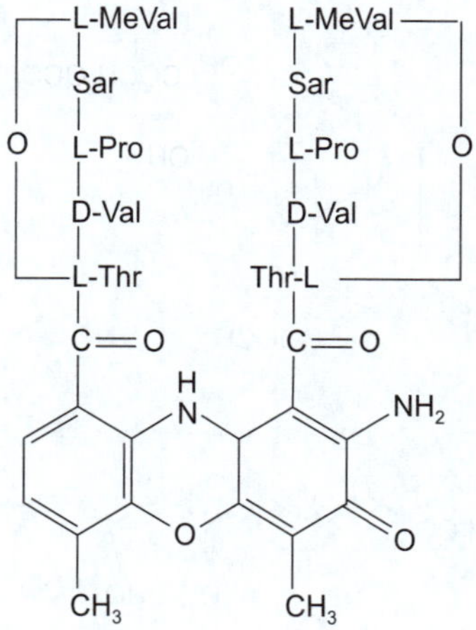

Plicamycin or mithramycin

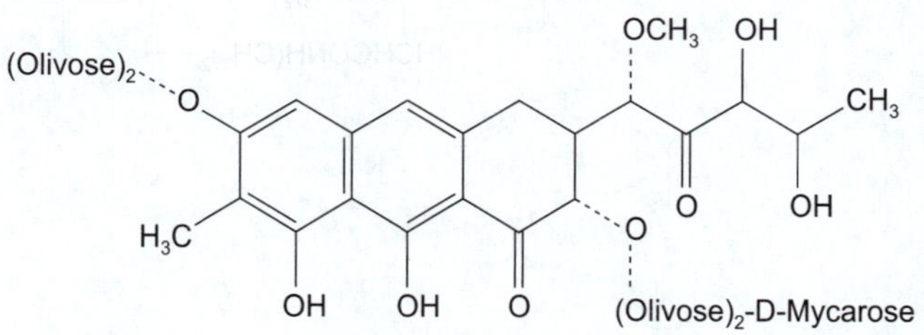

IV. Plant Products

a. **Vinca alkaloids**

Vinorelbine

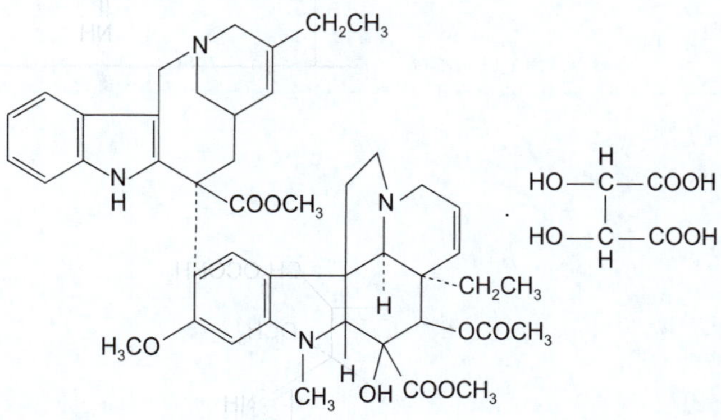

Vincristine, vinblastine

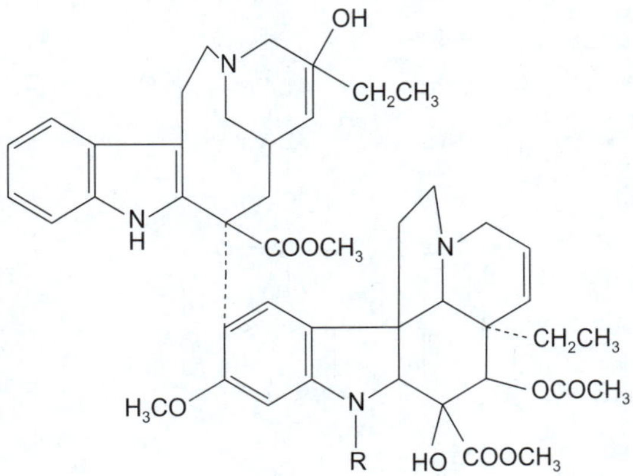

Vincristine, R = CHO

Vinblastine, R = CH_3

b. Camptothecin derivatives

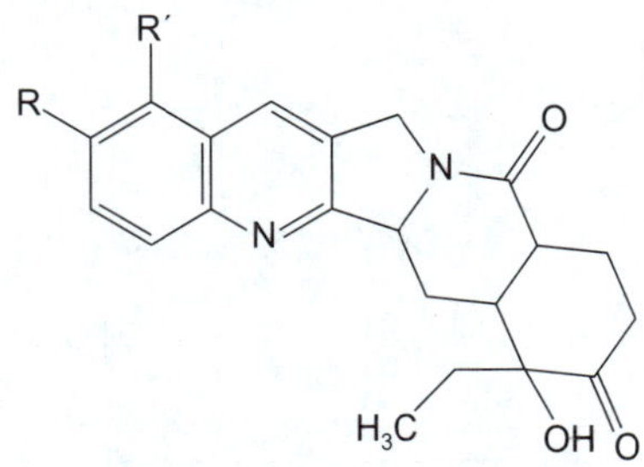

Name	***R***	***R′***
Camptothecin	–H	–H
Irinotecan	$-C_2H_5$	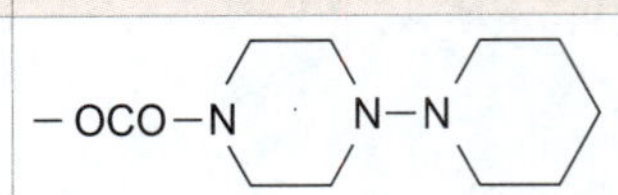
Topotecan	$-CH_2N(CH_3)_2$	–OH

c. Epipodophyllo toxins

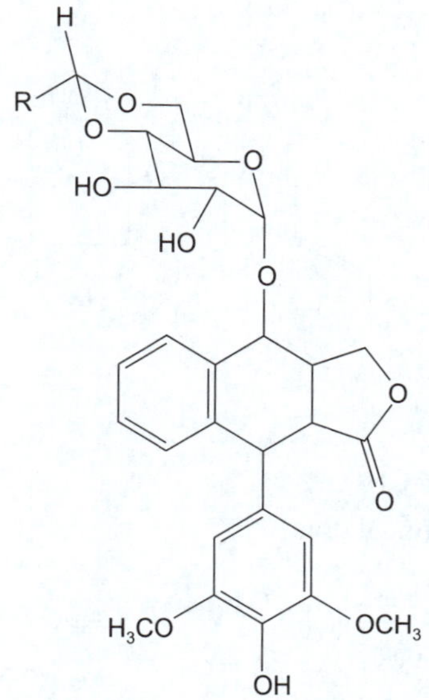

Etoposide, R = CH_3

Teniposide, R = 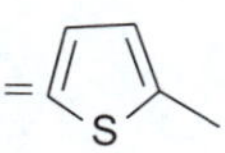

d. Taxol derivatives

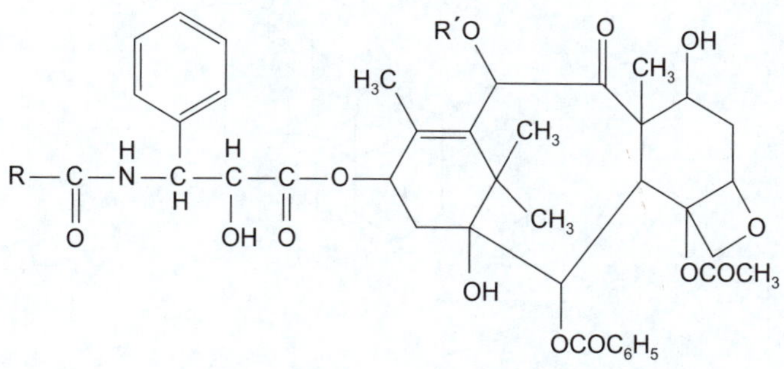

Name	R	R′
Paclitaxel	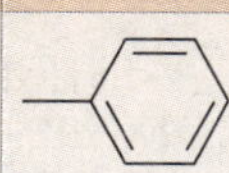	$-COCH_3$
Docetaxel	$(CH_3)_3CO-$	–H

V. Enzymes

Examples: L-Asparaginase, pegaspargase

VI. Hormones

a. Estrogenic derivatives

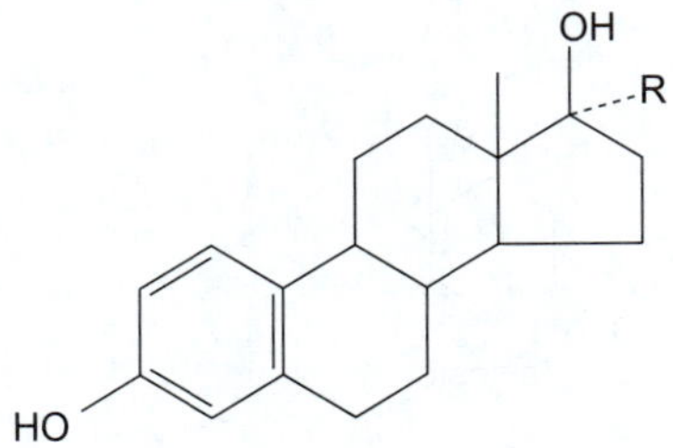

(i) 17-β-Estradiol, R = H

(ii) Ethinyl estradiol, R = —C≡CH

Diethylstilbesterol (non-steroidal drug)

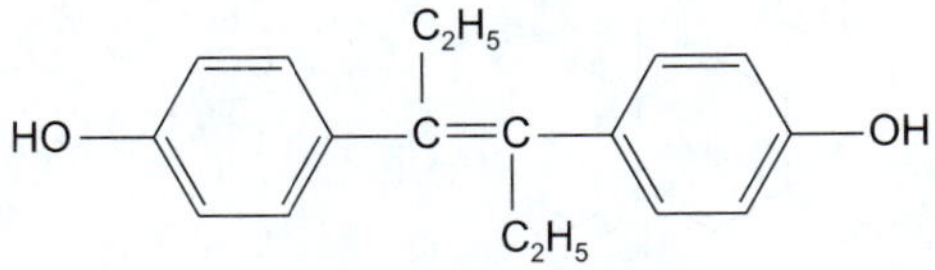

b. Progestine derivatives

Progesterone

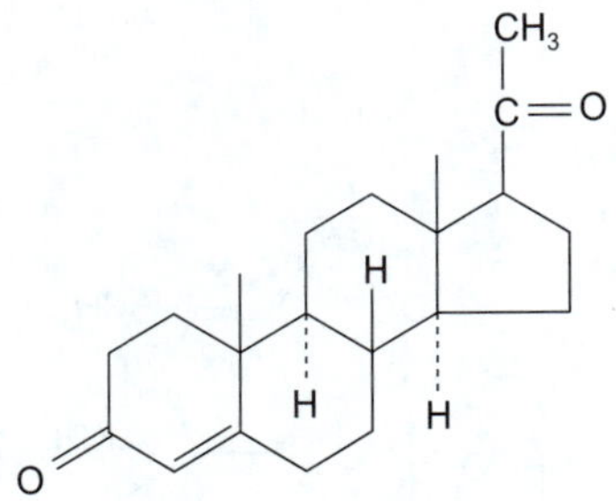

Progestins

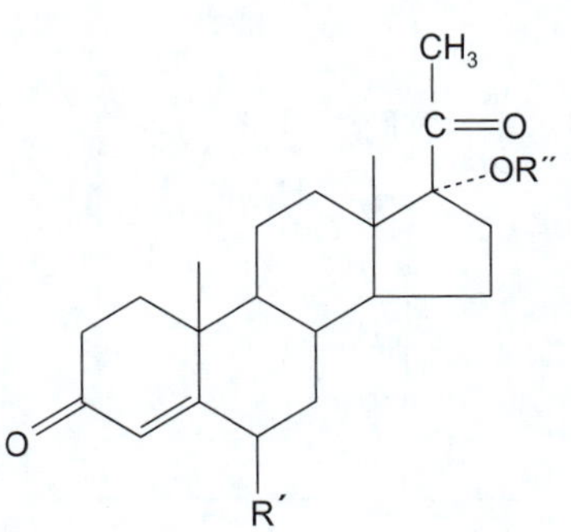

(i) Hydroxy progesterone caproate
R′ = –H, R″ = $-COC_5H_{11}$

(ii) Medroxy progesterone acetate
R′ = $-CH_3$, R″ = $-COCH_3$

c. Testosterone derivatives

Testosterone

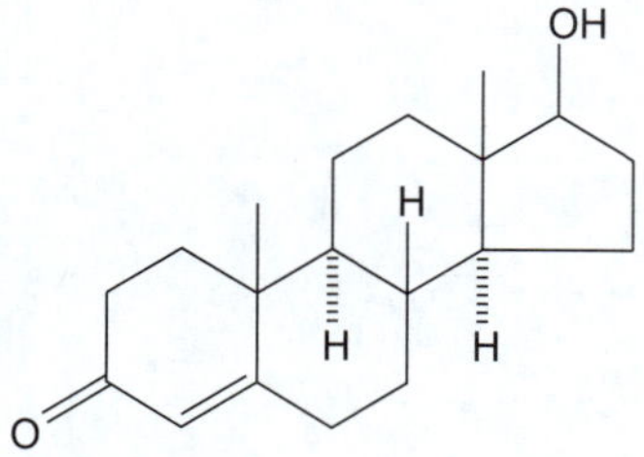

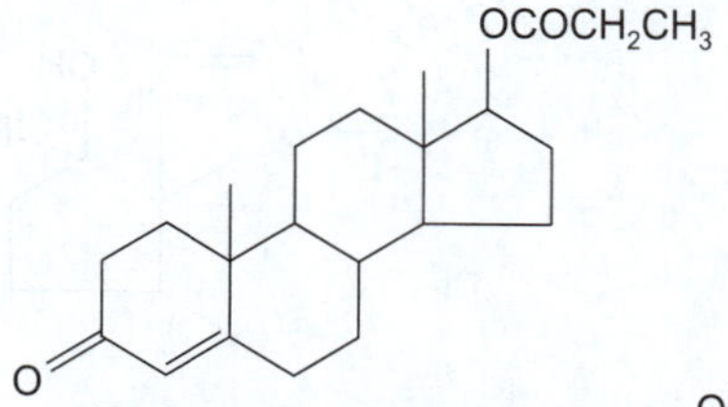

Testosterone propionate

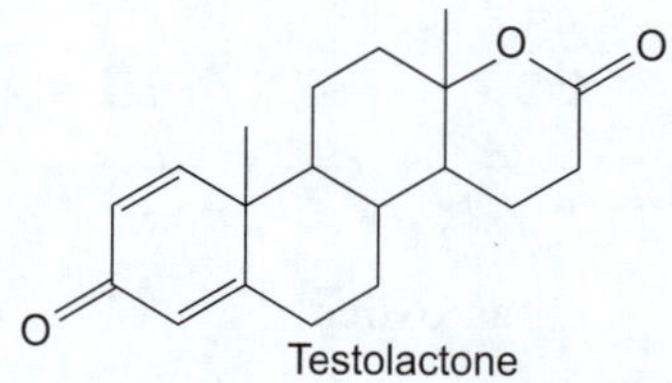

Testolactone

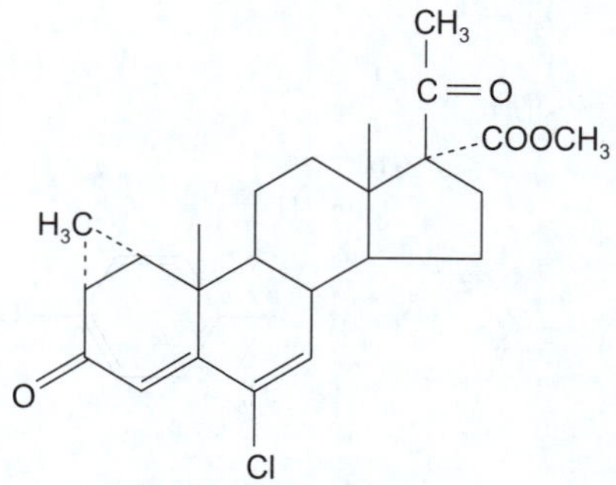

Cyproterone acetate

d. Steroidal anti-inflammatory agents

Prednisone

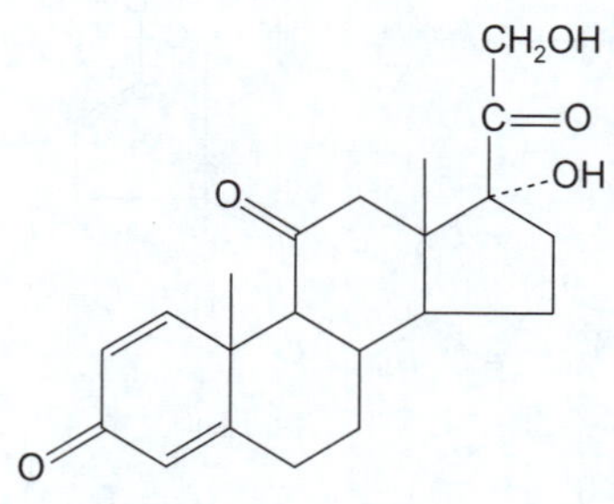

Flutamide (non-steroidal antiandrogen)

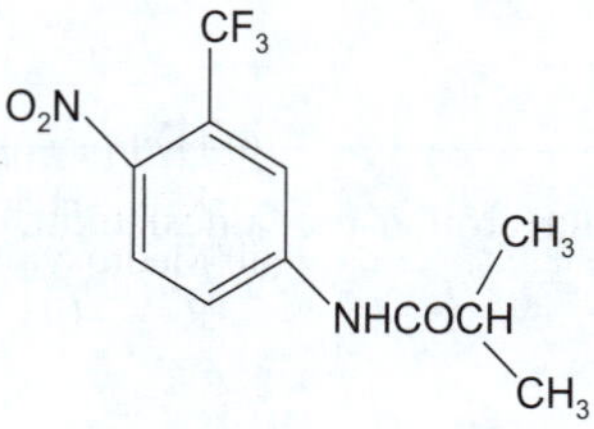

e. Miscellaneous agents

Mitotane

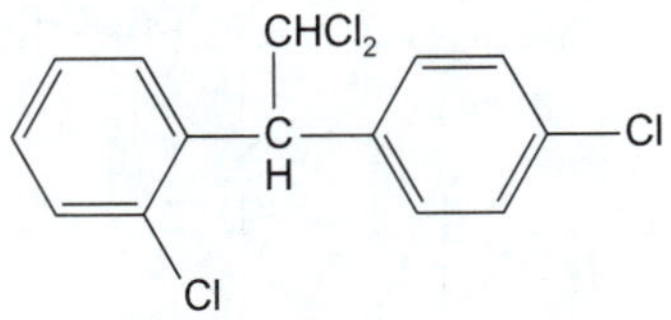

Tamoxifen

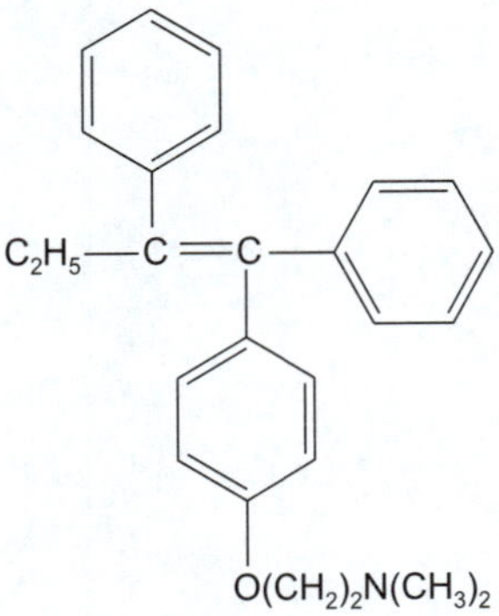

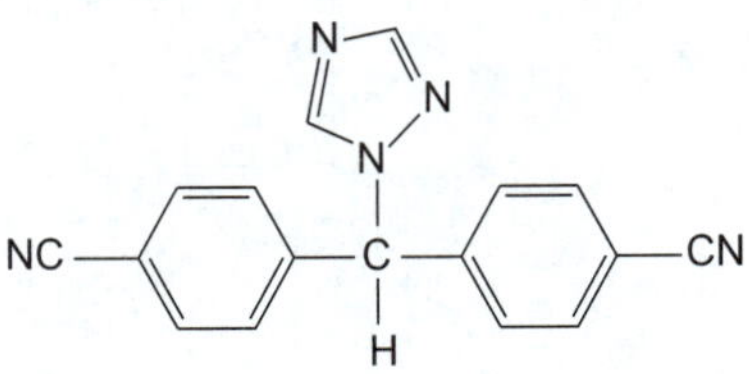

Letrozole

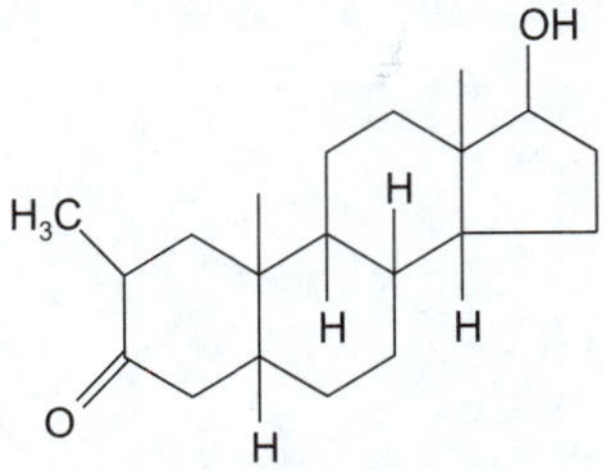

Dromostanolone

Pipobroman

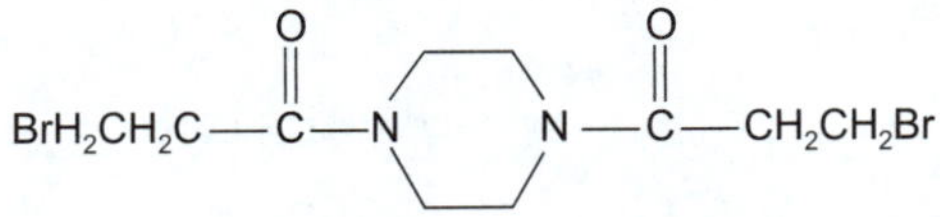

Aminoglutethimide

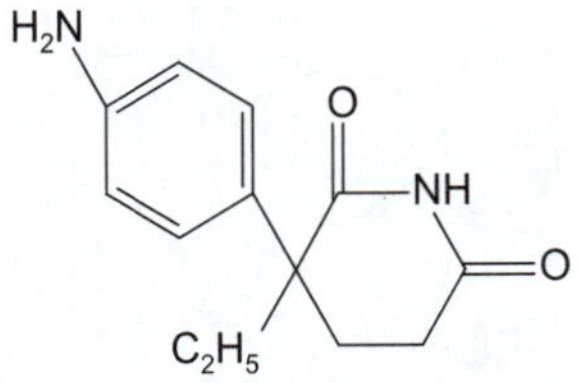

VII. Immunotherapy

Interferon α-2a; interferon α-2b; interferon α-n3; aldesleukin, diftitox, denileukin; and Bacillus-calmette-Guèrin (BCG)

VIII. Monoclonal Antibodies

Rituximab, gemtuzumab, ozogamicin

IX. Radiotherapeutic Agents

Chromic phosphate P-32; sodium phosphate P-32; sodium iodide I-131; strontium-89 chloride; samarium Sm-153, lexidronam

X. Cytoprotective Agents

Mesna, amifostine, dexrazoxane

XI. Miscellaneous

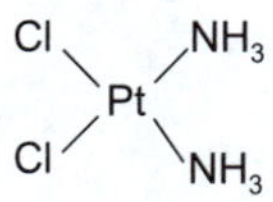

Cisplastin

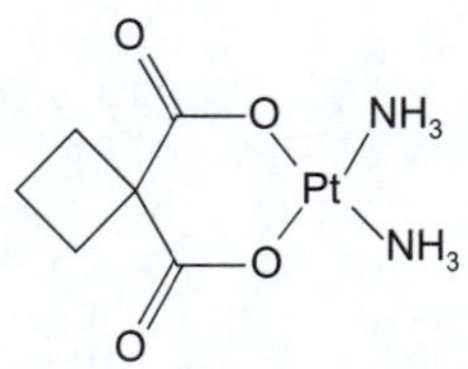

Carboplastin

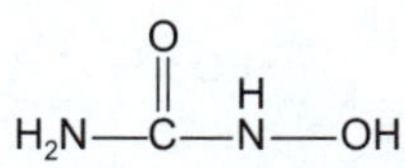

Hydroxy urea

$Ga(NO_3)_3 \cdot 9H_2O$

Gallium nitrate

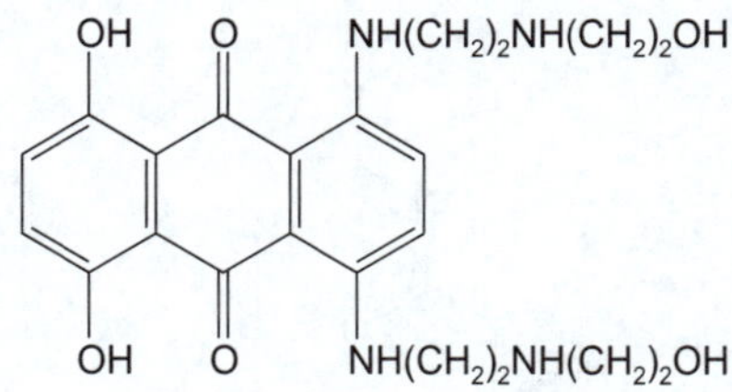

Mitoxantrone

XII. Newer Drugs

a. Pazopanib (Votrient)

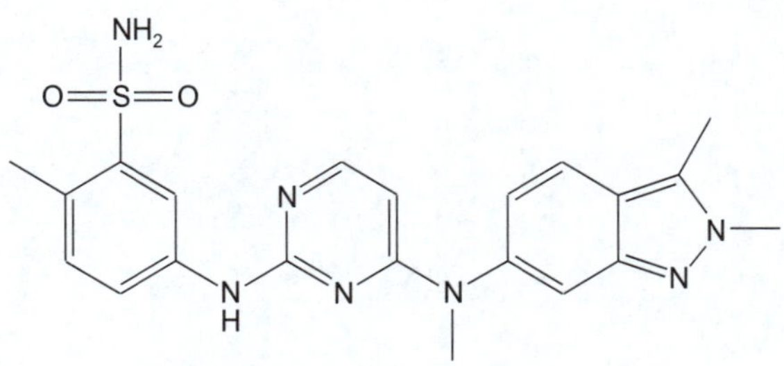

b. Sunitinib malate (Sutent)

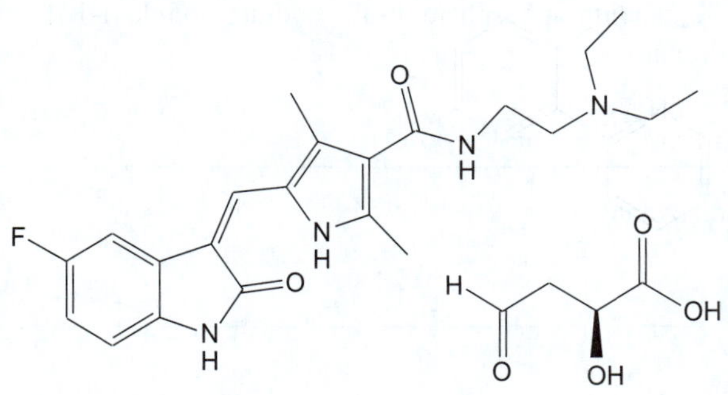

c. Everolimus (Afinitor)

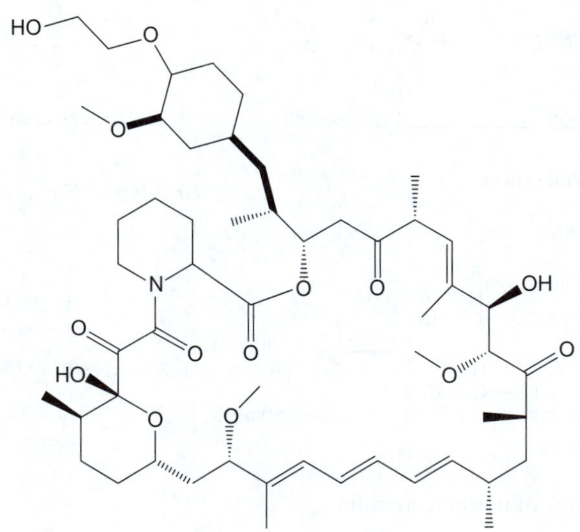

d. Vandetanib (Vandetanib)

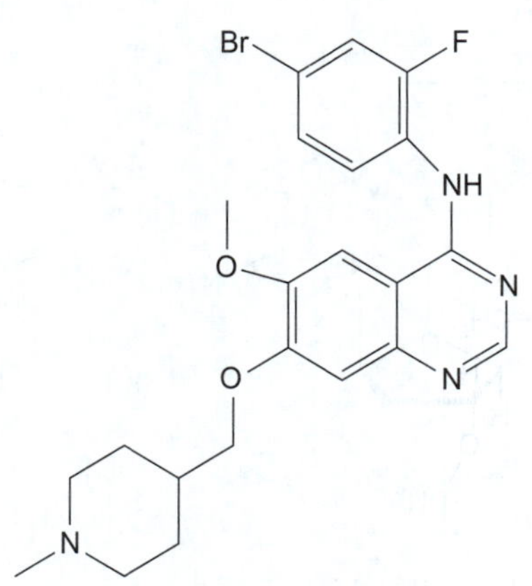

e. Vismodegib

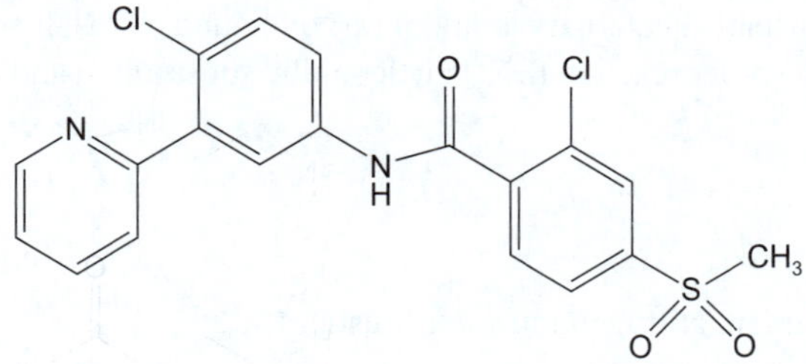

f. Trastuzumab

g. Eribulin mesylate

h. Pertuzumab (Perjeta)

SYNTHESIS AND DRUG PROFILE

I. Alkylating Agents

Step I: Intramolecular cyclization

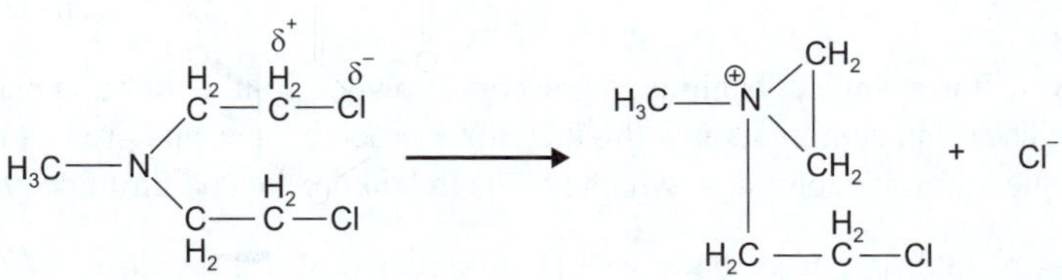

Step II: Nucleophilic attack of unstable aziridine

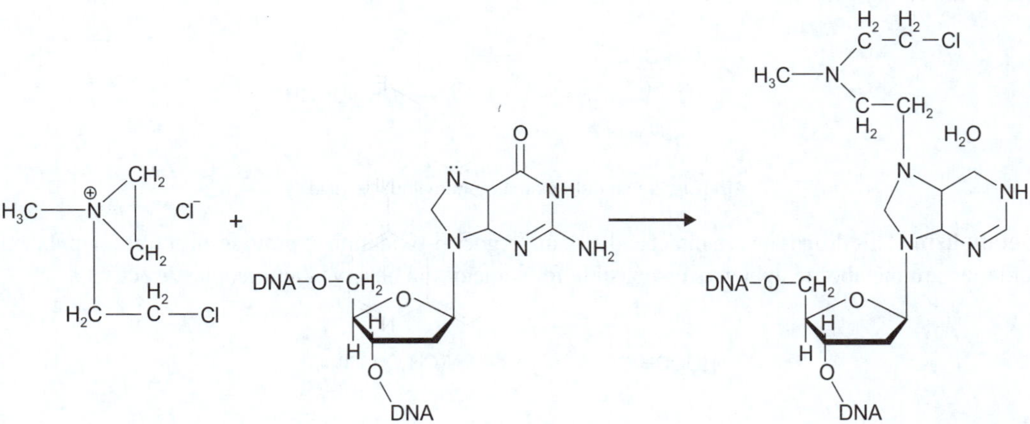

Mode of action: These compounds produce highly reactive carbonium ion intermediates that transfer alkyl group to cellular macromolecules by forming covalent bonds. It alkylates the 7th nitrogen atom of guanine residue in DNA, and results in cross-linking or abnormal base-pairing. Initially, one of the

2-chloro ethyl side chain undergoes a first-order (SN_1) intramolecular cyclization with the release of Cl^- and formation of highly reactive ethyleniminium intermediate (Step I). By this reaction, tertiary amine is converted to an unstable quaternary ammonium compound, which react by forming carbonium ion. This precedes a second-order reaction (SN_2) nucleophilic substitution and alkylates the 7th N atom in guanine (Step II).

a. Nitrogen Mustards

Mechlorethamine (Mustargen, Nitrogen mustard, Mustine)

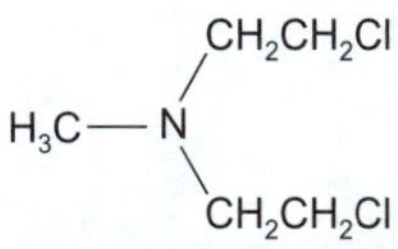

2,2′-Dichloro-N-methyl diethylamine

Synthesis

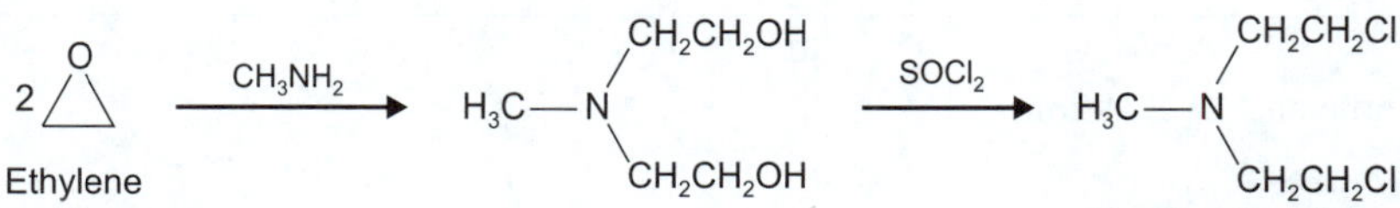

Properties and uses: It is a white crystalline hygroscopic powder, soluble in water and in alcohol. It is used in Hodgkin's disease in combination with vincristine, procarbazine, and prednisone. Most serious toxic reaction is bone marrow depression, which results in leukopenic and thrombocytopenia.

Dose: Single doses of 400 μg per kg body weight or a course of 4 daily doses of 100 μg per kg is normally administered by intravenous (IV) injection in a strength of 1 mg per ml in sodium chloride injection.

Chlorambucil (Leukaran)

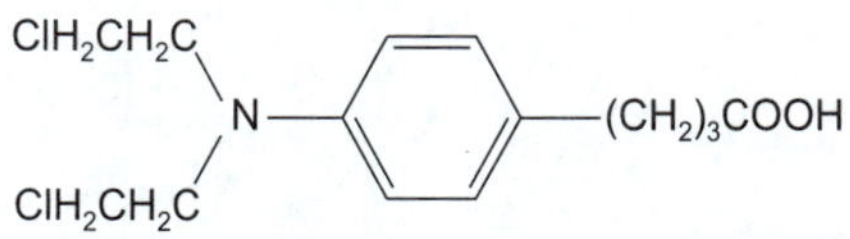

4[*p*-[*Bis*(2-chloroethyl)amino]phenyl]butyric acid

Metabolism: This drug is active intact and also undergoes β-oxidation to provide an active phenylacetic acid mustard metabolite, which is responsible for some of the observed antineoplastic activity.

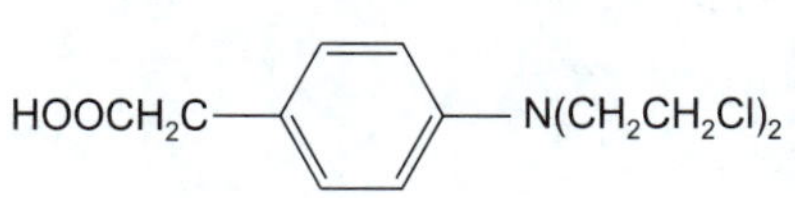

Synthesis

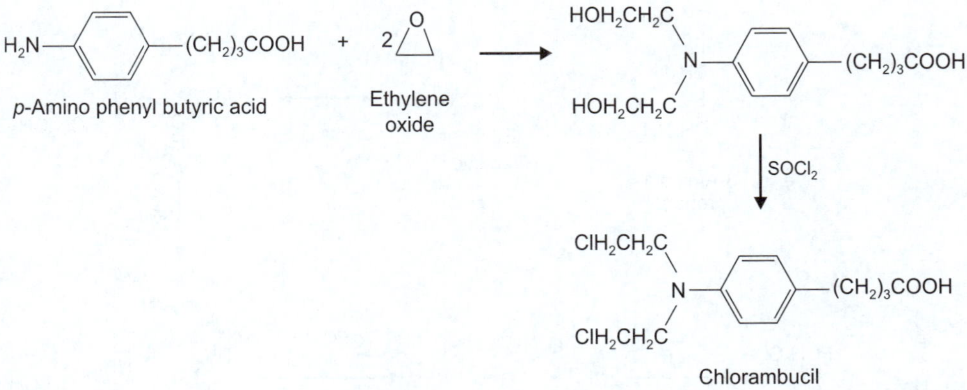

Properties and uses: Chlorambucil is a white crystalline powder, practically insoluble in water, and soluble in acetone and alcohol. It is used in the treatment of chronic lymphocytic leukaemia, macroglobulinaemia, lymphosarcoma, and Hodgkin's disease.

Assay: Dissolve the sample in acetone, add water, and titrate with 0.1 M sodium hydroxide, using phenolphthalein as indicator.

Dose: Usual oral doses are 100–200 µg per kg body weight daily (usually 4–10 mg as a single daily dose) for 4–8 weeks.

Dosage forms: Chlorambucil tablets IP, BP.

Ifosamide (Holoxan)

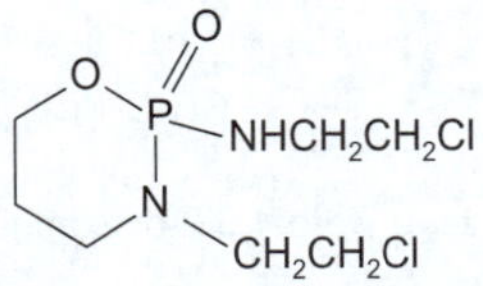

3-(2-Chloroethyl)-2-(2-chloroethyl)amino tetrahydro-2*H*-1,3,2-oxazaphosphorin-2-oxide

Properties and uses: Ifosamide is a white crystalline hygroscopic powder, soluble in water and methylene chloride. It is used for testicular cancer, leukaemia, ovarian, and breast carcinoma.

Assay: It is assayed by adopting liquid chromatography technique.

Synthesis

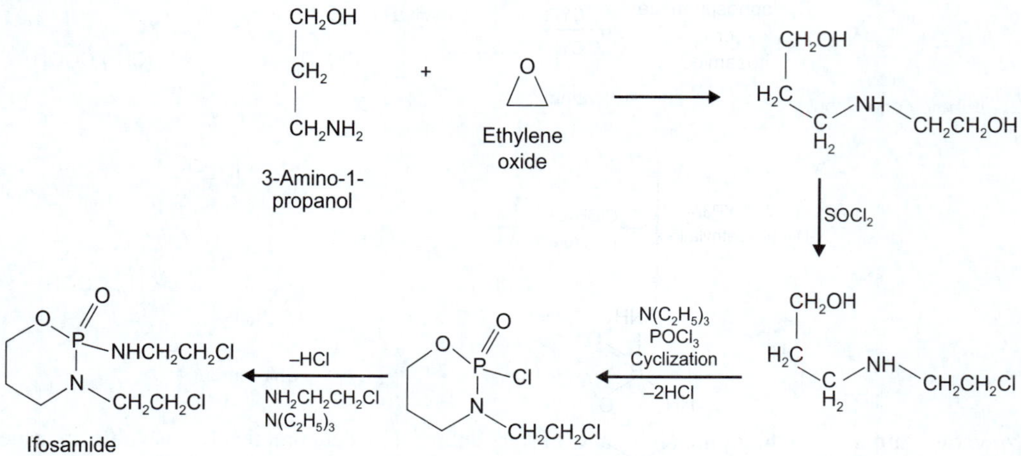

Dose: For the treatment of solid tumours of cervix, lungs, thymus, testes, and ovary; sarcoma; lymphoma of adults different licensed dosage regimens are available. Regimen 1: 8–12 g per m^2 divided over 3–5 days, repeat course every 2–4 weeks. Regimen 2: 6 g per m^2 divided over 5 days, repeat course every 3 weeks. Regimen 3: 5–6 g per m^2 (maximum, 10 g), given as a single 24 hrs infusion, repeat course every 3–4 weeks.

Cyclophosphamide (Cytoxan)

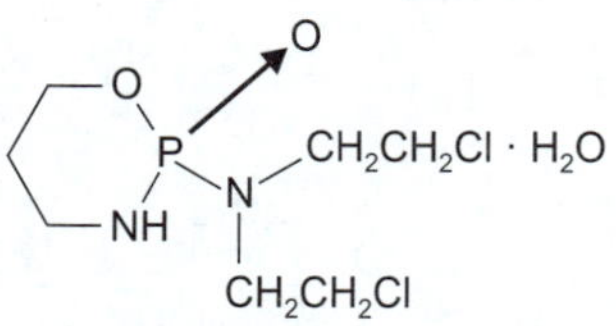

2-[*Bis*(2-chloroethyl)amino] tetrahydro-1,3,2-oxazaphosphorin-2-oxide monohydrate

Metabolism: The initial metabolic step is mediated primarily by CYP2B6 and involves hydroxylation of the oxazaphosphorine ring to generate a cabinolamine. CYP3A4 also catalyzes an inactivating N-dechloroethylation reaction, which yields nephrotoxic and neurotoxic chloroacetaldehyde.

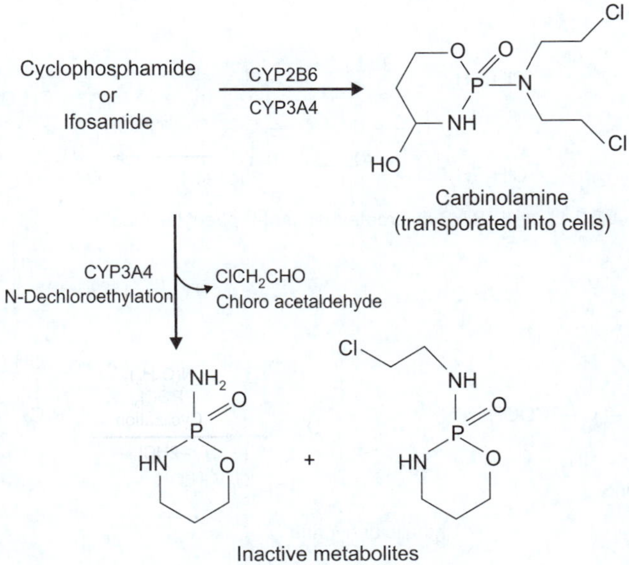

Synthesis

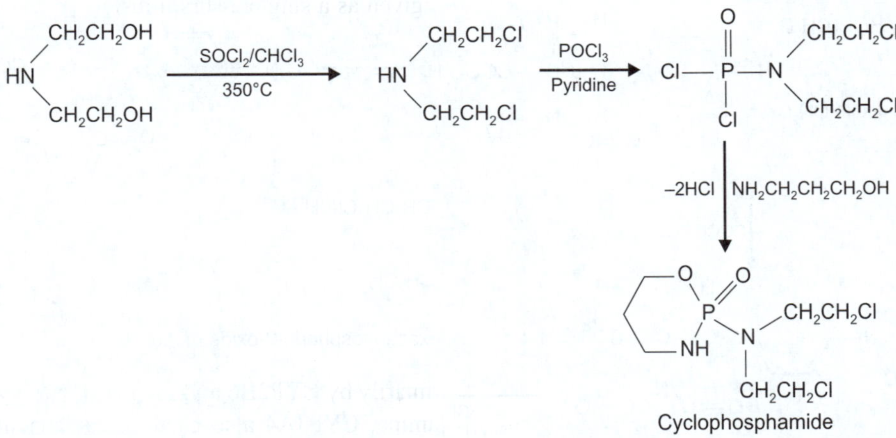

Properties and uses: Cyclophosphamide is a white crystalline powder, soluble in water and alcohol. It is one among the widely used anticancer drugs and it is superior to many alkylating agents. It is active against multiple myeloma chronic lymphocytic leukaemias, acute leukaemia of children, Hodgkin's disease, breast, ovarian cancer, and lung cancer.

Assay: Dissolve the sample in sodium hydroxide solution in ethylene glycol, boil under reflux, and rinse with water, add 2-propanol, dilute nitric acid, 0.1 M silver nitrate, and ferric ammonium sulphate solution and titrate with 0.1 M ammonium thiocyanate.

Dose: Initial adult dose of 40–50 mg per kg given intravenously in divided doses over 2–5 days and for children 2–8 mg per kg daily through IV injection.

Dosage forms: Cyclophosphamide injection IP, BP, cyclophosphamide tablets IP, BP.

Melphalan (Alkeran)

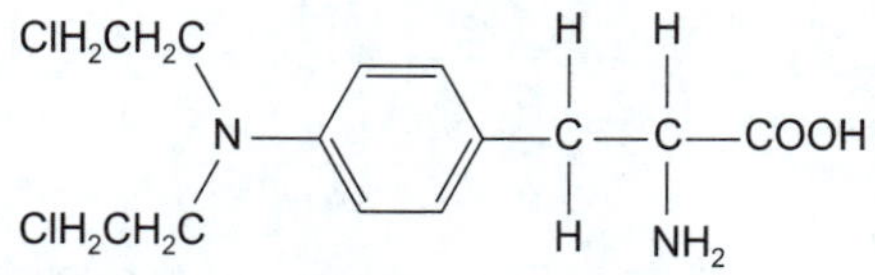

4-[*Bis*(2-chloroethyl)amino]-L-phenylalanine

Synthesis

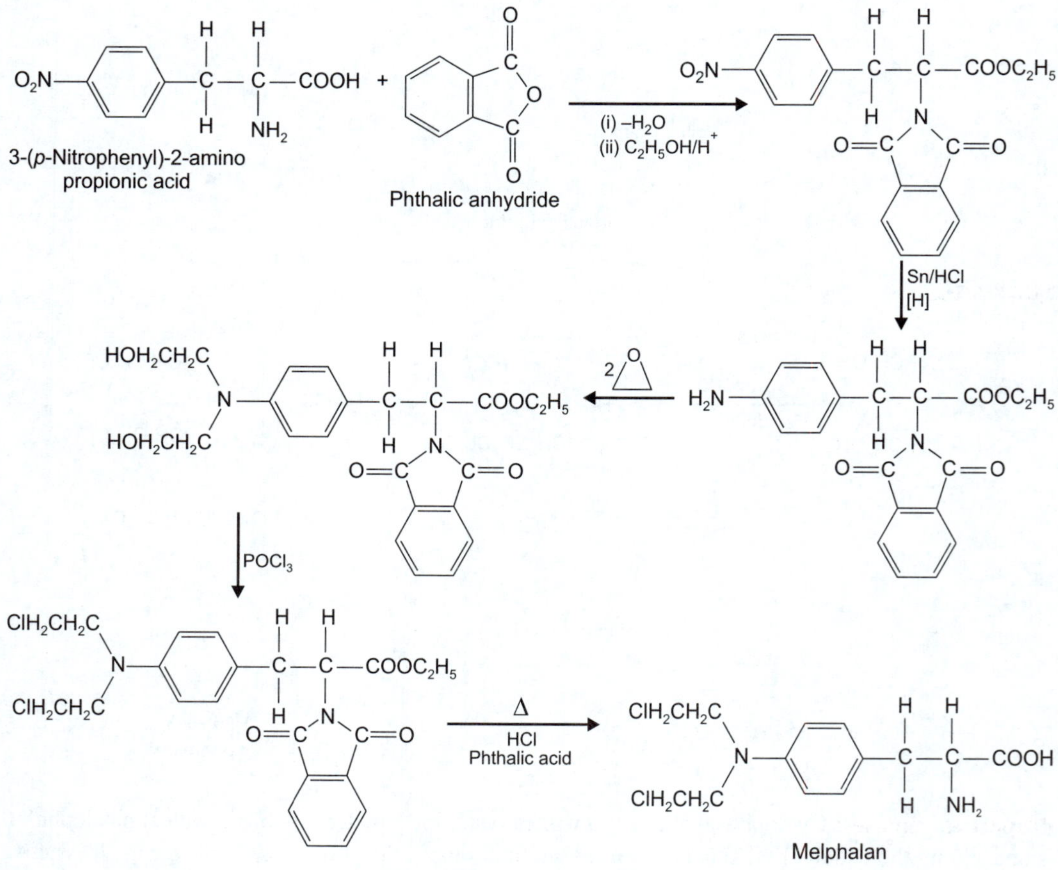

Properties and uses: Melphalan is a white powder, practically insoluble in water and ether, slightly soluble in methanol and dissolves in dilute mineral acids. Melphalan is active against multiple myeloma, breast, testicular, and ovarian carcinoma.

Assay: To the sample add 20% w/v solution of potassium hydroxide, heat on a water bath, add water and nitric acid, cool, and titrate with 0.1 M silver nitrate. Determine the end point potentiometrically.

Dose: Orally 150 µg per kg body weight daily for 4–7 days combined with prednisone 40–60 mg daily; 250 mg per kg daily for 4–5 days; or 6 mg daily by 2–3 weeks.

Dosage forms: Melphalan injection IP, BP, melphalan tablets IP, BP.

Estramustine

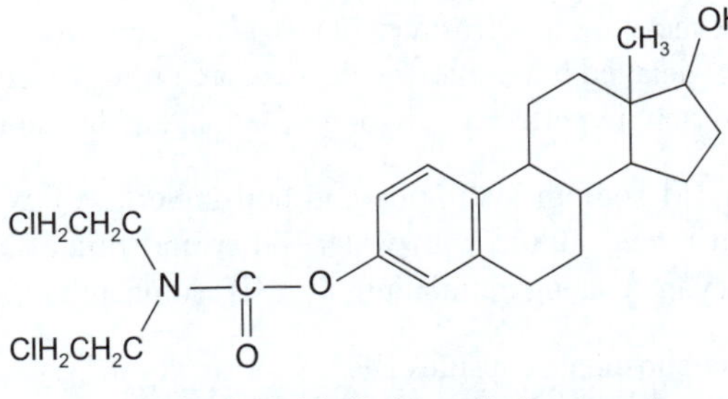

Estradiol-3-*bis*-(2-chloroethyl)carbamate

Synthesis

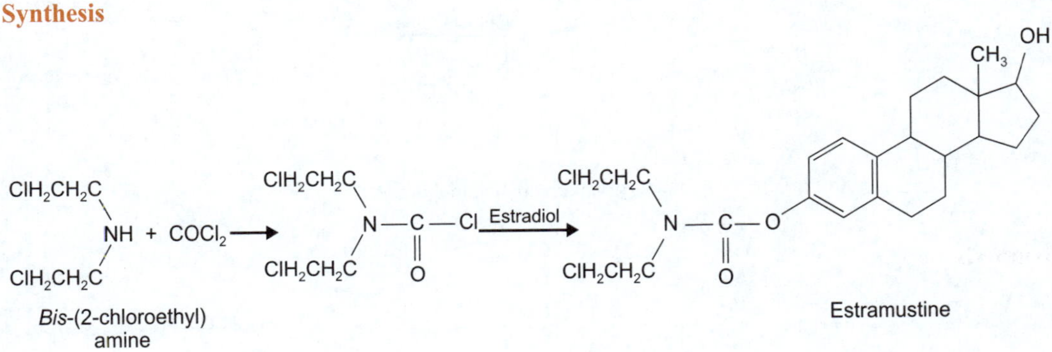

Metabolism: The resonance-stabilized mustard-like antineoplastic agent utilizes an oestradiol carrier to deliver to the steroid-dependent prostrate tissue selectively, and its use is limited to the palliative treatment of progressive prostrate cancer. In estramustine sodium phosphate, the essential 17 β-hydroxy group has been esterified with phosphoric acid, and the C-3 phenol has been carbamylated. The body still, however, transports the basic steroidal pharmacophore into the cells. The ionized sodium phosphate ester of the active 17 β-hydroxy group makes the compound water-soluble and to be able to distribute it in the blood. The ester is readily cleaved during absorption to provide the active 17 β-hydroxy group.

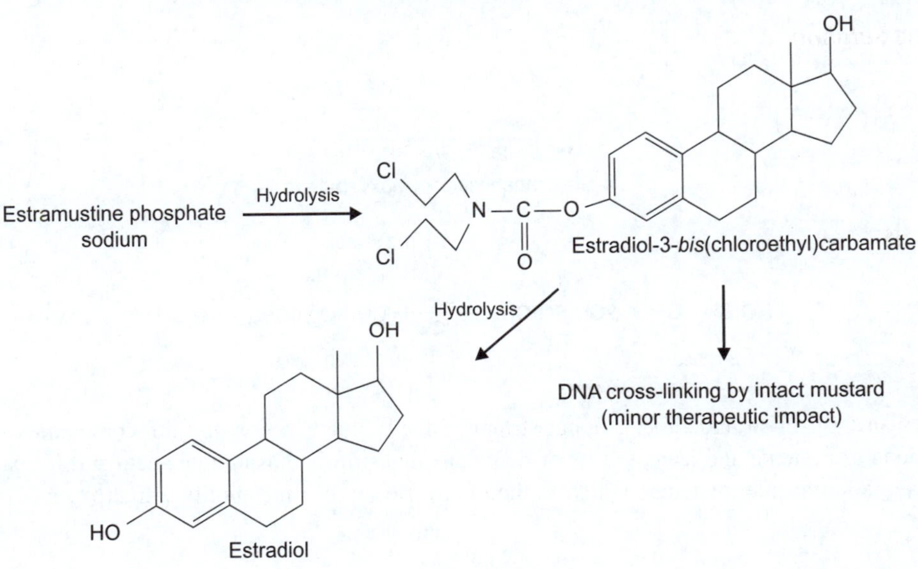

Properties and uses: Estramustine sodium phosphate is a white powder, soluble in water and in methanol, and very slightly soluble in absolute ethanol. It is an alkylating agent, which is approved for metastatic/progressive cancer of the prostate, but is also active for advanced breast cancer. It causes nausea and vomiting, delayed bone-marrow depression, mild gynecomastia, thrombophlobitis, occasional myocardial infarction, hypertension, hypoglycaemia, and hepatotoxicity.

Assay: To the sample, add 1M sodium hydroxide and boil under a reflux condenser. Cool and add 0.1 M silver nitrate and nitric acid, dilute with water. Filter and titrate the excess of silver nitrate with 0.1 M ammonium thiocyanate using ammonium iron(III) sulphate as indicator.

Dosage forms: Estramustine phosphate capsules BP.

Uracil Mustard

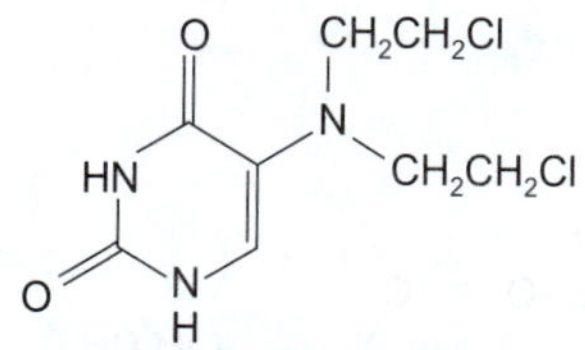

5-[*Bis*(2-chloroethyl)amino] uracil

Synthesis

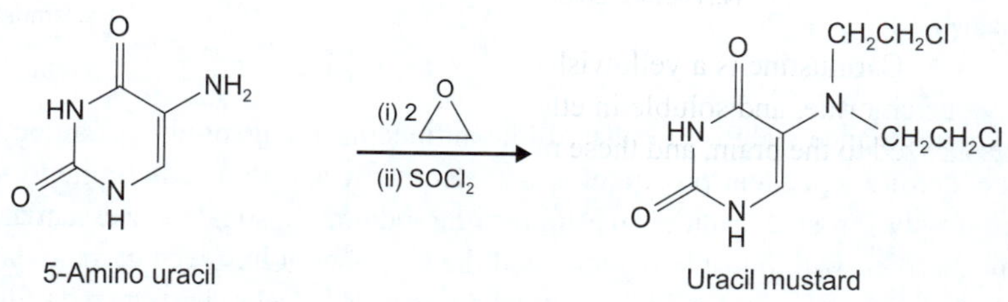

Properties and uses: It is an off-white crystalline powder, odourless, and soluble in water or alcohol. It is used for the treatment of prostrate cancer.

b. Alkyl Sulphones

Busulfan (Mylearn)

$$CH_3SO_2O(CH_2)_4OSO_2CH_3$$

1,4-*Bis*(methanesulphonyloxy) butane

Synthesis

$$\underset{\text{1,4-Butanediol}}{HO(CH_2)_4OH} + 2CH_3SO_2Cl \xrightarrow[-2HCl]{\text{Pyridine}} \underset{\text{Busulfan}}{CH_3SO_2O(CH_2)_4OSO_2CH_3}$$

Metabolism: Busulfan undergoes sulphur stripping due to interaction with thiol compounds such as glutathione or cysteine and leads to loss of two equivalents of methosulphonic acid and formation of cyclic sulphonium intermediates, which is then converted into a metabolite 3-hydroxythiolane-1,1-dioxide.

Properties and uses: Busulfan is a white crystalline powder, very slightly soluble in water and alcohol, soluble in acetone and acetonitrile. It is used in the treatment of chronic granulocytic leukaemia.

Assay: To the sample add water, boil under a reflux condenser, cool and titrate with 0.1 M sodium hydroxide using phenolphthalein as indicator until a pink colour is obtained.

Dose: For granulocytic leukaemia, the daily oral dose is 60 µg per kg body weight, up to a maximum single daily dose of 4 mg, and to be continued till the white cell count falls between 15,000 and 25,000 per mm^3.

Dosage forms: Busulfan tablets IP, BP.

c. Nitrosourea

Carmustine

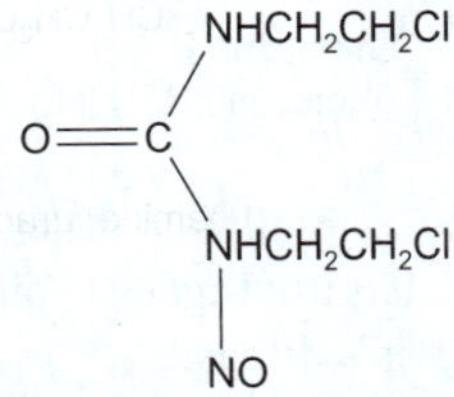

N,N′-*Bis*(2-chloroethyl)-N-nitrosourea

Properties and uses: Carmustine is a yellowish granular powder, very slightly soluble in water, very soluble in methylene chloride, and soluble in ethanol. It is used against brain tumours and leukaemia, which have metastasized to the brain, and these multiple states respond to a combination of carmustine and prednisone.

Synthesis

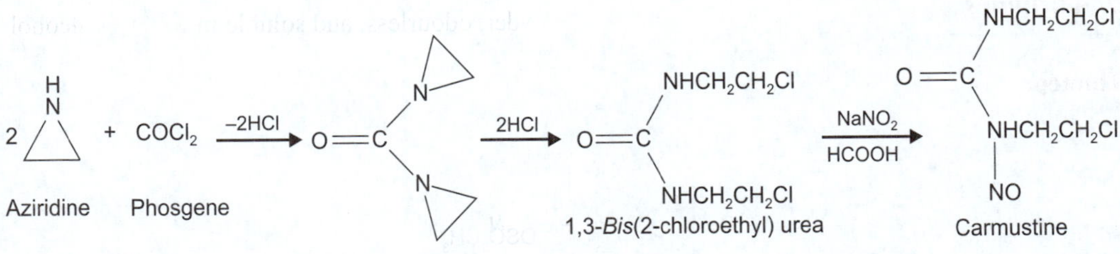

Assay: Dissolve the sample in ethanol, dilute with water, and measure the absorbance at the maxima at 230 nm using ultraviolet spectrophotometer.

Lomustine and Semustine (Ceenu, Cinu)

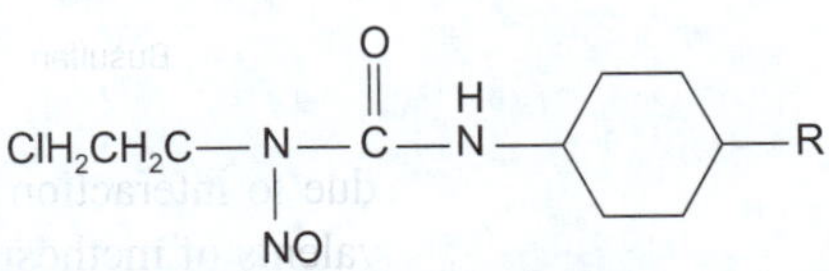

1-(2-Chloroethyl)-3-cyclohexyl-1-nitrosourea

Synthesis

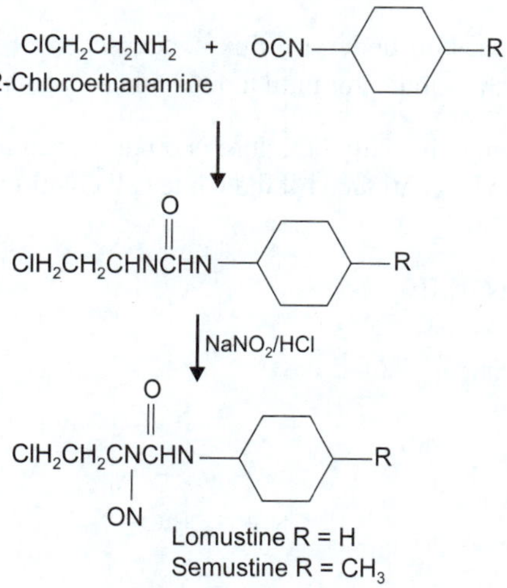

Properties and uses: Lomustine is a yellow crystalline powder, practically insoluble in water, soluble in acetone, methylene chloride, and alcohol. It is used against both primary and metastatic brain tumours and as secondary therapy in relapsed Hodgkin's disease.

Assay: Dissolve the sample in alcohol, add potassium hydroxide, and boil under a reflux condenser. Add water and nitric acid, cool and titrate with 0.1 M silver nitrate. Determine the end point potentiometrically. Perform a blank titration.

Dose: Usual dose is 130 mg/m^2 orally every 6 weeks.

Dosage forms: Lomustine capsules BP.

d. Aziridines

Thiotepa

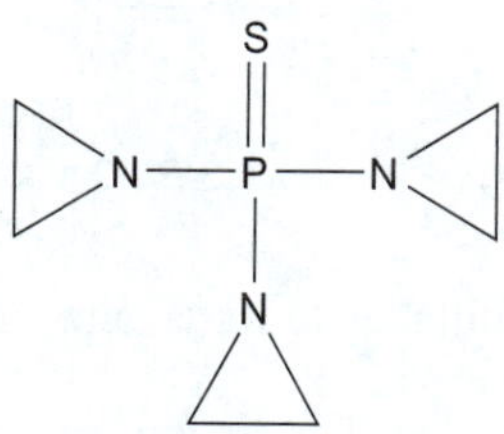

Tri-(1-aziridyl) phosphine sulphide

Synthesis

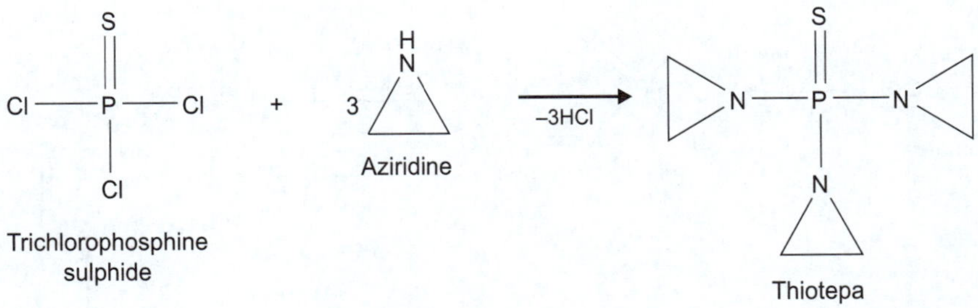

Metabolism: Thiotepa undergoes oxidative desulphuration forming an active cytotoxic metabolite known as triethylene phosphoramide (TEPA). Aziridine metabolism occurs with liberation of ethanolamine.

Properties and uses: Thiotepa exists as white crystalline flakes, freely soluble in water, chloroform, and ethanol. It is used as cytotoxic alkylating agent.

Assay: Transfer the sample to an iodine flask with the aid of 20% w/v solution of sodium thiosulphate and titrate immediately with 0.1 M hydrochloric acid, using methyl orange as indicator, until a faint red colour persists for 10 sec. Stopper the flask, allow to stand for 30 min, and titrate with 0.1 M sodium hydroxide using phenolphthalein as indicator. Subtract the volume of 0.1 M sodium hydroxide used from the volume of 0.1 M hydrochloric acid used.

Dosage forms: Thiotepa injection IP, BP.

Benzotepa

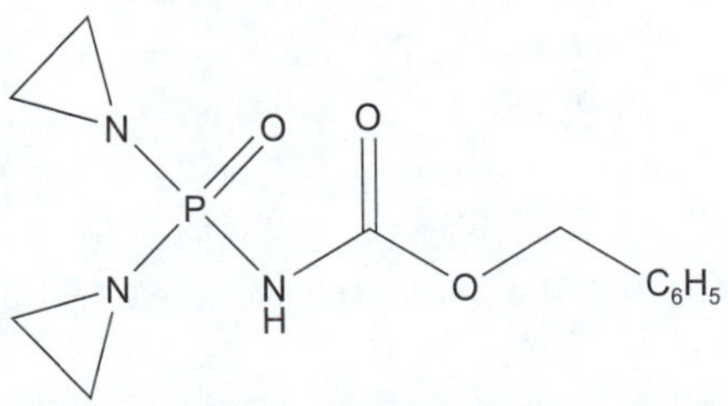

Benzyl di(aziridin-1-yl)phosphorylcarbamate

Synthesis

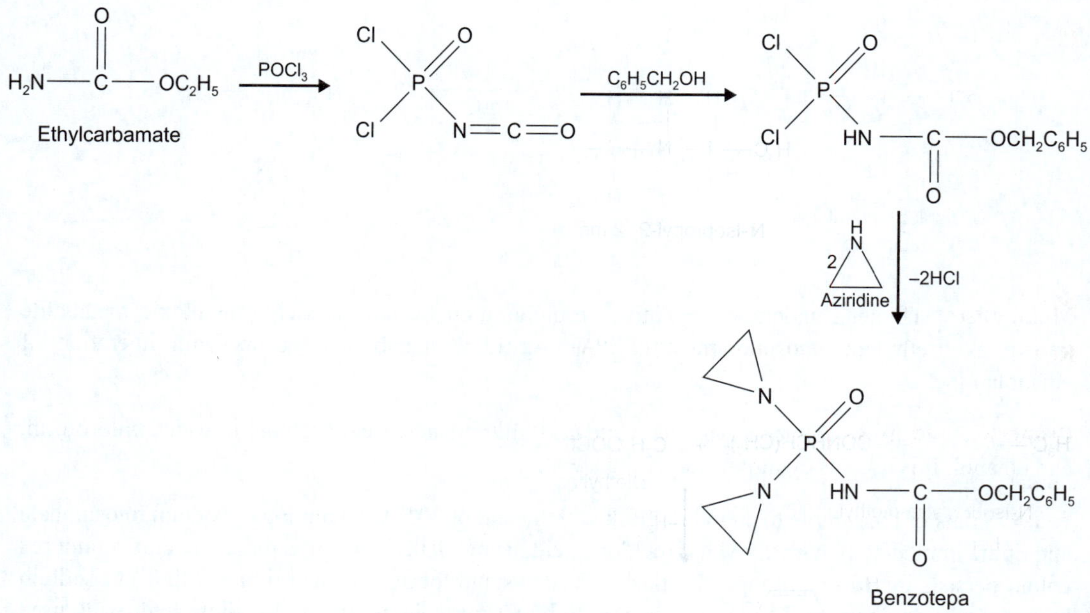

Altretamine

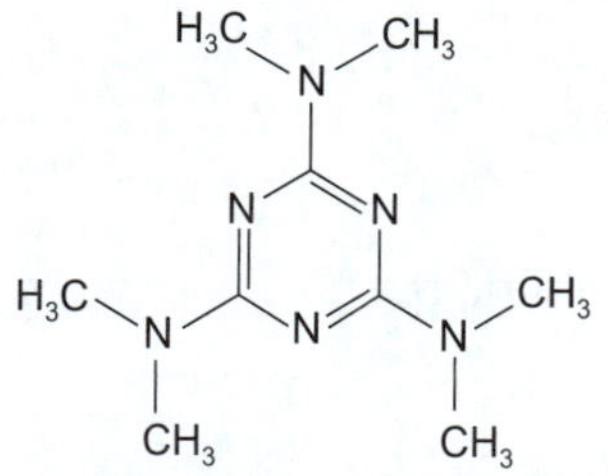

N^2,N^2,N^4,N^4,N^6,N^6-Hexamethyl-1,3,5-triazine-2,4,6-triamine

Synthesis

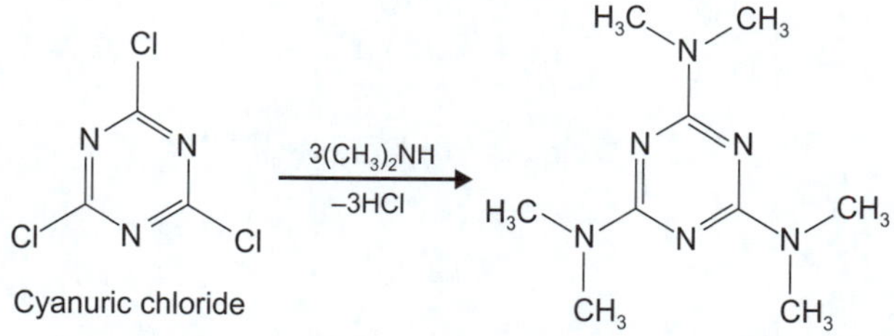

e. Methyl Hydrazines

Procarbazine

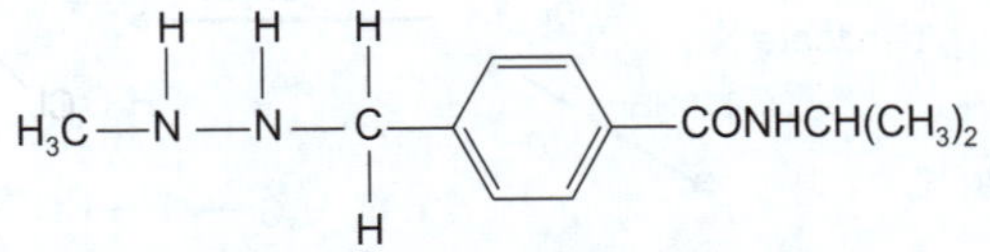

N-Isopropyl-2-(2-methyl hydrazine)-*p*-toluamide

Synthesis

Route I. From: N-Isopropyl-*p*-methyl benzamide

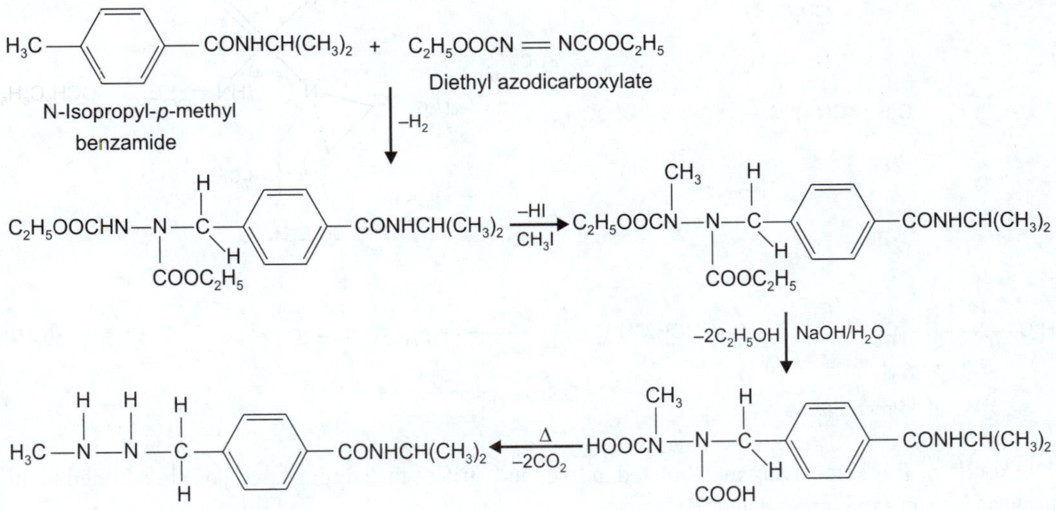

Route II. From: Methyl-4-methylbenzoate

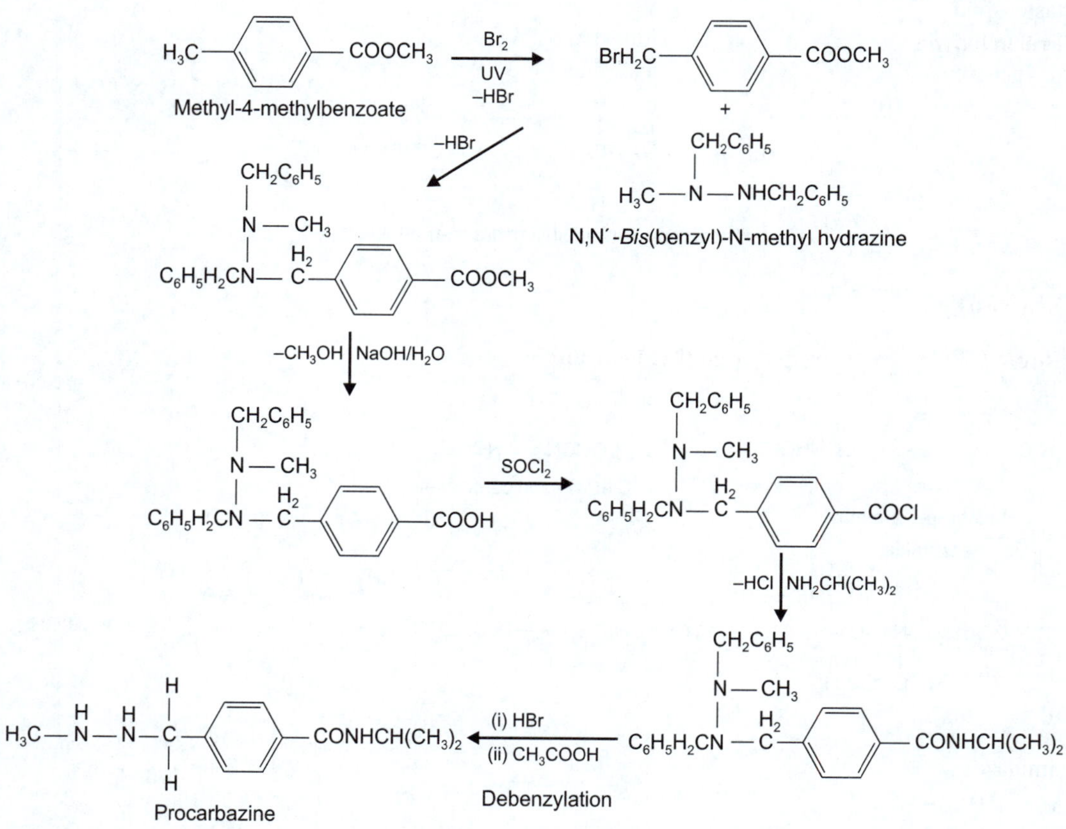

Metabolism: It is extensively metabolized in liver and 70% of the administered dose is excreted in the urine as N-isopropyl terephthalamine acid.

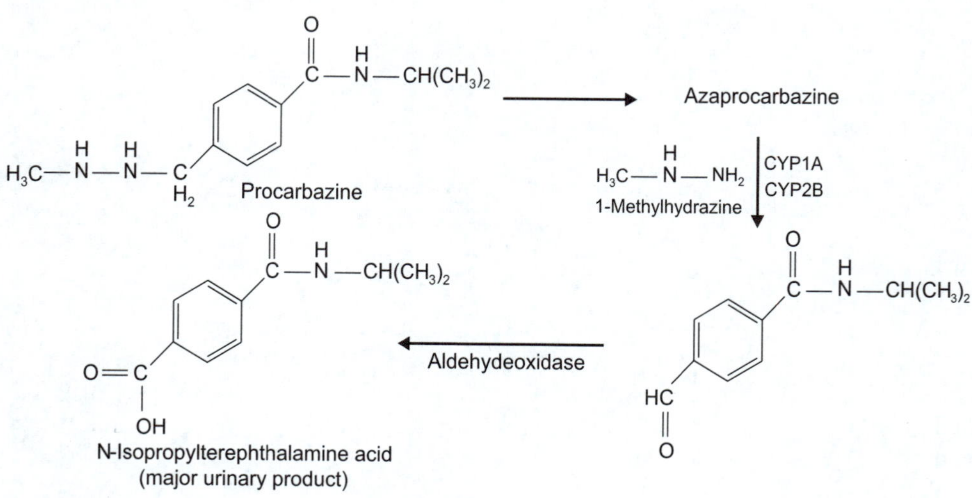

Properties and uses: It exists as white to pale yellow crystalline powder with a slight odour and a bitter taste, soluble in water or alcohol, slightly soluble in chloroform, but insoluble in ether. Solutions are acid to litmus, stable in light, slowly oxidized in air, and stable at room temperature (in the presence of oxygen, oxidation is accelerated by increased temperature).

Dacarbazine

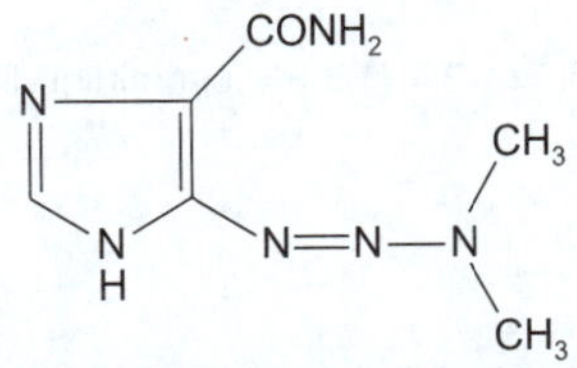

5-(3,3-dimethyl-1-triazenyl)-1*H*-imidazole-4-carboxamide

Synthesis

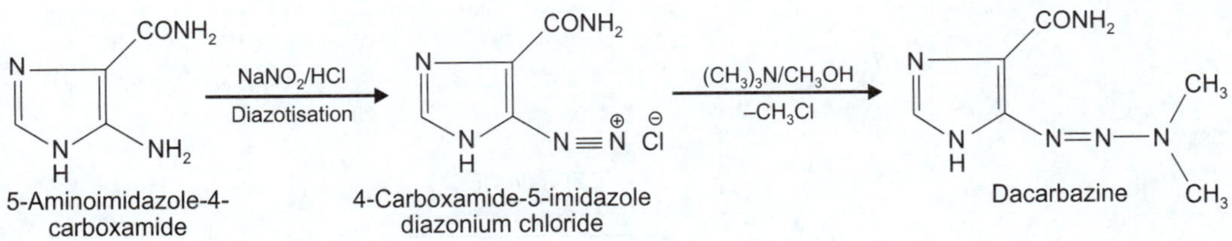

Metabolism: Approximately 40% of the drug is excreted unchanged, but both of the 5-amino imidazole-4- carboxamine and the carboxylic acid are seen in urine as metabolites.

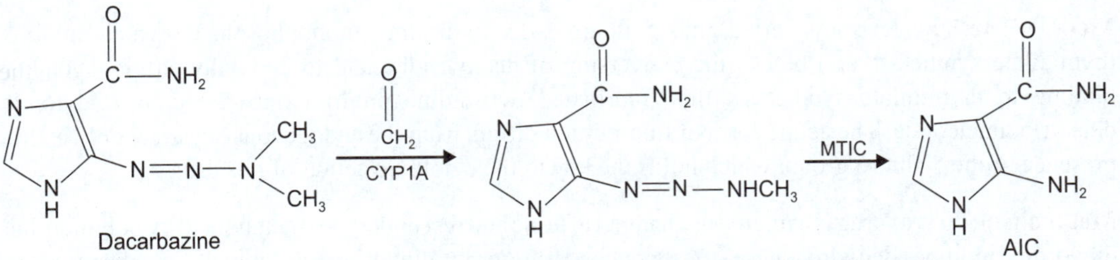

MTIC = 3-Methyl-(triazen-1-yl) imidazole-4-carboxamide

AIC = 5-Amino imidazole-4-carboxamide

Properties and uses: It is used as a cytotoxic agent, which is colourless to ivory coloured microcrystalline powder, soluble in water or alcohol.

II. Antimetabolites

Mode of action: These are analogues that resemble normal compounds of co-enzymes, which participate in the DNA synthesis and competitively inhibit the utilization of normal substrate or incorporates to make dysfunction.

a. Pyrimidine Analogues

The structural modification of these metabolites may be on the pyrimidine ring.

5-Fluorouracil

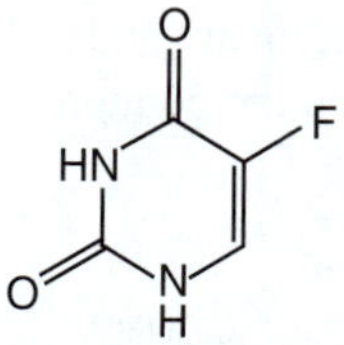

5-Flouoro-2,4-(1*H*,3*H*)pyrimidinedione

Synthesis

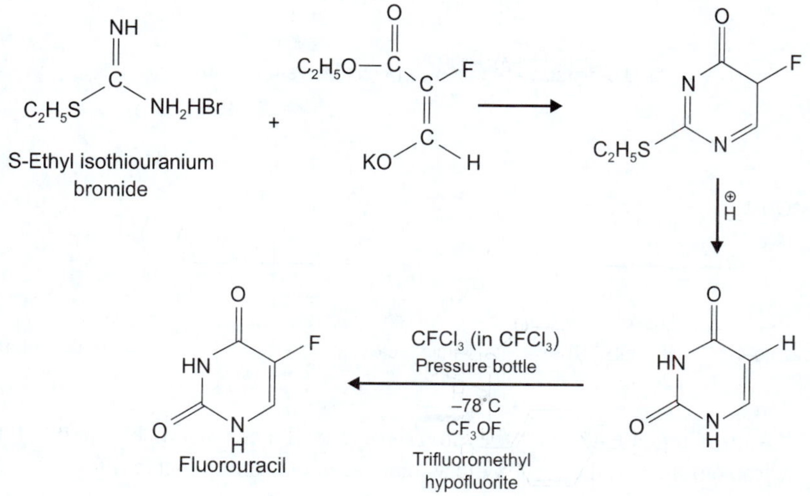

Mode of action: It is converted into 5-flouro-2-deoxy uridine monophosphate, which inhibits thymidilate synthetase and blocks the conversion of deoxyuridic acid to deoxythymidilic acid. For binding to thymidilate synthetase, this fluorinated pyrimidine prodrug must be converted to its deoxyribonucleotide. The active form of fluorouracil differs from the endogenous substrate only by the presence of the 5-fluoro group, which holds the key to the cytotoxic action of this drug.

Metabolism: 20% of drug is excreted unchanged in urine and rest undergoes metabolism by polymorphic dihydropyrimidine dehydrogenase to produce 5-fluoro-5,6-dihydrouracil, which is converted to α-fluorouridopropionic acid by dihydropyrimidinase and to α-fluoro-β-alanine by β-ureidopropionase.

Properties and uses: Fluorouracil is a white crystalline powder, sparingly soluble in water, and slightly soluble in alcohol. It is used topically in the treatment of pancancerous dermatoses, especially actinic keratosis, for which it is the treatment of choice, if the lesions are multiple, even if the lesions that are not clinically discernable respond. For this reason, the drug is applied to the entire affected area. Healing continues for 1 to 2 months after treatment. The drug does not affect non-keratotic lesion. It is a secondary immunosuppressive agent, and therefore, is not used in organ transplantation. It is the most active drug available for colorectal cancer. It is effective in the management of the breast, colon, pancreas, rectum, and stomach. It may have devastating bone marrow and gastrointestinal toxicity.

Assay: Dissolve the sample in dimethylformamide by gentle warming, cool and titrate with 0.1 M tetrabutylammonium hydroxide, using thymol blue as indicator.

Dosage forms: Fluorouracil injection IP, BP, fluorouracil cream BP.

Fluoxuridine

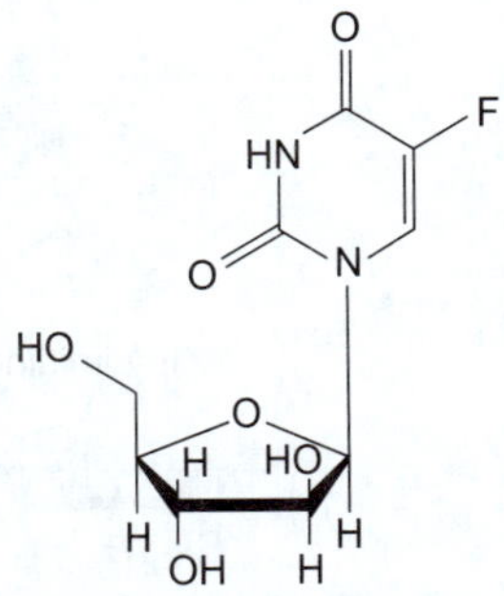

1-(2-Deoxy-D-ribofuranosyl)-5-fluorouracil

Synthesis

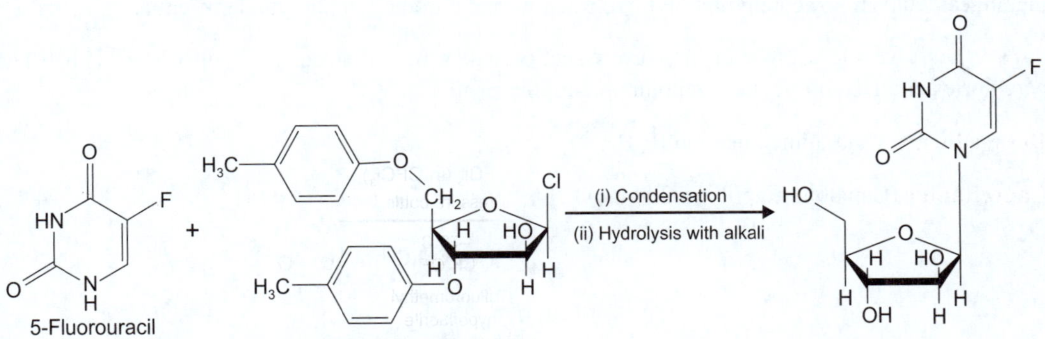

5-Fluorouracil

3,5-Di-o-p-tolyl-2-deoxyribosyl-1-chloride

Fluoxuridine

Metabolism: This deoxyribonucleoside prodrug is bioconverted via 2′-deoxyuridine kinase-mediated phosphorylation to the same active 5-fluoro-dUMP structure generated in the multistep biotransformation of fluorouracil.

Properties and uses: It is a white to off-white odourless powder, which is soluble in water, alcohol, or chloroform. Fluoxuridine is a prodrug of 5-fluorouracil. It is used for the palliation of gastrointestinal adenocarcinoma metastatic to the liver in patients who are considered incurable by surgery.

Cytarabine

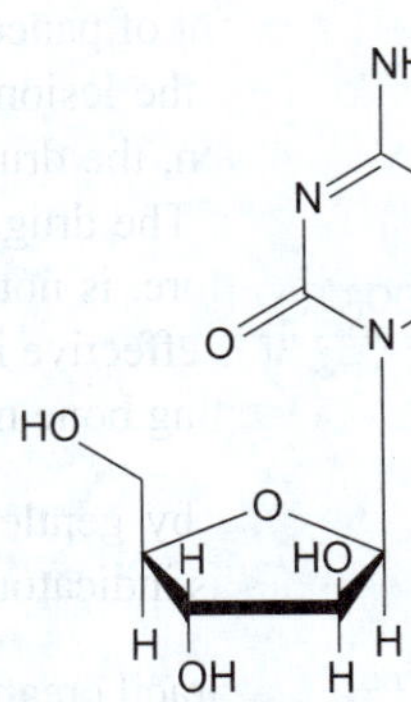

1-β-D-Arabinofuranosyl cytosine

Synthesis

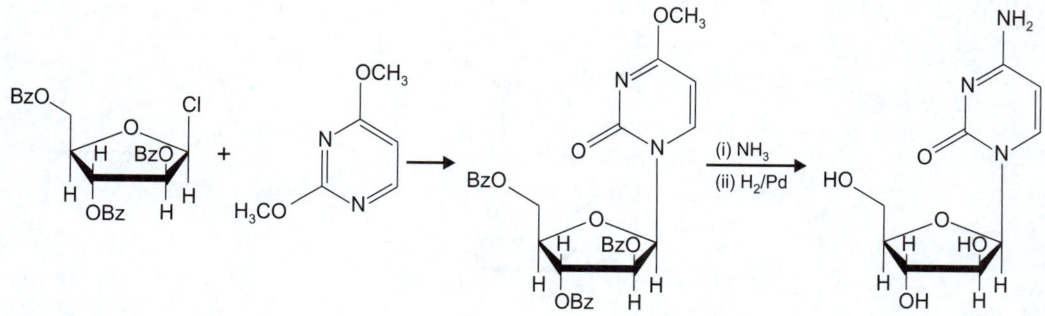

Cytarabine

Properties and uses: Cytarabine is a white crystalline powder, soluble in water, very slightly soluble in alcohol and methylene chloride. It is used for acute leukaemia, chronic myclocytic leukaemia, meningeal leukaemia, acute lympholytic leukaemia, and chronic lympholytic leukaemia.

Assay: Dissolve the sample in anhydrous acetic acid, warm, if necessary, and titrate with 0.1 M perchloric acid. Determine the end point potentiometrically.

Dosage forms: Cytarabine injection IP, BP.

Capecitabine (Captabin, Capiibine, Xabine)

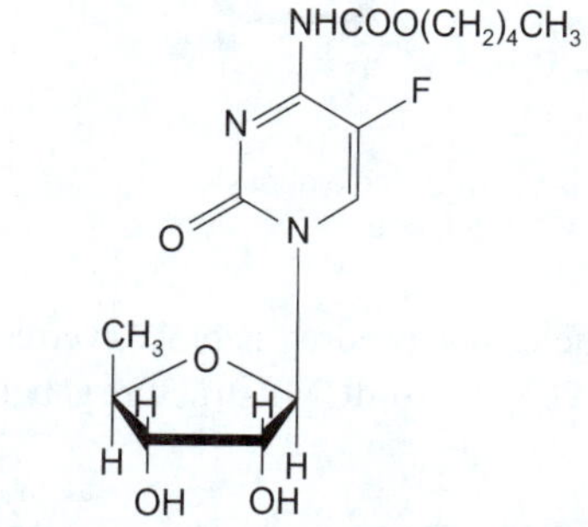

5′-Deoxy-5-fluoro-N4-(pentyloxycarbonyl) cytidine

Synthesis

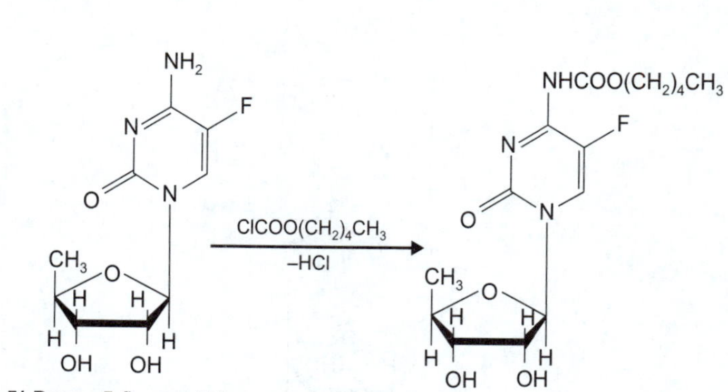

Capecitabine

Metabolism: The drug is actually another 5-fluorodeoxy uridine monophosphate prodrug. When given orally, it is extensively metabolized to fluorouracil, which is then converted to the active fluorinated deoxyribonucleotide.

Uses: It is used in acute granulocytic leukaemia of adults and children.

Dose: The dose for colorectal cancer and breast cancer for adults is 1.25 g per m^2 two times a day for 2 weeks followed by a 1-week rest period. Therapy is to be given in 3-week cycles. Recommended treatment duration for colorectal cancer is 6 months. May be used in combination with docetaxel at 75 mg per m^2 given as 1 hr IV infusion, once in every 3 weeks for the treatment of breast cancer.

Gastric cancer: The dose for adults, used in combination with platinum-based compound, 1 g per m^2 two times a day for 14 days followed by a 7-day rest period. First dose is given on the evening of day 1 and the last dose on the morning of day 15.

b. Purine Analogues

Mode of action: These drugs are converted into appropriate monoribonucleotides, which inhibit the conversion of inosine monophosphate to adenine and guanine nucleotides.

6-Mercaptopurine (Purinethol)

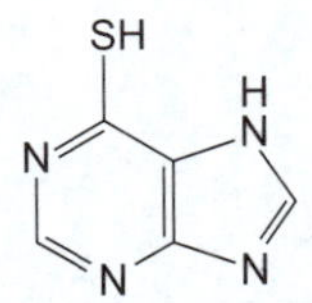

Purine-6-thiol

Properties and uses: Mercaptopurine is a yellow crystalline powder, practically insoluble in water, slightly soluble in alcohol, and dissolves in solutions of alkali hydroxides. It is used in the treatment of acute monocytic leukaemia.

Assay: Dissolve the sample in dimethylformamide and titrate with 0.1 M tetrabutylammonium hydroxide. Determine the end point potentiometrically.

Dose: The usual initial oral dose for children and adults is 2.5 mg per kg body weight daily, but the dose varies as per individual response and tolerance.

Synthesis

Route I. From: 7*H*-Purin-6-ol

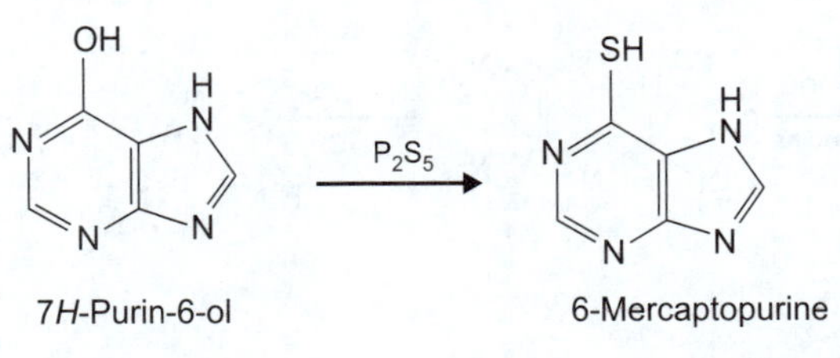

Route II. From: 6-Chloropyrimidine-4,5-diamine

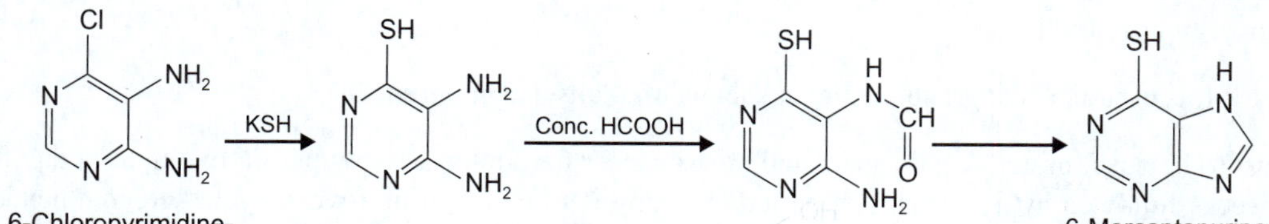

6-Chloropyrimidine-4,5-diamine

6-Mercaptopurine

Route III. From: Hypoxanthine

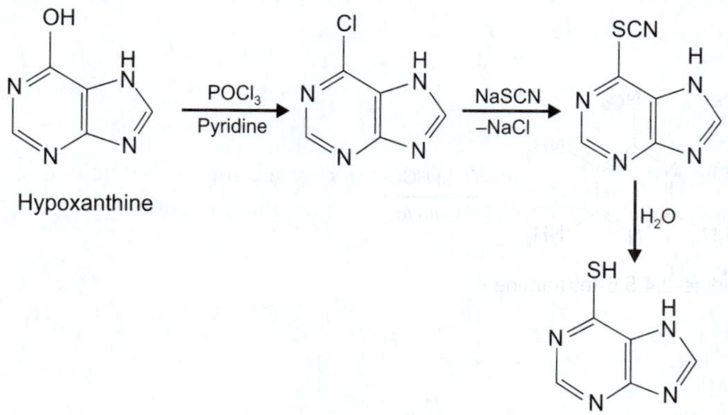

Hypoxanthine

6-Mercaptopurine

Dosage forms: Mercaptopurine tablets IP, BP, mercaptopurine oral suspension BP.

Thioguanine

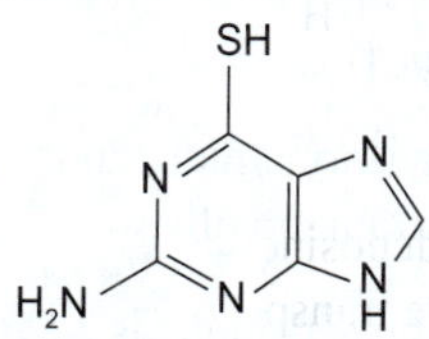

2-Amino purine-6-thiol

Synthesis

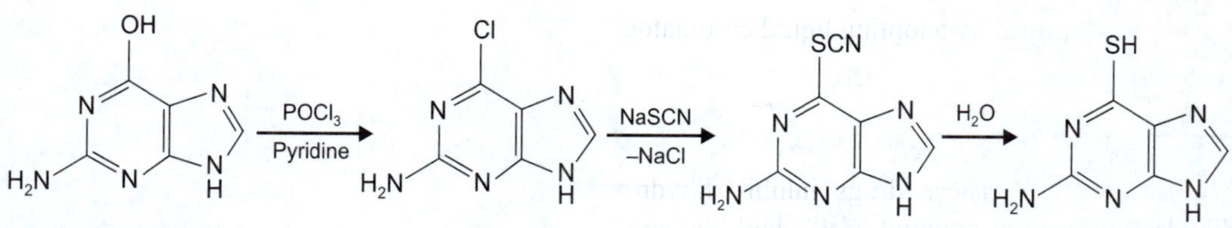

2-Amino-9-*H*-purin-6-ol

Thioguanine

Properties and uses: It is used in treating acute leukaemia, especially in combination with cytarabine. The adverse effects are bone marrow depression, leucopenia, thrombocytopenia, and bleeding.

Fludarabine

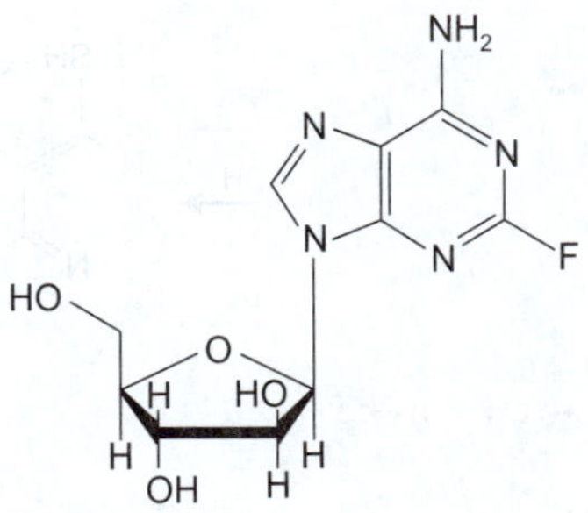

Synthesis

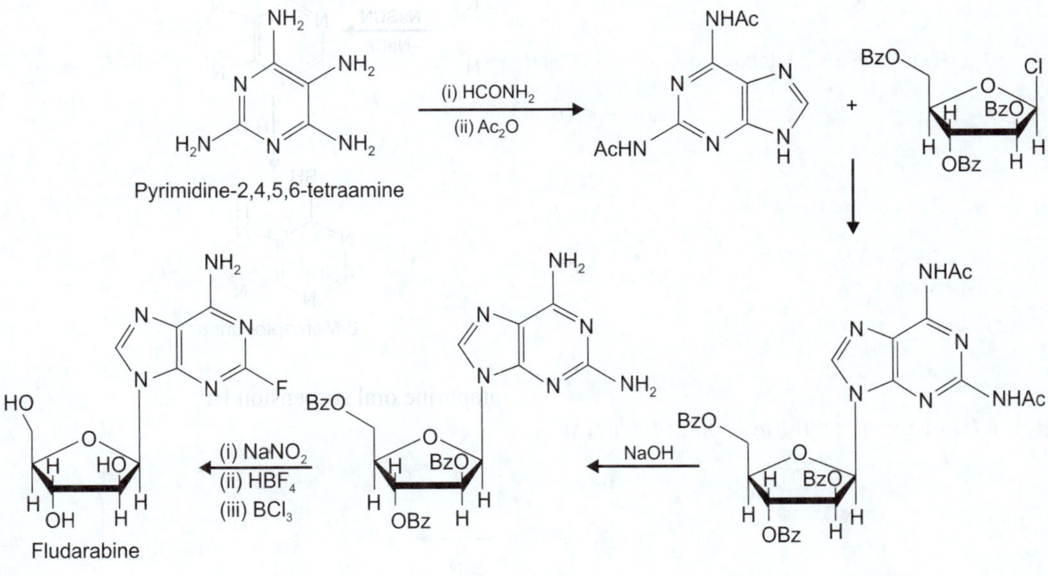

Metabolism: This is a 3-halogenated adenosine-based nucleoside, which undergoes conversion to active triphosphate nucleotides after active transport into the tumour cells.

Properties and uses: Fludarabine phosphate is a white crystalline hygroscopic powder, slightly soluble in water, soluble in dimethylformamide, and very slightly soluble in anhydrous ethanol. It shows activity against low-grade lymphoma and mycosis fungoides.

Assay: It is assayed by adopting liquid chromatography technique.

c. Folic Acid Analogues

Mode of action: These drugs inhibit dihydrofolate reductase (DHFRase), which converts the dihydrofolic acid to tetrahydrofolic acid, the co-enzyme required for one carbon transfer reaction in *de novo* purine synthesis and amino acid interconversion.

Methotrexate (Amethopterin)

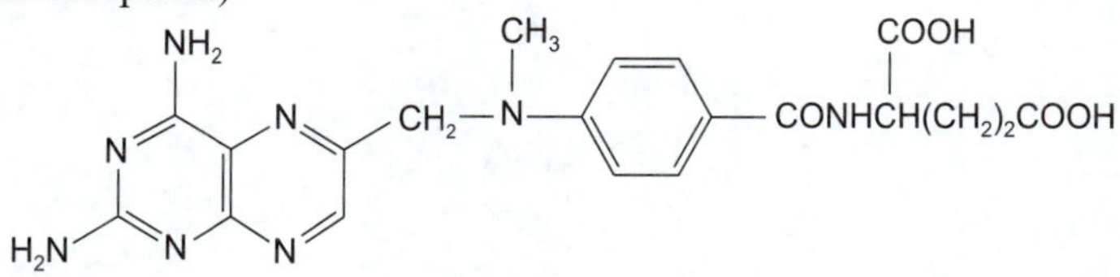

Synthesis

Route I. From: Pyrimidine-2,4,5,6-tetraamine

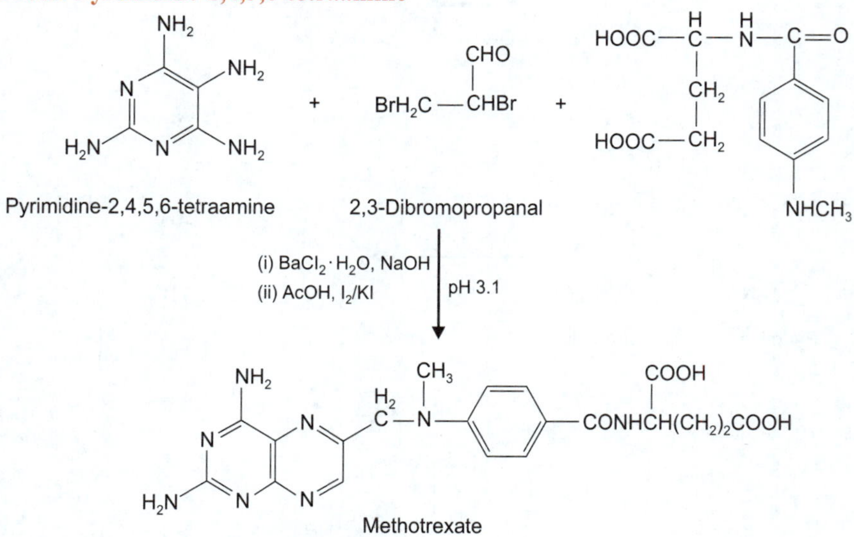

Route II. From: Pyrimidine-2,4,5,6-tetraamine

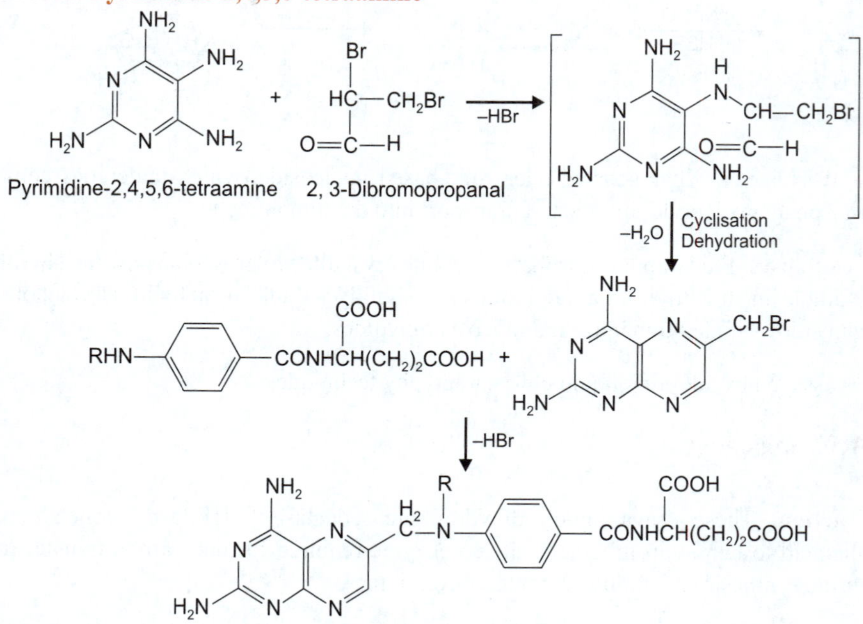

R = H (Aminopterin)
R = CH_3 (Methotrexate)

Properties and uses: Methotrexate is a yellow or orange crystalline hygroscopic powder, practically insoluble in water, ethanol, and methylene chloride. It dissolves in dilute mineral acids and dilute solutions of alkali hydroxides and carbonates. It is used for the treatment of acute lymphocytic leukaemia, acute lymphoblastic leukaemia, breast cancer, and epidermoid cancer of the head, neck, and lung cancer.

Assay: It is assayed by adopting liquid chromatography technique.

Dose: For the maintenance therapy of acute lymphoblastic leukaemia, the dose is 15–30 mg per m^2 body surface once or twice weekly either orally or intramuscularly, with other agents, such as mercaptopurine.

Dosage forms: Methotrexate injection IP, BP, methotrexate tablets IP, BP.

Azathioprine

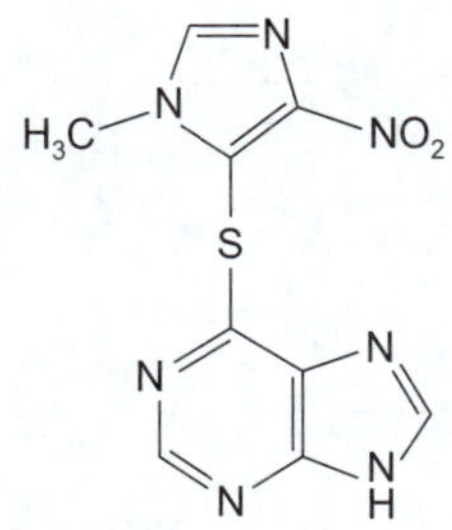

6-[(1-Methyl-4-nitro-1*H*-imidazol-5-yl)thio]-1*H*-purine

Synthesis

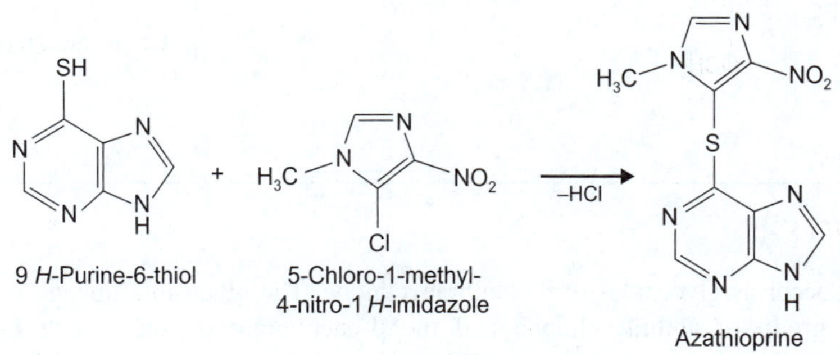

Properties and uses: Azathioprine is a pale-yellow powder, practically insoluble in water and alcohol. It is soluble in dilute solutions of alkali hydroxides and sparingly soluble in dilute mineral acids. It is used as an immunosuppressant.

Assay: Dissolve the sample in dimethylformamide and titrate with 0.1 M tetrabutylammonium hydroxide. Determine the end point potentiometrically.

Dosage forms: Azathioprine tablets BP.

Trimetrexate

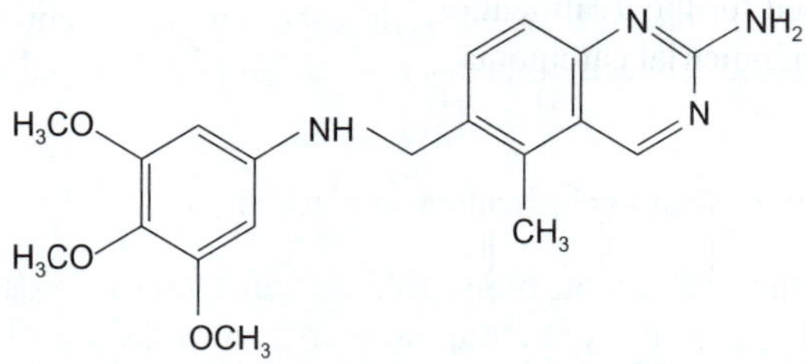

5-Methyl-6-((3,4,5-trimethoxyphenylamino)methyl)quinazoline-2,4-diamine

Synthesis

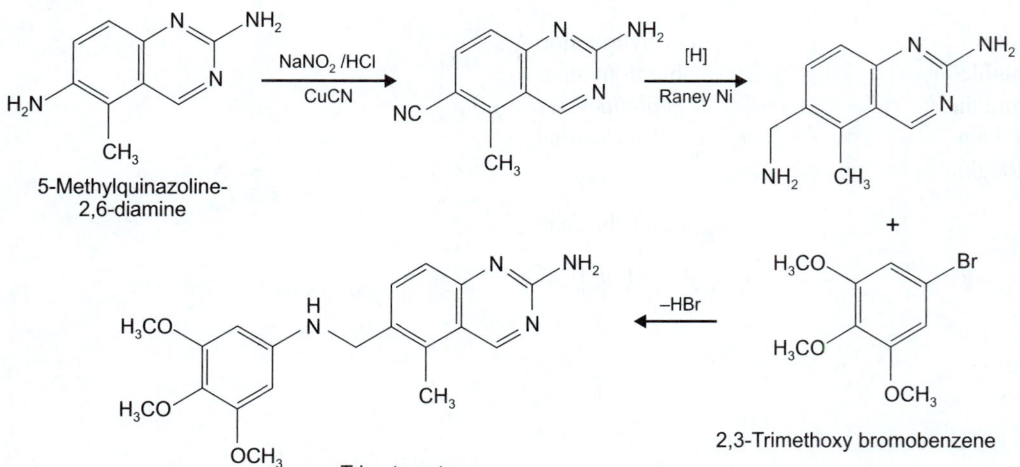

III. Antibiotics

a. Anthracyclines

Anthracyclines occur as glycosides of the anthracyclinone. The glycosidic linkage usually involves the-7-hydroxyl group of anthracyclinone and the β-enentiomer of sugar with L-configuration. Anthracyclinone refers to an aglycone containing the anthraquinone chromophore within a linear hydrocarbon skeleton related to that of tetracycline.

Daunorubicin

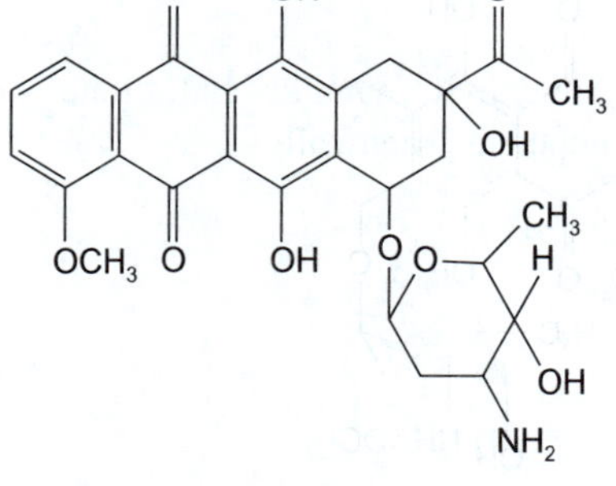

Properties and uses: Daunorubicin is obtained from the fermentation of *Streptomyces peuletiues*. This drug binds to the DNA and inhibits nucleic acid synthesis, mitosis, and promote chromosomal aberration. This drug is used for the treatment of acute myclocytic leukaemia, primary hepatocellular carcinomal, and ovarian endometrial carcinoma.

Doxorubicin

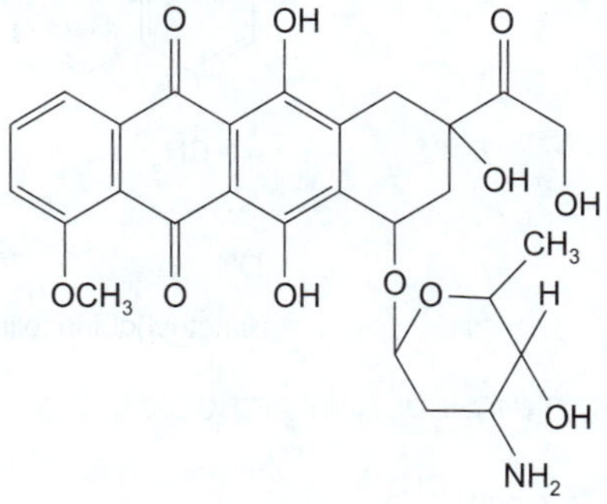

Properties and uses: Doxorubicin hydrochloride is an orange-red crystalline hygroscopic powder, soluble in water, and slightly soluble in methanol. Doxorubicin is 14-hydroxy daunorubicin obtained from the cultures of *Streptomyces peuletiues*. It is one of the most effective antitumour agent. It is used in the treatment of acute lymphocytic leukaemia, breast, lung, ovarian, thyroid, gastric carcinoma, and Hodgkin's disease.

Assay: It is assayed by adopting liquid chromatography technique.

Dosage forms: Doxorubicin HCl injection IP, doxorubicin HCl tablets IP, doxorubicin injection BP.

Idarubicin

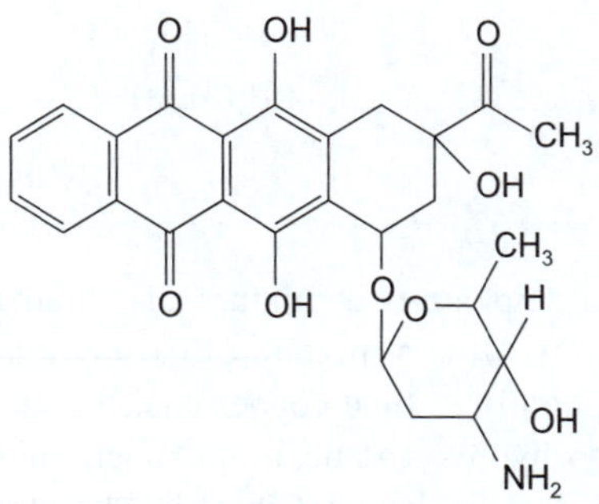

Properties and uses: Idarubicin is demethoxy daunorubicin. It is a synthetic analogue of naturally occurring anthracyclines. It is used in acute myelogeneous leukaemia and acute lymphocytic leukaemia.

Valrubicin

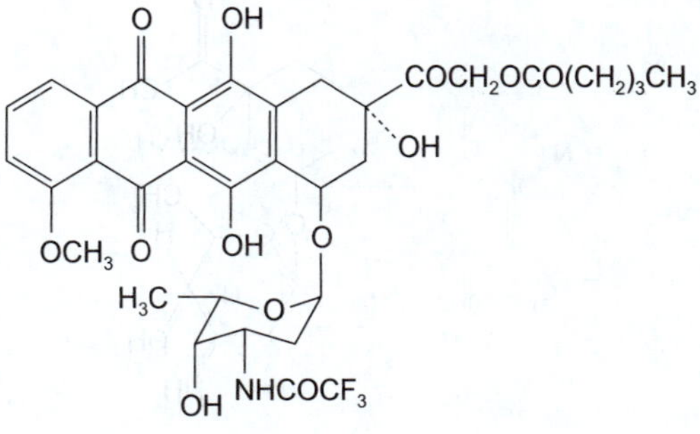

Properties and uses: Valrubicin is a derivative of doxorubicin in which the amino group has a trifluoro-acetyl substituent and 14-hydroxy group is converted to valerate ester.

Bleomycin sulphate

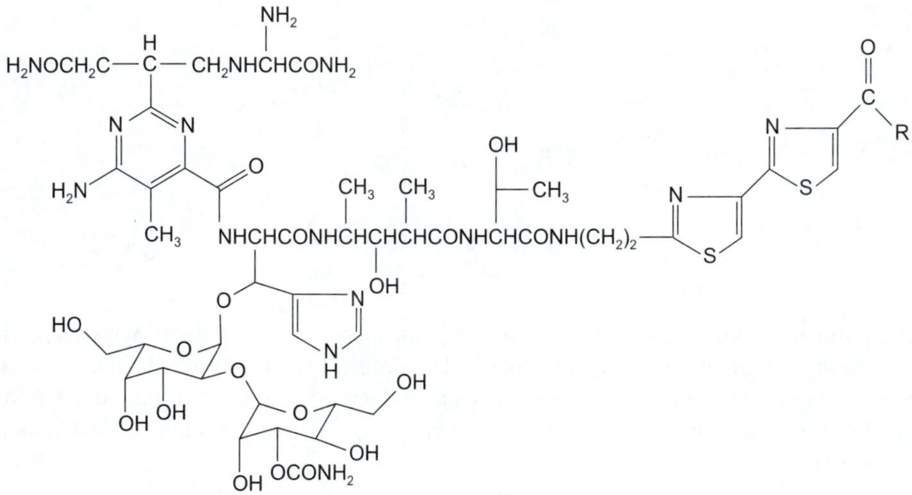

Name	*R*
Bleomycinic acid	–OH
Bleomycin A_2	$-NH(CH_2)_3\overset{\oplus}{S}(CH_3)_2$
Bleomycin B_2	$-NH(CH_2)_4NH-C(=NH)-NH_2$

Properties and uses: Bleomycin sulphate is a mixture of cytotoxic glycopeptidase isolated from the strain of *Streptomyces verticillers*. It is a mixture of closely related compounds with bleomycin A_2 and B_2, Bleomycins occurs naturally as blue copper chelates. Inside the cell, bleomycin forms a complex with Fe(II), gives rise to hydroxyl radical and superoxide radicals. These radicals cleave the phosphodiesterase bond of DNA. This degradation of DNA strands is thought to be a lethal event in cells. It is effective in the treatment of testicular carcinomas. It is also useful in the treatment of squamous cell carcinomas of the head, neck, oesophagus, skin, and the genitourinary tract, including the cervix, vulva, scrotum, and penis.

b. Mitomycin-C

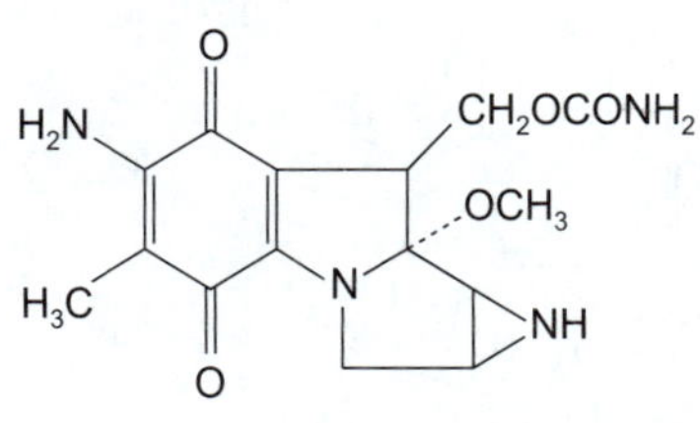

Properties and uses: Mitomycin exists as blue–violet crystals or crystalline powder, slightly soluble in water, freely soluble in dimethylacetamide, sparingly soluble in methanol, and slightly soluble in acetone. It is obtained from *Streptomyces eqespitosus*; it contains three different carcinostatic functions, quinone, carbamate, and aziridine. The molecule is unreactive in its natural state. After intracellular enzymatic or spontaneous chemical reduction of the quinone and loss of the methoxy group, mitomycin becomes a bifunctional or trifunctional alkylating agent. The drug inhibits DNA synthesis at the O^6 and N^7 positions of guanine. In addition, single-strand breakage of DNA is caused by mitomycin. It is used in gastric and pancreatic carcinoma.

Assay: It is assayed by adopting liquid chromatography technique.

Dactinomycin or Actinomycin D

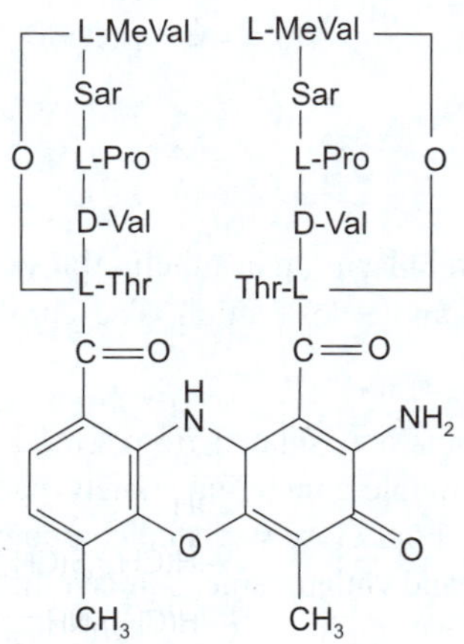

Properties and uses: It is obtained from the cultures of *Streptomyces antibioticus*. It consists of tricyclic phenoxazone ring in the quinone oxidation state and two identical polypeptide and intercalates into the double helical DNA. The main biochemical consequence of the intercalation of actinomycin into DNA is the inhibition of DNA and RNA synthesis, which in turn leads to depletion of protein and cell death.

Plicamycin (Mithramycin)

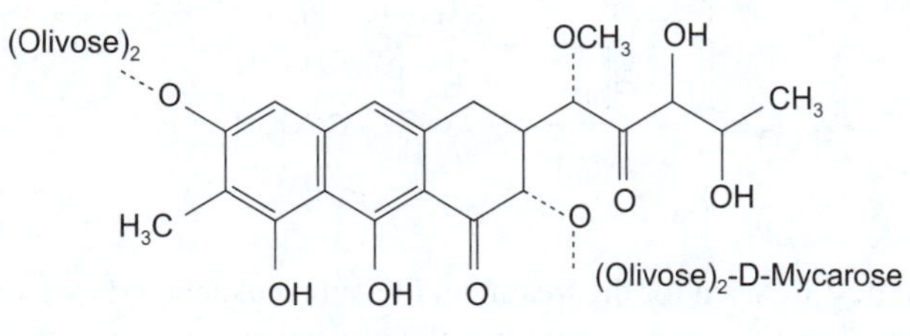

Properties and uses: It is an aureolic acid derivative obtained from *Stremyles plicatus* or *Streptomyces argillaceus*. It forms a complex with divalent metals, such as magnesium and calcium and such complex formation is required before binding with DNA. It inhibits DNA-dependent RNA polymerase, which leads to cell death. It is used in the treatment of embryonal tumours of the testes and metastic cancers.

IV. Plant Products

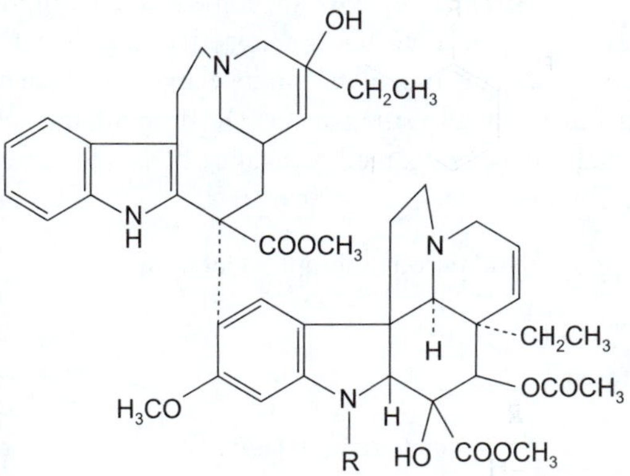

Vincristine R = CHO

Vinblastine R = CH_3

Mode of action: It binds to microtubular protein tubulin, prevents polymerization and assembly of microtubules, and causes mitotic spindle destruction. The chromosomes fail to move apart during mitosis and lead to metaphase arrest.

Properties and uses: Vinca alkaloids are isolated from *Catharanthus roseus*. They have complex structures composed of a dimeric indole-containing moiety named catharanthine and an indoline-containing moiety named vindoline. Four closely related compounds have antitumour activity, that is, vincristine, vinblastine, vinrosidine, and vinleurosine. Semisynthetic derivative vinorelbine is also used as an antitumour agent.

a. Vinorelbine

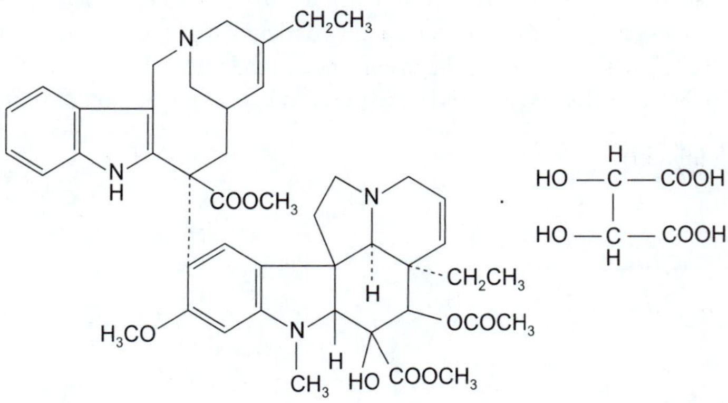

Properties and uses: They are used for the treatment of acute leukaemia, Hodgkin's disease, testicular cell tumour, lymphocytic lymphoma, histicytic lymphoma, and carcinoma of the breast.

b. Camptothecin derivatives

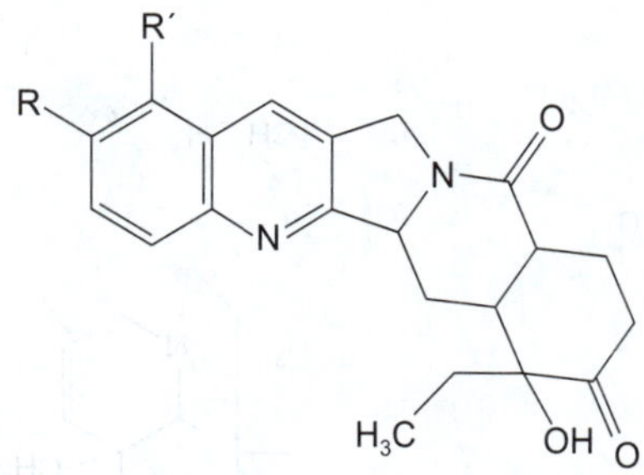

Name	*R*	*R′*
Camptothecin	–H	–H
Irinotican	$–C_2H_5$	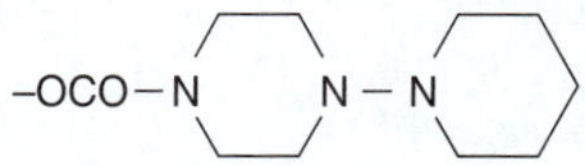
Topotecan	$–CH_2N(CH_3)_2$	–OH

Properties and uses: Camptothecin is a pentacyclic alkaloid originally isolated from *Camptotheca acuminata*. These drugs are used for the treatment of colorectal and ovarian cancers.

c. Epipodophyllotoxins

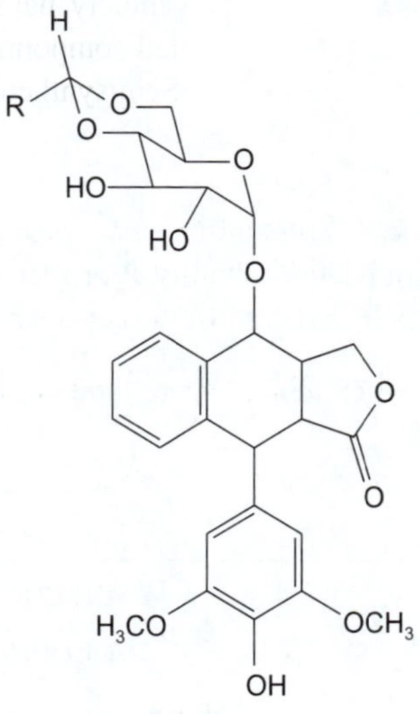

Etoposide R = CH_3

Teniposide R = 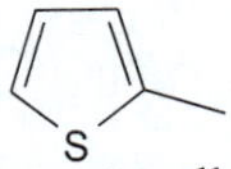

Mode of action: It arrests cells in G_2 phase and causes DNA breaks by affecting the DNA topoisomerase function and the resealing of DNA strand is prevented.

Properties and uses: Etoposide and teniposide are semisynthetic derivatives of podophyllotoxin. It is obtained as extracts of May apple plant. It is effective in the treatment of lung cancer, testicular cancer, and Hodgkin's disease.

d. Taxol derivatives

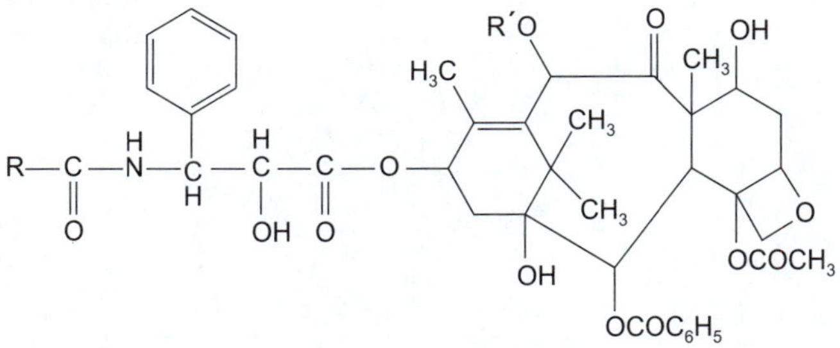

Name	*R*	*R$_1$*
Paclitaxel	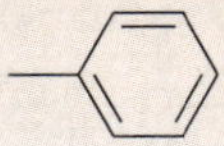	–COCH$_3$
Docetaxel	$(CH_3)_3CO$–	–H

Mode of action: This stabilizes the polymerization of tubulin and the depolymerization is prevented.

Properties and uses: The taxol derivative, paclitaxel, is isolated from the Western row tree, *Taxus brevifolia*. It is the first member of the taxane family used in cancer therapy. It is used for metastatic ovarian and breast cancer, lung, mouth, oesophageal, and bladder carcinomas.

V. Enzymes

L-Asparaginase

It is an enzyme isolated from *Escherichia coli* and *Erwinia carotovora*. The enzyme has a molecular mass of 130,000. It consists of four equivalent subunits. It breaks down asparagin to aspartic acid and ammonia. It is active against tumour cells having lost the capacity to synthesize asparagines.

Properties and uses: It is used to treat childhood acute lymphocytic leukaemia in combination with vincristine and prednisone.

VI. Hormones

Mitotane

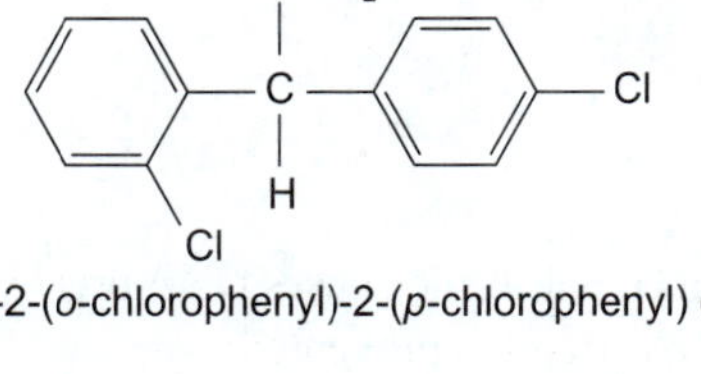

1,1-Dichloro-2-(*o*-chlorophenyl)-2-(*p*-chlorophenyl) ethane

Synthesis

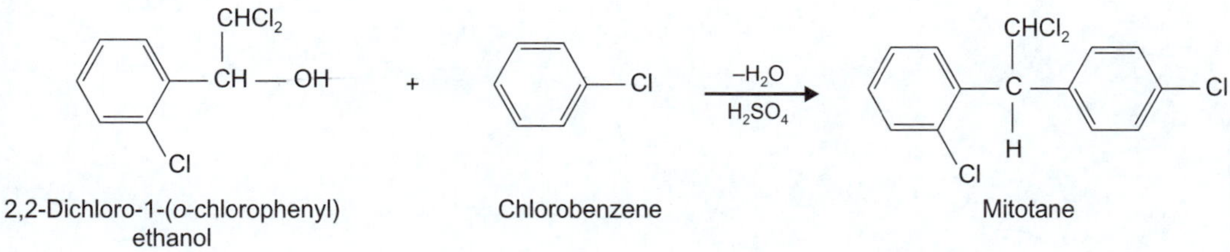

Properties and uses: It is indicated only for treating adrenal cortex carcinoma.

Diethylstilbesterol

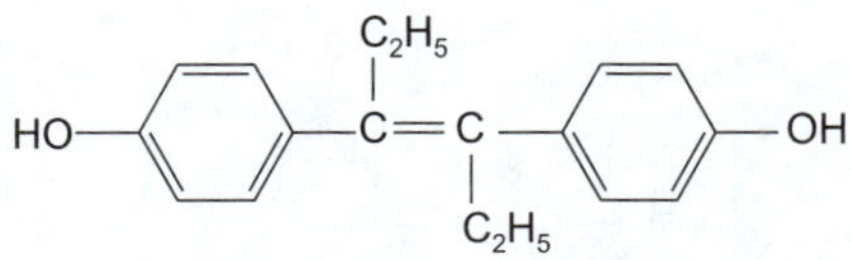

4,4′-(1,2-Diethyl-1,2-ethanediyl)*bis*-phenol

Synthesis

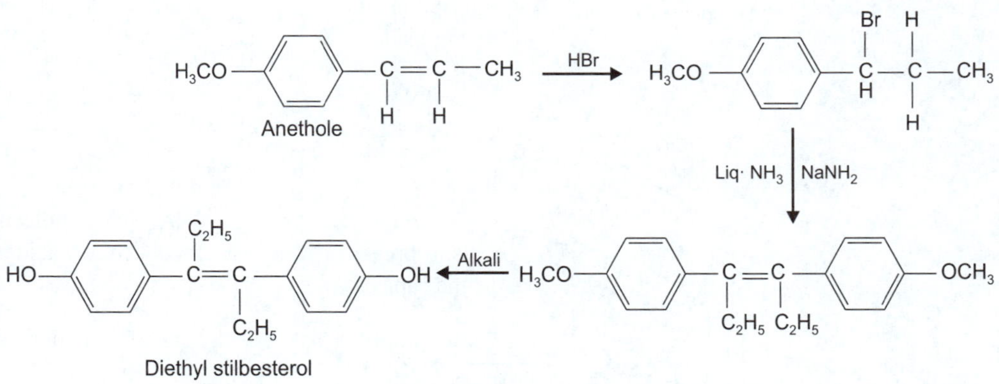

Properties and uses: Diethylstilbesterol is a white crystalline powder, practically insoluble in water, and soluble in alcohol and alkali hydroxides solutions. It is used for pallative therapy and produces relief in primary as well as metastatic prostrate carcinoma.

Assay: Dissolve the sample in ethanol and dilute with the same solvent. To the resulting solution, add dipotassium hydrogen phosphate solution. Prepare in the same manner, a reference solution using diethylstilbestrol reference standard. Irradiate with mercury lamp and measure the absorbance of the irradiated solutions at the maximum of 418 nm, using water as a blank.

Dosage forms: Diethylstilbestrol pessaries BP, diethylstilbestrol tablets BP.

Progesterone

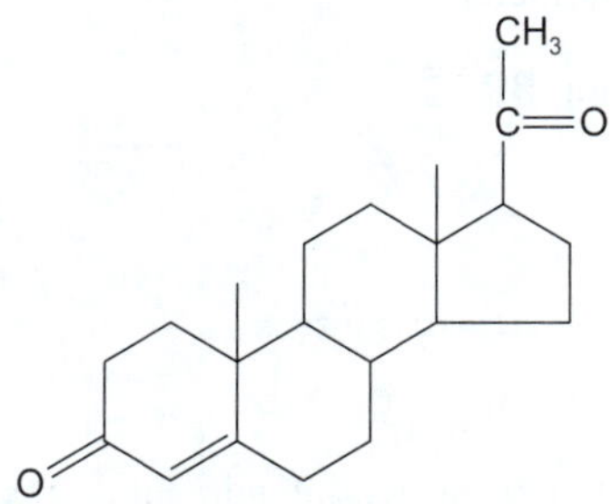

17-Acetyl-10,13-dimethyl-1,7,8,10,11,12,13,15,16,17-decahydro-2*H*-cyclopenta[*a*]phenanthren-3(6*H*,9,14*H*)*H*-one

Synthesis

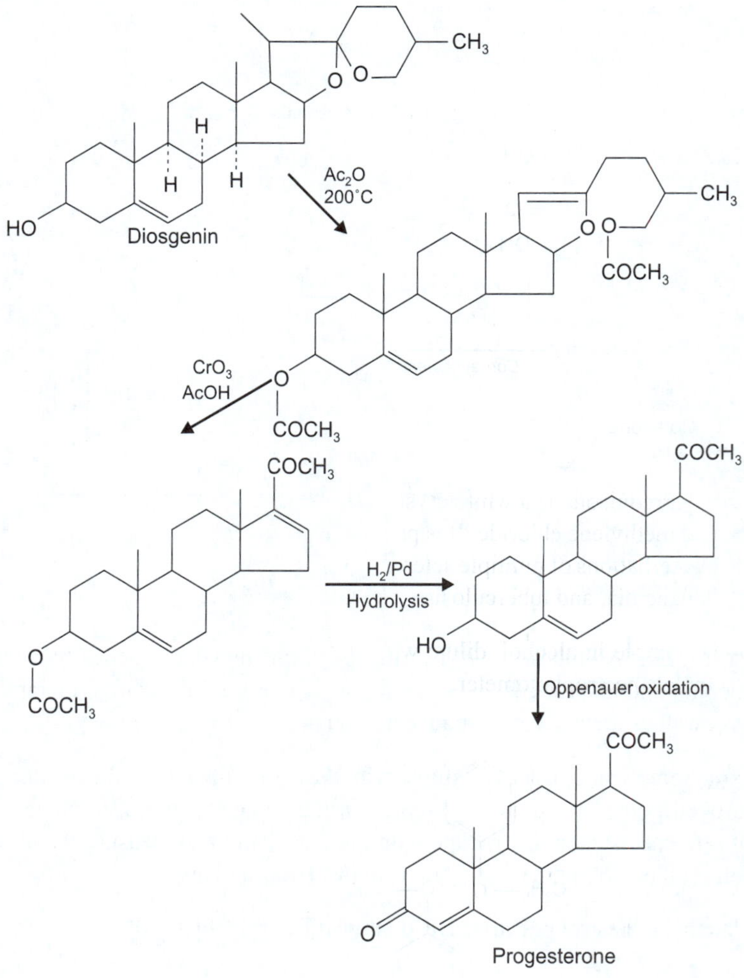

Properties and uses: Progesterone exists as white crystalline powder or colourless crystals, practically insoluble in water, soluble in ethanol, sparingly soluble in acetone and fatty oils. Progestins are pallative in 50% cases of advanced and metastatic endometrial carcinoma.

Assay: Dissolve the sample in alcohol, dilute with the same solvent, and measure the absorbance at 241 nm using ultraviolet spectrophotometer.

Dosage forms: Progesterone injection BP.

Prednisone

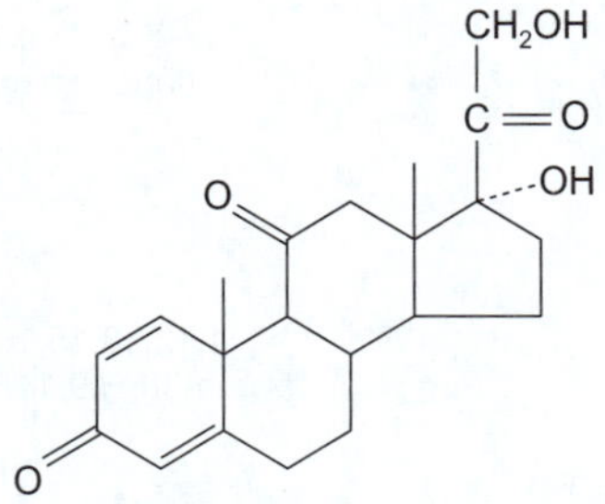

(17R)-17-Hydroxy-17-(2-hydroxyacetyl)-10,13-dimethyl-7,8,13,15,16,17-hexahydro-6*H*-cyclopenta[a]phenanthrene-3,11(9*H*,10*H*,12*H*,14*H*)-dione

Synthesis

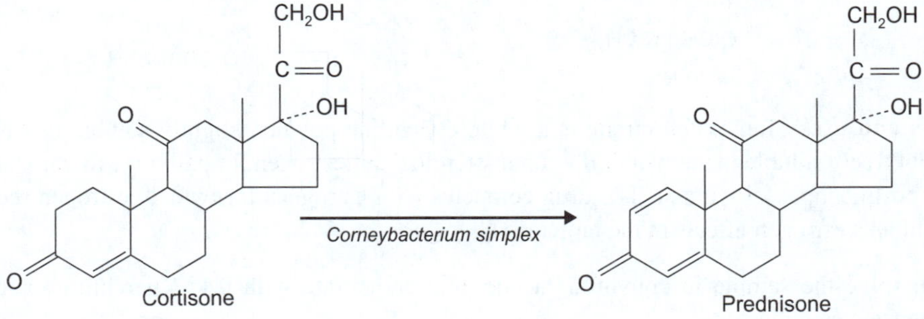

Properties and uses: Prednisone is a white crystalline powder, practically insoluble in water, slightly soluble in alcohol and methylene chloride. It is predominantly used in cancer chemotherapy, and in the treatment of acute exacerbations of multiple sclerosis. In paediatrics, it is widely used to treat nephrosis, rheumatic caslitis, leukaemia, and tuberculosis.

Assay: Dissolve the sample in alcohol, dilute with the same solvent, and measure the absorbance at 238 nm using ultraviolet spectrophotometer.

Tamoxifen

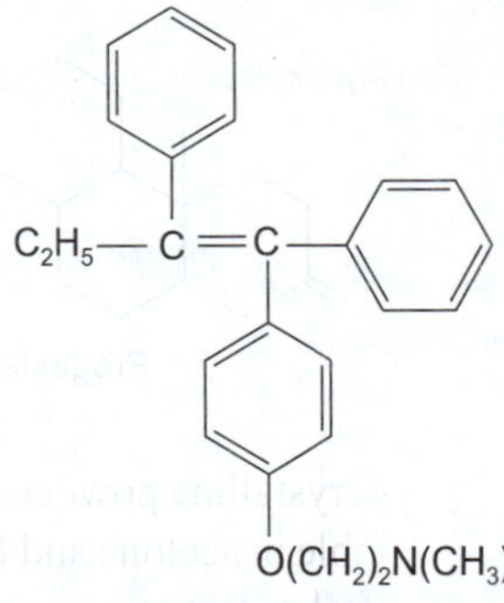

2-[4-(1,2-Diphenyl-1-butenyl)phenoxy]-N,N-dimethyl ethanamine

Synthesis

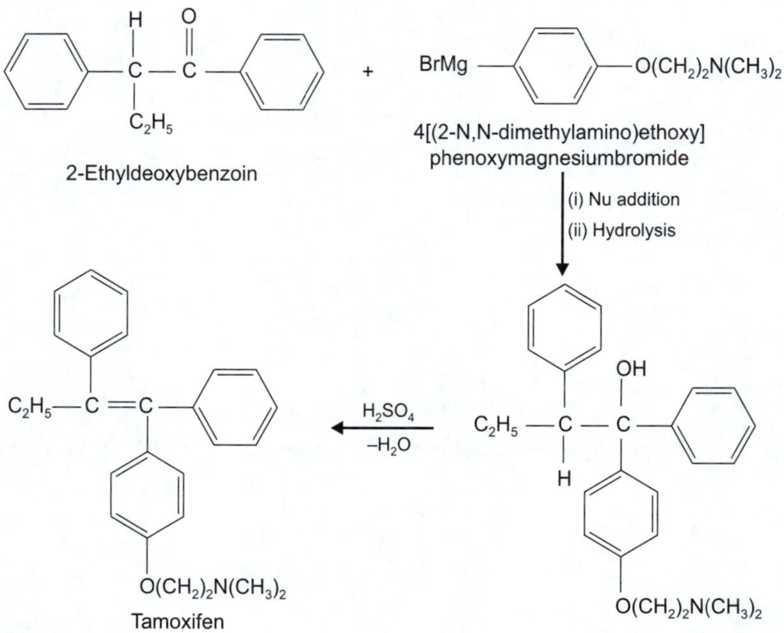

Properties and uses: Tamoxifen citrate is a white crystalline powder, slightly soluble in water and acetone, but freely soluble in methanol. It is a non-steroidal antiestrogen for palliative therapy of breast cancer in postmenopausal women. The drug competes with estrogens for cytosol estrogen receptors, and thus, blocks estrogen effects in the target tissue.

Assay: Dissolve the sample in anhydrous acetic acid and titrate with 0.1 M perchloric acid using naphtholbenzein as indicator.

Dosage forms: Tamoxifen citrate tablets IP, tamoxifen tablets BP.

Letrozole

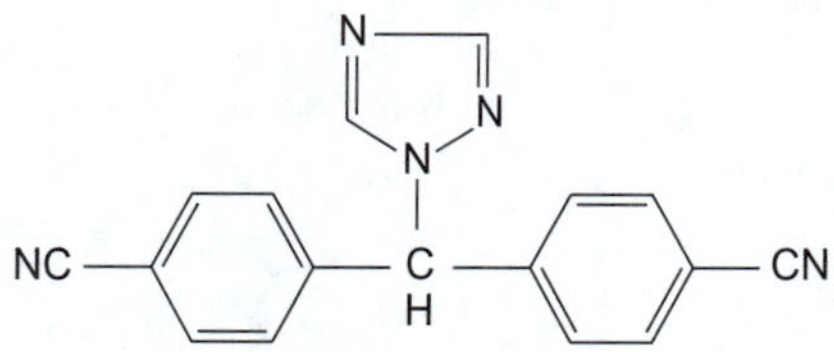

4,4'-(1*H*-1,2,4-triazol-1-yl-methylene)*bis* benzonitrile

Synthesis

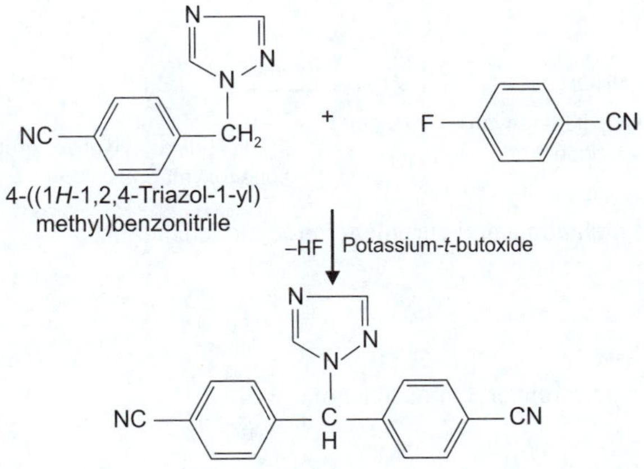

Letrozole

Properties and uses: Letrozole is a white or yellowish crystalline powder, practically insoluble in water, soluble in methylene chloride, and sparingly soluble in methanol. It is used for the treatment of breast carcinoma.

Assay: It is assayed by adopting liquid chromatography technique.

VII. Immunotherapy

Interferons

The interferons are a family of cytokines with broad-spectrum antiviral and anticancer activity making them biological responsive modifiers. Three types of naturally occurring interferons have been found:

1. Leukocytic interferons: Interferons α-2a produced by lymphocytes and macrophages.
2. Fibroblast interferons: Interferons α-n3 produced by fibroblast epithelial cell and macrophages.
3. Immune interferons: Interferons γ synthesized by CD4+, CD8+, and natural killer lymphocytes.

VIII. Miscellaneous

Hydroxy urea

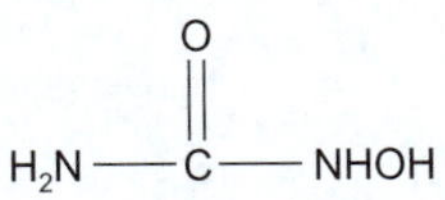

1-Hydroxy carbamide

Synthesis

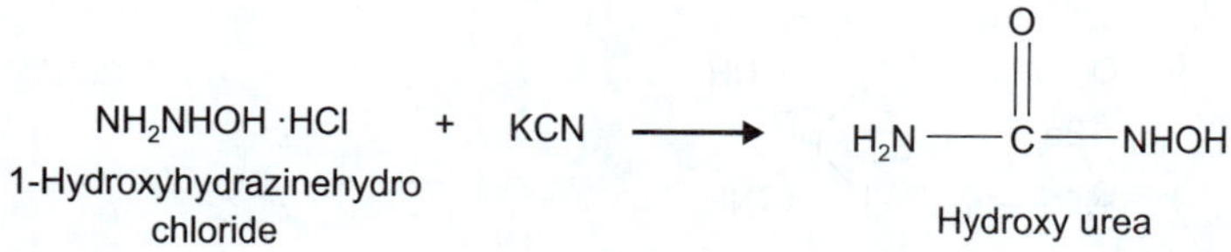

Uses: It is active against melanoma and chronic myelocytic leukaemia.

Gallium nitrate

$Ga(NO_3)_3 . 9H_2O$

Uses: It is used to treat cancer-related hypocalcaemia.

Cisplastin

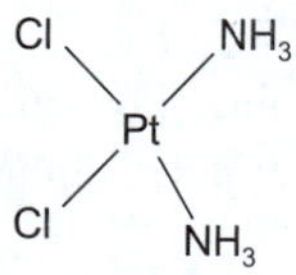

Cis-diamine dichloro platinum (CDDP)

Synthesis

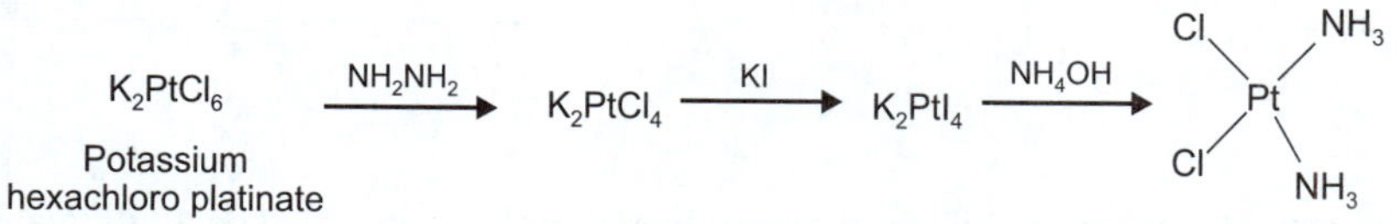

Cis -Diamine dichloro platinum

Properties and uses: Cisplatin is a yellow powder or yellow or orange-yellow crystals, slightly soluble in water, sparingly soluble in dimethylformamide, and practically insoluble in alcohol, used in testicular tumour.

Assay: It is assayed by adopting liquid chromatography technique.

Dosage forms: Cisplatin injection BP.

Carboplatin

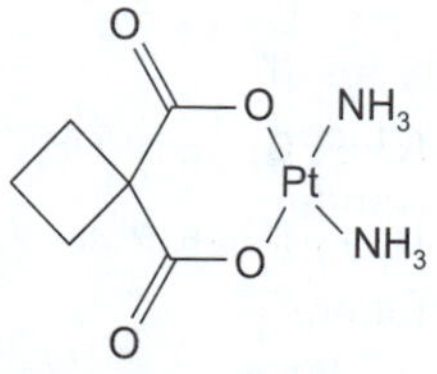

Cis-Diamine(1,1-cyclobutane dicarboxylato) platinum

Synthesis

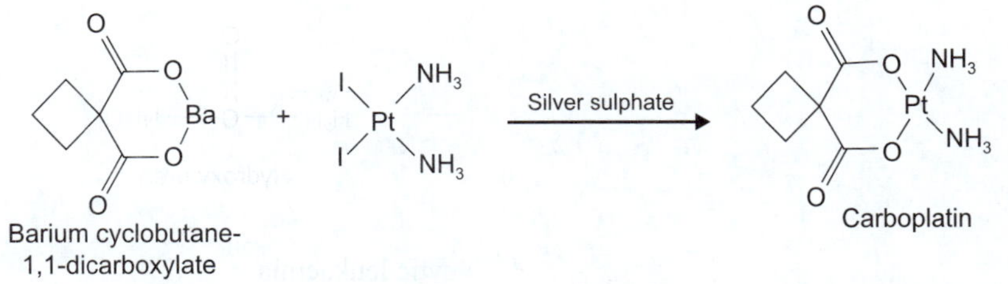

Properties and uses: Carboplatin is a colourless crystalline powder, sparingly soluble in water, very slightly soluble in acetone and alcohol. Food and Drug Administration (FDA) approved it for treatment of advanced ovarian cancer. It is cross-resistant with cisplatin in this tumour. Activity also has been reported in lung cancer, head and neck cancer, and testicular cancer. The usual dose-limiting toxicity is bone marrow suppression, especially, thrombocytopenia.

Assay: It is assayed by gravimetric method.

Dosage forms: Carboplatin injection BP.

IX. Newer Drugs

a. Pazopanib (Votrient)

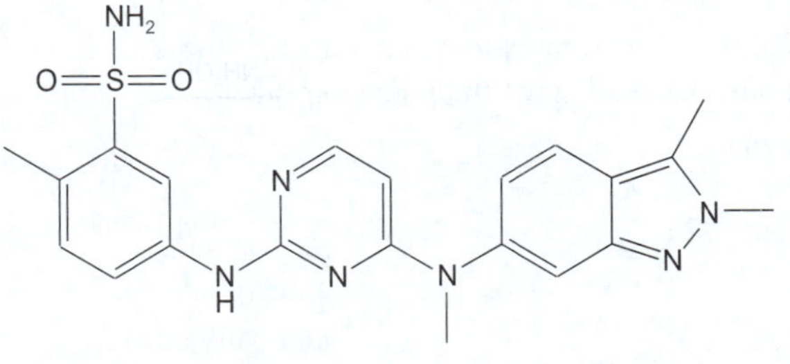

Mode of action: It is an inhibitor of vascular epidermal growth factor receptor (VEGFR) tyrosine kinase, acts at all three isoforms: VEGFR-1, VEGFR-2, and VEGFR-3. VEGF is a chemical signal, which is produced by cells that stimulates the growth of new blood vessels. It is part of the system that restores the oxygen supply to tissues when blood circulation is inadequate. When VEGF is overexpressed, it leads to disease. Solid cancers will not be able to grow without adequate blood supply. Therefore, the cancer that can express VEGF is able to grow and metastasize.

Properties and uses: It is used specifically for the treatment of patients who have advanced renal cell carcinoma. Adverse events associated with the use of pazopanib include diarrhoea, hypertension, hair colour change, nausea, fatigue, anorexia, vomiting.

Dose: It is supplied as a tablet formulated for oral administration. The initial dose is 800 mg orally once daily without food (at least 1 hour before or 2 hours after a meal). The dose should not exceed 800 mg.

b. **Sunitinib malate** (Sutent)

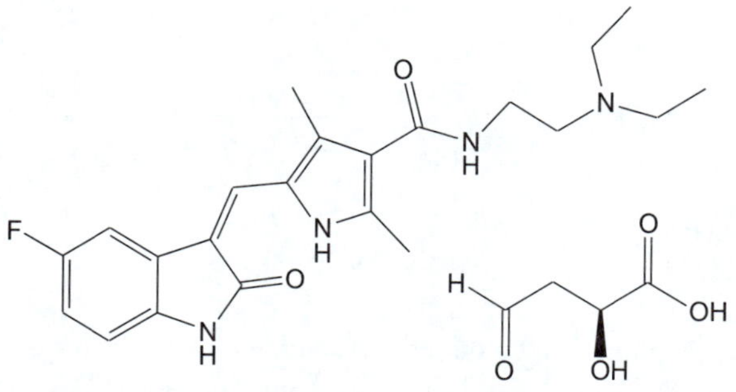

Mode of action: It is an oral multikinase inhibitor, which acts by blocking multiple molecular targets concerned with the growth, proliferation, and spread of cancer. Two targets for this drug are VEGFR and platelet-derived growth factor receptor (PDGFR), which are expressed by many types of solid tumours and are thought to play a crucial role in angiogenesis, the process by which tumours acquire blood vessels, nutrients, and oxygen needed for growth. This drug also inhibits other targets important to tumour growth, including KIT, FLT3, and RET.

Properties and uses: Sunitinib malate is specifically used for the treatment of progressive, well-differentiated pancreatic neuroendocrine tumours in patients with unresectable locally-advanced or metastatic disease. Undesirable effects associated with the use of this drug are fatigue, asthenia, diarrhea, nausea, stomatitis, vomiting, abdominal pain, hypertension, bleeding.

Dose: The recommended dose for pancreatic neuroendocrine tumours is 37.5 mg to taken orally once daily continuously without a scheduled off-treatment period.

c. **Everolimus** (Afinitor)

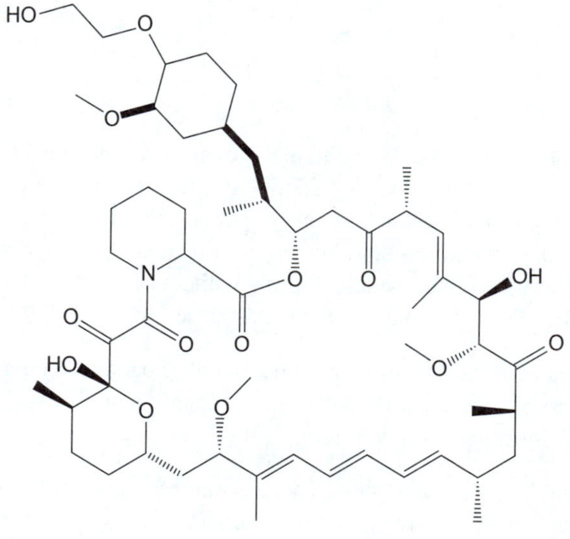

Mode of action: Everolimus is an inhibitor of mammalian target of rapamycin (mTOR). mTOR is a serine/threonine protein kinase that regulates cell growth, cell proliferation, cell motility, cell survival, protein synthesis, and transcription. In several human cancers, the mTOR pathway is dysregulated.

In *in vitro* and/or *in vivo* studies, inhibition of mTOR by this drug has been found to reduce cell proliferation, angiogenesis, and glucose uptake.

Properties and uses: It is specifically permitted in patients with unresectable, locally advanced, or metastatic disease for the treatment of progressive neuroendocrine tumours of pancreatic origin. Adverse actions associated with the use of this drug include stomatitis, rash, diarrhoea, fatigue, fever, and headache.

Dose: The suggested dose of everolimus for pancreatic cancer is 10 mg once daily.

d. Vandetanib (Vandetanib)

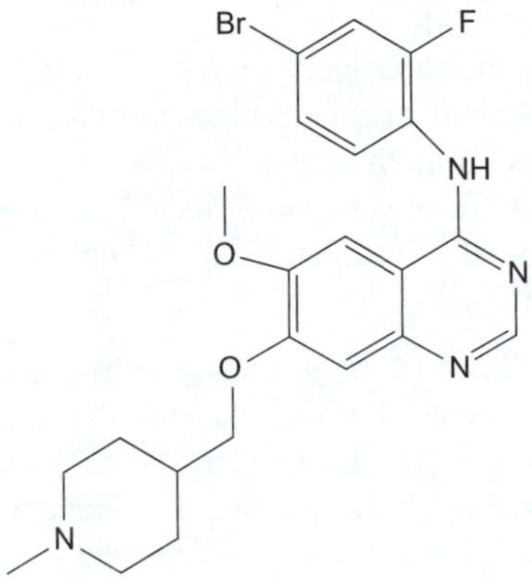

Mode of action: It is a kinase inhibitor. *In vitro* studies have shown that this drug inhibits the activity of tyrosine kinases including members of the epidermal growth factor receptor (EGFR) family, protein tyrosine kinase 6 (BRK), TIE2, members of the EPH receptors kinase family, vascular endothelial cell growth factor (VEGF) receptors, rearranged during transfection (RET), and members of the Src family of tyrosine kinases. In *in vitro* models of angiogenesis, this drug inhibits endothelial cell migration, proliferation, survival, and new blood vessel formation. It inhibits EGFR-dependent cell survival *in vitro*. Epidermal growth factor (EGF)-stimulated receptor tyrosine kinase phosphorylation in tumour cells and endothelial cells and VEGF-stimulated tyrosine kinase phosphorylation in endothelial cells are also inhibited. *In vivo* vandetanib administration reduced tumour cell-induced angiogenesis, tumour vessel permeability, and inhibited tumour growth and metastasis in mouse models of cancer.

Properties and uses: It is specifically used in the treatment of symptomatic or progressive medullary thyroid cancer in patients with unresectable locally-advanced or metastatic disease. Adverse events associated with the use of vandetanib may include hypertension, headache, fatigue, decreased appetite, and abdominal pain.

Dose: The suggested daily dose is 300 mg of vandetanib taken orally, with or without food. Until patients are no longer benefiting from treatment or an unacceptable toxicity occurs, treatment with vandetanib should be continued.

If vandetanib tablets cannot be taken whole, the tablets can be dispersed in a glass containing 2 ounces of non-carbonated water and stirred until the tablet is dispersed. Immediately, the dispersion should be swallowed. To ensure that the full dose is received, an additional 4 ounces of non-carbonated water should be mixed with any residues in the glass and swallowed.

e. **Vismodegib** (Erivedge)

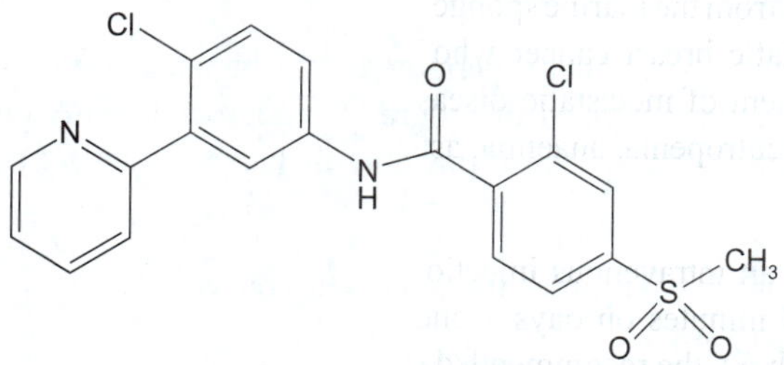

2-Chloro-N-(4-chloro-3-pyridin-2-ylphenyl)-4-methylsulfonylbenzamide

Mode of action: It is an inhibitor of the hedgehog (Hh) signalling pathway. It binds to and inhibits smoothened, a transmembrane protein involved in hedgehog signal transduction. Cellular development and division in several cell types, both through direct cellular activation and through secondary activation of multiple pathways of tissue generation, including angiogenesis and tissue growth, are promoted by the Hh pathway. In basal cell carcinoma, the pathway is typically overactivated through down regulation of Hedgehog inhibition.

Properties and uses: It is an inhibitor of the hedgehog (Hh) signalling pathway, approved for the treatment of adults with metastatic basal cell carcinoma, or with locally-advanced basal cell carcinoma which has recurred following surgery or who are not candidates for surgery, and who are not candidates for radiation. Adverse events associated with the use of vismodegib may include muscle spasms, dysgeusia, weight loss, alopecia, fatigue, nausea, diarrhea, decreased appetite, constipation and arthralgias.

Dose: 150 mg taken orally once daily until disease progression or until unacceptable toxicity.

f. **Trastuzumab** (Herceptin)

Mode of action: It is a humanized IgG1 kappa monoclonal antibody that selectively binds with high affinity to the extracellular domain of the human epidermal growth factor receptor 2 protein (HER2). HER2 is a cell membrane surface-bound receptor tyrosine kinase and is normally involved in the signal transduction pathways leading to cell growth and differentiation. HER2 is overexpressed in certain cancers. Trastuzumab binds to the extracellular juxtamembrane domain of HER2 and inhibits the proliferation and survival of HER2-dependent tumours.

Properties and uses: Trastuzumab is specifically used in combination with cisplatin and capecitabine or 5-fluorouracil, for the treatment of patients with HER2 overexpressing metastatic gastric or gastroesophageal junction enocarcinoma, who have not received prior treatment for metastatic disease. Adverse events with the use of trastuzumab for gastric cancer may include, neutropenia, diarrhea, fatigue, anaemia, stomatitis, weight loss, fever, thrombocytopenia.

Dose: Trastuzumab is supplied as a solution for intravenous administration. The recommended initial dose of trastuzumab for gastric cancer is 8 mg/kg as a 90 minute intravenous infusion followed by subsequent doses of 6 mg/kg as an intravenous infusion over 30–90 minutes every three weeks until disease progression.

g. **Eribulin mesylate** (Halaven)

Mode of action: Without affecting the shortening phase, it inhibits the growth phase of microtubules and sequesters tubulin into non-productive aggregates. Via a tubulin-based antimitotic mechanism, it exerts its effects leading to G2/M cell-cycle block, disruption of mitotic spindles, and, ultimately, apoptotic cell death after prolonged mitotic blockage.

Properties and uses: It is a non-taxane microtubule dynamics inhibitor and a synthetic analogue of halichondrin B (isolated from the marine sponge *Halichondria okadai*). The drug is used for the treatment of patients with metastatic breast cancer who have already received at least two chemotherapeutic regimens for the treatment of metastatic disease. Adverse events associated with the use of eribulin mesylate may include neutropenia, anaemia, asthenia/fatigue, alopecia, peripheral neuropathy, nausea, and constipation.

Dose: It is supplied as an intravenous injection. The recommended dose is 1.4 mg/m^2 administered intravenously over 2–5 minutes on days 1 and 8 of a 21-day cycle. For patients with mild hepatic impairment (Child-Pugh A), the recommended dose is 1.1 mg/m^2 administered intravenously over 2–5 minutes on days 1 and 8 of a 21-day cycle. For patients with moderate hepatic impairment (Child-Pugh B), the dose is 0.7 mg/m^2 administered intravenously over 2–5 minutes on Days 1 and 8 of a 21-day cycle. For patients with moderate renal impairment (creatinine clearance of 30–50 ml/min), the dose is 1.1 mg/m^2 administered intravenously over 2–5 minutes on days 1 and 8 of a 21-day cycle.

h. Pertuzumab (Perjeta)

Mode of action: Extracellular dimerization domain (subdomain II) of the human epidermal growth factor receptor 2 protein (HER2) is targeted by the drug and, thereby, blocks ligand-dependent heterodimerization of HER2 with other HER family members, including EGFR, HER3, and HER4. As a result of this, the drug inhibits ligand-initiated intracellular signalling through two major signal pathways, mitogen-activated protein (MAP) kinase and phosphoinositide 3-kinase (PI3K). Inhibition of these signalling pathways leads to cell growth arrest and apoptosis, respectively. The drug also mediates antibody-dependent cell-mediated cytotoxicity (ADCC). When administered in combination with herceptin, its antitumour activity is significantly augmented.

Properties and uses: It is a HER2/neu receptor antagonist compound, found to augment antitumour activity as a complement to herceptin, as the two medicines target different regions on the HER2 receptor. In combination with trastuzumab and docetaxel, it is specifically used for the first-line treatment of HER2$^+$ metastatic breast cancer. Adverse reactions associated with the use of pertuzumab in combination with trastuzumab and docetaxel may include diarrhoea, rash, alopecia, neutropenia, nausea, fatigue, and peripheral neuropathy.

Dose: Initial dose is 840 mg administered as a 60-minute intravenous infusion, followed every 3 weeks thereafter by 420 mg administered as a 30–60 minute intravenous infusion.

Acalabrutinib

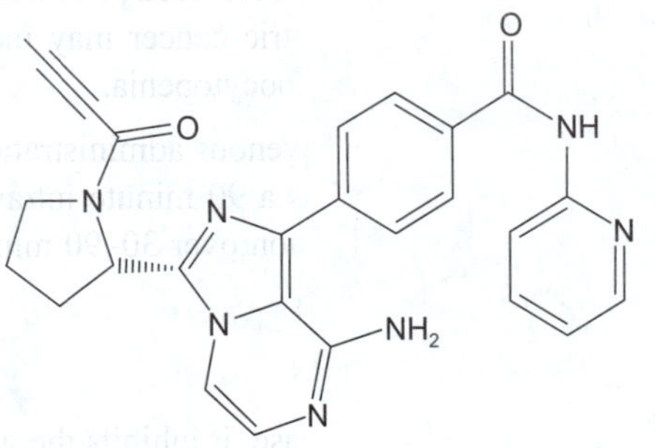

Uses:

It is an inhibitor of Bruton's tyrosine kinase (BTK) possess antineoplastic activity.

Abemaciclib

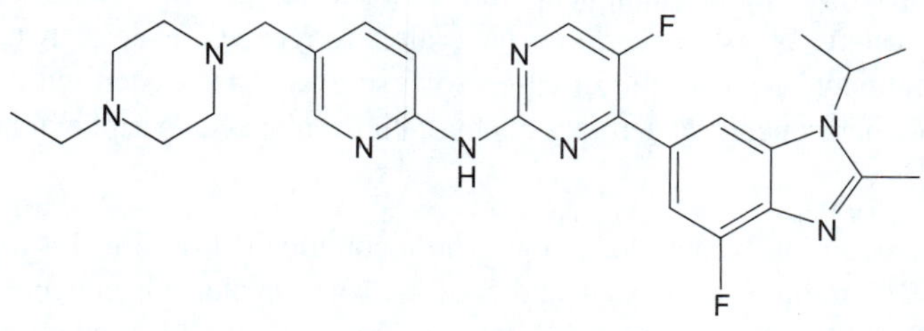

Uses:

It is an orally available cyclin-dependent kinase (CDK) inhibitor possessses antineoplastic activity.

Copanlisib

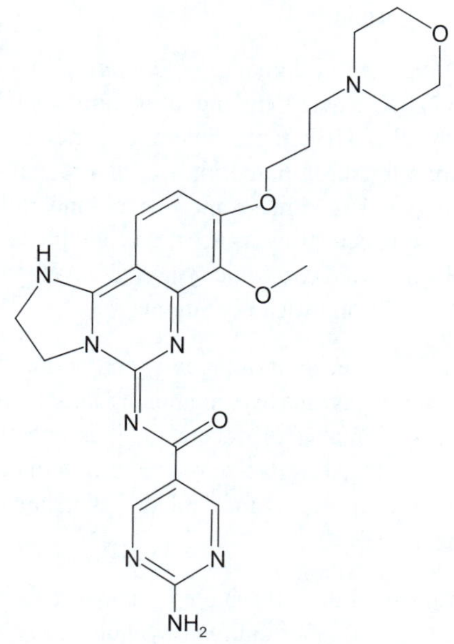

Uses:

It is used as an antineoplastic agent.

Neratinib

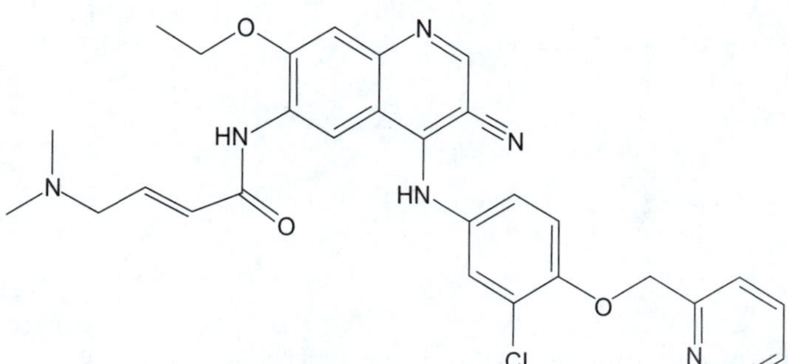

Uses:

It is a tyrosine kinase inhibitor and an antineoplastic agent.

Ribociclib

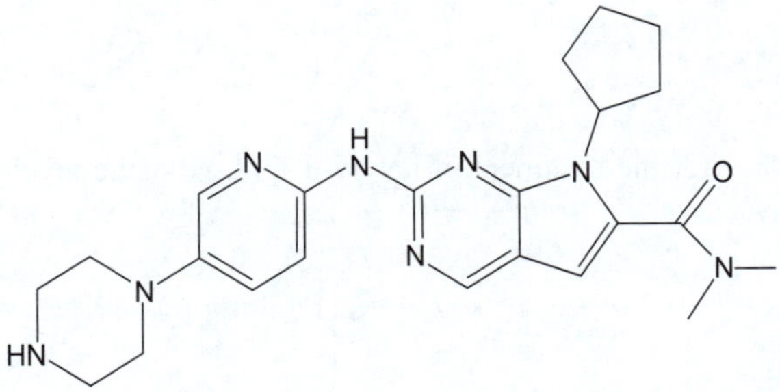

Uses: It is used for the treatment of certain kinds of breast cancer.

Gilteritinib

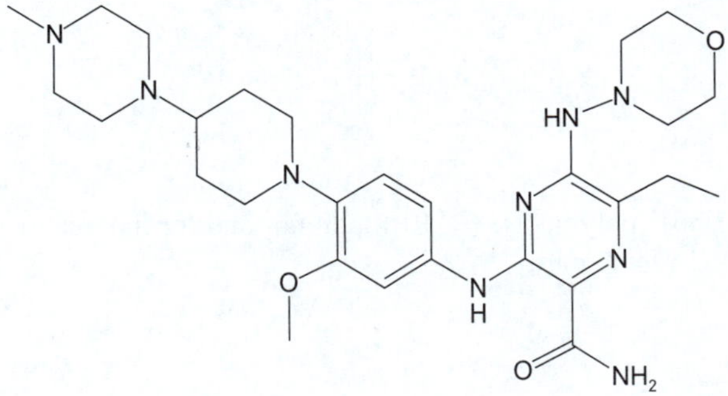

Uses:

1. It is a tyrosine kinase inhibitor and used as an anticancer drug.
2. It has been repurposed as a potential antiviral drug as a possible application in the treatment of COVID-19.

Larotrectinib

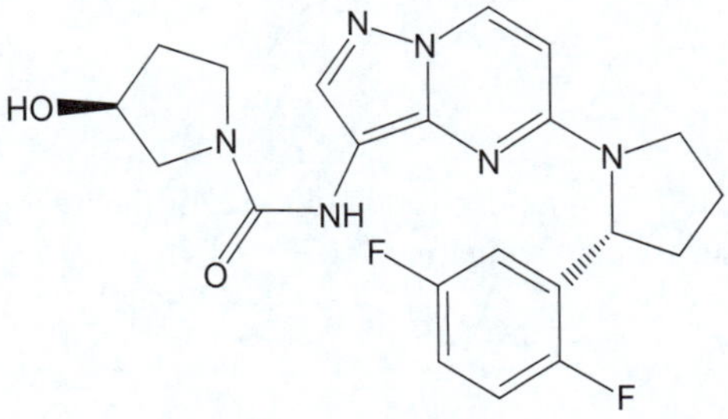

Uses: It is a tyrosine kinase inhibitor and used as an anticancer drug.

Glasdegib

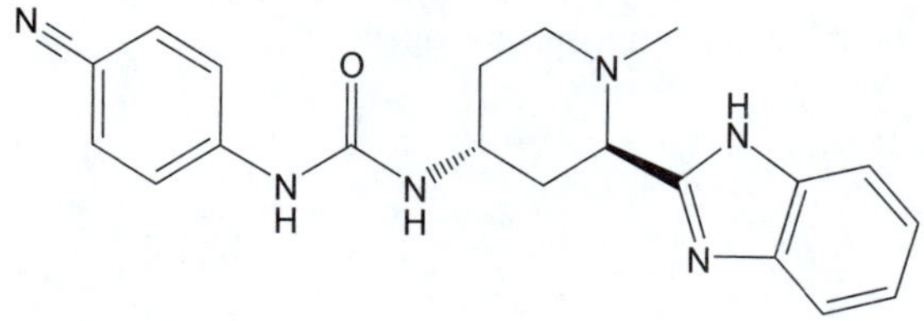

Uses: It is a drug of choice for the treatment of newly-diagnosed acute myeloid leukemia (AML) in adults older than 75 years.

Alazoparib

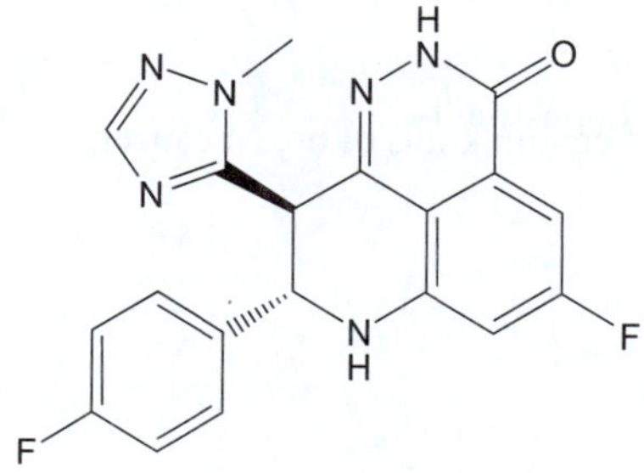

Uses: It is a poly-ADP ribose polymerase (PARP) inhibitor and for the treatment of advanced breast cancer with germline BRCA mutations.

Dacomitinib

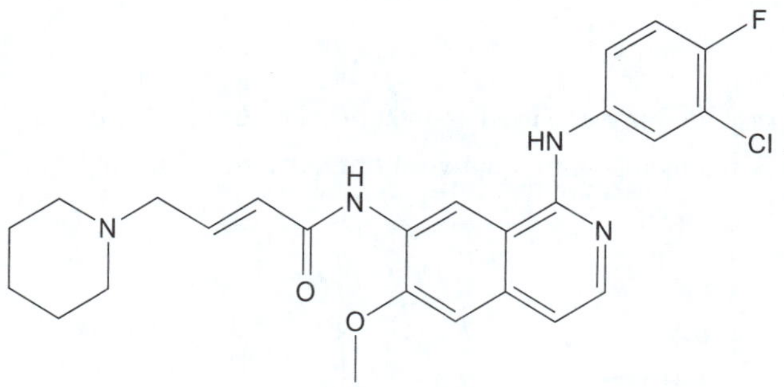

Uses: It is a narrow-spectrum tetracycline-derived antibiotic for the treatment of inflammatory lesions of non-nodular moderate-to-severe acne vulgaris.

Duvelisib

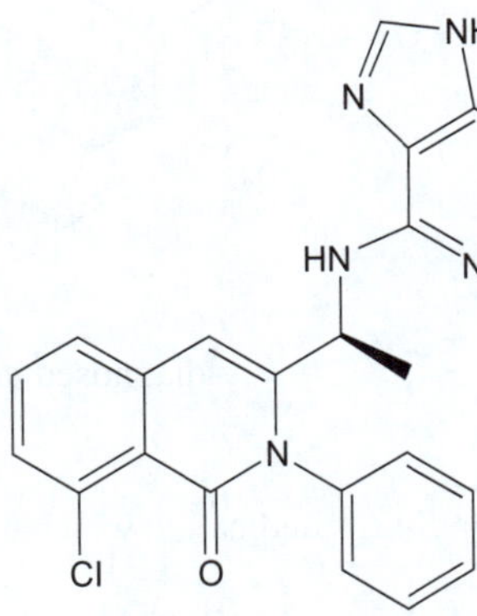

Uses: It is used for the treatment of non-small-cell lung carcinoma.

Ncorafenib

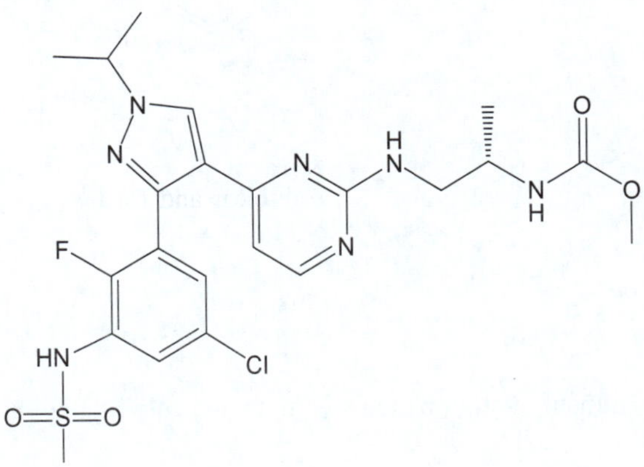

Uses: It is an anticancer agent used to treat certain kind of melanomas.

Binimetinib

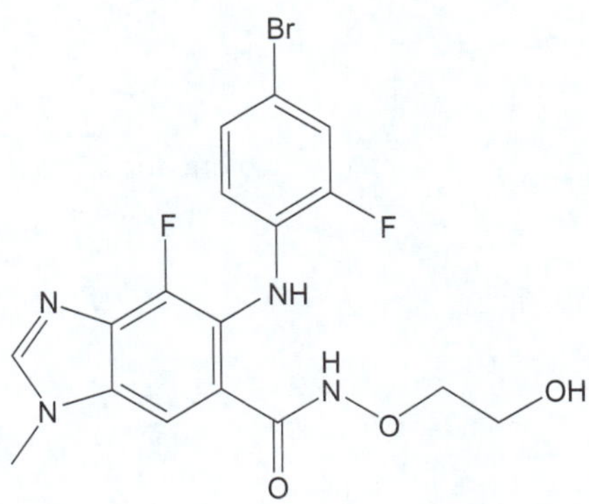

Uses: It is an anticancer agent.

Apalutamide

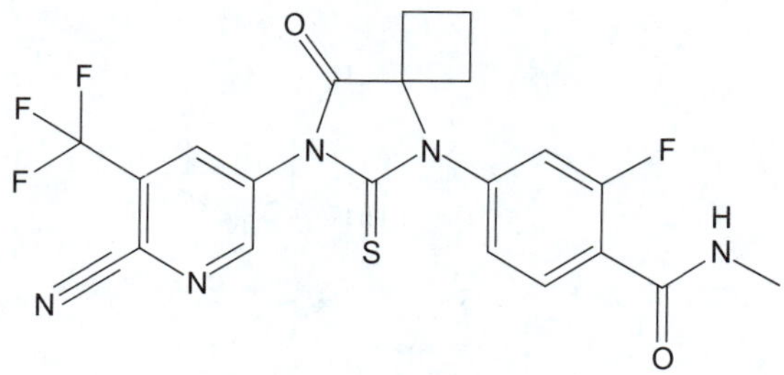

Uses: It is a non-steroidal antiandrogen (NSAA) medication which is used for the treatment of prostate cancer.

Zanubrutinib

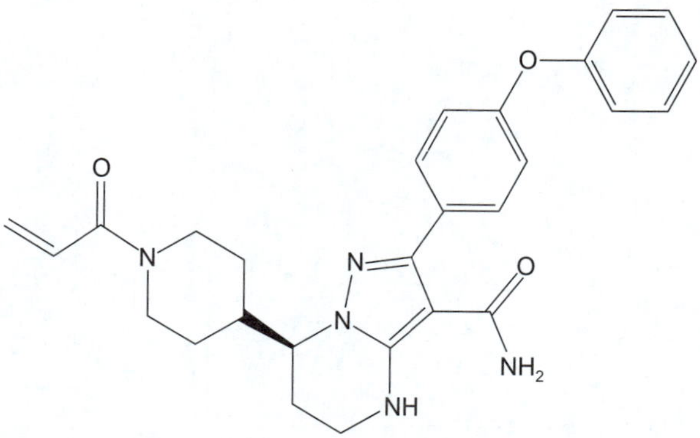

Uses: It is used for the treatment of adult patients with mantle cell lymphoma (MCL).

Fedratinib

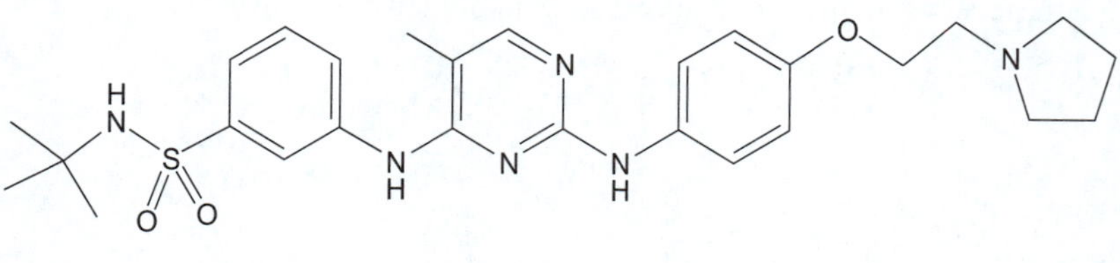

Uses: It is used as anticancer agent.

Entrectinib

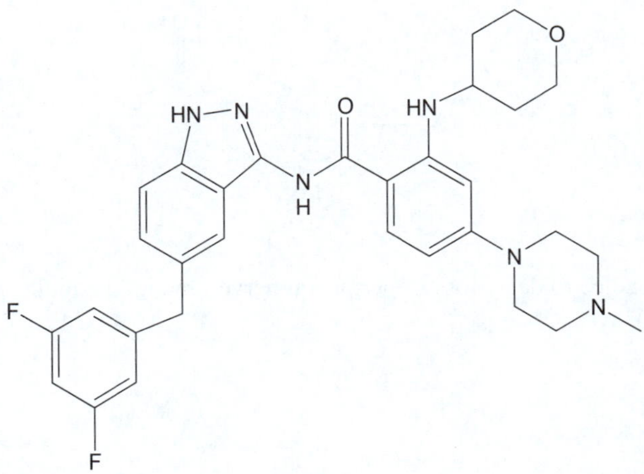

Uses: It is used as anticancer agent to treat non-small lung cancer.

Selinexor

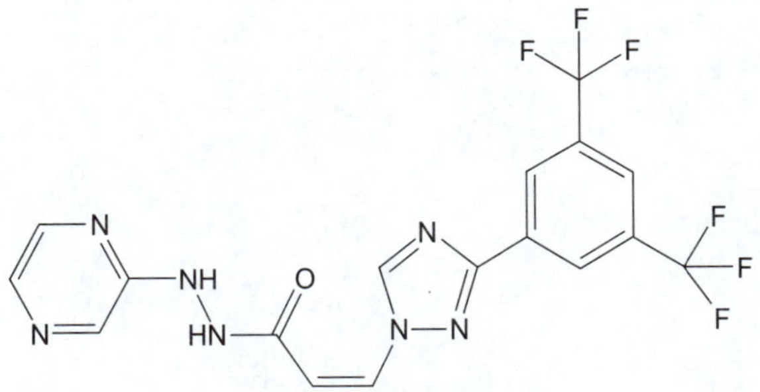

Uses: It is used as an anticancer agent.

Alpelisib

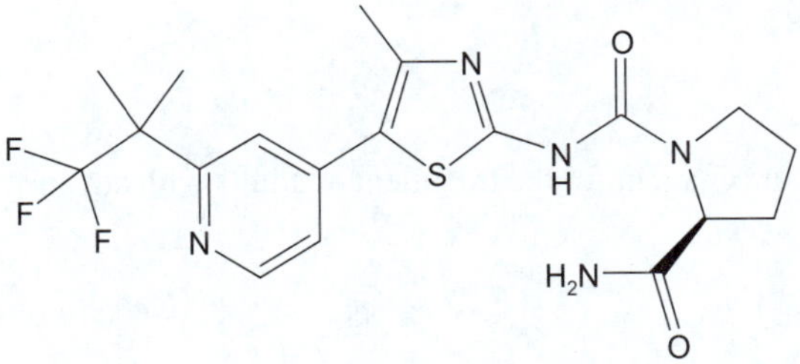

Uses: It is used as an anticancer agent to treat breast cancer.

Afamidis

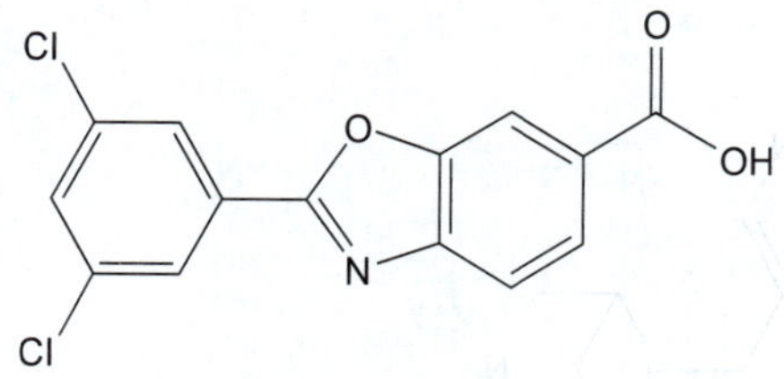

Uses: It is a drug of choice to delay loss of peripheral nerve function in adults with familial amyloid polyneuropathy (FAP).

Erdafitinib

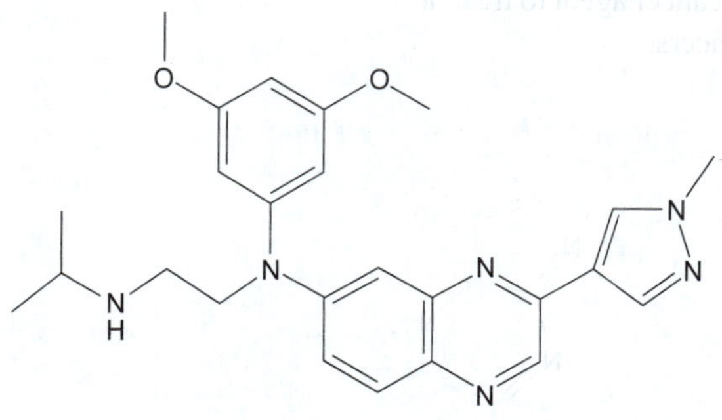

Uses: It is used as an anticancer agent.

Ripretinib

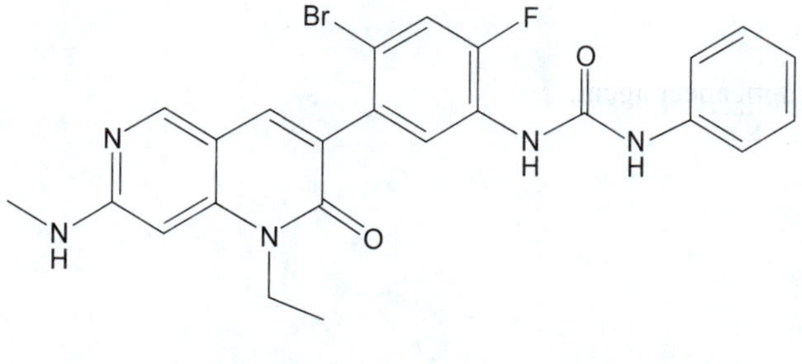

Uses: It is used as an anticancer agent for the treatment of adults with advanced gastrointestinal stromal tumor (GIST).

Selpercatinib

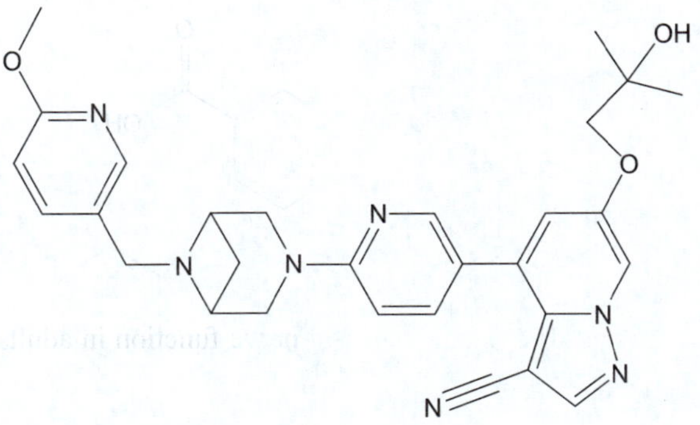

Uses: It is used as an anticancer agent to treat non-small cell lung cancer, medullary thyroid cancer, and other types of thyroid cancers.

Capmatinib

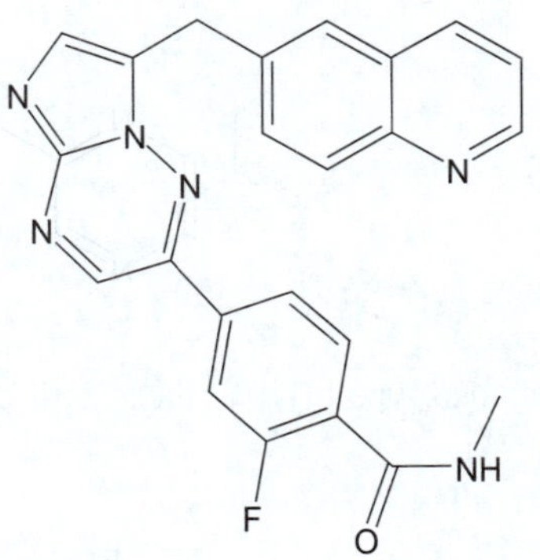

Uses: It is used as an anticancer agent.

Pemigatinib

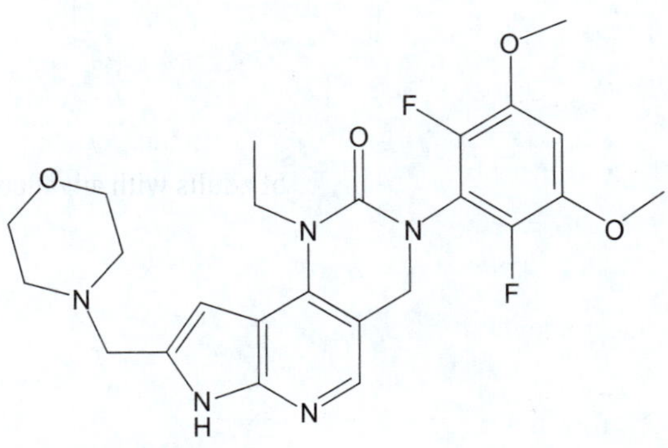

Uses: It is used as an anticancer agent to treat bile duct cancer.

Tucatinib

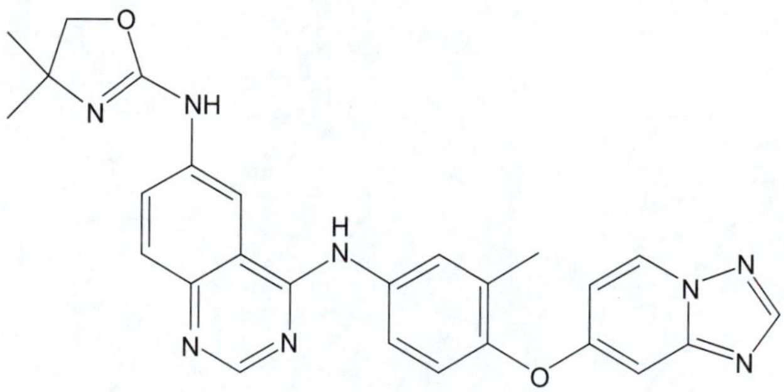

Uses: It is used as an anticancer agent to treat HER2-positive breast cancer.

Selumetinib

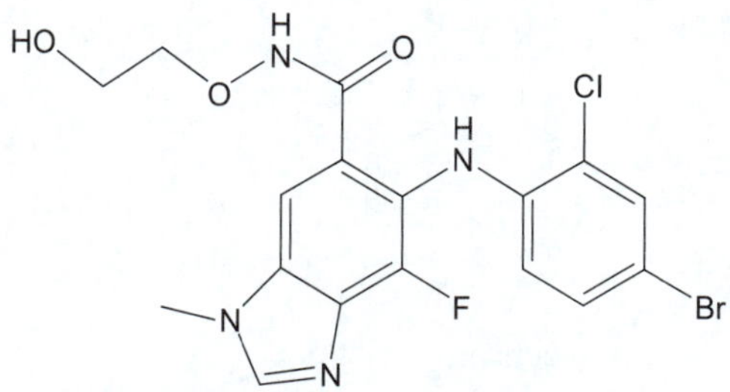

Uses: It is used to treat neurofibromatosis type 1 (NF1), the genetic disorders of nervous system causing tumours to grow on nerves.

Tazemetostat

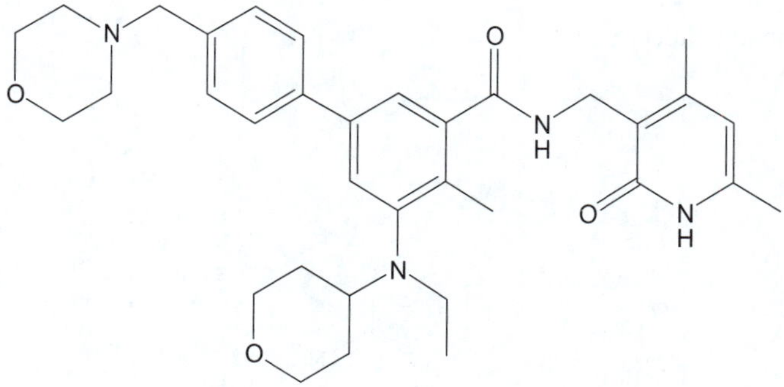

Uses: It is used as an anticancer agent.

Avapritinib

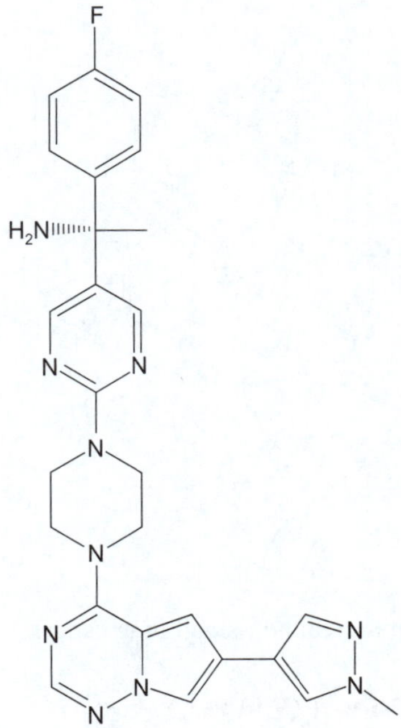

Uses: It is used for the treatment of cancers produced by mutation (anticancer agent).

Zanubrutinib

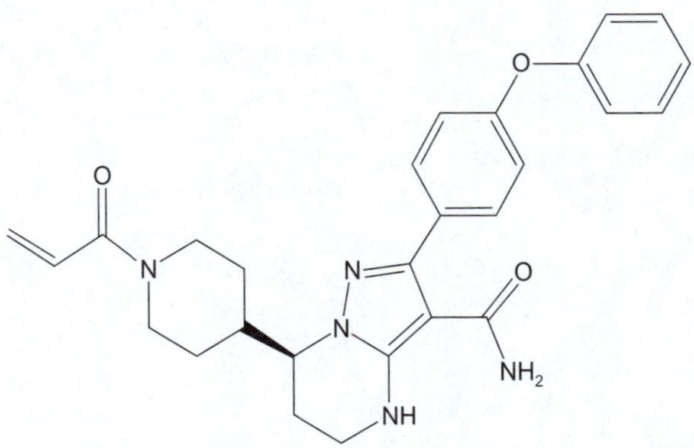

Uses: It is used for the treatment of adult patients with mantle cell lymphoma (MCL).

Fedratinib

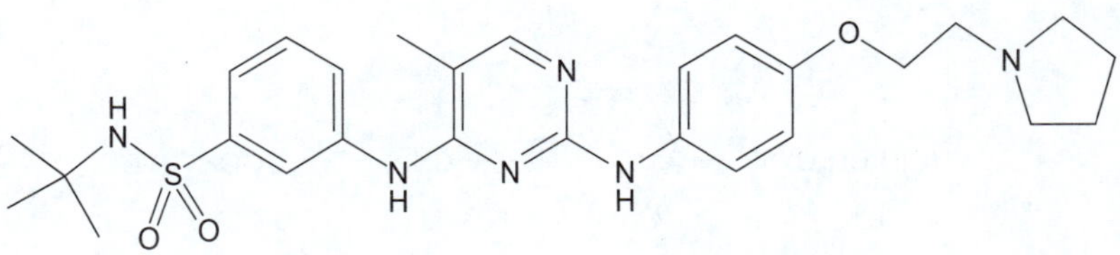

Uses: It is used as anticancer agent.

Entrectinib

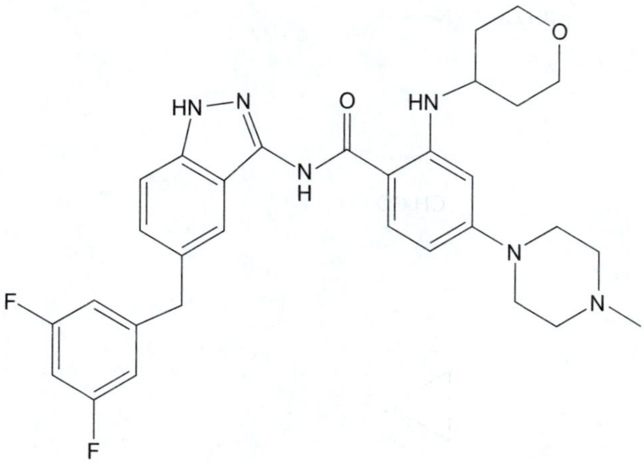

Uses: It is used as anticancer agent to treat non-small lung cancer.

CLASSIFICATION BASED ON PCI SYLLABUS

Alkylating Agents

Meclorethamine

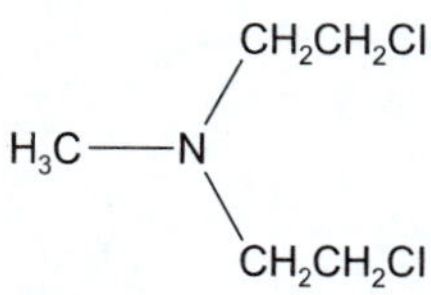

Cyclophosphamide

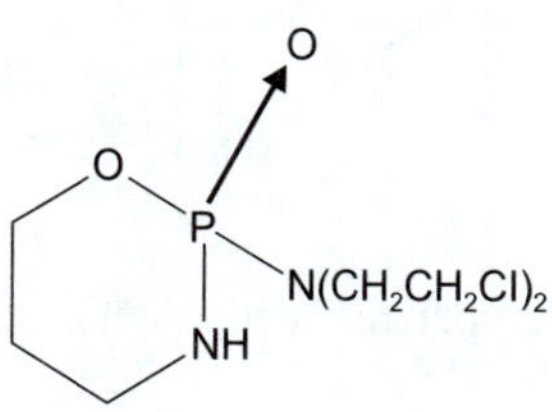

Melphalan

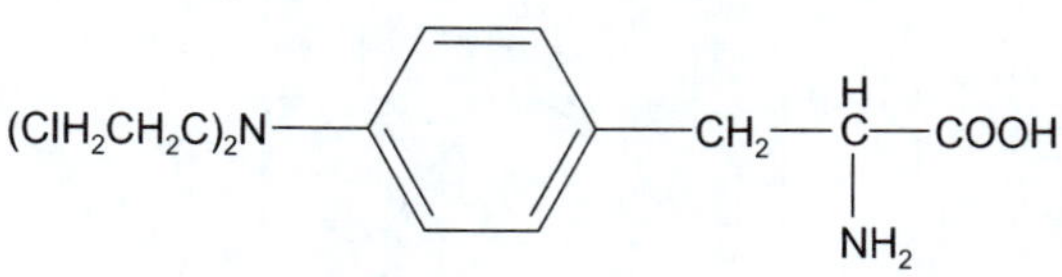

Chlorambucil

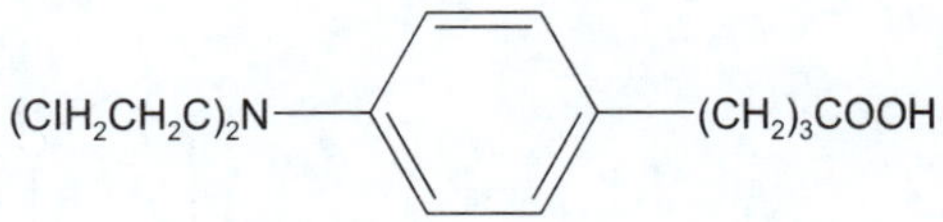

Busulfan

$CH_3SO_2O(CH_2)_4OSO_2CH_3$

Thiotepa

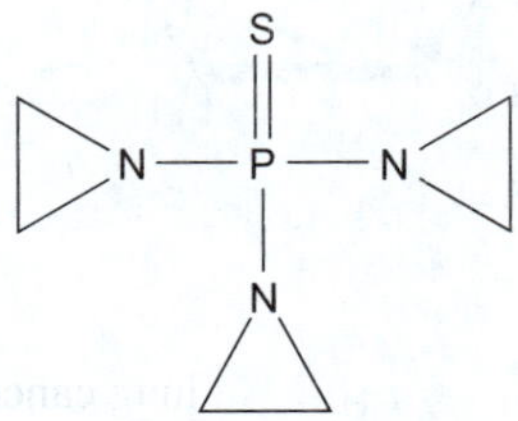

Antimetabolites

Mercaptopurine

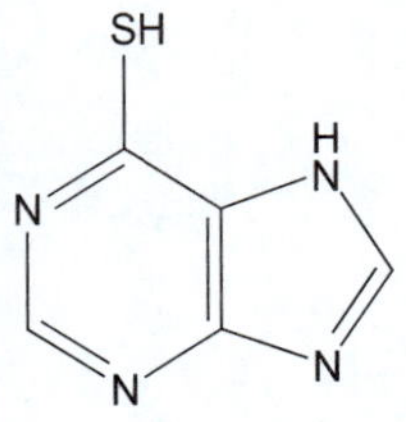

Thioguanine

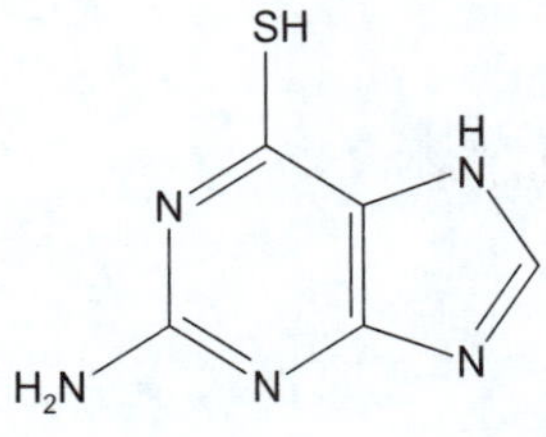

Fluorouracil

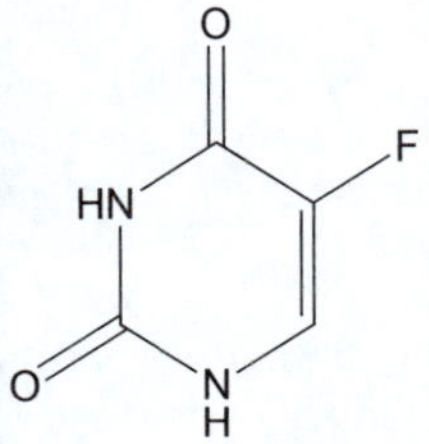

Floxuridine

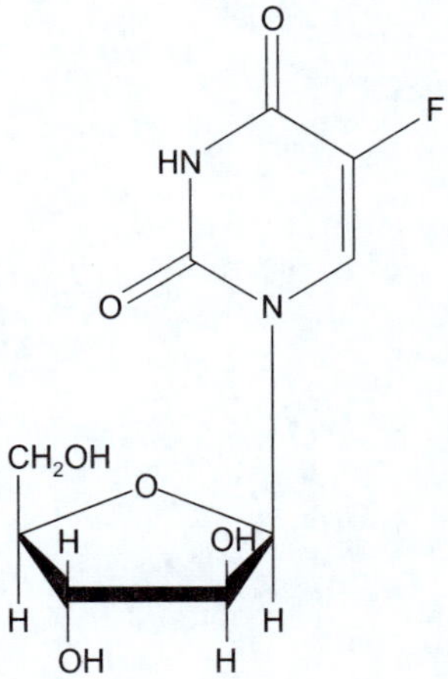

Cytarabine

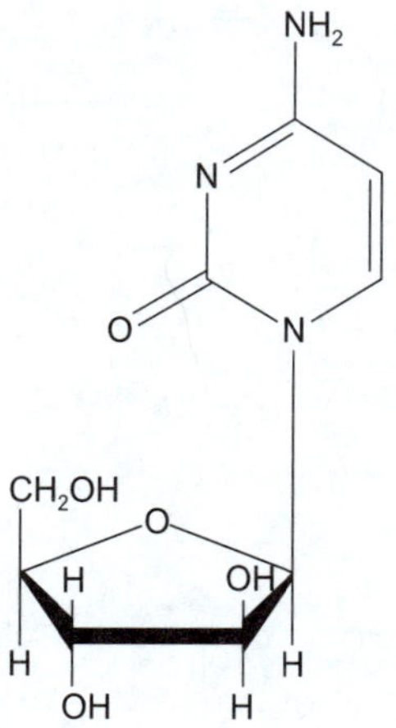

Methotrexate

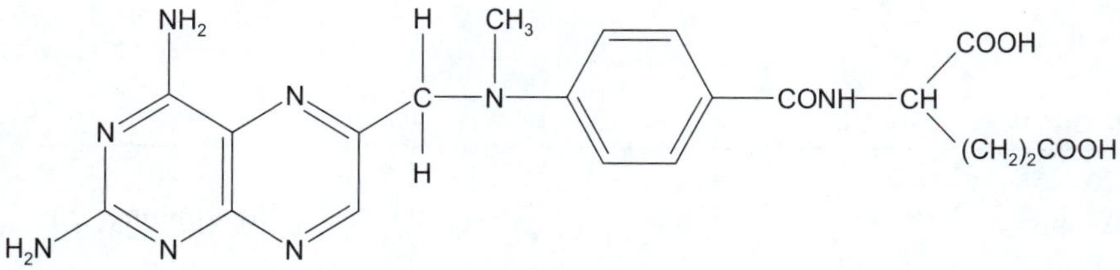

Azathiophrine

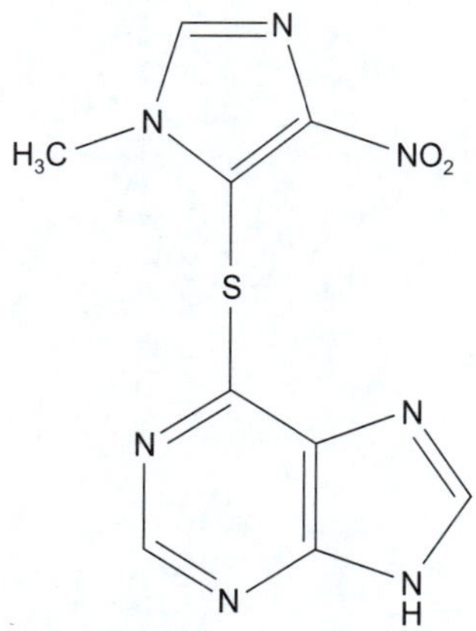

Antibiotics

Dactinomycin

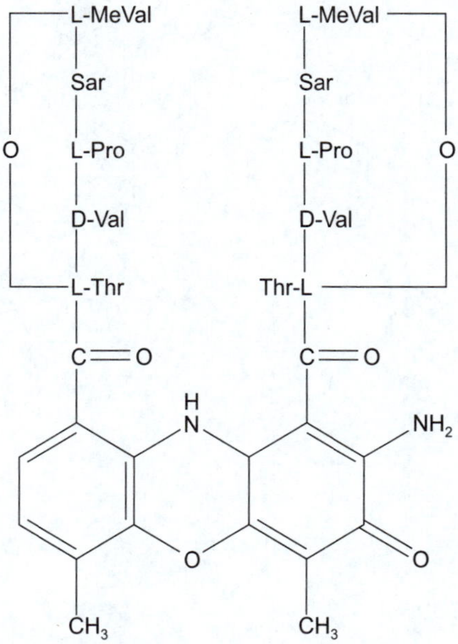

Daunorubicin

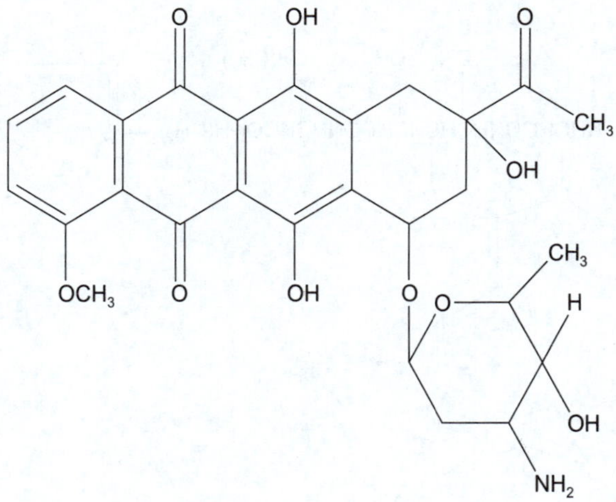

Doxorubicin

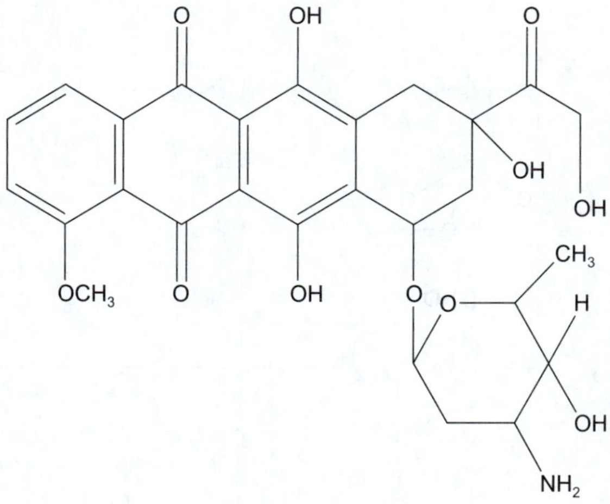

Bleomycin

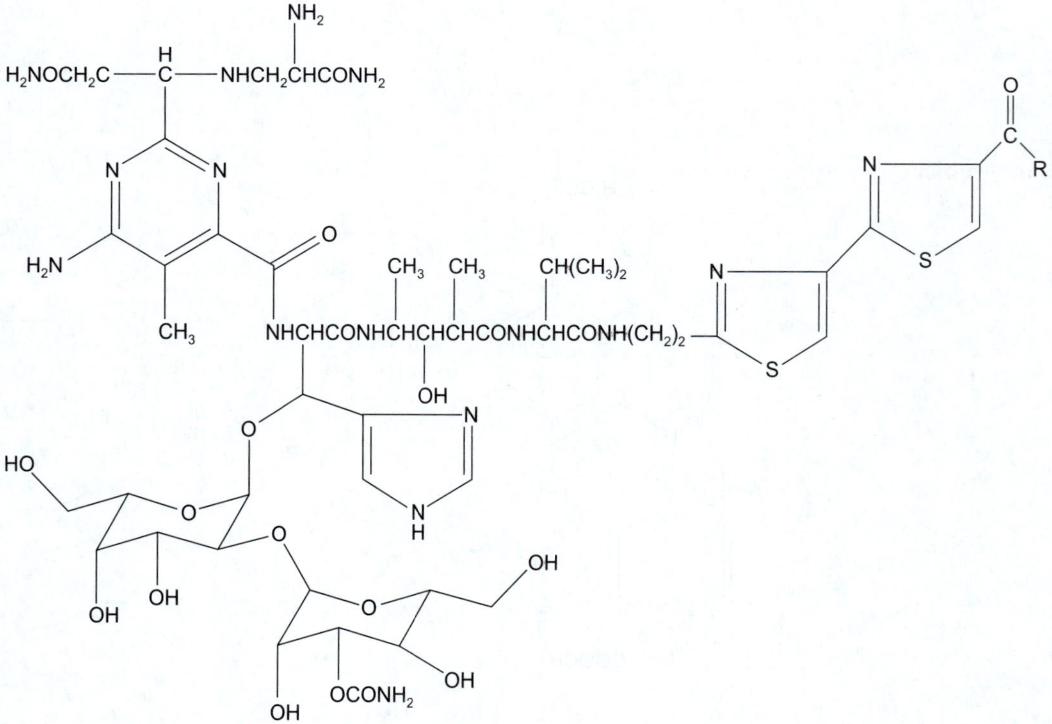

Bleomycin A_2, R = $-NH(CH_2)_3\overset{\oplus}{S}(CH_3)_2$

Bleomycin B_2, R = $-NH(CH_2)_4NH-C(=NH)-NH_2$

Plant Products

Etoposide

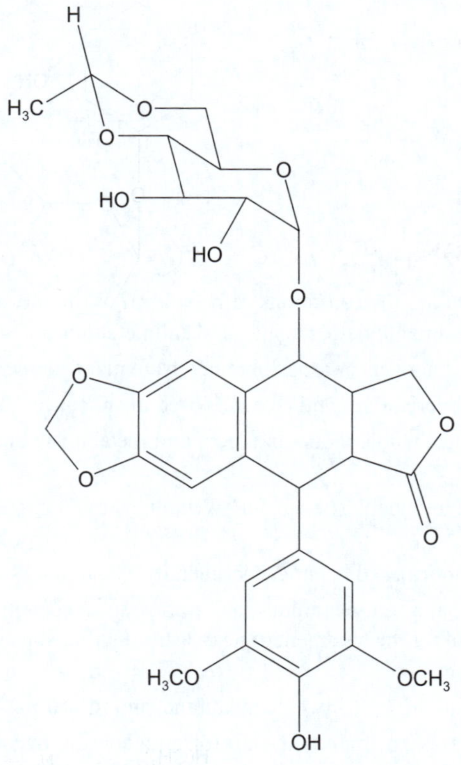

Vinblastin sulphate

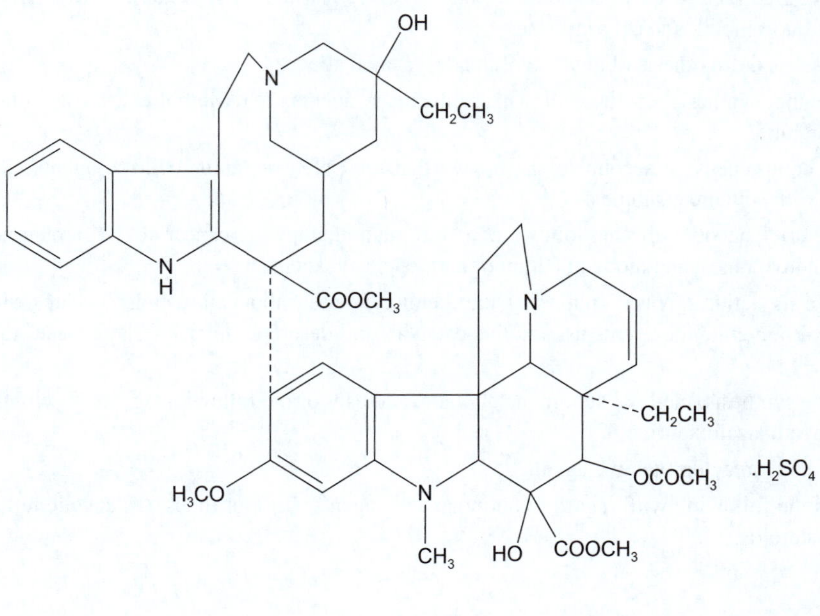

Miscellaneous

Cisplatin

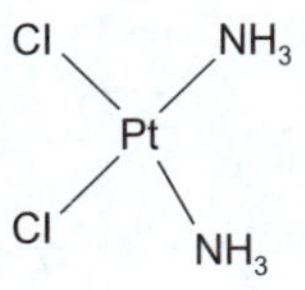

Mitotane

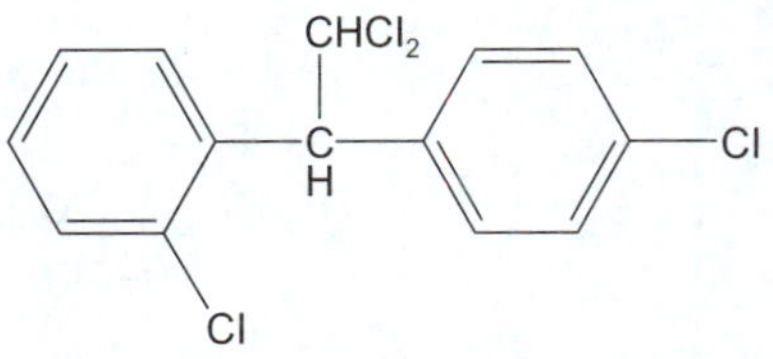

PROBABLE QUESTIONS

1. What is a neoplasm? What are the causations of neoplasm? Write the structure, name, synthesis, and uses of at least two drugs from alkylating agents and antimetabolites.
2. Describe in detail about the anticancer drugs obtained from plant source.
3. Write a brief note on taxol derivatives and enzymes used in anticancer therapy.
4. Write the structure, chemical name, mode of action, and metabolism and uses of any three anticancer drugs from different class.
5. How will you classify the antineoplastic agents? Write the structure, chemical name, and uses of two agents from each class.
6. Write an account on antibiotics used in anticancer therapy.
7. Mustards, methanesulphonates, ethylenimines, and nitrosoureas constitute four vital categories of the alkylating agents employed for the treatment of neoplasms. Outline the synthesis, metabolism, and uses of the following drugs:
   (a) chlorambucil, (b) busulfan, (c) trithylene melamine, and (d) carmustine.
8. Recognition of antibiotics as an important class of antineolastic agents. Justify the statement with reference to the following drugs: (a) dactinomycin and (b) daunorubicin.
   i. How would you classify 'antimetabolites'?
   ii. Give the structure, chemical name, and uses of the following: (a) Methotrexate, (b) meracaptopurine, (c) fluorouracil, and (d) azaserine.
   iii. Discuss the synthesis of any one of the drug stated above.
9. Outline the synthesis of the following anticancer agents: (a) Methotrexate, (b) lomustine, and (c) cytarabine.
10. Give a comprehensive account of hormones that are potent as antineoplastic agents. Support your answer with suitable examples.
11. Give a brief account of the following: (a) Immunotherapy in cancer and (b) pharmacokinetics, pharmacodynamics, and mode of action of antineoplastic agents.
12. What are alkylating agents. Explain with the chemical reaction about alkylating mechanism in anticancer therapy. Enumerate the agents used in this category and describe the synthesis and uses of any two of them.
13. Write the synthesis, mode of action, metabolism, and uses of the following agents: Cyclophosphamide, thiotepa, and azathiapurine.
14. Write a note on cytoprotective agents.
15. Discuss the following with regard to antineoplastic agents: (a) Pteridines, (b) acyclic tertiary amines, and (c) steroids.

SUGGESTED READINGS

1. Abraham DJ (ed). *Burger's Medicinal Chemistry and Drug Discovery* (6th edn). New Jersey: John Wiley, 2007.
2. Bruntan LL, Lazo JS, and Parker KL. *Goodman and Gilman's: The Pharmacological Basis of Therapeutics* (11th edn). New York: McGraw Hill, 2006.
3. *British Pharmacopoeia*. Medicines and Healthcare Products Regulatory Agency. London, 2008.
4. Capizzi RL and Agrawal K. 'Drugs useful in the chemotherapy of the acute leukaemia'. In *Handbook of Experimental Pharmacology*, Fisher JW (ed), Vol. 101, pp. 523–64. Berlin: Springer-Verlag, 1992.
5. Dimmock JR and Kumar P. 'Anticancer and cytotoxic properties of Mannich bases'. *Curr Med Chem* 4: 1–22, 1997.
6. Dimmock JR, Murthi NK, Hetherington M, Quail JW, Pugazhenthi U, Sudom AM, Chamankhah M, Rose P, Pass, E, Allen TM, Halleran S, Szydlowski J, Mutus B, Tannous M, Manavathu EK, Myers, TG, Clercq E De, and Balzarini J. 'Cytotoxic activities of Mannich bases of chalcones and related compounds'. *J Med Chem* 41: 1014– 1026, 1998.
7. Garnick MB, Griffin JD, Sack MJ, Blum RH, Israel M, and Frei E. 'Anthracycline'. In *Antibiotics in Cancer Chemotherapy*, Muggia FM, Young CW, and SK Carter (eds). The Hague: Martinus Nijhoff, 1982.
8. Gennaro AR. *Remington: The Science and Practice of Pharmacy* (21st edn). New York: Lippincot Williams and Wilkins, 2006.
9. Handchumacher RE. Cancer Chemotherapy–Examples of Current Progress and Future Perspective. In *IUPHAR, 9th International Congress of Pharmacology Proceedings* (Pt. 2.) W Paton, J Mitchell, and Turner P (eds). London: Macmillan, 1984.
10. *Indian Pharmacopoeia*. Ministry of Health and Family Welfare. New Delhi, 1996.
11. Klein E, Milgrom H, Stoll HL, Helm F, Walker HJ, and Holtermann OA. 'Topical 5-fluorouracil chemotherapy for pre-malignant and malignant epidermal neoplasma'. In *Cancer Chemotherapy* 11, Bradsky I and Kahn SB (eds). New York: Grune and Stratton, 1972.
12. Lednicer D and Mitscher LA. *The Organic Chemistry of Drug Synthesis*. New York: John Wiley, 1995.
13. Lemke TL and William DA. *Foye's Principle of Medicinal Chemistry* (6th edn). New York: Lippincott Williams and Wilkins, 2008.
14. Chabner BA and Collins JM (eds). *Cancer Chemotherapy: Principles and Practice*. Philadelphia: JB Lippincott, 1990.
15. Sartorelli AC and Johns DG (eds). 'Antineoplastic and immunosupressive agents (Pt II)'. *Handbook der experimentellen Pharmakologie*, Vol. 38, pp. 348–72. Berlin: Springer-Verlag, 1975.
16. Pandeya SN. 'Chelation in anticancer activity'. In *Textbook of Inorganic Medicinal Chemistry*, pp. 79–83. SG Publisher, 1998.
17. Reynolds EF (ed). *Martindale the Extra Pharmacopoeia* (31st edn). London: The Pharmaceutical Press, 1997.
18. Skipper HT and Schabel FM (ed). 'Quantitative and cytokinetic studies in experimental tumour models'. In *Cancer Medicine* (3rd ed), Holland JF and Frei E (eds). Philadelphia: Lea and Febiger, 1973.
19. Skoda J. 'Azapyrimidine nucleoside'. In *Antineoplastic and Immunosuppressive Agents* (Pt II), Sarterelli AC and John GD (eds). Berlin: Handbuch de Experimentellen Pharmakology, 1975.
20. Umezava H. 'Cancer drugs of microbial origin'. In *Methods in Cancer Res. XVI. Cancer Drug Development* (Pt A), Deveta VT Jr (ed). New York: Academic Press, 1979.
21. Zubrod CG. 'Historical pespectice of curative chemotherapy'. In *Oncology*, Clark RL, Cumely RW, Mcloy JE, and Lopeland M (eds). Being the Proceedings of the Tenth International Cancer Congress Year Book. Chicago, 1970.

CHAPTER 23

Antileprotic Drugs

INTRODUCTION

Leprosy is a chronic disease caused due to acid-fast bacillus called *Mycobacterium leprae* and produces nodules on the skin and causes loss of sensation. Once the organism enters into the body, it multiplies and produces antigen–antibody reaction and causes cell-mediated immunity, and produces allergic reaction by the metabolite of the microorganism and finally produces lepra reaction.

Categories of Leprosy

1. Tuberculoid leprosy
2. Lepromatous leprosy
3. Intermediate leprosy
4. Borderline leprosy

Lepromatous leprosy: Large number of organisms that are present in the affected area and induce lepra reaction.

Tuberculoid leprosy: It is characterized by skin molecules with clear centre and well-defined margin.

Intermediate leprosy: It is localized hypo-pigmentation with some sensory loss.

Borderline leprosy: It is an intermediate stage between tuberculoid leprosy and lepromatous leprosy.

CLASSIFICATION

Antileprotic drugs are classified into the following:

I. Sulphones
II. Benzpyrazine derivatives: Clofazimine
III. Plant drugs

I. Sulphones

Dapsone (Diaminodiphenyl sulphone, DDS)

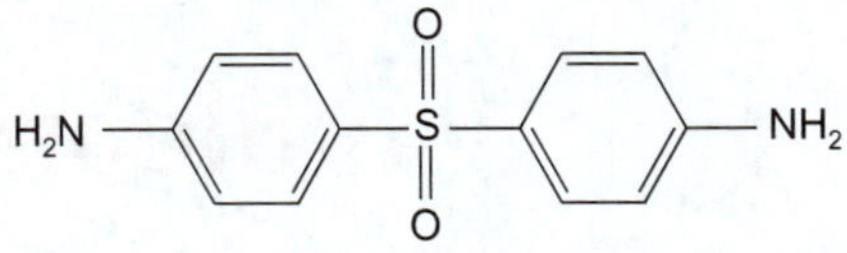

Acedapsone

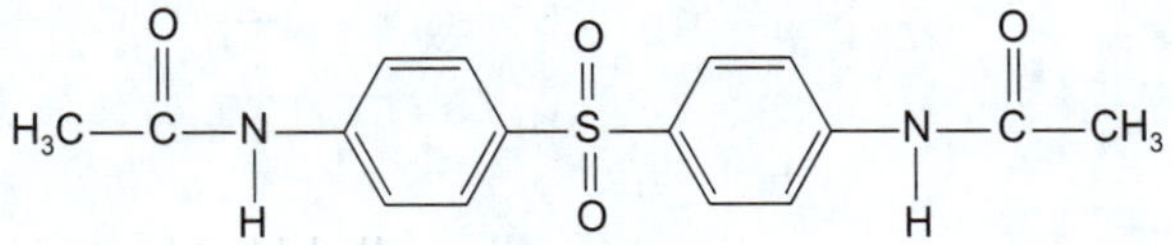

Solapsone sodium

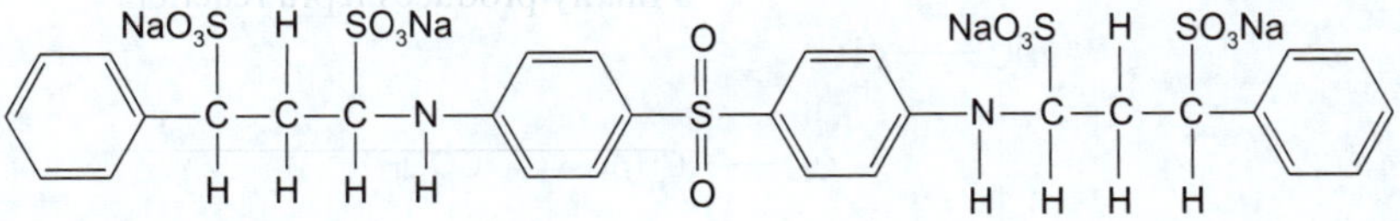

Sulfoxone sodium

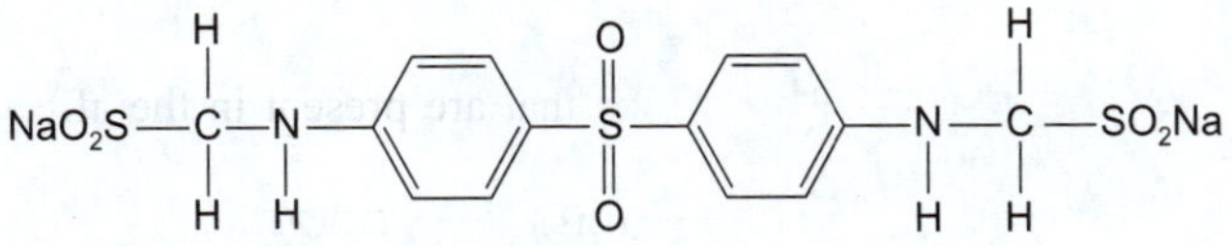

Gluco sulfone sodium

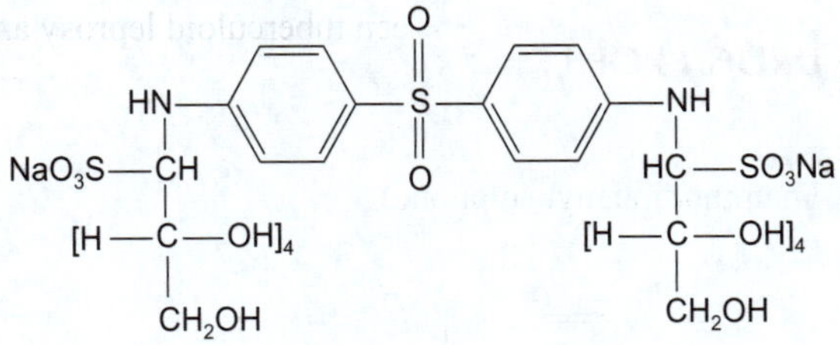

II. Dibenz Pyrazine Derivatives

Clofazimine (Lamprene)

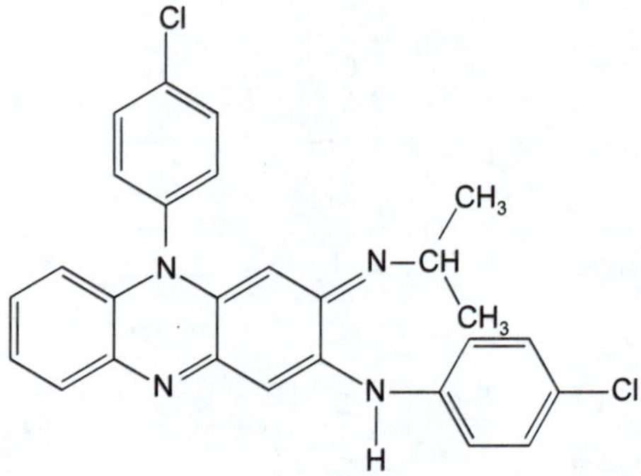

III. Plant Drug

i. Chaulmaogric acid

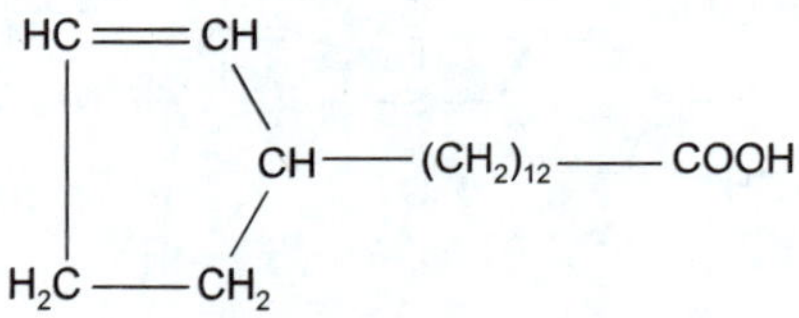

ii. Hydrocapric acid

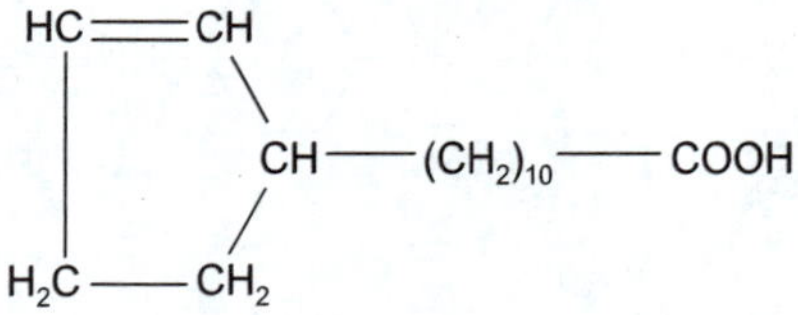

SYNTHESIS AND DRUG PROFILE

I. Sulphones

i. Dapsone (DDS, Diaminodiphenyl sulphone)

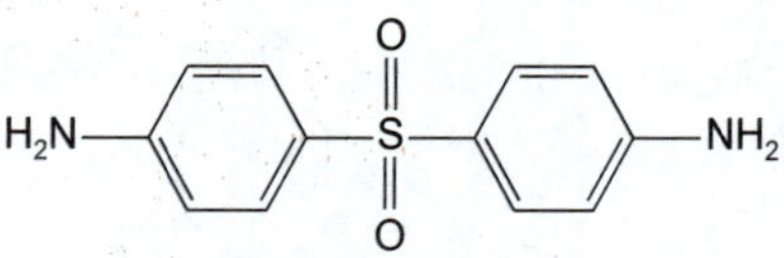

4-(4-Aminophenylsulfonyl)benzenamine

Synthesis

Route I. From: 4-Chloronitrobenzene

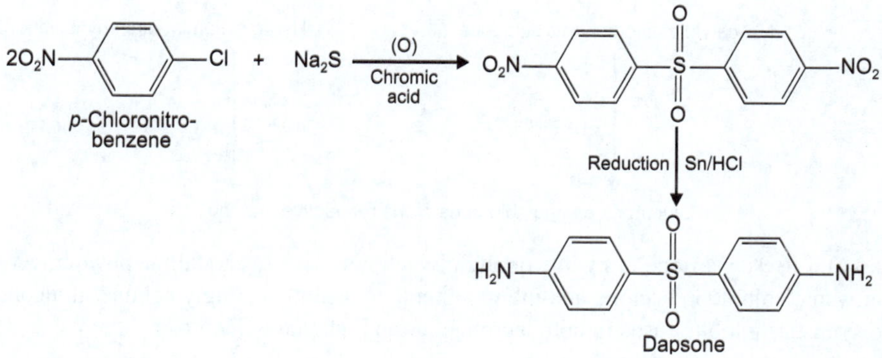

Route II. From: 4-Chloronitrobenzene

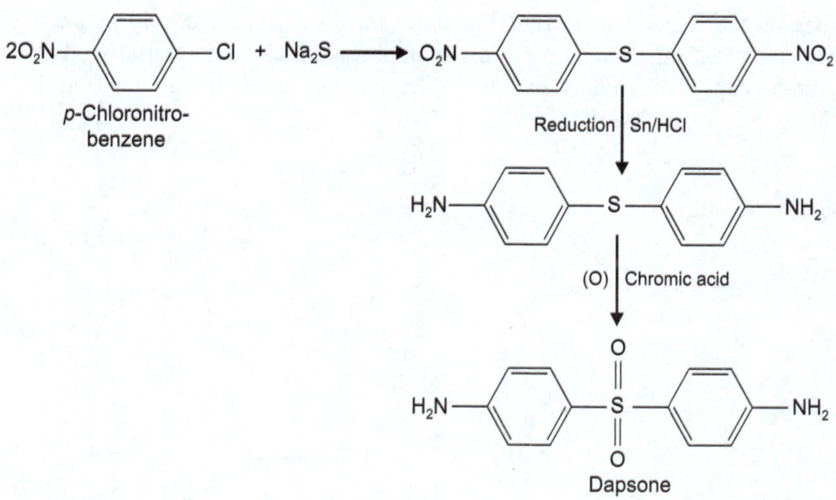

Metabolism: The major metabolic product of dapsone results from N-acetylation in the liver by N-acetyltransferase. It also undergoes N-hydroxylation to hydroxylamine derivative. These metabolic reactions are catalyzed by CYP3A4 isoforms. Neither of these compounds possesses significant leprostatic activity, although N-acetyldiamino-diphenyl sulphone may be deacetylated back to dapsone. Products found in the urine consist of small amounts of dapsone and the metabolites, that is, N-acetyldiamino-diphenyl sulphone and N-hydroxy-diamino-diphenyl sulphone, as well as glucuronide and sulphate of each of these substances.

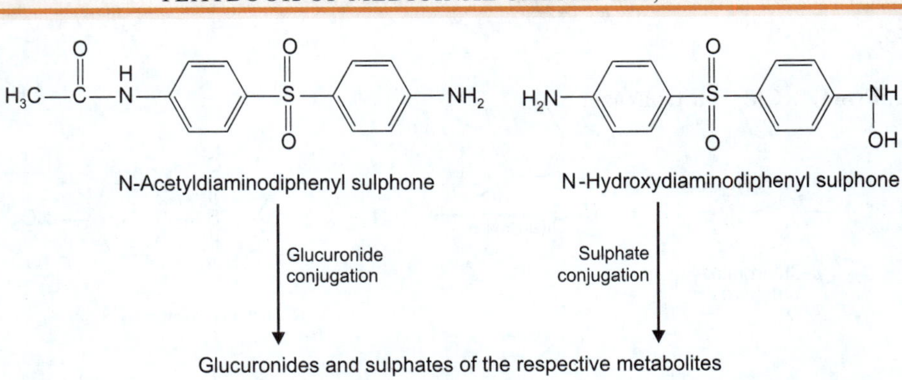

Properties and uses: Dapsone is a white or slightly yellowish-white crystalline powder, very slightly soluble in water, soluble in acetone and dilute mineral acids, but sparingly soluble in alcohol. It is a folic acid synthesis inhibitor used in both lepromatous and tuberculoid leprosy.

Assay: Dissolve the sample in dilute hydrochloric acid and add potassium bromide. Cool in ice and titrate against 0.1 N sodium nitrate. Determine the end point electrometrically.

Dose: The dose as tablets is 25 or 100 mg. For adults the dose consumed is 50 mg per day orally. For lepromatous leprosy, 100 mg dapsone + 600 mg rifampin and/or clofazimine 100 mg daily for at least 2 years followed by dapsone monotherapy. For borderline tuberculoid disease, dapsone 100 mg daily + rifampin 600 mg once monthly for 6 months.

Dosage forms: Dapsone tablets IP, BP.

ii. Solapsone sodium

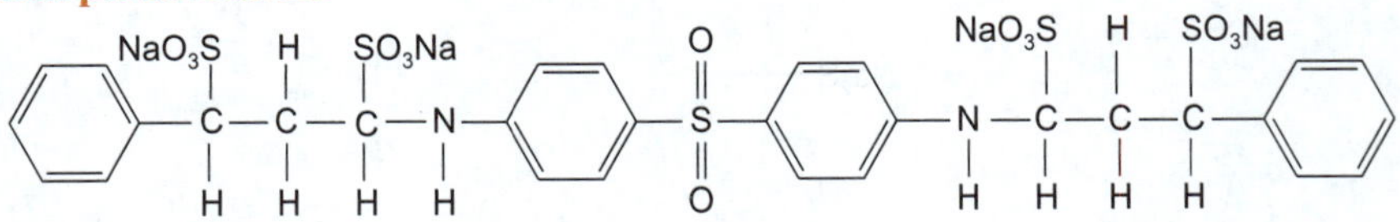

Synthesis

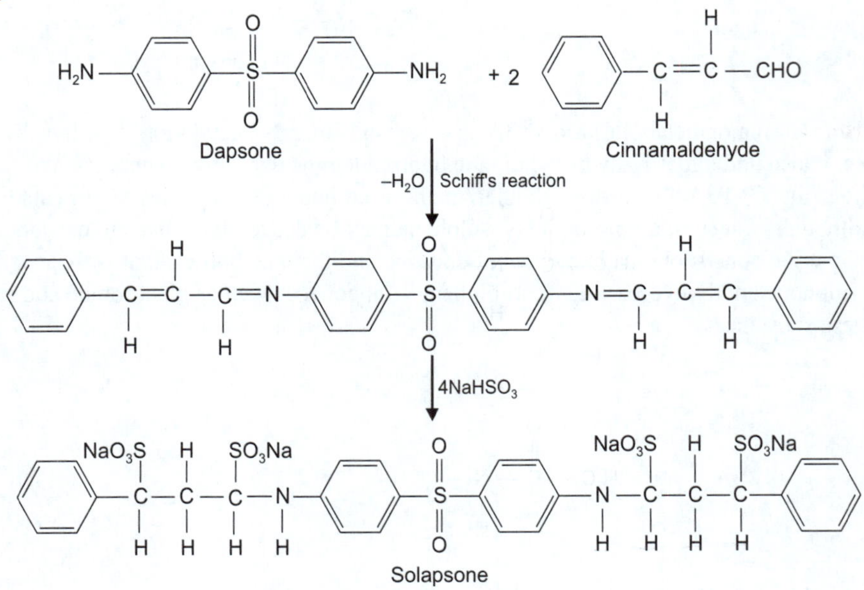

Acedapsone

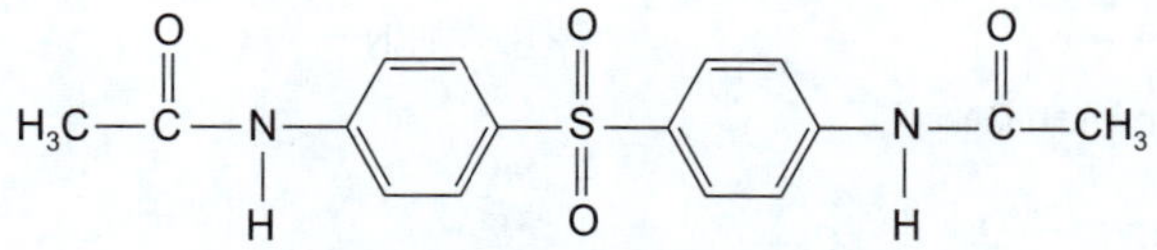

N,N-Di(acetyl amino diphenyl) sulphone

Synthesis

Route I. From: Dapsone

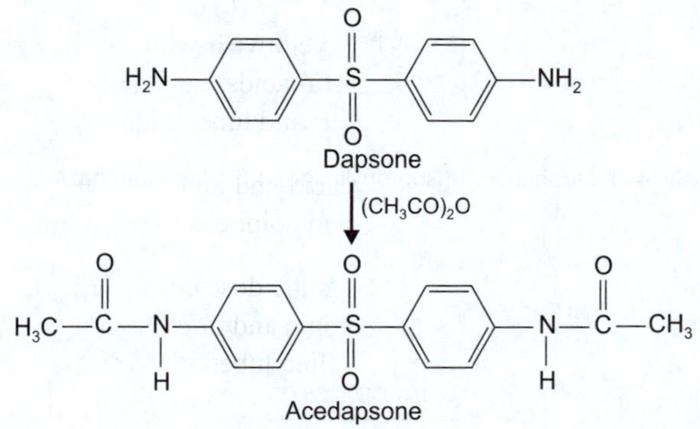

Route II. From: 4-Chloronitrobenzene

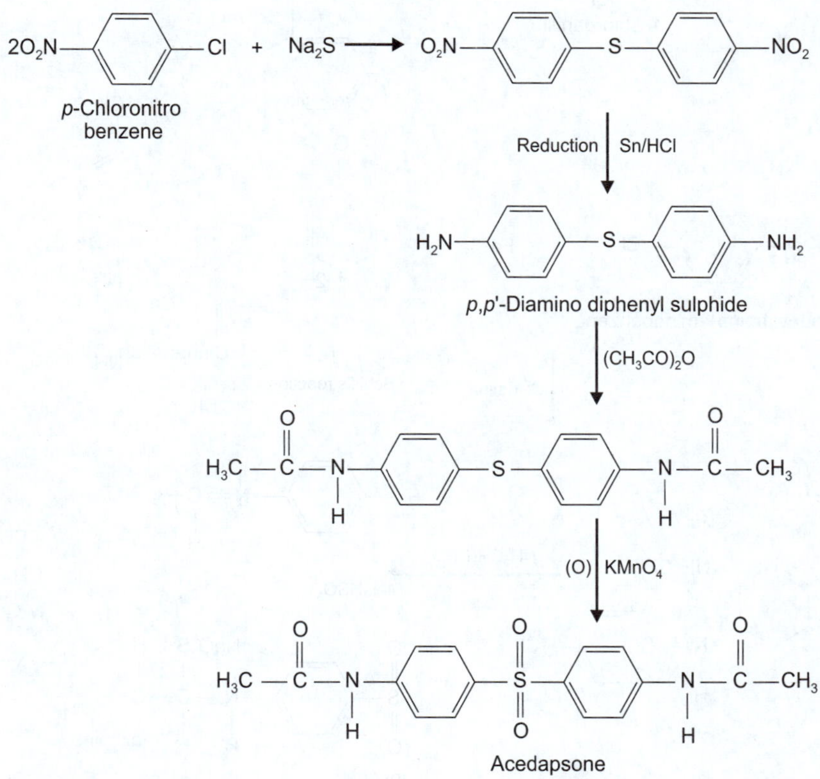

Properties and uses: Acedapsone (prodrug of dapsone) is used in the treatment of both lepromatous and tuberculoid type of leprosy.

II. Benzpyrazine derivatives

i. Clofazimine (Lamprene)

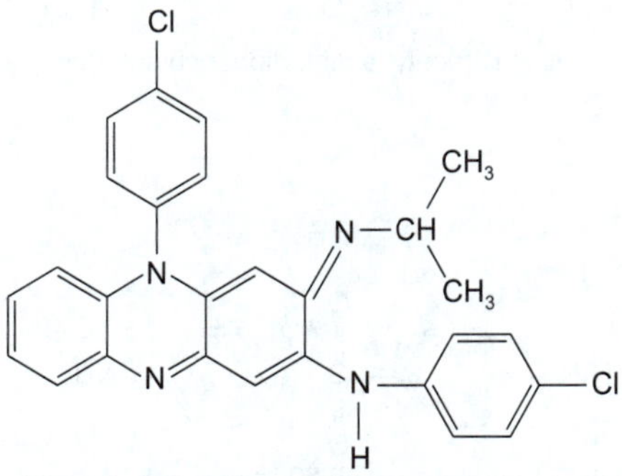

(Z)-N,5-*Bis*(4-chlorophenyl)-3-(isopropylimino)-3,5-dihydrophenazin-2-amine

Synthesis

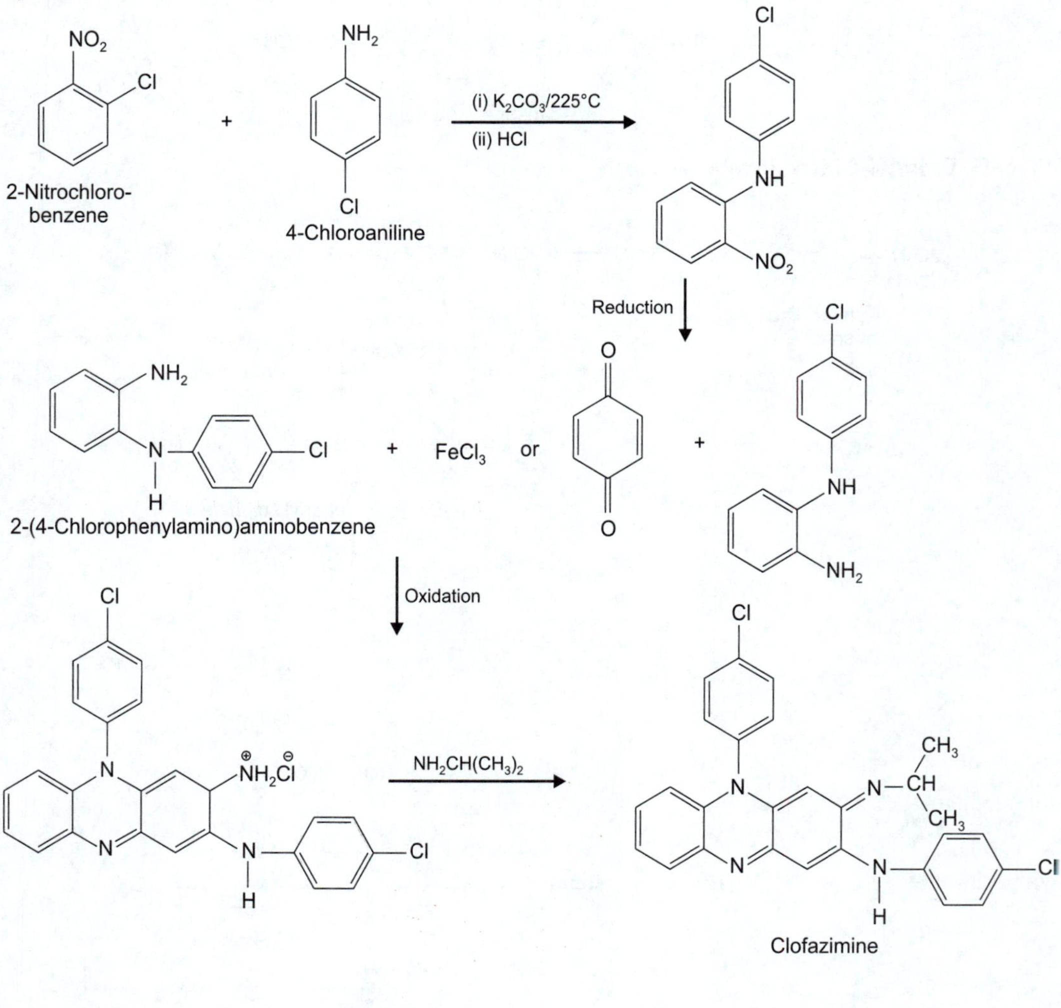

Metabolism: It is thought to undergo hydroxylic dehalogenation on the 4-chloroaniline, followed by sulphate conjugation. It also undergoes glucuronic acid conjugation.

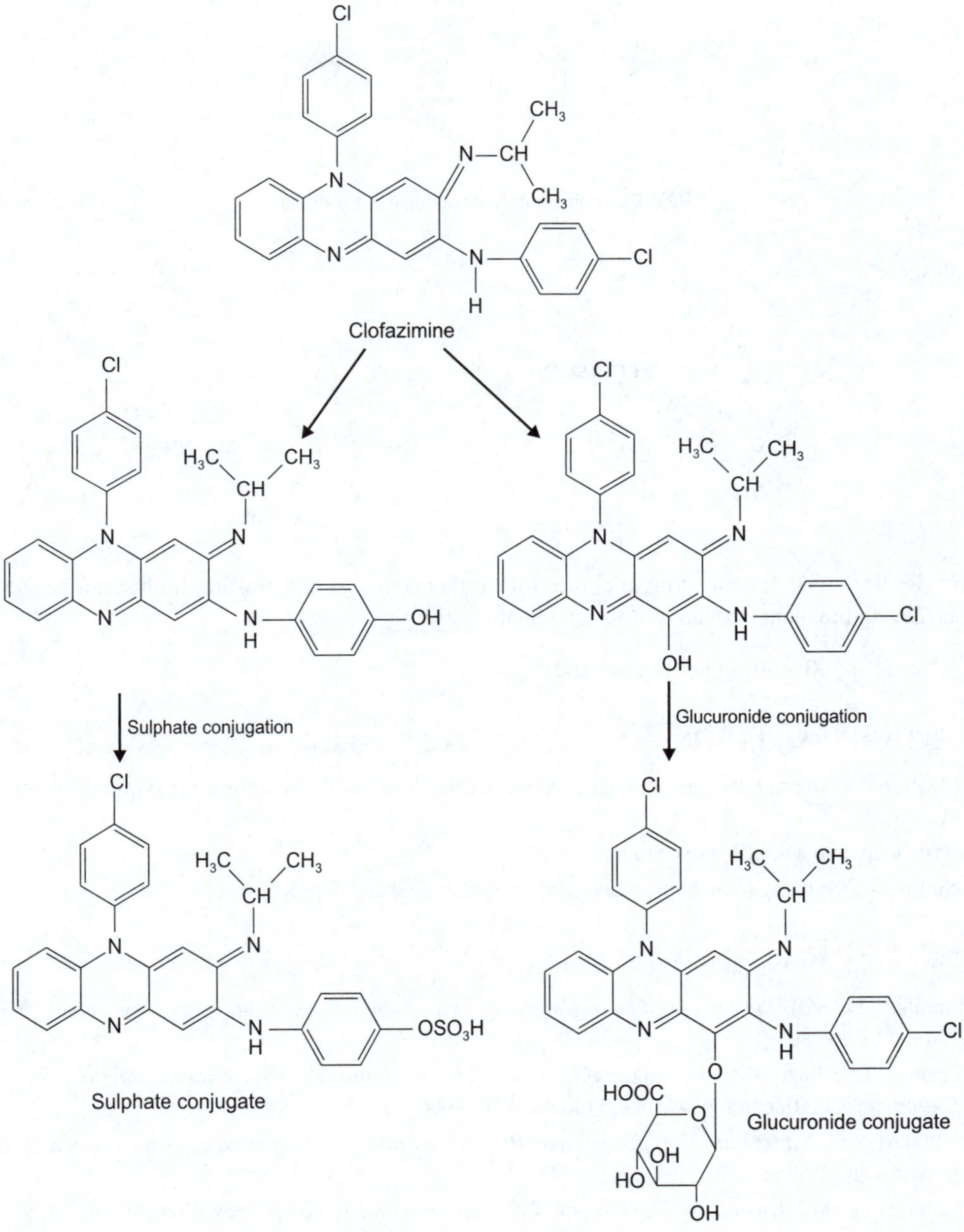

Properties and uses: Clofazimine is a reddish-brown fine powder, practically insoluble in water, soluble in methylene chloride, and very slightly soluble in ethanol. It is used as antileprotic drug.

Assay: Dissolve the sample in methylene chloride, add acetone and anhydrous acetic acid and titrate with 0.1 M perchloric acid. Determine the end point potentiometrically.

Dose: The dose orally is 100 mg daily.

Dosage forms: Clofazimine capsules IP, BP.

iv. Thalidomide (Thaloda, Thycad, Thalomid)

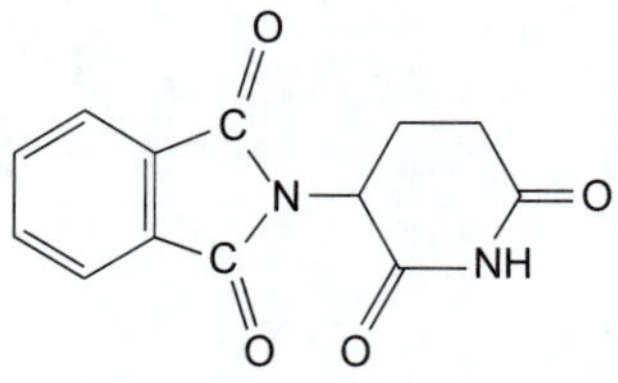

2-(2,6-Dioxopiperidin-3-yl)isoindoline-1,3-dione

Synthesis

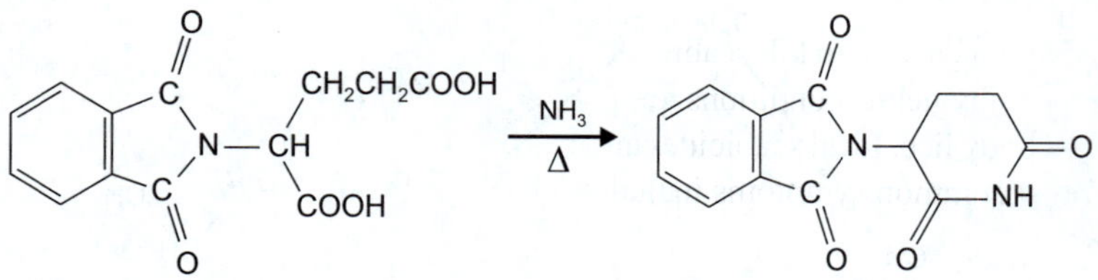

Properties and uses: It is the drug of choice for Erythema nodosum leprosum. It must not be used in women during pregnancy because of its teratogenic activity.

Dose: Doses of 100–300 mg per day are effective.

PROBABLE QUESTIONS

1. Mention the different categories of leprosy, classify the drugs used, and outline the synthesis of any two of them.
2. Write a note on sulphones used in leprosy.
3. Outline the synthesis, metabolism, and uses of clofazimine and dapsone.

SUGGESTED READINGS

1. Abraham DJ (ed). *Burger's Medicinal Chemistry and Drug Discovery* (6th edn). New Jersey: Wiley, 2007.
2. Bruntan LL, Lazo JS, and Parker KL. *Goodman and Gilman's: The Pharmacological Basis of Therapeutics* (11th edn). New York: McGraw Hill, 2006.
3. Gennaro AR. *Remington: The Science and Practice of Pharmacy* (21st edn). New York: Lippincot Williams and Wilkins, 2006.
4. Lednicer D and Mitscher LA. *The Organic Chemistry of Drug Synthesis*. New York: Wiley, 1995.
5. Lemke TL and William DA. *Foye's Principle of Medicinal Chemistry* (6th edn). New York: Lippincott Williams and Wilkins, 2008.

CHAPTER 24

Antiscabies an Antipedicular Age

Scabicides are compounds used to kill scabies and control the growth of *Sarcoptes scabiei*, an organism that thrives under unhygienic conditions or poor personal hygiene. Antipedicular agents used to eliminate head and body lice. Ideal scabicides and pediculicides must kill the adult parasites and destroy their eggs. The most common symptoms include itching and pimple like rashes.

DRUGS USED IN SCABIES AND PEDICULOSIS

Benzyl benzoate

It is a naturally occurring ester obtained from Peru balsam and other resins. It is also prepared synthetically from benzyl alcohol and benzoyl chloride.

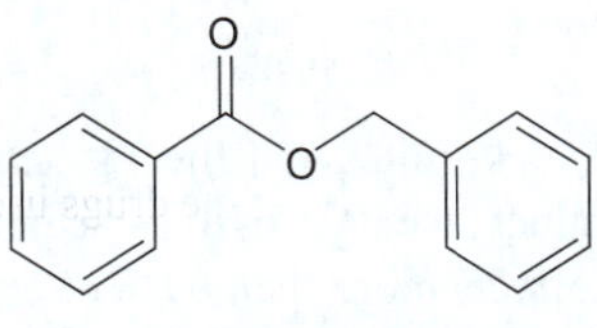

It is an effective scabicide when applied topically. Immediate relief from itching, probably results from its local anesthetic effect. However, a complete cure is frequently achieved with a single application of a 25% emulsion of benzyl benzoate in oleic acid stabilized by triethanolamine. This preparation is odourless, non-staining and non-irritating to the skin.

Lindane

It is 1,2,3,4,5,6-hexachloro cyclohexane or benzene hexachloride.

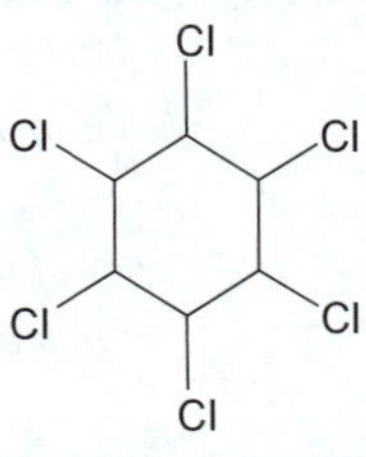

1,2,3,4,5,6- hexachloro cyclohexane or benzene hexachloride

It is prepared by chlorination of benzene, during the preparation, mixture of 5-isomers is obtained. The gamma isomer is responsible for the insecticidal activity. The action of lindane against insects is 3-fold and it is a direct contact poison, it has a fumigant effect and it acts as a stomach poison. Its toxicity in humans is less than that of DDT. It is used locally as a cream, lotion or shampoo for the treatment of scabies and pediculosis.

Crotamiton

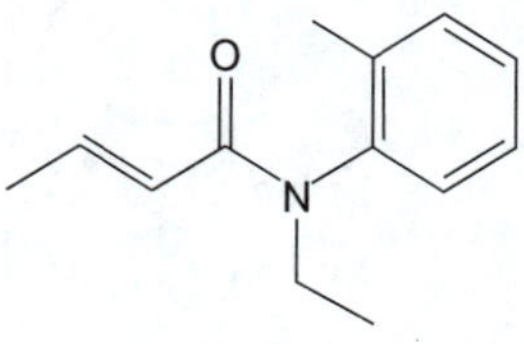

Crotamiton

It is available in 10% concentration lotion and a cream intended for the topical treatment of scabies. It is having antipruritic effect, probably because of its local anesthetic action.

Premethrin

It is a mixture consisting of 60% *trans* and 40% *cis* racemic isomers.

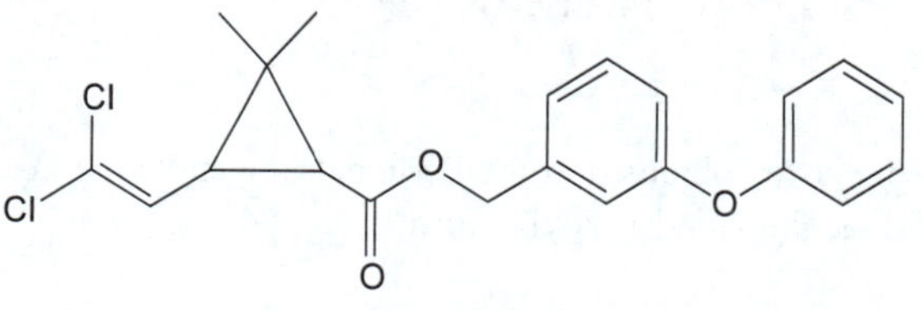

Premethrin

It exerts lethal action against lice, tick, mites and flies. It acts on the nerve cell membrane of the parasite and disrupts Na^+ channel conductance. It is used as pediculicide for the treatment of head lice. A single application of 1% solution effects more than 99% of cases. The most frequent side effect is pruritis which occurred in about 6% of the patients tested.

Abametapir

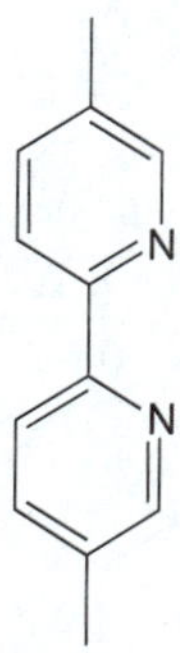

Abametapir

Uses: It is used for the treatment of head lice infestation.

SECTION VII

Miscellaneous

CHAPTER 25

Preservatives

Preservatives are added to various dosage forms and cosmetic preparations to prevent degradation. In parental and ophthalmic preparations, preservatives are used to maintain sterility in case of accidental contamination during use.

An ideal preservative would be effective at low concentrations against all possible microorganisms. It should be non-toxic and compatible with other constituents of the preparation and should be stable in the shelf life of the preparation. In some cases, combination of preservative agents can be used.

Maximum number of pharmaceutical preparations are easily liable to deterioration or consequent spoilage by microorganisms which challenge the hygiene of that preparation. Hence, all kind of pharmaceutical preparations stored for long-term period of time should be preserved properly. Along with this the pharmaceutical injectable preparations stored in vials are necessarily required specific concentration of antimicrobial agents to prevent the contamination during the withdrawal of dosages. Proper preservation of drugs/pharmaceutical preparations are achieved by using antimicrobial agents or preservatives.

PARA-HYDROXY BENZOIC ACID DERIVATIVES

Esters of *p*-hydroxy benzoic acid (parabenes) have distinct antifungal properties. They are less toxic to the human host because they undergo rapid hydrolysis *in-vivo* to *p*-hydroxy benzoic acid, which is quickly conjugated and excreted. This property makes them useful for liquid dosage forms. The preservative activity generally increases with molecular weight but methyl ester is most effective against moulds whereas propyl ester is most effective against yeast. The lipid soluble propyl ester is preferred for drugs in oil or lipophilic bases.

Methyl paraben

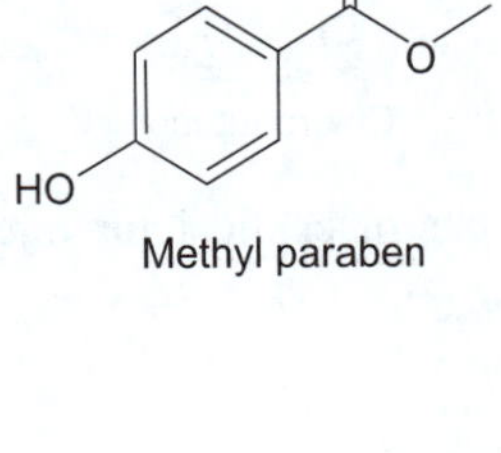

Methyl paraben

It is used against moulds growth.

Propyl paraben

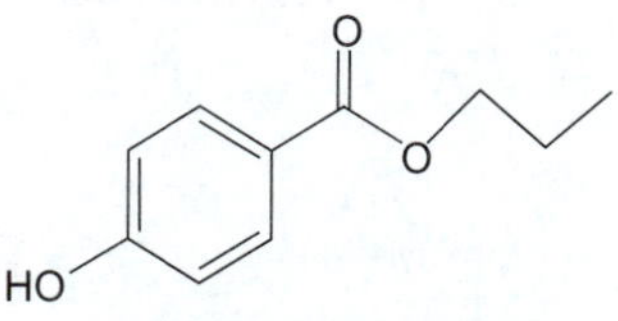

Propyl paraben

Primarily used to retard yeast growth.

Butyl paraben

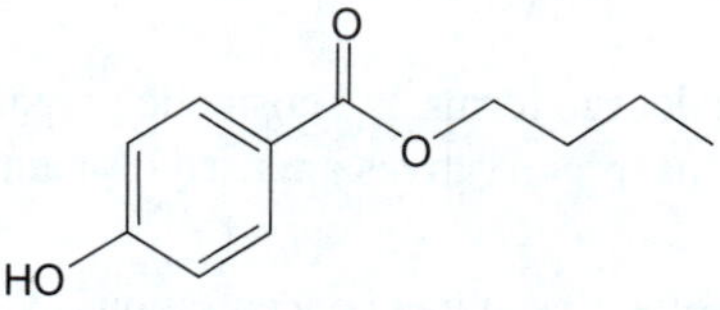

Butyl paraben

It is sparingly soluble in water but very soluble in alcohol and non-polar organic solvents.

Ethyl paraben

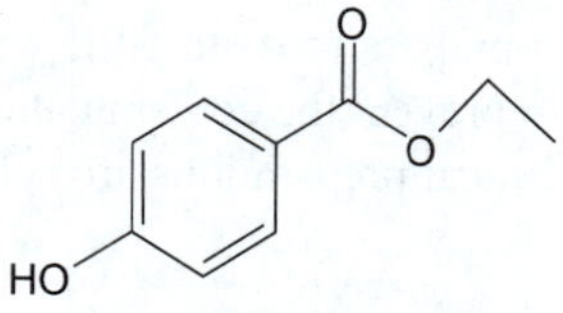

Ethyl paraben

It is insoluble in alcohol and most organic solvents but soluble in water.

Other Preservatives

Chlorobutanol

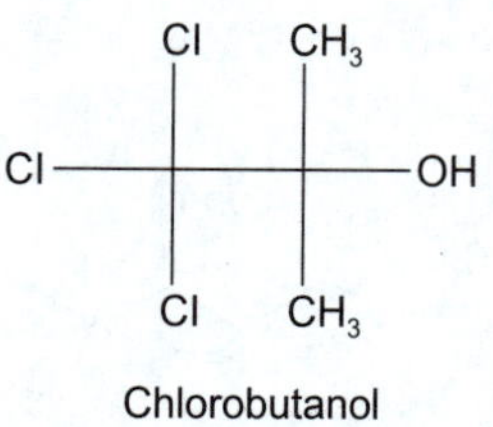

Chlorobutanol

It is used as a bacteriostatic agent in pharmaceutical for injection, ophthalmic use and intranasal administration.

Benzyl alcohol (Phenyl carbinol or phenyl methanol)

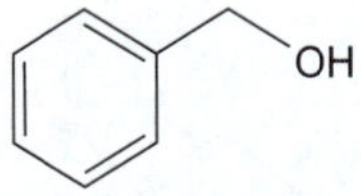

Benzyl alcohol (phenyl carbinol or phenyl methanol)

It is commonly used as preservatives in vials or injectable drugs in concentrations of 1–4% in water or saline solution. It has added advantage of having a local anesthetic action. It is commonly used in ointments and lotions as an antiseptic in the treatment of various skin diseases.

Phenyl ethyl alcohol

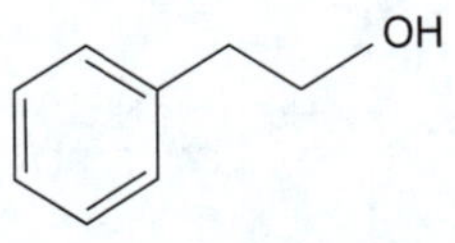

Phenyl ethyl alcohol

It is mainly used in perfumes.

Benzoic acid

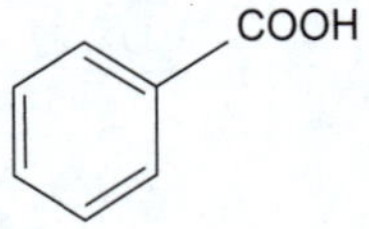

Benzoic acid

It is used externally as an antiseptic in lotions, ointments and mouthwashes. It is more effective as a preservative in foods and pharmaceutical products at low pH.

Sodium benzoate

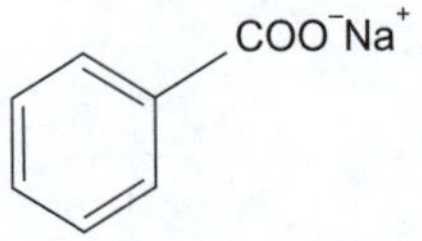

Sodium benzoate

Used as a preservative in acidic liquid preparations in which benzoic acid is released.

Sodium propionate

$CH_3CH_2COO^-Na^+$

Sodium propionate

It is an effective antifungal agent and is used as a preservative.

Sorbic acid

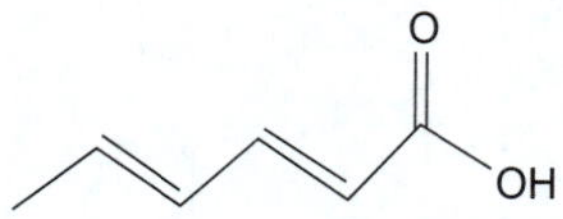

Sorbic acid

It is an effective antifungal preservative used to preserve syrups, elixirs, ointments and lotions containing components such as sugars which support mould growth.

Phenyl mercuric nitrate

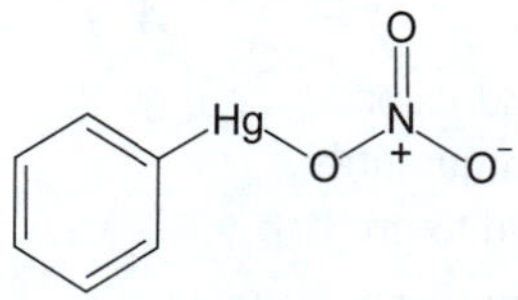

Phenyl mercuric nitrate

It is used to preserve injectable drugs against bacterial contamination. Disadvantage of organic mercurials is that their bacteriostatic efficacy is reduced in presence of serum.

CHAPTER 26

Diagnostic Agents

Diagnostic medical imaging of body and its parts include a group of techniques used in diagnosis and further treatment of disease. This technique utilizes electromagnetic radiation to pass through tissues and pass the internal information needed to produce an image of the particular tissue or organ.

All of the techniques are different by means of their diverge in their physical means, methods and the information that they can provide. All of these techniques give information, i.e. anatomical or functional, that is given in the form of image for interpretation by a trained and well-experienced physician.

Medical imaging starts with the discovery of X-ray by Roentgen in the year 1895. In olden days, X-rays used to produce images of chest and skeleton. But nowadays, the medical diagnostic imaging utilizes the following techniques.

1. Nuclear medicines or decaying radioactive traces
2. Computed tomography (CT) ionizing radiations.
3. Magnetic resonance imaging (MRI)—radiowaves
4. Ultrasound—high-frequency sound waves

Nowadays, these imaging techniques support the physician to perform interventional procedures such as organ biopsy or abscess drainage.

Diagnostic agents are the substances used to examine the body in order to detect impairment of its normal functions. Usually, these agents find no other use in medicine.

The degree of usefulness of these agents is determined by the following factors.

1. Solubility
2. Mode and rate of excretion
3. Metabolism
4. Chemical configuration and chemical composition

Generally, they are divided into two classes:

1. **Clinical diagnostic chemicals:** For determining normal and pathological products in urine, blood, faeces and other body fluids.
2. **Diagnostic agents:** They are applied directly in the body. The diagnostic agents are further divided into three groups:
   i. *Radio-opaque substances:* They cast a shadow film and also useful in fluoroscopic examination. Example: Barium sulphate.
   ii. Compounds for testing functional capacity.
   iii. Compounds modifying physiological actions.

Let us discuss diagnostic chemicals/drugs in detail.

Certain substances are retained or excreted almost exclusively only by a specific organ. Thus depending upon the property of retention or excretion, this impairment in the organ function can be searched out. For example, phenol tetrachlorophthalein, when administered parenterally, it is found to be excreted only in the bile, hence the failure in removing the dye through the bile is indicative of impaired functioning of the organ.

1. **Drugs used to test kidney function:** To test kidney function, the bladder is completely emptied before the dye is administered. This is done under aseptic conditions by introducing a catheter into the bladder.

   Example:

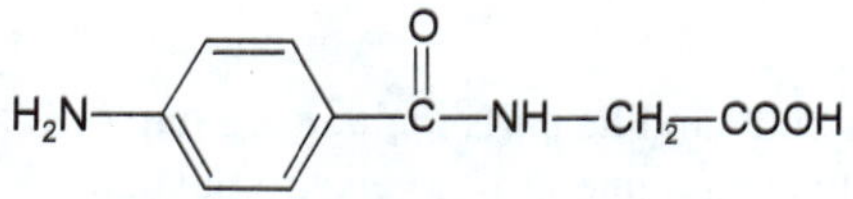

p-Amino hippuric acid

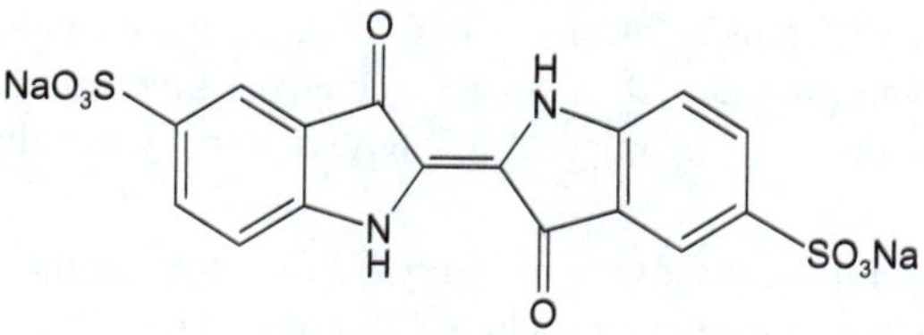

Indigotin disulfonate sodium

2. **Drugs used to test liver function:** Liver is the main site for metabolic and detoxifying enzymes of the body. Agents whose excretion depends exclusively upon liver function are used to detect the liver dysfunction. The role of clearance of such agents from the plasma becomes a measure of the excretory capacity of the liver.

   Example:

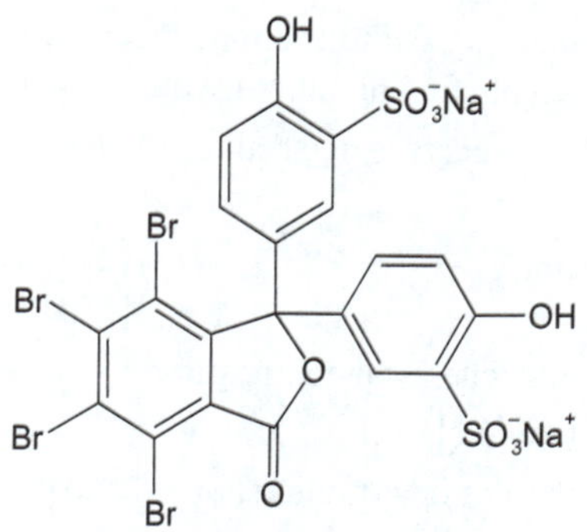

Sulfobromophthalein sodium

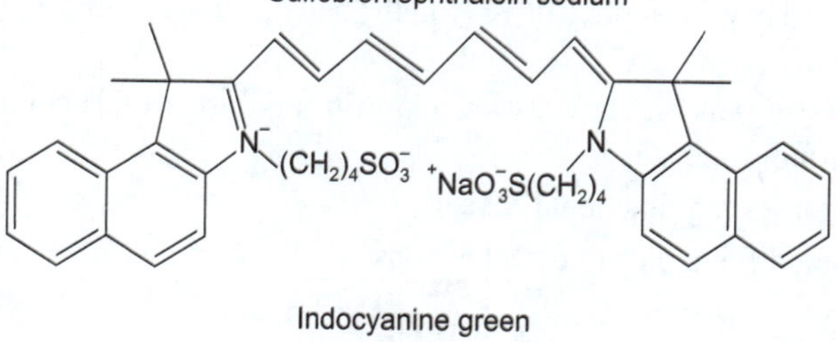

Indocyanine green

3. **Agents used to test gastric function:** Many gastric stimulants are used to gather the evidence of hyper or hyposecretion of gastric acid. Proof for the absence of gastric acid in the stomach is necessary in the diagnosis of pernicious anaemia, while oversecretion of gastric acid confirms the case of peptic ulcer. The gastric stimulants mainly used to test gastric function includes alcohol, caffeine, pentagastrine, histamine, etc. For example, pentagastrin is used for diagnosis or pernicious anaemia, gastric carcinoma, atropic gastritis or hypersecretion of gastric acid.

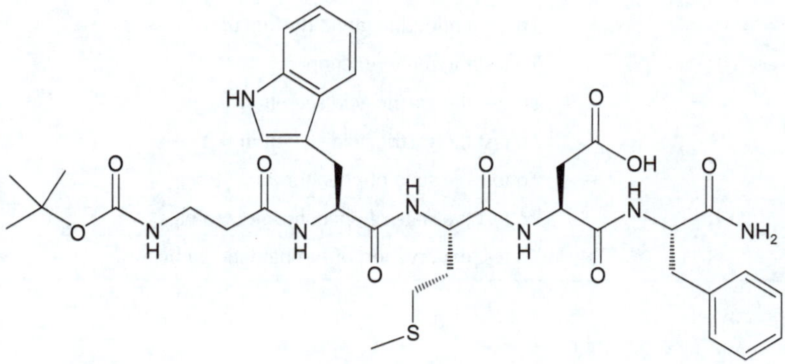

Pentagastrin

4. **Agents used to test cardiac function:** Evans blue and indocyanine green are used to determine blood volume and cardiac output.

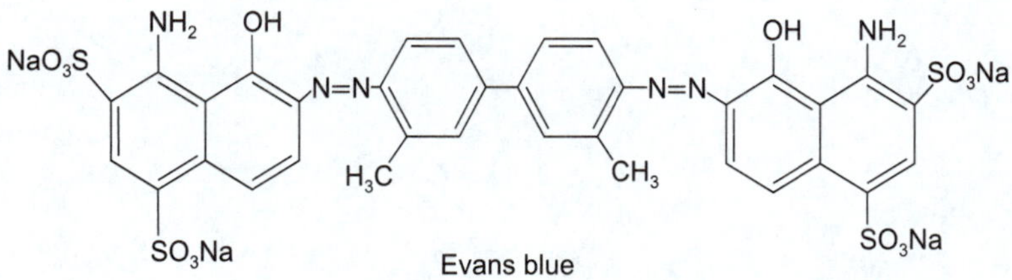

Evans blue

5. **Miscellaneous diagnostic chemicals:** Metyrapone is used to determine residual pituitary function in patients with hypopituitarism.

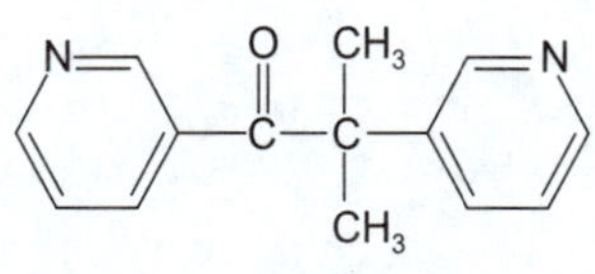

Metyrapone

Fluorescein sodium is used for ophthalmological studies.

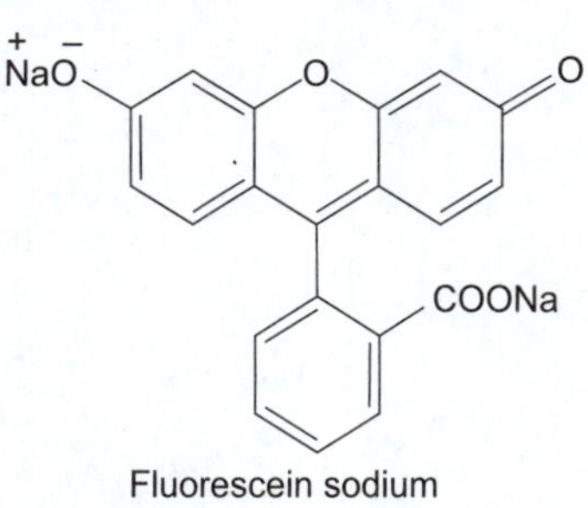

Fluorescein sodium

Diagnostic drugs:

Following are commonly used diagnostic drugs to test the presence of specific disease state of the organ.

Drug	*Diagnostic use*
L-arginine	To test growth hormone secretion response
Dexamethasone	To test endocrine gland dysfunction
Mannitol	To test the renal function
Histamine	To test the gastric acid secretion
Pentagastrin	To test the gastric acid secretion
Phentolamine	To test the state of pheochromocytoma
Tyramine	To test the state of pheochromocytoma
Norepinephrine	To test denervation of sympathetic pathways

Index